PRINCIPLES OF

MEDICAL BIOCHEMISTRY

GERHARD MEISENBERG, PH.D.
Department of Biochemistry
Ross University School of Medicine
Roseau, Commonwealth of Dominica, West Indies

WILLIAM H. SIMMONS, PH.D.
Department of Molecular and Cellular Biochemistry
Loyola University School of Medicine
Maywood, Illinois

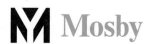 Mosby

St. Louis Baltimore Boston Carlsbad Chicago Minneapolis New York Philadelphia Portland
London Milan Sydney Tokyo Toronto

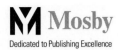

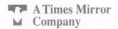

Publisher: Richard Furn
Editors: Emma Underdown and Bev Copland
Developmental Editor: Rebecca Gruliow
Editorial Assistant: Kim Davis
Project Manager: Chris Baumle
Production Editor: Marian Hall
Designer: Emily Betsch
Manufacturing Manager: William A. Winneberger, Jr.
Cover design: Carolyn O'Brien
Cover images: © Tony Stone Images

Printed in the United States of America
Composition by Progressive Information Technologies, Inc.
Printing/binding by Von Hoffmann Press, Inc.

Mosby, Inc.
11830 Westline Industrial Drive
St. Louis, Missouri 63146

Library of Cataloging in Publication Data

Meisenberg, Gerhard.
   Principles of medical biochemistry / Gerhard Meisenberg, William H. Simmons.
     p.   cm.
   Includes bibliographical references and index.
   ISBN 0-8151-4410-5
   1. Biochemistry. 2. Clinical biochemistry. I. Simmons, William H., Ph. D. II. Title
   [DNLM: 1: Biochemistry. 2. Molecular Biology. QU 34 M515p 1998]
   QP514.2.M45   1998
   572'.024'61—dc21
   DNLM/DLC
   for Library of Congress   98-2505
                                                        CIP

98 99 00 01 02 / 9 8 7 6 5 4 3 2

Preface

This book is an outgrowth of our experience in teaching biochemistry to first-year medical students. It is therefore designed for students who have had at least 1 year of biology and 1 year of chemistry at the undergraduate level and who are learning biochemistry concurrently with other subjects in the preclinical medical sciences. Although it is written primarily for students of medicine, it also is useful for veterinary, dental, and pharmacy students, and it is equally suitable as an undergraduate text for students in premedical programs.

We are writing this book at a time when our understanding of the biochemical basis of health and disease is growing in leaps and bounds. Fascinating as this growth of knowledge is for the biochemist, it can be daunting for the student: how can a medical student possibly acquire the vast amount of relevant knowledge about biochemistry and molecular biology? Which aspects of this ever-growing field really are important for the medical practitioner? Our approach is a modest one: we simply explain how things work in the body and how derangements in these processes can cause disease. The best approach to biochemistry for the medical student is quite different from the way biochemistry is taught to prospective biochemists. The Ph.D. biochemist has to employ a magnifying-glass approach to molecular structure and reactions. His concern is the detailed description of molecular structure and the structure-function relationship for individual proteins and other biomolecules. The medical student, in contrast, has to take the bird's-eye view: rather than analyzing structures and reactions in ever more detail, his concern is the living entity of the human body. Whereas the biochemist asks "How does this enzymatic reaction proceed?" the physician asks "What is the importance of this reaction for the normal functioning of the body, and what happens when it goes wrong?"

Medical students often fail to see the relationship between the inhumanly logical world of biochemistry textbooks and the real world out there, the world of patients and doctors and people like you and me. We have to cultivate the interface between these two worlds, going back and forth between them with ease, linking the unfamiliar with the familiar. Throughout this book we adopt the strategy of presenting the varied aspects of human biochemistry in the context of their function rather than as abstract chemical entities. This is followed by descriptions of situations in which these functions are disrupted.

This is a comprehensive text of medical biochemistry; this accounts for its large size. Nevertheless, we tried to de-emphasize those aspects of biochemistry that have little immediate relevance for medical practice while emphasizing those that do. There is, for example, precious little about the history of biochemistry and about the experimentation that led to our present knowledge. When methods are presented in some detail, they are presented because they currently are or soon will be important in medical practice, not because of their importance in biochemical research. You will find chapters about such medically relevant topics as DNA technology (Chapter 10), lipoproteins (Chapter 20), vitamins and minerals (Chapter 24), plasma proteins (Chapter 25), and the molecular biology of cancer (Chapter 28).

Although the book is littered with descriptions of a variety of diseases, we did not include formal case studies in the main body of the text. We do, however, have a collection of case studies at the end of the book. They are separate because most of them elaborate on material from more than one chapter. Indeed, they touch on material that the student is likely to encounter in basic medical courses other than biochemistry, reaching from basic anatomy and physiology to medical ethics. This, after all, is the value of case studies: to apply knowledge acquired in separate contexts to the type of problem that the physician is likely to see in the workplace.

Contents

PART FIVE:
INTEGRATION   511

Chapter 25   Plasma Proteins   511

Chapter 26   Extracellular Messengers   547

PRINCIPLES OF
MEDICAL BIOCHEMISTRY

PART ONE

PRINCIPLES OF MOLECULAR STRUCTURE AND FUNCTION

Chapter 1

Introduction to Biomolecules

Biochemistry is concerned with our bodies' chemical components—their properties, functions, synthesis, transport, and degradation. Therefore, the first question facing the student of biochemistry is: what are the components of the human body? Table 1.1 shows the approximate composition of the "textbook" 75-kg adult. Of the components listed, the **triglyceride** content is the most variable, depending on the amount of adipose tissue. Triglycerides are the most important storage form of metabolic energy. **Protein** is a major component of all tissues, but most people have more than half of it in their muscles. Proteins are responsible for most of the specialized functions of living tissues. **Carbohydrates** are far less abundant than proteins. Some carbohydrates serve structural functions in the extracellular tissue spaces. Others, including glucose and the storage polysaccharide

glycogen, are important as substrates for the generation of metabolic energy. Soluble inorganic salts are present throughout the body, in both the intracellular and extracellular fluids. And the insoluble salts, most of them related to calcium phosphate, form the inorganic matrix of bone.

In this chapter, we introduce the principles of molecular structure, the types of noncovalent interactions between biomolecules, and the structural features of the major classes of biomolecules.

WATER: THE SOLVENT OF LIFE

Water is by far the most important constituent of the human body (Table 1.1). All other components of living systems are in intimate contact with water, and all biochemical reactions take place in an aqueous environment. Interactions with water are

TABLE 1.1

Approximate composition of a 75-kg adult

Substance	Content (%)
Water	60
Inorganic salt, soluble	0.7
Inorganic salt, insoluble*	5.5
Protein	16
Triglyceride (fat)†	13
Membrane lipids	2.5
Carbohydrates	1.5
Nucleic acids	0.2

* In bones.
† In adipose tissue.

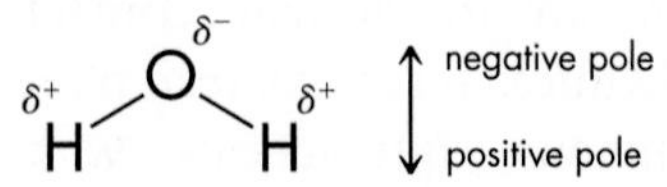

FIG. 1.1

Hydrogen bonds (· · ·) between water molecules.

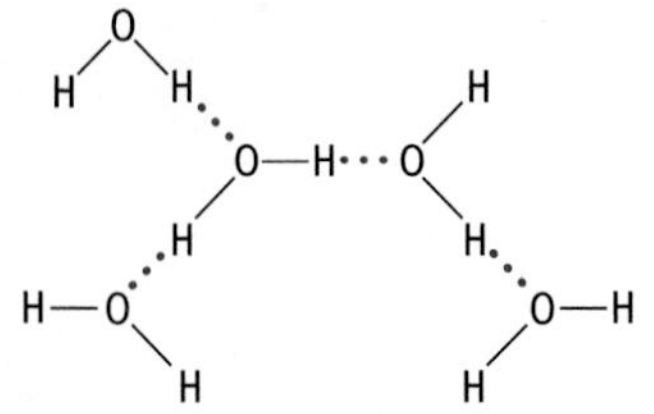

FIG. 1.2

Solution of sodium chloride in water: the ions are surrounded by noncovalently bound water molecules, which form a hydration shell.

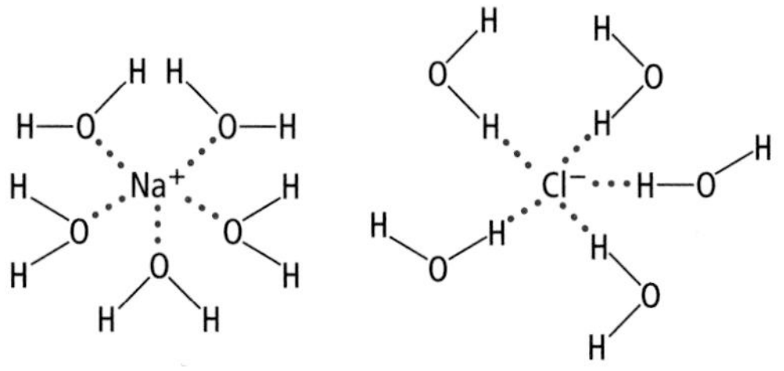

important for the properties of biomolecules. These interactions determine the higher-order structures of such macromolecules as proteins and nucleic acids, and they are essential for the formation of supramolecular aggregates, including biological membranes and a variety of fibrous structures. Therefore we can understand the properties of biomolecules only if we are familiar with the solvent in which they function.

Water molecules contain polarized bonds

The structure of water is simplicity itself: two hydrogen atoms are bonded to an oxygen atom at an angle of 105°:

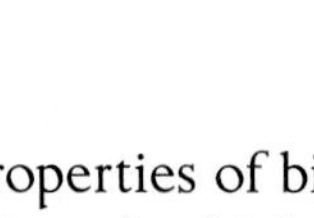

This simple molecule has a distinguishing feature: the binding electron pairs are displaced toward the oxygen atom, providing the oxygen with a high electron density and leaving the hydrogen atoms electron deficient. The oxygen is said to have a partial negative charge (δ^-), and the hydrogens have partial positive charges (δ^+). Therefore, *the water molecule forms a dipole*:

The dipolar nature of water has momentous consequences. Unlike charges attract each other; therefore, the hydrogens of a water molecule are attracted by the oxygens of other water molecules, forming **hydrogen bonds** (Fig. 1.1). Unlike the covalent bonds that hold together the hydrogen and oxygen atoms within the individual water molecules, *hydrogen bonds are weak*, forming and breaking continuously. Nevertheless, *these bonds shape the physical properties of water*. They are, for example, responsible for its abnormally high boiling point.

The water in the fluid compartments of the body always contains inorganic **cations** (positively charged ions), such as sodium and potassium, and **anions** (negatively charged ions), such as chloride and phosphate. These ions are kept in solution by **ion-dipole interactions** (Fig. 1.2): the cations associate with the oxygen atoms, and the anions associate with the hydrogen atoms of the water molecules. Although ion-dipole interactions are weak, noncovalent interactions that break and reform continuously, ions always are surrounded by a **hydration shell** of noncovalently bound water molecules.

TABLE 1.2

Typical ionic compositions of extracellular (interstitial) and intracellular fluids

Ion	Concentration (mM) in: Extracellular fluid	Cytoplasm
Na^+	137	10
K^+	4.7	141
Ca^{2+}	2.4	10^{-4}*
Mg^{2+}	1.4	31
Cl^-	113	4
$HPO_4^{2-}/H_2PO_4^-$	2	11
HCO_3^-	28†	10†
Organic acids, phosphate esters	1.8	100
pH	7.4	6.5 – 7.5

* Cytoplasmic concentration. Concentrations in mitochondria and endoplasmic reticulum are much higher.
† The lower HCO_3^- concentration in the intracellular space is caused by the lower intracellular pH, which affects the equilibrium
$$HCO_3^- + H^+ \rightleftharpoons H_2CO_3 \rightleftharpoons CO_2 + H_2O.$$

Table 1.2 shows the typical ionic compositions of intracellular (cytoplasmic) and extracellular (interstitial) fluids. Interestingly, the relative abundances of the different ions in extracellular fluid resemble those of seawater — a silent reminder of our distant evolutionary origins.

Water contains hydronium ions and hydroxyl ions

Water molecules can dissociate reversibly into hydroxyl ions and hydronium ions:

1

$$H_2O + H_2O \rightleftharpoons H_3O^+ + OH^-$$

Hydronium ion · Hydroxyl ion

In pure water, only a minute proportion of the molecules is in the H_3O^+ and OH^- forms:

2

$$[H_3O^+] = [OH^-] = 10^{-7}M$$

These concentrations are expressed as molar concentrations (mol/liter, mol/L, or M). *One mole of a*

TABLE 1.3

Relationship among pH, $[H^+]$, and $[OH^-]$

pH	$[H^+]$*	$[OH^-]$*
4	10^{-4}	10^{-10}
5	10^{-5}	10^{-9}
6	10^{-6}	10^{-8}
7	10^{-7}	10^{-7}
8	10^{-8}	10^{-6}
9	10^{-9}	10^{-5}
10	10^{-10}	10^{-4}

* $[H^+]$ and $[OH^-]$ are measured in mol/liter (M).

substance is its molecular weight in grams. Water, for example, has a molecular weight close to 18; therefore, 18 g of water are equal to 1 mol. For the sake of simplicity, the hydronium ion concentration $[H_3O^+]$ usually is expressed as the **proton concentration,** or the **hydrogen ion concentration** $[H^+]$, disregarding the fact that the proton actually is attached to the free electron pair of a water molecule.

In aqueous solutions, the product of proton (i.e., hydronium ion) concentration and hydroxyl ion concentration is a constant:

3

$$[H^+] \times [OH^-] = 10^{-14}\,M^2$$

The proton concentration $[H^+]$ of an aqueous solution, which is otherwise measured in moles/liter, usually is expressed as the **pH value,** which is defined as *the negative logarithm of the hydrogen ion concentration:*

4

$$pH = -lg[H^+]$$

Using Equations 3 and 4, we can predict the H^+ and OH^- concentration at any given pH value (Table 1.3).

The pH value of an aqueous solution is related to the presence of **acids** and **bases.** According to the **Brønsted definition,** in aqueous solutions *an acid is a substance that releases a proton, and a base is a substance that binds a proton.* The typical example of an acidic group is the carboxy group, which is the distinguishing feature of the organic acids:

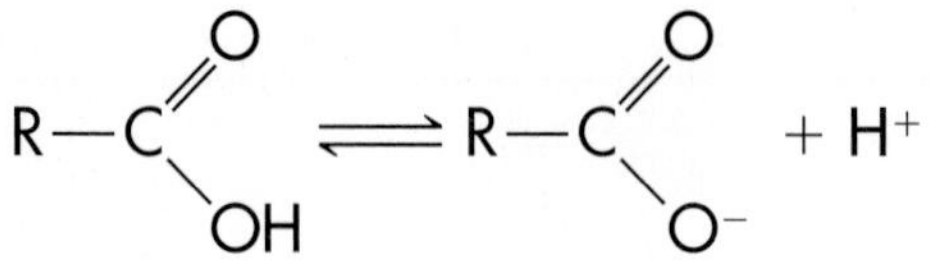

Carboxylic acid
(protonated form)   Carboxylate anion
(deprotonated form)

The protonation–deprotonation reaction is reversible, and the carboxylate anion therefore fits the definition of a Brønsted base. It is called the **conjugate base** of the acid.

Amino groups are the major basic groups in biomolecules:

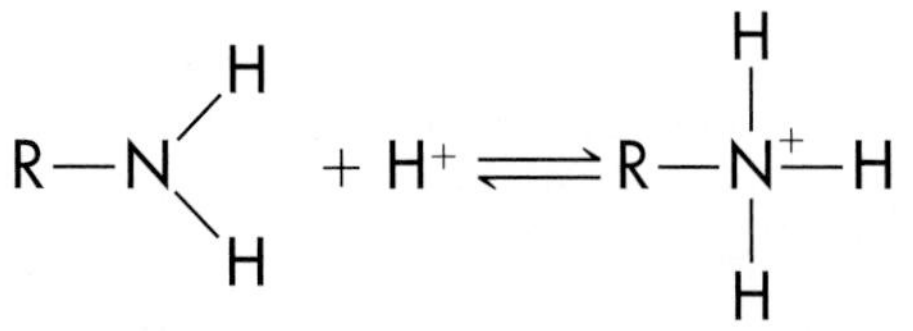

Amine
(deprotonated form)   Ammonium salt
(protonated form)

In this case, the amine is the base and the ammonium salt is its **conjugate acid**. The most important acidic groups in biomolecules are **carboxy groups, phosphate esters**, and **phosphodiesters**. These groups are deprotonated and are negatively charged at pH 7. **Sulfhydryl groups** and **phenolic hydroxy groups** are weakly acidic. They become deprotonated only at pH values much greater than 7. **Aliphatic (nonaromatic) amino groups**, including the primary, secondary, and tertiary amines, are basic. They are protonated and are positively charged at pH 7. **Aromatic amines** are only weakly basic. They become protonated at pH values much less than 7.

Ionizable groups are characterized by their pK values

The equilibrium of a protonation/deprotonation reaction is described by the **dissociation constant** (K_D). For the reaction

$$R—COOH \rightleftharpoons R—COO^- + H^+$$

the dissociation constant K_D is defined as

5

$$K_D = \frac{[R—COO^-] \times [H^+]}{[R—COOH]}$$

This can be rearranged to

6

$$[H^+] = K_D \times \frac{[R—COOH]}{[R—COO^-]}$$

The dissociation constant corresponds to the equilibrium constant, which is discussed in Chapter 4. The molar concentrations in this equation are the concentrations observed at equilibrium.

Because the hydrogen ion concentration $[H^+]$ is expressed most conveniently as the pH value, we can bring Equation 6 into the negative logarithm:

7

$$pH = pK - \lg \frac{[R—COOH]}{[R—COO^-]}$$
$$= pK + \lg \frac{[R—COO^-]}{[R—COOH]}$$

The pK value is defined as *the negative logarithm of the dissociation constant*. The pK value is a property of an individual ionizable group. If, therefore, a molecule has more than one ionizable group, as in the case of the amino acids (see Chapter 2), it has more than one pK value.

Equation 7 is called the **Henderson–Hasselbalch equation**. It can be used to determine which proportion of an ionizable group is in the protonated or deprotonated state at a given pH. If, for example, the pH value (which can be varied experimentally) equals the pK value (which is a fixed property of the group), the Henderson-Hassel-balch equation yields a value of zero for $\lg[R—COOH]/[R—COO^-]$. Therefore, $[R—COOH]/[R—COO^-] = 1$. We see now that *the pK value corresponds to that pH value at which the ionizable group is half-protonated*. The pK value is a measure for the "strength" of an acidic or basic group. At pH values less than the pK value (high $[H^+]$), ionizable groups are mostly protonated; at pH values greater than the pK (low H^+), the groups are mostly deprotonated (Table 1.4).

TABLE 1.4

Protonation state of a carboxy group and an amino group at different pH values

	Carboxy group		Amino group	
pH	% of group protonated (R—COOH)	% of group deprotonated (R—COO⁻)	% of group protonated (R—NH₃⁺)	% of group deprotonated (R—NH₂)
pK + 3	0.1	99.9	0.1	99.9
+ 2	1	99	1	99
+ 1	10	90	10	90
pH = pK	50	50	50	50
pK − 1	90	10	90	10
− 2	99	1	99	1
− 3	99.9	0.1	99.9	0.1

COVALENT BONDS AND NONCOVALENT INTERACTIONS

Complexity is a hallmark of biochemistry: more than a million chemically different molecules are present in the human body, and most of these are proteins and nucleic acids with high molecular weights (>10,000 Da) and well-defined structures. (Fortunately, students need not memorize them all.) Despite their complexity, however, most biomolecules contain not more than 3 to 6 different elements out of the 92 that are available in nature. Carbon (C), hydrogen (H), and oxygen (O) are always present. Many biomolecules also contain nitrogen (N), and sulfur (S) and phosphorus (P) are present in some. The atoms within a molecule are held together by **covalent bonds.** Covalent bonds are produced by the sharing of electrons between the participating atoms. The atoms in biomolecules are arranged in a limited number of functional groups (Table 1.5). Whereas the strong, stable covalent bonds establish the overall structure of the molecules, **noncovalent interactions** provide weak attractive forces between atoms, either within a molecule or between different molecules.

Bonds are formed by reactions between functional groups

Living cells construct **macromolecules** ("large molecules") from small building blocks. The bonds between these building blocks are formed—formally at least—by reactions between two functional

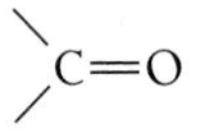

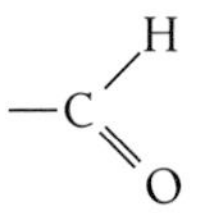

TABLE 1.5

Functional groups in biomolecules

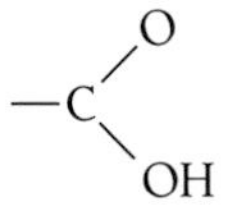

1. Hydrocarbon groups
—CH₃	Methyl
—CH₂—CH₃	Ethyl
—CH₂—	Methylene
—CH=	Methine

2. Oxygen-containing groups
R—OH	Hydroxy (alcoholic)
—OH (phenolic ring)	Hydroxy (phenolic)
\C=O	Keto
—C(H)(=O)	Aldehyde
—C(=O)OH	Carboxy

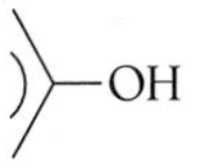

   Keto and Aldehyde grouped as Carbonyl.

3. Nitrogen-containing groups
—NH₂	Primary amine
\NH	Secondary amine
\N—	Tertiary amine
—N±—	Quaternary ammonium salt

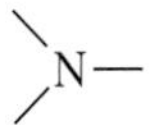

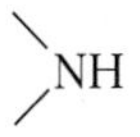

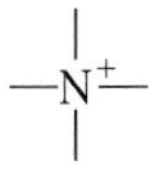

4. Sulfur-containing group
   | —SH | Sulfhydryl group |

TABLE 1.6

Important bonds in biomolecules

Bond	Structure	Formed from	Occurs in
Ether	$R_1{-}O{-}R_2$	$R_1{-}OH + HO{-}R_2$	Methyl ethers, some membrane lipids
Carboxylic ester	$R_1{-}\overset{\overset{O}{\|}}{C}{-}O{-}R_2$	$R_1{-}\overset{\overset{O}{\|}}{C}{-}OH + HO{-}R_2$	Triglycerides, other lipids
Acetal	$\begin{matrix} R_2{-}O & & O{-}R_3 \\ & C & \\ R_1 & & H \end{matrix}$	$R_1{-}\overset{O}{\underset{H}{C}}{-}OH + HO{-}R_3$	Di-, oligo-, and polysaccharides (glycosidic bonds)
Mixed anhydride*	$R{-}\overset{\overset{O}{\|}}{C}{-}O{-}\overset{\overset{O^-}{\|}}{\underset{O}{P}}{-}O^-$	$R{-}\overset{\overset{O}{\|}}{C}{-}OH + HO{-}\overset{\overset{O^-}{\|}}{\underset{O}{P}}{-}O^-$	Some metabolic intermediates
Phosphoanhydride*	$R{-}O{-}\overset{\overset{O^-}{\|}}{\underset{O}{P}}{-}O{-}\overset{\overset{O^-}{\|}}{\underset{O}{P}}{-}O^-$	$R{-}O{-}\overset{\overset{O^-}{\|}}{\underset{O}{P}}{-}OH + HO{-}\overset{\overset{O^-}{\|}}{\underset{O}{P}}{-}O^-$	Nucleotides; most important: ATP
Phosphate ester	$R{-}O{-}\overset{\overset{O^-}{\|}}{\underset{O}{P}}{-}O^-$	$R{-}OH + HO{-}\overset{\overset{O^-}{\|}}{\underset{O}{P}}{-}O^-$	Many metabolic intermediates, phosphoproteins
Phosphodiester	$R_1{-}O{-}\overset{\overset{O^-}{\|}}{\underset{O}{P}}{-}O{-}R_2$	$R_1{-}OH + HO{-}\overset{\overset{O^-}{\|}}{\underset{O}{P}}{-}OH + HO{-}R_2$	Nucleic acids, phospholipids
Unsubstituted amide	$R{-}\overset{\overset{O}{\|}}{C}{-}NH_2$	$R{-}\overset{\overset{O}{\|}}{C}{-}OH + H{-}N\overset{H}{\underset{H}{\big<}}$	Asparagine, glutamine
Substituted amide	$R_1{-}\overset{\overset{O}{\|}}{C}{-}\overset{}{\underset{H}{N}}{-}R_2$	$R_1{-}\overset{\overset{O}{\|}}{C}{-}OH + H{-}\overset{}{\underset{H}{N}}{-}R_2$	Polypeptides (peptide bond)
Thioester*	$R_1{-}\overset{\overset{O}{\|}}{C}{-}S{-}R_2$	$R_1{-}\overset{\overset{O}{\|}}{C}{-}OH + HS{-}R_2$	Acetyl-CoA, other "activated" acids
Thioether	$R_1{-}S{-}R_2$	$R_1{-}SH + HO{-}R_2$	Methionine

* "Energy-rich" bonds.

groups, and bond formation is accompanied by the release of water. This type of reaction is called a **condensation reaction.** Conversely, bonds can be cleaved by the addition of water, in a reaction type called **hydrolysis.** The most important examples of bonds are listed in Table 1.6.

Bond formation is an **endergonic** (energy-requiring) process (see Chapter 4), and therefore *the construction of large molecules from small ones requires metabolic energy.* Bond cleavage by hydrolysis, however, is **exergonic** (energy-producing) and does not require metabolic energy. The digestive enzymes, for example, which catalyze hydrolytic bond cleavages (see Chapter 14), work perfectly well in the lumen of the gastrointestinal tract, where neither adenosine triphosphate (ATP) nor other forms of usable energy are available.

Some bonds contain more energy than others. Most ester, ether, acetal, and amide bonds require between 1 and 5 kcal/mol for their formation, and the same amount of energy is released during their hydrolysis. **Anhydride bonds** and **thioester bonds,** however, have energy contents greater than 5 kcal/mol. They are classified, rather arbitrarily, as **energy-rich bonds.**

Isomeric forms are common in bio-molecules

Isomers are chemically different molecules with identical composition. Three different types of isomers can be distinguished in biomolecules:

1. **Positional isomers** differ in the positions of functional groups within the molecule.

Examples:

2-Phosphoglycerate

3-Phosphoglycerate

Glyceraldehyde

Dihydroxyacetone

2. **Geometric isomers** differ in the arrangement of substituents at a rigid portion of the molecule.

The *cis-trans* isomers of carbon–carbon double bonds (see also Chapter 11, Figure 11.8) are a typical example:

cis double bond   *trans* double bond

The two forms are not interconvertible because there is no rotation around the double bond, and all substituents (H, R_1, and R_2) are fixed in the same plane. Also, ring systems show geometric isomerism, with substituents facing to either one or the other surface of the ring. Geometric isomers are called **diastereomers.**

3. **Optical isomers** differ in the orientation of substituents around an asymmetric carbon. An asymmetric carbon is characterized by the presence of four *different* substituents. If only one asymmetric carbon is present in the molecule, the resulting isomers are mirror images. Such isomers are called **enantiomers.** They are related to each other like the left hand and the right hand, and therefore, the phenomenon of optical isomerism often is called **chirality** (Gr. χειρ, "hand").

Unlike positional and geometric isomers, which differ in their melting point, boiling point, solubility, and crystal structure, *enantiomers have identical physicochemical properties.* They can be distinguished only by the direction in which they turn the plane of polarized light. If more than one asymmetric carbon is present in the molecule, the resulting isomers are not mirror images, and they have different physicochemical properties. In this case, the isomeric forms are geometric isomers. Optical isomers commonly are represented in the **Fisher projection,** in which the substituents above and below the asymmetric carbon face behind the plane of the paper, and those on the left and right face to the front:

The carbon is placed in the center of a tetrahedron whose corners are formed by the four substituents.

For example:

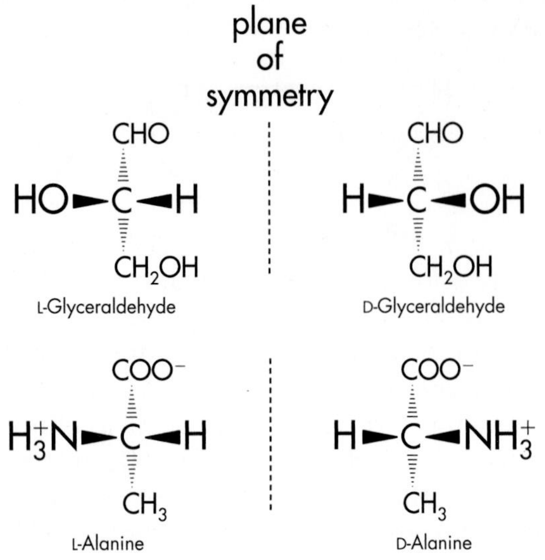

plane
of
symmetry

CHO

HO—C—H

CH₂OH

L-Glyceraldehyde

CHO

H—C—OH

CH₂OH

D-Glyceraldehyde

COO⁻

H_3^+N—C—H

CH₃

L-Alanine

COO⁻

H—C—NH_3^+

CH₃

D-Alanine

Most importantly, *even enantiomers differ in their biological properties*: binding interactions between chiral biomolecules are stereospecific (selective for one or the other enantiomer), and the enzymes that catalyze chemical reactions in the body readily distinguish among different optical isomers (see page 57).

Biomolecules form a variety of noncovalent interactions

Whereas the atoms within the molecules are held together by covalent bonds, *interactions between molecules are mediated by noncovalent interactions*. The principal noncovalent interactions are:

1. **Dipole–dipole interactions.** These also are known as **hydrogen bonds**, because they usually involve a hydrogen atom that is bound covalently to an electronegative atom such as oxygen or nitrogen. The **electronegativity** is the tendency of an atom to attract electrons. For the atoms commonly encountered in biomolecules, the rank order of electronegativity is

$$O > N > S \geq C \geq H$$

Examples of groups that are capable of hydrogen bond formation are the oxygen-containing groups and the primary and secondary amino groups shown in Table 1.5.

See Box 1.1 for examples (see also Fig. 1.1).

2. **Electrostatic interactions,** or **salt bonds,** are formed by the attractive force between a negatively charged ion (anion) and a positively charged ion (cation).

An example is the salt bond between a carboxylic acid and a primary amine:

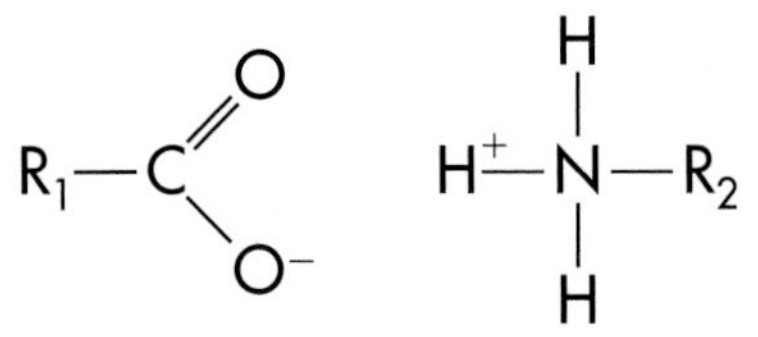

$$R_1-C \overset{O}{\underset{O^-}{\big|\big|}} \qquad H^+\!-\!\overset{H}{\underset{H}{N}}\!-\!R_2$$

BOX 1.1

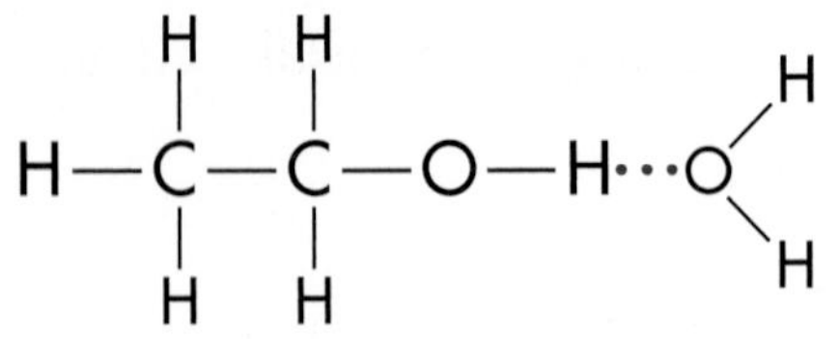

Hydrogen bond between
ethanol and water

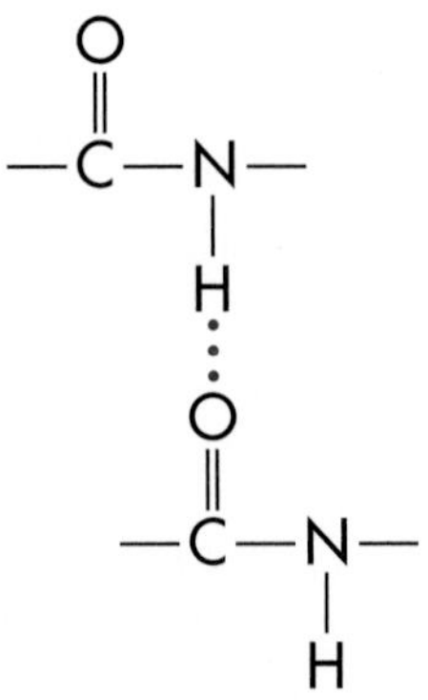

Hydrogen bond between
two peptide bonds

Introduction to Biomolecules Principles of Molecular Structure and Function

3. **Ion–dipole interactions** are formed between an ion and a polarized bond. An example is shown in Figure 1.2.

4. **Hydrophobic interactions** are formed in aqueous solutions between molecules or portions of molecules that do not positively interact with water. Hydrophobic interactions are not based on an attractive force between the interacting groups but rather on the fact that *an interface between a hydrophobic structure and water is energetically unfavorable*: it limits the ability of the water molecules to form hydrogen bonds with their neighbors. The molecules have to reorient themselves to maximize the hydrogen bonds with neighboring water molecules, thereby attaining a more ordered state, and this ordered state is energetically unfavorable (see Chapter 4). The association of the hydrophobic groups is favored because *it decreases the aqueous-hydrophobic interface*.

5. **Van der Waals forces** are important whenever two molecules approach each other (Fig. 1.3). A weak attractive force prevails at moderate distances, but a strong repulsive force is observed at close proximities. The attractive van der Waals force is the result of induced dipoles in the molecules; the repulsive force is caused by electrostatic repulsion between the electron shells of neighboring atoms. The van der Waals forces determine how tightly the molecules are packed. The attractive force prevents "empty spaces"; the repulsive force prevents overcrowding.

Noncovalent interactions are important because *they determine the biological properties of biomolecules:*

a. *Noncovalent interactions with water molecules are required for water solubility.* Substances that contain polarized bonds and are able to form hydrogen bonds with water molecules often are water soluble. The same is true for charged molecules that form ion–dipole interactions with water. If a molecule can exist in either a charged or an uncharged state, *the charged form is more water soluble*. Molecules with large hydrophobic portions often are insoluble in water.

b. *Noncovalent interactions form higher-order structures in macromolecules.* These interactions are formed between different portions of the same molecule: they are intramolecular. Proteins (see Chapter 2) and nucleic acids (Chapter 6) have elaborate higher-order structures, which are essential for their biological properties.

c. *Molecules can bind to each other by noncovalent interactions.* Examples include the binding of substrates to enzymes (see Chapter 4), of antibodies to antigens (Chapter 25), and of hormones to their receptors (Chapter 27).

FIG. 1.3

Attractive and repulsive van der Waals forces. At the van der Waals contact distance (arrow), the opposing forces cancel each other.

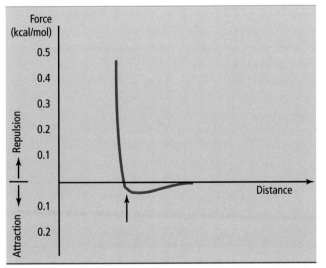

THE MAJOR CLASSES OF BIOMOLECULES

Having reviewed some general aspects of molecular structure, we now will briefly introduce the structures of the major classes of biomolecules, namely, the triglycerides, carbohydrates, proteins, and nucleic acids. More detailed information about these structures will be presented in later chapters.

Triglycerides consist of fatty acids and glycerol

The **triacylglycerols**, better known as **triglycerides** in the medical literature, are the major storage form of metabolic energy in the human body.

They consist of glycerol and fatty acids. **Glycerol** is a trivalent alcohol:

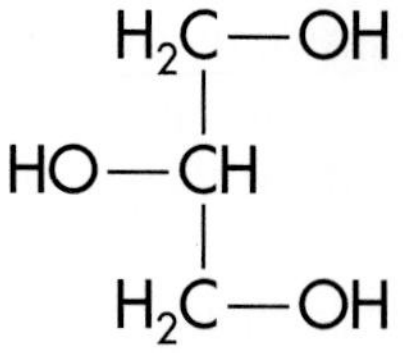

$$H_2C-OH$$
$$HO-CH$$
$$H_2C-OH$$

Glycerol

Fatty acids consist of a long hydrocarbon chain with a carboxy group at one end. In most cases, the chain length is between 16 and 20 carbons. See Box 1.2 for an example.

Palmitic acid also can be written as shown in Box 1.3. It is an example of a **saturated fatty acid. Unsaturated fatty acids** have at least one carbon–carbon double bond. For example:

$$H_3C-(CH_2)_5-CH=CH-(CH_2)_7-COOH$$

Palmitoleic acid

Fatty acids have pK values between 4.7 and 5.0, and therefore, they are mostly in the deprotonated ($-COO^-$) form at pH 7.

In the triglycerides, all three hydroxy groups of glycerol are esterified with a fatty acid as shown in Box 1.4. Although the ester bonds have a limited potential for hydrogen bond formation, *the triglycerides are insoluble in water* because of the long hydrocarbon chains of their fatty acid residues.

The **monoacylglycerols (monoglycerides)** and **diacylglycerols (diglycerides)** have only one or two fatty acids, respectively, bound to glycerol. The positions of the fatty acids are specified in their names (R, R_1, R_2 = hydrocarbon chains of the fatty acids) as shown in Box 1.5.

BOX 1.2

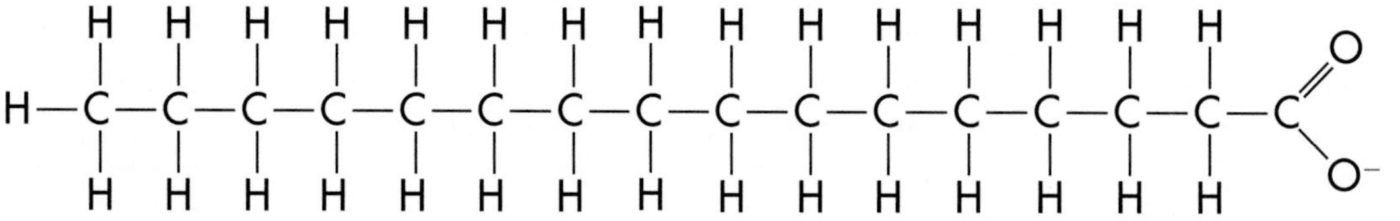

Palmitic acid

BOX 1.3

$$H_3C-(CH_2)_{14}-COOH \quad \text{or}$$

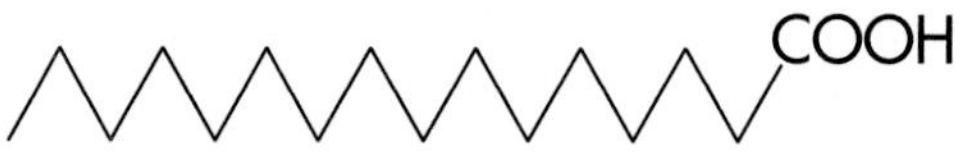

BOX 1.4

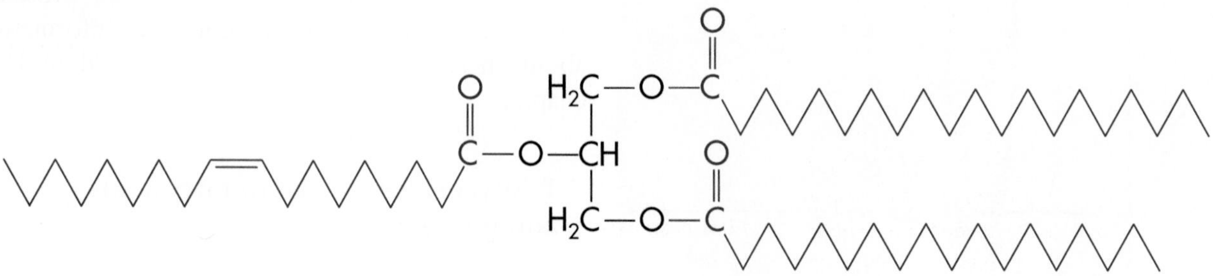

Triglyceride

Substances with strong hydrophobic properties, including the mono-, di-, and triglycerides, are called **lipids,** irrespective of their specific molecular architecture.

Monosaccharides have either a keto group or an aldehyde group

The **monosaccharides,** which are the building blocks of all carbohydrates, contain a variable number of carbons. Each carbon carries a hydroxy group, except for one that forms a carbonyl group. Monosaccharides are distinguished by the number of carbons and by the nature of the carbonyl group, which is either an aldehyde or a keto group as shown in Box 1.6.

Examples include D-glyceraldehyde and dihydroxyacetone:

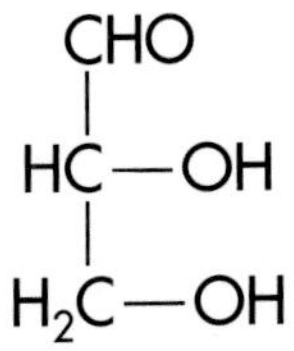

$$
\begin{array}{ll}
\text{CHO} & \text{H}_2\text{C—OH} \\
\text{HC—OH} & \text{C=O} \\
\text{H}_2\text{C—OH} & \text{H}_2\text{C—OH}
\end{array}
$$

D-Glyceraldehyde (an aldotriose) 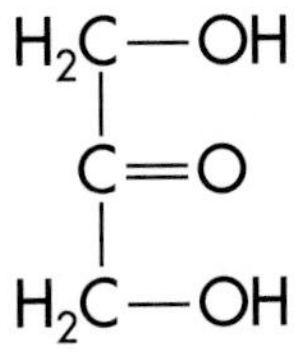   Dihydroxyacetone (a ketotriose)

BOX 1.5

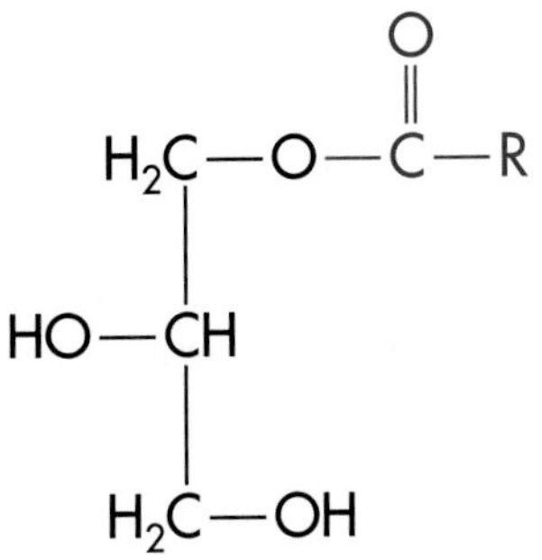

1-Monoacylglycerol 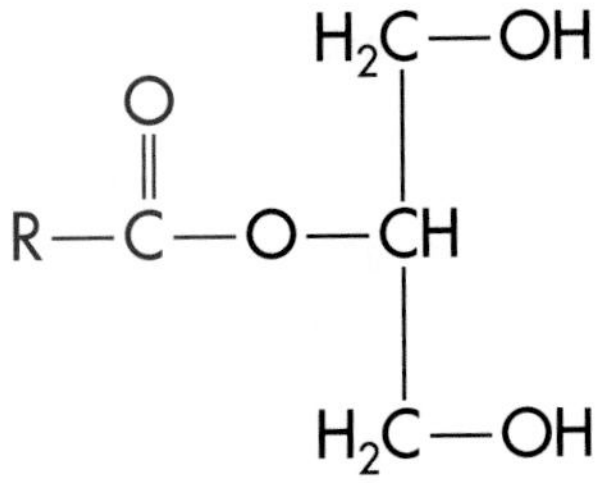   2-Monoacylglycerol 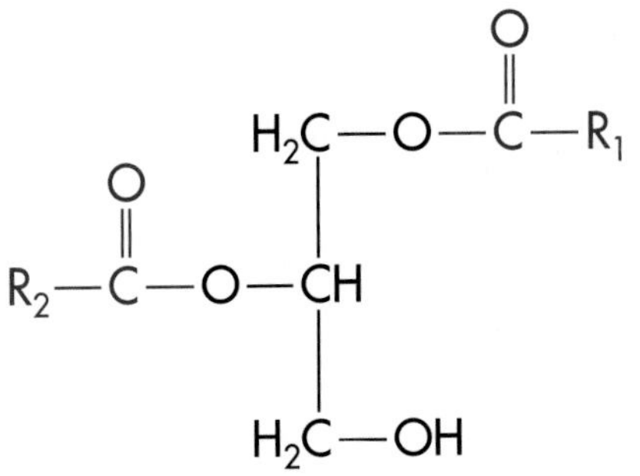   1,2-Diacylglycerol

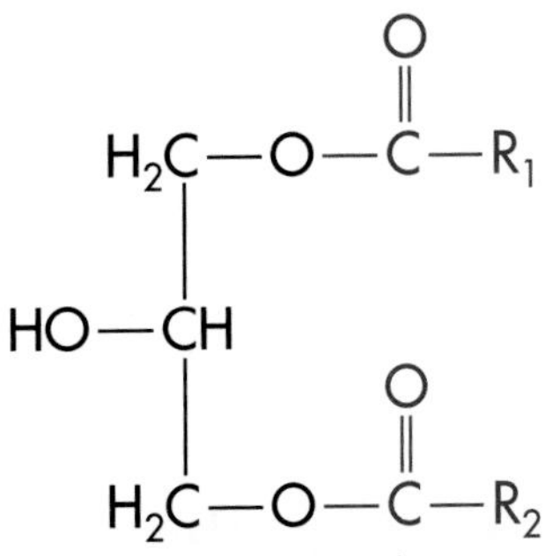

1,3-Diacylglycerol

BOX 1.6

Triose: 3-carbon sugar
Tetrose: 4-carbon sugar
Pentose: 5-carbon sugar
Hexose: 6-carbon sugar
Heptose: 7-carbon sugar
etc.

Aldose: Monosaccharide with an aldehyde group

Ketose: Monosaccharide with a keto group

BOX 1.7

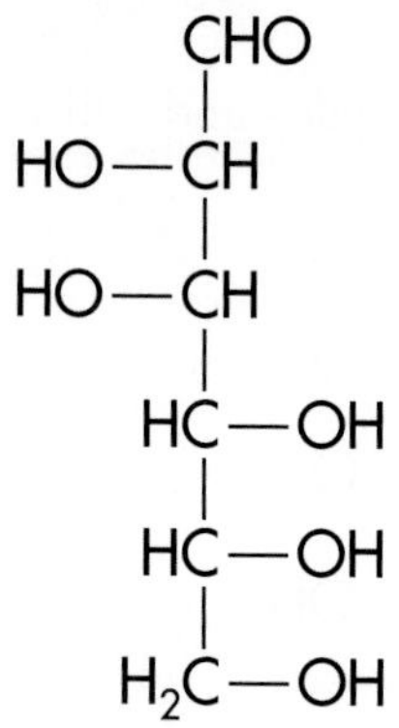

D-Mannose

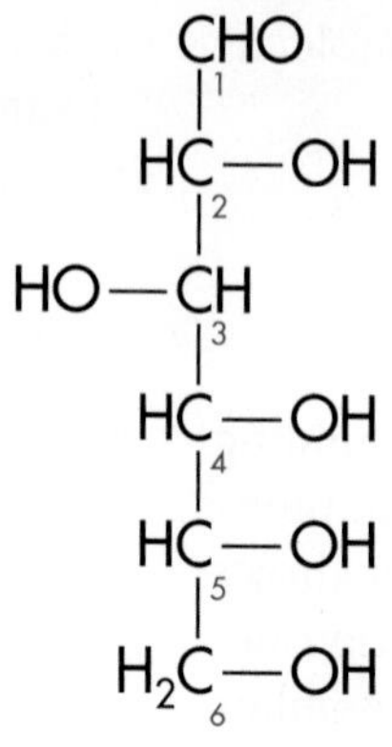

D-Glucose

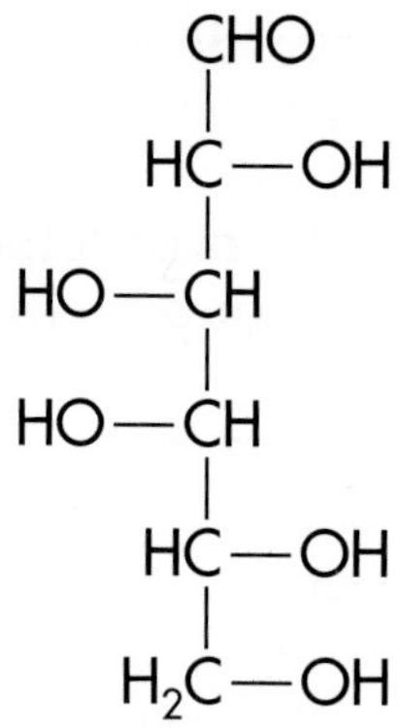

D-Galactose

The most important monosaccharide is D-glucose, an aldohoxose:

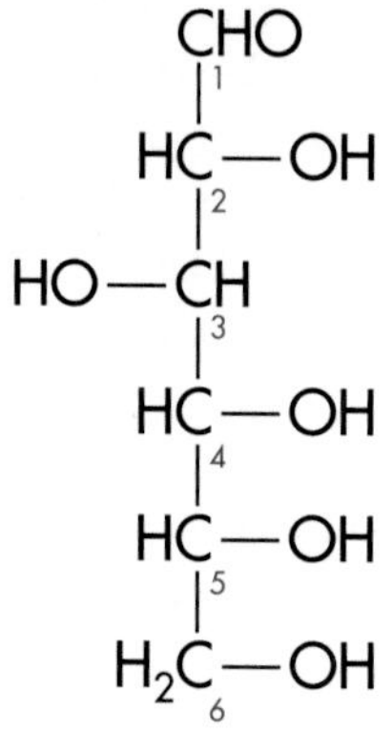

D-Glucose

The carbons of the monosaccharides are conveniently numbered, starting with the aldehyde carbon or, for ketoses, the terminal carbon closest to the keto carbon. By convention, the "D" in D-glyceraldehyde and D-glucose refers to the orientation of substituents at the carbon farthest removed from the carbonyl carbon (C-2 and C-5, respectively).

When we examine the structure of D-glucose, we find not less than four asymmetric carbons: carbons 2, 3, 4, and 5 all have four different substituents. We can therefore construct 16 optical isomers. There are, indeed, aldohexoses that differ in the orientation of the substituents at one or more of their asymmetric carbons.

Examples are shown in Box 1.7. These three sugars are not mirror images of each other. Therefore, they are not enantiomers but diastereomers, and they have different physical and chemical properties. Monosaccharides differing in the orientation of substituents around one of their asymmetric carbons are called **epimers.** D-Mannose is a C-2 epimer, whereas D-galactose is a C-4 epimer of glucose.

Monosaccharides form ring structures

Most monosaccharides spontaneously form ring structures in which the aldehyde (or keto) group forms a hemiacetal (or hemiketal) bond with one of the hydroxy groups. If the ring contains five atoms, it is called a **furanose** ring; if it contains six atoms, it is called a **pyranose** ring. The ring structures are written either in the **Fisher** projection or in the **Haworth** projection as shown in Box 1.8.

In aqueous solutions, only 1 of 40,000 glucose molecules is in the open-chain form. When the ring structure forms, carbon 1 of glucose becomes asymmetric. Therefore we can form two isomers, α-D-glucose and β-D-glucose. These two isomers, which differ only in the arrangement of the substituents around the carbonyl carbon, are not called epimers but rather **anomers.** In glucose, carbon 1 (the aldehyde carbon) is the **anomeric carbon.** In fructose, carbon 2 (the keto carbon) is anomeric. Unlike the epimers, which are stable under ordinary conditions, anomers interconvert spontaneously. This process is called **mutarotation.** It is

BOX 1.8

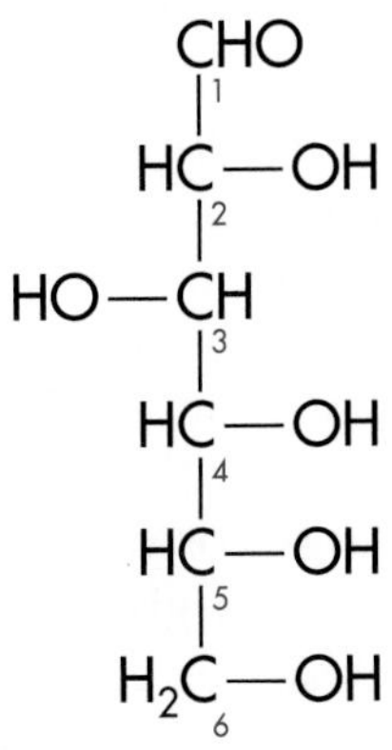

D-Glucose
(open-chain form)

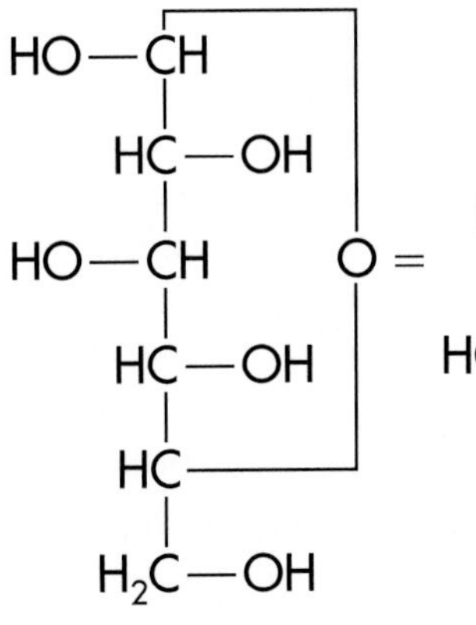

β-D-Glucopyranose
(modified Fisher projection)

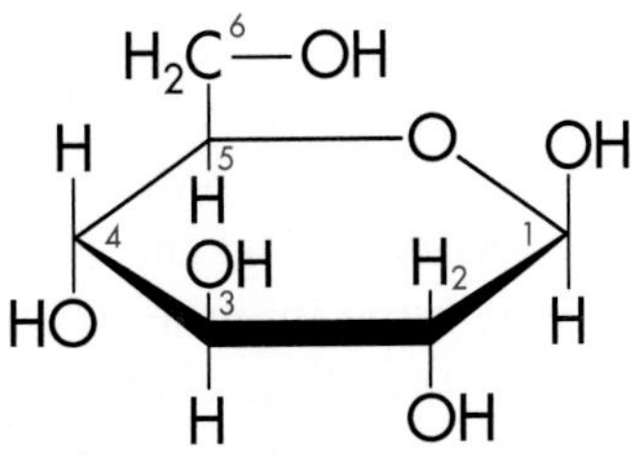

β-D-Glucopyranose
(Haworth projection)

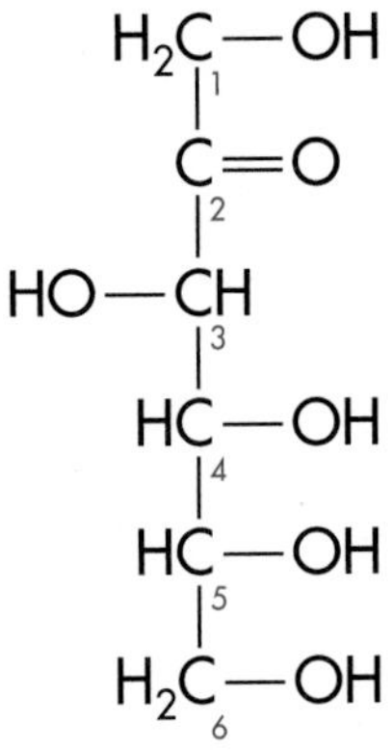

D-Fructose
(open-chain form)

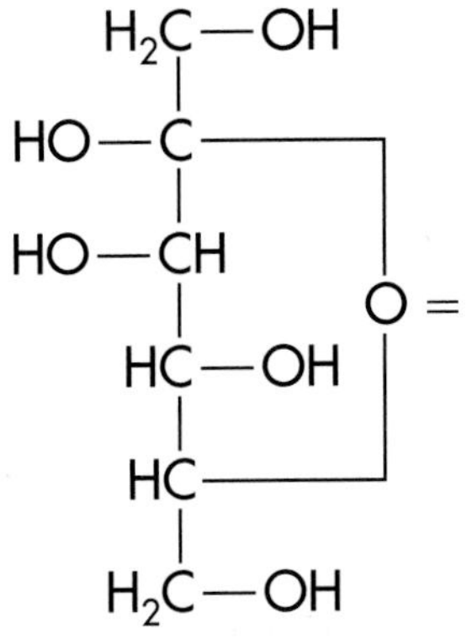

β-D-Fructofuranose
(modified Fisher projection)

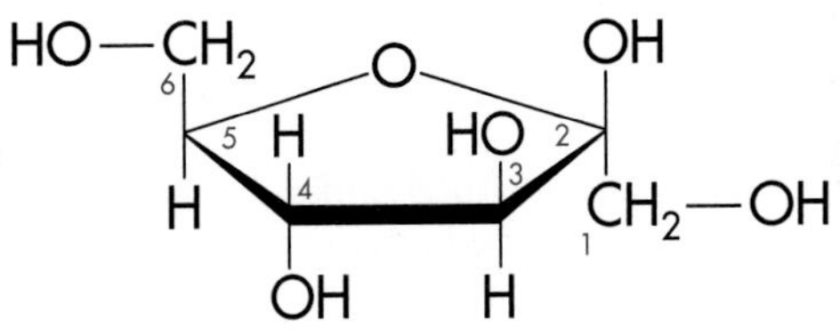

β-D-Fructofuranose
(Haworth projection)

BOX 1.9

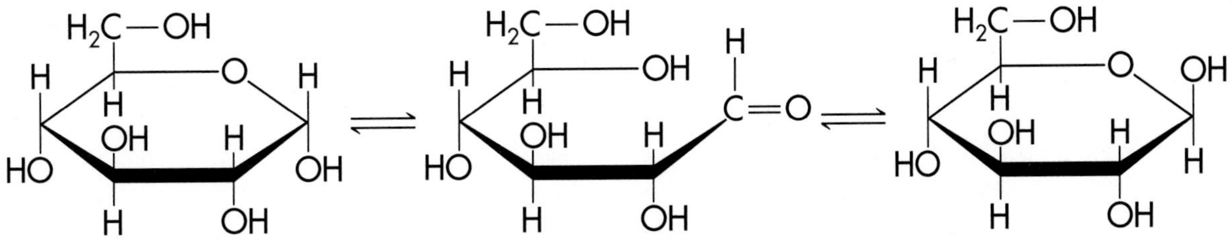

α-D-Glucopyranose
(34%)

D-Glucose
open-chain form
(0.0025%)

β-D-Glucopyranose
(66%)

caused by the occasional opening and reclosure of the ring as shown in Box 1.9. The equilibrium between the α and β anomers, with approximately 34% of the glucose molecules in the α-form and 66% in the β-form, is reached within several hours in neutral solutions, but mutarotation is accelerated greatly in the presence of acids or bases.

Complex carbohydrates are formed by glycosidic bonds

Complex carbohydrates are held together by glycosidic bonds between monosaccharides. *The glycosidic bonds in carbohydrates are acetal or ketal bonds involving the anomeric carbon (the aldehyde or keto carbon, respectively) of one of the participating monosaccharides.* The anomeric carbon can form the glycosidic bond in either the α or the β configuration. Bond formation eliminates mutarotation, and therefore, two different products can be formed. Maltose and cellobiose, for example (Fig. 1.4), differ only in the orientation of their 1,4-glycosidic bonds.

Structures formed from two monosaccharides are called **disaccharides.** If three, four, five, or six monosaccharides are present, the products are called tri-, tetra-, penta-, and hexasaccharides, respectively. **Oligosaccharides** (Gr. ὀλίγος, "a few") contain a few monosaccharides, and **polysaccharides** (Gr. πολύς, "many") contain many monosaccharides (Fig. 1.5).

Glycosidic bonds also can be formed between the anomeric carbon of a monosaccharide and a noncarbohydrate. In glycoproteins (see Chapter 2), for example, oligosaccharides are bound by glycosidic bonds to the side chains of amino acid residues. If the sugar is bound to its partner through an oxygen atom, the bond is called **O-glycosidic**; if it is bound through a nitrogen, it is called **N-glycosidic.**

Monosaccharides, disaccharides, and oligosaccharides, ordinarily known as "sugars," are water soluble because of their high hydrogen-bonding potential. Polysaccharides, however, often are insoluble because of their large size, which increases the opportunities for intermolecular interactions.

FIG. 1.4

Structures of some common disaccharides. Conventionally, the nonreducing end of the disaccharide is written on the left side, the reducing end on the right side.

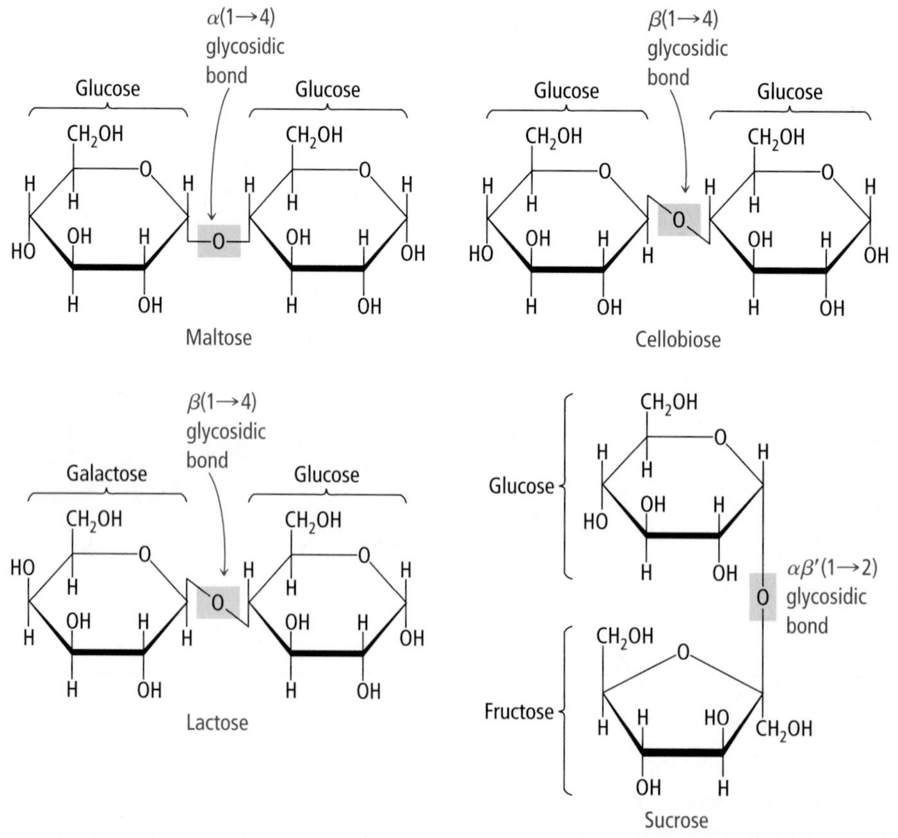

Monosaccharides have reducing properties that depend on their carbonyl group. *Once engaged in the formation of a glycosidic bond, the carbonyl group loses its reducing properties.* Of the disaccharides shown in Fig. 1.4, for example, only sucrose is not a reducing sugar because both of the anomeric carbons participate in the glycosidic bond. The other disaccharides have a reducing end and a nonreducing end.

FIG. 1.5

Structures of some common polysaccharides. **A,** *Amylose* is an unbranched polymer of glucose residues in α-1,4 glycosidic linkage. Together with amylopectin—a branched glucose polymer with a structure resembling that of glycogen—it forms the starch granules in plants. **B,** Like amylose, *cellulose* is an unbranched polymer of glucose residues. As a major component in the cell walls of plants, it is the most abundant biomolecule on earth. The marked difference in the physical and biological properties between the two polysaccharides is caused by the presence of β-1,4 rather than α-1,4 glycosidic bonds in cellulose. **C,** *Glycogen* is the storage polysaccharide of animals and humans. Like amylose, it contains chains of glucose residues in α-1,4 glycosidic linkage. Unlike amylose, however, the molecule is branched: some glucose residues in the chain form a third glycosidic bond, using their hydroxy group at carbon 6.

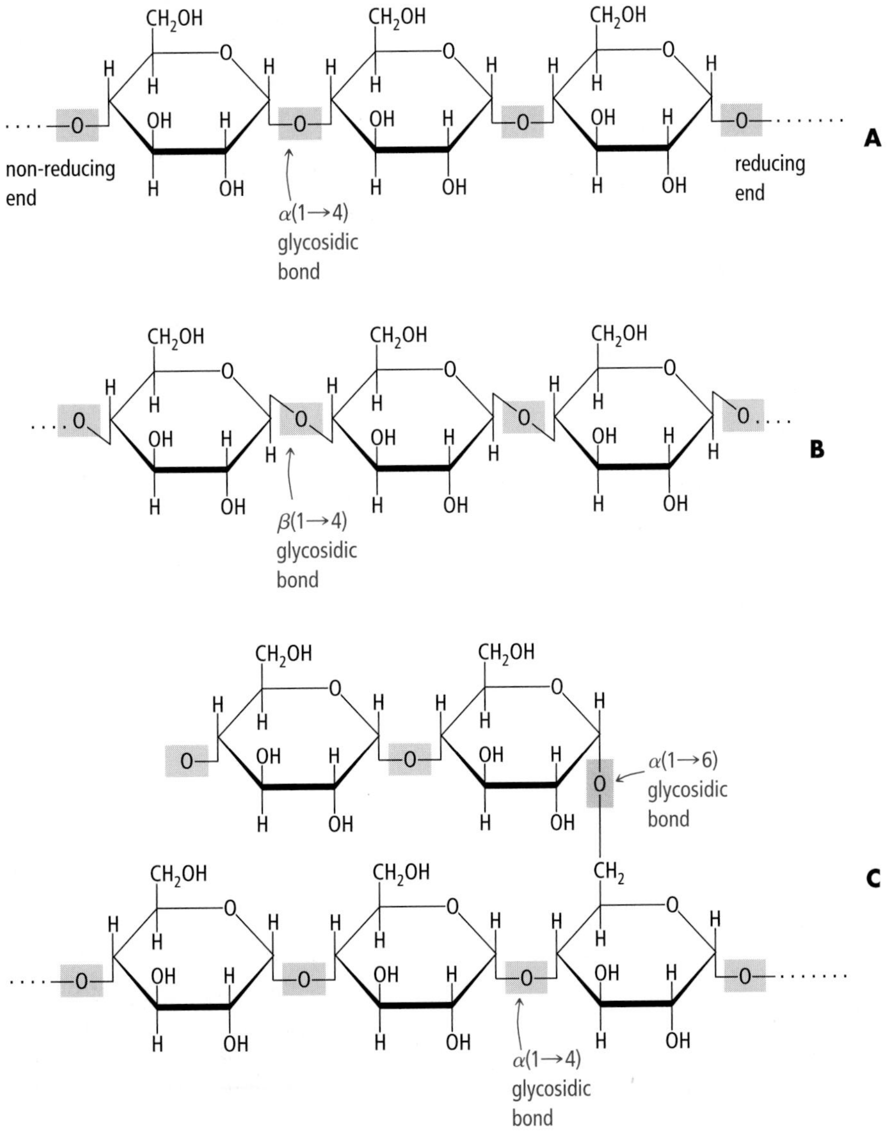

Polypeptides are formed from amino acids

Polypeptides are constructed from 20 different amino acids. All amino acids have a **carboxy group** and an **amino group,** both bound to the same carbon. This carbon, called the **α-carbon,** also carries a hydrogen atom and a fourth group, the **side chain,** which differs in the 20 amino acids. The general structure of the amino acids can therefore be depicted as:

$$
\begin{array}{ccc}
\text{COO}^- & & \text{COO}^- \\
\text{H}_3^+\text{N} \blacktriangleright \text{C} \blacktriangleleft \text{H} & \text{or} & \text{H} \blacktriangleright \text{C} \blacktriangleleft \text{NH}_3^+ \\
\text{R} & & \text{R} \\
\text{L-Amino acid} & & \text{D-Amino acid}
\end{array}
$$

where R (residue) is the variable side chain. The asymmetric nature of the α-carbon gives rise to D and L isomers, but *only the L-amino acids occur in polypeptides.*

Dipeptides are formed by a reaction between the carboxy group of one amino acid and the amino group of another amino acid. The substituted amide bond thus formed is called the **peptide bond** as shown in Box 1.10. Chains of "a few" amino acids are called **oligopeptides,** and chains of "many" amino acids are called **polypeptides** as shown in Box 1.11.

Nucleic acids are formed from nucleotides

There are two types of nucleic acid, **ribonucleic acid (RNA)** and **deoxyribonucleic acid (DNA).** These nucleic acids consist of three kinds of building blocks:

1. A **pentose sugar,** which is ribose in RNA and 2-deoxyribose in DNA:

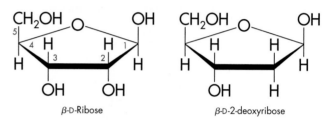

β-D-Ribose   β-D-2-deoxyribose

2. **Phosphate,** which is bound to hydroxy groups in ribose or 2-deoxyribose.

3. Heterocyclic bases, which include the purine bases **adenine** and **guanine** and the pyrimidine bases **cytosine, uracil,** and **thymine.** The pyrimidines have a single six-membered

---

BOX 1.10

$$
\underset{\substack{| \\ \text{H}_3^+\text{N}-\text{CH}-\boxed{\text{COO}^-}}}{\overset{\text{R}_1}{}} + \underset{\substack{\boxed{\text{H}_3^+\text{N}}-\text{CH}-\text{COO}^-}}{\overset{\text{R}_2}{}} \longrightarrow \underset{\text{Dipeptide}}{\text{H}_3^+\text{N}-\text{CH}-\overset{\text{O}}{\text{C}}-\underset{\text{H}}{\text{N}}-\text{CH}-\text{COO}^-}
$$

H₂O

peptide bond

Dipeptide

BOX 1.11

$$
\text{H}_3^+\text{N}-\underset{\text{R}_1}{\text{CH}}-\underset{\text{H}}{\overset{\text{O}}{\text{C}}}-\text{N}-\underset{\text{R}_2}{\text{CH}}-\underset{\text{H}}{\overset{\text{O}}{\text{C}}}-\text{N}-\underset{\text{R}_3}{\text{CH}}-\underset{\text{H}}{\overset{\text{O}}{\text{C}}}-\text{N}-\underset{\text{R}_4}{\text{CH}}-\underset{\text{H}}{\overset{\text{O}}{\text{C}}}-\text{N}-\underset{\text{R}_5}{\text{CH}}-\underset{\text{H}}{\overset{\text{O}}{\text{C}}}-\text{N}-\underset{\text{R}_6}{\text{CH}}-\text{COO}^-
$$

A hexapeptide (an oligopeptide cantaining six amino acids)

FIG. 1.6

Structures of some nucleosides and nucleotides. A prime (') is used for the numbering of the carbons in the sugar, to distinguish it from the numbering of the ring carbons and nitrogens in the bases. **A,** Examples of ribonucleosides. **B,** Examples of deoxyribonucleosides. **C,** Examples of nucleotides.

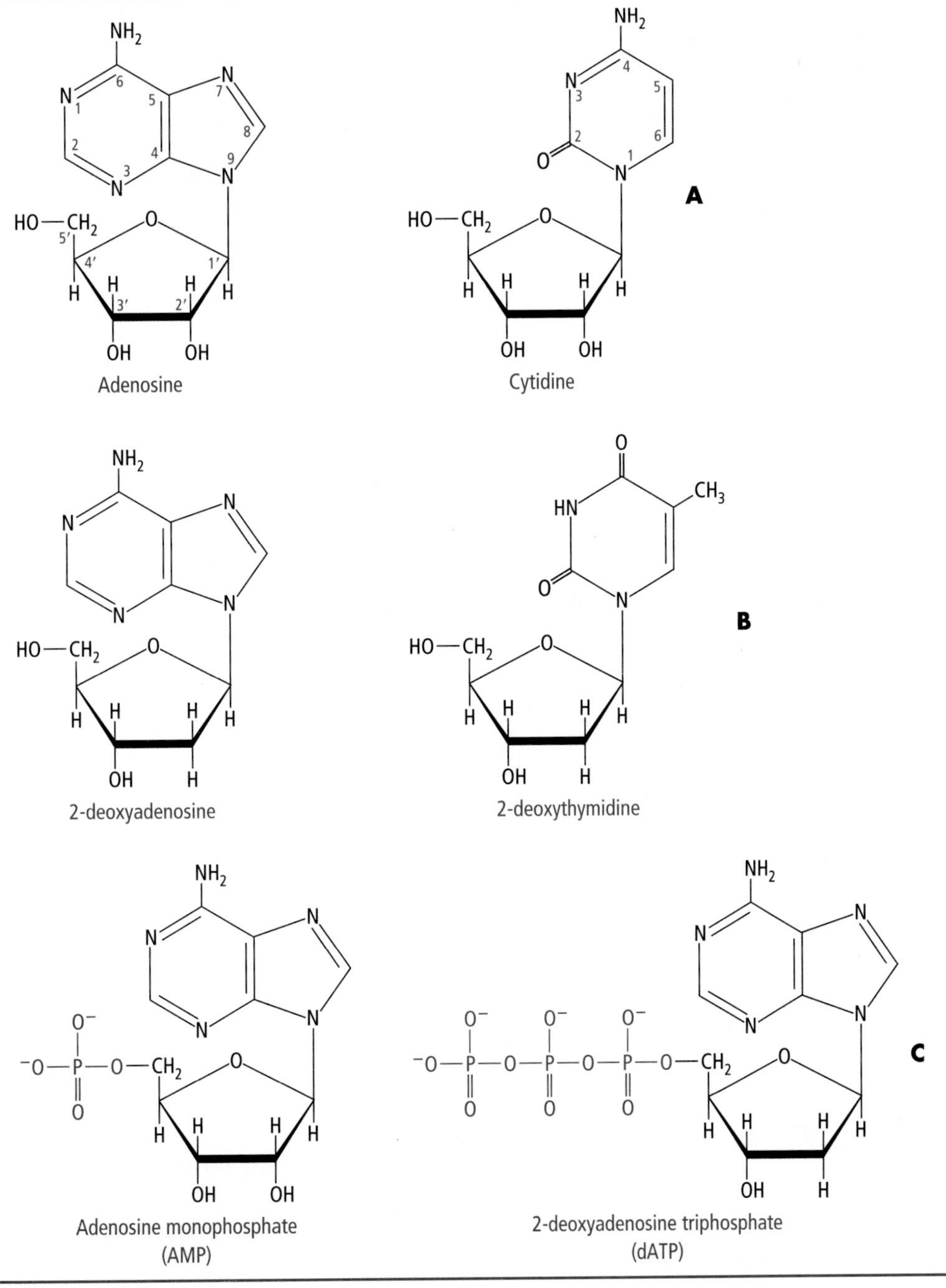

Adenosine

Cytidine

A

2-deoxyadenosine

2-deoxythymidine

B

Adenosine monophosphate
(AMP)

2-deoxyadenosine triphosphate
(dATP)

C

ring; the purines consist of two condensed rings:

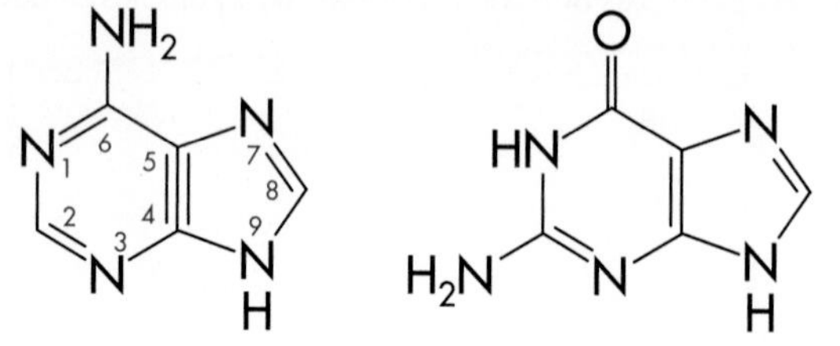

Adenine

Guanine

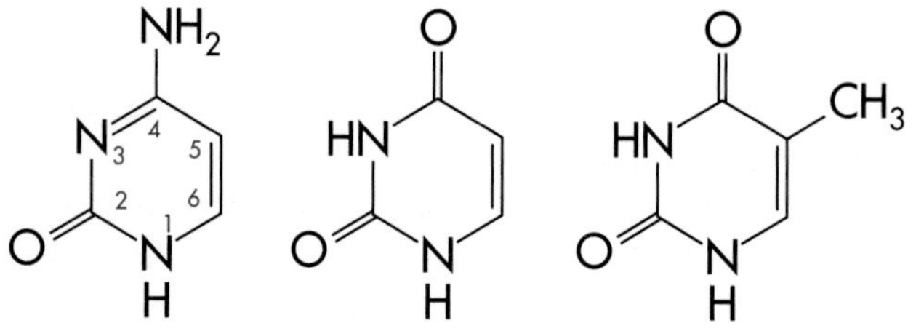

Cytosine

Uracil

Thymine

Nucleosides are formed from a heterocyclic base that is bound to C-1 of ribose or 2-deoxyribose by an N-glycosidic bond (Fig. 1.6). They are characterized as ribonucleosides and deoxyribonucleosides, respectively.

Nucleotides have the structure of the nucleosides, but they possess one, two, or three phosphate groups bound to carbon 5 of the sugar. They are named as phosphate derivatives of the nucleosides. Thus, adenosine monophosphate (AMP), adenosine diphosphate (ADP), and adenosine triphosphate (ATP) contain one, two, and three phosphate residues, respectively.

Nucleic acids are polymers of nucleoside monophosphates. The phosphate group forms a phosphodiester bond between the 5′ and 3′ hydroxy groups of adjacent ribose or 2-deoxyribose residues (Fig. 1.7). Most nucleic acids are very large. They often contain thousands—or, in the case of deoxyribonucleic acid (DNA), many millions—of nucleotides.

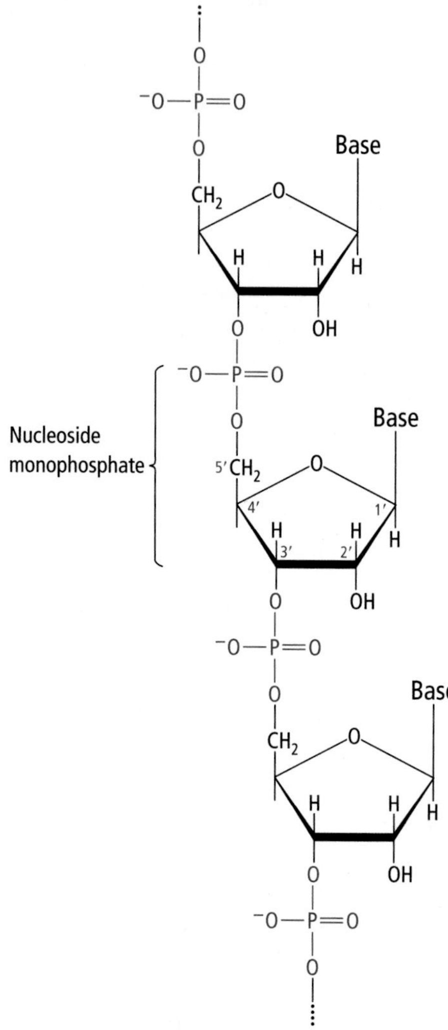

Most biomolecules are polymers

In biochemistry, we encounter a bewildering diversity of structure and function, and this diversity stems from the large size of most biomolecules. The carbohydrates, polypeptides, and nucleic acids illustrate a common principle by which large molecular size and structural diversity are generated: simple-

FIG. 1.7

Structure of ribonucleic acid (RNA). Deoxyribonucleic acid (DNA) has a similar structure, but it contains 2-deoxyribose instead of ribose. The nucleic acids are polymers of nucleoside monophosphates.

Nucleoside monophosphate

structured building blocks are linked covalently into long chains (Table 1.7). The macromolecules formed in this way are called **polymers** (Gr. πόλυς, "many," and μέρος, "part"), and their building blocks are called **monomers** (Gr. μόνος, "single"). Structural diversity is possible because not only is the chain length of the polymers variable, but more than one kind of monomer can be used. Polypeptides, for example, are constructed from 20 different amino acids, and DNA and RNA each contain four different bases, which can be arranged in unique sequences.

TABLE 1.7

Composition of biopolymers

Monomer	Polymer	Bond type
Monosaccharides	Polysaccharides	O-glycosidic bond
Amino acids	Polypeptides	Peptide bond
Nucleoside monophosphates	Nucleic acids	Phosphodiester bond

SUMMARY

All biochemical processes take place in aqueous solutions, and the properties of biomolecules are, therefore, largely determined by their interactions with water. Water solubility is determined by the ability of a molecule to form hydrogen bonds or ion–dipole interactions with the surrounding water molecules. Hydrophobic interactions, however, make the molecules insoluble in water. These interactions are noncovalent, and they are far weaker than the covalent bonds that hold together the atoms within the molecules.

According to their building blocks, we can distinguish several classes of biomolecules. The triglycerides consist of glycerol and three fatty acids; the carbohydrates consist of monosaccharides held together by glycosidic bonds; proteins consist of polypeptides, and polypeptides are chains of amino acids held together by peptide bonds. The nucleic acids consist of nucleoside monophosphates. With the exception of the triglycerides, these molecules are hydrophilic. Polysaccharides, polypeptides, and nucleic acids are polymers: they are long chains of monomeric building blocks held together by covalent bonds.

Many biomolecules have ionizable groups. Molecules with free carboxy groups or covalently bound phosphate carry negative charges at neutral pH, and those with aliphatic amino groups carry positive charges. These charges make the molecules water soluble, and they permit the formation of salt bonds with inorganic ions and with other biomolecules. The tendency of each ionizable group to accept or donate protons (positively charged hydrogen ions) is described by its pK value. If the pK value is known, we can predict which percentage of an ionizable group is in the protonated or deprotonated form at any given pH.

QUESTIONS

1. This molecule (2,3-bisphosphoglycerate, BPG) is present in red blood cells, where it binds noncovalently to hemoglobin. Which functional groups in hemoglobin can make the strongest noncovalent interactions with BPG at a "physiological" pH value of 7.0?

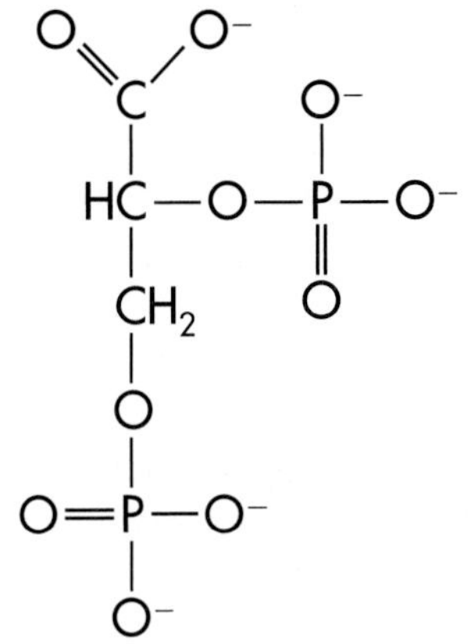

   A. Sulfhydryl groups
   B. Alcoholic hydroxy groups
   C. Hydrocarbon groups
   D. Amino groups
   E. Carboxy groups

2. Lipid-soluble molecules can diffuse freely through biological membranes, but nonphysiological substances that interact strongly with water do not penetrate across membranes. The molecule shown here is acetylsalicylic acid (aspirin). What can you

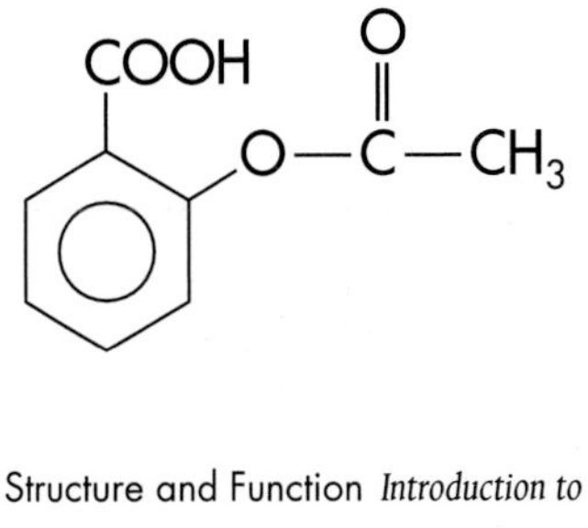

predict about the diffusion of aspirin across biological membranes?

  A. It diffuses equally well at all pH values.
  B. It diffuses more easily at pH 8 than at pH 2.
  C. It diffuses more easily at pH 2 than at pH 7.
  D. It diffuses more easily at pH 7 than at pH 2 or pH 10.

3. Inorganic phosphate, which is a major anion in the intracellular space, has three acidic functions with pK values of 2.3, 6.9, and 12.3, as shown in Box 1.12. In skeletal muscle fibers, the intracytoplasmic pH is approximately 7.1 at rest and 6.6 during vigorous anaerobic exercise. What does this mean for inorganic phosphate in muscle tissue?

  A. Phosphate molecules absorb protons when the pH decreases during anaerobic exercise.
  B. On average, the phosphate molecules carry more negative charges during anaerobic contraction than at rest.
  C. Phosphate molecules release protons when the pH decreases during anaerobic exercise.
  D. The most abundant form of the phosphate molecule in the resting muscle fiber carries one negative charge.

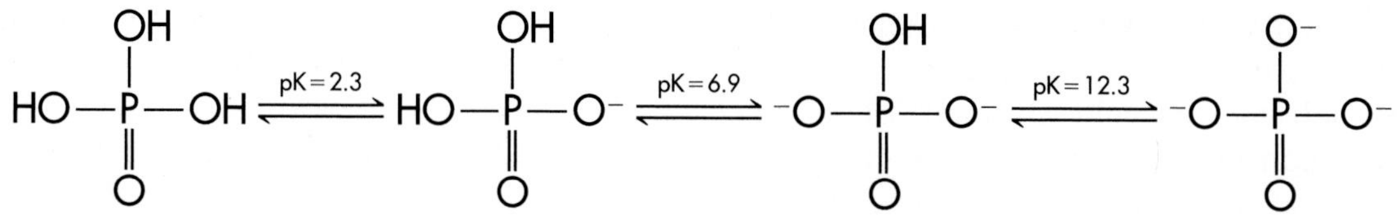

Chapter 2

Introduction to Protein Structure

All of the important properties of living cells depend on proteins. The maintenance of cell structure requires structural proteins, which are either constituents of the cellular membranes or form fibrous structures within the cell; metabolic activity depends on enzyme proteins, which catalyze chemical reactions; and gene expression requires numerous proteins that cooperate with nucleic acids in such processes as DNA replication, RNA synthesis, and protein synthesis. We can appreciate the roles of proteins for the cell only if we understand the structural features of proteins that enable them to perform this variety of tasks.

Proteins consist of polypeptides, which are polymers formed from 20 different amino acids. Held together by **peptide bonds,** the amino acids form long, unbranched chains that contain usually more than 100 and often more than 1000 amino acids. Some proteins consist of a single polypeptide; others are formed from two or more polypeptides held together either by covalent bonds or by noncovalent interactions. Some proteins contain a nonpolypeptide group as well. In these proteins, the nonpolypeptide group is called the **prosthetic group,** and the polypeptide is called the **apoprotein.** A prosthetic group often is employed when the biological function of the protein requires a functional group that is not available in any of the 20 amino acids. The most important element of diversity, however, is the variability of the amino acid sequence: from 20 different amino acids we can construct 20^2 (400) different dipeptides, 20^3 (8000) different tripeptides, and 20^4 (160,000) different tetrapeptides. A polypeptide with 100 amino acids can have 20^{100} different amino acid sequences.

In this chapter, we are concerned with the structures and properties of the 20 amino acids that occur in proteins, with the levels of protein structure, and with the physicochemical properties of proteins.

THE AMINO ACIDS

Proteins are constructed from 20 different amino acids, and their properties depend on the properties of the functional groups in these amino acids. Therefore, we will introduce the structures and properties of the amino acids first, before proceeding to the principles of protein structure.

Amino acids are zwitterionic structures

The general structure of the amino acids is simple enough: a carboxy group, an amino group, a hydrogen atom, and a variable side chain designated as R (residue) are bound to a central carbon, the α-carbon:

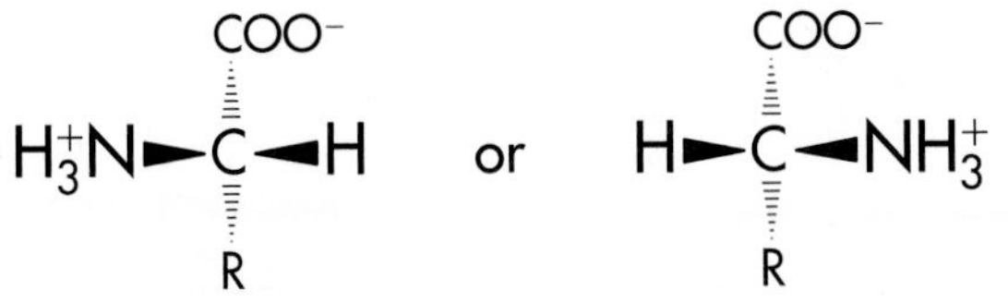

$$
\begin{array}{ccc}
\text{COO}^- & & \text{COO}^- \\
| & & | \\
\text{H}_3^+\text{N}\!-\!\text{C}\!-\!\text{H} & \text{or} & \text{H}\!-\!\text{C}\!-\!\text{NH}_3^+ \\
| & & | \\
\text{R} & & \text{R} \\
\text{L-Amino acid} & & \text{D-Amino acid}
\end{array}
$$

BOX 2.1

$$\underset{\text{pH} = 1.0}{\overset{\displaystyle \text{COOH}}{\underset{\displaystyle \text{CH}_3}{\text{H}_3^+\text{N}-\overset{\displaystyle |}{\underset{\displaystyle |}{\text{C}}}-\text{H}}}} \rightleftharpoons \underset{\text{pH} = 6.1}{\overset{\displaystyle \text{COO}^-}{\underset{\displaystyle \text{CH}_3}{\text{H}_3^+\text{N}-\overset{\displaystyle |}{\underset{\displaystyle |}{\text{C}}}-\text{H}}}} \rightleftharpoons \underset{\text{pH} = 11.0}{\overset{\displaystyle \text{COO}^-}{\underset{\displaystyle \text{CH}_3}{\text{H}_2\text{N}-\overset{\displaystyle |}{\underset{\displaystyle |}{\text{C}}}-\text{H}}}}$$

pK of α-carboxy = 2.3   pK of α-amino = 9.9

Because of their position on the α-carbon, the carboxy and amino groups are called the **α-carboxy group** and the **α-amino group,** respectively. The side chain R differs in the 20 amino acids.

Of the two optical isomers, *only the L-amino acids are found in proteins.* D-Amino acids are rare in nature, although they do occur in some bacterial products.

Both the α-carboxy group and the α-amino group are ionizable. In all natural amino acids, the α-carbon has a pK close to 2.0, whereas the pK of the α-amino group is near 9 or 10. Therefore, we encounter three different protonation states at different pH values, as illustrated for the amino acid alanine in Box 2.1.

FIG. 2.1

Titration curve of the amino acid alanine. The two level segments are caused by the buffering capacity of the carboxy group (at pH 2.3) and the amino group (at pH 9.9).

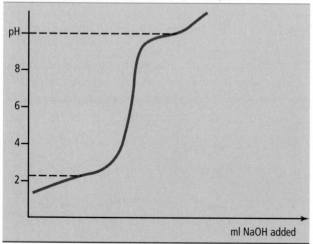

At pH values less than the pK of the α-carboxy group, alanine is mostly in a positively charged, that is, cationic form. At pH values greater than the pK of the α-amino group, the molecule is mostly in a negatively charged (anionic) form. At pH values between the pK values of the two groups, however, the predominant form of the molecule carries both a positive and a negative charge. This form is called a **zwitterion** (German *Zwitter*, "hermaphrodite"). The **isoelectric point (pI)** is defined as *the pH value at which the number of positive charges equals the number of negative charges.* For a simple amino acid such as alanine, the pI is halfway between the pK values of the two ionizable groups.

A **titration curve** is obtained by treating an acidic solution of an amino acid with increasing amounts of a strong base, or by treating an alkaline solution with a strong acid (Fig. 2.1). At pH values close to the pK value of an ionizable group, the pH changes little in response to the addition of base or acid: at these pH values, the ionizable groups buffer the pH because they release and absorb protons as the pH value is increased or decreased, respectively. *Any ionizable group buffers the pH of the solution at pH values close to its pK.*

Some amino acids have an additional acidic or basic group in their side chains. These amino acids have two different zwitterionic forms (Fig. 2.2). The pI of the acidic amino acids (monoamino, dicarboxylic acids) is halfway between the pK values of the two acidic groups, and the pI of the basic amino acids (diamino, monocarboxylic acids) is halfway between the pK values of the two basic groups. The titration curve of an acidic or basic amino acid shows three rather than two buffering areas.

FIG. 2.2

Prevailing ionization states of the amino acids aspartate (**A**) and lysine (**B**) at different pH values. The isoelectric points of aspartate and lysine are 2.95 and 10.0, respectively.

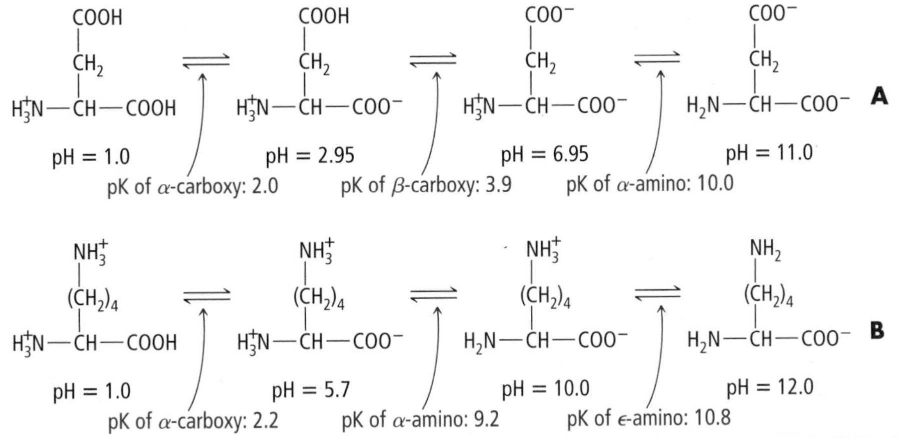

Amino acid side chains form many noncovalent interactions

The properties of the amino acids are, in large part, determined by the functional groups in their side chains and by the noncovalent interactions that they can form (Fig. 2.3 and Table 2.1). Some amino acids—including the branched-chain aliphatic amino acids valine, leucine, and isoleucine; the aromatic amino acids phenylalanine, tyrosine, and tryptophan; and the sulfur amino acids cysteine and methionine—have hydrophobic side chains. The side chains of others, such as serine, asparagine, and glutamine, are hydrophilic even though they are uncharged. Also, some amino acids have an acidic or basic group in their side chains that can assume a negative or positive charge at physiologic pH values (Table 2.2).

Some amino acid side chains also can form covalent bonds in proteins. The cysteine sulfhydryl group, for example, can form disulfide bonds (see next section), and the side chains of serine, threonine, and asparagine can form glycosidic bonds with carbohydrates.

PROTEIN STRUCTURE

Polypeptides are linear, unbranched polymers of amino acids, and their covalent structure can be described in terms of their amino acid sequence. There is, however, more to protein structure than just the sequence of amino acids. The long, threadlike polypeptides in the proteins form numerous noncovalent interactions, both with other polypeptides and between different parts of the same polypeptide. These interactions cause the polypeptide to bend, twist, wind, and coil into a highly ordered structure that is stable under physiologic conditions. The resulting **higher-order structure** is essential for the biological properties of the proteins.

Peptide bonds and disulfide bonds form the primary structure of proteins

The amino acids in the polypeptides are held together by **peptide bonds**. A **dipeptide** is formed by a condensation reaction between the α-carboxy and α-amino groups of two amino acids. See Box 2.2 for an example.

Oligopeptides consist of "a few" (3 to approximately 50) amino acids, and **polypeptides** are chains of "many" amino acids held together by peptide bonds as in Box 2.3. Each peptide has an **amino terminus**, conventionally written on the left side, and a **carboxy terminus**, written on the right side. In some peptides the terminal amino or carboxy

TABLE 2.1

Noncovalent interactions and covalent bonds formed by amino acid side chains in proteins

Type	Amino acid	Abbreviation*		Hydrophobic interactions	Hydrogen bonds†	Salt bonds‡	Covalent bonds
Small	Glycine	Gly	G	(+)	−	−	−
	Alanine	Ala	A	+	−	−	−
Branched chain	Valine	Val	V	++	−	−	−
	Leucine	Leu	L	+++	−	−	−
	Isoleucine	Ile	I	+++	−	−	−
Hydroxy	Serine	Ser	S	+	+	−	⎫ Phosphate ester O-glycosidic bond in glycoproteins
	Threonine	Thr	T	++	+	−	⎭
Sulfur	Cysteine	Cys	C	++	−	(+)	Disulfide bond
	Methionine	Met	M	+++	−	−	−
Aromatic	Phenylalanine	Phe	F	+++	−	−	−
	Tyrosine	Tyr	Y	++	+	−	Phosphate ester
	Tryptophan	Trp	W	++	+	−	−
Acidic and derivatives	Aspartate	Asp	D	−	++	+++	−
	Asparagine	Asn	N	−	+++	−	N-glycosidic bond
	Glutamate	Glu	E	+	++	+++	−
	Glutamine	Gln	Q	+	+++	−	−
Basic	Lysine	Lys	K	++	++	+++	−
	Arginine	Arg	R	+	+++	+++	−
	Histidine	His	H	−	+++	+	−
Imino	Proline	Pro	P	++	−	−	−

* The amino acids are abbreviated by either a three-letter code or a one-letter code.
† Hydrogen bonds formed by the side chain in the uncharged state.
‡ In the pH 6 to 8 range.

BOX 2.2

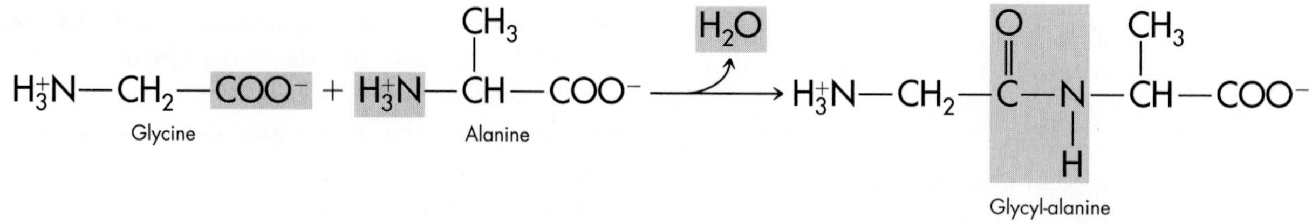

$H_3^+N—CH_2—COO^-$ + $H_3^+N—CH(CH_3)—COO^-$ → (H$_2$O) → $H_3^+N—CH_2—C(=O)—N(H)—CH(CH_3)—COO^-$

Glycine   Alanine   Glycyl-alanine

group is modified structurally. The amino terminus, for example, may be acetylated, or the carboxy terminus may be amidated as shown in Box 2.4. Although formed from an acidic and a basic group, the peptide bond is not ionizable. However, it can form hydrogen bonds, and therefore, peptides and proteins tend to be water soluble. Proteins do carry numerous positive and negative charges, but these

TABLE 2.2

pK values of some amino acid side chains*

Amino acid	Side chain		pK
	Protonated form	Deprotonated form	
Glutamate	$-(CH_2)_2-COOH$	$-(CH_2)_2-COO^-$	4.3
Aspartate	$-CH_2-COOH$	$-CH_2-COO^-$	3.9
Cysteine	$-CH_2-SH$	$-CH_2-S^-$	8.3
Tyrosine	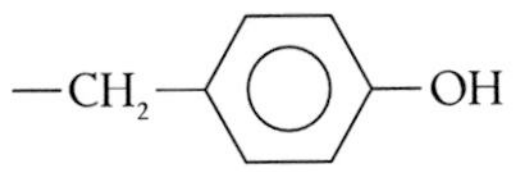 $-CH_2-$⟨benzene ring⟩$-OH$	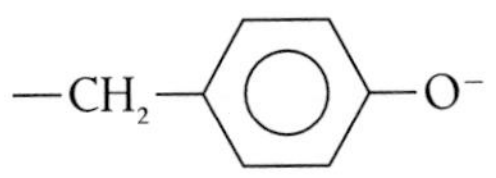 $-CH_2-$⟨benzene ring⟩$-O^-$	10.1
Lysine	$-(CH_2)_4-NH_3^+$	$-(CH_2)_4-NH_2$	10.8
Arginine	$-(CH_2)_3-NH-\overset{\overset{+}{NH_2}}{\underset{\parallel}{C}}-NH_2$	$-(CH_2)_3-NH-\overset{NH}{\underset{\parallel}{C}}-NH_2$	12.5
Histidine	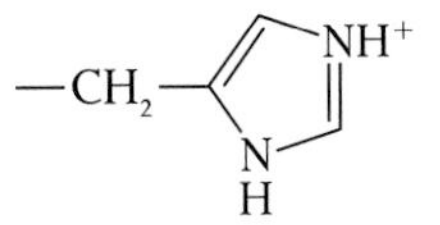 $-CH_2-$⟨imidazole-NH$^+$⟩	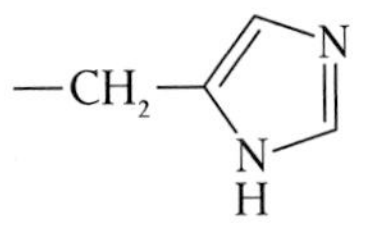 $-CH_2-$⟨imidazole-N⟩	6.0
α-Carboxy (free amino acid)			1.8 − 2.4
α-Amino (free amino acid)			≈9.0 − 10.0
Terminal carboxy (peptide)			≈3.0 − 4.5
Terminal amino (peptide)			≈7.5 − 9.0

* In proteins, the side chain pK values may differ by more than one pH unit from those in the free amino acids.

BOX 2.3

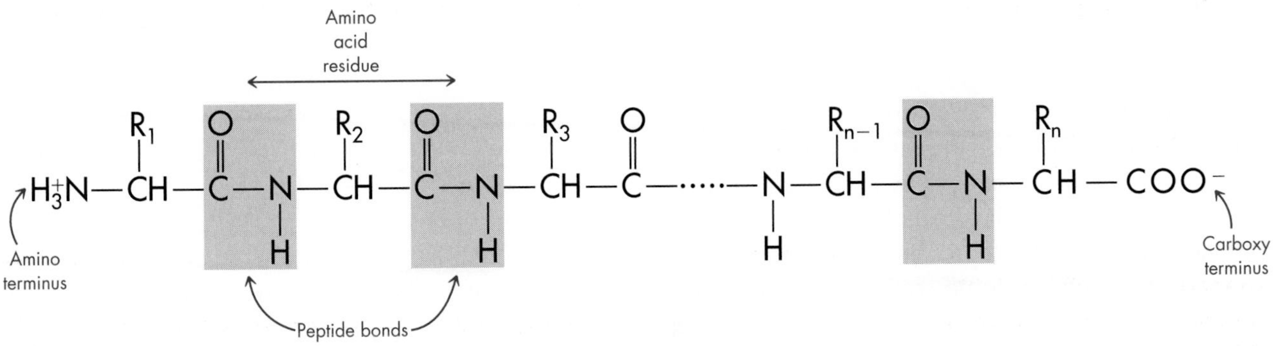

Amino
acid
residue

$H_3^+N-CH-\underset{\parallel}{\overset{R_1}{C}}-\underset{H}{\overset{O}{N}}-CH-\underset{\parallel}{\overset{R_2}{C}}-\underset{H}{\overset{O}{N}}-CH-\overset{R_3}{\overset{O}{C}}-\cdots-\underset{H}{N}-CH-\underset{\parallel}{\overset{R_{n-1}}{C}}-\underset{H}{\overset{O}{N}}-\overset{R_n}{CH}-COO^-$

Amino
terminus

Peptide bonds

Carboxy
terminus

BOX 2.4

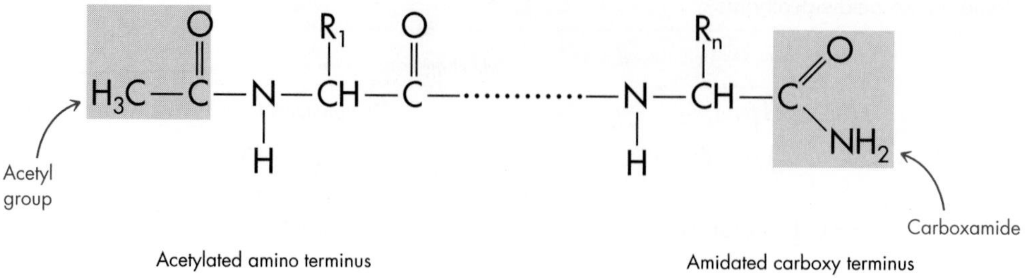

Acetyl group

Acetylated amino terminus

Carboxamide

Amidated carboxy terminus

BOX 2.5

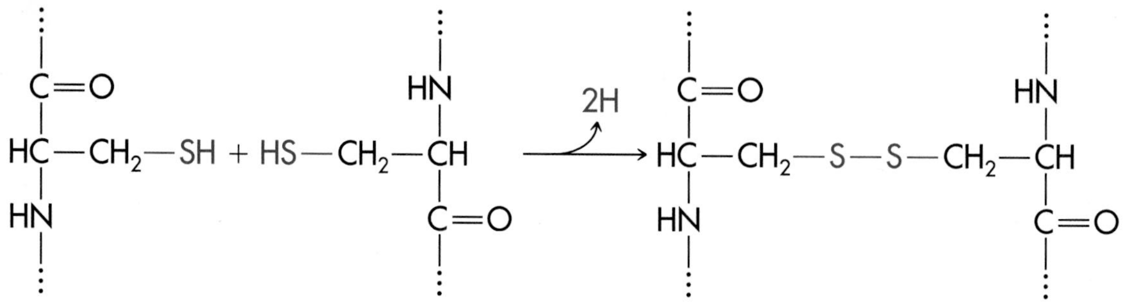

are present on the side chains of the basic and acidic amino acids: lysine, arginine, and, to some extent, histidine contribute positive charges, whereas the glutamate and aspartate side chains are negatively charged at pH 7. The pK values of the amino acid side chains in proteins are similar to those in the free amino acids (see Table 2.2), and therefore the pI of a protein can be predicted from the relative abundances of the acidic and basic amino acid residues.

Many, but not all, proteins contain **disulfide bonds.** These bonds are formed between the side chains of two cysteine residues as shown in Box 2.5. Because disulfide bond formation is accompanied by the removal of hydrogen, it is considered an oxidation. Disulfide bonds are formed in the endoplasmic reticulum (ER), and therefore *they are present in most secreted proteins and membrane proteins that are processed through this organelle* (see Chapter 8), but not in cytoplasmic proteins. The bonds can be formed between cysteine residues in the same polypeptide (intrachain) or in different polypeptides (interchain).

The enzymatic degradation of disulfide bond–containing proteins yields **cystine,** a dimer of cysteine that occurs in tissues and body fluids together with the other amino acids as shown in Box 2.6. The covalent structure of the protein, specified by its amino acid sequence and the positions of the disulfide bonds, is called its **primary structure.**

The peptide bond is rigid

In most peptide bonds, except those formed by the nitrogen of proline, the two atoms of the peptide bond have four substituents: a hydrogen, an oxygen, and two α-carbons. The peptide bond is described conventionally as a single bond:

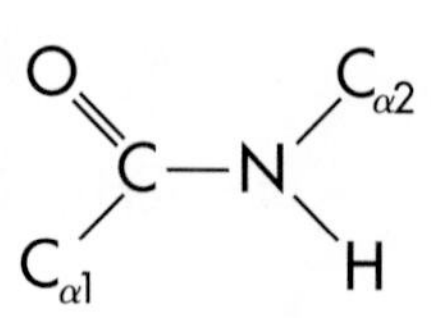

A C—N single bond, like a C—C single bond, should show free rotation. In this case, the triangular plane formed by the O=C—$C_{\alpha 1}$ portion should

FIG. 2.3

Structures of the amino acids in proteins.

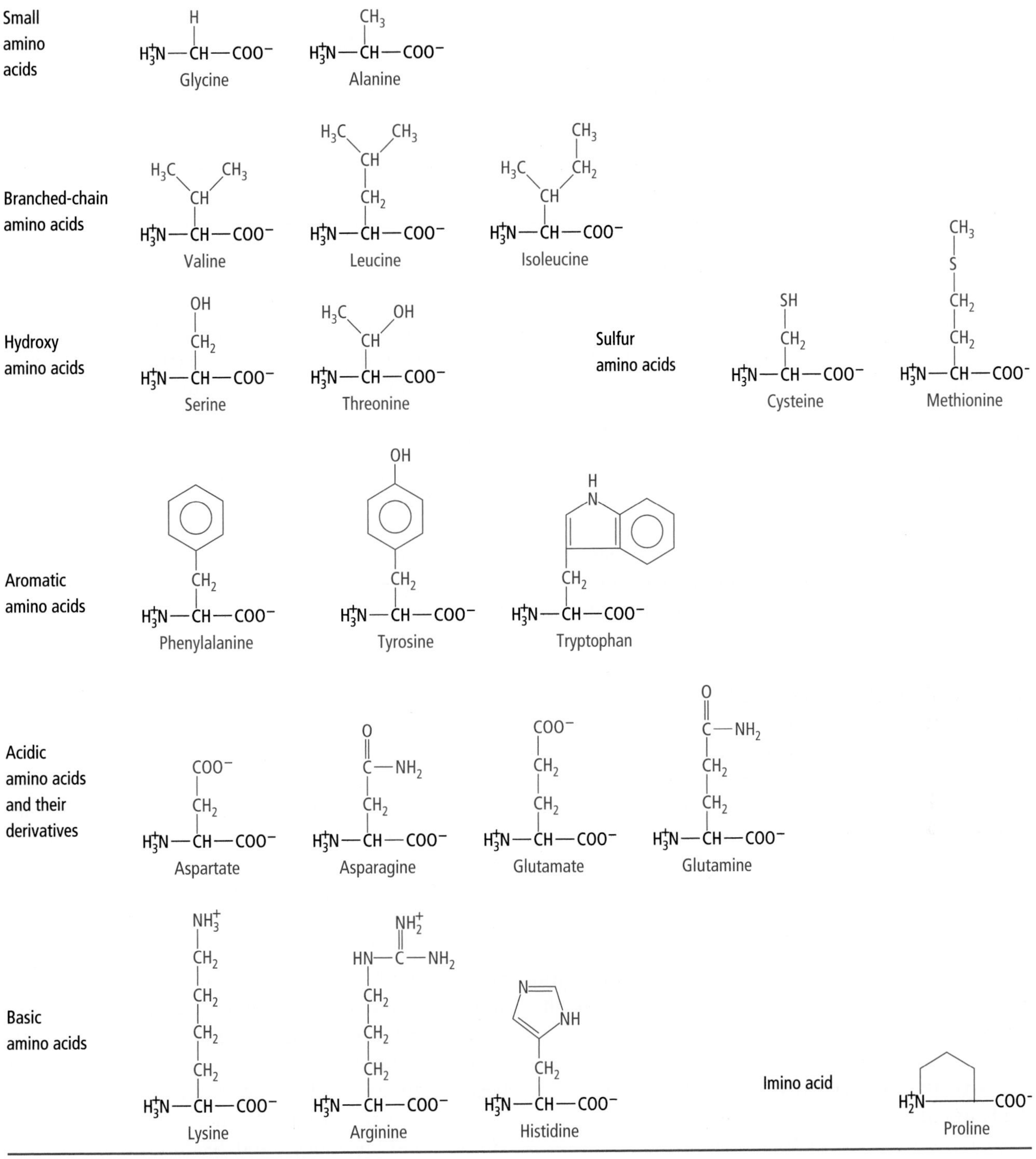

Small amino acids

Glycine

Alanine

Branched-chain amino acids

Valine

Leucine

Isoleucine

Hydroxy amino acids

Serine

Threonine

Sulfur amino acids

Cysteine

Methionine

Aromatic amino acids

Phenylalanine

Tyrosine

Tryptophan

Acidic amino acids and their derivatives

Aspartate

Asparagine

Glutamate

Glutamine

Basic amino acids

Lysine

Arginine

Histidine

Imino acid

Proline

BOX 2.6

$$\begin{array}{c}
\vdots \\
| \\
C=O \\
| \\
HC-CH_2-S-S-CH_2-CH \\
| \\
HN \\
| \\
\vdots
\end{array}
\quad
\begin{array}{c}
\vdots \\
| \\
HN \\
| \\
\\
| \\
C=O \\
| \\
\vdots
\end{array}
\quad
\xrightarrow[\text{enzymes}]{\text{Proteolytic}}
\quad
\begin{array}{c}
COO^- \\
| \\
HC-CH_2-S-S-CH_2-CH \\
| \\
NH_3^+
\end{array}
\quad
\begin{array}{c}
NH_3^+ \\
| \\
\\
| \\
COO^-
\end{array}$$

be able to rotate out of the plane of the $C_{\alpha2}$—N—H portion. However, the peptide bond actually is a resonance hybrid of two structures:

$$\begin{array}{ccc}
O & \diagup C_{\alpha2} & \qquad O^- \diagup C_{\alpha2} \\
\diagdown C-N & & \diagdown C=N \\
C_{\alpha1} \quad H & & C_{\alpha1} \qquad H^+
\end{array}$$

Its "real" structure is halfway between these two extremes. The partial double bond character of the peptide bond is important for its rotational freedom: like C=C double bonds (see Chapter 11, Fig. 11.8), C=N double bonds do not rotate. Indeed, *the peptide bond is rigid, and its four substituents are all fixed in the same plane.* The natural peptide bonds are in the *trans* configuration, with the two α-carbons opposite each other.

Aside from the peptide bond, the polypeptide backbone contains bonds between the α-carbon and the peptide bond carbon and between the α-carbon and the nitrogen. These bonds are true single bonds, with the expected rotational freedom (Fig. 2.4). Rotation around the nitrogen-α-carbon bond is measured as the φ (phi) angle, and rotation around the peptide carbon-α-carbon bond as the ψ (psi) angle.

Proteins have complex higher-order structures

Because two of the three bonds in the polypeptide backbone are able to rotate, polypeptides can bend themselves into a variety of shapes and assume unique **higher-order structures**. In **globular proteins**, the polypeptide folds itself into a compact shape. Most globular proteins are water soluble, but others are integrated into the structures of cellular membranes. Hemoglobin and myoglobin (see Chapter 3), enzymes (see Chapter 4), membrane proteins (see Chapter 11), and plasma proteins (see Chapter 25) are globular proteins. **Fibrous proteins** are long and threadlike, and most serve structural functions. Keratin, the protein of hair, fingernails, and the horny layer of the skin (see Chapter 12), is a fibrous protein, as is collagen, which forms fibers in the extracellular matrix of connective tissues (see Chapter 13).

The α-helix and β-pleated sheet are the most common secondary structures in proteins

A **secondary structure** is a regular, repetitive folding pattern that is formed when all the φ angles and all the ψ angles in a polypeptide are the same. Only a limited number of secondary structures are energetically possible.

In the **α-helix** (Fig. 2.5), the atoms of the polypeptide backbone are wound in a right-handed spiral. The term "right-handed" refers to the direction of the turn: if the thumb of the right hand pushes along the helix axis, the flexed fingers describe the twist of the polypeptide backbone. The α-helix is very compact: each full turn has 3.6 amino acid residues, and each amino acid is advanced 1.5 Å along the helix axis. Therefore, a complete turn advances by 3.6 × 1.5 = 5.4 Å. This is called the **pitch** of the helix.

The α-helix is maintained by hydrogen bonds that are formed between the peptide bonds. Each peptide bond

FIG. 2.4

Geometry of the peptide bond. The φ and ψ angles are variable. (© Irving Geis.)

- ● α-Carbon
- ● Carbonyl carbon
- ● Hydrogen
- ● Nitrogen
- ● Oxygen
- ○ Side chain

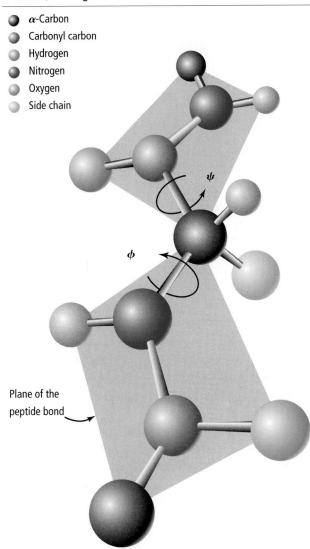

Plane of the
peptide bond

FIG. 2.5

Structure of the α-helix.

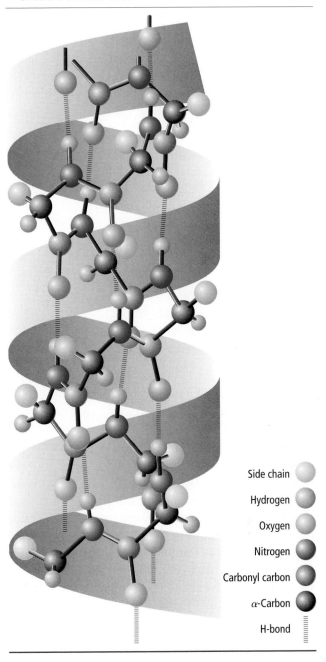

- ○ Side chain
- ○ Hydrogen
- ○ Oxygen
- ● Nitrogen
- ● Carbonyl carbon
- ● α-Carbon
- ⦙ H-bond

C=O is hydrogen bonded to the peptide bond N—H four amino acid residues ahead of it. Each C=O and each N—H in the main chain is hydrogen bonded. Moreover, these hydrogen bonds are colinear: the N, H, and O form a nearly straight line, and this is, energetically speaking, the most favorable alignment for hydrogen bonds. We should be aware, however, that even the cooperative action of many hydrogen bonds can be disrupted easily in an aqueous environment, where water molecules compete with the atoms of the polypeptide chain for hydrogen bond formation. The strength of an intramolecular hydrogen bond in the α-helix is similar to that of the hydrogen bonds between water molecules.

The amino acid side chains face outward, away from the helix axis. The side chains are not essential for helix formation, although their interactions can stabilize or destabilize the helix. Proline, which cannot rotate around its C—N bond, fits poorly

FIG. 2.6

Structure of the parallel and antiparallel β-pleated sheets. **A,** The parallel β-pleated sheet. **B,** The antiparallel β-pleated sheet.

FIG. 2.7

Structure of the β-turn. Note the abrupt reversal in the direction of the polypeptide main chain.

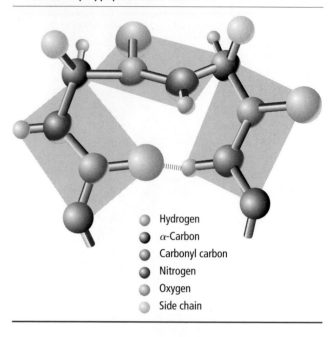

- ⬤ Hydrogen
- ⬤ α-Carbon
- ⬤ Carbonyl carbon
- ⬤ Nitrogen
- ⬤ Oxygen
- ⬤ Side chain

into the α-helix. Also glycine destabilizes the α-helix. This amino acid is small and flexible, and therefore it can assume many energetically favorable conformations other than the α-helix.

The α-helix is common in both fibrous and globular proteins. Many fibrous proteins, including myosin, tropomyosin, and α-keratin (Chapter 12), contain long, uninterrupted α-helices. In globular proteins, on the other hand, short stretches of α-helix are interrupted by nonhelical segments (see Chapter 3, Fig. 3.2).

The polypeptides that form the **β-pleated sheet** (Fig. 2.6) are almost fully extended, with a rise of 3.5 Å per amino acid residue. The formation of intrachain hydrogen bonds between the peptide bonds, as in the α-helix, is sterically impossible because the C=O and N—H bonds are arranged almost perpendicular to the axis of the polypeptide. Instead, *hydrogen bonds are formed between the peptide bond C=O and N—H groups of polypeptides that lie side by side.* The interacting polypeptides are aligned either parallel or antiparallel. Either they belong to two different chains or they are different sections of the same polypeptide. More than two polypeptides can form a β-pleated sheet, giving rise to large, blanket-like structures. Like the α-helix, the β-pleated sheet occurs in both fibrous and globular proteins.

The **β-turn** (Fig. 2.7) is a sharp bend or hairpin loop that abruptly changes the direction of the polypeptide. Like the α-helix and β-pleated sheet, it is formed by main-chain hydrogen bonds. It often is found in antiparallel β-pleated sheets where the polypeptide bends back on itself.

Globular proteins have a hydrophobic core

The term **tertiary structure** refers to the overall folding pattern of the polypeptide. In most globular proteins, short sections of secondary structure, usually less than 30 amino acids in length, alternate with irregularly folded sequences (Fig. 2.8). The portions without secondary structure allow the polypeptide to curl itself into a compact shape. The noncovalent interactions that stabilize the tertiary structure differ from those in the classical sec-

FIG. 2.8

Structure of globular protein domains containing both α-helical and β-pleated sheet structures. Note that each α-helical or β-pleated sheet structure is formed from only a short section of the polypeptide. These elements of secondary structure are separated by nonhelical portions. Each ribbon represents a β-pleated sheet with the arrow indicating the N-terminal to C-terminal direction.

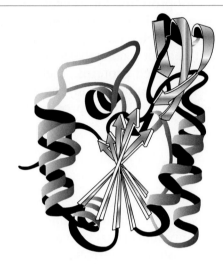

Phosphoglycerate Kinase domain 2

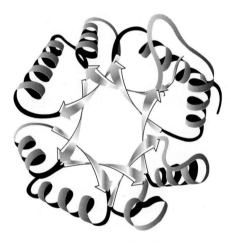

Pyruvate Kinase domain 1

ondary structures: although both the α-helix and the β-pleated sheet are stabilized by hydrogen bonds between the peptide bonds, *the major cohesive forces in tertiary structures are hydrophobic interactions between amino acid side chains.* In water-soluble globular proteins, the surface is occupied by hydrophilic side chains, whereas nonpolar residues form a hydrophobic core.

Long polypeptides often fold themselves into more than one compact globular unit. The different globular parts of these polypeptides are called **domains.** The domains are connected by more extended, flexible parts of the polypeptide chain. Domains usually are formed from between 100 and 400 amino acid residues, and different domains may have different biological functions. We know, for example, enzyme proteins whose different domains have different catalytic activities.

Quaternary structures are formed by interactions between different polypeptides (**subunits**). Therefore, only proteins that consist of more than one polypeptide have a quaternary structure. In some of these proteins, the subunits are held together only by noncovalent interactions, but others are stabilized by interchain disulfide bonds.

The higher-order structure forms while the polypeptide is synthesized

Three important events take place during protein synthesis: *the formation of the peptide bonds, the establishment of the higher-order structure, and the formation of additional covalent bonds.* The first step is peptide bond formation. **Ribosomes** synthesize polypeptides by the sequential addition of amino acids, starting from the amino terminus (see Chapter 6). As the growing polypeptide emerges from the ribosome, it folds itself into its higher-order structure. This takes place immediately, even before the ribosome has finished its work: protein folding is **cotranslational** (translation = ribosomal peptide bond synthesis). In most cases, protein folding requires only noncovalent interactions within the polypeptide itself, and therefore the native (original) folding pattern of the polypeptide should be its thermodynamically most favorable conformation. This rule is not without exceptions: helper proteins called **chaperones** are required for the proper folding of at least some proteins. In these cases, the final conformation of the protein is not necessarily its thermodynamically most favorable state.

During protein folding, cysteine residues that are far removed in the amino acid sequence may be brought into close proximity. With the help of an enzyme in the endoplasmic reticulum, disulfide bonds are formed from these cysteine residues. Disulfide bonds, therefore, do not establish the higher-order structure. They only stabilize the

FIG. 2.9

Examples of posttranslational modifications in proteins. **A,** A phosphoserine residue. Aside from serine, threonine and tyrosine also can form phosphate bonds in proteins. **B,** An N-acetylgalactosamine residue bound to a serine side chain. Serine and threonine form O-glycosidic bonds in glycoproteins. **C,** An N-acetylglucosamine residue bound to an asparagine side chain by an -N-glycosidic bond. These "N-linked" carbohydrates are also common in glycoproteins. **D,** Some enzymes contain covalently bound prosthetic groups. As a coenzyme (see Chapter 5), the prosthetic group participates in the enzymatic reaction. This example shows biotin, which is bound covalently to a lysine side chain.

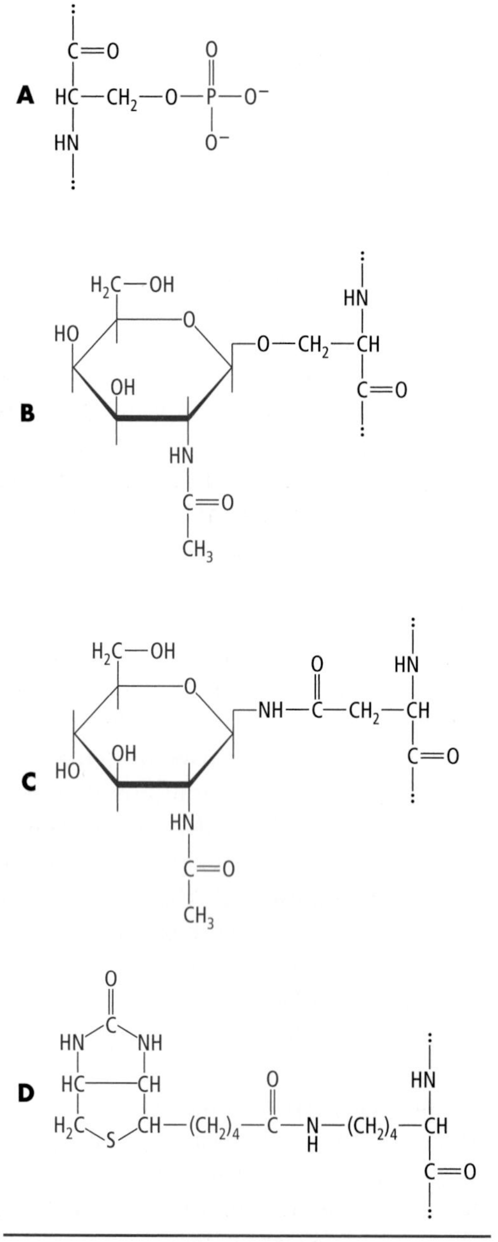

structure that already has been formed by noncovalent interactions.

Posttranslational modifications other than disulfide bond formation also are common. Many proteins contain carbohydrate or phosphate groups covalently bound to amino acid side chains (Fig. 2.9). Other proteins contain noncovalently bound molecules. **Lipoproteins,** for example, are noncovalent aggregates of lipids and proteins held together by hydrophobic interactions (see Chapter 20). Proteins that contain a nonpolypeptide component are called **conjugated proteins.** Their polypeptide component is the **apoprotein;** the bound nonpolypeptide group is called the **prosthetic group.**

THE PHYSICAL PROPERTIES OF PROTEINS

Proteins vary greatly in such physicochemical characteristics as water solubility, buffering capacity, chemical stability, and crystal structure. These properties depend on molecular weight, amino acid composition, and, above all, the higher-order structure of the protein. In the following sections we will review the typical properties of proteins and introduce some laboratory techniques that exploit these properties.

Proteins lose their biological activities when their higher-order structure is destroyed

The peptide and disulfide bonds in proteins are covalent bonds that are stable under ordinary conditions. **Peptide bonds** can be hydrolyzed under mild conditions in the presence of proteolytic enzymes, but in the absence of enzymes they can be cleaved only by heating with strong acids or bases. **Disulfide bonds,** if present, can be cleaved by reducing or oxidizing agents as shown in Box 2.7. The noncovalent interactions that maintain the higher-order structure of proteins are far weaker than the covalent bonds. Indeed, *the higher-order structure of proteins can be destroyed by ordinary heating.* Most proteins suffer **heat denaturation** within a few minutes at temperatures somewhere between 50°C and 80°C. At these temperatures, the highly ordered, neatly folded polypeptide is converted to a messy tanglework known as a **random coil.**

BOX 2.7

$$\text{C}=\text{O} \quad \text{HC}-\text{CH}_2-\text{S}-\text{S}-\text{CH}_2-\text{CH} \quad \text{HN} \xrightarrow[\text{Reduction}]{[\text{H}]} \text{C}=\text{O} \quad \text{HC}-\text{CH}_2-\text{SH} + \text{HS}-\text{CH}_2-\text{CH} \quad \text{HN}$$

Oxidation [Ȯ]

$$\text{C}=\text{O} \quad \text{HC}-\text{CH}_2-\overset{\text{O}}{\underset{\text{O}}{\overset{\|}{\underset{\|}{\text{S}}}}}-\text{O}^- + {}^-\text{O}-\overset{\text{O}}{\underset{\text{O}}{\overset{\|}{\underset{\|}{\text{S}}}}}-\text{CH}_2-\text{CH} \quad \text{HN}$$

Denaturation leads to a complete loss of the protein's biological function. Stated another way, *the biological functions of proteins depend on their higher-order structures.* The physical properties also are changed drastically by denaturation. Water-soluble proteins, in particular, become insoluble. The boiling of an egg is a familiar example of this phenomenon.

If the native conformation of the protein is indeed its thermodynamically most stable state, denaturation should be reversible. Under well-controlled laboratory conditions, renaturation is indeed possible for many small proteins. Larger proteins, however, do not readily renature, and under real-world conditions *protein denaturation generally is irreversible*: the boiled egg does not become unboiled when kept in the cold.

Proteins can be denatured by many treatments other than heating: many **detergents** and **organic solvents** denature proteins by disrupting hydrophobic interactions. Being nonpolar, they insinuate themselves between the side chains of hydrophobic amino acids. Strong **acids** and **bases** denature proteins because they change their charge pattern. In a strong acid, the protein loses its negative charges, and in a strong base, it loses its positive charges. This deprives the protein of intramolecular salt bonds that normally help to stabilize its higher-order structure. Also, the counterions that become bound to the protein surface under these conditions can interfere with the higher-order structure. The addition of **trichloroacetic acid (TCA)** is a standard procedure for the removal of proteins from serum or other biological samples: the proteins denature, become insoluble, and can be removed by centrifugation. High concentrations of some small hydrophilic agents with high hydrogen-bonding potential, such as **8M urea** or **6M guanidine hydrochloride**, also can denature proteins. They do so by disrupting the hydrogen bonds between water molecules. For this reason, the extent to which water molecules assume a more "ordered" position at an aqueous/nonpolar interface is reduced, and the hydrophobic interactions within the protein are weakened.

$$\underset{\text{Urea}}{\text{H}_2\text{N}-\overset{\text{O}}{\overset{\|}{\text{C}}}-\text{NH}_2} \qquad \underset{\text{Guanidine hydrochloride}}{\text{H}_2\text{N}-\overset{\overset{\text{NH}_2^+}{\|}}{\text{C}}-\text{NH}_2 \quad \text{Cl}^-}$$

Even many heavy metal ions, such as lead, cadmium, and mercury, denature proteins. These metals bind to carboxylate groups and, in particular, to sulfhydryl groups in many proteins. This affinity for functional groups in proteins is the basis for their toxicity.

We can only be astounded at the fragility of life: an increase of the body temperature by more than 5°C or 6°C, for example, is fatal, and the blood pH has to be maintained between 7.0 and 7.7 at all times. These subtle changes in the physical environment do not affect covalent bonds, but *they disrupt noncovalent interactions*. It is because of the weakness and vulnerability of noncovalent interactions that we had to evolve sophisticated regulatory mechanisms for the maintenance of a constant internal environment.

The solubility of proteins depends on pH and salt concentration

Fibrous proteins form insoluble fibers, and many globular membrane proteins are insoluble because they are integrated firmly into the structure of the membrane. Most globular proteins, however, are water soluble. Their solubility depends on the salt concentration: it is higher in a moderately concentrated salt solution (1–10% salt) than in distilled water because salt ions prevent electrostatic interactions between different protein molecules (Fig. 2.10, A, B). Excess salt, however, precipitates proteins because most of the water molecules become tied up in the hydration shells of the salt ions.

FIG. 2.10

Effects of salt and pH on protein solubility. **A,** Protein in distilled water. Salt bonds between protein molecules cause the molecule to aggregate. The protein becomes insoluble. **B,** Protein in 5% sodium chloride (NaCl): salt ions bind to the surface charges of the protein molecules, thereby preventing intermolecular salt bonds. **C,** The effect of pH on protein solubility: the formation of intermolecular salt bonds is favored at the isoelectric point. At pH values greater or less than the pI, the electrostatic interactions between the molecules are mainly repulsive.

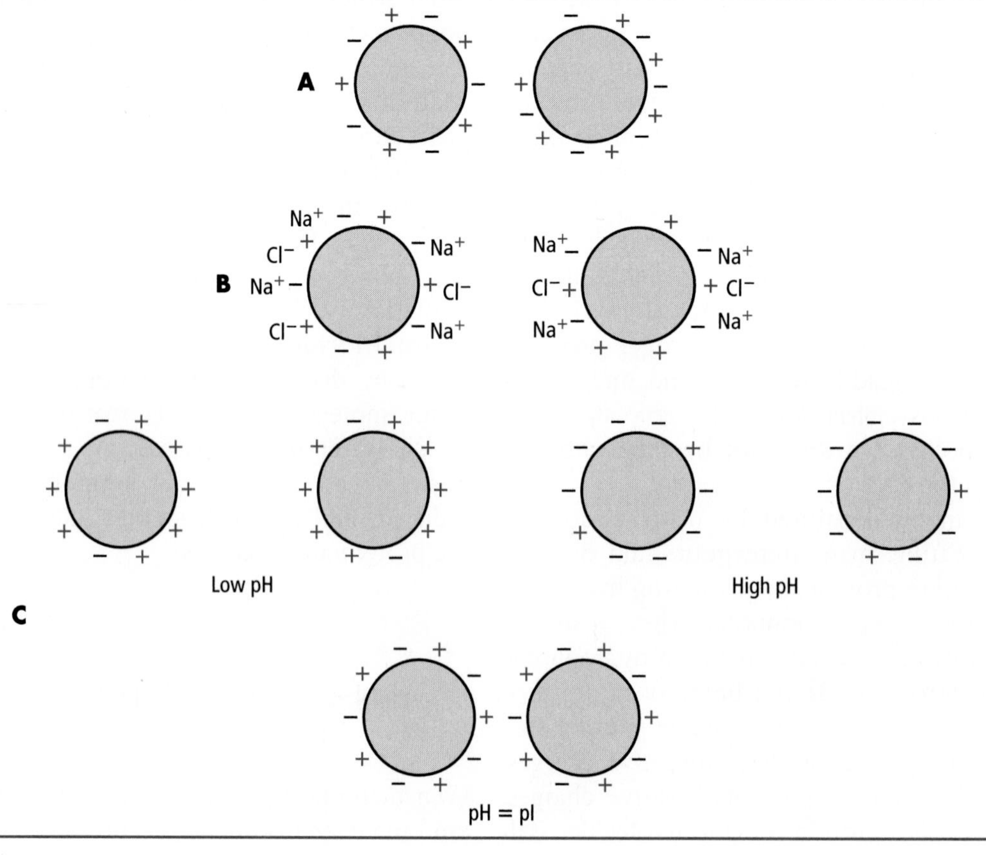

Effectively, the salt ions compete with the protein molecules for the available solvent. Similarly, water-miscible organic solvents like ethanol or acetone compete for water molecules, thereby precipitating proteins without denaturing them. Therefore *in the laboratory, proteins can be precipitated either by high salt concentration or by the addition of water-miscible organic solvents*. Unlike denaturation, precipitation is reversible and does not permanently destroy the protein's biological properties.

The pH value also affects the water solubility: *the solubility of proteins is minimal at their isoelectric point (pI)*. Because they carry equal numbers of positive and negative charges at their pI, the proteins have a maximal opportunity for the formation of intermolecular salt bonds (Fig. 2.10, C).

Proteins absorb UV radiation

Protein solutions do not absorb visible light and therefore are uncolored unless the protein contains a colored prosthetic group, such as the heme group or a flavin (Chapter 5). Proteins do, however, absorb ultraviolet (UV) radiation with two absorption maxima at 190 and 280 nm (Fig. 2.11). The absorbance peak at 190 nm is caused by the peptide bonds, and the peak at 280 nm is caused by aromatic amino acid side chains. The peak at 280 nm is more useful in laboratory practice because it is relatively specific for proteins. Nucleic acids, however, have an absorbance peak at 260 nm, which overlaps the 280 nm peak of proteins.

Proteins can be separated by their charge or their molecular weight

Proteins can be purified and isolated by many methods. In **dialysis,** a protein solution containing salts or other low-molecular-weight contaminants is enclosed in a bag of porous cellophane (Fig. 2.12). The pores in the cellophane membrane permit the passage of small molecules and inorganic ions, but not of the large protein molecules. By suspending the bag in a stirred buffer solution, the low-molecular-weight contaminants are removed. The dialysis of kidney patients is based on the same principle: the patient's blood is passed along semipermeable membranes through which low-molecular-weight waste products are removed while plasma proteins and blood cells are retained. The blood, of course, is not dialyzed against distilled water but against a solution with physiologic concentrations of nutrients and inorganic ions.

Electrophoresis is the most common method for protein separation in the clinical laboratory. It is based on the movement of charged proteins in an electrical field. Cellulose acetate foil, starch gel, or other carrier materials can be used (Fig. 2.13, A). At pH values greater than the isoelectric point (pI), the protein carries an excess of negative charges and moves to the anode. At pH values less than the pI, positive charges prevail and the protein moves to

---

FIG. 2.11

Typical UV absorbance spectra of proteins and nucleic acids. The protein absorbance peak at 280 nm is caused by the aromatic side chains of tyrosine and tryptophan. Nucleic acids absorb at 260 nm because of the aromatic character of their purine and pyrimidine bases.

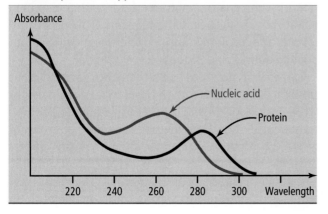

FIG. 2.12

The use of dialysis for protein purification. Only small molecules and inorganic ions can pass through the porous membrane.

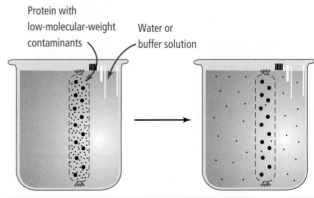

FIG. 2.13

Protein separation by electrophoresis. **A,** On a wet cellulose acetate foil, the proteins are separated according to their net change. If, as in this case, an alkaline pH is used, the proteins are negatively charged and move to the anode.
B, Electrophoresis in a cross-linked polyacrylamide gel. Although small molecules can move in the field, larger ones "get stuck" in the gel. Under suitable pH conditions, this method separates on the basis of molecular weight rather than charge.

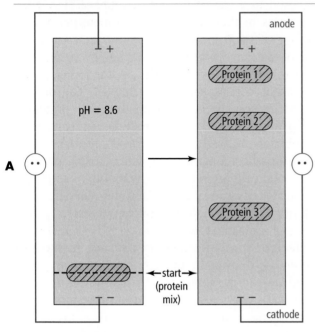

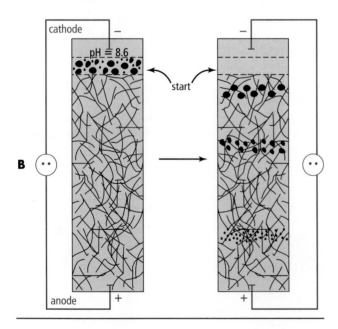

the cathode. At the isoelectric point, the net charge is zero and it does not move.

Electrophoresis is the standard method for the separation of plasma proteins and isoenzymes (Chapter 25), and for the detection of structurally abnormal proteins (Chapter 9). If a structurally abnormal protein differs from its normal counterpart by a single amino acid substitution, *the electrophoretic mobility is changed only if the charge pattern is changed.* If, for example, a glutamate residue is replaced by aspartate, the electrophoretic mobility is unchanged because these two amino acid residues carry the same charge. If, however, glutamate is replaced by an uncharged amino acid such as valine, one negative charge is removed and the two proteins can be separated by electrophoresis.

Electrophoresis can be performed in a cross-linked polyacrylamide or agarose gel, which impairs the movement of large molecules but not that of small molecules. Under pH conditions at which all proteins move to the same pole, they are separated mainly according to their molecular weight rather than their charge (Fig. 2.13, *B*). This method often is used in the presence of a reducing agent such as mercaptoethanol, which cleaves disulfide bonds, and a strong detergent that denatures proteins while keeping the polypeptides in solution.

Both the amino acid sequence and the higher-order structure are known for many proteins

The covalent structure of proteins can be determined by chemical methods. For **amino acid analysis,** the peptide bonds in the protein are hydrolyzed by boiling in 6 N hydrochloric acid (HCl) for 24 hours. The amino acids are then separated by chromatographic methods and determined quantitatively with suitable reagents. This procedure reveals the protein's amino acid composition, but not the amino acid sequence.

Large polypeptides also can be cleaved into smaller fragments. Proteolytic enzymes are particularly useful for this. Trypsin, for example, cleaves only peptide bonds formed by the carboxy group of lysine or arginine, whereas chymotrypsin cleaves only the bonds on the carboxy side of hydrophobic amino acid residues (see Chapter 14). The short fragments generated in this way are more manageable in sequencing studies than the large polypeptide from which they were derived.

Sequence analysis itself is performed by **Edman degradation** (Fig. 2.14). In each degradation cycle, the N-terminal amino acid is converted to a fluorescent derivative, the phenylthiohydantoin (PTH) amino acid. The peptide is shortened by one amino acid, and the whole procedure can be repeated.

The amino acid sequences of more than a thousand polypeptides have been determined by classical sequencing studies. The sequences of many more proteins are becoming known by an entirely different approach: because the amino acid sequences of polypeptides are encoded by genes (see Chapter 6), the base sequence of the gene predicts the amino acid sequence of its polypeptide. In many cases, genes have been sequenced (see Chapter 10) and the amino acid sequence of the encoded poly-

peptide has been deduced, even in cases in which the polypeptide never has been isolated. Efforts at sequencing the entire human genome are under way, and we may soon know the amino acid sequences of all our proteins.

The chemical synthesis of proteins is far more difficult than their structural analysis. Although polypeptides with more than 100 amino acids have been synthesized by chemists, only small oligopeptides can be produced cost effectively in large quantities. This limitation is deplorable because many naturally occurring proteins—for example, protein hormones and blood-clotting factors—are useful therapeutic agents. Alternatively, these proteins can be produced by genetically engineered microorganisms. The latter approach, which has become increasingly important in recent years, is discussed in Chapter 10.

FIG. 2.14

Edman degradation, the principal method for protein sequencing. The phenylthiohydantoin (PTH) amino acid is a fluorescent derivative that can be identified by chromatographic methods. The reactions can be repeated, shortening the polypeptide by one amino acid during each cycle.

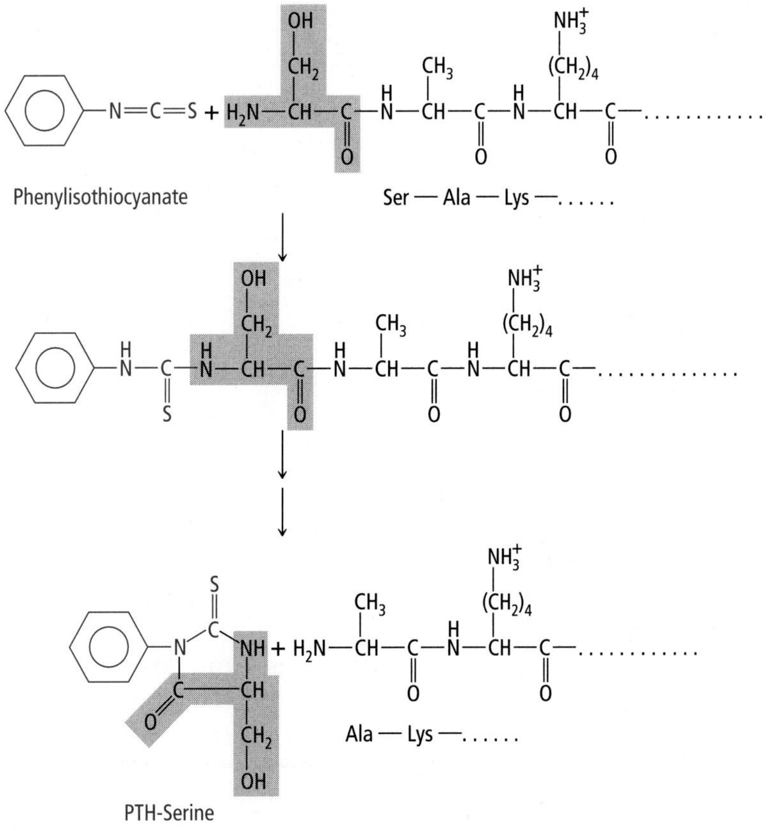

The higher-order structures of proteins can be analyzed by **X-ray diffraction.** This method is based on the scattering of X-rays that are passed through a protein crystal. The scattered X-rays form a diffraction pattern, and the analysis of this diffraction pattern yields information about the relative positions of atoms in the crystal. The structures of the α-helix and the β-pleated sheet, for example, were determined by Pauling and Corey during the 1940s and 1950s by a combination of X-ray diffraction and molecular model building.

SUMMARY

Proteins consist of 20 different amino acids, held together by peptide bonds. Both the amino acid side chains and the peptide bonds form noncovalent interactions in proteins. The covalent structure of the protein is called its primary structure. It is specified by the amino acid sequence and the positions of additional covalent bonds. The secondary structure is a regular, repetitive folding pattern of the polypeptide. The most important secondary structures are the α-helix and the β-pleated sheet. Both of these are stabilized by hydrogen bonds between the peptide bonds. The tertiary structure is the overall folding pattern of the polypeptide. It is stabilized mostly by hydrophobic interactions between amino acid side chains. Some proteins consist of more than one polypeptide (subunit). Their subunit composition and interactions are referred to as the quaternary structure. Many proteins contain disulfide bonds, a type of covalent bond formed by cysteine side chains. Disulfide bonds are either within the polypeptide (intrachain) or between polypeptides (interchain). Nonpolypeptide components also are common in proteins. They are referred to as prosthetic groups; the polypeptide component is called the apoprotein.

The noncovalent higher-order structure of proteins can be destroyed by heating, detergents, nonpolar organic solvents, heavy metals, and strong acids or bases. This is called denaturation, and it leads to a complete loss of the protein's biological properties. Laboratory methods are available for the measurement of the protein concentration in biological samples. Proteins also can be purified by methods that separate them on the basis of either molecular weight or charge. The structure of proteins can be determined by chemical and physical methods. Both the primary structures and the higher-order structures are known for many proteins.

Further Reading

Blaber M, Zhang X-j, Matthews BW: Structural basis of amino acid α helix propensity. *Science* 260, 1637−1640, 1993.

Branden C, Tooze J: *Introduction to protein structure*. Garland, New York, 1991.

Franks F, editor: *Characterization of proteins*. Humana Press, Totowa, NJ, 1988.

Hamaguchi K: *The protein molecule: conformation, stability and folding*. Springer Verlag, Berlin, 1992.

Kamoun PP: Denaturation of globular proteins by urea: breakdown of hydrogen or hydrophobic bonds? *Trends Biochem Sci* 13, 424−425, 1988.

Scopes RK: *Protein purification: principles and practice, 3rd ed.* Springer Verlag, New York, 1994.

Thomas PJ, Bao-He Qu B-H, Pedersern PL: Defective protein folding as a basis of human disease. *Trends Biochem Sci* 20(11), 456−459, 1995.

QUESTIONS

1. The component of a water-soluble globular protein that is most likely to be present in the center of the molecule rather than on its surface is
   A. A glutamate side chain
   B. A histidine side chain
   C. A phenylalanine side chain
   D. A phosphate group covalently linked to a serine side chain
   E. An oligosaccharide covalently linked to an asparagine side chain

2. The structure shown here is an oligopeptide that is acetylated at its amino end and amidated at its carboxy end, making the terminal groups unionizable.

   Acetyl-Ala-Glu-His-Ser-Lys-Gly-amide

This oligopeptide has an isoelectric point close to

A. 4.3
B. 5.1
C. 6.0
D. 8.4
E. 10.8

3. Protein A has a molecular weight of 55,000 and a pI of 4.8; protein B has a molecular weight of 84,000 and a pI of 4.9. The most promising method for the separation of these two proteins is

A. Electrophoresis in a cross-linked poly-acrylamide gel
B. X-ray diffraction
C. Dialysis
D. Paper electrophoresis
E. Distillation

4. Human serum contains approximately 7% protein. Essentially all of these proteins are globular proteins with pK values close to 4 or 5. In the test tube, these proteins will form an insoluble precipitate after all of the following treatments *except*

A. Boiling the serum for 5 minutes
B. Adding sodium chloride to a concentration of 35%
C. Adjusting the pH to 4.5
D. Boiling the serum with 6 N hydrochloric acid for 10 hours

Chapter 3

Oxygen Transporters:

Hemoglobin and Myoglobin

Our bodies require approximately 500 g of molecular oxygen per day. The transport of this amount from the lungs to the extrapulmonary tissues is problematic: at an oxygen partial pressure of 90 torr, which prevails in the lung capillaries, only 2.8 mL (4.1 mg) of O_2 can dissolve physically in 1 L of plasma. This limits the amount that can be transported in physical solution to not more than 30 g per day. Actually, however, our blood contains 150 g of the oxygen-binding protein hemoglobin per liter. With this hemoglobin concentration, 1 L of blood can dissolve 280 mg of oxygen, approximately 70 times more than hemoglobin-free blood plasma.

Two proteins in the body are designed specifically for the reversible binding of molecular oxygen. **Hemoglobin** is the oxygen carrier in red blood cells: it brings oxygen from the lungs to the extrapulmonary tissues. **Myoglobin** is found in muscle tissue, where it stores oxygen for times of strenuous exercise.

The binding of oxygen to these proteins, known technically as **oxygenation**, is reversible:

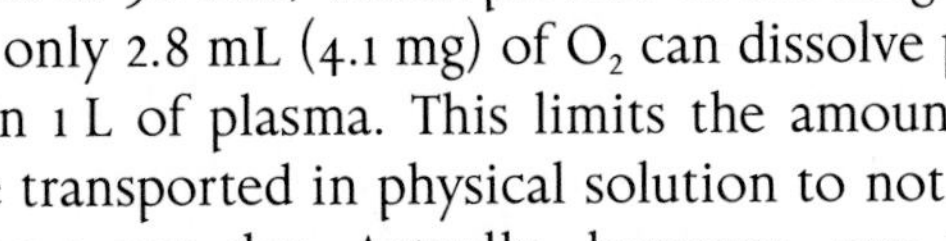

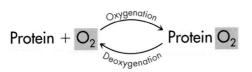

Therefore *oxygen binds to the oxygen-binding proteins when it is plentiful and is released when oxygen is scarce.*

The heme group is the oxygen-binding site of hemoglobin and myoglobin

None of the functional groups in the common amino acids has any binding affinity for molecular oxygen. Therefore the oxygen-binding proteins have to employ a nonpolypeptide component, the **heme group,** as their oxygen-binding site.

Heme consists of a porphyrin, called **protoporphyrin IX,** with a ferrous iron chelated in its center (Fig. 3.1). Protoporphyrin IX contains four five-membered nitrogen-containing rings, known as **pyrrole rings,** held together by methine ($-CH=$) bridges and decorated with methyl ($-CH_3$), vinyl ($-CH=CH_2$), and propionate ($-CH_2-CH_2-COO^-$) side chains. The porphyrin ring system contains conjugated double bonds (double bonds alternating with single bonds) that absorb visible light. *These double bonds are responsible for the color of our blood.* The color is affected by the oxygenation state: oxygenated hemoglobin is red, and deoxyhemoglobin is blue. Therefore, oxygen deficiency, or **hypoxia,** can be recognized as a blue discoloration of the lips and other mucous membranes. This is called **cyanosis.**

The most important part of the heme group is its iron. Like other heavy metals, ionized iron can form coordinate bonds with the free electron pairs of oxygen or nitrogen atoms. In heme, the iron is bound to the nitrogens of the four pyrrole rings.

FIG. 3.1

Structure of the heme group in hemoglobin and myoglobin. Note that the upper part of the group is hydrophilic because of the charged propionate side chains, whereas the lower part is hydrophobic. The conjugated double bonds in the ring system are responsible for its color. Oxyhemoglobin is red, deoxyhemoglobin blue.

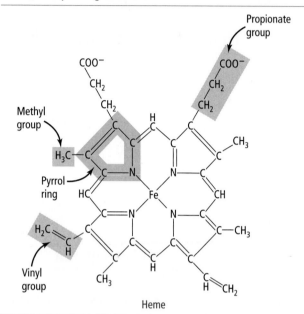

Heme

Both in hemoglobin and in myoglobin, the iron forms a fifth bond with a nitrogen atom in a histidine side chain of the apoprotein. This histidine is called the **proximal histidine.** A sixth coordinate bond can be formed with molecular oxygen:

His

Iron can exist in a ferrous (Fe^{2+}) and a ferric (Fe^{3+}) state. Ferric iron is the more oxidized form because it can be formed from ferrous iron by the removal of an electron:

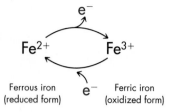

Fe^{2+} Fe^{3+}

Ferrous iron (reduced form)   Ferric iron (oxidized form)

The heme iron in hemoglobin and myoglobin is always in the ferrous state. Even during oxygen binding, it is not oxidized to the ferric form: it becomes oxygenated but not oxidized.

Myoglobin is a tightly packed globular protein

Myoglobin is a simple-structured substance, with a single polypeptide chain of 153 amino acids and a tightly bound heme group (molecular weight = 17,000 dalton, or 17 kDa). The primary structures of at least two dozen mammalian myoglobins have been determined thus far. Because of its small size, myoglobin has been a pet subject for structural studies using X-ray diffraction (see Chapter 2). These studies have revealed a globular protein with dimensions of roughly $2.5 \times 3.5 \times 4.5$ nm (Fig. 3.2). *Approximately 75% of the amino acid residues in the polypeptide participate in the formation of α-helical structures.* Eight α-helices are present, with lengths ranging from 7 to 23 amino acids. These α-helices are connected by nonhelical sequences. Starting from the amino-terminus, the eight α-helices are designated by capital letters A through H. The positions of the amino acid residues are specified by the helix letter and by their position within the helix. The proximal histidine, for example, which is in position 93 of the polypeptide, is designated His F8 because it is the eighth amino acid in the F helix.

Many of the α-helices are amphipathic: hydrophobic amino acid residues are clustered on one edge and hydrophilic residues on the other (Fig. 3.3). The hydrophobic edge faces inward to the center of the molecule. Indeed, *the interior of myoglobin is filled with tightly packed nonpolar side chains, and hydrophobic interactions are the major stabilizing force in the tertiary structure.* The surface of myoglobin, however, is occupied mainly by hydrophilic amino acid side chains, which make the molecule water soluble.

The heme group is tucked between the E helix and the F helix. One half of it is embedded between the two helices, held in place by hydrophobic inter-

FIG. 3.2

Tertiary structures of myoglobin and the β-chain of hemoglobin, as revealed by X-ray diffraction. Only the α-carbons are shown. The amino acid residues are designated by their position in one of the eight helices (A through H, starting from the amino terminus) or nonhelical linkers. The proximal histidine F8, for example, is the eighth amino acid in the F helix, counting from the amino end.

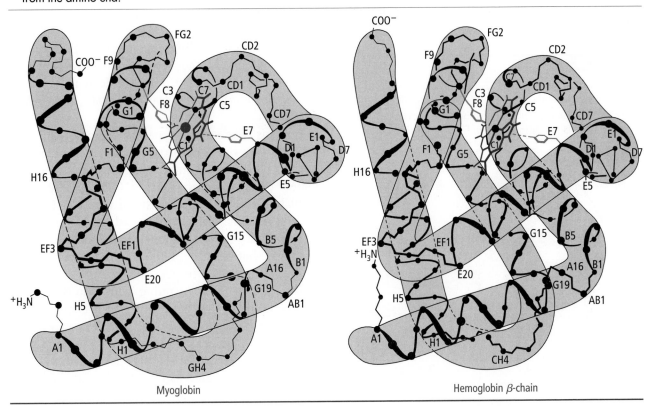

Myoglobin

Hemoglobin β-chain

actions with amino acid side chains. The half containing the two negatively charged propionate groups (Fig. 3.1), however, is exposed to the surrounding water. Next to the heme iron, on the side opposite the proximal histidine, we find another histidine side chain, the **distal histidine** (His E7). The cavity between the distal histidine and the heme iron is just large enough to allow the access of an oxygen molecule.

Like most other intracellular proteins, *myoglobin contains no disulfide bonds*, and its tertiary structure is maintained only by noncovalent forces. When the pH is decreased to 3.5 and urea is added, the heme group dissociates from the apoprotein and the α-helical structure is lost. After removal of the urea (by dialysis—see Chapter 2) and restoration of a physiological pH, however, the protein renatures spontaneously and the heme group binds in the correct orientation. This experiment demonstrates that *the native conformation of myoglobin is its thermodynamically most favorable state* and that the information inherent in its primary structure is sufficient for proper folding.

The red blood cells are specialized for oxygen transport

All the hemoglobin in the blood is enclosed in the erythrocytes (red blood cells, RBCs). Erythrocytes are released from the bone marrow and circulate for approximately 120 days before they are scavenged by phagocytic cells in the spleen and other tissues. Unlike all other cells in our body, *they have no nucleus* and therefore are unable to divide or to synthesize proteins. Their hemoglobin is inherited from their nucleated precursors in the bone marrow. They also lack mitochondria, and therefore, they do not consume any of the oxygen they transport. They cover their modest energy needs by the anaerobic metabolism of glucose to lactic acid. Erythrocytes are "bags" filled with hemoglobin at a concentration of not less than 33%, physically dissolved in the cytoplasm.

The hemoglobin concentration of whole blood, as well as the percentage of the blood volume occupied by the blood cells (the **hematocrit**, Table 3.1), are diagnostically important. Patients with an abnormally low hemoglobin concentration are said to have **anemia**.

The hemoglobins are tetrameric proteins

The most important difference between hemoglobin and myoglobin is the subunit structure: myoglobin consists of a single polypeptide with its heme group, but *hemoglobin has four polypeptides, each with its own heme*.

Humans have several types of hemoglobin (Table 3.2). All types consist of two pairs of nonidentical chains, with a total molecular weight of approximately 65,000. **Hemoglobin A (HbA)** is the major adult hemoglobin and consists of two α chains and two β chains. The **minor adult hemoglobin (HbA$_2$)** and **fetal hemoglobin (HbF)** also have two α chains, but instead of the β chains they have δ chains and γ chains, respectively.

The α chains have 141 amino acids. The β, γ, and δ chains, collectively called the "non-α chains," have 146 amino acids. *All of these chains are structurally related*: the β and δ chains differ in 10 and the β and γ chains in 39 of their 146 amino acids. The α and β chains are not related as closely: they are identical in 64 of their amino acids.

Although hemoglobin chains are distant relatives of myoglobin, only 28 amino acids are identical in α chains, β chains, and myoglobin. These conserved amino acids include the proximal and distal histidines and some of the other amino acids contact-

---

FIG. 3.3

Axial view of the E-helix in sperm whale myoglobin. This helix is an example of an amphipathic helix. The only hydrophilic amino acid on the otherwise hydrophobic edge of the helix is the distal histidine E7.

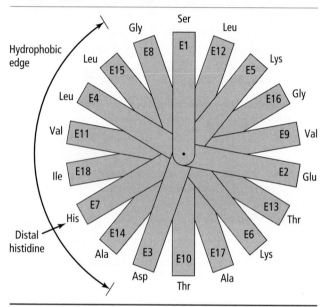

TABLE 3.1

Characteristics of red blood cells (RBCs) and hemoglobin

Diameter of RBCs	7.3 μm
Life span of RBCs	120 days
Number of RBCs	4.2−5.4 million/ mm³ (female)
	4.6−6.2 million/ mm³ (male)
Intracorpuscular hemoglobin concentration	33%
Hematocrit*	38%−46% (female)
	42%−53% (male)
Hemoglobin in whole blood	12%−15% (female)
	14%−17% (male)

* Hematocrit = the percentage of the blood volume occupied by blood cells; measured by centrifugation of whole blood.

TABLE 3.2

The most important human hemoglobins*

Type	Subunit structure	Importance
Major adult (HbA)	$\alpha_2\beta_2$	97% of adult hemoglobin
Minor adult (HbA$_2$)	$\alpha_2\delta_2$	2%-3% of adult hemoglobin
Fetal (HbF)	$\alpha_2\gamma_2$	Major hemoglobin in second and third trimesters of pregnancy

* See also Chapter 9.

ing the heme group. Many of the nonconserved amino acid positions are "conservative" substitutions: the alternative amino acids, although different, have similar physicochemical properties.

The subunits of hemoglobin have folding patterns that are surprisingly similar to the tertiary structure of myoglobin (Fig. 3.2). As in myoglobin, the heme group is tucked between the E and F helices. Most importantly, the immediate environment of the heme iron is the same in each case, with the proximal histidine (His F8) bound on one side and the distal histidine (His E7) guarding the entrance on the opposite side. Overall, *hemoglobin looks like four myoglobin molecules glued together.* Like myoglobin, the individual hemoglobin subunits have hydrophobic cores, and most of their surface is formed by hydrophilic amino acid residues. Like myoglobin, hemoglobin has no disulfide bonds, and the glue between the subunits consists only of noncovalent interactions.

Myoglobin and the hemoglobins, which form the globin family of proteins, demonstrate that very similar higher-order structures and biological properties can be achieved by polypeptides with widely differing amino acid sequences.

Methemoglobin is a nonfunctional, oxidized form of hemoglobin

The heme iron of hemoglobin (and myoglobin) binds molecular oxygen only in the ferrous (Fe^{2+}) state. Its oxidation to the ferric (Fe^{3+}) form results in **methemoglobin,** which is useless as an oxygen transporter. Normally, less than 1% of the total hemoglobin is in the form of methemoglobin, but *oxidizing chemicals cause excessive methemoglobin formation.* These chemicals include many aniline dyes, aromatic nitro compounds, and inorganic and organic nitrites. Fortunately, the red blood cell can defend itself against excessive methemoglobin formation:

1. *Erythrocytes contain reducing substances* such as ascorbic acid (see Chapter 24) and glutathione (Chapter 17), which destroy many oxidizing agents before they have the opportunity to react with hemoglobin.
2. *The binding of heme to the apoprotein creates a protective environment for the iron.* When heme is dissociated from the apoprotein, it rapidly becomes oxidized

to **hemin** by molecular oxygen, and hemin binds a hydroxyl ion to form **hematin.** Occasionally, patients are encountered who suffer from congenital (present at birth) methemoglobinemia because of a structural abnormality in the heme-binding pocket of the α or β chain. The replacement of the proximal histidine by a tyrosine residue, for example, causes methemoglobinemia.
3. *The enzyme methemoglobin reductase reduces methemoglobin back to normal hemoglobin,* using NADH (see Chapter 5) as a reductant. Individuals with a deficiency of methemoglobin reductase (a rare genetic defect) have congenital methemoglobinemia.

Methemoglobinemia is treated with methylene blue, which reduces the ferric iron back to the ferrous state.

Carbon monoxide competes with oxygen for binding to the heme iron

Carbon monoxide (CO), a product of incomplete combustion, is present in cigarette smoke, automobile exhaust, and many other sources. A small amount even is formed in the human body (see Chapter 22). Like molecular oxygen, *carbon monoxide binds to the ferrous iron in hemoglobin and myoglobin.* CO has a 200-fold-higher affinity for heme than O_2 does, and therefore, even a low concentration of CO is sufficient to displace O_2 from its binding site on the heme iron and cause serious poisoning.

Despite its high affinity for heme, *carbon monoxide binding is reversible:* in a normally breathing patient with carbon monoxide poisoning, oxygen gradually displaces the carbon monoxide from its binding site on the heme iron, leading to a slow recovery in the course of several hours. The interaction between carbon monoxide and oxygen at the heme iron is an example of **competitive antagonism:** both ligands compete for the same binding site, displacing each other. The outcome depends on the relative affinities and concentrations of the ligands. Because CO has a 200-fold-higher binding affinity than O_2, a CO concentration of only 1/200th of the O_2 concentration is sufficient to convert half of the oxyhemoglobin to CO-hemoglobin. Therefore *carbon monoxide poisoning can be overcome by elevated oxygen partial pressure,* and hyperbaric oxygen is the treatment of choice.

Acute CO poisoning is seen in patients who have inhaled car exhaust gas with suicidal intent, and in people trapped in a burning building. Throbbing headache, confusion, and fainting on exertion occur when 30% to 50% of the heme groups are occupied by carbon monoxide, and a CO saturation of 80% is rapidly fatal. *Patients with carbon monoxide poisoning are not cyanosed,* because CO-hemoglobin has a bright cherry-red color. Chronic exposure occurs in smokers, who have 4% to 8% of their hemoglobin in the CO form. Because this impairs oxygen transport, smoking should be discouraged in all patients who suffer from poor tissue oxygenation, particularly patients with angina pectoris (myocardial ischemia).

Oxygenated and deoxygenated hemoglobins have different quaternary structures

The quaternary structure of hemoglobin depends on its oxygenation state. In deoxyhemoglobin, the subunits are held together by eight salt bonds between the polypeptides, in addition to a number of hydrogen bonds and other noncovalent interactions. On oxygenation, the salt bonds break and a new set of hydrogen bonds forms. Overall, the interactions between the subunits in oxyhemoglobin are weaker than in the deoxy form. Therefore, the conformation of deoxyhemoglobin is called the **T conformation** (tense, or taut), and that of oxyhemoglobin is called the **R conformation** (relaxed) (Fig. 3.4).

How can oxygen binding change the conformation of the protein? The bond distances between the heme iron and the five nitrogens with which it is complexed shorten when oxygen binds. This distorts the shape of the heme group and exerts a pull on the F helix, to which the proximal histidine (F8) belongs. The interactions with the other subunits are destabilized, and the shape of the whole molecule is shifted in the direction of the R conformation.

The most important biological difference between the T and R conformations is their oxygen-binding affinity: *the R conformation binds oxygen 150 to 300 times more tightly than the T conformation.*

Proteins that, like hemoglobin, can assume alternative higher-order structures are called **allosteric proteins.** *The alternative conformations of an allosteric protein interconvert spontaneously, and their equilibrium is*

FIG. 3.4

Simplified model for the transition from T to R conformation during successive oxygenations of hemoglobin. Partially oxygenated hemoglobin spends most of its time in intermediate conformational states. Actually, different conformations ranging from "pure" T to "pure" R exist in equilibrium in each oxygenation state.

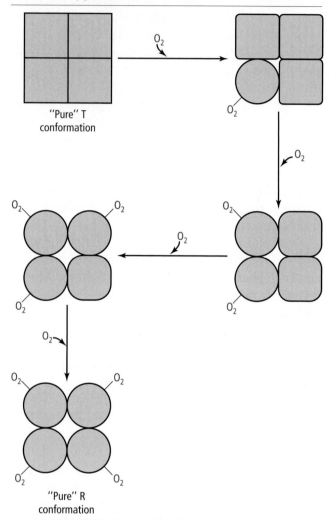

"Pure" T conformation

"Pure" R conformation

affected by ligand binding. A **ligand** (Latin *ligare*, "to bind") is any small molecule that binds reversibly to a protein.

Cooperativity of oxygen binding to hemoglobin leads to a sigmoidal oxygen-binding curve

The **oxygen-binding curve** describes the fractional saturation of the heme groups at various oxygen

FIG. 3.5

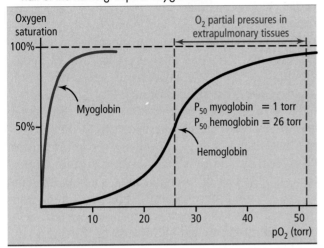

Oxygen-binding curves of hemoglobin and myoglobin. The P_{50} is defined as the oxygen partial pressure at which one half of the heme groups is oxygenated.

has a higher oxygen affinity. The same process is repeated after binding of the second and third oxygen molecules. Effectively, *oxygen binding to a heme group in hemoglobin increases the oxygen affinities of the remaining heme groups.* This effect is called **positive cooperativity.**

How does cooperativity affect the efficiency of hemoglobin as an oxygen transporter? Without cooperativity, an eighty-one fold increase of the pO_2 would be required to raise the oxygen saturation from 10% to 90%. For hemoglobin, however, a 4.8-fold increase is sufficient to do the same. This means that hemoglobin can readily bind oxygen in the lungs and then easily give it up in the tissue capillaries. Thus, hemoglobin is approximately 96% saturated in the lung capillaries (pO_2 = 90 torr) but only 33% saturated in the capillaries of working muscle (pO_2 = 20 torr). Less oxygen is extracted in the capillaries of other tissues, so the mixed venous blood still is 60% to 70% oxygenated. Although this oxygen is useless under ordinary conditions, it can keep us alive for a few minutes after acute respiratory arrest.

partial pressures. The oxygen partial pressure (pO_2) is approximately 100 torr in the lung alveoli, 90 torr in the lung capillaries, and between 20 and 60 torr in the capillaries of various tissues. The lowest oxygen partial pressure is found in the capillaries of contracting muscle, where it may decrease to 20 torr during heavy exercise.

Figure 3.5 shows that *myoglobin binds oxygen far tighter than hemoglobin:* the oxygen partial pressure required for half-saturation of myoglobin (its P_{50}) is only 1 torr, whereas hemoglobin requires 26 torr. *This difference in oxygen affinities facilitates the transfer of oxygen from the blood to the tissue.*

The shapes of the oxygen-binding curves differ as well: the myoglobin curve is a rectangular hyperbola. This has to be expected for a simple equilibrium reaction of the type

$$Mb + O_2 \rightleftharpoons Mb \cdot O_2$$

The binding curve of hemoglobin, however, is sigmoidal. Why? In the completely deoxygenated form, hemoglobin is predominantly in the T conformation, which has a very low oxygen affinity. This accounts for the flat part of the curve below approximately 10 torr. With increasing oxygen partial pressure, however, the first heme becomes oxygenated nevertheless. Oxygenation of the first heme shifts the structure of the hemoglobin molecule in the direction of the R conformation, which

BPG is a negative allosteric effector of oxygen binding to hemoglobin

2,3-Bisphosphoglycerate (BPG) is a small organic molecule that is present in red blood cells at a concentration of approximately 5 mM, roughly equimolar with hemoglobin:

Most BPG is noncovalently bound to hemoglobin in a stoichiometry of one molecule of BPG per hemoglobin molecule. Positioned in a central cavity between the subunits, it forms salt bonds with positively charged amino acid residues in the two β chains.

BPG binds only to the T conformation of hemoglobin—not to the R conformation. The result is a stabilization of the T conformation, which has a low oxygen-binding affinity (Fig. 3.6). Therefore, the observed effect is *a decreased oxygen-binding affinity*.

BPG is a physiologically important regulator of oxygen binding to hemoglobin. The BPG concentration in red blood cells increases during hypoxic conditions, including lung diseases, severe anemia, and adaptation to high altitude. This increase barely affects oxygenation in the lung capillaries, but *it enhances the unloading of oxygen in the tissues whose oxygen partial pressures are in the steep part of the oxygen-binding curve* (Fig. 3.7).

BPG is characterized as a **negative allosteric effector** with respect to oxygen binding to hemoglobin. (A **positive allosteric effector** would increase the oxygen-binding affinity.)

As an allosteric effector, BPG affects the oxygen affinity by binding to a site distant from the oxygen-binding site, acting through a conformational change in the protein. In allosteric proteins, interactions between different ligands, such as BPG and O_2, are called **heterotropic effects**. Interactions between identical ligands, as in the cooperativity of oxygen binding, are called **homotropic effects**.

Allosteric interactions between different ligand binding sites are not unique to hemoglobin. Many proteins are allosteric. The activities of many enzymes, for example, are regulated by positive or negative allosteric effectors (see Chapter 4). *Most allosteric proteins consist of more than one subunit, and the subunit interactions are affected by ligand binding.*

FIG. 3.6

Effect of 2,3-BPG on the equilibrium between the T and R conformations of hemoglobin. The salt bonds between 2,3-BPG and the β-chains stabilize the T conformation.

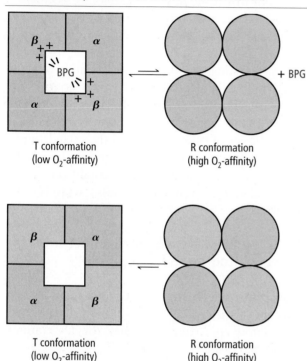

Fetal hemoglobin has a higher oxygen-binding affinity than adult hemoglobin

In adult hemoglobin (HbA), BPG forms salt bonds with the amino termini of the β chains and with the side chains of Lys EF6 and His H21 in the β chains. In the γ chains of fetal hemoglobin (HbF), His H21 is replaced by a serine residue that is not able to form a salt bond. Therefore, *BPG binds less tightly to HbF than to HbA*; this, in turn, reduces the effect of BPG on the oxygen affinity. At physiologic BPG concentration, the P_{50} of HbF is only 20 torr, compared with 26 torr for HbA. *This facilitates the transfer of oxygen from the maternal blood to the fetal blood in the capillaries of the placenta.*

The Bohr effect facilitates oxygen delivery

The oxygen-binding affinity of hemoglobin is reduced not only by BPG, but by a low pH value as well. This phenomenon, known as the **Bohr effect,** is important in actively metabolizing tissues.

FIG. 3.7

Effect of 2,3-BPG on the oxygen-binding affinity of hemoglobin (Hb).

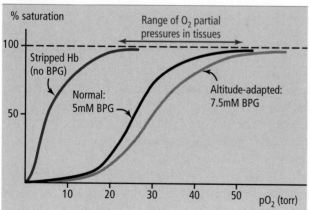

Carbon dioxide is an end product of oxidative metabolism, and in aqueous solution it forms carbonic acid:

$$CO_2 + H_2O \rightleftharpoons H_2CO_3 \rightleftharpoons HCO_3^- + H^+$$

Lactic acid also is formed in places where oxygen is needed, particularly in exercising muscle and in ischemic tissues (see Chapter 16).

The protons produced by these processes reduce oxygen binding because *oxygenated hemoglobin is more acidic than deoxyhemoglobin*: oxygen binding releases protons according to the equation

$$\text{Hemoglobin} + O_2 \rightleftharpoons \\ \text{Hemoglobin} \cdot O_2 + 0.7\,H^+$$

An increase in the proton concentration, as occurs in exercising muscle, shifts the equilibrium of this reaction to the left, favoring the release of oxygen from hemoglobin. Most of the approximately 0.7 protons that are released during the binding of each oxygen molecule are released as a result of pK changes of those groups that participate in the formation of the intersubunit salt bonds in the T but not the R conformation. The equilibrium of the reaction

$$Hb \cdot O_2 + 0.7\,H^+ \rightleftharpoons Hb + O_2$$

is defined by the dissociation constant K_D (see also Chapter 4):

$$K_D = \frac{[Hb] \times [O_2]}{[Hb \cdot O_2] \times [H^+]^{0.7}}$$

This equation can be rearranged to:

$$\frac{[Hb]}{[Hb \cdot O_2]} = K_D \times \frac{[H^+]^{0.7}}{[O_2]}$$

We see that at a constant oxygen partial pressure ($[O_2]$), an increase of the hydrogen ion concentration ($[H^+]$) favors the deoxygenated state [Hb].

Carbon dioxide also decreases the oxygen affinity of hemoglobin. This effect is mediated by the covalent binding of CO_2 to the terminal amino groups of the α and β chains, resulting in the formation of **carbamino hemoglobin:**

$$\text{Hemoglobin---NH}_2 + CO_2 \rightleftharpoons$$

$$\text{Hemoglobin---NH---}\overset{\overset{\displaystyle O}{\|}}{C}\text{---O}^- + H^+$$

This reaction is reversible and proceeds spontaneously, without the need for an enzyme. Carbamino hemoglobin has a lower oxygen affinity than unmodified hemoglobin. Like the pH effect, the CO_2 effect ensures that *oxygen is released preferentially in actively metabolizing tissues, where it is most needed.*

Most carbon dioxide is transported as bicarbonate

The transport of carbon dioxide is not problematic. CO_2 has a higher water solubility than oxygen, and

---

FIG. 3.8

The major mechanism of carbon dioxide transport. Note that all processes are reversible. Their direction is determined by the concentrations of the involved substances. **A,** in the extrapulmonary tissues; **B,** in the lung capillaries.

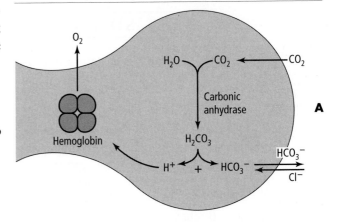

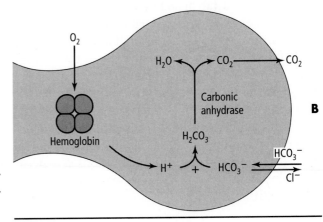

therefore, a significant portion can be transported physically dissolved in the plasma. Carbamino hemoglobin and the carbamino derivatives of plasma proteins also transport some of the CO_2.

Approximately 80% of the CO_2, however, is transported in the form of inorganic bicarbonate (Fig. 3.8). The CO_2 produced in extrapulmonary tissues diffuses passively across the erythrocyte membrane. In the cell, it encounters **carbonic anhydrase,** a highly active enzyme (see Chapter 4, Table 4.1) that rapidly establishes an equilibrium among CO_2, H_2O, and carbonic acid. Most of the carbonic acid, in turn, dissociates spontaneously into a proton and the bicarbonate anion. While the proton is bound by hemoglobin as part of the Bohr effect, the bicarbonate is released from the cell in exchange for a chloride ion. This exchange, which requires a specific ion channel in the membrane, is called the **chloride shift.** The bicarbonate now is transported to the lungs, physically dissolved in the plasma. In the lung capillaries, all the previously described processes proceed in the opposite direction.

SUMMARY

We require oxygen-binding proteins because molecular oxygen is poorly soluble in our body fluids. Hemoglobin is the oxygen-binding protein in erythrocytes, and myoglobin binds oxygen in muscle tissue. Both proteins employ heme as a prosthetic group. Myoglobin consists of a single polypeptide with a noncovalently bound heme group, and hemoglobin has four polypeptides, each with its own heme. Adult hemoglobin (HbA) has two α chains and two β chains, and fetal hemoglobin (HbF) has two α chains and two γ chains. Myoglobin has a far higher oxygen-binding affinity than the hemoglobins, and HbF has a somewhat higher affinity than HbA. Hemoglobin can be poisoned by oxidizing agents that oxidize the ferrous heme iron to the ferric state, and by carbon monoxide, which occupies the oxygen-binding site on the heme iron. Hemoglobin (but not myoglobin) has allosteric properties. There is positive cooperativity between the heme groups, leading to a sigmoidal oxygen-binding curve; BPG and protons are negative allosteric effectors that decrease the oxygen-binding affinity.

QUESTIONS

1. A pharmaceutical company tries to develop a drug that improves tissue oxygenation by increasing the percentage of oxygen that is released from hemoglobin during its passage through the capillaries of extrapulmonary tissues. This drug, it is hoped, will become a popular doping agent for athletes. The company should try a drug that
   A. Binds to the heme iron
   B. Inhibits the degradation of BPG, thereby increasing its concentration in erythrocytes
   C. Binds to ion channels in the RBC membrane, thereby increasing the intracellular pH value
   D. Binds to the R conformation of hemoglobin but not the T conformation
   E. Induces the synthesis of hemoglobin γ chains in adults

2. A worker in a chemical factory loses consciousness within a few minutes after falling into a vat containing nitrobenzene, an aromatic nitro compound. This very well may be caused by an action of nitrobenzene on hemoglobin, most likely
   A. Competitive inhibition of oxygen binding
   B. Oxidation of the heme iron to the ferric state
   C. Reductive cleavage of disulfide bonds between the hemoglobin subunits
   D. Hydrolysis of peptide bonds in hemoglobin α and β chains
   E. Inhibition of hemoglobin synthesis

3. The oxygen-binding curve of hemoglobin is sigmoidal because
   A. The binding of oxygen to a heme group increases the oxygen affinities of the other heme groups.
   B. The heme groups of the α chains have a higher oxygen affinity than the heme groups of the β chains.
   C. The distal histidine allows the hemoglobin molecule to change its conformation in response to an elevated carbon dioxide concentration.
   D. The subunits are held in place by interchain disulfide bonds.
   E. The solubility of the hemoglobin molecule changes with its oxidation state.

Chapter 4

Enzymatic Reactions

During its normal metabolic activity, the cell uses hundreds of different nutrients that serve as starting materials, or **substrates,** of metabolic processes. Thousands of metabolic intermediates are formed from these nutrients, and all of them have to be channeled through appropriate metabolic pathways. We can, indeed, imagine the cell as a test tube in which thousands of chemical reactions take place simultaneously and in a highly ordered fashion.

Most metabolic reactions would not proceed at any significant rate if their substrates simply were mixed in a test tube by an overoptimistic chemist. Because chemical reaction rates are temperature dependent, our chemist possibly could force the reaction by increasing the temperature. He also could try a nonselective catalyst, for example, a strong acid or a strong base. Our bodies, of course, are not in this lucky situation because the body temperature and the pH values of the various cellular organelles have to be kept within narrow limits.

The body depends on highly selective catalysts called **enzymes.** By definition, a catalyst is a substance that accelerates a chemical reaction without being consumed in the process. Because it is regenerated at the end of each catalytic cycle (Fig. 4.1), a single molecule of the catalyst can convert a large number of substrate molecules into product molecules. Therefore only a small amount of the catalyst is needed.

THERMODYNAMICS

Chemical reactions have thermodynamic and kinetic properties. The thermodynamic properties are related to the energy balance and the equilibrium of the reaction, and the kinetic properties describe its rate (velocity). *Enzymes affect only the kinetics but not the thermodynamics of chemical reactions.* Before analyzing enzyme kinetics, we have to consider some of the thermodynamic aspects that are common to all chemical reactions.

The reaction equilibrium can be described by the equilibrium constant

In theory, *all chemical reactions are reversible.* The reaction equilibrium can be determined experimentally by allowing the reaction to proceed to completion and then measuring the concentrations of the reactants. The position of the equilibrium is described by the **equilibrium constant** (K_{equ}), defined as the *ratio of product to substrate concentrations at equilibrium.* For a simple reaction

$$A \rightleftharpoons B$$

the equilibrium constant is

$$K_{equ} = \frac{[B]}{[A]}$$

FIG. 4.1

The catalytic cycle. The substrate has to bind to the enzyme to form a noncovalent enzyme-substrate complex (Enzyme · Substrate). The actual reaction takes place while the substrate is bound to the enzyme. Note that the enzyme is regenerated at the end of the catalytic cycle.

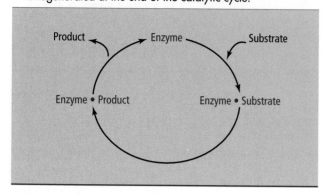

[B] and [A] are the molar concentrations of product B and substrate A at equilibrium.

If more than one substrate or product participates, *their concentrations must be multiplied*. For the reaction

$$A + B \rightleftharpoons C + D$$

the equilibrium constant is

$$K_{equ} = \frac{[C] \times [D]}{[A] \times [B]}$$

The example of the alcohol dehydrogenase (ADH) reaction shows us a practical application. The balance of this reaction is

1

$$H_3C—CH_2OH + NAD^+ \rightleftharpoons$$
Ethanol

$$H_3C—CHO + NADH + H^+$$
Acetaldehyde

NAD^+ is a coenzyme that functions as a hydrogen acceptor in this reaction (see Chapter 5). The equilibrium constant of the reaction is approximately

2

$$K_{equ} = \frac{[Acetaldehyde] \times [NADH] \times [H^+]}{[Ethanol] \times [NAD^+]}$$
$$= 10^{-11}M$$

What are the relative concentrations of acetaldehyde and ethanol at equilibrium if [NADH] = [NAD$^+$] and pH = 7.0? From Equation (2) we obtain

3

$$\frac{[Acetaldehyde]}{[Ethanol]} = 10^{-11}M \times \frac{[NAD^+]}{[NADH]} \times \frac{1}{[H^+]}$$
$$= 10^{-11} \times 1 \times 10^7$$
$$= 10^{-4}$$

We have 10,000 times more ethanol than acetaldehyde at equilibrium.

Under aerobic conditions, however, the cellular concentration of NAD$^+$ always is much higher than that of NADH. If we assume that the cellular concentration of [NAD$^+$] is 1000 times higher than [NADH], Equation 3 assumes the numerical values of

$$\frac{[Acetaldehyde]}{[Ethanol]} = 10^{-11} \times 1000 \times 10^7$$
$$= 10^{-1}$$
$$= \frac{1}{10}$$

The pH value also is important. At pH 8.0 and an [NAD$^+$]/[NADH] ratio of 1000, for example, Equation 3 yields

$$\frac{[Acetaldehyde]}{[Ethanol]} = 10^{-11} \times 1000 \times 10^8$$
$$= 10^0$$
$$= 1$$

This example shows that *a reaction can be driven in the direction of product formation if the concentration of one of the substrates is increased or that of one of the products is decreased.*

To adapt the equilibrium constant to physiologic conditions, we use a "biological equilibrium constant," K'_{equ}. In the definition of K'_{equ} we assign a value of 1.0 to the water concentration if water is a reactant, and a value of 1.0 to a proton concentration of 10^{-7} mol/L if protons participate in the reaction. The K'_{equ} of the alcohol dehydrogenase reaction, for example, is not

10^{-11} mol/L but 10^{-4} mol/L. At pH 8.0 in the previous example, the proton concentration would be given a numerical value of 10^{-1}.

The free energy change is the driving force for chemical reactions

During chemical reactions, heat either is released or absorbed. The change in the heat content of the reacting system is characterized as ΔE. It is measured either in kilocalories per mole (kcal/mol) or in kilojoules per mole (kJ/mol; 1 kcal = 4.184 kJ). By convention, *a negative sign of ΔE indicates that heat is released, and a positive sign indicates that heat is absorbed.* A more general description of energy changes is the **enthalpy change, ΔH**:

4

$$\Delta H = \Delta E + P \times \Delta V$$

where P is the pressure and ΔV is the volume change. $P \times \Delta V$ is the work done by the system. This value may be quite substantial in such work-performing devices as a car motor, but in the human body the volume changes (ΔV) are negligible, and therefore $\Delta H \approx \Delta E$. A negative sign of ΔH signifies an **exothermic reaction;** a positive sign means an **endothermic reaction.** *The enthalpy change corresponds to the difference in the total chemical bond energies between the substrates and the products.*

ΔH is not the only determinant of the reaction equilibrium, and some endothermic reactions do occur spontaneously. The change in **entropy,** designated as ΔS, also is important. *Entropy is a measure for the randomness or disorderliness of the system.* A cluttered desk often is cited as an example of a system of high entropy. *A positive ΔS means that the system becomes more disordered during the reaction.* The entropy change and the enthalpy change are combined in the **free energy change, ΔG:**

5

$$\Delta G = \Delta H - T \times \Delta S$$

where T is the absolute temperature measured in kelvin.

ΔG is the most important thermodynamic function because *it is the driving force of the reaction.* Like ΔE and ΔH (Equation 4), it is measured in kilocalo-

ries per mole (kcal/mol) or kilojoules per mole (kJ/mol). *A negative sign of ΔG indicates an **exergonic reaction**, one that proceeds spontaneously and forms product from substrate. A positive sign of ΔG indicates an **endergonic reaction,** which can proceed only in the backward direction. At equilibrium, ΔG equals zero.*

Equation 5 shows that a reaction can be driven either by a decrease in enthalpy (negative ΔH) or by an increase in entropy (positive $T \times \Delta S$): *the preferred conditions in nature are low enthalpy and high entropy.* The $T \times \Delta S$ part of Equation 5 is small in most biochemical reactions. Entropy-driven processes are, however, important in biological systems. *Diffusion is an entropy-driven process* (Fig. 4.2, A). In this case, the enthalpy change ΔH equals zero, and according to Equation 5, it can occur only when ΔS is positive: it proceeds spontaneously until the molecules are distributed randomly throughout the system. This is the state of maximal entropy.

The human body is a highly ordered system: it has low entropy. This is thermodynamically unfavorable, and therefore *biochemical reactions have to antagonize the tendency for increasing entropy* (positive $T \times \Delta S$ in Equation 5). This is possible only by the use of exothermic reactions, in which the enthalpy of the system decreases (negative ΔH in Equation 5): *we have to use chemical bond energy to maintain the low-entropy state of our bodies.* In the example shown in Fig. 4.2, B and C, the cell has to use chemical bond energy, obtained from ATP hydrolysis (ATP $\rightarrow$ ADP + P_i, negative ΔH), to establish a sodium gradient across the membrane (negative $T \times \Delta S$ for sodium "pumping"). In the absence of the chemical bond energy in ATP, the gradient dissipates, the entropy of the system increases, and the cell dies.

The standard free energy change is related to the equilibrium constant

The "real" free energy change ΔG is not a property of the reaction as such but *it is affected by the relative reactant concentrations.* To obtain a convenient energetic expression that predicts the equilibrium of the reaction, we have to define the **standard free energy change, $\Delta G^{o\prime}$.** This is the *free energy change under standard conditions.* Standard conditions are defined as a concentration of 1 mol/L for all reactants (except protons) and a pH value of 7.0. As in

FIG. 4.2

Diffusion as an entropy-driven process. **A**, In a hypothetical two-compartment system, molecules diffuse until their concentrations are equal. This is the state of maximal entropy. **B**, The living cell maintains a gradient of sodium ions across its plasma membrane. The cell can maintain this gradient, which represents a low-entropy state, only by "pumping" sodium out of the cell. The pump is fueled by the chemical bond energy in ATP. **C**, The dead cell lacks ATP: it cannot maintain its sodium gradient. Without the chemical bond energy of ATP, a high-entropy state develops spontaneously, with intracellular [Na$^+$] = extracellular [Na$^+$].

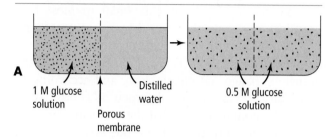

A 1 M glucose solution   Distilled water   Porous membrane   0.5 M glucose solution

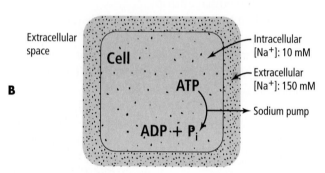

B Extracellular space   Cell   ATP   ADP + P$_i$ Intracellular [Na$^+$]: 10 mM   Extracellular [Na$^+$]: 150 mM   Sodium pump

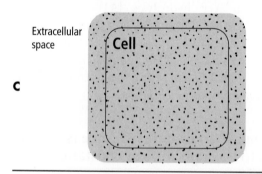

C Extracellular space   Cell

the real free energy change ΔG by the equation

6

$$\Delta G = \Delta G^{0\prime} + R \times T \times \log_e \frac{[C] \times [D]}{[A] \times [B]}$$
$$= \Delta G^{0\prime} + R \times T \times 2.303 \times \lg \frac{[C] \times [D]}{[A] \times [B]}$$

where R is the gas constant and T is the absolute temperature measured in kelvin. The numerical value of R is 1.987×10^{-3} kcal $\times$ mol^{-1} $\times$ K^{-1}. At 25°C (298 K), the values for Equation 6 are

7

$$\Delta G = \Delta G^{0\prime} + 1.987 \times 10^{-3} \times 298 \times 2.303 \times \lg \frac{[C] \times [D]}{[A] \times [B]}$$

8

$$= \Delta G^{0\prime} + 1.364 \times \lg \frac{[C] \times [D]}{[A] \times [B]}$$

At equilibrium, ΔG equals zero and therefore Equation 8 yields

9

$$\Delta G^{0\prime} = -1.364 \times \lg \frac{[C] \times [D]}{[A] \times [B]}$$

The reactant concentrations under the logarithm are now the equilibrium concentrations. Their ratio corresponds to the "biological" equilibrium constant K'_{equ}:

10

$$\frac{[C] \times [D]}{[A] \times [B]} = K'_{equ}$$

By substituting Equation 10 into Equation 9, we obtain

11

$$\Delta G^{0\prime} = -1.364 \times \lg K'_{equ}$$

There is a negative logarithmic relationship between the $\Delta G^{0\prime}$ and the equilibrium constant K'_{equ} of the reaction. With

the definition of K'_{equ}, the water concentration is given a value of 1.0.

Considering the reaction

$$A + B \longrightarrow C + D$$

the standard free energy change $\Delta G^{0\prime}$ is related to

TABLE 4.1

Relationship between the equilibrium constant K'_{equ} and the standard free energy change $\Delta G^{o'}$.

K'_{equ}	$\Delta G^{o'}$ [kcal/mol]
10^{-5}	6.82
10^{-4}	5.46
10^{-3}	4.09
10^{-2}	2.73
10^{-1}	1.36
1	0
10	-1.36
10^2	-2.73
10^3	-4.09
10^4	-5.46
10^5	-6.82

TABLE 4.2

Approximate turnover numbers of some enzymes

Enzyme	Turnover number [sec^{-1}]*
Carbonic anhydrase	600,000
Catalase	80,000
Acetylcholinesterase	25,000
Triose phosphate isomerase	4,400
α-Amylase	300
Lactate dehydrogenase (muscle)	200
Chymotrypsin	100
Aldolase	11
Lysozyme	0.5
Fructose 2,6-bisphosphatase	0.1

* Turnover numbers are measured at saturating substrate concentrations. They depend on the assay conditions, including temperature and pH.

Equation (11), we can calculate one if the other is known (Table 4.1). A negative sign of $\Delta G^{o'}$ indicates that the product concentration is higher than the substrate concentration at equilibrium, whereas a positive sign indicates that the substrates are favored over the products.

ENZYME KINETICS

Enzymes can change only the reaction rate—not the equilibrium—of the catalyzed reaction. In the following sections, the effect of enzymatic catalysis on the reaction rate at different substrate concentrations, as well as the effects of temperature, pH, and various inhibitors on enzymatic reactions are described.

Enzymes are highly selective biocatalysts

Generally, *almost all known enzymes are proteins.* There is no compelling chemical reason for this, and indeed we know of a small number of ribonucleic acid (RNA) molecules that possess enzymatic activity. These catalytic RNAs are called **ribozymes.** Most of them play specialized roles in gene expression, but they do not seem to be involved in metabolic reactions. *The "typical" enzyme is a globular protein* that either is dissolved in the cytoplasm or in a cellular organelle, or is bound to a membrane. Some

enzymes perform outdoor work. They catalyze reactions in the interstitial space, in the vascular space, or, as in the case of the digestive enzymes (see Chapter 14), in an external compartment.

Enzymes are useful because they are very selective, both for the substrate and for the reaction type. Typically, each individual reaction requires its own enzyme, and whether a reaction proceeds depends on the presence or absence of the enzyme. If, for example, an enzyme is lacking because of a genetic defect, only one reaction is blocked.

Enzymes not only are selective, but are powerful as well. They often accelerate the reaction rate many billion- or even trillionfold. Most enzyme-catalyzed reactions would not proceed at a noticeable rate at all without the enzyme. The **turnover number** describes the catalytic power of an enzyme. It is defined as *the number of substrate molecules converted to product by one enzyme molecule per second.* Table 4.2 shows the turnover numbers of some enzymes.

Rate constants are useful to describe reaction rates

The rate (velocity) of a chemical reaction can be described by a rate constant k. In an uncatalyzed reaction in which only one substrate reacts

$$A \xrightarrow{k} B$$

the reaction rate is defined by

12

$$V = k \times [A]$$

For a reversible reaction, we have to consider the forward reaction and the backward reaction separately:

• $$A \underset{k_{-1}}{\overset{k_1}{\rightleftarrows}} B$$

13

$$V_{\text{forward}} = k_1 \times [A]$$

14

$$V_{\text{backward}} = k_{-1} \times [B]$$

At equilibrium, V_{forward} equals V_{backward}, and therefore the net reaction is zero:

15

$$k_1 \times [A] = k_{-1} \times [B]$$

16

$$\frac{[B]}{[A]} = \frac{k_1}{k_{-1}} = K_{\text{equ}}$$

Equation 16 shows that *the equilibrium constant K_{equ}, previously defined as $[B]/[A]$ at equilibrium (see the thermodynamics section of this chapter), also is the ratio of the two rate constants.*

If we consider only the forward reaction, Equation 12 describes a **first-order reaction**. In a first-order reaction, *the reaction rate is directly proportional to the substrate concentration*: if the substrate concentration [A] is doubled, the reaction rate V is doubled as well. One-substrate reactions typically follow first-order kinetics. A classical example for a first-order reaction is the decay of a radioactive isotope.

If two substrates participate, we are likely to find a **second-order reaction**: the reaction rate depends on the concentrations of both substrates. For

$$A + B \overset{k}{\longrightarrow} C + D$$

we obtain

17

$$V = k \times [A] \times [B]$$

*A **zero-order reaction** is independent of the substrate concentration*: no matter how many substrate molecules are present in the test tube, only a fixed number are converted to product per second:

18

$$V = k$$

Zero-order kinetics are observed only in catalyzed reactions in which the substrate concentration is high and the amount and turnover number of the catalyst, rather than the substrate availability, are the limiting factors.

Enzymes decrease the free energy of activation

Reactions are thermodynamically possible when the free energy content of the products is lower than that of the substrates. In these cases the ΔG of the reaction has a negative sign; but not all reactions that are thermodynamically possible actually occur at a perceptible rate. This is because *the substrate has to be converted to a **transition state** before the product can be formed.* The transition state is structurally intermediate between the substrate and the product, but its free energy content is higher. Therefore it is unstable; once formed, it decomposes almost immediately to form either substrate or product.

In the example given in Fig. 4.3, the reaction is exergonic because the free energy content of the product is lower than that of the substrate. The uncatalyzed reaction does not occur at a perceptible rate, however, because the substrate has to be converted to the transition state first. *The free energy difference between the substrate and the transition state is called the **free energy of activation** (ΔG_{act}).* This energy has to be supplied by the kinetic energy of the reacting molecules. For this reason, *the rate of chemical reactions is increased by increased temperature.*

The free energy of activation is an energy barrier that prevents chemical reactions. Therefore, a condition can exist that is not the most favorable state thermodynamically but is maintained because the activation energy is too high. This state is called **metastable.** The human body is metastable in an oxygen-containing atmosphere: although CO_2 and H_2O are thermodynamically more stable than the complex organic molecules that form our bodies, we are not spontaneously oxidized because the free energy of activation is too high.

FIG. 4.3

Energy profile of a reaction. The enzyme facilitates the reaction by decreasing the free energy content of the transition state. —— Uncatalyzed reaction; —— catalyzed reaction. ΔG_{act}, free energy of activation.

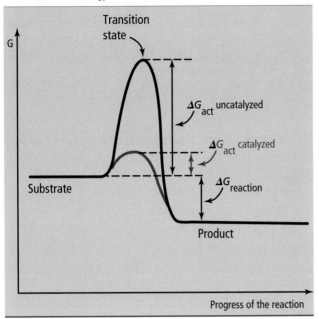

FIG. 4.4

The two models of enzyme-substrate binding. **A**, The lock-and-key model. *S*, substrate. **B**, The induced-fit model.

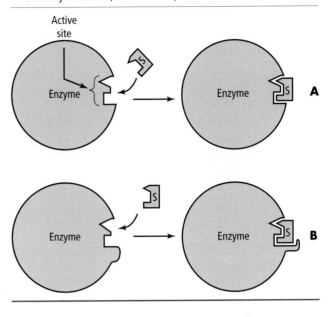

The enzyme forms favorable interactions with the transition state of the reaction. It stabilizes the transition state, decreases its free energy content, and decreases the free energy of activation. This allows the reaction to proceed at acceptable temperatures. *Enzymes increase the rate of the reaction by decreasing the free energy of activation.*

Enzymes accelerate both the forward and the backward reactions, and *the equilibrium constant remains unchanged.* Also $\Delta G^{o\prime}$ is unchanged.

The enzyme-substrate complex is formed by noncovalent interactions

Enzymatic reactions proceed stepwise:

$$E + S \rightleftharpoons E \cdot S \rightleftharpoons E \cdot P \rightleftharpoons E + P$$

where E = free enzyme; S = free substrate; P = free product; E·S = enzyme-substrate complex; and E·P = enzyme-product complex.

In the first step, the formation of the **enzyme-substrate complex** (E·S), the substrate binds noncovalently to a binding site on the surface of the enzyme protein. This site, the **active site** of the enzyme, contains the functional groups for substrate binding and for catalysis. It typically includes amino acid residues that are far apart in the covalent structure of the polypeptide. This is not surprising, because enzymes are globular proteins with intricate folding patterns. If a prosthetic group participates in the reaction as a coenzyme, it is present in the active site as well.

According to the **lock-and-key model,** the substrate and the active site bind each other because their surfaces are complementary (Fig. 4.4, *A*). Frequently, however, substrate binding induces a conformational change in the active site that facilitates further enzyme-substrate interactions. This is known as **induced fit** (Fig. 4.4, *B*). Functional groups of the enzyme protein that participate in catalysis rather than in initial substrate binding can be brought to the substrate by induced fit.

The geometry of enzyme-substrate binding is essential for the enzyme's **substrate specificity:** only a molecule that is able to bind correctly to the enzyme can be a substrate. Most enzymes have a rather tight substrate specificity. *If the substrate is optically active, generally only one of the isomers is admitted.* This is to be expected because the enzyme, being

FIG. 4.5

A three-point attachment is the minimal requirement for stereoselectivity. In this hypothetical example, the enzyme-substrate complex is formed by a salt bond, a hydrogen bond, and a hydrophobic interaction. The substrate binds whereas its enantiomer *(shown below)* is not able to form an enzyme-substrate complex.

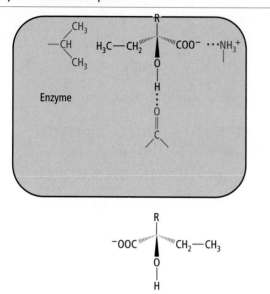

formed only from L-amino acids, is optically active itself. A three-point attachment, as shown schematically in Fig. 4.5, is the minimal requirement for stereoselectivity.

Many enzymatic reactions can be described by Michaelis–Menten kinetics

In Michaelis–Menten kinetics, we analyze enzymatic reactions under simplified assumptions:

- *The reaction has only one substrate.*
- *The molar concentration of the substrate is much higher than that of the enzyme.*
- *We consider only the initial reaction rate*, at a time when the product concentration still is negligibly low. Therefore, we can disregard the backward reaction.
- *We follow the course of the reaction for a very short time*, neglecting the changes in substrate and product concentrations that take place as the reaction proceeds.

The detailed steps of the reaction are

$$E + S \; \underset{\textstyle ①}{\rightleftharpoons} \; E \cdot S \; \underset{\textstyle ②}{\rightleftharpoons} \; E \cdot P \; \underset{\textstyle ③}{\rightleftharpoons} \; E + P$$

Assuming a low product concentration, we can neglect the rates of the backward reactions in steps ② and ③. In addition, we can lump steps ② and ③ together to yield

$$E + S \; \underset{k_{-1}}{\overset{k_1}{\rightleftharpoons}} \; E \cdot S \; \xrightarrow{k_2} \; E + P$$

The velocity or rate (V) of product formation, which corresponds to the rate of the overall reaction, is

19

$$V = k_2 \times [E \cdot S]$$

Is there an upper limit to V? There is, because the enzyme-substrate complex (E·S) is formed from the free enzyme. Its concentration cannot be higher than that of the total enzyme (E_T). Therefore the maximal reaction rate (V_{max}) is

20

$$V_{max} = k_2 \times [E_T]$$

We also can describe the tightness of binding between the enzyme and the substrate by defining the **"true" dissociation constant** of the enzyme-substrate complex. The true dissociation constant is the equilibrium constant (compare Equation 13 with Equation 16) for the reaction $E \cdot S \rightleftharpoons E + S$:

21

$$K_D = \frac{[E] \times [S]}{[E \cdot S]} = \frac{k_{-1}}{k_1}$$

The enzyme-substrate complex not only can decompose back to free enzyme and free substrate, but it can undergo catalysis as well. Under steady-state conditions, the concentration of the enzyme-substrate complex is constant, and its rate of formation is balanced by its rate of decomposition. For

$$E + S \; \underset{k_2}{\overset{k_1}{\rightleftharpoons}} \; E \cdot S \; \xrightarrow{k_2} \; E + P$$

we obtain

22

$$k_1 \times [E] \times [S] = \underbrace{k_{-1} \times [E \cdot S]}_{\text{Rate of dissociation of } E \cdot S \text{ to } E + S} + \underbrace{k_2 \times [E \cdot S]}_{\text{Rate of product formation}}$$

which yields

23

$$k_1 \times [E] \times [S] = (k_{-1} + k_2) \times [E \cdot S]$$

and

24

$$\frac{[E] \times [S]}{[E \cdot S]} = \frac{k_{-1} + k_2}{k_1} = K_m$$

This is the definition of the **Michaelis constant,** K_m. It is similar to the true dissociation constant of the enzyme-substrate complex, which is defined as k_{-1}/k_1 (see Equation 21). Indeed, in most enzymatic reactions the catalytic rate constant k_2 (also called k_{cat}) is much smaller than k_{-1}.

The meaning of K_m becomes clear when we remodel Equation 24 to yield

25

$$\frac{[E]}{[E \cdot S]} = \frac{K_m}{[S]}$$

or

26

$$[E \cdot S] = [E] \times \frac{[S]}{K_m}$$

We see that K_m is indicated in moles per liter. We also see that *when the substrate concentration [S] equals* K_m, *the concentration of the enzyme-substrate complex E·S equals that of the free enzyme E.* The sum of the latter two concentrations is that of the total enzyme molecules in the system (E_T):

27

$$[E] + [E \cdot S] = [E_T]$$

or

28

$$[E] = [E_T] - [E \cdot S]$$

We saw previously, in Equation 19, that the reaction rate is proportional to the concentration of the enzyme-substrate complex. Therefore *the Michaelis constant* K_m *is not only the substrate concentration at which the enzyme is half-saturated with its substrate, but also that at which the reaction rate is half-maximal.*

To obtain the Michaelis−Menten equation, we first combine Equations 25 and 28:

29

$$\frac{[E_T] - [E \cdot S]}{[E \cdot S]} = \frac{K_m}{[S]}$$

This becomes

30

$$\frac{[E_T]}{[E \cdot S]} - 1 = \frac{K_m}{[S]}$$

and

31

$$\frac{[E_T]}{[E \cdot S]} = \frac{K_m}{[S]} + 1 = \frac{K_m}{[S]} + \frac{[S]}{[S]} = \frac{K_m + [S]}{[S]}$$

By combining Equations (19) and (20), we obtain

32

$$\frac{V_{max}}{V} = \frac{[E_T] \times k_2}{[E \cdot S] \times k_2} = \frac{[E_T]}{[E \cdot S]}$$

We can now combine Equations 31 and 32 to obtain the **Michaelis−Menten equation:**

33

$$\frac{V_{max}}{V} = \frac{K_m + [S]}{[S]}$$

or

34

$$V = V_{max} \times \frac{[S]}{K_m + [S]}$$

K_m and V_{max} can be determined graphically

The derivation of K_m and V_{max} is not just a joyful intellectual exercise for the student−these kinetic

FIG. 4.6

Relationship between reaction rate (V) and substrate concentration ([S]) in a typical enzymatic reaction.

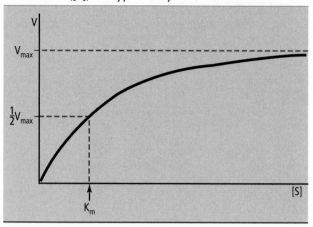

FIG. 4.7

A Lineweaver–Burk plot for a typical enzymatic reaction. It is derived from the equation $\dfrac{1}{V} = \dfrac{1}{V_{max}} + \dfrac{K_m}{V_{max}} \times \dfrac{1}{[S]}$

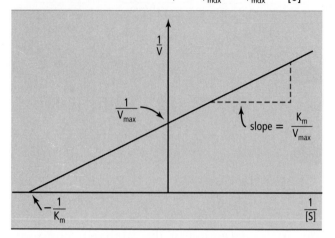

properties are useful for describing reaction rates at various substrate concentrations. The curve shown in Fig. 4.6 can easily be obtained experimentally by incubating a fixed amount of the enzyme with different substrate concentrations and measuring the reaction rates.

We see immediately that the enzymatic reaction shows **saturation kinetics:** at high substrate concentrations, the reaction rate does not increase indefinitely but approaches the maximal reaction rate V_{max}. *At substrate concentrations far higher than the Michaelis constant K_m, the reaction shows zero-order kinetics.* Almost all enzyme molecules are present as the enzyme-substrate complex, and the reaction rate is no longer limited by substrate availability, but by the amount and turnover number of the enzyme.

The Michaelis constant K_m can be determined graphically as that point on the x axis that corresponds to $1/2\ V_{max}$ on the y axis. *At substrate concentrations far below the K_m, the reaction rate is related almost linearly to the substrate concentration, and the reaction shows first-order kinetics.*

In a double-reciprocal plot, known as the **Lineweaver–Burk plot** (Fig. 4.7), the relationship between $1/V$ and $1/[S]$ describes a straight line. This line corresponds to the equation

35

$$\frac{1}{V} = \frac{1}{V_{max}} + \frac{K_m}{V_{max}} \times \frac{1}{[S]}$$

which is obtained by turning the Michaelis–Menten

equation (Equation 34) upside down. The intersection of this line with the y axis is $1/V_{max}$, and its intersection with the x axis is $-1/K_m$.

The transition from first-order to zero-order kinetics with increasing substrate concentration can be compared with the ticket sales in a bus terminal. When passengers are scarce, the number of tickets sold per minute depends directly on the number of passengers: tickets are sold according to first-order kinetics. However, during rush hour, when a line forms, the rate of ticket sales is limited not by passenger availability but by the turnover number of the ticket clerk: no matter how long the line, it progresses at a constant rate V_{max}. Tickets now are sold according to zero-order kinetics.

Substrate half-life can be determined for first-order but not for zero-order reactions

We can distinguish between first-order and zero-order kinetics when we observe the rate at which the substrate disappears or the product appears over time. In an "irreversible" reaction in which the rate of the backward reaction is so low that it can be neglected, we obtain the relationships shown in Fig. 4.8. In this graph, the reaction rate corresponds to the slope of the curve. The rate of the first-order reaction—but not of the zero-order reaction—declines over time because less and less substrate is available. *The **half-life** is the time period during which*

FIG. 4.8

The disappearance of the substrate is traced for a zero-order reaction (━━━) and a first-order reaction (━━━). The half life, $T_{\frac{1}{2}}$, is defined as that time period during which half of the substrate is converted to product in the first-order reaction.

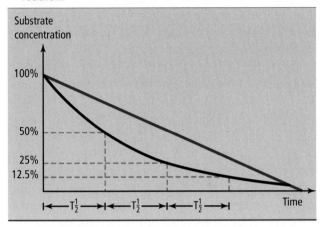

FIG. 4.9

Blood alcohol concentration after the ingestion of 120 g of ethanol. The linear decrease of the alcohol level 2 to 10 hours postingestion shows that a zero-order reaction limits the rate of alcohol metabolism.

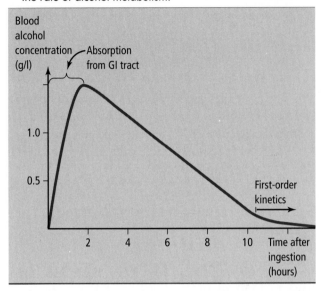

one half of the substrate is consumed. It can be determined for a first-order reaction but not for a zero-order reaction.

Drug metabolism illustrates the effect of substrate concentration. In most cases, the drug concentration in the metabolizing tissues (often the liver) is far below the K_m of the enzyme. Therefore, drug metabolism follows first-order kinetics, and a half-life can be determined — most conveniently by monitoring the blood level of the drug over time.

The metabolism of alcohol is different: its levels in blood and tissue are so high after a few drinks that the metabolizing enzyme, alcohol dehydrogenase (ADH, see the thermodynamics section in this chapter), is saturated almost completely. Therefore the reaction becomes more or less independent of the substrate concentration: no matter how drunk the subject is, only approximately 10 g of alcohol can be metabolized per hour. Therefore, the decrease of the blood alcohol level initially is not asymptotic but linear. Only at very low alcohol levels, when the enzyme is no longer saturated, do we see a transition from zero-order to first-order kinetics (Fig. 4.9).

k_{cat}/K_m predicts the ezyme activity at low substrate concentrations

V_{max} is directly proportional to the total enzyme concentration (see Equation 20), and therefore

enzyme activities are determined most conveniently at saturating substrate concentrations whenever the investigator is interested in the amount of the enzyme. This is, for example, done when serum enzymes are determined for diagnostic purposes in the clinical laboratory (see Chapter 25). Enzyme activities often are expressed as **international units (IU)**. One IU is defined as the amount of enzyme that converts 1 μmol of substrate to product per minute. The V_{max} of an enzyme depends on temperature, pH, and other factors; therefore, the incubation conditions have to be specified.

Under physiologic conditions, most enzymes are not saturated with their substrate. Therefore the catalytic rate constant k_{cat} (k_2) and the enzyme concentration (see Equation 20) are not sufficient to predict the actual reaction rate. At very low substrate concentrations, the k_{cat}/K_m ratio is the best predictor of the actual reaction rate. We can see this when we combine Equations 19 and 26:

36

$$V = \frac{k_2}{K_m} \times [E] \times [S]$$

At substrate concentrations far below K_m, almost all the enzyme molecules are present as free enzyme rather than enzyme-substrate complex, and

$$[E] \approx [E_T]$$

Therefore (k_2 is k_{cat}), and Equation 36 yields

37

$$V \approx \frac{k_{cat}}{K_m} \times [E_T] \times [S]$$

We see now that *under conditions of very low substrate concentration, the reaction rate is directly proportional to the enzyme concentration* $[E_T]$, *substrate concentration* $[S]$, *and* k_{cat}/K_m. The reaction is first order because of the linear relationship between V and $[S]$.

Each substrate has its own Michaelis constant

In most two-substrate reactions, both substrates have to bind to the active site of the enzyme to form a ternary complex. In other cases, the reaction proceeds by a **ping-pong mechanism:**

$$E + S_1 \longrightarrow E \cdot S_1 \longrightarrow E^* + P_1$$
$$E^* + S_2 \longrightarrow E^* \cdot S_2 \longrightarrow E + P_2$$

In this case, the enzyme itself becomes modified chemically in a first reaction during which the first substrate is converted to product. In the second reaction, the enzyme is regenerated to its original state. A typical example of this mechanism will be encountered in the transamination reactions (see Chapter 21), in which an amino group from the first substrate becomes covalently bound to the prosthetic group of the enzyme from which it is transferred to the second substrate.

Irrespective of the reaction mechanism, *separate* K_m *values can be determined for the two substrates of the reaction.* This can be done experimentally by using a saturating concentration of one substrate while varying that of the other.

Allosteric enzymes do not obey Michaelis-Menten kinetics

Not all enzymes show simple Michaelis–Menten kinetics. Allosteric enzymes, in particular, yield aberrant shapes of the $V/[S]$ graph in Fig. 4.6. Figure 4.10 shows a sigmoidal relationship reminiscent of the oxygen-binding curve of hemoglobin (Fig. 3.5). This suggests an allosteric enzyme with more than one active site and positive cooperativity between the active sites. This curve would not yield a straight line in the Lineweaver–Burk plot. *Allosteric effectors increase or decrease the activity of the enzyme by binding to regulatory sites distant from the substrate-binding site.*

Allosteric enzymes often are found in strategic locations in metabolic pathways, where their activities are regulated physiologically by positive or negative effectors. Typical allosteric effectors of metabolic enzymes include metabolites such as citrate and coenzymes such as ADP and ATP. The second messengers of hormones also regulate intracellular enzymes by allosteric actions. In most allosteric enzymes, the binding of a positive or negative allosteric effector increases or decreases the affinity of the enzyme for its substrate. Less commonly, the V_{max} is changed with little or no change in the substrate affinity.

Some enzymes also are regulated by covalent modifications, most commonly by the *phosphorylation and dephosphorylation of serine, threonine, and, occasionally, tyrosine side chains.* These enzymes are actually allosteric enzymes in which the equilibrium between the more-active and the less-active conformation is affected not only by reversibly binding allosteric effectors but also by phosphorylation/dephosphorylation (Fig. 17.16 in Chapter 17, for example).

FIG. 4.10

Plot of velocity (V) against substrate concentration ($[S]$) for an allosteric enzyme with positive cooperativity. *A*, Enzyme alone; *B*, enzyme + positive allosteric effector; *C*, enzyme + negative allosteric effector.

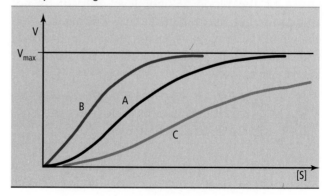

Enzyme activity depends on temperature and pH

The rate of chemical reactions increases with increased temperature. The magnitude of this increase depends on the free energy of activation ΔG_{act}: the greater ΔG_{act} is, the greater the temperature dependence. The **Q_{10} value** is the factor by which the reaction is accelerated when the temperature is increased by 10°C. Uncatalyzed reactions usually have Q_{10} values between 2 and 5. In enzymatic reactions, which have a rather low ΔG_{act}, Q_{10} values between 1.7 and 2.5 are most common. At very high temperatures, however, typically somewhere between 50°C and 70°C, enzymes become irreversibly denatured. Therefore, under ordinary assay conditions *an optimum curve is observed* that declines steeply at high temperatures (Fig. 4.11).

The temperature dependence of enzymatic reactions is at least partially responsible for the increased metabolic rate during fever. Presumably, it also is responsible for the fact that we cannot tolerate body temperatures greater than 42°C. The most sensitive enzymes already may denature at temperatures greater than this. Protein denaturation is a time-dependent process, and an enzyme that survives a temperature of 45°C for some minutes may well denature gradually in the course of several hours.

Hypothermia is tolerated far better than hyperthermia, and most individual cells can survive temperatures as cold as 0°C. In peripheral parts of the body, the temperature can decrease to close to 0°C

on a cold winter day. This blocks nerve conduction and muscular activity, but it does not cause irreversible damage unless the tissue water freezes. *The metabolic rate is, of course, depressed at low temperatures,* and therefore a slowdown in the vital functions of the brain and myocardium limits our tolerance to hypothermia. Also, a vicious cycle develops when decreased enzymatic activity limits heat production during hypothermia, thereby decreasing the body temperature even more.

Hypothermia can improve the ability of tissues to tolerate hypoxia because it decreases oxygen consumption. This effect can be exploited during open-heart surgery when the blood flow has to be interrupted for brief time periods. Also, organs used for transplantation keep best in the cold.

Enzymatic reactions also depend on the pH value, but the pH-dependence is quite different for different enzymes (Fig. 4.12). The reason for this pH-dependence is that *enzymatic catalysis requires ionizable groups in the active site of the enzyme* whose protonation state depends on the pH (see the last section of this chapter). Substrate binding is sometimes mediated by electrostatic interactions, which depend on the correct protonation state of groups both on the substrate and on the enzyme. In addition, extreme pH values always are likely to denature the enzyme.

The pH values of tissues and body fluids are tightly regulated. Deviations of more than 0.5 pH unit from the normal blood pH of 7.4 are rapidly fatal. Furthermore, the intracellular compartments have tightly regulated pH values that ensure the proper activity levels of their enzymes. The cytoplasm of

FIG. 4.11

Temperature dependence of a typical enzymatic reaction.

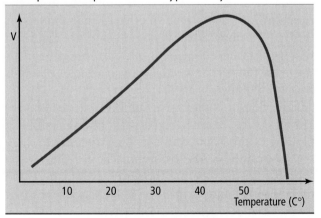

FIG. 4.12

pH dependence of some enzymes.

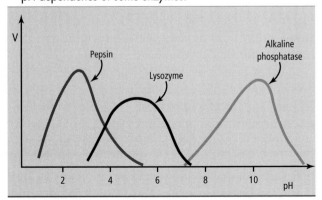

BOX 4.1

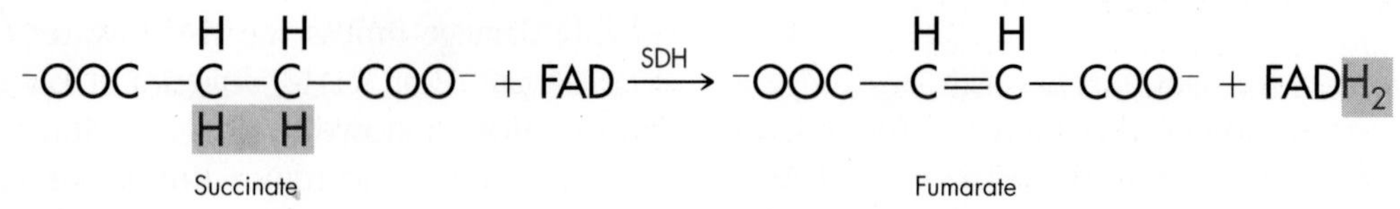

$$^-OOC - \underset{\underset{H}{|}}{\overset{\overset{H}{|}}{C}} - \underset{\underset{H}{|}}{\overset{\overset{H}{|}}{C}} - COO^- + FAD \xrightarrow{\text{SDH}} \; ^-OOC - \underset{}{\overset{\overset{H}{|}}{C}} = \underset{}{\overset{\overset{H}{|}}{C}} - COO^- + FADH_2$$

Succinate   Fumarate

most cells has a pH value of 6.5 to 7.0. The mitochondrial matrix has a pH value of 7.5 to 8.0, and the lysosomes are mildly acidic, with pH values between 4.5 and 5.5. Lysosomal enzymes generally have pH optima in the acidic range.

Different types of reversible enzyme inhibition can be distinguished kinetically

We already have encountered the principle of **competitive inhibition** as the mechanism of carbon monoxide poisoning (see Chapter 3): CO impairs oxygen binding to hemoglobin because it competes for the same binding site. Likewise, *a competitive enzyme inhibitor impairs substrate binding because it binds to the active site of the enzyme itself.* Competitive inhibitors are related structurally to the normal substrate of the enzyme. A classic example is the inhibition of succinate dehydrogenase (SDH) by malonate. This mitochondrial enzyme catalyzes the reaction shown in Box 4.1. The reaction is competitively inhibited by malonate:

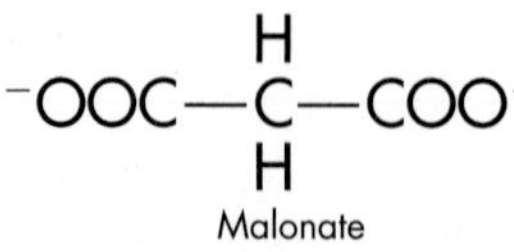

$$^-OOC - \underset{\underset{H}{|}}{\overset{\overset{H}{|}}{C}} - COO^-$$

Malonate

Malonate binds to the enzyme by the same electrostatic interactions as the normal substrate succinate, but it cannot be converted to a product.

In other cases, the inhibitor can be converted to a product: *two alternative substrates can compete for the same enzyme.* A clinically important example is encountered in methanol poisoning (Fig. 4.13). Methanol sometimes is swallowed accidentally by people who read "methyl alcohol" on a label and think it is the real stuff. Methanol, however, can be fatal because it is converted to formaldehyde and formic acid,

FIG. 4.13

Role of alcohol dehydrogenase (ADH) in the metabolism of methanol and ethanol. The two substrates compete for the enzyme. Therefore, ethanol inhibits the formation of toxic formaldehyde and formic acid from methanol.

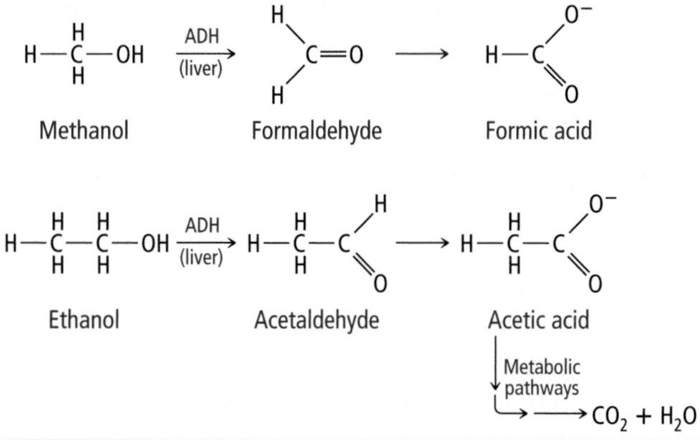

toxic metabolites that can accumulate to high concentrations.

The first enzyme of methanol metabolism, alcohol dehydrogenase (ADH), metabolizes ethanol as well. Fortunately, the ethanol metabolites are less toxic than the methanol metabolites and do not accumulate because they are metabolized quickly to carbon dioxide and water. When ethanol is administered to a patient with methanol poisoning, the formation of the toxic methanol metabolites is delayed because ethanol competes with methanol for the enzyme: the patient is drunk, but alive. This is one of the very few situations in which ethanol is a useful therapeutic agent.

How does a competitive inhibitor affect enzyme kinetics? $V_{\max}$ *remains unchanged* because inhibitor binding is reversible and can be overcome by high concentrations of the substrate. The binding of the substrate to the enzyme, however, is impaired, and the apparent binding affinity is decreased. *This effect is reflected in an increased* K_m (Fig. 4.14).

FIG. 4.14

The effects of inhibitors on enzymatic reactions. *A,* Uninhibited enzyme: *B,* enzyme + competitive inhibitor; *C,* enzyme + noncompetitive inhibitor; *D,* enzyme + uncompetitive inhibitor. For noncompetitive inhibition, it is assumed that the inhibitor binds equally well to the free enzyme and the enzyme-substrate complex (see text). The kinetic effects of irreversible inhibitors resemble those shown here for the noncom-petitive inhibitor. *A,* Reaction rate (*V*) plotted against substrate concentration ([S]). *B,* In the Lineweaver–Burk plot, the effects of inhibitors on V_{max} and K_m are reflected in changes of the intercepts with the y and x axis, respectively.

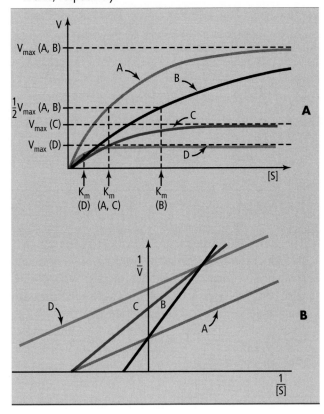

than it does to the enzyme-substrate complex, or vice versa.

In **uncompetitive inhibition,** the inhibitor binds only to the enzyme-substrate complex, not to the free enzyme, a behavior opposite to that of a competitive inhibitor. This rather unusual type of inhibition *reduces both K_m and V_{max}.* In contrast to competitive inhibitors, which are most effective at low substrate concentrations, *uncompetitive inhibitors work best when the substrate concentration is high.*

Product inhibition by high concentrations of the reaction product is, in most cases, competitive: the formation of the enzyme-product complex competes with the formation of the enzyme-substrate complex. *Product inhibition is very common in metabolic reactions, where it often is important as a physiologic mechanism of feedback inhibition.*

Covalent modification can inhibit enzymes irreversibly

Competitive, noncompetitive, and uncompetitive inhibitors bind noncovalently to the enzyme. Therefore, their actions are reversible, and enzyme activity is restored fully once the inhibitor is removed. In vitro, reversible inhibitors can be removed by extensive dialysis (see Chapter 2), and in the body, they are subject to metabolic inactivation or renal excretion. In **irreversible inhibition,** however, *the inhibitor forms a covalent bond with the enzyme.* This type of inhibition cannot be relieved by simple removal of the inhibitor, but only by the synthesis of new enzyme.

The principle of irreversible inhibition is illustrated best by the **organophosphorus compounds** (Fig. 4.15). These toxins are used extensively as insecticides, and some have been developed as "nerve gases" for chemical warfare. They are neurotoxic, both in humans and in insects, because they react with acetylcholinesterase, the enzyme that degrades acetylcholine at cholinergic synapses (see Chapter 26). The active site of acetylcholinesterase contains a serine residue that forms a transient covalent bond with the substrate during catalysis. *The organophosphates react covalently and irreversibly with this serine residue.* Without its essential serine hydroxy group, the enzyme is dead. Acetylcholine accumulates and causes fatal derangements in both the central and peripheral nervous systems.

Some inhibitors reduce enzyme activity by binding to the enzyme protein at a site distant from the substrate-binding site. Inhibitors of this type are unrelated structurally to the substrate. In classical **noncompetitive inhibition,** the binding of the inhibitor does not prevent substrate binding. The catalytic activity, however, either is reduced or lost completely in the presence of the bound inhibitor. *If the noncompetitive inhibitor binds equally well to the free enzyme and the enzyme-substrate complex, it reduces V_{max} without affecting K_m* (Fig. 4.14). However, different kinetic effects are observed if the noncompetitive inhibitor binds more tightly to the free enzyme

FIG. 4.15

Mechanism of action of the "nerve gas" sarin, a typical organophosphorus compound. The lethal dose (LD_{50}) of sarin in humans is approximately 0.01 mg/kg.

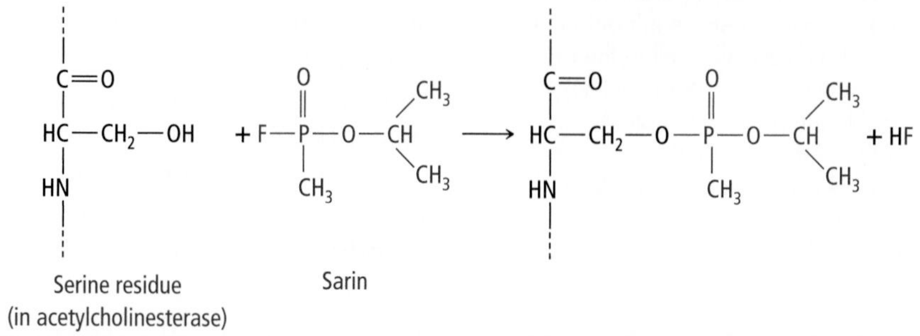

Serine residue
(in acetylcholinesterase)   Sarin

BOX 4.2

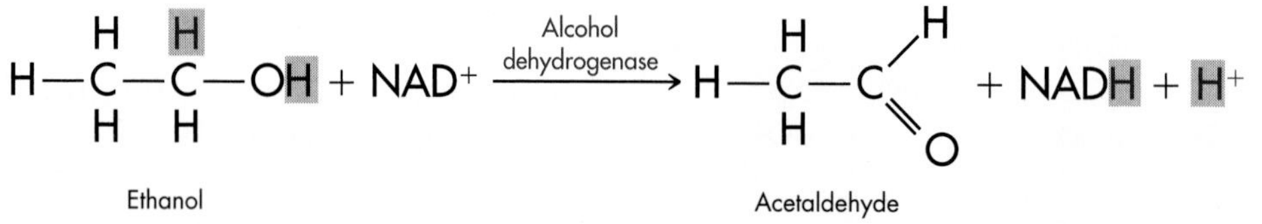

Ethanol   Acetaldehyde

REACTION TYPES AND REACTION MECHANISMS

Enzymes are highly selective for both their substrate and their reaction type. These selectivities depend on interactions between enzyme and substrate that are established both during the formation of the enzyme-substrate complex and later in the course of the reaction. To increase the reaction rate, in particular, we need multiple interactions between enzyme and substrate that facilitate the formation of the transition state and lower the free energy of activation.

Enzymes are classified according to their reaction type

Enzymes are grouped into six classes on the basis of their reaction type:

1. **Oxidoreductases** catalyze oxidation-reduction reactions. These include *electron transfers, hydrogen transfers, and reactions in which molecular oxygen participates.*

The **dehydrogenases** are the most common oxidoreductases. *They transfer hydrogen between a substrate and a coenzyme,* most commonly NAD, NADP, FAD, or FMN (see Chapter 5). These enzymes are named according to the substrate from which the hydrogen is removed. See Box 4.2 for an example.

Oxygenases use molecular oxygen as a substrate. The **dioxygenases** use both oxygen atoms of O_2 to oxidize their substrate; the **monooxygenases** use one oxygen atom to oxidize their substrate and the other one to oxidize a reduced coenzyme. Most **hydroxylases** are monooxygenases:

$$\text{Substrate—H} + O_2 + \text{NADPH} + H^+ \longrightarrow$$
$$\text{Substrate—OH} + \text{NADP}^+ + H_2O$$

Peroxidases use hydrogen peroxide or an organic peroxide as one of their substrates. Technically, **catalase** is a peroxidase. It degrades hydrogen peroxide to molecular oxygen and water:

$$H_2O_2 \longrightarrow H_2O + \tfrac{1}{2}O_2$$

BOX 4.3

$$\underset{\text{Glycerol}}{\underset{\displaystyle \begin{array}{c} H_2C\!-\!OH \\ | \\ HO\!-\!CH \\ | \\ H_2C\!-\!OH \end{array}}{}} + ATP \xrightarrow{\text{Glycerol}\atop\text{kinase}} \underset{\substack{\text{Glycerol} \\ \text{3-phosphate}}}{\begin{array}{c} H_2C\!-\!OH \\ | \\ HO\!-\!CH \\ | \\ H_2C\!-\!O\!-\!\overset{\displaystyle O^-}{\underset{\displaystyle O}{P}}\!-\!O^- \end{array}} + ADP$$

BOX 4.4

$$R_1\!-\!\overset{\displaystyle H}{\underset{\displaystyle H}{C}}\!-\!\underset{\displaystyle OH}{CH}\!-\!R_2 \rightleftharpoons R_1\!-\!CH\!=\!CH\!-\!R_2 + H_2O$$

2. **Transferases** *transfer a group from one molecule to another.* The **kinases**, which transfer phosphate from ATP or some other nucleoside triphosphate to a second substrate, are typical examples. These enzymes are named according to the substrate to which the phosphate is transferred. See Box 4.3 for an example.

   Other examples of transferases include the **phosphorylases**, which cleave bonds by the addition of inorganic phosphate; the **glycosyl transferases**, which transfer an "activated" monosaccharide to an acceptor molecule; the **transaminases**, which transfer amino groups; and the **peptidyl transferase** of the ribosome (Chapter 6).

3. **Hydrolases** *cleave bonds by the addition of water.* They are grouped according to their substrates, such as peptidases, esterases, lipases, phospholipases, glycosidases, or phosphatases. The digestive enzymes (Chapter 14) and the lysosomal enzymes are hydrolases.

   The cleavage specificities of those hydrolytic enzymes that act on polymeric substrates are indicated by the prefixes endo- (Greek, "inside") and exo- ("outside"). An endoglycosidase, for example, cleaves a polysaccharide anywhere, even at sites far removed from the ends. Conversely, an exoglycosidase cleaves only the glycosidic bond next to the end, releasing a monosaccharide. Similarly, we distinguish between endo- and exopeptidases and endo- and exonucleases. These enzymes cleave peptide bonds in polypeptides and phosphodiester bonds in nucleic acids, respectively.

4. **Lyases** *remove a group nonhydrolytically,* forming a double bond. Examples are the **dehydratases** as shown in Box 4.4 and **decarboxylases**:

$$R\!-\!\overset{\displaystyle O}{\underset{\displaystyle OH}{C}} \longrightarrow R\!-\!H + O\!=\!C\!=\!O$$

   Many lyase reactions proceed in the opposite direction, creating a new bond and obliterating a double bond in one of the substrates. These enzymes often are called **synthases.**

5. **Isomerases** *catalyze the interconversion of positional, geometric, or optical isomers.* See Box 4.5.

6. **Ligases** *couple the hydrolysis of a phosphoanhydride bond in ATP or some other energy-rich compound to the for-*

mation of a bond. These enzymes often are called **synthetases.** Glutamine synthetase is an example as shown in Box 4.6. **DNA ligase** and the **aminoacyl-tRNA synthetases** (Chapter 6) are further examples. The biotin-dependent carboxylases (Chapter 16) also are classified as ligases.

Four mechanisms account for enzymatic catalysis

We can distinguish four general mechanisms that are encountered frequently in the "black box" of enzymatic catalysis:

1. The **entropy effect,** also known as "proximity effect," is based on the *approximation of substrates in a two-substrate reaction.* In the absence of the enzyme, a reaction takes place only when two substrate molecules collide with sufficient kinetic energy to reach the transition state. Not only is sufficient kinetic energy required, but the collision has to occur in exactly the right geometric orientation—certainly a rare event in a dilute solution and at a low temperature, conditions in which most molecules do not have enough kinetic energy anyway. The enzyme, however, binds the substrates to its active site in the correct geometric orientation, thereby increasing the frequency of productive collisions.
2. **Steric stabilization of the transition state** is important when the conformation of the transition state differs from that of the substrate. The reaction is facilitated when *the binding interactions with the enzyme are energetically more favorable in the conformation of the transition state than in that of the substrate.* This decreases the free energy content of the transition state to a greater extent than that

BOX 4.5

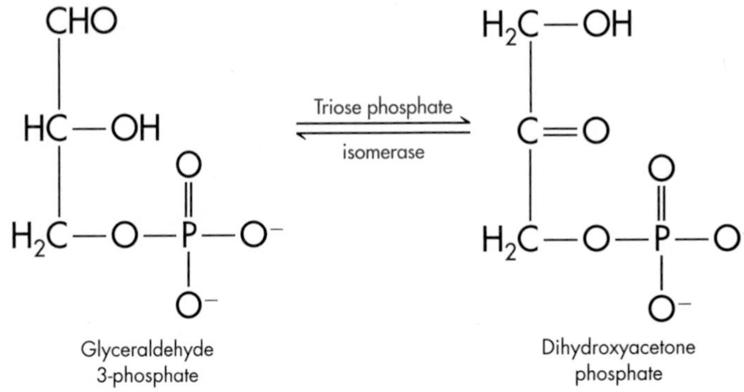
CHO
HC—OH
H2C—O—P—O⁻
Triose phosphate
isomerase
H2C—OH
C=O
Glyceraldehyde
3-phosphate
Dihydroxyacetone
phosphate

BOX 4.6

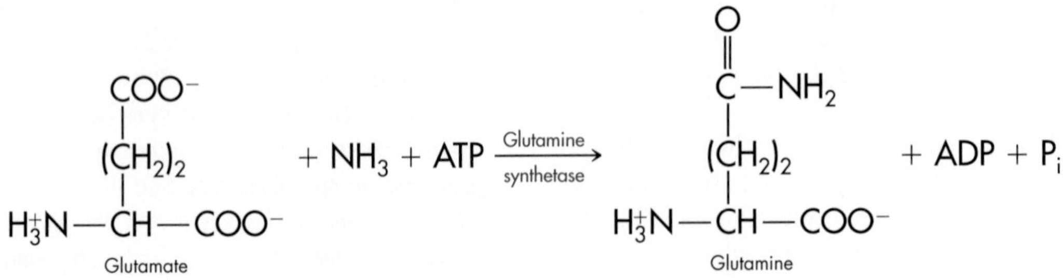
COO⁻
(CH2)2
H3N—CH—COO⁻
+ NH3 + ATP
Glutamine
synthetase
C—NH2
+ ADP + Pi
Glutamate
Glutamine

of the substrate, and ΔG_{act} is reduced. This effect is sometimes called as "substrate strain" because the enzyme effectively bends the substrate into the shape of the transition state.

3. **General acid-base catalysis** occurs in almost all enzymatic reactions. In most cases, it is effected by *ionizable groups on the enzyme that act as proton donors or proton acceptors.* In other cases, electron pair donors or acceptors, known respectively as Lewis bases and Lewis acids, participate in the reaction.

Whereas protons that are donated or abstracted by the enzyme during the formation of the transition state participate directly in the reaction, electrostatic interactions and ion-pair interactions between the transition state and the enzyme stabilize the transition state and decrease its free energy content. We realize at this point that *any favorable noncovalent interaction between the enzyme and the transition state of the reaction decreases the free energy of activation and increases the reaction rate.*

General acid−base catalysis is the most important reason for the pH-dependence of enzymatic reactions. The ionizable groups that participate in this type of catalysis have to be in the correct protonation state. If, for example, the reaction requires a deprotonated glutamate side chain with a pK of 4.0 as a general base and a protonated histidine side chain with a pK of 6.0 as a general acid, only pH values between 4.0 and 6.0 will allow high reaction rates.

4. **Covalent catalysis** is based on the formation of a *transient covalent bond between enzyme and substrate during catalysis.* Covalent catalysis, for example, is used by the serine proteases, which bind part of their substrate covalently to a serine side chain.

Lysozyme uses a combination of substrate strain and general acid-base catalysis

Lysozyme is an endoglycosidase, and its substrate is **peptidoglycan,** a bacterial cell wall polysaccharide with an alternating sequence of *N*-acetylglucosamine and *N*-acetylmuramic acid. These polysaccharide chains are cross-linked covalently by short oligopeptides (Fig. 4.16). Peptidoglycan is responsible for the mechanical strength of bacterial cell walls, and in its absence, the cell is destroyed by osmotic forces.

Lysozyme is present in tears, saliva, and other external body secretions in humans and also in the lysosomes of phagocytic cells. In secretions, it stands in the first line of defense against potentially pathogenic bacteria, and in phagocytic cells, it participates in the intracellular digestion of bacteria. Many other natural sources also contain lysozyme,

FIG. 4.16

Structure of peptidoglycan, the substrate of lysozyme. NAG, *N*-acetylglucosamine; NAM, *N*-acetylmuramic acid.

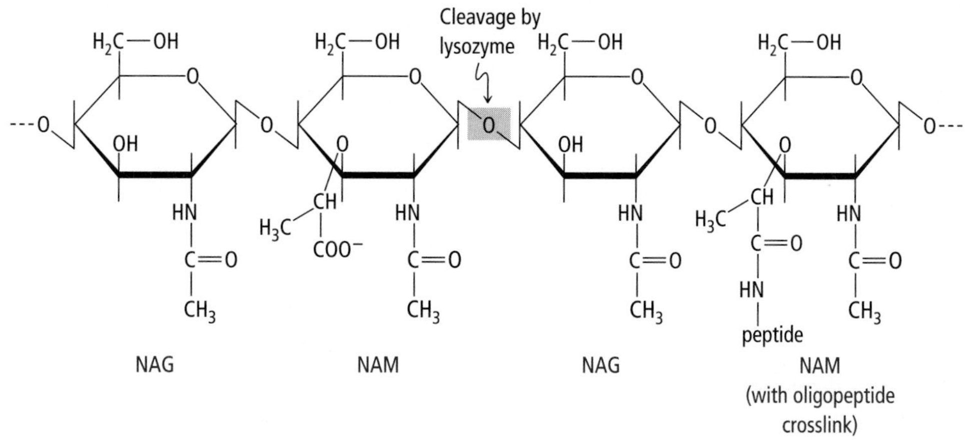

and the enzyme from egg white has been used extensively for biochemical studies.

Lysozyme is a humble creature, with a single polypeptide chain of 129 amino acids and no prosthetic group. Like myoglobin (see Chapter 3), it has a compact tertiary structure that is maintained mostly by hydrophobic interactions in the center of the molecule. There is little α-helical structure and some β-pleated sheet, but most of the polypeptide is devoid of secondary structure. The substrate-binding site is formed by a cleft in the surface of the enzyme. *Not less than six sugar residues of the substrate bind in this cleft by hydrogen bonds and van der Waals interactions.*

The monosaccharide rings of the substrate can assume alternative conformations, of which the chair conformation is energetically the most favorable (Fig. 4.17, A). During the formation of the enzyme-substrate complex, five of the six binding monosaccharide residues can form their interactions with the enzyme in their preferred chair conformation. *One of them, however, binds only in the less-favored half-chair conformation.* It is the glycosidic bond formed by C-1 of this distorted sugar residue that is

---

FIG. 4.17

The lysozyme reaction. **A**, During the formation of the enzyme-substrate complex, one of the monosaccharides in the substrate is distorted from its normal chair conformation into the energetically less-preferred half-chair conformation. **B**, A highly reactive carbocation is an intermediate in the lysozyme reaction. Note that the half-chair conformation is the preferred conformation of the carbocation. Also, the carbocation is stabilized by a salt bond with a deprotonated aspartate side chain.

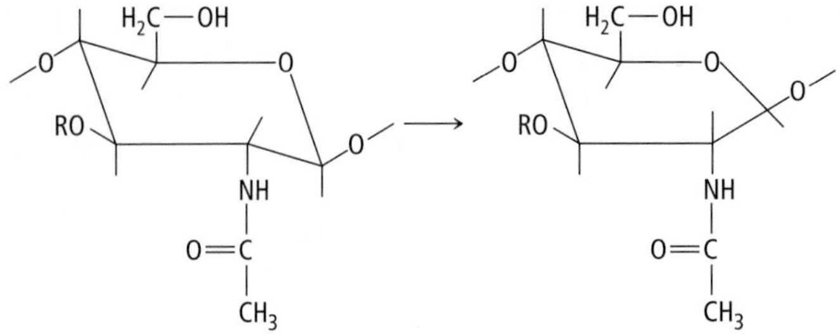

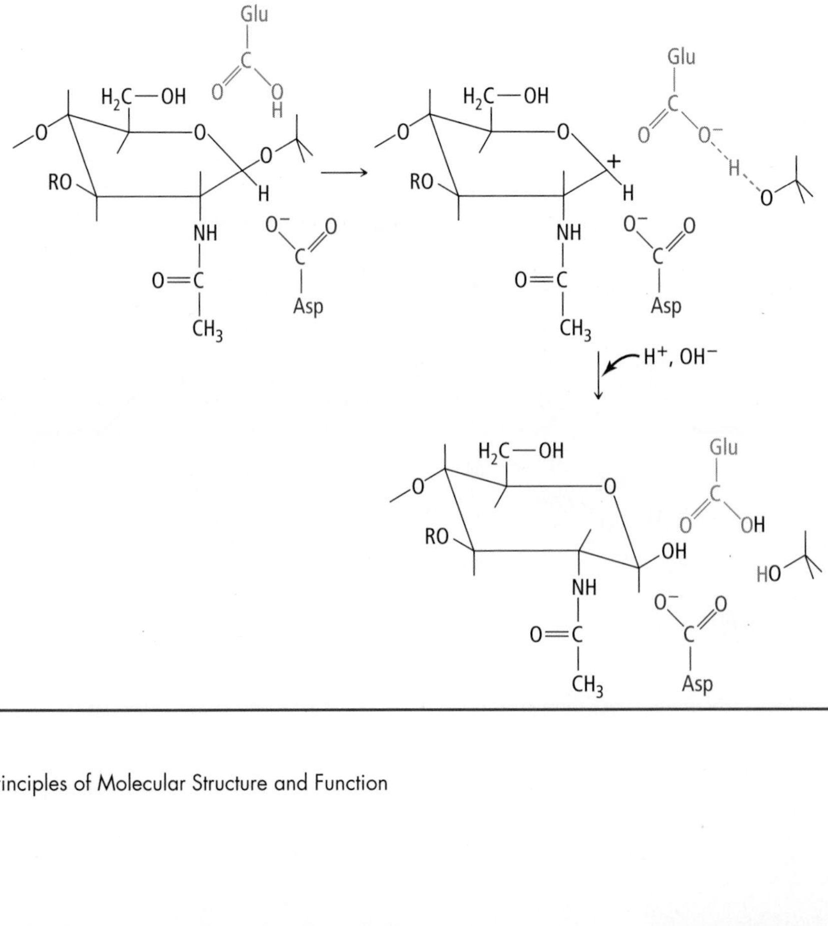

cleaved by lysozyme. In the enzyme-substrate complex, a glutamate and an aspartate side chain are positioned on opposite sides of this bond. The aspartate side chain is deprotonated at pH values greater than 4, and the glutamate side chain, which is in a nonpolar environment, has an unusually high pK value of approximately 6.

During the reaction (Fig. 4.17, *B*), *the protonated glutamate side chain donates its proton to the glycosidic bond.* The bond is cleaved, and an unstable carbocation forms at C-1 of the sugar. This is the transition state of the reaction. Unlike the original monosaccharide residue, the carbocation prefers the half-chair conformation, which already is present in the enzyme-substrate complex. We see how the geometry of enzyme-substrate binding favors the transition state over the substrate. In addition, *the transition state is stabilized by a salt bond with the aspartate side chain.* Despite these favorable interactions with the enzyme, however, the carbocation is extremely short-lived and reacts almost immediately with a hydroxyl ion or a water molecule.

The lysozyme reaction demonstrates the use of *substrate strain* and *general acid-base catalysis* in an enzymatic reaction. Predictably, the pH optimum of the reaction is between 4 and 6, the approximate pK values of the catalytically important aspartate and glutamate side chains.

Chymotrypsin forms a transient covalent bond during catalysis

Peptide bonds can be cleaved by four different mechanisms:

1. **Carboxyl proteases** (not to be confused with the "carboxypeptidases," see Chapter 14), which include pepsin and some lysosomal enzymes, have two acidic amino acid side chains in their active sites. One of these has to be protonated and the other one deprotonated during catalysis. The pH optima of these enzymes are in the acidic range.
2. **Metalloproteases** contain a metal ion in the active site that participates in catalysis. The best-known examples are the zinc-containing pancreatic carboxypeptidases (see Chapter 14).
3. **Serine proteases** are the largest group. They include the pancreatic enzymes trypsin, chymotrypsin, and elastase (see Chapter 14), as well

as thrombin and the other proteases of the blood clotting system (Chapter 25). They contain a serine residue that forms a covalent bond during catalysis.
4. **Thiol proteases** have a catalytic mechanism similar to the serine proteases, but it is a cysteine sulfhydryl group rather than a serine hydroxy group that reacts with the substrate.

The pancreatic serine protease **chymotrypsin** consists of three disulfide-bonded polypeptides with a total of 241 amino acids (see Chapter 14). Like most enzymes, it is a tightly packed globular protein. There is very little α-helix, but considerable portions are arranged in antiparallel β-pleated sheet structures.

Like lysozyme, chymotrypsin contains no prosthetic group. *The most important amino acid residue in the active site is a serine residue, Ser-195.* The susceptible ("scissile") bond of the substrate is placed on the hydroxy group of this serine residue during the formation of the enzyme-substrate complex. The substrate binds to the active site by hydrogen bonds between peptide bonds in the substrate and the enzyme. Indeed, a stretch of the substrate binds to the active site in the conformation of an antiparallel β-pleated sheet. A more specific interaction is formed by the side chain of the amino acid whose carboxy group contributes to the scissile bond: this side chain fits into a hydrophobic pocket of the enzyme. For this reason, *chymotrypsin prefers peptide bonds that are formed by the carboxy group of large hydrophobic amino acids.*

The catalytic mechanism outlined in Fig. 4.18 requires a deprotonated histidine residue, His-57, and a deprotonated aspartate residue, Asp-102, besides Ser-195. These three amino acids, which are separated extensively in the primary structure, are hydrogen bonded to each other in the active site, forming a "catalytic triad."

Catalysis by chymotrypsin is actually a sequence of two reactions. In the first reaction, the peptide bond in the substrate is cleaved and one of the fragments is bound covalently to the serine side chain to form an **acyl-enzyme intermediate.** In the second reaction, this acyl-enzyme intermediate is cleaved hydrolytically. In both reactions, a negatively charged **tetrahedral intermediate** is encountered as a transition state. These tetrahedral intermediates are stabilized by hydrogen bonds with two N—H

FIG. 4.18

Catalytic mechanism of chymotrypsin, a typical serine protease.

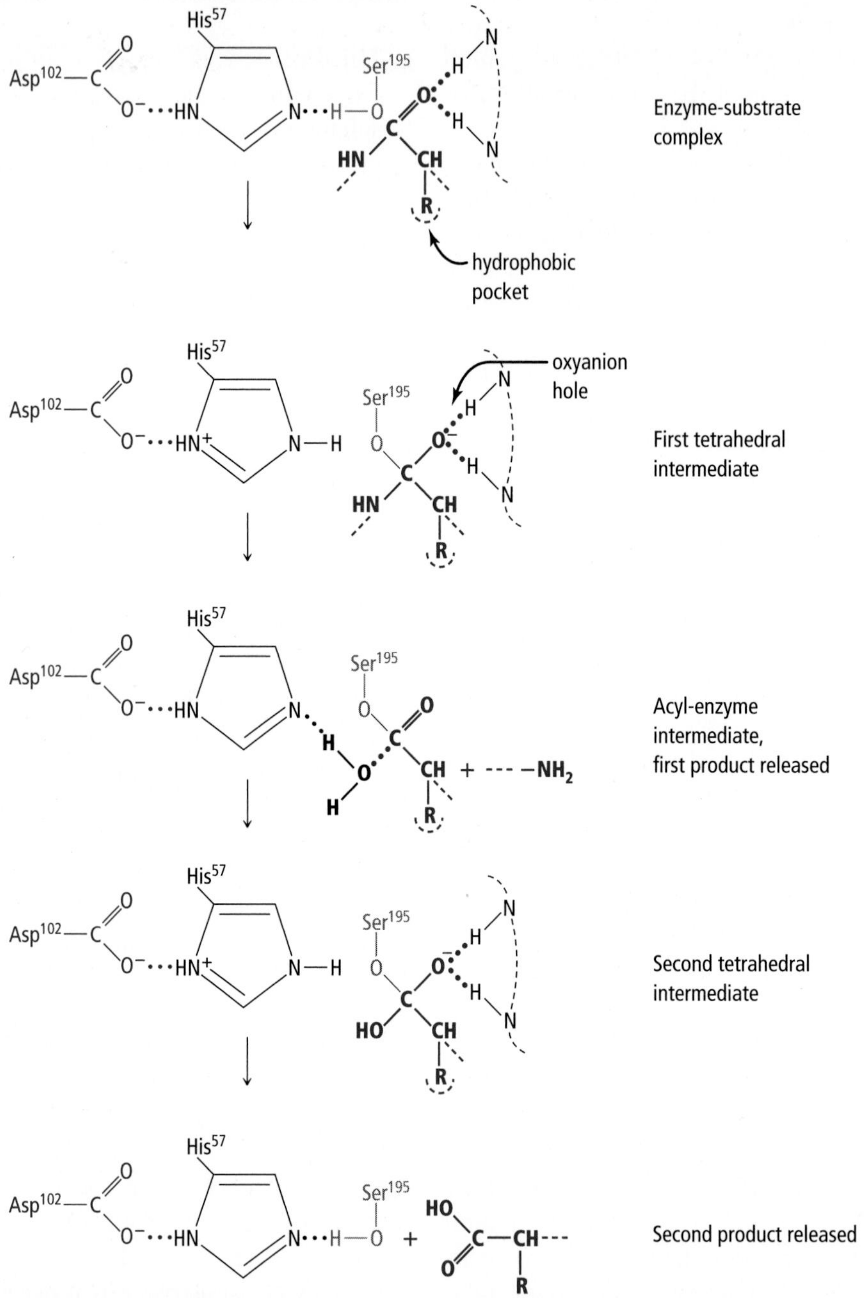

Enzyme-substrate complex

hydrophobic pocket

First tetrahedral intermediate

oxyanion hole

Acyl-enzyme intermediate, first product released

Second tetrahedral intermediate

Second product released

groups in the main chain of the enzyme, which form an "oxyanion hole." This stabilization of the transition state by favorable interactions in the oxyanion hole is reminiscent of lysozyme, in which an unstable carbocation is stabilized by a salt bond with an aspartate side chain (Fig. 4.17, B).

The histidine side chain is required for the forma-tion of the transition state as well: to form the neg-atively charged tetrahedral intermediate, *a proton has to be transferred from the hydroxy group of Ser-195 to His-57.* Asp-102 remains negatively charged throughout the catalytic cycle. Its negative charge increases the proton affinity of His-57 by an electrostatic interac-tion with its protonated form.

FIG. 4.19

Energy profile for the reaction of a serine protease.

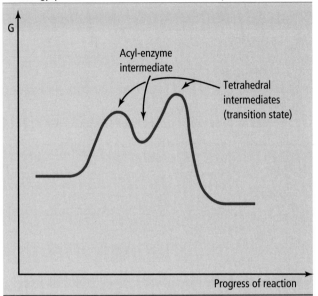

The covalent acyl-enzyme intermediate does not qualify as a transition state. Unlike a transition state, it does not occupy a peak but rather a valley in the energy profile of the reaction (Fig. 4.19).

All known mammalian serine proteases are structurally homologous to varying extents. Like the hemoglobin and myoglobin chains (see Chapter 3), the serine proteases form a "family" whose members are related through a common evolutionary ancestry. They all possess the same "catalytic triad," and a number of amino acid residues around Ser-195 and His-57 are invariant. The substrate-binding sites, however, are different. Trypsin, for example, contains an aspartate residue in its substrate-binding pocket, which forms a salt bond with positively charged amino acid side chains. Therefore, trypsin does not cleave the peptide bonds of hydrophobic amino acids, but those on the carboxy side of lysine and arginine.

SUMMARY

All chemical reactions proceed to an equilibrium state that can be described by the equilibrium constant. The position of the equilibrium, in turn, depends on the relative free energy contents of the substrates and products. Therefore, the equilibrium can be predicted from the standard free energy change of the reaction. Enzymes cannot affect the free energy change or the equilibrium of the reaction; they only can increase the reaction rate.

Enzymatic catalysis requires the initial noncovalent binding of the substrate to the active site of the enzyme to form an enzyme-substrate complex. The reaction itself is catalyzed by interactions between functional groups in the active site and the substrate. All chemical reactions, both catalyzed and uncatalyzed, have to proceed through a transition state, and interactions between substrate and enzyme facilitate the formation of the transition state and decrease its free energy content. The enzymatic reaction is accelerated relative to the uncatalyzed reaction because of the greater ease with which the transition state is reached.

Enzymes show saturation kinetics: at very low substrate concentrations, the reaction rate increases almost linearly with increasing substrate concentration and the reaction shows first-order kinetics. At very high substrate concentrations, the reaction rate cannot be increased by further increases of the substrate concentration, and the reaction shows zero-order kinetics. At high substrate concentrations, most of the enzyme molecules are present in the form of the enzyme-substrate complex.

The specific enzyme activity can be expressed as the turnover number. This is the number of substrate molecules that an enzyme molecule converts to product per second. The Michaelis constant K_m, however, is related to the affinity between enzyme and substrate. It is expressed in moles per liter and corresponds to the substrate concentration at which one half of the enzyme molecules are present in the form of the enzyme-substrate complex and the reaction rate is half-maximal.

The rate of enzymatic reactions increases with increasing temperature, typically with a doubling of the reaction rate for a temperature increase of about 10°C. Enzymatic reactions also depend on the pH, because most enzymes use ionizable groups for catalysis, and these groups have to be in the proper ionization state. Enzymes also can be inhibited specifically, and various types of enzyme inhibition can be distinguished according to the mode of interaction between enzyme and inhibitor and the kinetic consequences of this interaction.

QUESTIONS

1. During a drug screening program, you find that one of your agents decreases the activity of the enzyme monoamine oxidase. A fixed dose of the chemical reduces the catalytic activity of the enzyme at all substrate concentrations, with a decrease in V_{max}. The K_m is unaffected. This inhibitor is
    A. Definitely a competitive inhibitor
    B. Definitely a noncompetitive inhibitor
    C. Definitely an irreversible inhibitor
    D. Either a competitive or an irreversible inhibitor
    E. Either a noncompetitive or an irreversible inhibitor

2. The irreversible enzymatic reaction

Oxaloacetate + Acetyl-CoA $\longrightarrow$
$$\text{Citrate} + \text{CoA—SH}$$

is inhibited by high concentrations of its own product citrate. This product inhibition can be overcome, and a normal V_{max} can be restored, when the oxaloacetate concentration is raised, but not when the acetyl-CoA concentration is raised. This observation suggests that citrate is
    A. An irreversible inhibitor reacting with the oxaloacetate-binding site of the enzyme
    B. A competitive inhibitor binding to the acetyl-CoA-binding site of the enzyme
    C. A competitive inhibitor binding to the oxaloacetate-binding site of the enzyme
    D. A noncompetitive inhibitor of the enzyme

3. An enzymatic reaction works best at pH values between 6 and 8. This is compatible with the assumption that the reaction mechanism requires two ionizable amino acid side chains in the active site of the enzyme, possibly
    A. Protonated glutamate and deprotonated aspartate
    B. Protonated histidine and deprotonated lysine
    C. Protonated glutamate and deprotonated histidine

    D. Protonated arginine and deprotonated lysine
    E. Protonated cysteine and deprotonated histidine

Questions 4, 5, and 6 refer to the following scenario:

A biotechnology company has cloned four different forms of the enzyme money synthetase, which catalyzes the reaction

Garbage + ATP $\longrightarrow$
$$\text{Money} + \text{ADP} + \text{Phosphate} + \text{H}^+$$

The K_m values of these enzymes for garbage and the V_{max} values are:

Enzyme 1: $K_m = 0.1$ mM, $V_{max} = 5.0$ mmol/min
Enzyme 2: $K_m = 0.3$ mM, $V_{max} = 2.0$ mmol/min
Enzyme 3: $K_m = 1.0$ mM, $V_{max} = 5.0$ mmol/min
Enzyme 4: $K_m = 3.0$ mM, $V_{max} = 20$ mmol/min

4. Which of the four enzymes is fastest at a saturating ATP concentration and a garbage concentration of 0.01 mM?
    A. Enzyme 1
    B. Enzyme 2
    C. Enzyme 3
    D. Enzyme 4

5. Which of the four forms of money synthetase is fastest at a saturating ATP concentration and a garbage concentration of 10 mM?
    A. Enzyme 1
    B. Enzyme 2
    C. Enzyme 3
    D. Enzyme 4

6. If the money synthetase reaction is freely reversible, which of the following manipulations would be best to favor money formation over garbage formation and to increase the [Money]/[Garbage] ratio at equilibrium?
    A. Decrease the pH value.
    B. Add another enzyme that destroys ADP.
    C. Use a very low concentration of ATP.
    D. Increase the temperature.
    E. Add a noncompetitive inhibitor.

Chapter 5

Coenzymes

The examples of lysozyme and chymotrypsin in the previous chapter showed that many enzymes can catalyze their reactions without the help of a nonpolypeptide component, using only their amino acid residues for catalysis. Some enzymatic reactions, however, require a nonpolypeptide cofactor, a **coenzyme.**

The time-honored name "coenzyme" is applied to two different types of cofactors that function either as **cosubstrates** or as true **prosthetic groups.** A cosubstrate is a promiscuous molecule that associates with the active site of the enzyme only transiently, for the purpose of the reaction. Cosubstrates are changed chemically during the reaction. After completion of the reaction, the chemically modified cosubstrate dissociates away and is free to participate in other enzymatic reactions. A prosthetic group, in contrast, is monogamous: it is bonded permanently to the active site of its enzyme, either covalently or noncovalently.

Some coenzymes can be synthesized in the body de novo ("from scratch"), but others contain a vitamin as part of their structure or have vitamin character themselves. Enzymatic reactions that require a vitamin-derived coenzyme are inhibited when the vitamin is in short supply.

Individual coenzymes are concerned with specific reaction types such as hydrogen transfer, methylation, or carboxylation. Thus, the testwise student often can predict the coenzyme of an enzymatic reaction from the reaction type.

ATP has two energy-rich bonds

The generation of metabolic energy is a must for any living cell, and we have to obtain this energy from the oxidation of carbohydrates, fat, protein, and, in some individuals, ethanol. *Energy is required to drive endergonic biosynthetic reactions, active membrane transport, and muscle contraction.*

A central question in bioenergetics is: how does the cell manage to couple a large number of different exergonic reactions to the multitude of energy-demanding processes? Nature has solved this problem by a very simple trick: *exergonic reactions are used for the synthesis of the energy-rich compound **adenosine triphosphate (ATP)**, and the chemical bond energy of ATP drives the energy-dependent processes.* Thus, ATP is used as the energetic currency of the cell (Fig. 5.1).

FIG. 5.1

The function of ATP as the "energetic currency" of the cell.

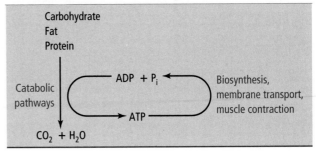

75

FIG. 5.2

Sequential hydrolysis of ATP.

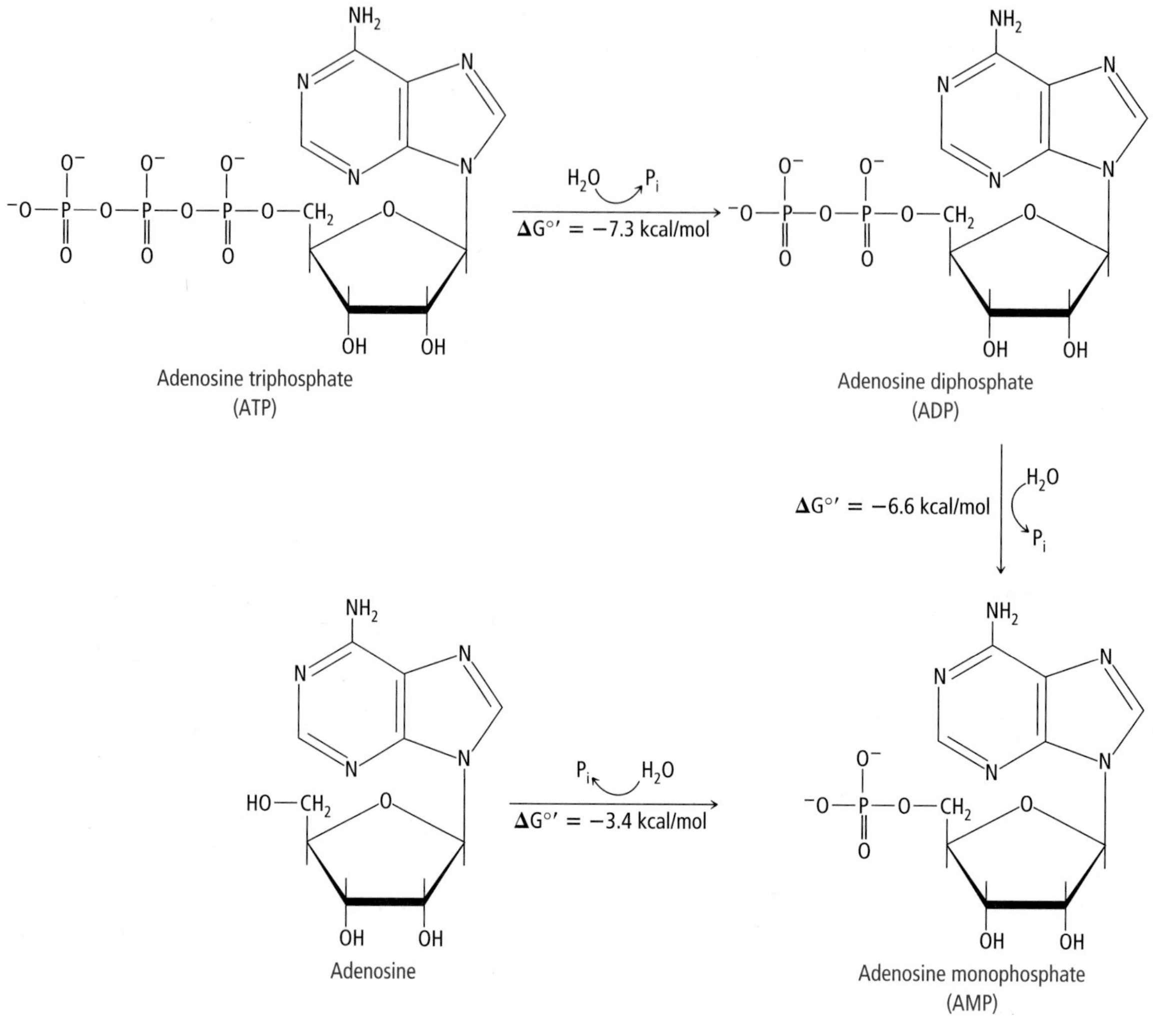

Adenosine triphosphate
(ATP)

H_2O P_i

$\Delta G^{\circ\prime} = -7.3$ kcal/mol

Adenosine diphosphate
(ADP)

$\Delta G^{\circ\prime} = -6.6$ kcal/mol

H_2O

P_i

Adenosine

P_i H_2O

$\Delta G^{\circ\prime} = -3.4$ kcal/mol

Adenosine monophosphate
(AMP)

To understand the function of ATP, we first have to examine its structure (Fig. 5.2). Chemically, ATP is an ordinary ribonucleotide (see Chapter 1), one of the building blocks for RNA synthesis. It does not contain a vitamin, and the whole molecule can be synthesized from simple precursors (see Chapter 23). Its most important part is made up of three phosphate residues that are bound to carbon 5 of ribose and complexed with a magnesium ion (Fig. 5.3).

The first phosphate is linked to ribose by a phosphate ester bond, but *the two bonds that link the phosphates to each other are energy-rich phosphoanhydride bonds.* The free energy changes shown in Fig. 5.2 apply to standard conditions. The actual free energy change

FIG. 5.3

Magnesium complexes formed by ATP. Mg^{2+}-ATP complexes are the actual substrates of ATP-dependent enzymes.

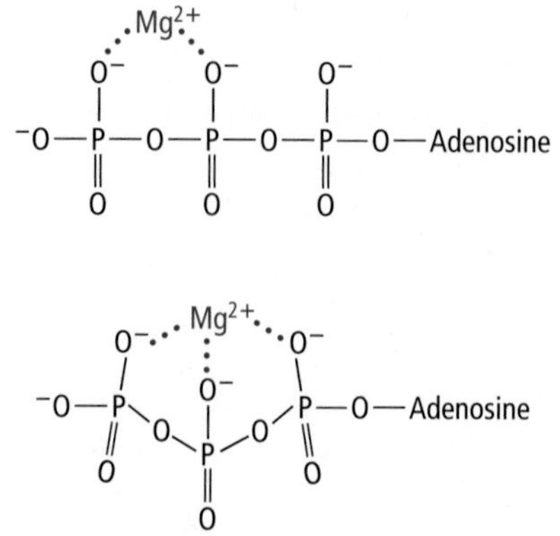

BOX 5.1

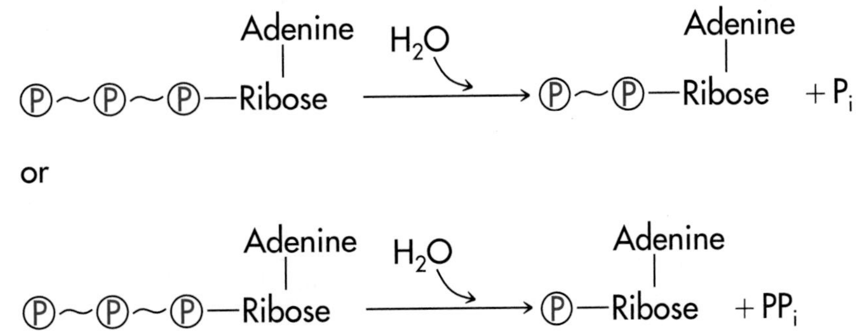

Adenine
|
(P)~(P)~(P)—Ribose $\xrightarrow{\text{H}_2\text{O}}$ (P)~(P)—Ribose $+ \text{P}_i$
                Adenine
                |

or

Adenine
|
(P)~(P)~(P)—Ribose $\xrightarrow{\text{H}_2\text{O}}$ (P)—Ribose $+ \text{PP}_i$
                Adenine
                |

BOX 5.2

$$-O-\overset{\overset{\displaystyle O^-}{|}}{\underset{\underset{\displaystyle O}{||}}{P}}-O-\overset{\overset{\displaystyle O^-}{|}}{\underset{\underset{\displaystyle O}{||}}{P}}-O^- \xrightarrow[\text{H}_2\text{O}]{\text{Pyrophosphatase}} -O-\overset{\overset{\displaystyle O^-}{|}}{\underset{\underset{\displaystyle O}{||}}{P}}-OH + HO-\overset{\overset{\displaystyle O^-}{|}}{\underset{\underset{\displaystyle O}{||}}{P}}-O^-$$

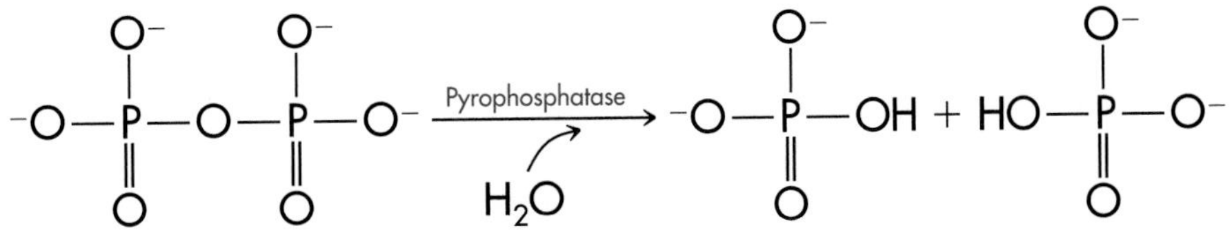

for the hydrolysis of ATP to ADP + P_i depends on pH, ionic strength, and the concentrations of ATP, ADP, phosphate, and magnesium. It is close to -11 or -12 kcal/mol under "real-cell" conditions.

In the structures of ATP and other high-energy phosphates, the phosphate bond often is written $\sim$(P) (squiggle P):

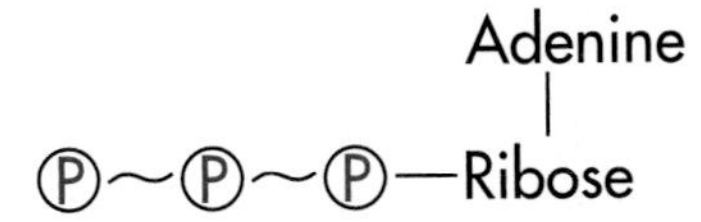

Adenine
|
(P)~(P)~(P)—Ribose

In energy-demanding reactions, ATP can be hydrolyzed in two ways as shown in Box 5.1. P_i is inorganic phosphate, and PP_i is inorganic pyrophosphate, a product that still contains an energy-rich phosphoanhydride bond:

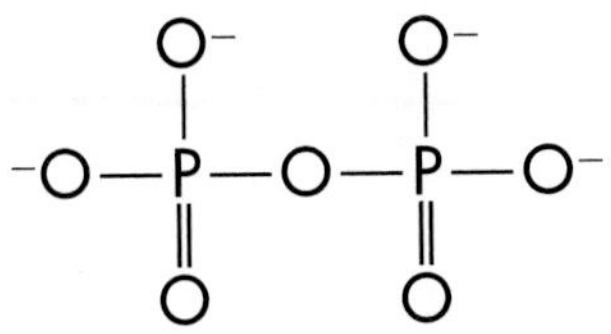

$$-O-\overset{\overset{\displaystyle O^-}{|}}{\underset{\underset{\displaystyle O}{||}}{P}}-O-\overset{\overset{\displaystyle O^-}{|}}{\underset{\underset{\displaystyle O}{||}}{P}}-O^-$$

Both cleavages release approximately the same amount of free energy. In the cell, however, the hydrolysis to AMP and pyrophosphate supplies more energy because pyrophosphate is removed rapidly from the reaction equilibrium by hydrolysis as shown in Box 5.2. Several cellular enzymes have pyrophosphatase activity. The more common cleavage reaction, however, is the hydrolysis to ADP + P_i.

ATP is the phosphate donor in phosphorylation reactions

Table 5.1 lists the most important processes in which ATP either supplies energy or is used as a biosynthetic precursor. Only phosphorylation reactions and the coupling to endergonic reactions will be considered here.

The term **phosphorylation** refers to the covalent attachment of a phosphate group to a substrate, most commonly by the formation of a phosphate ester bond. Let us assume that the cell wants to convert glucose to glucose 6-phosphate, a simple phosphate ester as shown in Box 5.3. We can try to

BOX 5.3

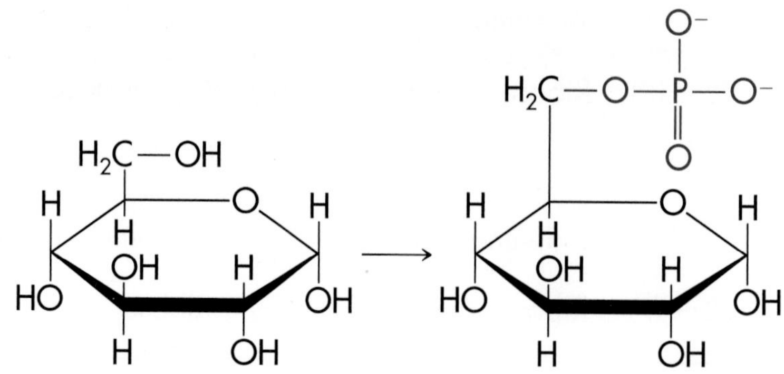

Glucose → Glucose 6-phosphate

TABLE 5.1

Uses of adenosine triphosphate (ATP)

Process	Function
RNA synthesis	Precursor
Phosphorylation	Phosphate donor
Coupling to ender-gonic reactions	Energy source
Active membrane transport	Energy source
Muscle contraction Ciliary motion	Energy source

synthesize this product by reacting free glucose with inorganic phosphate:

$$\text{Glucose} + P_i \xrightarrow{\text{Glucose 6-phosphatase}} \text{Glucose 6-phosphate} + H_2O$$

The enzyme glucose 6-phosphatase really exists, but the reaction has a $\Delta G^{o\prime}$ value of $+3.3$ kcal/mol. This corresponds to an equilibrium constant K_{equ} of approximately 4×10^{-3} L/mol. At an intracellular phosphate concentration of 10 mM, there would be approximately 25,000 molecules of glucose for each molecule of glucose 6-phosphate!

A more promising approach for the synthesis of glucose 6-phosphate would be the use of ATP as a source of the phosphate group:

$$\text{Glucose} + \text{ATP} \xrightarrow{\text{Hexokinase}} \text{Glucose 6-phosphate} + \text{ADP}$$

This reaction has a $\Delta G^{o\prime}$ value of -4.0 kcal/mol. Note that the difference in the $\Delta G^{o\prime}$ values of the hexokinase and glucose 6-phosphatase reactions corresponds to the free energy content of the phosphoanhydride bond in ATP (7.3 kcal/mol). Now the equilibrium constant is close to 10^3, and if the cellular ATP concentration is 10 times higher than the ADP concentration, we have 10,000 molecules of glucose 6-phosphate for each molecule of glucose at equilibrium!

ATP hydrolysis can be coupled to endergonic reactions

Not only phosphorylation reactions are driven in the desired direction by ATP. For example, the reaction shown in Box 5.4, which occurs in the mitochondria (see Fig. 16.12), has a $\Delta G^{o\prime}$ value of -8.5 kcal/mol and therefore is essentially irreversible in the direction of citrate formation. In the cytoplasm, however, we find the enzyme ATP-citrate lyase, which couples this reaction to ATP synthesis:

$$\text{Acetyl-CoA} + \text{Oxaloacetate} + \text{ADP} + P_i \longrightarrow \text{Citrate} + \text{Coenzyme A} + \text{ATP}$$

The $\Delta G^{o\prime}$ of this reaction is -1.2 kcal/mol. This value is the sum of the free energy changes for

BOX 5.4

$$\underset{\text{Acetyl-CoA}}{H_3C-\overset{\overset{\displaystyle O}{\|}}{C}-S-CoA} + \underset{\text{Oxaloacetate}}{O=\overset{\displaystyle}{\underset{\underset{\displaystyle H_2C-COO^-}{|}}{C}}-COO^-} + H_2O \xrightarrow[\text{synthase}]{\text{Citrate}} \underset{\text{Citrate}}{HO-\overset{\overset{\displaystyle H_2C-COO^-}{|}}{\underset{\underset{\displaystyle H_2C-COO^-}{|}}{C}}-COO^-} + \underset{\text{Coenzyme A}}{HS-CoA} + H^+$$

citrate formation (-8.5 kcal/mol) and ATP synthesis ($+7.3$ kcal/mol). The reaction is now reversible and, under suitable conditions, can proceed in the direction of citrate cleavage: *ATP hydrolysis enables the cell to cleave citrate into oxaloacetate and acetyl-CoA.*

The adenine nucleotides are in equilibrium

Adenosine triphosphate is not a tightly bound prosthetic group, but rather a cosubstrate that can diffuse freely, or be transported, from ATP-synthesizing to ATP-consuming enzymes. Its cellular concentration may be as high as 5 mM (2.5 g/L) in some tissues. The lifespan of an ATP molecule is approximately 2 minutes, and although its total body content is only about 100 g, *approximately 60 kg are produced and consumed every day.*

In the cell, the three adenine nucleotides are in equilibrium through the **adenylate kinase** reaction (adenylate = AMP):

$$ATP + AMP \xrightleftharpoons{\text{Adenylate kinase}} 2\ ADP$$

The energy status of the cell can be described as the [ATP]/[ADP] ratio, or as the **energy charge:**

$$\text{Energy charge} = \frac{[ATP] + \frac{1}{2}[ADP]}{[ATP] + [ADP] + [AMP]}$$

The energy charge can vary between 0 and 1. Healthy cells always maintain a high energy charge, with [ATP]/[ADP] ratios of 5 to 200 in different cell types. The energy charge is decreased when ATP synthesis is impaired, as in hypoxia (oxygen defi-ciency), or when ATP consumption is increased, as during muscle contraction. *When the energy charge is zero, the cell is dead.*

GTP, UTP, and CTP participate in enzymatic reactions as well

All cells contain guanosine triphosphate (GTP), uridine triphosphate (UTP), and cytidine triphosphate (CTP), besides ATP. Guanosine triphosphate rather than ATP is used as an energy source in some reactions, most notably in the ribosomal steps of protein synthesis (see Chapter 6). Uridine triphosphate is used to activate monosaccharides for the synthesis of complex carbohydrates (Chapter 17), and CTP plays a similar role in phospholipid synthesis (Chapter 19). The mono-, di-, and triphosphate forms are in equilibrium through kinase reactions:

$$\left. \begin{array}{l} GMP \\ UMP \\ CMP \end{array} \right\} + ATP \xrightleftharpoons[]{\text{Nucleoside monophosphate kinases}} \left. \begin{array}{l} GDP \\ UDP \\ CDP \end{array} \right\} + ADP$$

and

$$\left. \begin{array}{l} GDP \\ UDP \\ CDP \end{array} \right\} + ATP \xrightleftharpoons[]{\text{Nucleoside diphosphate kinase}} \left. \begin{array}{l} GTP \\ UTP \\ CTP \end{array} \right\} + ADP$$

FIG. 5.4

Structures of nicotinamide adenine dinucleotide (NAD⁺) and nicotinamide adenine dinucleotide phosphate (NADP⁺). **A,** Structures of the coenzymes. NAD⁺: R = −H; NADP⁺: R = −PO₃²⁻. **B,** The reversible hydrogenation of the nicotinamide portion in NAD⁺/NADH and NADP⁺/NADPH.

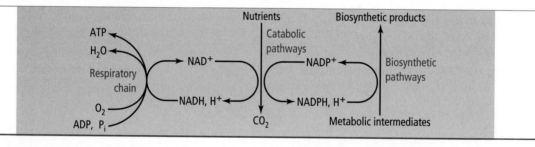

FIG. 5.5

Metabolic functions of NAD and NADP.

Some coenzymes participate in dehydrogenase reactions

Redox reactions are reactions in which *electrons are transferred from one substrate to another,* either alone or together with protons. *The cosubstrates **NAD** and **NADP** are specialized for the transfer of hydrogen (hydrogen = electron + proton) in dehydrogenase reactions.* In both coenzymes (Fig. 5.4), nicotinamide is the hydrogen-carrying part of the molecule. The additional phosphate in NADP does not affect the hydrogen transfer potential, but it is important for recognition by

enzymes. *Most dehydrogenases are quite discriminating, using either NAD or NADP only.*

NAD⁺ acquires two electrons and a proton during catabolic, oxidative reactions and *feeds them into the respiratory chain of the mitochondria,* where they are oxidized to water by molecular oxygen (see Chapter 16). NADP⁺ also accepts electrons in catabolic pathways, but *it feeds them into biosynthetic pathways* in which reduced products such as fatty acids or cholesterol are produced from more oxidized metabolic intermediates (Fig. 5.5).

Some dehydrogenases do not use NAD or NADP

FIG. 5.6

FMN and FAD as hydrogen carriers. **A,** Structures of the coenzymes. The structure formed from the dimethylisoalloxazine ring and ribitol is called riboflavin (vitamin B_2). **B,** Hydrogen transfer by the dimethylisoalloxazine ring of FMN and FAD.

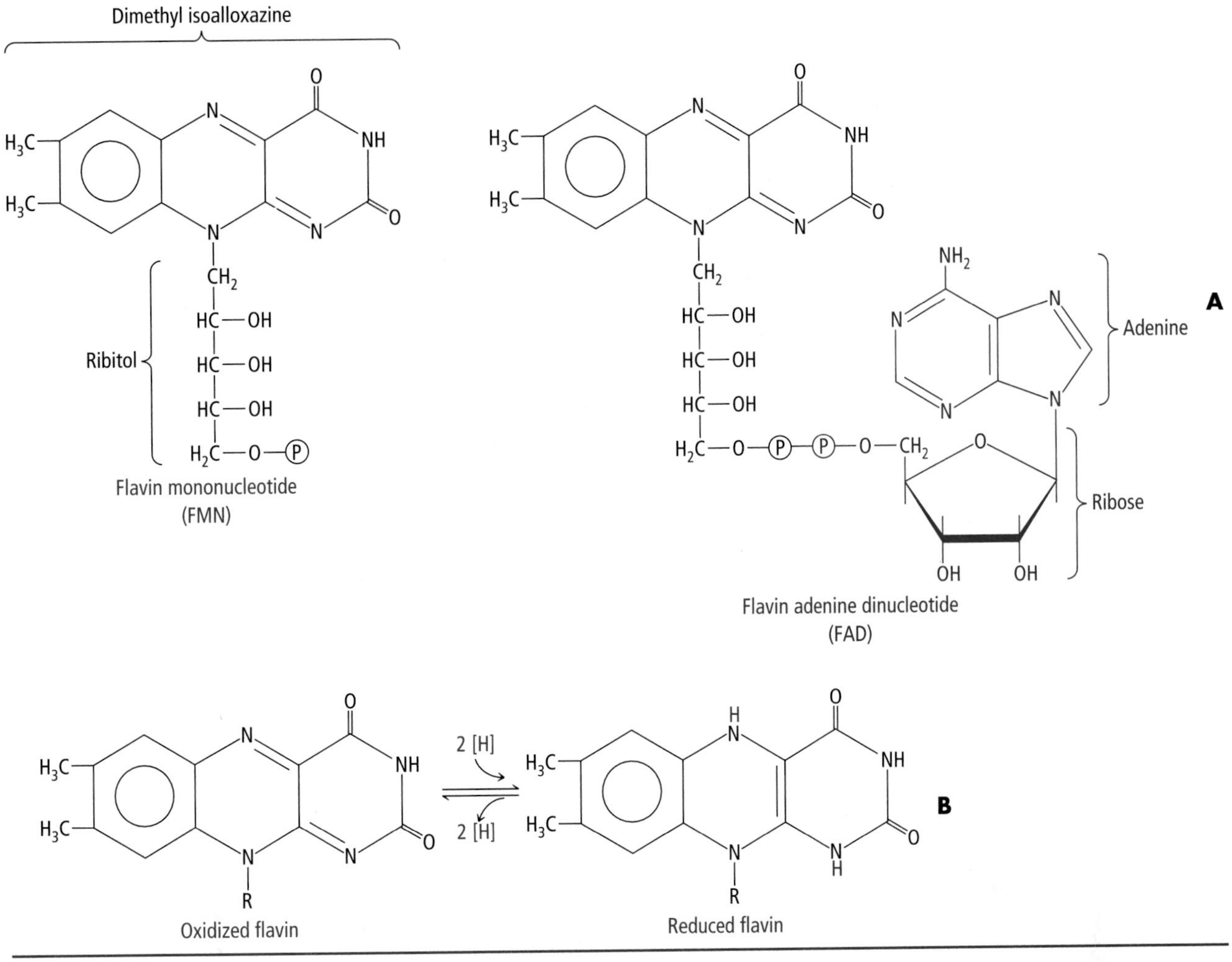

Flavin mononucleotide
(FMN)

Flavin adenine dinucleotide
(FAD)

Oxidized flavin

2 [H]

2 [H]

Reduced flavin

but flavin adenine dinucleotide (**FAD**) or flavin mononucleotide (**FMN**). These coenzymes contain an isoalloxazine ring that accepts and donates hydrogen (Fig. 5.6). Unlike NAD and NADP, *the flavin coenzymes are bound tightly to the apoprotein, either noncovalently or by a covalent bond.* These proteins are called **flavoproteins** (Latin *flavus,* "yellow") because of the yellow color of the oxidized flavin coenzymes.

Coenzyme A is used to activate organic acids

Coenzyme A (Fig. 5.7) is a *soluble carrier of acyl groups.* The business end of the molecule is a sulfhydryl

group, which forms thioester bonds with many organic acids. Therefore its structure can be abbreviated as CoA-SH, and its acid derivatives, or acyl-CoAs, are written as:

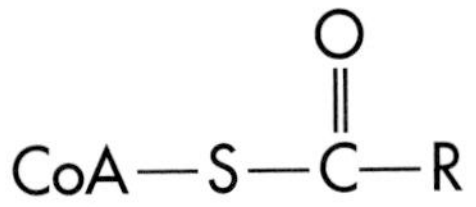

$$CoA-S-\overset{\overset{\displaystyle O}{\|}}{C}-R$$

Typical examples are acetyl-CoA and palmitoyl-CoA as shown in Box 5.5. The thioester bonds in these derivatives are energy rich, with a free energy content between 7 and 8 kcal/mol. *CoA-thioesters are used for biosynthetic reactions in which the acid is transferred from coenzyme A to an acceptor molecule.* Acetylation reactions (the "A" in coenzyme A stands for "acetyla-

FIG. 5.7

The structure of coenzyme A.

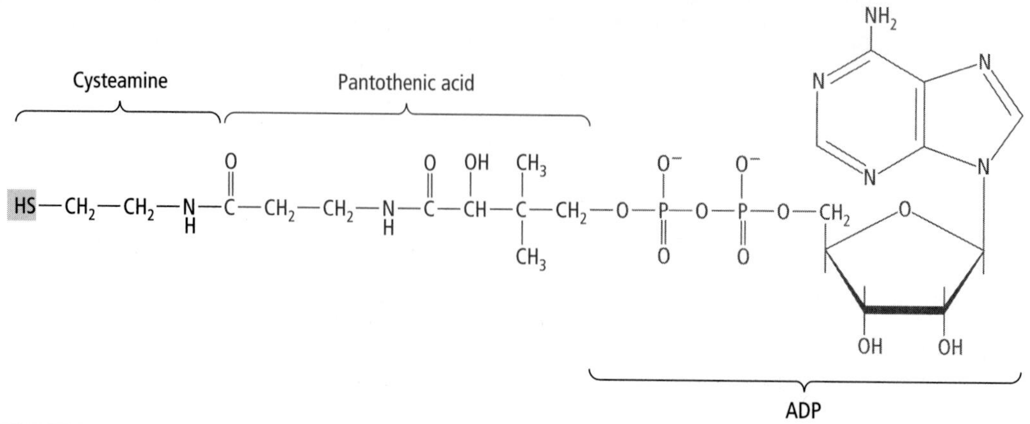

BOX 5.5

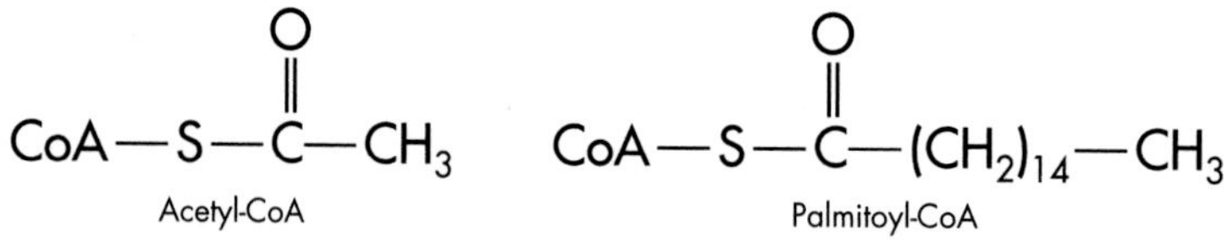

FIG. 5.8

S-Adenosyl methionine (SAM) as a methyl group donor. **A,** Structure of the coenzyme. **B,** Formation of a methoxy group in a SAM-dependent methylation.

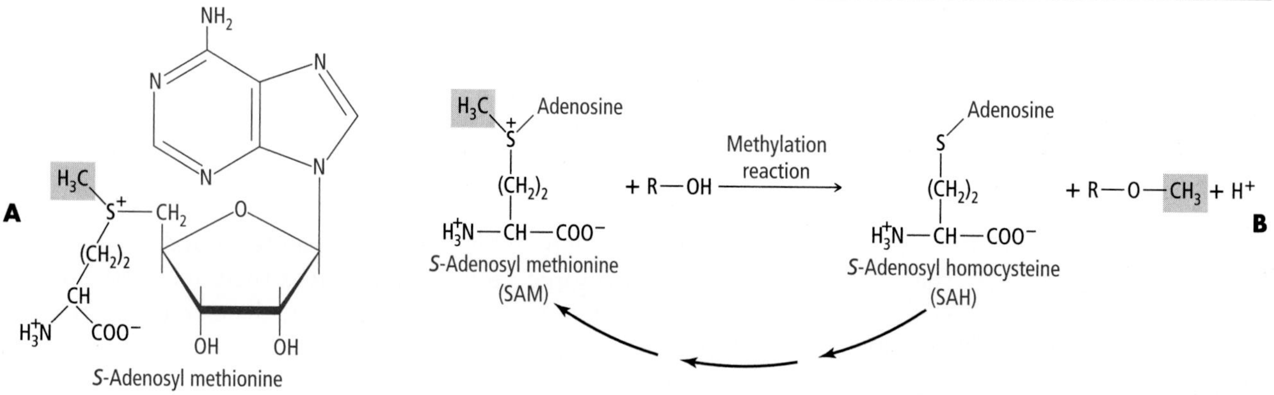

tion") and the synthesis of triglycerides (see Chapter 18) and other fatty acid-containing lipids proceed through CoA-activated intermediates. Indeed, the acyl group in a CoA-derivative is activated for biosynthetic reactions in much the same way that the terminal phosphate of ATP is activated for phosphorylation reactions.

S-adenosyl methionine is an important methyl group donor

Methylations are reactions in which a methyl (CH_3) group is transferred to an acceptor molecule. The methyl group donor for most biological methylations is **S-adenosyl methionine (SAM)** (Fig. 5.8).

TABLE 5.2

Summary of the most important coenzymes

Coenzyme	Present as	Functions in	Vitamin*
Adenosine triphosphate (ATP)	Cosubstrate	Energy-dependent reactions	—
Guanosine triphosphate (GTP)	Cosubstrate	Energy-dependent reactions	—
Uridine triphosphate (UTP)	Cosubstrate	Activation of monosac-charides	—
Cytidine triphosphate (CTP)	Cosubstrate	Phospholipid synthesis	—
NAD and NADP	Cosubstrate	Hydrogen transfers	Niacin
Flavin adenine dinucleotide (FAD) and flavin mononucleotide (FMN)	Prosthetic group	Hydrogen transfers	Riboflavin
Coenzyme A	Cosubstrate	Acylation reactions	Pantothenic acid
S-Adenosyl methionine (SAM)	Cosubstrate	Methylation reactions	—
Heme	Prosthetic group	Electron transfers	—
Biotin	Prosthetic group	Carboxylation reactions	Biotin
Tetrahydrofolate (THF)	Cosubstrate	One-carbon transfers	Folic acid
Pyridoxal phosphate (PLP)	Prosthetic group	Amino acid metabolism	B_6
Thiamine pyrophosphate (TPP)	Prosthetic group	Carbonyl transfers	Thiamine (B_1)
Lipoic acid	Prosthetic group	Oxidative decar-boxylations	—

* The vitamins are discussed in Chapter 24.

By donating its methyl group, SAM is converted to S-adenosyl homocysteine (SAH); SAH, in turn, can be converted back to SAM (see Chapter 21). Like coenzyme A, SAM is a cosubstrate rather than a prosthetic group.

Several other coenzymes participate in specific types of enzymatic reactions. These coenzymes (Table 5.2) will be discussed in the context of those metabolic reactions in which they participate.

Many enzymes require a metal ion

Alkali metals such as sodium (Na^+) and potassium (K^+) are required by many enzymes to maintain their active conformation. Transition metals such as iron (Fe), zinc (Zn), copper (Cu), and manganese (Mn), however, often are found in the active site, where they participate in catalysis. In some reactions, a tightly bound metal ion functions as an electron carrier by reversibly changing its oxidation state:

$$Fe^{3+} \overset{e^-}{\underset{e^-}{\rightleftharpoons}} Fe^{2+}$$

$$Cu^{2+} \overset{e^-}{\underset{e^-}{\rightleftharpoons}} Cu^{+}$$

In other cases, the metal acts as a Lewis acid, or electron pair acceptor. This occurs, for example, in the carbonic anhydrase reaction as shown in Box 5.6. Binding to the zinc ion increases the electron density on the oxygen of the water molecule, thereby activating it for a nucleophilic attack on the carbon of CO_2.

BOX 5.6

$$CO_2 + H_2O \rightleftharpoons H_2CO_3$$

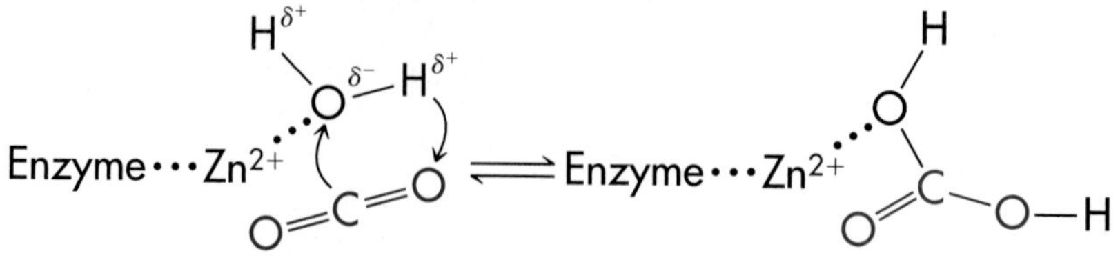

SUMMARY

Some—but not all—enzymatic reactions require the participation of a nonpolypeptide component called a coenzyme. Some coenzymes are tightly bound prosthetic groups; others are soluble cosubstrates. Coenzymes contain structural features that enable them to function in specific reaction types. The cosubstrate ATP contains two energy-rich phosphoanhydride bonds that are used in phosphorylation reactions and that permit the molecule to act as the energetic currency of the cell, driving endergonic reactions. The coenzymes NAD, NADP, FMN, and FAD are hydrogen carriers in many dehydrogenase reactions. S-Adenosyl methionine (SAM) is a methyl group donor, and coenzyme A is used to activate organic acids for biosynthetic reactions. Many enzymes also contain a metal ion in their active site that participates in catalysis.

QUESTIONS

1. Protein kinases are enzymes that phosphorylate amino acid side chains of proteins in ATP-dependent reactions. A protein kinase can be classified as a(n)
   A. Oxidoreductase
   B. Hydrolase
   C. Isomerase
   D. Lyase
   E. Transferase

2. Cyanide is a potent inhibitor of cell respiration that prevents the oxidation of all nutrients. Therefore, cyanide definitely will reduce the cellular concentration of
   A. Heme groups
   B. AMP
   C. Coenzyme A
   D. ATP
   E. S-Adenosyl methionine

3. This reaction has a standard free energy change $\Delta G^{o\prime}$ of -0.8 kcal/mol.

Succinyl-CoA + GDP + P$_i$ $\longrightarrow$
　　　　　Succinate + CoA-SH + GTP

If the free energy content of a phosphoanhydride bond in GTP is 7.3 kcal/mol, what would be the standard free energy change of the reaction

Succinyl-CoA + H$_2$O $\longrightarrow$
　　　　　Succinate + CoA-SH

   A. -8.1 kcal/mol
   B. $+6.5$ kcal/mol
   C. $+8.1$ kcal/mol
   D. -6.5 kcal/mol
   E. $+0.8$ kcal/mol

PART TWO

GENETIC INFORMATION: DNA, RNA, AND PROTEIN SYNTHESIS

Chapter 6

DNA, RNA, and Protein Synthesis:

The Central Dogma of Molecular Biology

What a cell looks like and what it does are determined by its proteins. Its structure depends on proteins in its membranes and in the cytoskeleton. Enzyme proteins are in charge of metabolic activities, and many other cell functions, such as motility and excitability, depend on specialized proteins as well. Our bodies can synthesize close to 100,000 different polypeptides, each with its own unique amino acid sequence. The polypeptides are synthesized by ribosomes in the cytoplasm, but their amino acid sequence has to be specified by the DNA in the chromosomes. Therefore instructions have to be sent from the chromosome to the ribosome. These instructions are car-ried by **messenger RNA (mRNA)**. Gene expression requires two important steps (Fig. 6.1):

1. During **transcription**, which takes place in the nucleus, an mRNA molecule is synthesized, the structure of which mirrors that of a segment of DNA.
2. During **translation**, which is the task of the ribosome, the structure of the mRNA specifies the amino acid sequence of a polypeptide.

The functional unit of the genetic databank is the **gene.** *A gene is a length of DNA that directs the synthesis of a polypeptide.* Genes consist of a transcribed sequence, called the **transcription unit,** and regula-

FIG. 6.1

Expression of genetic information. In all organisms, the DNA of the gene is first copied into a single-stranded molecule of messenger RNA (mRNA). This process is called transcription. During ribosomal protein synthesis, the base sequence of the mRNA is used to specify the amino acid sequence of a polypeptide. This is called translation. **A,** In prokaryotic cells, translation follows immediately on transcription. **B,** Eukaryotic cells have a nuclear membrane. Therefore transcription and translation take place in different compartments: transcription in the nucleus and translation in the cytoplasm.

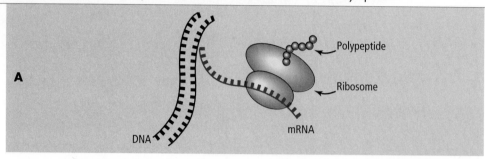

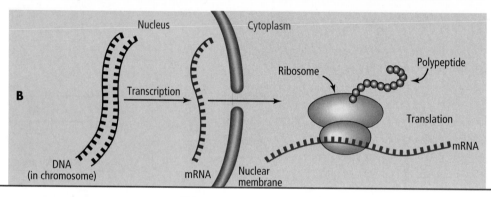

tory sites (Fig. 6.2). The **chromosome** is a much larger structure, consisting of a DNA molecule with hundreds or even thousands of genes.

As it is expressed, the genetic message is amplified: a single gene can be transcribed into thousands of mRNA molecules, and each mRNA can be translated into thousands of polypeptides. A red blood cell (RBC), for example, contains 5×10^8 copies of the hemoglobin β-chain, but the nucleated RBC precursors have only two copies of the β-chain gene!

DNA STRUCTURE AND DNA REPLICATION

DNA does not only direct the synthesis of proteins. It also is able to replicate itself, producing two daughter molecules that are identical to the parent molecule. The continuity of life is based on this unique ability of DNA. Indeed, we can view the living cell as *an artificial environment, created by DNA for the benefit of its own replication.* In the following sections,

we introduce the structure of DNA and the mechanism of its replication.

DNA structure and the principles of gene expression are the same in all organisms

Living things are grouped into two major branches based on their cell structure: the **prokaryotes,** which include the bacteria, actinomycetes, and blue-green algae, and the **eukaryotes,** which include the protozoa and the different phyla of plants and animals. The major distinguishing feature of eukaryotic cell structure is *the compartmentalization of the cell into organelles by intracellular membranes.* The most important differences between prokaryotes and eukaryotes are summarized in Fig. 6.3 and Table 6.1.

Three features are common to all living cells:

1. *All cells are surrounded by a plasma membrane.* This is a flimsy, fluid, flexible structure (see Chapter 11)

FIG. 6.2

Chromosomes and genes. **A,** Protein-coding genes consist of a transcribed sequence (▓) which is preceded by a regulatory region (■). Outside the genes are untranscribed spacers (░), which usually are very short in prokaryotes. The chromosomal DNA is very large, containing many hundreds or thousands of genes on a single, double-stranded molecule. **B,** Many prokaryotic genes are lined up in large transcription units that are transcribed into a single polycistronic mRNA. The ribosome translates the polycistronic mRNA into several polypeptides. A single regulatory region controls the transcription of all genes in the transcription unit.

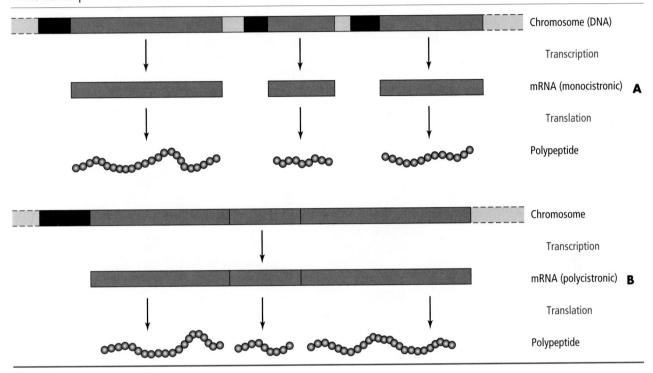

that forms a diffusion barrier between the cell and its environment.

2. *All cells display metabolic activity,* with energy-generating and energy-consuming processes.

3. *All cells store genetic information in the form of DNA,* and the information flow during gene expression is from DNA to RNA to protein.

In this chapter, we introduce the principles of molecular genetics in prokaryotes. The corresponding processes in eukaryotes (described in Chapter 8) are similar but often are more complex. Also, less detail is known about the eukaryotic system than about the prokaryotic system.

DNA contains four bases

DNA is a polymer of nucleoside monophosphates (Fig. 6.4, *B*; see also Chapter 1 for the general structure of nucleotides). Its backbone is formed by al-

TABLE 6.1

Typical differences between prokaryotic and eukaryotic cells

Property	Prokaryotes	Eukaryotes
Typical size	$0.4-4\ \mu m$	$5-50\ \mu m$
Nucleus	−	+
Membrane-bounded organelles	−	+
Cytoskeleton	−	+
Endo- and exocytosis	−	+
Cell wall	+ (some −)	+ (plants) − (animals)
No. of chromosomes	1 (+ plasmids)	>1
Ploidy	Haploid	Haploid or diploid
Histones	−	+
Introns	−	+
Ribosomes	70S	80S

FIG. 6.3

Typical elements of prokaryotic and eukaryotic cell structure. *R*, Ribosomes; *ER*, endoplasmic reticulum; *L*, lysosome; *P*, peroxisome; *EV*, endocytotic vesicle; *SV*, secretory vesicle; *G*, Golgi apparatus; *Mit*, mitochondrion. **A,** Typical bacterial (prokaryotic) cell. **B,** Typical human (eukaryotic) cell.

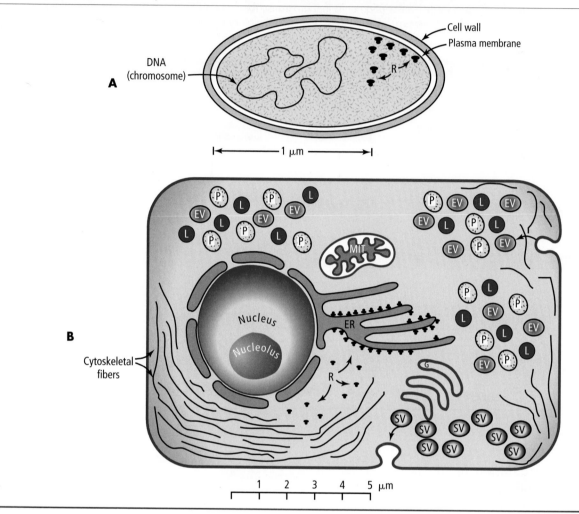

ternating phosphate and 2-deoxyribose residues, held together by phosphodiester bonds (Fig. 6.5). Carbons 3 and 5 of 2-deoxyribose participate in these bonds, whereas carbon 1 forms a β-N-glycosidic bond with nitrogen 1 of a pyrimidine base or with nitrogen 9 of a purine base.

The two ends of a DNA strand are not equivalent: at one end we find a free hydroxy group at C-5 of the terminal 2-deoxyribose, and at the other end is a free hydroxy group at C-3. The carbons of 2-deoxyribose are numbered by a prime (') to distinguish them from the carbons and nitrogens of the bases, and therefore we speak of the 5' end and the 3' end of the DNA strand. *Nucleic acids have a polarity,* which reminds us of the polarity of polypeptides with their amino terminus and carboxy terminus (see Chapter 2). By convention, the 5' terminus of a DNA (or RNA) strand is written at the left end of the sequence, the 3' terminus at the right end. The sequence itself can be written as a sequence of the bases. Thus, the tetranucleotide in Fig. 6.5 is written as ACTG, not GTCA.

Even a simple oligonucleotide shows us that *the variability of DNA structure rests in its base sequence.* With four different bases we can construct 4^2 (16) different dinucleotides and 4^3 (64) different trinucleotides; 4^{100} possibilities exist for a sequence of 100 nucleotides.

FIG. 6.4

The building blocks of DNA. **A,** Structures of the four bases, 2-deoxyribose, and phosphate. A and G are purines; C and T are pyrimidines. **B,** Structure of 2-deoxy-AMP (dAMP), one of the four 2-deoxyribonucleoside monophosphates in the repeat structure of DNA. Note that a nitrogen of the base is bound by a β-N-glycosidic bond to C-1 of 2-deoxyribose, while C-5 forms a phosphate ester bond.

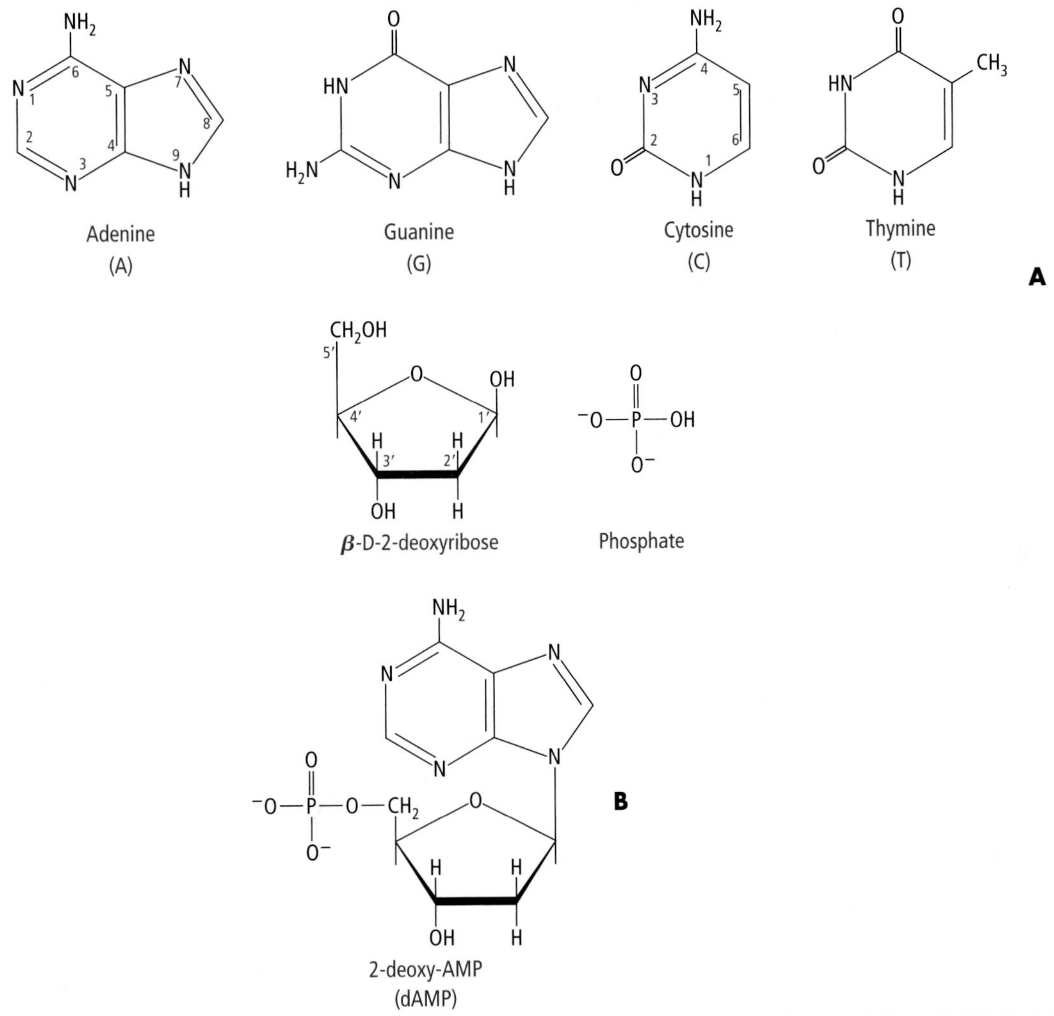

Adenine (A) Guanine (G) Cytosine (C) Thymine (T)

β-D-2-deoxyribose   Phosphate

2-deoxy-AMP (dAMP)

The Watson-Crick double helix is the principal higher-order structure of DNA

The DNA of living cells is always present in a double-stranded form. Its major higher-order structure is the famous **double helix,** which was proposed by James Watson and Francis Crick in 1953, based largely on X-ray diffraction studies. The most prominent features of the Watson-Crick double helix (Figs. 6.6 and 6.7) are:

1. *The two strands of the double helix have opposite polarity.* Opposite polarity is not a unique feature of the DNA double helix, but it occurs whenever DNA or RNA forms base-paired structures.

2. *The 2-deoxyribose/phosphate backbones of the two strands form two ridges on the surface of the molecule. The phosphate groups are negatively charged at physiologic pH values.*

3. *The bases face inward to the helix axis, but their edges are exposed to the aqueous environment. They form the lining of two grooves that are framed by the ridges of the sugar-phosphate backbone. Because the N-glycosidic bonds are not exactly opposite each other (Fig. 6.8), the two grooves are of unequal*

FIG. 6.5

Structure of the (2-deoxy-) tetranucleotide ACTG. The DNA strands in chromosomes are far larger, with lengths of many million nucleotide units. *A,* Adenine; *C,* cytosine; *T,* thymine; *G,* guanine.

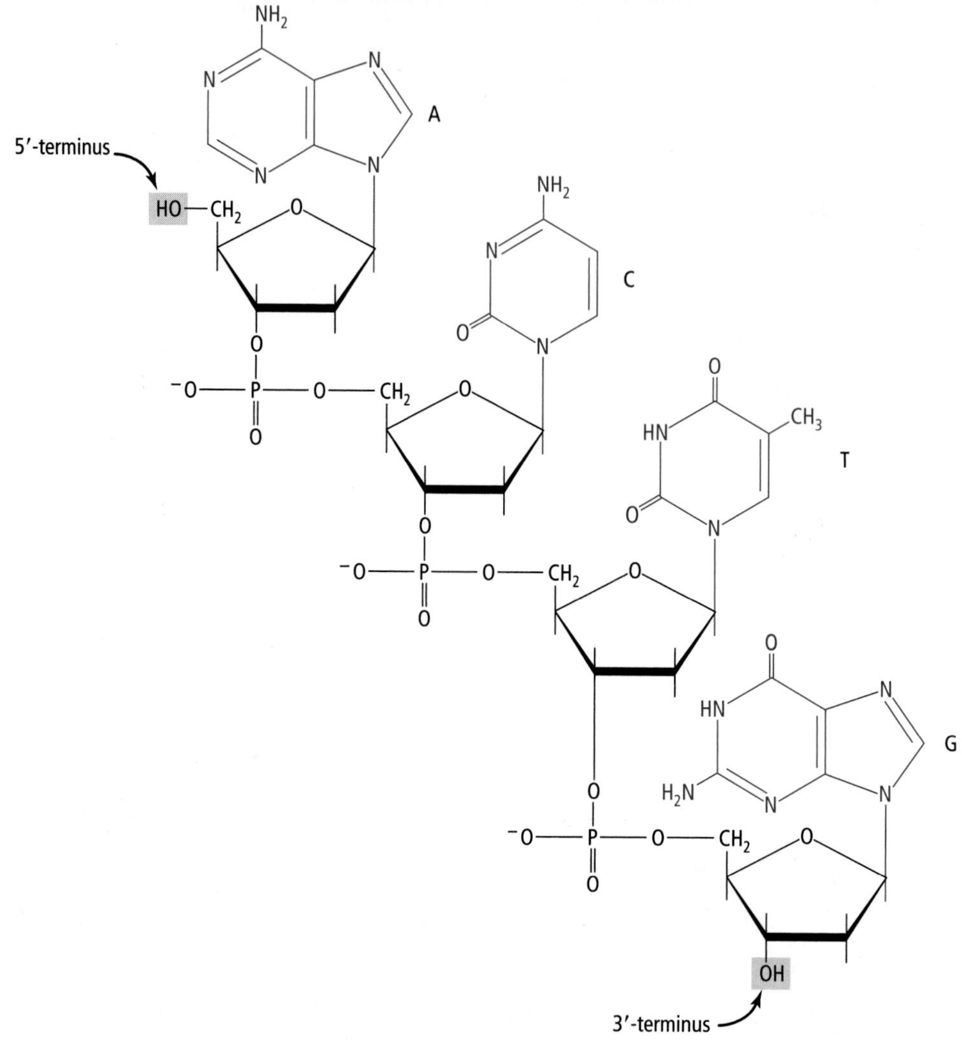

size. They are called the **major groove** and the **minor groove**.

4. *In each of the two strands, successive bases lie flat, one on top of the other,* like a stack of pancakes on a platter. There is no water between successive bases, and the heterocyclic rings form numerous van der Waals interactions. This **base stacking** is the strongest noncovalent force in the double helix. The bases are planar structures that can form hydrogen bonds only in the plane of their ring systems. They scarcely are able to form hydrogen bonds perpendicular to this plane, and therefore, their flat surfaces are hydrophobic.

5. *Bases in opposite strands interact by hydrogen bonds.* These interactions are very specific: adenine (A) always pairs with thymine (T), and guanine (G) always pairs with cytosine (C). Each A-T base pair is held together by two hydrogen bonds, each G-C pair by three. Because of the specificity of base pairing, double-stranded DNA molecules always contain equal molar amounts of A and T and of G and C. Most importantly, *the base sequence of one strand predicts exactly that of the opposite strand.* DNA replication and DNA repair would not be possible without this complementarity of base sequence.

FIG. 6.6

Schematic view of the DNA double strand. Note that the strands are antiparallel and that only A-T and G-C base pairs are permitted. Therefore the base sequence of one strand predicts the base sequence of the opposite strand.

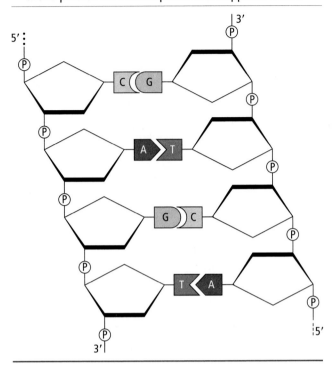

FIG. 6.7

Space-filling model of the Watson-Crick double helix (B-DNA).

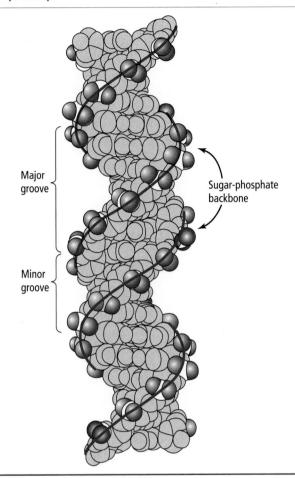

6. *The double strand is wound into a right-handed helix* with approximately 10 base pairs per turn. Each full turn of the helix advances approximately 3.4 nm along the helix axis. Because of electrostatic repulsion between the phosphate groups, the double helix prefers a stiff, extended shape but also can be bent and twisted without major distortions of the regional structure.

A-DNA and Z-DNA are alternative higher-order structures

Although the vast majority of the DNA in living cells is present as the Watson-Crick double helix, also known as **B-DNA**, there are two other possible conformations (Table 6.2). **A-DNA,** which does not occur in living cells, is formed from B-DNA by dehydration. It is somewhat thicker and more compact than B-DNA. In **Z-DNA** (the Z stands for "zigzag"), the sugar-phosphate backbone zigzags in a left-handed helix that is thinner and more stretched out than B-DNA and A-DNA. It requires a sequence of alternating purines and pyrimidines. Small regions of Z-DNA appear to be present in eukaryotic chromosomes, but their function, if any, is enigmatic.

DNA can be denatured

Like other noncovalent structures, *the Watson-Crick double helix is unstable at high temperatures.* When the temperature is increased gradually, this process of heat denaturation, also called **melting,** begins in areas with a high A-T content. A-T base pairs are separated more easily than G-C base pairs because they are held together by only two rather than three hydrogen bonds. Because of the cooperativity of strand interactions, however, the whole molecule is converted to a single-stranded **random coil** over a narrow temperature range (Figs. 6.9 and 6.10). The **melting temperature** (T_m) is defined as the tem-

FIG. 6.8

Cross sections through an A-T and a G-C base pair in the DNA duplex. The A-T base pair is held together by two hydrogen bonds (- - -), the G-C base pair by three.

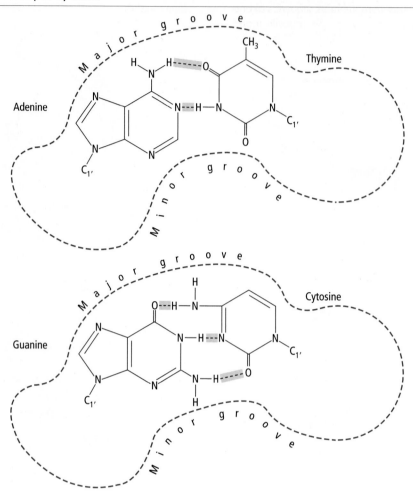

TABLE 6.2

Comparison of A-DNA, B-DNA, and Z-DNA

Property	A-DNA	B-DNA	Z-DNA
Helix sense	Right	Right	Left
Base pairs/turn	11	10	12
Rise/base pair*	2.6Å	3.4 Å	3.7 Å
Helix pitch*	28.6 Å	34 Å	44.4 Å
Widest diameter*	25.5 Å	23.7 Å	18.4 Å
Major groove	Narrow, very deep	Wide and deep	Wide and flat
Minor groove	Wide and shallow	Narrow and deep	Very narrow

* One angstrom (Å) is 0.1 nm or 10^{-10} meter.

FIG. 6.9

Melting of DNA. (© 1997 Wiley-Liss.)

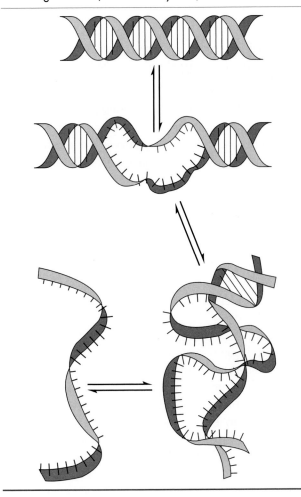

FIG. 6.10

Melting of DNA, monitored by the increase of UV absorbance at 260 nm. The melting temperature increases with increased GC content of the DNA. It is also affected by ionic strength and pH. The melting temperature is the temperature at which the increase in UV absorbance is half-maximal.

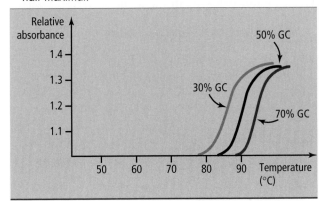

perature at which half of the double-stranded structure is lost. At physiologic pH and ionic strength, the melting temperature of DNA is between 85°C and 95°C.

Heat denaturation affects the physical properties of the DNA. The viscosity of DNA solutions decreases on melting because the single strands are far more flexible than the stiff, resilient double helix; also, the UV absorbance at 260 nm, which is caused by the heterocyclic bases, increases by approximately 37% because the base stacking interactions are disrupted.

DNA also can be denatured by a decrease of the salt concentration and by extreme pH values. A variety of chemical agents that interfere with hydrogen bonding or base stacking are effective denaturants as well. Treatment with formamide, for example, of-

ten is used as an alternative to heat denaturation in the laboratory.

When cooled slowly to 5°C to 20°C below the melting temperature, DNA molecules renature spontaneously. This is called **annealing.** Although small DNA molecules anneal almost instantaneously, seconds to minutes are required for large molecules.

DNA is supercoiled

Many naturally occurring DNA molecules are circular. When a linear duplex is unwound partially by one or several turns before it is linked into a circle, the resulting circle is strained torsionally. This strain can be relieved either by partial strand separation or by supercoiling of the duplex around its own axis—much as a telephone cord twists around itself. This kind of supertwist is called a **negative supertwist.** The opposite situation, in which the helix is overwound, is called a **positive supertwist.** *Most cellular DNAs are supertwisted negatively.* They have approximately 5% to 7% fewer right-handed turns than expected from the number of their base pairs. *This underwound condition facilitates the unwinding of the double helix during DNA replication and transcription.*

The supertwisting of DNA is regulated by enzymes that are known collectively as **topoisomerases.** These enzymes cleave a phosphodiester bond either in one strand or in both strands, thus creating a molecular swivel. After rotation of the

DNA around its axis, the nick is sealed by the enzyme (Fig. 6.11). Some topoisomerases only relax positive or negative supertwists. This is a passive process that requires no external energy source. However, others actively pump positive or negative supertwists into previously relaxed DNA. These enzymes require energy in the form of ATP.

DNA replication is semiconservative

The structure of the DNA duplex predicts the mechanism of its replication: the two strands can be separated from each other without the breakage of co-

valent bonds, and the base sequence of one strand exactly predicts that of the other strand. The basic events during DNA replication, as shown in Fig. 6.12, are therefore simple:

1. *The duplex separates into two single strands.*
2. *A new complementary strand is synthesized for each of the two single strands.*

The first step requires *ATP-dependent enzymes that unwind the helix and separate the strands:* the second step requires *an enzyme that synthesizes a new complementary strand for each of the two parental strands.* Strand separation and DNA synthesis occur in close succession. The unwinding of the parental duplex creates the **replication fork,** and *it is at the replication fork where the new DNA is synthesized.* The mechanism of DNA replication is known as **semiconservative replication** because one of the two strands in the daughter molecule is always old, whereas the other one is newly synthesized.

DNA is synthesized by DNA polymerases

The best-known system of DNA replication is that of *Escherichia coli (E. coli),* an intestinal bacterium that has enjoyed the steady affection of generations of molecular biologists. The key enzymes of DNA replication in *E. coli,* as in all other cells, are the **DNA polymerases.** *The DNA polymerases synthesize the new DNA strand stepwise, nucleotide by nucleotide, in the* $5' \rightarrow 3'$ *direction.* The precursors are the deoxyribonucleoside triphosphates dATP, dGTP, dCTP, and dTTP, and the phosphodiester bond is formed by linking the proximal phosphate of the nucleotide to the

---

FIG. 6.11

Relaxation of positive supertwists in DNA by a topoisomerase.

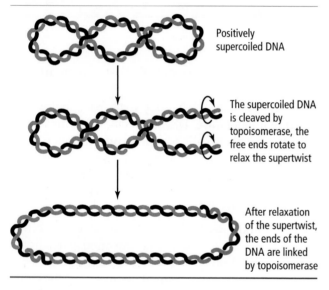

Positively supercoiled DNA

The supercoiled DNA is cleaved by topoisomerase, the free ends rotate to relax the supertwist

After relaxation of the supertwist, the ends of the DNA are linked by topoisomerase

---

FIG. 6.12

The semiconservative mechanism of DNA replication.

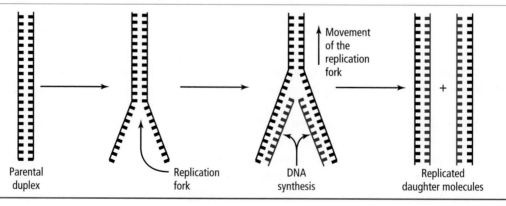

Parental duplex — Replication fork — DNA synthesis — Movement of the replication fork — Replicated daughter molecules

3'-hydroxy group at the end of the growing strand (Fig. 6.13). The second and third phosphates of the nucleotide form pyrophosphate, which is cleaved rapidly to inorganic phosphate by cellular pyrophosphatases. The hydrolysis of pyrophosphate makes the polymerization reaction irreversible.

The DNA polymerases require a single-stranded DNA as a template. For this reason, the parental DNA duplex has to be unwound before the DNA polymerase can set to work. While synthesizing the new strand in the $5' \rightarrow 3'$ direction, the enzyme moves along the template strand in the $3' \rightarrow 5'$ direction. DNA polymerases are "literate" enzymes. They can read the base sequence of their templates, and they even have enough common sense to incorporate only those bases in the new strand that pair correctly with the base in the template strand. Therefore *the new strand is exactly complementary to the template strand.*

FIG. 6.13

Template-directed synthesis of DNA by DNA polymerases.

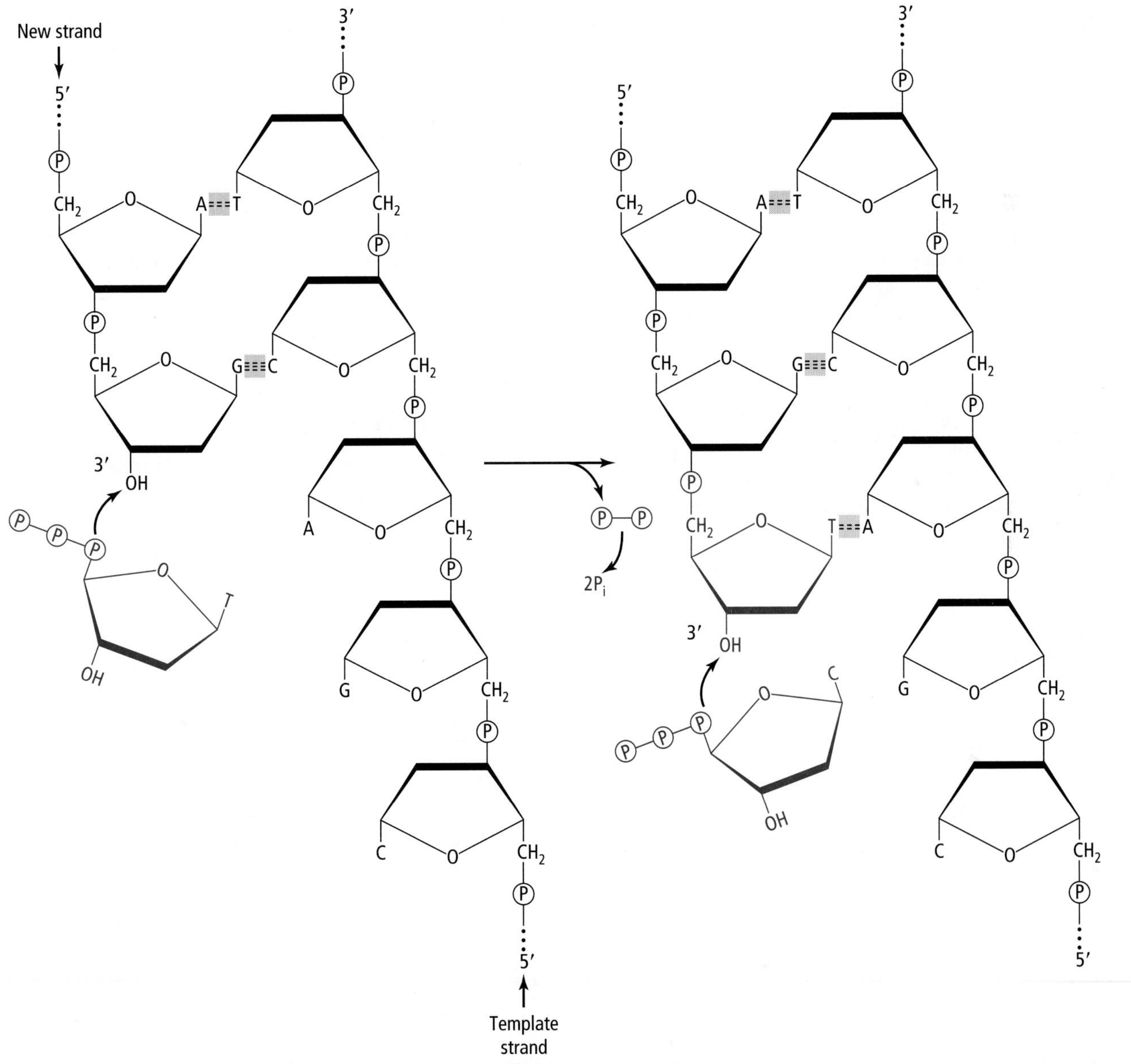

Bacterial DNA polymerases have exonuclease activities

A **nuclease** is a hydrolytic enzyme that cleaves phosphodiester bonds in a nucleic acid. DNAses cleave DNA, and RNAses cleave RNA. Nucleases that cleave internal phosphodiester bonds are called **endonucleases,** and those that cleave bonds at the ends are called **exonucleases.** Some exonucleases cleave only at the 5′ end of the strand; others cleave only at the 3′ end. Nucleases also are specific for either single-stranded or double-stranded substrates. Some are more or less nonselective for the bases in their substrate, whereas others cleave only very specific sequences.

All bacterial DNA polymerases have a **3′-exonuclease activity**, which is required for proofreading: nobody is perfect, and even the smartest DNA polymerase sometimes makes a mistake by incorporating the wrong nucleotide in the new strand. This can be deadly because a change of the base sequence, known as a **mutation,** can result in the synthesis of a faulty protein. Fortunately the enzyme can correct this type of error by removing the mismatched base from the 3′ terminus (Fig. 6.14). The polymerase replaces the mismatched base with the correct one, and replication can continue. *This proofreading mechanism reduces the error rate from 1 in 10⁴ or 1 in 10⁵ to approximately 1 in 10⁷.*

Most bacterial DNA polymerases have a **5′-exonuclease activity** as well (Fig. 6.14). This activity is not required for proofreading, but it removes damaged DNA during DNA repair (see Chapter 9.1) and erases the RNA primer during DNA replication.

E. coli has three different DNA polymerases, each designed for different tasks. They differ, in particular, in their affinity for the DNA template and in the number of nucleotides that are polymerized before the enzyme dissociates from the template. This property is described as **processivity.**

Poly I has a low processivity: its affinity for DNA is low, and therefore it tends to fall off its template after polymerizing only a few dozen nucleotides. It functions mostly in DNA repair (see Chapter 9) and plays only an accessory role in DNA replication.

Poly III *is the major enzyme of DNA replication. It clamps tightly to its template and polymerizes hundreds of thousands of nucleotides without interruption, at a rate of almost 1000 nucleotides per second.* Because the chromosome of *E. coli* has only approximately 4 million base pairs,

FIG. 6.14

Exonuclease activities of bacterial DNA polymerases. The products of these cleavages are nucleoside 5′-monophosphates. **A,** 3′-Exonuclease activity: only mismatched bases are removed from the 3′ end of the newly synthesized DNA strand. This activity is required for proofreading. **B,** 5′-Exonuclease activity: base-paired nucleotides are removed from the 5′ end. This activity is required to erase the RNA primer during DNA replication and to remove damaged portions of DNA during DNA repair.

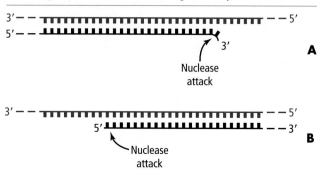

the enzyme may well replicate the whole chromosome in one sitting. The cell does not have more than approximately 10 poly III molecules at the time of DNA replication, so the high processivity is required for speedy and efficient DNA replication. **Poly II** has an intermediate processivity. It is thought to participate in some types of DNA repair.

Unwinding proteins create a single-stranded template for DNA replication

E. coli has a single circular chromosome with a total length of 1.3 mm — approximately 1000 times the diameter of the cell. Its replication is initiated at a single site, known as **oriC.** The 245-base-pair sequence of oriC is recognized by proteins that initiate the unwinding of the double helix. This unwinding creates two replication forks that move in opposite directions. *Unwinding and DNA synthesis proceed bidirectionally until the two replication forks meet at the opposite side of the chromosome* (Figs. 6.15 and 6.16). This process takes approximately 30 minutes.

Strand separation is an ATP-dependent process that requires a **helicase.** At least nine helicases have been described in *E. coli*, and one of them, the dnaB protein, is the major strand-separating protein during DNA replication. Once separated, the strands associate with a single-stranded DNA binding protein **(SSB protein),** which prevents reaggregation.

FIG. 6.15

Replication of the circular chromosome of *E. coli*. Replication proceeds bidirectionally from a single replication origin (oriC). – – – and · · · indicate new strands.

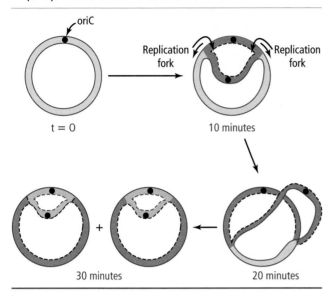

FIG. 6.16

Replication fork of *E. coli*.

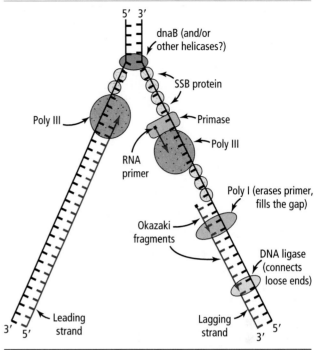

DNA gyrase also is required. This topoisomerase acts on the double-stranded DNA ahead of the moving replication fork. *It relaxes positive supertwists passively and induces negative supertwists by an ATP-dependent mechanism.* Without the gyrase, the unwinding at the replication fork soon would result in overwinding of the remaining unseparated DNA. Gyrase, helicase, and SSB protein are known collectively as **unwinding proteins.**

One of the new DNA strands is synthesized discontinuously

None of the known DNA polymerases can assemble the first nucleotides of a new chain. This task is left to a specialized RNA polymerase, the **primase.** This enzyme synthesizes a small piece of RNA, only approximately five nucleotides long, in the replication fork. *This small RNA, base-paired with the template strand, is the primer for poly III.*

The next problem concerns the direction of DNA synthesis. Overall, the synthesis of new DNA has to follow the movement of the replication fork, but the DNA polymerases synthesize only in the $5' \rightarrow 3'$ direction, reading their template $3' \rightarrow 5'$. Because the parental double strand is antiparallel, only one of the new DNA chains, the **leading strand,** can be synthesized by a poly III molecule, which simply

travels with the replication fork. The other strand, the **lagging strand,** has to be synthesized piecemeal. In the wake of the moving replication fork, the primase comes into action repeatedly, followed by poly III. This produces DNA fragments of approximately 1000 nucleotides that originally contain the RNA primer at their $5'$ end. They are called **Okazaki fragments.** The RNA primer is removed soon by the $5'$-exonuclease activity of poly I, and the gaps are filled by its polymerase activity.

Poly I cannot connect the loose ends of two Okazaki fragments. To do so requires a **DNA ligase,** which links the phosphorylated $5'$ terminus of one fragment with the free $3'$ terminus of another. To provide the energy for this bond formation, the bacterial enzyme hydrolyzes the phosphoanhydride bond in NAD (see Chapter 5), whereas the corresponding eukaryotic enzyme hydrolyzes ATP (Fig. 6.17).

RNA AND THE GENETIC CODE

All cellular RNAs are copied from a DNA template in the process of **transcription,** but only messenger RNA (**mRNA**) contains instructions for protein synthesis. Whereas its own base sequence is a faithful copy of the gene from which it was transcribed, the relationship between its base sequence and the amino acid sequence of the polypeptide is defined by the **genetic code.** Ribosomal RNA (**rRNA**) is not translated, but it plays structural and enzymatic roles as a constituent of the ribosome. The **transfer RNAs (tRNAs)** are small cytoplasmic RNAs that bind amino acids covalently and deliver them to the ribosome for protein synthesis (see Table 6.3). Only 3% of all cellular RNA in *E. coli* is mRNA, although approximately one third of the RNA synthesized in this organism is mRNA. The reason for this discrepancy is the short lifespan of bacterial mRNA—on the order of a few minutes. Human mRNAs, however, live for an average of 10 hours before they succumb to cellular nucleases.

RNA can base-pair like DNA

There are only two strictly chemical differences between DNA and RNA: RNA contains ribose instead

---

FIG. 6.17

Reaction of DNA ligase. The two DNA strands have to be base-paired with a complementary strand in a DNA duplex. *NMN,* Nicotinamide mononucleotide (contains nicotinamide + ribose + phosphate).

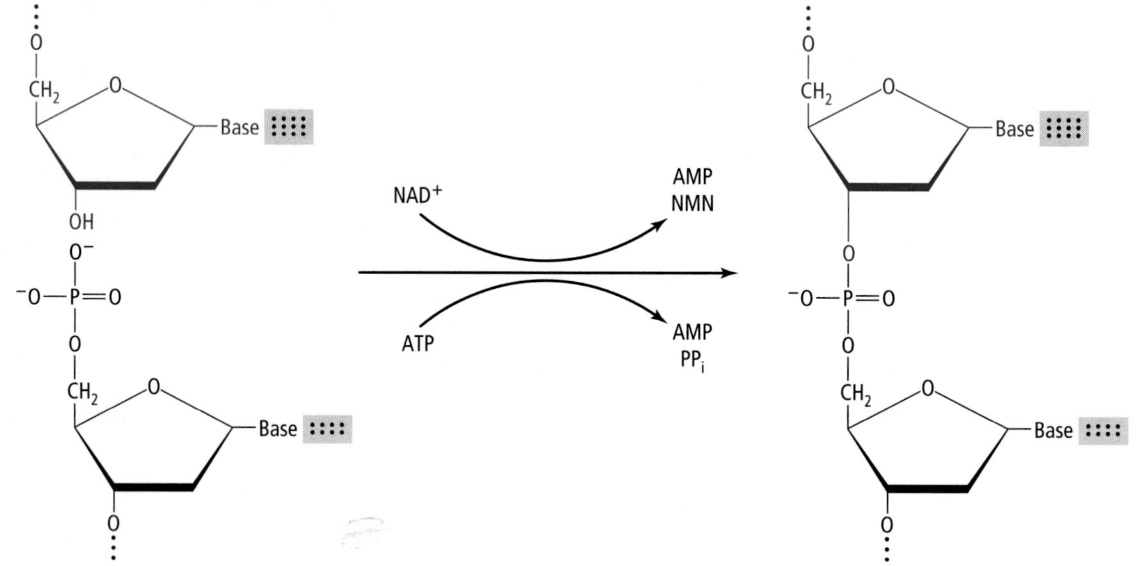

TABLE 6.3

Properties of ribosomal RNA (rRNA), transfer RNA (tRNA), and messenger RNA (mRNA)

Property	rRNA	tRNA	mRNA
Relative abundance	Most abundant	Less abundant	Least abundant
Mol wt (in *E. coli*)	1.2×10^6 0.55×10^6 3.6×10^4	$2-3 \times 10^4$	Heterogeneous
Location (in eukaryotes)	Ribosomes, nucleolus	Cytoplasm	Nucleus, cytoplasm
Function	Structure of ribosomal subunits, peptidyl transferase activity	Brings amino acids to the ribosome	Transmits information for protein synthesis

of 2-deoxyribose and uracil instead of thymine (see Table 6.4). Thymine and uracil are distinguished only by a methyl group, and because this methyl group does not participate in base pairing (Fig. 6.7), *both uracil and thymine pair with adenine.*

Although base-pairing is possible, the 2'-hydroxy group prevents the formation of a classical Watson-Crick double helix. Nevertheless, *RNA can form a double helix similar to that of A-DNA* (see Table 6.2). Moreover, hybrids between a DNA strand and an RNA strand form a double helix resembling A-DNA. Although RNA can form a double helix, *all cellular RNAs are single stranded.* Most RNA molecules (see Fig. 6.27) contain both unpaired portions and base-paired regions in which complementary sequences within the same strand form a double helix. True double-stranded RNA does occur as the genetic material of some viruses (see Chapter 7).

The sigma subunit of bacterial RNA polymerase is required for the specific initiation of transcription

All cellular RNA in bacteria is synthesized by **RNA polymerase.** The complete enzyme, known as the **RNA polymerase holoenzyme,** has the subunit structure α_2, β, β', σ (see Table 6.5). The σ subunit is bound only loosely to the other subunits. It is not required for the catalytic activity, and the **RNA polymerase core enzyme** (α_2, β, β') still is able to synthesize RNA, even at an increased rate.

Before starting transcription, RNA polymerase has to find the gene. Genes possess a recognition site immediately upstream of the transcribed sequence, to which the RNA polymerase has to bind before it can initiate transcription. This recognition site is called the **promoter.** How does the enzyme find the promoter? The holoenzyme binds nonselectively and with moderately high affinity to double-stranded DNA and slides along the double helix. Once it encounters a promoter, the enzyme stops moving. The transcriptional initiation complex thus formed is called the **closed complex.** The **open complex** is formed when the enzyme separates the DNA double helix on a length of approximately 18 base pairs, starting at a conserved AT-rich sequence approximately 10 base pairs upstream of the transcriptional start site. Strand separation is essential because *transcription, like DNA replication, requires a non − base-paired template strand.*

RNA polymerase binds the promoter through its σ subunit. The sigma subunit does not participate in the elon-

---

TABLE 6.4

Differences between DNA and RNA

Property	DNA	RNA
Sugar	2-Deoxyribose	Ribose
Bases	A, G, C, T	A, G, C, U
Strandedness in vivo	Double strand	Single strand
Typical size	Often $>10^6$ base pairs	60-20,000 bases
Function	Genetic information	Gene expression

TABLE 6.5

Comparison of the bacterial DNA polymerases and RNA polymerase

Property	DNA polymerase I	DNA polymerase III	RNA polymerase
Subunit structure	Single polypeptide	8 Subunits	$\alpha_2 \beta\beta'\sigma$
Mol wt	$\approx 103,000$	$\approx 170,000^*$	$\approx 450,000$
Substrates	dATP, dGTP, dCTP, dTTP	dATP, dGTP, dCTP, dTTP	ATP, GTP, CTP, UTP
Direction of synthesis	$5' \rightarrow 3'$	$5' \rightarrow 3'$	$5' \rightarrow 3'$
Template required	DNA	DNA	DNA
Primer required	Yes	Yes	No
Speed (bases/sec)	$10-20$	$600-1,000$	≈ 20
3'-Exonuclease activity	Yes	Yes	No
5'-Exonuclease activity	Yes	Yes	No

*Core enzyme ($\alpha + \epsilon + \vartheta$ subunits) only. Several other polypeptides are associated with this core enzyme in vivo.

FIG. 6.18

Consensus sequence for promoters in *E. coli*. All of these promoters are recognized by the major sigma subunit of *E. coli*. Some belong to *E. coli* genes, others to bacteriophages infecting *E. coli*. Only the base sequence of the coding strand (nontemplate strand) is shown. Colored bases to the right of the TATAAT consensus indicate start of transcription.

P$_R$	CGGCATGATA	TTGACT	TATTGAATAAAATTGGG TAAATTTGACTCAACG
T7Al	AAAAGAG	TTGACT	TAAAGTCTAACCTATAG GATACTTACAGCCAT
lac	ACCCCAGGC	TTTACA	CTTTATGCTTCCGGCTCGTATGTTGTGTGGAATT
araC	GCCGTGATTATAGACAC	TTTTGT	TACGCGTTTT TGTCATGGCTTTGGTC
trp	AAATGAGC	TGTTGACAA	TTAATCATCGAACTAG TTAACTAGTACGCAAG
bioB	CATAATCGAC	TTGTAAAC	CAAATTGAAAAGATT TAGGTTTACAAGTCTA
tRNA$_{tyr}$	CAACGTAACAC	TTTACAG	CGGCGCGTCATTTGA TATGATGCGCCCCGCT
Str	TGTATATTTC	TTGACAC	CTTTTCGGCATCGCCC TAAAATTCGGCGTCCT
Tet	ATTCTCATGT	TTGACAG	CTTATCATCGATAAGC TTTAATGCGGTAGTTT
Consensus sequence		TTGACA	TATAAT

gation phase of RNA synthesis, but rather dissociates away from the core enzyme after the formation of approximately 10 phosphodiester bonds. The dissociation of the σ subunit marks the transition from the initiation to the elongation phase of transcription: without the σ subunit, the core enzyme no longer has a specific affinity for the promoter. It is free to vacate the promoter and to travel along the base sequence of the gene.

Although they are all recognized by the same σ subunit, the promoters of different genes look surprisingly different. The binding site extends over approximately 60 base pairs and includes the first 10 to 12 bases of the transcribed sequence. Sequences that are reasonably well conserved in the promoters of different genes are clustered approximately 10 base pairs and 35 base pairs upstream of the transcriptional start site. Even these regions are not identical in different promoters, but we can deduce a **consensus sequence** of the most commonly encountered bases (Fig. 6.18).

Why do different genes have different promoters? The reason is that different genes have to be transcribed at different rates. Some are transcribed up to 10 times per minute, whereas others are transcribed only once every 10 or 20 minutes. Rate-limiting factors in transcription are the initial binding of the RNA polymerase holoenzyme to the promoter and the transition from the closed to the open initiation complex. These processes depend on the base sequence of the promoter. In general, *the more the promoter resembles the consensus sequence, the higher the rate of transcription.*

DNA is faithfully copied into RNA

RNA synthesis resembles DNA synthesis in most respects. Like the DNA polymerases, *RNA polymerase uses nucleoside triphosphates as precursors.* ATP, GTP, CTP, and UTP are required, and synthesis proceeds in the $5' \rightarrow 3'$ direction while the DNA template is read $3' \rightarrow 5'$ (Fig. 6.19). RNA polymerase, however, unlike the DNA polymerases, can do without a primer. It starts a new chain simply by placing a ribonucleoside triphosphate in the first position (Fig. 6.20).

Only one strand of the duplex DNA is read. This strand, which is complementary to the RNA, is called the *template strand.* The opposite strand, which has the same base sequence as the RNA transcript (T replacing U), is the **coding strand.** The speed of transcription in *E. coli* is on the order of 10 to 20 nucleotides incorporated per second, 50 times slower than DNA replication.

Like the DNA polymerases, RNA polymerase is lacking in creative spirit. It functions as a copy machine, faithfully transcribing a DNA sequence into an RNA sequence. *It has a 1000 times higher error rate than poly III,* though, with misincorporation frequencies on the order of 1 in 10,000. RNA polymerase has no nuclease activities, and it does not proofread its product. The high error rate can be tolerated because RNA is synthesized and degraded continuously; thus, the damage caused by a single faulty RNA molecule is slight.

The most important principle that we have encountered so far is that *all nucleic acid synthesis requires a DNA template.* Cellular organisms draw the informa-

FIG. 6.19

The elongation phase of transcription. RNA polymerase separates the double helix on a length of about 18 base pairs to form a "transcription bubble." Only one of the two DNA strands is used as a template.

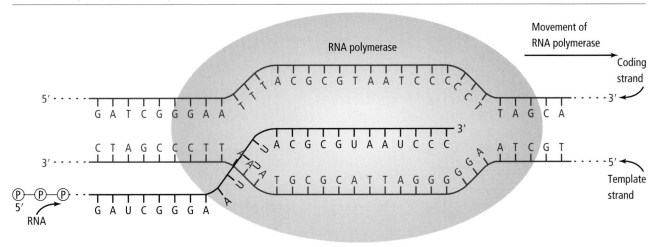

Transcription is terminated when the RNA forms a hairpin loop

How does RNA polymerase terminate transcription? Like the promoters, transcriptional termination sites look different in different genes. One consistent feature, however, is the presence of a twofold axis of symmetry: the base sequence of one DNA strand traced in one direction from the symmetry axis is the same as that of the opposite strand traced in the opposite direction (Fig. 6.21). A sequence of this type is called a **palindrome.** A palindrome is a word or sentence that reads the same in both directions, as in MADAM, I'M ADAM or A MAN—A PLAN—A CANAL—PANAMA. When a palindrome is transcribed, the RNA transcript forms a **hairpin loop** by internal base pairing. The hairpin loop often is rich in GC base pairs, which interact more strongly than AU base pairs. This GC-rich sequence often is followed by a U-rich sequence.

Transcription can be inhibited by drugs

Chemotherapeutic agents are used in the living organism to kill such undesirable life forms as pathogenic bacteria, fungi, parasites, and cancer cells. A good chemotherapeutic drug must be selective: it has to perform its mission without collateral damage to normal cells. As a rule of thumb, bacteria can be killed more easily in the human body than fungi or parasites because they are more different from our own cells than the eukaryotic pathogens; cancer cells are the most difficult to eradicate because they are too similar to the normal somatic cells from which they are derived.

Transcription can be inhibited in several ways. **Rifampicin** inhibits transcription by tight binding to the β subunit of bacterial RNA polymerase, but the major eukaryotic RNA polymerases (see Chapter 8) are not affected. Bacteria are not killed immediately by this treatment, but they become unable to grow: the drug is not **bactericidal** but **bacteriostatic.** Rifampicin is used for the treatment of several bacterial infections, including tuberculosis. Unfortunately the bacteria can become resistant to rifampicin by a point mutation that changes the structure of the rifampicin-binding site on the β subunit. With continued treatment, the resistant mutants are selected rapidly until the whole bacterial population is resistant, and the drug becomes useless.

Actinomycin D (Fig. 6.22) inhibits transcription by an entirely different mechanism. This drug contains a planar phenoxazone ring system that becomes intercalated (sandwiched) between two GC base pairs in double-stranded DNA, and two

FIG. 6.20

Formation of the first phosphodiester bond during transcription. The nucleotide at the 5′ terminus of the RNA remains in the 5′-triphosphate form. Compare this with the mechanism of DNA synthesis shown in Fig. 6.13.

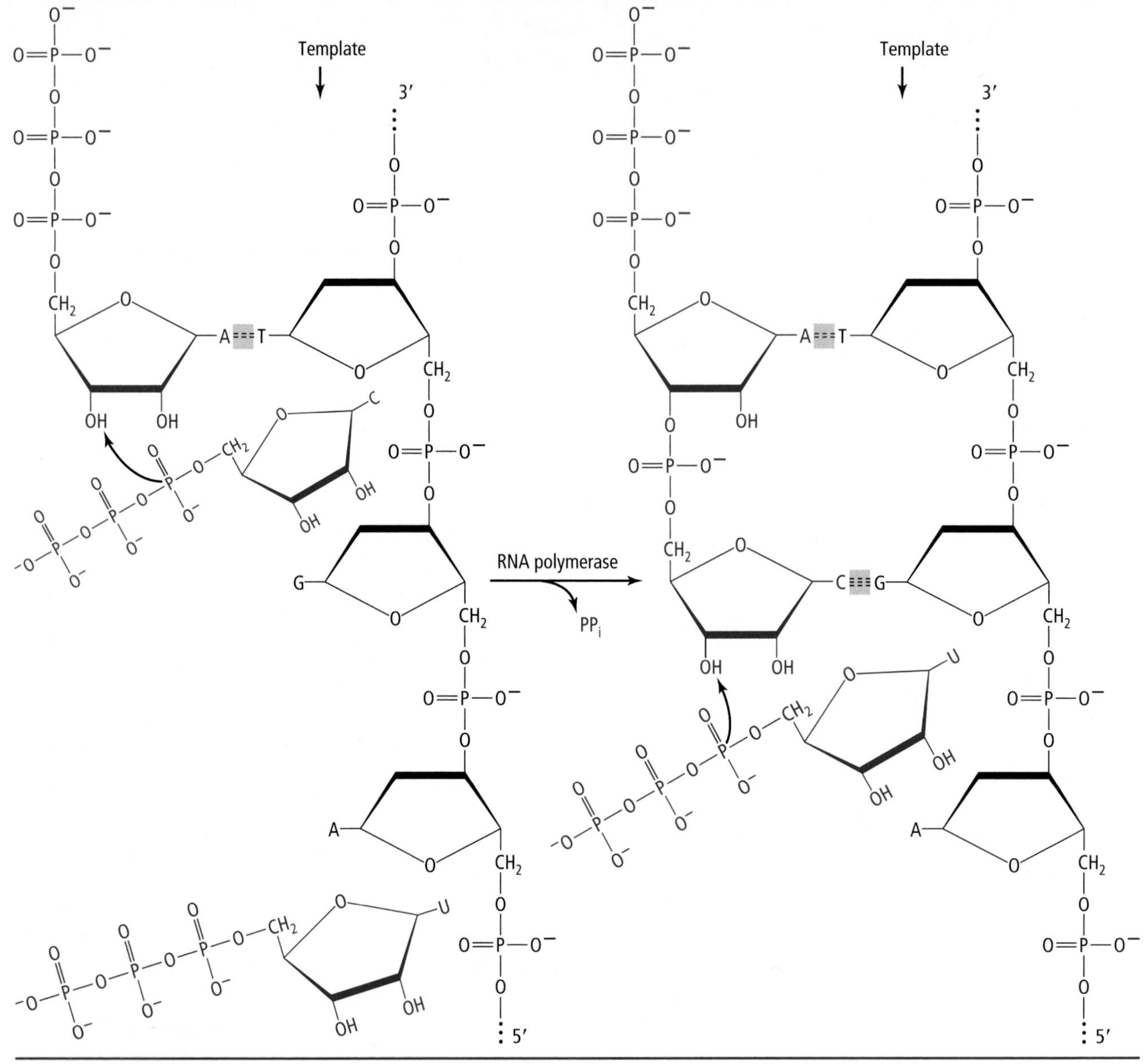

oligopeptide tails in the molecule clamp the drug to the minor groove of the double helix. RNA polymerase cannot transcribe past the bound drug. DNA has the same structure in all organisms. Therefore actinomycin D is toxic for eukaryotes as well as prokaryotes, and it cannot be used for the treatment of bacterial infections. However, for unknown reasons it is very effective in the treatment of Wilms' tumor (nephroblastoma), a rare childhood tumor.

Some RNAs are chemically modified after transcription

Chemical modifications of RNA after its synthesis by RNA polymerase are known collectively as **post-transcriptional processing**. Of the three major RNA types, **mRNA** is processed extensively in eukaryotes (see Chapter 8) but rarely in prokaryotes.

The **ribosomal RNAs** are derived from a single large precursor, both in prokaryotes and in eukary-

FIG. 6.21

Termination sequence of a viral gene that is transcribed by the bacterial RNA polymerase. **A,** Sequence of the DNA double strand. **B,** The RNA transcript forms a hairpin loop.

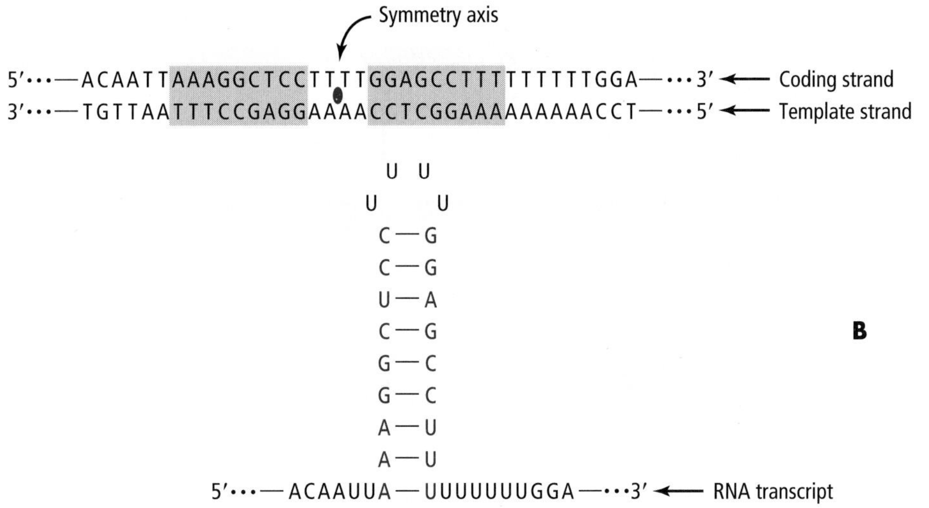

Symmetry axis

```
5'···—ACAATTAAAGGCTCCTTTTGGAGCCTTTTTTTTTGGA—···3' ← Coding strand      A
3'···—TGTTAATTTCCGAGGAAAACCTCGGAAAAAAAAACCT—···5' ← Template strand
```

```
          U  U
        U      U
        C — G
        C — G
        U — A
        C — G
        G — C
        G — C
        A — U
        A — U
5'···—ACAAUUA—UUUUUUUGGA—···3' ←  RNA transcript
```

B

FIG. 6.22

Structure of actinomycin D.

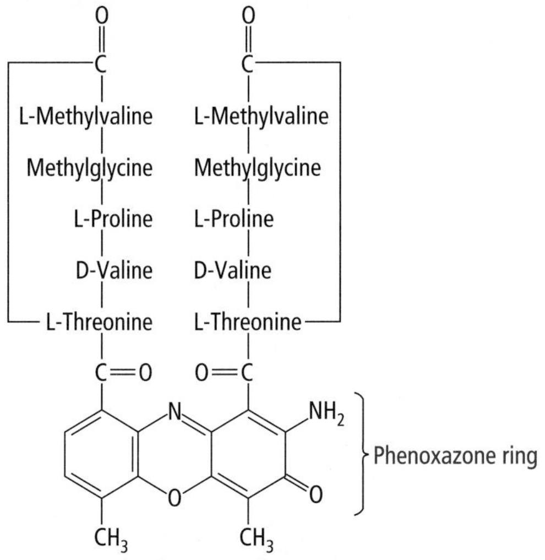

```
      O              O
      ‖              ‖
      C              C
  |       |      |       |
  | L-Methylvaline    L-Methylvaline |
  |       |      |       |
  | Methylglycine     Methylglycine |
  |       |      |       |
  | L-Proline       L-Proline |
  |       |      |       |
  | D-Valine        D-Valine |
  |       |      |       |
  L-Threonine      L-Threonine
      |              |
      C=O        O=C
```

Phenoxazone ring

mechanism of synthesis guarantees that the three rRNAs are produced in equimolar amounts. Bacterial rRNA contains some methylated bases as well, and eukaryotic rRNA contains some methylated ribose residues (Fig. 6.24). The methylating enzymes use S-adenosylmethionine (SAM, see Chapter 5) as a methyl group donor.

Most **tRNA** genes of E. coli are integrated into larger transcription units with other tRNA genes and sometimes with rRNA or protein-coding genes. A large transcript is produced from which the tRNA is modeled by the concerted action of various endo- and exonucleases. A great variety of unusual or chemically modified bases also occur in tRNA, both in prokaryotes and in eukaryotes (Fig. 6.24).

The genetic code defines the relationship between the base sequence of the mRNA and the amino acid sequence of the polypeptide

Obviously, a single base cannot specify an amino acid in a polypeptide, because mRNA has only four bases and polypeptides contain 20 amino acids. A sequence of two bases can specify 4^2 (16) amino acids, and a sequence of three bases can specify 4^3 (64) amino acids.

In fact, the genetic code is a triplet code in which a sequence of three bases on the mRNA, the **codon,** specifies an

otes (Fig. 6.23). Approximately seven transcription units for rRNA are present in the genome of E. coli, and each of them contains the sequences of the 5S, 16S, and 23S rRNAs. Some of these rRNA genes contain the sequences of one or several tRNAs as well. The large transcript that is synthesized initially by RNA polymerase is cleaved into the three rRNAs (+ tRNAs) by specific endonucleases. The bacterial ribosome contains one copy of each rRNA, and this

FIG. 6.23

Processing of rRNA precursors in prokaryotes and eukaryotes. **A,** In *E. coli.* **B,** In *Homo sapiens.*

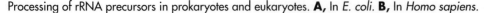

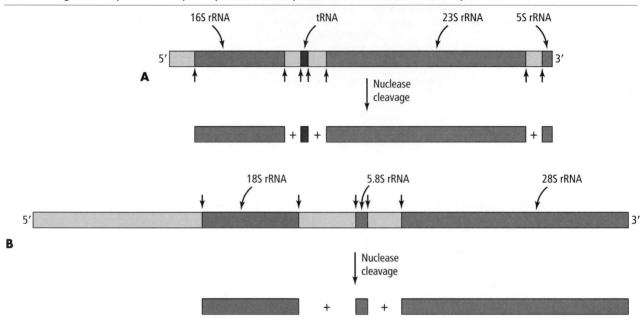

amino acid. This sequence of codons is translated by the ribosome in the $5' \rightarrow 3'$ direction, the same direction in which the mRNA itself is synthesized by RNA polymerase. *As the ribosome walks along the mRNA in the $5' \rightarrow 3'$ direction, it synthesizes the polypeptide in the amino $\rightarrow$ carboxy terminal direction.*

The genetic code (Fig. 6.25) has some prominent properties:

1. *It is colinear.* The sequence of amino acids in the polypeptide—from the amino end to the carboxy end—corresponds exactly to the sequence of their codons in the mRNA, read from the 5' to the 3' end.
2. *It is nonoverlapping and commaless.* Within the coding sequence the codons are aligned without overlap and without empty spaces in between. Each base belongs to one and only one codon.
3. *It contains 61 amino acid–coding codons and the three stop codons, UAA, UAG, and UGA.* One of the amino acid–coding codons, AUG, also serves as a start codon.
4. *It is unambiguous.* Each codon specifies one—and only one—amino acid.
5. *It is degenerate.* More than one codon may code for one amino acid.
6. *It is universal.* With the minor exception of the start codon AUG, which determines N-formyl methionine in prokaryotes and methionine in eukaryotes, the code is identical in prokaryotes and eukaryotes. Some minor variations, however, do occur in the very small genomes of mitochondria and chloroplasts, as well as in ciliated protozoa (Table 6.6).

The near-universality of the genetic code shows that *all surviving life on earth is descended from a common ancestor.* It is hard to imagine how a complex and seemingly arbitrary system like the genetic code could have been invented independently by different proto-cells. The universality of the code is interesting not only for the philosopher but also for the genetic engineer. It implies, for example, that *coding sequences of eukaryotic genes that are introduced artificially into prokaryotic cells can be expressed correctly.*

We have to address one last question: if there are three possible **reading frames** for a colinear, nonoverlapping, and commaless triplet code, how does the ribosome recognize the correct base triplet as a codon? The answer is that the ribosome locates the initiation codon AUG in the 5'-terminal region of the mRNA. It then reads successive base triplets as codons until it reaches a stop codon, which signals the end of the polypeptide. This im-

FIG. 6.24

Some posttranscriptional modifications in tRNA and rRNA. Hypoxanthine is introduced into tRNA by replacement of adenine. The other unusual bases shown here are produced by the enzymatic modification of existing bases.

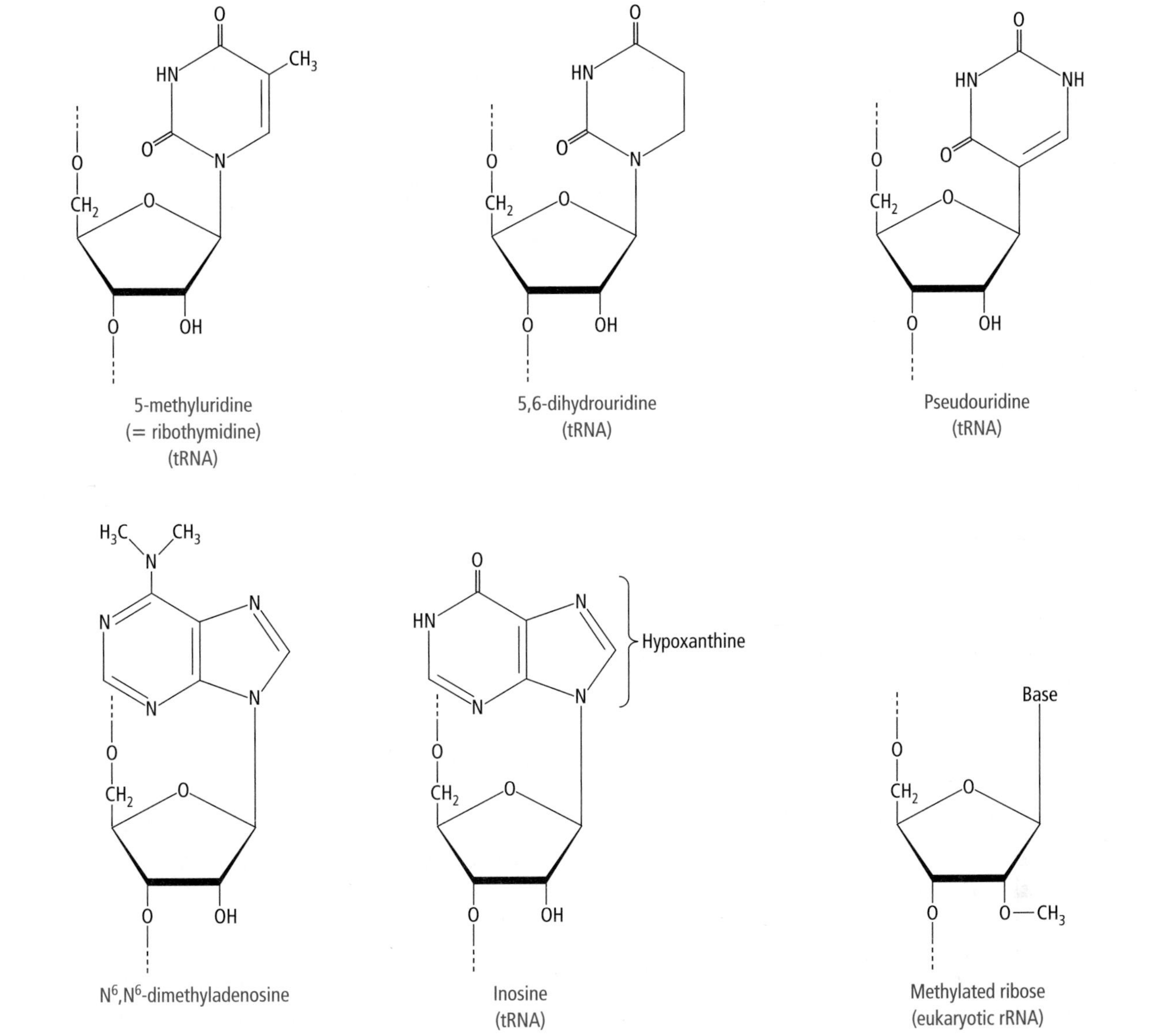

5-methyluridine
(= ribothymidine)
(tRNA)

5,6-dihydrouridine
(tRNA)

Pseudouridine
(tRNA)

N^6,N^6-dimethyladenosine

Inosine
(tRNA)

Methylated ribose
(eukaryotic rRNA)

plies that *the 5' and 3' ends of the mRNA are not translated* (Fig. 6.26).

PROTEIN SYNTHESIS

Transcription is simple: a sequence of four different bases simply is copied into another sequence of four different bases. Also, the bases in the template strand interact specifically, by base pairing, with the bases in the RNA transcript. Translation is far more difficult because there are no specific binding interactions between bases and amino acids. Therefore the mechanism of translation is complex, requiring not only mRNA and precursor amino acids but a whole specialized organelle — the ribosome.

tRNA is the adapter molecule in protein synthesis

The tRNAs are small, soluble RNAs, containing 70 to 90 nucleotides. Although their base sequences

TABLE 6.6

Variations of the genetic code

Codon	Standard code	Tetrahymena (a ciliate)	Mitochondria			
			Human	Yeast	Insects (Drosophila)	Plants (Maize)
UGA	Stop	Stop	Trp	Trp	Trp	Stop
UAA, UAG	Stop	Gln	Stop	Stop	Stop	Stop
AUA	Ile	Ile	Met	Met	Met	Ile
AGA, AGG	Arg	Arg	Stop	Arg	Ser	Arg
CUA, CUG, CUC, CUU	Leu	Leu	Leu	Thr	Leu	Leu

FIG. 6.25

The genetic code.

UUU ⎤ Phe UUC ⎦ UUA ⎤ Leu UUG ⎦	UCU ⎤ UCC ⎥ Ser UCA ⎥ UCG ⎦	UAU ⎤ Tyr UAC ⎦ UAA ⎤ Stop UAG ⎦	UGU ⎤ Cys UGC ⎦ UGA Stop UGG Trp
CUU ⎤ CUC ⎥ Leu CUA ⎥ CUG ⎦	CCU ⎤ CCC ⎥ Pro CCA ⎥ CCG ⎦	CAU ⎤ His CAC ⎦ CAA ⎤ Gln CAG ⎦	CGU ⎤ CGC ⎥ Arg CGA ⎥ CGG ⎦
AUU ⎤ AUC ⎥ Ile AUA ⎦ AUG Met (Start)	ACU ⎤ ACC ⎥ Thr ACA ⎥ ACG ⎦	AAU ⎤ Asn AAC ⎦ AAA ⎤ Lys AAG ⎦	AGU ⎤ Ser AGC ⎦ AGA ⎤ Arg AGG ⎦
GUU ⎤ GUC ⎥ Val GUA ⎥ GUG ⎦	GCU ⎤ GCC ⎥ Ala GCA ⎥ GCG ⎦	GAU ⎤ Asp GAC ⎦ GAA ⎤ Glu GAG ⎦	GGU ⎤ GGC ⎥ Gly GGA ⎥ GGG ⎦

vary widely, all tRNAs share some common structural and functional features (Fig. 6.27):

1. *The molecule is folded into a cloverleaf structure with three base-paired stems and three loops.*
2. *The 3′ terminus always ends with the sequence CCA. This part of the molecule can form a covalent bond with an amino acid.*
3. *One of the three non−base-paired loops of the cloverleaf contains the* **anticodon.** The three bases of the anticodon pair with the codon on the mRNA during ribosomal protein synthesis.

The other two leaflets of the cloverleaf are the **dihydrouridine loop** and the **TψC loop** (thymine−pseudouracil−cytosine), named after conserved bases in their structures. A variable loop also is present in most tRNAs. These structures participate in recognition by the aminoacyl-tRNA synthetases and in binding to the ribosome.

Amino acids are activated by an ester bond with the 3′-terminus of the tRNA

There are nearly 60 different tRNAs in the cell, and each of them presents only one amino acid to the ribosome. The amino acid derivative of the tRNA, the **aminoacyl-tRNA,** is formed by a soluble cytoplasmic **aminoacyl-tRNA synthetase.**

The balance of the activation reaction (Fig. 6.28) is

$$\text{Amino acid} + \text{tRNA} + \text{ATP} \rightleftharpoons$$
$$\text{Aminoacyl-tRNA} + \text{AMP} + \text{PP}_i$$

The reaction is reversible because the ester bond between amino acid and tRNA is almost as energy rich as a phosphoanhydride bond in ATP. Nevertheless it is driven to completion by the subsequent hydrolysis of inorganic pyrophosphate to inorganic phosphate, which removes pyrophosphate from the reaction equilibrium.

FIG. 6.26

The reading frame of mRNA and the importance of the start-and-stop codons. **A,** The determination of the reading frame. The ribosome identifies the start codon AUG, then reads successive base triplets as codons. The cotranscriptional initiation of translation depicted here is specific for prokaryotes. **B,** The overall structure of mRNA. mRNAs have a 5'-untranslated sequence upstream of the start codon and a 3'-untranslated sequence downstream of the stop codon. The 5'-untranslated region is required for the initial binding of the mRNA to the ribosome during the initiation of translation.

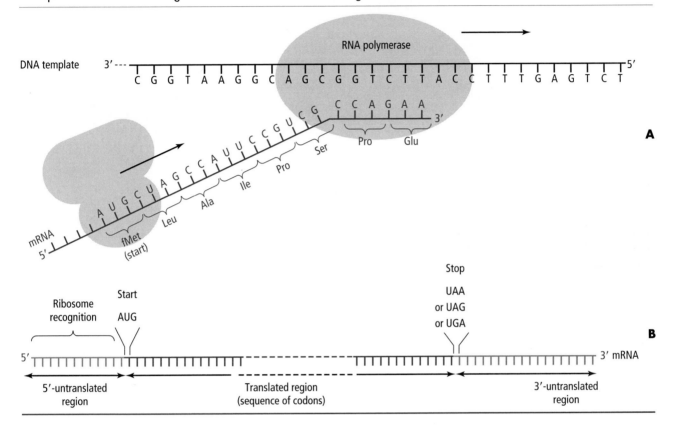

Many tRNAs recognize more than one codon

There are only 20 different aminoacyl-tRNA synthetases in bacterial cells, each of them specific for 1 of the 20 amino acids. If an amino acid can be bound to more than one tRNA, the same enzyme can recognize all acceptor tRNAs.

During protein synthesis, *the codon of the mRNA base-pairs with the anticodon of the tRNA in an antiparallel orientation.* Assuming strict Watson-Crick base pairing, we can therefore expect at least 61 different tRNAs for the 61 amino acid-coding codons. Actually, however, some protein-synthesizing systems can do with less. Mammalian mitochondria, for example, have no more than 22 different tRNAs.

This is possible because pairing between the third codon base and the first anticodon base does not always follow the strict rules of Watson-Crick base pairing: U at the 5' end of the anticodon can pair not only with A but also with G, and a G in the first anticodon position pairs either with C or with U. Also, in several tRNAs the first anticodon base is hypoxanthine (the corresponding nucleoside is called inosine), and this base can pair with A, U, or C. This freedom of base pairing is called **wobble.**

Part of the degeneracy of the genetic code is the result of wobble. As seen in Fig. 6.25, codons specifying the same amino acid usually differ in the third codon base. This is the "wobble position," and in many cases, the alternative codons are read by the same tRNA.

FIG. 6.27

Structure of a typical tRNA (yeast tRNA^Phe). Note the wide separation between the amino acid binding site ("acceptor stem") and the anticodon. Modified nucleosides: m^6A, 6-methyladenosine; m^5C, 5-methylcytidine; Cm, 2'-O-methylcytidine; m^7G, 7-methylguanosine; m^2G, 2-methylguanosine; m^2G, 2,2-dimethylguanosine; Gm, 2'-O-methylguanosine; UH_2, dihydrouridine; ψ^2, pseudouridine; Y, "hypermodified" purine. **A,** The "cloverleaf" structure. Conserved bases are indicated by dark color. **B,** The tertiary structure. The three stem-loop structures of the cloverleaf are shown in color. (© 1976 American Association for the Advancement of Science.)

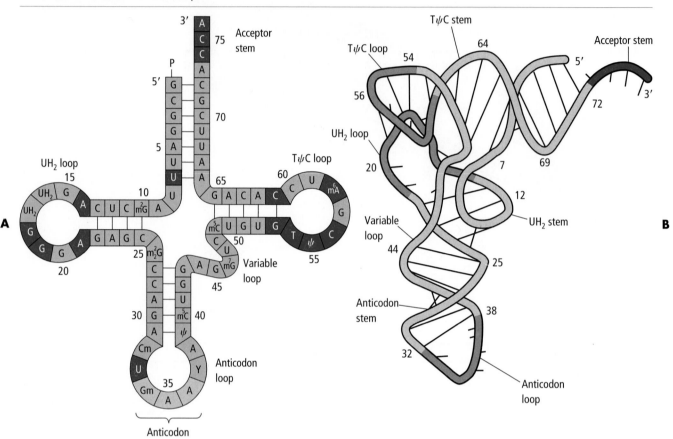

Ribosomes are the workbenches for protein synthesis

Although they enjoy the prestigious status of organelles, ribosomes are not surrounded by a membrane and do not form a separate cellular compartment. They simply are large, catalytically active ribonucleoprotein particles. In bacteria, they are either free-floating in the cytoplasm or attached to the plasma membrane, whereas in eukaryotes, they are either free in the cytoplasm or bound to the membranes of the endoplasmic reticulum (ER). In addition, the mitochondria of eukaryotes and, in plants, the chloroplasts, have their own

ribosomes. *E. coli* contains approximately 16,000 ribosomes; a typical eukaryotic cell has more than 1 million.

Ribosomes consist of a large subunit and a small subunit. According to their sedimentation rate in the ultracentrifuge, bacterial ribosomes are characterized as 70S ribosomes, with a 30S and a 50S subunit. Eukaryotic ribosomes—at least those in the cytoplasm and on the ER—are somewhat larger: an 80S ribosome is formed from a 40S and a 60S subunit. The ribosomal subunits are held together loosely by noncovalent interactions. In vitro, they aggregate at high Mg^{2+}/K^+ ratios but dissociate at low Mg^{2+} concentrations. In the cell, protein-

FIG. 6.28

Activation of the amino acid for protein synthesis. The activation reactions are catalyzed by highly selective aminoacyl-tRNA synthetases in the cytoplasm. The aminoacyl-tRNA is the immediate substrate for ribosomal protein synthesis.

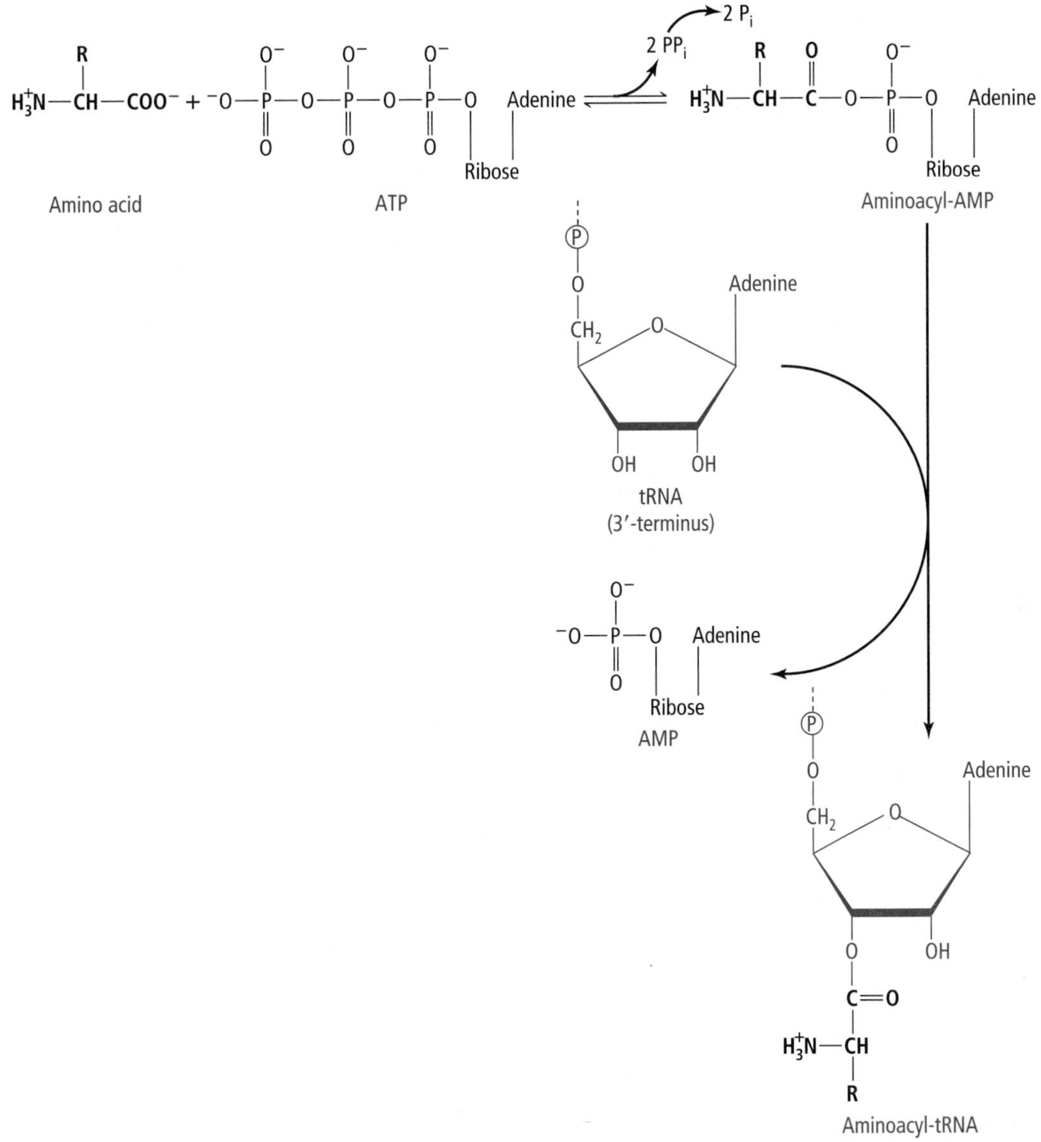

synthesizing ribosomes always are present as 70S or 80S particles, whereas inactive ribosomes exist as individual subunits.

The composition of bacterial and eukaryotic ribosomes is summarized in Table 6.7. Each ribosomal RNA molecule and (with one exception) each ribosomal protein is present in only one copy per ribosome. The components are held together noncovalently, and ribosomal subunits can be assembled in the test tube from the purified ribosomal proteins and RNAs.

Following are some features of ribosomal protein synthesis:

1. *During initiation of protein synthesis, the ribosome binds to a site near the 5′ terminus of the mRNA.*

2. *mRNA is read in the 5′ → 3′ direction; the polypeptide is synthesized in the amino → carboxy terminal direction.*

3. *The ribosome has two binding sites for tRNAs. These*

TABLE 6.7

Features of prokaryotic and eukaryotic ribosomes

Property	E. coli	H. sapiens (cytoplasmic)*
Diameter (nm)	20	25
Mass (kDa)	2700	4200
Sedimentation coefficient†		
Complete ribosome	70S	80S
Small subunit	30S	40S
Large subunit	50S	60S
RNA content	65%	50%
Protein content	35%	50%
rRNA, small subunit	16S	18S
rRNAs, large subunit	5S, 23S	5S, 5.8S, 28S
No. of proteins		
Small subunit	21	34
Large subunit	34	50

* For mitochondrial ribosomes, Chapter 8
† S, Svedberg unit, which describes the behavior of particles in the ultracentrifuge. Higher S values are associated with heavier particles, but they are not additive.

sites are occupied by an aminoacyl-tRNA and a peptidyl-tRNA during the elongation phase of protein synthesis.

4. *The ribosome possesses the enzymatic activity for peptide bond formation.*

5. *Energy-dependent steps in ribosomal protein synthesis require GTP rather than ATP.*

6. *Some steps in protein synthesis require the help of soluble cytoplasmic proteins,* which are known as **initiation factors, elongation factors,** and **termination factors.**

7. *Each ribosome synthesizes only one polypeptide at a time, but an mRNA molecule is read simultaneously by many ribosomes.* Ribosomes lined up on an mRNA can be seen under the electron microscope. These structures are called **polyribosomes** or **polysomes.**

The initiation complex contains formylmethionyl-tRNA

During the initiation phase of protein synthesis *the ribosome has to associate with mRNA and the initiator tRNA.* Translation starts at the initiation codon AUG, which is at least 25 nucleotides away from the

5′ terminus of the mRNA. In the initiation complex, AUG base-pairs with the anticodon of the **initiator tRNA,** which carries the modified amino acid N-formylmethionine (fmet). *Bacterial proteins always are synthesized with formylmethionine at their amino terminus.* In some proteins, this amino terminus is retained, but more commonly it is deformylated or the fmet is removed by a proteolytic cleavage.

Initially, the small (30S) ribosomal subunit associates with mRNA and the initiator tRNA to form the **30S initiation complex** (Fig. 6.29). In this complex, part of the 5′ untranslated region of the mRNA base-pairs with the 3′ end of the 16S RNA in the small ribosomal subunit. The most important sequence motif of the mRNA in this region is the **Shine-Delgarno sequence,** a purine-rich sequence (consensus sequence: AGGAG) approximately 10 nucleotides upstream of the initiation codon. Another specific interaction is the base pairing between the initiation codon and the anticodon of the fmet-tRNA. The initiation complex also contains three initiation factors, **IF1, IF2,** and **IF3.** IF1 and IF3 increase the rate of dissociation of the ribosomal subunits and maintain the dissociated state, respectively. IF2, which contains a bound GTP molecule, is required for the binding of the fmet-tRNA to the 30S initiation complex.

The **70S initiation complex** is formed when the 50S ribosomal subunit binds to the 30S initiation complex. The initiation factors are released while the bound GTP is hydrolyzed to GDP and inorganic phosphate.

The part of the ribosomal surface to which the initiator tRNA is bound is called the **P site** (for peptidyl-tRNA) because it is occupied by a peptidyl-tRNA during the elongation phase. A second tRNA-binding site, the **A site** (for aminoacyl-tRNA, or acceptor), still is empty. It accepts incoming aminoacyl-tRNA molecules during the elongation phase.

Polypeptides grow stepwise in the amino to carboxy terminal direction

The elongation cycle starts with the placement of an aminoacyl-tRNA in the A site (Fig. 6.30). This is not a passive process; the aminoacyl-tRNA is placed by **elongation factor Tu (EF-Tu).** Like IF2, EF-Tu is a GTP-binding protein, and it is a ternary complex of

FIG. 6.29

Formation of the 70S initiation complex in prokaryotes.

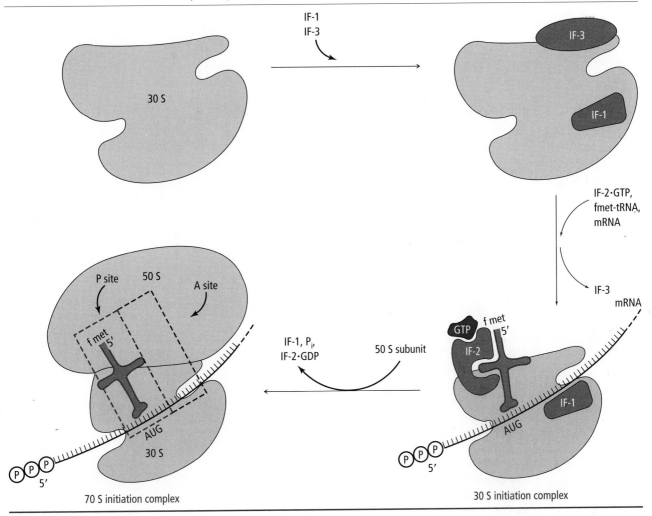

30 S

IF-1
IF-3

IF-3

IF-1

IF-2·GTP,
fmet-tRNA,
mRNA

IF-3

mRNA

P site   50 S   A site

f met
5'

IF-1, P$_i$,
IF-2·GDP

50 S subunit

GTP   f met
5'

IF-2

IF-1

AUG

AUG

30 S

30 S

P P P
5'

P P P
5'

70 S initiation complex

30 S initiation complex

EF-Tu, GTP, and the aminoacyl-tRNA that binds to the ribosome. EF-Tu is important for the specificity of placement: if the anticodon does not base-pair with the mRNA codon, the complex quickly dissociates from the ribosome. If codon and anticodon match, however, the bound GTP is hydrolyzed to GDP and phosphate, the EF-TU-GDP complex vacates the ribosome, and the aminoacyl-tRNA remains in the A site, ready for peptide bond formation.

The first peptide bond is formed by breakage of the ester bond between fmet and its tRNA and the *transfer of fmet to the amino group of the amino acid residue on the aminoacyl-tRNA in the A site* (Fig. 6.31). This reaction requires no external energy source, because the free energy content of the ester bond in the fmet-tRNA (≈ 7 kcal/mol) exceeds that of the pep-

tide bond (≈ 1 kcal/mol). The **peptidyl transferase** of the large ribosomal subunit that catalyzes peptide bond formation is not a ribosomal protein; rather, *it is an enzymatic activity of the 23S RNA in the large ribosomal subunit.* The 23S rRNA behaves, therefore, as an RNA enzyme, or **ribozyme.**

Peptide bond formation leaves a free tRNA in the P site and a peptidyl-tRNA in the A site. In the next step, called **translocation,** *the tRNA leaves the P site and the peptidyl-tRNA moves from the A site into the P site.* Codon-anticodon pairing is uninterrupted during translocation, and therefore *the ribosome moves along the mRNA by three bases.* Translocation requires the GTP-binding elongation factor **EF-G,** and it is accompanied by the hydrolysis of the bound GTP (Fig. 6.30).

FIG. 6.30

The first elongation cycle of ribosomal protein synthesis.

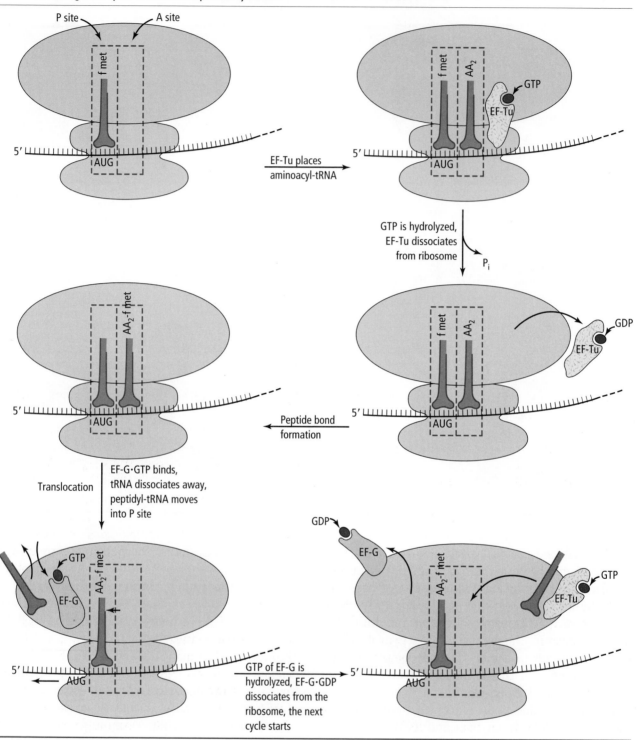

FIG. 6.31

Formation of the first peptide bond in the peptidyl transferase reaction.

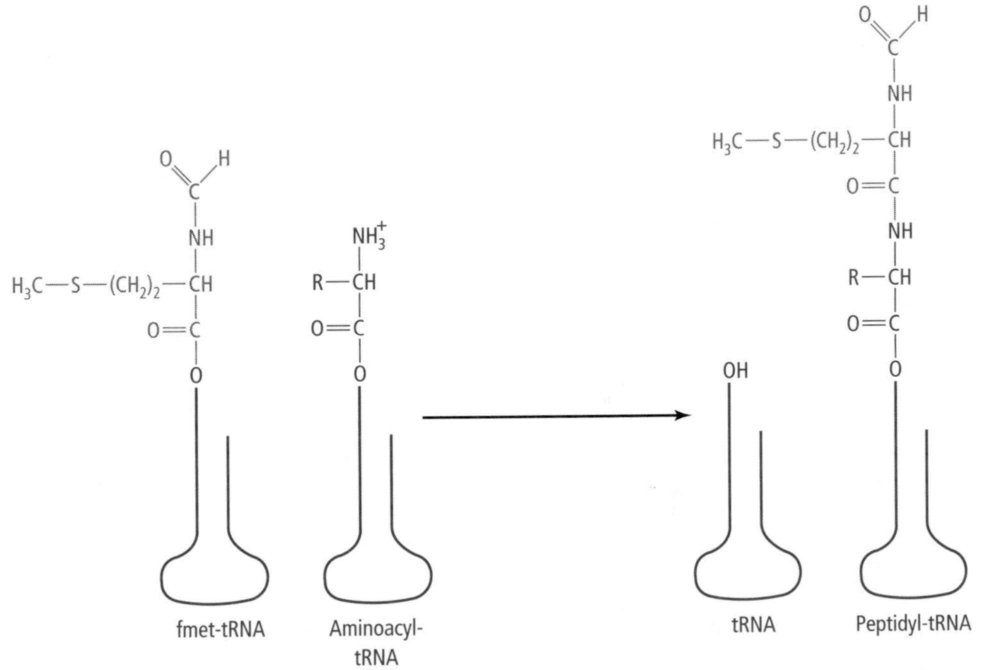

fmet-tRNA   Aminoacyl-tRNA   →   tRNA   Peptidyl-tRNA

The ribosome synthesizes polypeptides at a rate of approximately 15 amino acids per second. This is comparable with the speed of RNA synthesis ($\approx$ 20 nucleotides per second; see Table 6.5).

Stop codons are recognized by termination factors

The stop codons UAA, UAG, and UGA do not have matching tRNAs. Instead, one of two **termination factors** (also called **release factors**) binds to the stop codon. RF1 binds to UAA and UAG; RF2 binds to UAA and UGA. A third termination factor, RF3, contains bound GTP. It associates with RF1 or RF2 on the ribosome, and this complex changes the specificity of the peptidyl transferase: rather than forming a new peptide bond, it hydrolyzes the bond between the peptide and its tRNA.

Protein synthesis is energetically expensive

Ribosomal protein synthesis requires GTP for the formation of the initiation complex, for placement of the aminoacyl-tRNAs, for translocation, and pos-

sibly for termination. During each elongation cycle, there is a recurrent expense of two GTPs for placement and translocation. In addition, two high-energy phosphate bonds in ATP are required for the formation of the aminoacyl-tRNA. Therefore *four high-energy bonds are consumed for the synthesis of each peptide bond.* In rapidly growing bacterial cells, protein synthesis may consume 30% to 50% of the total metabolic energy, but the human body spends only about 5% of its basal metabolic rate for this purpose.

Many antibiotics inhibit protein synthesis

Growth and long-term survival are not possible without active protein synthesis. Antibiotic inhibitors of ribosomal protein synthesis have been invented by many microorganisms for chemical warfare against their competitors. These antibiotics bind to various sites on the ribosome and interfere with individual steps in protein synthesis (see Table 6.8). Because of the structural differences between prokaryotic and eukaryotic ribosomes (see Table 6.7), most of these antibiotics are selective for either prokaryotes or eukaryotes.

TABLE 6.8

Some antibiotic inhibitors of ribosomal protein synthesis

Drug	Target organisms	Ribosomal subunit bound	Effect on protein synthesis
Streptomycin	Prokaryotes	30S	Inhibits initiation, causes misreading of mRNA
Tetracycline	Prokaryotes	30S	Inhibits aminoacyl-tRNA binding
Chloramphenicol	Prokaryotes	50S	Inhibits peptidyl transferase
Cycloheximide	Eukaryotes	60S	Inhibits peptidyl transferase
Erythromycin	Prokaryotes	50S	Inhibits translocation
Puromycin	Prokaryotes, eukaryotes	50S, 60S	Terminates elongation

The inhibition of protein synthesis prevents cell growth, but most bacteria can survive for considerable periods without protein synthesis. Therefore *most ribosomally acting antibiotics are not bactericidal but bacteriostatic* (streptomycin is an exception). As in the case of rifampicin, bacteria can become resistant to ribosomally acting antibiotics by mutations that affect the target of drug action. Streptomycin resistance, for example, results from mutations in the gene for S12, a protein of the small ribosomal subunit to which this antibiotic binds. Even streptomycin-dependent bacterial mutants could be selected in the laboratory!

REGULATION OF GENE EXPRESSION

Some proteins are synthesized at all times. These proteins are called **constitutive. Inducible** proteins, however, are synthesized only under certain conditions.

Bacteria have to adjust their metabolic activities to the nutrient supply. For example, the cell can obtain its metabolic energy from such alternative sources as glucose, lactose, sucrose, various organic acids, and amino acids. In a cup of milk, for example, which contains lactose as its principal carbohydrate, the bacterium needs the enzymes of lactose degradation but not those for the degradation of sucrose. If, however, the bacterium falls into a glass of lemonade, which contains sucrose but not lactose, the enzymes of sucrose degradation are useful, but those of lactose metabolism are not.

The enzymes of biosynthetic pathways are required only when the end product of the pathway is not available from external sources. The enzymes of tryptophan synthesis, for example, are required only when the cell has to grow on a tryptophan-free medium.

Multicellular eukaryotes like us require regulated gene expression not only for metabolic adjustments to a fluctuating nutrient supply but also for cell and tissue differentiation. *All cells of our body have the same genes, but different cells make different proteins.* Hemoglobin, for example, is synthesized only in the bone marrow, and protein hormones are made only in specialized endocrine glands. *These differences are the result of cell-specific gene expression.*

The following sections will introduce the principles of transcriptional regulation in prokaryotes. The corresponding processes in eukaryotes will be discussed in Chapter 8.

A repressor protein regulates the transcription of the *lac* operon in *E. coli*

The disaccharide lactose can be used by *E. coli* for the generation of metabolic energy. After its transport across the plasma membrane by the membrane carrier **lactose permease**, lactose is cleaved to free glucose and galactose by the enzyme **β-galactosidase** (Fig. 6.32). A third protein, **β-galactoside transacetylase**, is not required for lactose catabolism, but it acetylates several other β-galactosides. It probably is concerned with the removal of nonmetabolizable β-galactosides from the cell. These three proteins are inducible: in the absence of lactose the cell contains only approximately 10 molecules of β-galactosidase, but several thousand molecules are

FIG. 6.32

The β-galactosidase reaction. A small percentage of the substrate is not hydrolyzed but rather is isomerized to 1,6-allolactose in a minor side reaction.

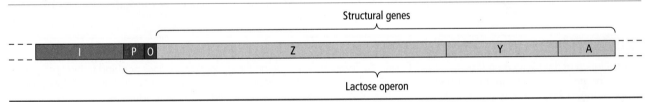

Lactose

−H₂O

Galactose + Glucose

1,6-Allolactose

FIG. 6.33

Structure of the lactose *(lac)* operon of *E. coli*. Promoter *(P)*, operator *(O)*, and structural genes are contiguous in all bacterial operons; the regulatory gene *(I)* may or may not be located next to the operon. *Z*, Gene for β-galactosidase; *Y*, gene for lactose permease; *A*, gene for β-galactoside transacetylase.

Structural genes

| I | P | O | Z | Y | A |

Lactose operon

present when lactose is the only carbon source. The levels of the permease and the transacetylase parallel exactly those of β-galactosidase.

The clue to this phenomenon was provided by gene mapping: *the genes for the three proteins are contiguous on the bacterial chromosome, and they are transcribed into a single polycistronic mRNA.* Therefore a single promoter is sufficient for the transcription of all three genes. The ribosome can synthesize three different polypeptides from this mRNA, because the coding sequence of each gene ends with a stop codon. At a short distance, the stop codons of the first two genes are followed by an internal start codon at which the synthesis of the next polypeptide is initiated.

Between the three protein-coding genes, or **structural genes**, and their shared promoter is an **operator** (Fig. 6.33; also see Fig. 6.36), a short regulatory DNA sequence that binds the ***lac* repressor.** There is some overlap between the RNA polymerase-binding site (promoter) and the binding site for the *lac* repressor (operator). Therefore *the RNA polymerase is unable to bind to the promoter when the operator is occupied by the* lac *repressor.*

The *lac* repressor is a tetrameric protein with four identical subunits, encoded by a separate gene that is transcribed constitutively at a low rate. In the absence of lactose, the *lac* repressor binds tightly to the operator and prevents the transcription of the structural genes. In the presence of lactose, however, a small amount of 1,6-allolactose is formed.

This minor side product of the β-galactosidase reaction (Fig. 6.32) binds tightly to the *lac* repressor, changing its conformation by an allosteric mechanism. The repressor-allolactose complex no longer binds to the operator, and the structural genes can be transcribed. 1,6-Allolactose functions as an **inducer** of the *lac* operon. The **operon** is defined as *the functional unit of promoter, operator, and structural genes.* In the case of the *lac* operon, the regulatory gene immediately precedes the operon, but this is not necessarily the case in other operons.

In many anabolic operons the product of the pathway acts as a corepressor

The tryptophan (*trp*) operon of *E. coli* codes for a set of five polypeptides that are required for the synthesis of tryptophan. The bacteria also can obtain their tryptophan—at far lesser expense—from the nutrient medium. Therefore *the energetically expensive biosynthetic pathway is required only when external tryptophan is not available.*

The arrangement of promoter, operator, and structural genes is essentially the same as in the *lac* operon (Fig. 6.34). There is, however, one important functional difference: the repressor of the *trp* operon, a dimer of identical subunits, is by itself unable to bind to the operator. *It becomes an active repressor only after binding tryptophan.* The operon is, therefore, transcribed only in the absence of tryptophan when the biosynthetic enzymes are actually needed. In this system the repressor protein is called an **aporepressor,** and tryptophan acts as a **corepressor.** This regulatory strategy is typical for anabolic operons.

Glucose regulates the transcription of many catabolic operons

When grown on a medium that contains both glucose and lactose, *E. coli* metabolizes glucose first. The levels of β-galactosidase and of the other products of the *lac* operon are very low during this period, and *the enzymes of lactose metabolism are induced only when glucose is depleted* (Fig. 6.35). This metabolic pattern is advantageous because glucose is metabolized more easily than lactose. The thrifty bacterium saves the expense for the synthesis of lactose-metabolizing enzymes by metabolizing glucose first. Not only the *lac* operon but also many other catabolic operons are repressed in the presence of glucose. This phenomenon is called **catabolite repression** (Fig. 6.36).

Catabolite repression is mediated by **cyclic AMP**

FIG. 6.34

Regulation of the tryptophan *(trp)* operon of *E. coli*. **A,** Tryptophan is absent: the aporepressor does not bind to the operator, and the structural genes are transcribed. *P,* Promoter; *O,* operator. **B,** Tryptophan is abundant: the "holorepressor" (aporepressor + tryptophan) binds to the operator. The binding of RNA polymerase is prevented, and the structural genes are not transcribed.

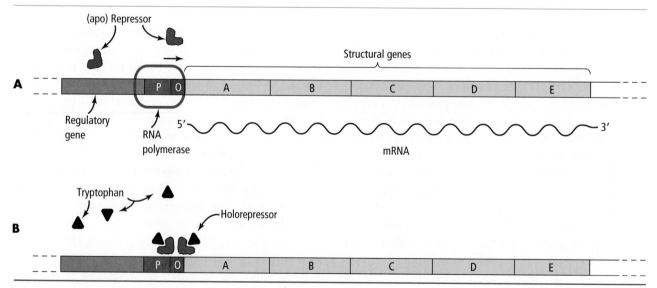

FIG. 6.35

Growth of *E. coli* bacteria on a mixture of glucose and lactose.

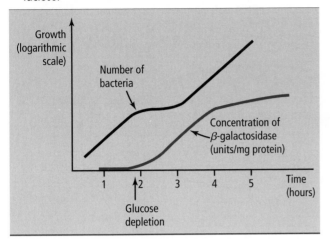

(cAMP). This regulatory metabolite serves as a second messenger of hormone action in animals and humans (see Chapter 26), but in bacteria it is regulated by glucose: *the intracellular cAMP level is low when glucose is plentiful and high when it is scarce.*

When glucose is depleted and cAMP is abundant, cAMP binds to a **catabolite activator protein (CAP),** a dimer of two identical 22-kDa subunits. CAP alone does not bind specifically to regulatory DNA sites, but *the CAP-cAMP complex binds tightly to the promoters of many catabolic operons,* including the *lac* operon. The binding sites for RNA polymerase and the CAP-cAMP complex are juxtaposed (Fig. 6.37, A), and the DNA-bound CAP-cAMP complex provides additional sites of interaction for RNA polymerase, thereby facilitating its binding to the promoter and the initiation of transcription.

FIG. 6.36

The mechanism of catabolite repression. The promoter of the *lac* operon is intrinsically weak and permits a high rate of transcription only when the CAP-cyclic AMP (cAMP) complex is bound to the DNA of the promoter. The cAMP level is low in the presence of glucose but rises in the absence of glucose when the cAMP-forming enzyme adenylate cyclase is activated. The catabolite activator protein *(CAP)* binds the promoter only when it is complexed with cAMP.

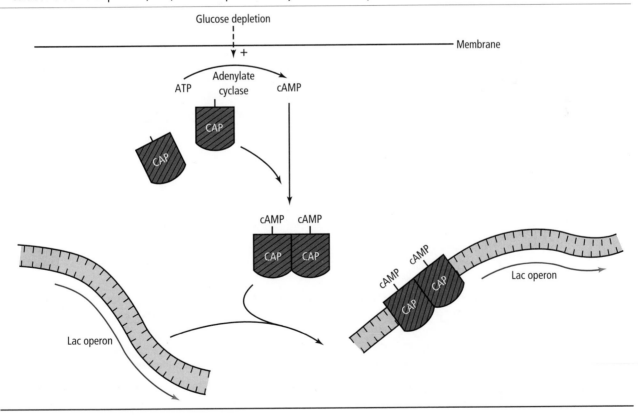

FIG. 6.37

Regulation of the lactose operon. **A,** The binding sites for RNA polymerase, repressor, and CAP-cAMP. **B,** Lactose absent, glucose present: RNA polymerase cannot start transcription. **C,** Lactose present, glucose present: weak binding of RNA polymerase to the promoter. **D,** Lactose present, glucose absent: strong binding of RNA polymerase to the promoter; high rate of transcription.

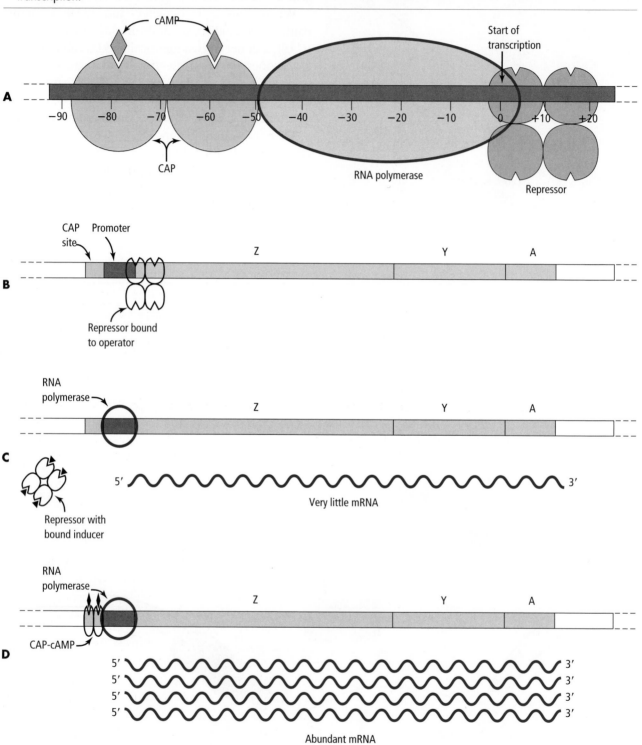

Transcriptional regulation is based on protein-DNA interactions

After encountering a few examples of transcriptional regulation in prokaryotes, we can point out some general features:

1. *The classical operon model applies only to prokaryotes.* The protein-coding genes of eukaryotes rarely are transcribed into a polycistronic mRNA, and functionally related genes may indeed be widely separated from each other. The genes for hemoglobin α chains and β chains, for example, are on different chromosomes (see Chapter 9).

2. *Transcription is controlled by proteins that bind to regulatory DNA sequences in the vicinity of the transcriptional initiation site.* The proteins can recognize these sites because the edges of the DNA bases are exposed in the major and minor grooves of the double helix. The regulatory proteins are allosteric, with binding and nonbinding conformations.

3. *Regulatory DNA-binding proteins often are controlled by small molecules such as 1,6-allolactose, cAMP, and tryptophan.* However, other control mechanisms are possible. These include interactions with other regulatory proteins and covalent modification by phosphorylation/dephosphorylation.

4. *The binding of a protein to a regulatory DNA sequence can either increase or decrease the rate of transcription.* These effects are called **positive control** and **negative control,** respectively. The stimulation of transcription by CAP-cAMP is an example of positive control, and the actions of the *lac* repressor and the *trp* repressor are examples of negative control.

5. *Most transcriptional regulators are either dimers (CAP, trp repressor) or larger oligomers (lac repressor) with identical or slightly different subunits.* Their structures are therefore symmetric. The symmetry of the proteins is reflected in the DNA sequences to which they bind: we find stretches of **dyad symmetry,** with the same kind of palindromic sequences that we encountered in transcriptional termination sites (Figs. 6.21 and 6.38). The oligomeric nature of DNA-binding regulatory proteins facilitates allosteric changes in their conformation, and their responses to effector molecules may be accentuated by positive cooperativity between binding sites on different subunits.

FIG. 6.38

Incomplete palindromic sequences in the binding sites of the *lac* repressor, the *trp* repressor, and the CAP-cAMP complex. Most transcriptional regulators bind their cognate DNA sites in a dimeric form, each subunit interacting with one leg of the palindrome left and right of the symmetry axis. **A,** The *lac* operator. **B,** The *trp* operator. **C,** The CAP-cAMP binding site of the *lac* operon.

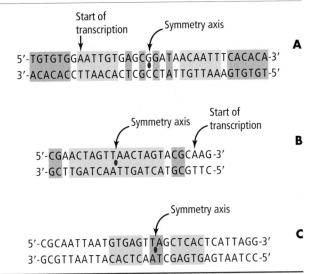

SUMMARY

The heritable characters of the cell are laid down in the base sequence of its DNA. DNA as it occurs in cells is a large, double-stranded molecule with an alternating sequence of 2-deoxyribose and phosphate in each strand, and the four bases adenine (A), guanine (G), cytosine (C), and thymine (T). The bases in opposite strands interact, forming A-T base pairs and G-C base pairs. Therefore the base sequence of one strand predicts the base sequence of the opposite strand. DNA can be replicated to form two identical daughter molecules. This requires the unwinding of the parental double strand and the synthesis of new complementary strands, with one of the old strands always used as a template. The new strands are synthesized by DNA polymerases, using deoxyribonucleoside triphosphates as precursors.

Gene expression requires the synthesis of RNA by RNA polymerase in a process called transcription. Like DNA replication, transcription requires a DNA template. The functional unit of gene expression is the gene, which is defined as the length of DNA coding for a polypeptide, or for a functional RNA in the case of the genes for ribosomal RNA (rRNA) and transfer RNA (tRNA). The RNA transcript of a protein-coding gene is called a messenger RNA (mRNA).

The set of rules by which the base sequence of the mRNA is translated into the amino acid sequence of the polypeptide is called the genetic code. Amino acids are specified by base triplets called codons. There are 61 amino acid-coding codons and three stop codons. The amino acid-coding codons are recognized by tRNAs during protein synthesis, and each tRNA presents an amino acid to the ribosome. During protein synthesis, the ribosome walks along the mRNA in the $5' \rightarrow 3'$ direction while polymerizing the polypeptide in the amino $\rightarrow$ carboxy terminal direction.

Gene expression is regulated. Genes contain regulatory DNA sequences near the transcriptional start site that bind regulatory proteins. The enhancement of transcription by a DNA-binding protein is called positive control, and the inhibition of transcription is called negative control.

Further Reading

Adams RLP, Knowler JT, Leader DP: *The biochemistry of the nucleic acids*, 11th ed. Chapman and Hall, London, 1992.

Arustein HRV, Cox RA: *Protein biosynthesis*. Oxford University Press, Oxford, 1992.

Sinden RR: *DNA structure and function*. Academic Press, New York, 1994.

QUESTIONS

1. The base triplet 5'-GAT-3' on the template strand of DNA is transcribed into mRNA. The anticodon that recognizes this sequence during translation is
   A. 5'-GAT-3'
   B. 5'-GAU-3'
   C. 5'-UAG-3'
   D. 5'-AUC-3'
   E. 5'-ATC-3'

2. The high fidelity of DNA replication in *E. coli* would not be possible without
   A. The high processivity of DNA polymerase III
   B. The σ subunit of DNA polymerase I
   C. The 5'-exonuclease activity of DNA polymerase III
   D. The 3'-exonuclease activity of DNA polymerase III
   E. The extremely high accuracy of the aminoacyl-tRNA synthetases

3. Stop codons are present
   A. On the coding strand of DNA, where they signal the end of transcription
   B. On the template strand of DNA, where they signal the end of transcription
   C. On the mRNA, where they signal the end of translation
   D. On the tRNA, where they signal the end of translation
   E. On termination factors, where they signal the end of translation

4. As a result of a mutation, an *E. coli* cell produces an aberrant aminoacyl-tRNA synthetase that attaches not leucine but isoleucine to one of the leucine-tRNAs. The result of this kind of mutation would be
   A. A disruption of codon-anticodon pairing during protein synthesis
   B. Premature chain termination during ribosomal protein synthesis
   C. Impaired initiation of ribosomal protein synthesis
   D. Inability of the aminoacyl-tRNA to bind to the ribosome
   E. A change in the genetic code

5. Like lactose, the pentose sugar arabinose can be used as a source of metabolic energy by *E. coli*. The most reasonable prediction for the regulation of the arabinose-catabolizing enzymes would be that
   A. Enzymes of arabinose catabolism are induced when glucose is plentiful.
   B. A repressor protein prevents the synthesis of arabinose-catabolizing enzymes in the absence of arabinose.
   C. The catabolite activator protein prevents the synthesis of arabinose-catabolizing enzymes in the absence of arabinose.
   D. Arabinose is likely to act as a corepressor, which is required for the binding of the repressor to the operator.
   E. Arabinose affects the synthesis of arabinose-catabolizing enzymes by increasing the cellular cyclic AMP level.

Chapter 7

Viruses

Cellular organisms have three prominent properties:

1. **Structure.** All living cells are surrounded by a plasma membrane that forms the boundary between the cell and its environment.
2. **Metabolism.** Cells generate metabolic energy, which is used for the synthesis of cellular macromolecules and for the maintenance of cell structure.
3. **Replication.** Cells possess genetic information in the form of DNA, and this information is replicated faithfully during each cycle of cell division.

Viruses have dispensed with the first two attributes of life: they do not form a cellular structure, and they do not generate metabolic energy. They do have nucleic acid–based genetic information, but replication is possible only in a host cell. *All viruses are obligatory intracellular parasites*, and we encounter them as the causative agents of many diseases, ranging from the common cold to acquired immunodeficiency syndrome (AIDS). In this chapter we introduce the life cycles and reproductive strategies of the major types of viruses.

Viruses can replicate only in a host cell

Viruses are villains not by choice but by necessity. Like other life forms, they have genetic information enshrined in a nucleic acid genome. However, they have no ribosomes to translate their genes into protein, and they lack the machinery for the generation of metabolic energy. To reproduce despite their many handicaps, they have to invade a host cell and appropriate its metabolic energy and protein-synthesizing machinery.

Outside the host cell, the virus exists as an inert virus particle, the **virion.** The virion is a package of genetic information wrapped in a protein coat. *Any kind of nucleic acid may form the viral genome:* some viruses have double-stranded DNA; others have single-stranded DNA, single-stranded RNA, or double-stranded RNA. Viruses are genetic paupers, with anywhere between 3 and 250 genes. *E. coli*, in contrast, has approximately 2000 genes, and humans have 50,000 to 100,000.

The nucleic acid genome is enclosed by a protein coat or **capsid.** The capsid is formed from a small number of different proteins that occur in a large number of copies and are arranged in a regular, crystalline structure. On a weight basis, most viruses contain far more protein than nucleic acid. The protein coat protects the nucleic acid from physical insults and enzymatic attack. It also is required for the virus to recognize and invade the host cell. Many animal viruses not only consist of nucleic acid and protein coat, which make up the **nucleocapsid,** but also are surrounded by an **envelope.** The viral envelope is a piece of host-cell membrane appropriated by the virus. It is studded with viral proteins, the **spike proteins** (Fig. 7.1).

Once it has entered its host cell, the viral nucleic acid is replicated. The viral genes, now stripped of their protein coat, direct the synthesis of viral proteins. Some of these proteins are enzymes for viral replication; others are the building blocks for the capsid or appear as spike proteins in the viral envelope.

FIG. 7.1

Sizes and structures of some typical viruses. **A,** Papilloma (wart) virus: a nonenveloped DNA virus of ikosahedral shape (spherical symmetry). **B,** Adenovirus: another nonenveloped DNA virus. **C,** Rabies virus: an enveloped RNA virus. **D,** Influenza virus: an enveloped RNA virus containing eight segments of ribonucleoprotein with helical symmetry.

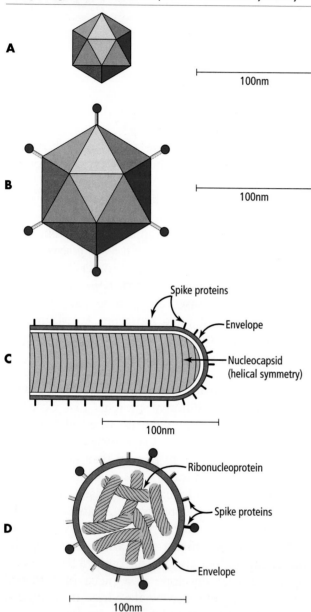

FIG. 7.2

Structure of bacteriophage T$_4$, one of the most complex DNA viruses known. Its capsid consists of approximately 40 different proteins.

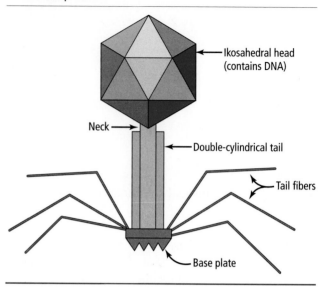

Bacteriophage T$_4$ destroys its host cell in the lytic pathway

The life cycle of a DNA virus can be exemplified by bacteriophage T$_4$. **Bacteriophages** ("bacteria-eaters") are viruses that replicate in bacterial hosts, and T$_4$ is specialized on *E. coli*. T$_4$ is a large virus, with a linear, double-stranded DNA chromosome carrying approximately 150 genes. Its architecture is quite complex (Fig. 7.2), with a compact head that contains the tightly packed DNA, a short neck, a cylindrical tail consisting of two coaxial hollow tubes, a base plate, and six spidery tail fibers. The capsid is built from approximately 40 different polypeptides, each of them present in numerous copies.

The first step in viral infection is **adsorption:** the tail fibers bind noncovalently to a surface component of the bacterial cell that functions as a **virus receptor.** Adsorption is followed by **penetration:** the sheath of the tail contracts, its inner core penetrates the cell wall, and the viral DNA is injected into the host cell. With the exception of a few nucleic acid-associated proteins, *the entire protein coat remains outside* (Fig. 7.3).

The expression of the viral genes is timed: some of them are transcribed immediately by the bacterial RNA polymerase. One of these "immediate-early" genes encodes a DNAse that degrades the host-cell chromosome. The viral DNA contains hydroxymethyl cytosine instead of cytosine and therefore is not attacked by this DNAse. During the later stages of the infection, viral proteins substitute for

FIG. 7.3

Reproduction of bacteriophage T$_4$ in its host *E. coli* by the lytic pathway.

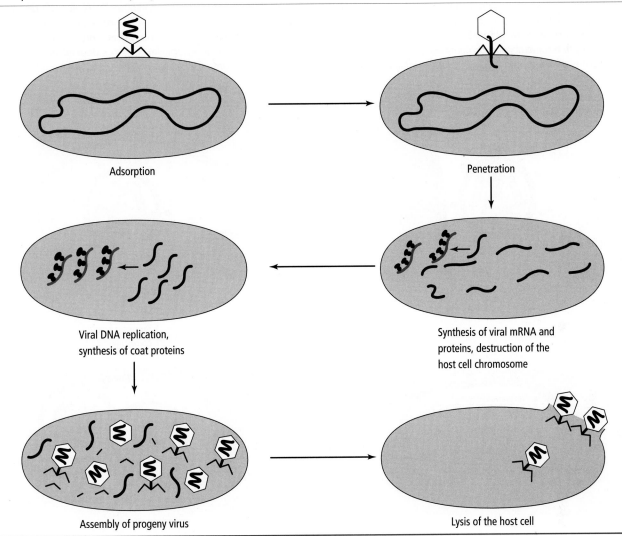

Adsorption

Penetration

Viral DNA replication,
synthesis of coat proteins

Synthesis of viral mRNA and
proteins, destruction of the
host cell chromosome

Assembly of progeny virus

Lysis of the host cell

the σ subunit of bacterial RNA polymerase (see Chapter 6) and direct the transcription of the "delayed-early" and "late" viral genes. The promoters of these genes are not recognized by the bacterial σ subunit.

The early viral proteins include enzymes for nucleotide synthesis, DNA replication, and DNA modification. The late proteins include the viral coat proteins. At this time, *new virus particles are assembled from the replicated viral DNA and the newly synthesized coat proteins.* A phospholipase and lysozyme are synthesized close to the end of the infectious cycle, and these enzymes destroy the bacterial plasma membrane and cell wall. This mode of virus replication is called the **lytic pathway** because it is accompanied by the lysis (destruction) of the host cell. The entire cycle takes some 20 minutes, and approximately 200 progeny viruses are released from the lysed host cell.

All DNA viruses substitute their own DNA for the host-cell DNA

Using lytic infection by the T$_4$ bacteriophage as a reference point, we can highlight some of the prominent features of viral infection:

FIG. 7.4

Two strategies for the uptake of an enveloped virus into its host cell. An initial noncovalent binding between a viral spike protein and the host-cell membrane is essential in both cases. **A,** Uptake of influenza virus, an enveloped RNA virus. Endocytosis is triggered by binding of the virus to the cell surface. The fusion of the viral envelope with the membrane of the endosome is facilitated by the low pH ($\approx$5.0) of this organelle. **B,** Uptake of human immunodeficiency virus (a retrovirus) is triggered by binding to the membrane glycoprotein CD4. The uptake of the nucleocapsid into the cytoplasm does not depend on endocytosis but is effected by direct fusion of the viral envelope with the plasma membrane. Only CD4-positive cells can be infected by this virus.

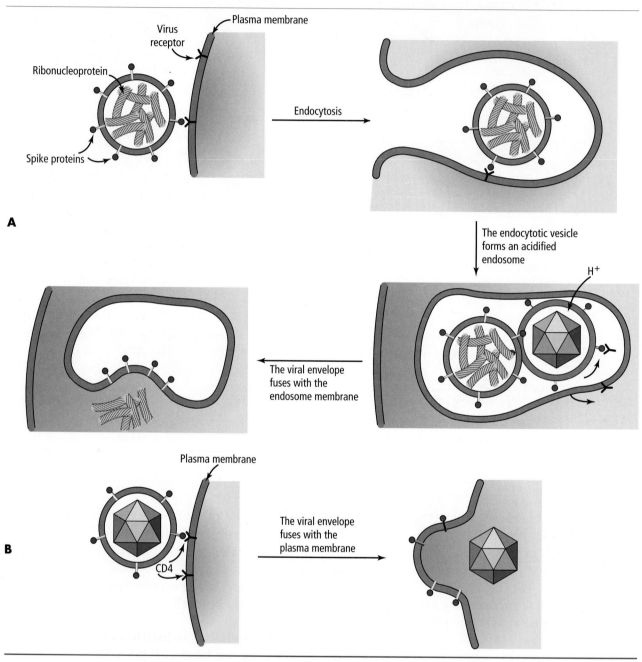

1. *Infection is initiated by specific binding of the virus to the surface of its host cell.* This requires viral surface proteins that either are part of the capsid or, in enveloped viruses, are embedded in the envelope as spike proteins. The viral surface proteins have to interact with a component of the host-cell surface that acts as a **virus receptor.** Only cells that possess the virus receptor can be infected. In the human body, viral infections often can be combatted by antibodies that coat the viral surface proteins, thereby preventing their binding to the host cell.

2. *T_4 and some other bacteriophages are constructed like syringes that inject their nucleic acid into the host cell.* Animal and human viruses use different strategies. Some of them trigger an endocytotic response after binding to the cell surface; some enveloped viruses simply fuse their envelope with the plasma membrane of the host cell, releasing the nucleocapsid into the host-cell cytoplasm. In these cases, uncoating of the viral nucleic acid occurs within the host cell (Fig. 7.4).

3. *Many viruses inhibit vital processes of the host cell,* but animal viruses usually do not go to the extreme of cutting their host's DNA to pieces.

4. *DNA viruses (and indeed all viruses) abuse the host-cell ribosomes for the synthesis of their own proteins.* DNA replication and transcription of the smaller viruses also rely mostly on host-cell enzymes, but the larger viruses, such as T_4, synthesize many of the required proteins themselves.

5. *The viruses of eukaryotes replicate either in the nucleus or in the cytoplasm.* Most DNA viruses replicate in the nucleus, where they can take advantage of the host's DNA and RNA polymerases and of other proteins of DNA replication and transcription, but most RNA viruses replicate in the cytoplasm.

6. *Virus-infected human cells do not always die of the infection.* Unlike T_4-infected *E. coli*, the infected cells shed virus particles continuously. The envelope of enveloped viruses is acquired from either the nuclear membrane or the plasma membrane when the virus buds out of its host cell.

λ Phage can integrate its DNA into the host-cell chromosome

Like T_4 phage, λ phage is a double-stranded DNA virus that is able to replicate in the lytic pathway. Like T_4, it is constructed as a syringe that injects its DNA into the host cell. The genome of λ phage, which contains approximately 40 genes, consists of a linear, double-stranded DNA molecule (48,502 base pairs) with single-stranded ends of 12 nucleotides each. These single-stranded ends have complementary base sequences (Fig. 7.5). After entering the host cell, these single-stranded ends anneal (i.e., base-pair), and the viral DNA is linked into a circle by a bacterial DNA ligase. Lytic infection can proceed as described earlier for T_4 phage.

Unlike bacteriophage T_4, however, λ phage can choose an alternative lifestyle: rather than destroy-

---

FIG. 7.5

Circularization of λ phage DNA. This event takes place immediately after the entry of the viral DNA into the host cell and does not require virally encoded proteins. The circular DNA is then either replicated in the lytic pathway or integrated into the bacterial chromosome.

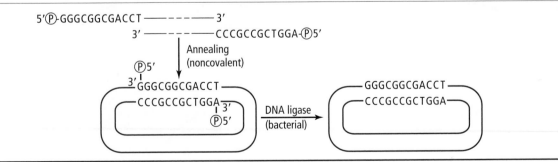

ing its host cell by brute force, λ phage DNA can integrate itself into a specific site of the host-cell chromosome, between the galactose and biotin operons. *The viral DNA is now part of the host-cell chromosome,* and it is replicated during each cycle of cell division. This mode of virus replication is called the **lysogenic pathway** (Fig. 7.6). The integrated virus DNA is called a **prophage,** and the bacterium is characterized as **lysogenic.**

The integration of the viral DNA requires a virally encoded **integrase.** Another delayed-early gene, which becomes activated under the same conditions as the integrase gene, codes for the λ **repressor.** *This protein maintains the lysogenic state by preventing the transcription of all phage genes except its own.* It even makes the lysogenic bacterium resistant to reinfection by λ phage because the genes of any incoming λ phage become repressed as well.

The lysogenic state can be maintained for hundreds or thousands of cell generations, but the viral genes, although dormant in the prophage of the repressor, can be reactivated. *Whenever the concentra-*

FIG. 7.6

The lysogenic pathway of λ phage.

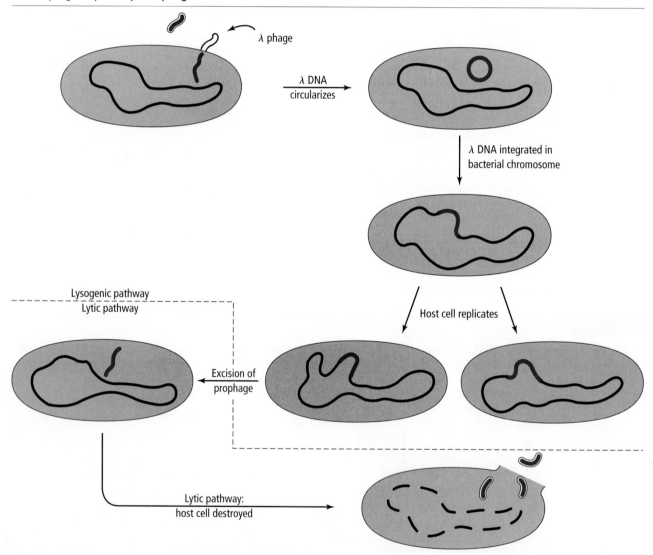

tion of the repressor falls below a critical limit, the genes of the lytic pathway become derepressed. One of the derepressed genes, the *xis* gene, codes for an excisionase that, in cooperation with the integrase protein, dissects the prophage out of the bacterial chromosome. Another gene, the *cro* gene, codes for a regulatory protein that switches the synthesis of the λ repressor off, thereby tilting the balance entirely toward the lytic pathway. Indeed, it is the alternative expression of either the λ repressor gene or the *cro* gene that determines whether the phage proceeds on the lysogenic or the lytic pathway.

The lysogenic state typically is terminated when the bacterium is exposed to UV radiation or other DNA-damaging stimuli. Under these conditions, a cellular protease is activated that degrades the λ repressor, thereby effecting the switch from the lysogenic to the lytic pathway. Like rats leaving a sinking ship, the virus leaves its troubled host.

RNA viruses require an RNA-dependent RNA polymerase

The genome of RNA viruses is either double stranded or single stranded. Only one of the two strands in a double-stranded RNA virus, the +

FIG. 7.7

The replicative cycle of a +-stranded animal RNA virus. ▇▇▇, + Strand; ▇▇▇ , − strand.

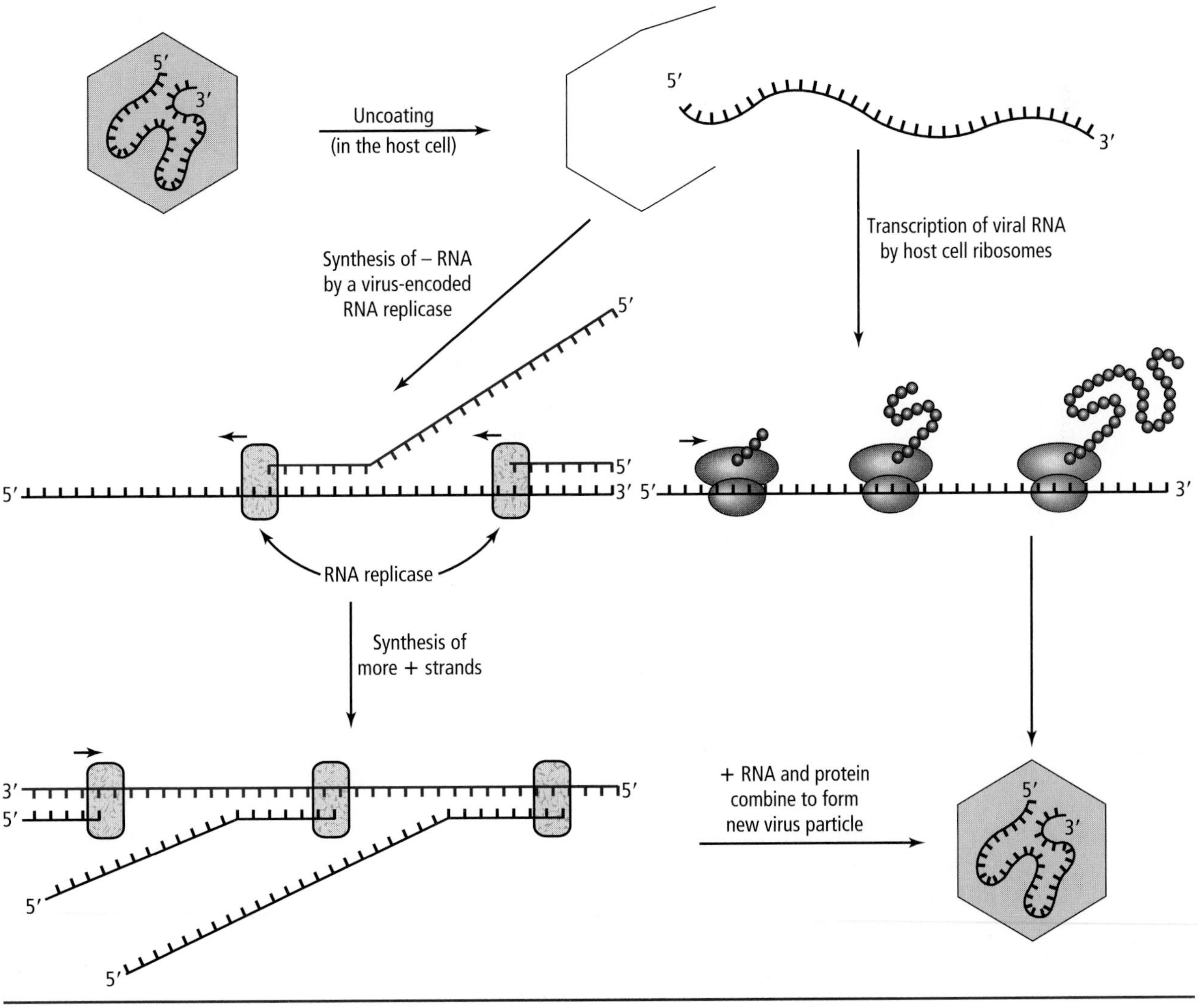

strand, can serve as an mRNA. The − strand is complementary to the + strand. In double-stranded RNA viruses as well as in those single-stranded RNA viruses whose genomic RNA is a + strand (or several + strands), the viral genes can be translated immediately without the need for initial RNA replication (Fig. 7.7).

The viral genome is replicated by an **RNA-dependent RNA polymerase,** also known as **RNA replicase.** This enzyme is not present in healthy cells, where all nucleic acid synthesis is DNA dependent, and therefore it has to be encoded by the virus itself. The viral RNA replicases are "sloppy" enzymes. Like the bacterial RNA polymerase, they do not possess a proofreading 3′-exonuclease activity, so their error frequency is high—on the order of one error for every 10,000 nucleotides. Therefore *RNA viruses have high mutation rates,* and they often manage to elude the host defenses by "inventing" new antigenic variants.

Those RNA viruses whose genomic RNA is a − strand have to synthesize + strands first, before they can produce viral proteins. Therefore they must carry at least one copy of the RNA replicase in the virion.

Retroviruses transcribe their genomic RNA into DNA

The retroviruses are a rather uniform group of viruses that infect eukaryotic hosts. Their genome consists of two identical copies of a + RNA, with a length close to 10,000 nucleotides, which is enclosed by an ikosahedral capsid. The nucleocapsid, in turn, is covered by an envelope that is derived from the plasma membrane. Because of the mechanism of reverse transcription, as shown in Fig. 7.8, the final double-stranded DNA is longer than the genomic RNA: it ends in repeat sequences left and right that are known as **long terminal repeats (LTRs).** The LTRs are required for the integration of the retroviral cDNA into the host-cell chromosome. The upstream LTR serves as a promoter and enhancer for transcriptional initiation, whereas the downstream LTR contains a polyadenylation site for transcriptional termination (see Chapter 8).

Like the RNA replicases, the reverse transcriptases do not proofread their products. Therefore *retro-*

viruses are plagued by high mutation rates, and new antigenic variants appear rapidly. This genetic instability poses a severe problem both for the immune system—which tries to combat retroviral infections—and for the scientist who tries to develop vaccines for these diseases. A vaccine for the AIDS virus, for example, still is not in sight because of the high mutation rate of the *env* gene. The reverse transcriptase of the AIDS virus is approximately 10 times less accurate than most other reverse transcriptases.

With the help of a virally encoded integrase, *the cDNA produced by the reverse transcriptase is integrated into the host-cell DNA as a* **DNA provirus.** The viral genes are transcribed (by a host-cell RNA polymerase) only after their integration into the host-cell genome. Transcription produces genomic virus RNA, and the translation of the viral RNA by host-cell ribosomes supplies the structural proteins of the virus particle. In most retroviral infections, the cell survives but produces virus particles for the rest of its lifetime. In AIDS, however, the infected cells die sooner or later. The body's main defense against retroviral infections, as against most other viral infections, is the destruction of any infected cell by T lymphocytes. Virus-infected cells are recognizable by the immune system because they display viral spike proteins on their surface (Fig. 7.9).

Plasmids are small "accessory chromosomes" or "symbiotic viruses" of bacteria

In addition to their single chromosome, most prokaryotes (and some lower eukaryotes) contain **plasmids,** small, semiindependent genetic elements consisting of a circular DNA double strand. Plasmids have anywhere between 2000 and 200,000 base pairs, and they may be present in 1 to 20 copies in the cell. Their replication is controlled by plasmid genes, which maintain an adequate copy number of the plasmid throughout the cell generations.

Plasmids carry genes that are transcribed and translated, but in contrast to the chromosomal genes *the plasmid genes are dispensable in most situations.* Toxin production, antibiotic resistance, the ability to degrade unusual metabolic substrates, and genetic recombination are some typical abilities conferred by plasmids. Most important in medicine are the **R factors** (R for resistance), which carry genes for

FIG. 7.8

Reverse transcription of retroviral RNA. *PB*, Primer-binding sequence; *LTR*, long terminal repeat; ▬, RNA; ▬, − DNA strand; ▭, + DNA strand.

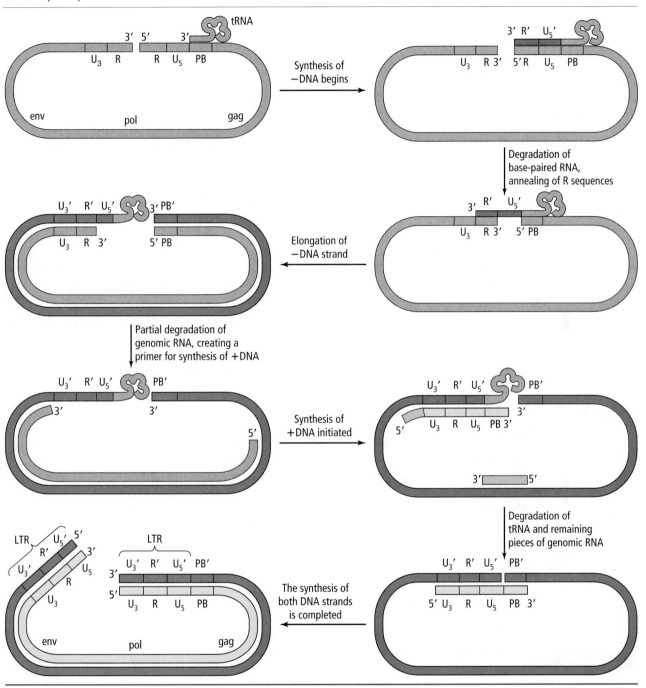

antibiotic resistance. Most of these resistance genes encode drug-inactivating enzymes. Penicillin, for example, is readily degraded by a plasmid-encoded **β-lactamase**, also known as **penicillinase** (Fig. 7.10). The lucky bacterium carrying this plasmid enjoys complete resistance to penicillin. R factor–containing bacteria have been selected by the widespread use of antibiotics and are now a major problem for the treatment of many bacterial infections.

FIG. 7.9

The life cycle of a retrovirus. The viral reverse transcriptase converts the viral RNA *(blue)* into a double-stranded DNA *(dark blue)*, which becomes integrated into the host-cell genome.

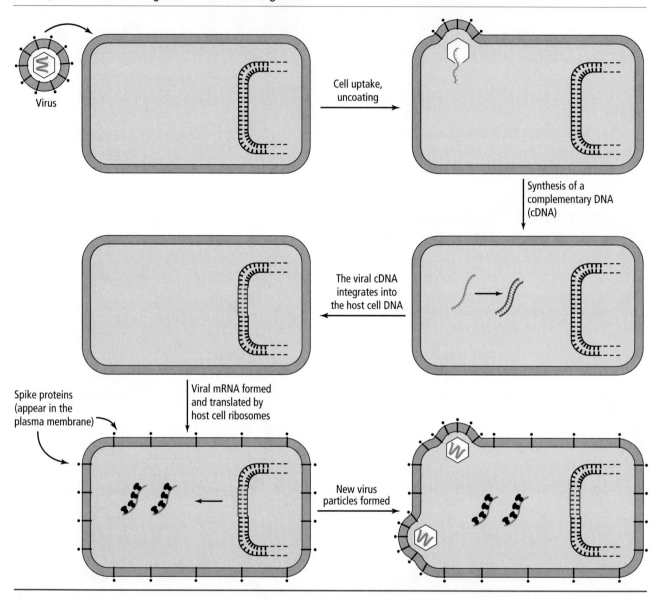

Virus

Cell uptake, uncoating

Synthesis of a complementary DNA (cDNA)

The viral cDNA integrates into the host cell DNA

Spike proteins (appear in the plasma membrane)

Viral mRNA formed and translated by host cell ribosomes

New virus particles formed

FIG. 7.10

The action of β-lactamase ("penicillinase") on penicillin G. The gene for this enzyme is often found on R-factor plasmids.

Penicillin G

β-lactamase

H_2O

Inactive product

FIG. 7.11

Cell-to-cell transfer of the F factor during conjugation in *E. coli.*

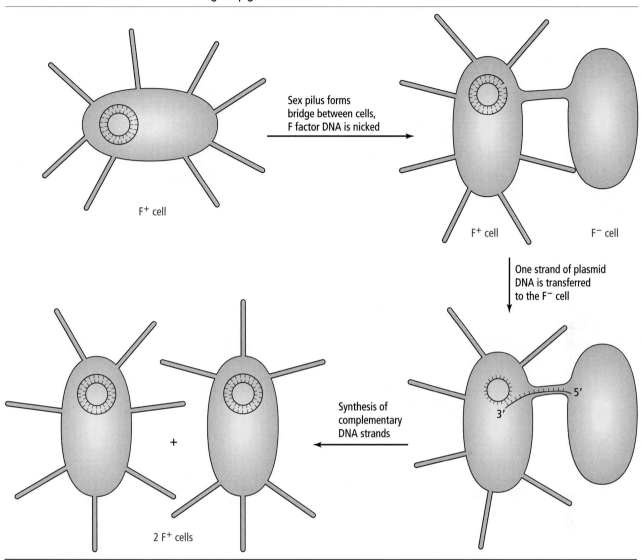

Sex pilus forms
bridge between cells,
F factor DNA is nicked

F⁺ cell

F⁺ cell   F⁻ cell

One strand of plasmid
DNA is transferred
to the F⁻ cell

Synthesis of
complementary
DNA strands

3′   5′

+

2 F⁺ cells

Some plasmids are transmissible

Some of the larger plasmids can transfer themselves from one bacterium to another. A classic example of this type of plasmid is the **F factor** (F for fertility) of *E. coli*. This large plasmid (94,500 base pairs) carries a set of approximately a dozen genes that are required for the formation of sex pili, hairlike processes protruding from the cell surface in all directions. Once an F factor–bearing cell (the F⁺ cell) encounters a cell without F factor (an F⁻ cell), a delicate bridge is formed between the cells by one of the sex pili. At this point, one of the two DNA strands of the plasmid is nicked, the DNA duplex unravels, and one of the strands worms its way into the F⁻ cell (Fig. 7.11). This step is followed by the synthesis of a new complementary DNA strand both in the F⁺ cell and in the ex-F⁻ cell. This type of DNA transfer is called **conjugation.**

The F factor behaves as an infectious agent that can spread in the bacterial population. Its genes are of no immediate benefit for the bacterium, but it facilitates the exchange of genetic information between the cells: occasionally, the F factor acquires genes from the bacterial chromosome and transfers them into the F⁻ cell together with its own genes. In rare cases, it becomes integrated into the bacterial chromosome and pulls a complete copy of the chromosome into the recipient cell during conjugation.

Some self-transmissible plasmids carry not only genes for their own replication and for conjugation but also useful genes. *Some R-factor plasmids are self transmissible,* and therefore *drug resistance often is transmissible,* both within a bacterial species and, occasionally, even between different species.

Bacteria also can exchange genetic information by transformation and transduction

Bacteria can acquire new DNA not only by conjugation. In **transformation,** a piece of foreign DNA is taken up by the bacterium and becomes integrated into the chromosome by homologous recombination (Fig. 7.12). Transforma-tion is not particu-

larly efficient because large DNA molecules do not easily cross the plasma membrane, but the permeability of the bacterial cell envelope for DNA can be increased in vitro by treating the recipient bacterium with high concentrations of calcium chloride.

In **transduction,** a bacteriophage carries a fragment of host-cell DNA from cell to cell. The host-cell DNA is packaged erroneously into a virus particle, and the virus injects bacterial DNA instead of (or in addition to) viral DNA into the next host cell.

Jumping genes can change their position in the genome

Most genes occupy a fixed position within the genome, but *some genes can move from one place to*

FIG. 7.12

Transfer of DNA between bacterial cells. The three mechanisms of DNA transfer shown here are collectively known as "parasexual" processes. **A,** Transformation. **B,** Transduction. **C,** Conjugation.

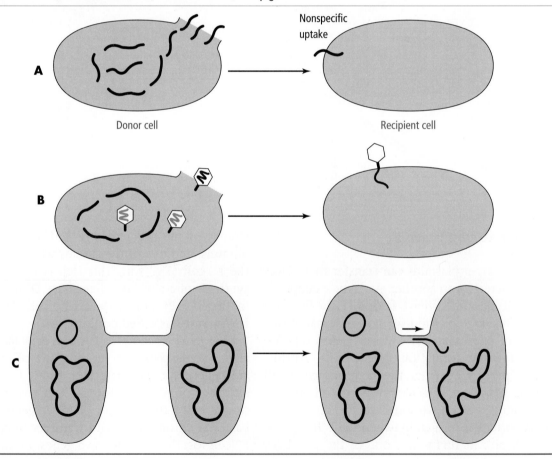

Donor cell   Recipient cell

another. The mobile DNA sequences of prokaryotes include insertion sequences and transposons.

An **insertion sequence** is a segment of DNA, typically between 750 and 1500 base pairs long, that is framed by inverted repeats of between 9 and 41 base pairs. Most insertion sequences are present in 5 to 30 copies in the cell. These copies are identical or nearly so, including the inverted repeats at their ends. The inverted repeats are flanked by short (4–12 base pairs), direct repeats that differ in the different copies of the insertion sequence.

Insertion sequences contain a single gene that encodes a **transposase**, a protein with several enzymatic activities required for transposition. Transposition can occur in two forms: in **conservative transposition**, the insertion sequence vacates its old position to settle in a new place. In **duplicative transposition**, however, the insertion

FIG. 7.13

A hypothetical mechanism for the duplicative transposition of a bacterial insertion sequence.

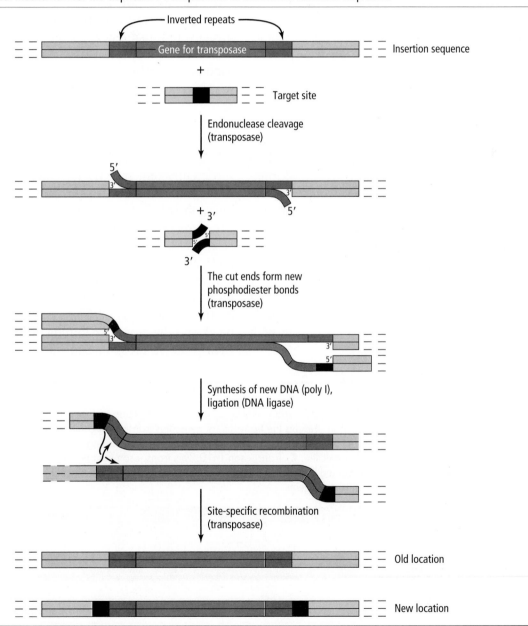

sequence replicates, and one of the replication products stays in its old location while the other one moves to a new site (Fig. 7.13).

The mechanism of transposition is poorly understood. *The transposase is specific for the inverted terminal repeats of its own insertion sequence*, and it therefore cannot transpose unrelated insertion sequences with different inverted repeats. The direct repeats are thought to be target site duplications that arise because the transposase makes staggered cuts in the DNA of the target site. Transposition is a rare event, occurring perhaps once every 1000 or 10,000 cell generations.

Like the insertion sequences, **transposons** are flanked by inverted repeats and contain the gene for their own transposase. Unlike insertion sequences, however, *they also contain useful genes*, for example, antibiotic-resistance genes. In many transposons, the flanking sequences are insertion sequences themselves (Fig. 7.14). Indeed, *any gene that becomes flanked by two insertion sequences becomes transposable*.

Transposon genes can be shuttled among the bacterial chromosome, plasmids, and bacteriophages, and they can be transmitted from cell to cell by conjugation, transduction, or transformation. However, the mobility of these genes is of no immediate advantage to the bacterium, and the transposition event easily can cause a crippling mutation when the mobile element jumps into an important gene. Therefore mobile elements are thought to be **selfish DNA**. Those mobile elements that contain antibiotic-resistance genes or other useful genes can be considered autonomous genetic elements that live in a symbiotic relationship with their host cell.

Genetic recombination requires the cutting and joining of DNA

In the previous sections, we discussed situations in which different DNA molecules become covalently linked. This process is called **recombination.**

There are two types of genetic recombination. **Site-specific recombination** depends on an enzyme that recognizes specific sequences either on one or on both DNA molecules. The integration of the λ phage DNA, for example, is effected by a viral integrase that recognizes both the phage DNA and the target site on the bacterial chromosome; the retroviral integrase is specific for the LTRs of the retroviral cDNA; and transposase recognizes the inverted terminal repeats of its transposon.

General recombination, also known as **homologous recombination**, requires no specific DNA sequence; *it depends on sequence identity or similarity between the recombining molecules*. Foreign DNA that is acquired by transformation or transduction, for example, can be integrated into the bacterial chromosome by homologous recombination—if it is sufficiently similar to the chromosomal DNA.

The molecular mechanism of homologous recombination is best known for *E. coli*, in which a number of recombination proteins have been identified (Fig. 7.15). In this system, a complex of the recB, recC, and recD proteins acts as an endonuclease and helicase to generate single-stranded DNA while the recA protein catalyzes the invasion of a DNA duplex by the single-stranded DNA. After a second strand break and the crosswise joining of the loose ends by DNA ligase, a cross-shaped intermediate called the

---

FIG. 7.14

Examples of mobile elements in bacteria. **A,** An insertion sequence: a gene for transposase that is flanked by inverted terminal repeat sequences ( ). **B,** Transposon Tn3. Besides the transposase gene, this transposon contains a gene for a repressor that regulates the expression of the transposase gene, and a gene for the penicillin-degrading enzyme β-lactamase. Bacteria carrying this transposon are resistant to penicillin. **C,** Transposon Tn10. This transposon contains a gene for tetracycline resistance (*tet-R* gene). Unlike Tn3, it is not framed by simple inverted repeats but rather by two identical insertion sequences (IS10L), each of them containing a transposase gene.

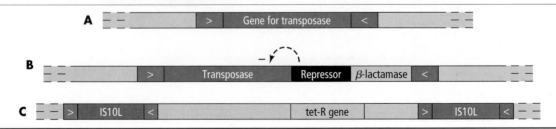

FIG. 7.15

The hypothetical mechanism of homologous recombination. This type of recombination results in a reciprocal exchange between two duplex DNA molecules. The proteins required for recombination (recBCD, recA, ruvC) have been described in *E. coli*. Proteins with equivalent functions are thought to exist in other organisms as well, both prokaryotes and eukaryotes. **A,** Formation of the Holliday intermediate. The Holliday intermediate itself can undergo further branch migration (not shown). **B,** Resolution of the Holliday intermediate.

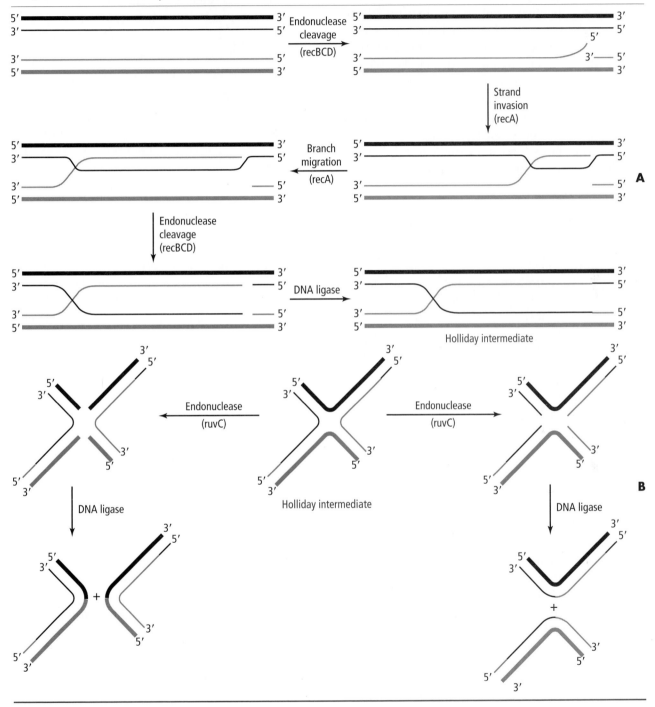

Holliday intermediate (named after Robin Holliday, who proposed this structure in 1964) is formed. This intermediate is resolved by the successive action of an endonuclease (ruvC in *E. coli*) and DNA ligase.

Homologous recombination is not limited to prokaryotes. In higher eukaryotes like us, *it occurs during prophase of meiosis I*, when homologous chromosomes exchange portions of DNA by this mechanism. The correct alignment of the homologous sequences (achieved with the help of recA in *E. coli*) is essential, and mispairing leads to major deletions and duplications. Gene duplications, in particular, which are very important in eukaryotic evolution, result from homologous recombination between misaligned chromosomes during meiosis.

Further Reading

Joklik WK: Structure, components and classification of virus. In: Joklik WK, Willett HP, Amos DB, Wilfert CM, editors: *Zinsser microbiology*, 20th ed., pp. 749-782. Appleton & Lange, Norwalk 1992.

Kreuzer KN: Bacteriophage. In: Joklik WK, Willett HP, Amos DB, Wilfert CM, editors: *Zinsser microbiology*, 20th ed., pp. 906-929. Appleton & Lange, Norwalk 1992.

Alcamo IE: *Fundamentals of microbiology*, 4th ed., pp. 317-353. Benjamin/Cummings, Redwood City 1994.

Shinohara A, Ogawa T: Homologous recombination and the roles of double-strand breaks. *Trends Biochem Sci* 20, 387-391, 1995.

Litrak S: *Retroviral Reverse Transcriptases*. Chapman and Hall, 1996.

SUMMARY

Viruses are infectious particles that consist of nucleic acid and protein. Although they have no cellular structure and no metabolism, they can replicate within a host cell by exploiting the host's enzymes, metabolic energy, and ribosomes. DNA viruses substitute their own genomic DNA for the host-cell DNA, directing the synthesis of viral mRNA and viral proteins. RNA viruses substitute their own RNA for the host's mRNA, directing the synthesis of viral proteins without the need for transcription. Finally, retroviruses synthesize a DNA copy of their genomic RNA and integrate this copy into the host-cell genome.

Prokaryotic cells contain a whole zoo of semiautonomous genetic elements. Plasmids are small, circular DNA duplexes that function as accessory chromosomes. Some plasmids behave as infectious agents, transmitting themselves from cell to cell by conjugation. Insertion sequences and transposons are mobile DNA sequences on the bacterial chromosome and on plasmids. They encode a transposase that catalyzes their movement into new genomic locations. Some viruses, plasmids, and mobile elements facilitate the exchange of genetic information between cells. This involves genetic recombination, the joining of two DNA molecules from different sources into a single molecule. Recombination occurs both in prokaryotes and in eukaryotes and requires specific enzyme systems.

QUESTIONS

1. To infect a new host cell, a virus has to bind specifically to a "virus receptor" on the surface of the host cell. In the case of the AIDS virus (a retrovirus), this initial interaction involves the viral
   A. Spike proteins
   B. Reverse transcriptase
   C. Capsid proteins
   D. RNA

2. The Holliday intermediate is a cruciform structure that appears as an intermediate in
   A. The integration of λ phage into the bacterial chromosome
   B. The integration of a retroviral cDNA into the host-cell genome
   C. Homologous recombination
   D. The replication of bacteriophage T_4
   E. The duplicative transposition of a bacterial insertion sequence

3. An inhibitor of reverse transcriptase would be useful in
   A. Preventing λ phage from integrating into the host-cell chromosome
   B. Preventing lytic infection by T_4 bacteriophage
   C. Inhibiting homologous recombination between two DNAs
   D. Curing rabies, a disease caused by an RNA virus
   E. Curing AIDS, a disease caused by a retrovirus

Chapter 8

The Human Genome and Its Expression

The crucial processes of DNA replication and gene expression, as described in Chapter 6, are the same in all living things on earth. All cells use double-stranded DNA as a genetic library, replicate their DNA, and express their genetic information through an RNA intermediate. Nevertheless, these processes are executed differently in prokaryotes and eukaryotes. In this chapter, we introduce the specific features of eukaryotic genes and their expression.

THE ARCHITECTURE OF THE HUMAN GENOME

Eukaryotic cells not only are much larger than their poor prokaryotic cousins, they also are equipped with far more DNA. Even a lowly unicellular eukaryote such as yeast has four to five times more DNA than the bacterium *E. coli* in its haploid genome. Fruit flies have 40 times, and humans 900 times, more DNA than *E. coli*, and amphibians have 5000 to 40,000 times more. *The haploid human genome contains approximately 3.9 billion base pairs*, with a stretched-out length of 130 cm of Watson-Crick double helix. During mitosis, this wealth of DNA is packaged in 23 chromosomes, with lengths of a few micrometers each.

The size of the individual DNA molecules is impressive, too: *each chromosome contains one and only one double-stranded DNA molecule* with a length of several centimeters. Unlike the bacterial chromosome, which is circular (see Chapter 6), *eukaryotic DNA is linear*. A typical human chromosome carries between 1000 and 6000 protein-coding genes, which are separated by vast expanses of noncoding DNA. In the following sections, we introduce the structural features of the human chromosomes and genes and the different types of noncoding DNA sequences.

Chromatin consists of DNA and histones

Chromatin is a nucleoprotein complex that is conspicuous in histologic preparations by its affinity for such basic dyes as hematoxylin and fuchsin. It occurs in two forms: **euchromatin** has a loose structure; **heterochromatin** is condensed more tightly and is deeper staining. *Only euchromatin is thought to contain actively transcribed genes.*

Chromatin consists of approximately 50% DNA and 50% **histones.** *The histones are small basic proteins that are bound noncovalently to DNA*, mostly by electrostatic interactions with the negatively charged phosphate groups of the nucleic acid. There are only five types of histones in eukaryotic cells (Table 8.1). With the exception of histone H1, whose structure varies in different species and even in different tissues of the same organism, the histones are well conserved throughout the phylogenetic tree. Thus, the amino acid sequences of histones H3 and H4 from pea seedlings and calf thymus differ in only four and two amino acid positions, respectively. Evidently the histones were invented early during

TABLE 8.1

The five types of histones

Type	Size (amino acids)	Location
H1	215	Linker
H2A	129	Nucleosome core
H2B	125	Nucleosome core
H3	135	Nucleosome core
H4	102	Nucleosome core

evolution* and serve the same essential function in all eukaryotic organisms.

Histones are subject to a number of posttranslational modifications, including the acetylation of lysine side chains, phosphorylation of serine side chains, methylations, and ADP-ribosylation. Most of these modifications are physiologically reversible. They are thought to prepare chromatin for DNA replication and transcription.

The nucleosome is the structural unit of chromatin

Under the electron microscope, chromatin looks like "beads on a string." The beads are the **nucleosomes,** little discs with a diameter of approximately 11 nm. Figure 8.1 shows the general structure of nucleosomes: their core consists of two copies each of histones H2A, H2B, H3, and H4, with approximately 146 base pairs of DNA wound around this histone core in a left-handed orientation. The nucleosomes are connected by a variable length of DNA, frequently 50 to 60 base pairs, which is associated with a single molecule of histone H1. Histone H1 participates in the formation of higher-order chromatin structures.

Nucleosomes are present both in euchromatin and in heterochromatin. Their structure loosens or unfolds during transcription, as evidenced by a greater sensitivity of the histones to sulfhydryl reagents and of the DNA to nucleases. Covalent modifications of the histones, possibly in the form

---

* We do not mean to imply an intentional act. Applying the rule of parsimony (also known as "Ockham's razor"), biologists assume that there is no purpose in evolution. However, some theologians disagree with this line of thought.

of acetylation of lysine side chains, are thought to be required to open the nucleosome for the transcriptional machinery.

The packaging of DNA into nucleosomes is only the first step in the condensation of genomic DNA. In a second step, the nucleosomes are coiled into a helical or solenoidal structure with a diameter of 30 nm (Fig. 8.1, B). These two packaging operations achieve a fortyfold reduction in the length of the genomic DNA. Although this may be sufficient for the dispersed chromatin of the interphase nucleus, a further 200-fold condensation is required for the formation of fully condensed chromosomes. This is achieved with the help of **scaffold proteins,** to which long loops of DNA are attached (Fig. 8.1, C).

Eukaryotic DNA replication starts from many origins

The important events in DNA replication are similar in prokaryotes and eukaryotes, but eukaryotic replication forks move at a pace of only 100 base pairs per second, 10 times slower than in E. coli. Considering the large size of eukaryotic DNA molecules, this creates a problem: with only one origin, the replication of the largest human chromosome would take 3 weeks! Actually, however, *human chromosomal DNA has multiple sites of origin for replication,* approximately one every 10,000 to 100,000 base pairs, and DNA replication therefore does not take much longer in humans than in bacteria.

The eukaryotic DNA polymerases, summarized in Table 8.2, are not characterized as well as their prokaryotic counterparts. As in prokaryotes, the tasks of replication and repair are performed by separate enzymes, and even the synthesis of the leading and the lagging strand appear to be performed by different enzymes.

Most human DNA does not code for proteins

Most of the 4.2 million base pairs in the bacterium E. coli code for proteins—a total of approximately 2000 polypeptides. Some fast-growing unicellular eukaryotes such as yeast also use most of their DNA for protein coding. In higher eukaryotes, however, only a small fraction of the total DNA codes for proteins. *The human genome encodes 50,000 to 100,000*

FIG. 8.1

Structure of chromatin. **A,** The nucleosome. **B,** Formation of the 30-nm fiber. **C,** Attachment of the 30-nm fiber to the central protein scaffold of the chromosome. Each loop of 30-nm fiber from one scaffold attachment to the next measures approximately 0.4 to 0.8 μm and contains 45,000 to 90,000 base pairs. (© 1980 W. H. Freeman & Co.)

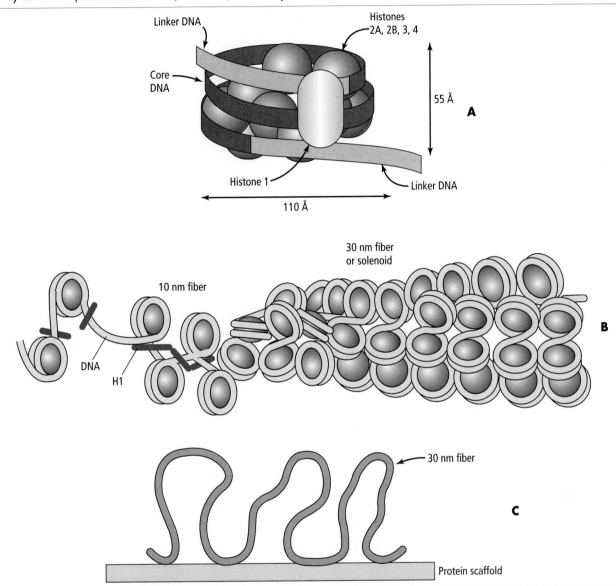

polypeptides, but no more than 3% to 4% of our 3.9 billion base pairs are required for this task.

Most of the remaining 96% to 97% consists of untranscribed sequences between the genes. Other noncoding sequences are present *within* the genes. Most of our genes are patchworks of **exons**, whose transcripts are processed to a mature mRNA, and untranslated intervening sequences called **introns**. *Introns are transcribed together with the exons, but they are removed by nuclear enzyme systems before the mRNA reaches the ribosome.* After the removal of the introns, the exons form a single, continuous coding sequence. Some genes have only one or two introns; others have several dozen. The total length of the introns may far exceed that of the exons (see Fig. 8.6 for an example). Very few eukaryotic genes, including the histone genes, are intronless. Most of the noncoding DNA in the untranscribed spacers and in the

TABLE 8.2

Properties of the eukaryotic DNA polymerases

Polymerase	Location	Mol wt	3'-Exonuclease activity	Primase activity	Processivity	Function
α	Nucleus	335,000*	−	+	Low	Replication of lagging strand (?)
δ	Nucleus	170,000†	+	−	High	Replication of leading strand (?)
ε	Nucleus	256,000‡	+	−	High	Repair ?
β	Nucleus	37,000	−	−	Low	Repair, possibly recombination
γ	Mitochondria	160,000-300,000§	+	−		Replication (+ repair ?) of mitochondrial DNA

* With catalytic subunit of MW 165,000.
† With catalytic core of MW 125,000.
‡ With catalytic core of MW 215,000.
§ With catalytic subunit of MW 125,000.

introns serves no obvious function. This **junk DNA** may differ considerably between different species and even between different individuals of the same species.

The introns are, in most cases, not required for proper gene expression, but they are important for the evolution of eukaryotic genes. *Different structural and functional domains of a polypeptide often are encoded by separate exons.* The immunoglobulin chains, for example, consist of several globular domains with similar amino acid sequences and tertiary structures, and each of these domains is encoded by its own exon (see Chapter 25). This is most likely the result of **exon duplication.** Another well-established example of exon duplication is the connective tissue protein fibronectin (see Chapter 13), which consists of repetitive "modules," with each module encoded by its own exon. In other cases, exons from different genes appear to have combined to form a new functional gene. This is called **exon shuffling.** Some of the fibronectin modules, for example, have relatives in the genes for prothrombin, factor XII, and other proteins of the blood-clotting system. *The exons appear to be the actual building blocks from which the multitude of eukaryotic genes has been assembled in the course of evolution.*

Mitochondria have their own DNA

More than 99% of the DNA in human cells resides in the nucleus, but a small amount is present in the mitochondria as well. This **mitochondrial DNA (mtDNA)** is a circular double strand with a length of 16,569 base pairs. It occurs in 4 to 10 copies in each mitochondrion.

mtDNA is genetically active, coding for a total of 13 polypeptides, 22 tRNAs, and 2 rRNAs (12S and 16S). The protein-coding genes are transcribed by a mitochondrial RNA polymerase, and they are translated by mitochondrial ribosomes that are structurally different from those in the cytoplasm.

Why do mitochondria have their own protein-synthesizing machinery? It is believed that more than 1.5 billion years ago, an aerobic prokaryotic cell established a symbiosis with an anaerobic eukaryote. In the course of time, *the prokaryote, living within the eukaryotic cell, evolved (or degenerated) into the present-day mitochondria.* During this time, most of the original prokaryotic (or promitochondrial) genes were transferred to the nucleus, leaving the mitochondria with a rudimentary but still functional protein-synthesizing system. The transfer of genetic material from the mitochondrion to the nucleus was advantageous because the mitochondrial DNA is exposed to oxidative stress, which results in a high mutation rate, whereas the nucleus is conspicuously free from oxidative enzymes (see Chapter 16). Also, the mitochondrial DNA is for the most part maternally inherited and has little opportunity for genetic recombination. Thus, *our genome is of hybrid origin, descended in part from a primordial eukaryote and in part from a symbiotic prokaryote.*

This **endosymbiont hypothesis** is supported amply by biochemical similarities between mitochondria and prokaryotes. The sequences of rRNA in mitochondria and bacteria, for example, are clearly related. A similar origin can be traced for the chloroplasts of plants, which are descended from a photosynthetic prokaryote.

Gene families originate by gene duplication and divergent evolution

Most protein-coding genes are present in only one copy in the haploid genome. Occasionally, however, we find **duplicated genes,** with two identical or near-identical copies close together on the same chromosome. *Some genes that code for very abundant RNAs or proteins are present in multiple copies.* In most cases, identical or near-identical copies of the gene are arranged in tandem, head-to-tail over long stretches of DNA, separated by untranscribed spacers. Examples in humans include the rRNA genes ($\approx$ 200 copies), the 5S rRNA gene ($\approx$ 2000 copies), the histone genes (20–50 copies), and most of the tRNA genes.

In other cases, two or more similar but not identical genes are present in the genome, usually close together on the same chromosome. The α- and β-like globin gene clusters (Chapter 9) are the classic examples of such **gene families.** Gene families arise during evolution by the duplication of a primordial gene, followed by divergent evolution of the duplication products.

Pseudogenes are unexpressed DNA sequences with sequence homology to a functional gene. A pseudogene arises when a gene duplicates and one of the duplication products becomes defunct as a result of crippling mutations that prevent transcription or translation. Pseudogenes still have the intron-exon structure of the functional gene from which they were derived, and they usually are located close to their functional counterpart on the chromosome.

The genome contains many short tandem repeats

Approximately 70% of our DNA, including the genes, consists of unique or nearly unique sequences. The remaining 30% of the sequences are repetitive. **Simple-sequence DNA** consists of short sequences—between two and a dozen base pairs—that are repeated many times in tandem. *The centromeres and telomeres of the chromosomes contain the largest agglomerations of simple-sequence DNA.* The centromeres are equipped with short oligonucleotide sequences, usually not more than 5 to 10 base pairs long, that are repeated more than a million times in the genome. Different chromosomes contain different repeat sequences. The ends of mammalian chromosomes are formed by the **telomeres,** which consist of the repeat sequence (TTAGGG)$_n$. This sequence is repeated in tandem between 500 and 5000 times in each telomere.

Most of the simple-sequence DNA outside the centromeres and telomeres occurs in the form of simple repeats, with two to five base pairs in the repeat unit. These units are repeated from a few times to approximately 50 times in any one location, and the same repeat may be present at many different sites. The most abundant repeat is an AC sequence that occurs in 50,000 to 100,000 locations throughout the genome. Repeats of three, four, or five bases are common as well, although they are not as numerous as the dinucleotide repeats. Most of them are present in the junk DNA of introns and untranscribed spacers; their functions, if any, are not known.

After partial endonuclease digestion, the centromeric and telomeric DNA can be separated from bulk genomic DNA by density gradient centrifugation. The repetitive DNA thus isolated is called **satellite DNA.** Likewise, DNA fragments consisting of simple tandem repeats outside the centromeric and telomeric regions can be isolated as **minisatellites** and **microsatellites.**

Telomere erosion is a normal feature of cellular aging

Unlike bacterial chromosomes, eukaryotic chromosomes contain a linear DNA, and the replication of this linear DNA poses a special problem: at the end of the chromosome, the leading strand can be extended to the very end of the template. The lagging strand, however, is synthesized in the opposite direction and requires the repeated synthesis of a small RNA primer. Even in the unlikely case that the last primer is at the very end of the template strand, the removal of this primer would leave a gap that cannot be filled by DNA polymerase (Fig. 8.2, *A*).

This problem is solved by **telomerase.** This enzyme acts at the end of the telomere, where it

FIG. 8.2

The terminal replication problem of telomeric DNA in eukaryotic chromosomes. **A,** The problem: one of the daughter chromosomes is incompletely replicated because DNA replication proceeds only in the 5'→ 3' direction, and the replication of the lagging strand ends at the site of the last RNA primer. **B,** The solution: telomerase elongates the overhanging 3' end of the incompletely replicated telomere. This is followed by the synthesis of the complementary strand. Although the mechanism of complementary strand synthesis is not firmly established, it is most likely effected by the regular mechanism of DNA replication, with the combination of primase and DNA polymerase activities. **C,** The hypothetical mechanism of telomere extension by telomerase.

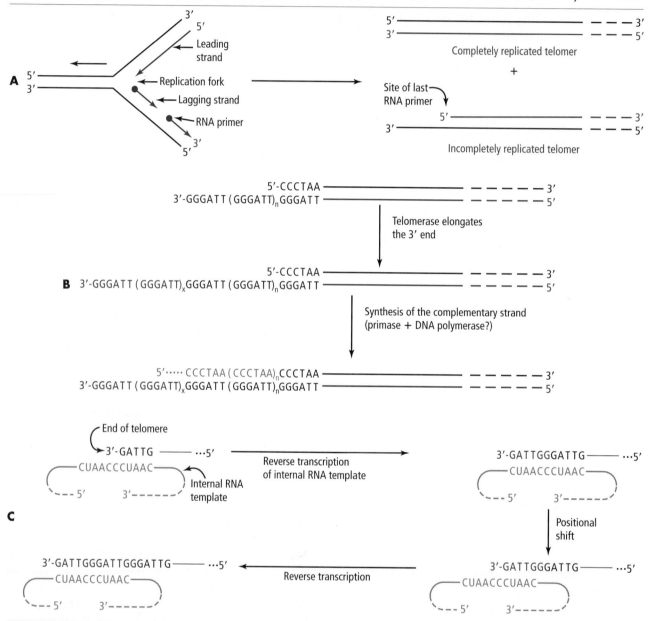

elongates the overhanging 3' end of the template DNA strand, adding the correct TTAGGG sequence of the telomere repeat. This new DNA has to be synthesized without the benefit of a DNA template, and therefore *the template has to be provided by the telomerase itself.* This template is a 150-nucleotide RNA that is an integral part of the enzyme. One section of this RNA is complementary to the repeat sequence at the 3' end of the telomere and can be used as a template for the synthesis of new telomeric DNA (Fig.

8.2, C). Once the 3' end has been extended, a new complementary strand is synthesized.

Telomerase is required for immortality. In the human body, only germline cells are immortal, whereas somatic cells have a finite lifespan. Moreover, only germline cells—not somatic cells—express telomerase. Cultured fibroblasts, for example, inevitably die after a few dozen mitotic divisions. Their life expectancy in culture depends on the age of the body from which they were taken: on average, the fibroblasts of an infant survive longer in culture than those of an aged individual. The best predictor of fibroblast lifespan, however, is not the chronological age of the donor but the average length of the telomeric DNA: *fibroblasts with long telomeres can look forward to a long life, but those with short telomeres will die soon.*

The implications of this are intriguing: in germline cells, the telomeres are maintained by the action of telomerase. The telomeres of sperm cells, for example, are longer than those of somatic cells. The expression of telomerase, however, tapers off during embryonic development, and the telomeres gradually shorten after this fateful event. *The cell loses its viability after a predictable number of cell divisions when the first telomeres are eroded.* Without their protective telomeres, the chromosomes are prone to haphazard chromosomal rearrangements, which in turn lead to unbalanced karyotypes in the progeny cells. More commonly, however, aged cells with undersized telomeres respond to this situation by growth arrest and programmed cell death, long before the telomeres have actually disappeared. These mechanisms will be discussed in Chapter 28.

Besides germline cells, *cancer cells express telomerase and are immortal* (see Chapter 28). This suggests that the lack of telomerase in somatic cells is not only a curse that seals our earthly fate, but also a protective mechanism that reduces the likelihood of malignant transformation: to become malignant, a somatic cell not only has to escape the controls that normally limit its growth; it also has to find ways to derepress its telomerase.

Some DNA sequences are copies of functional RNAs

The genome contains not only pseudogenes, which are the degenerate descendants of functional dupli-cated genes, but also **processed pseudogenes.** A processed pseudogene is clearly related to a normal gene, but unlike a true pseudogene *it consists only of exon sequences,* with an oligo-A tract of 10 to 50 nucleotides at the 3' end. This whole structure is framed by direct repeats of between 9 and 14 base pairs (Fig. 8.3). Unlike true pseudogenes, processed pseudogenes are not located in the immediate vicinity of their functional counterparts.

Processed pseudogenes arise during evolution by the reverse transcription of a cellular RNA (Fig. 8.3). Mature eukaryotic mRNAs possess a poly-A tail at their 3' end that, to a variable extent, is included in the reverse transcript and that accounts for the oligo-A tract at the 3' end of the processed pseudogene. The direct repeats are thought to arise as a target site duplication during the insertion of the reverse transcript into the genomic DNA, perhaps by a mechanism similar to that postulated for bacterial insertion sequences and transposons (see Chapter 7). The insertion of a reverse transcript into the genome is called **retroposition,** and processed pseudogenes are characterized as **nonviral retroposons.** Having lost their promoter during retroposition, processed pseudogenes are rarely, if ever, transcribed.

Viral retroposons are the relics of retroviral genomes. They betray their origin by the presence of sequences that are related to the viral *gag, pol,* and *env* genes, and by remnants of the long terminal repeats (see Chapter 7). These sequences are no longer infectious because they have accumulated mutations that prevent the synthesis of viral proteins and the production of infectious virions. Therefore *viral retroposons are the dead bodies of retroviruses, left to rot in the genomic soil.*

Some repetitive DNA sequences are mobile

The human genome is inhabited not only by functional genes and their derivatives, simple tandem repeats, and lots of undistinguished junk DNA, but also by repetitive sequences that occur in approximately 1000 to 500,000 copies each. This moderately repetitive DNA includes **short interspersed elements (SINEs),** with lengths of up to a few hundred base pairs, and **long interspersed elements (LINEs),** which measure up to some thousand base pairs.

FIG. 8.3

The origin of a processed pseudogene. ▬, Exons; ▬, introns.

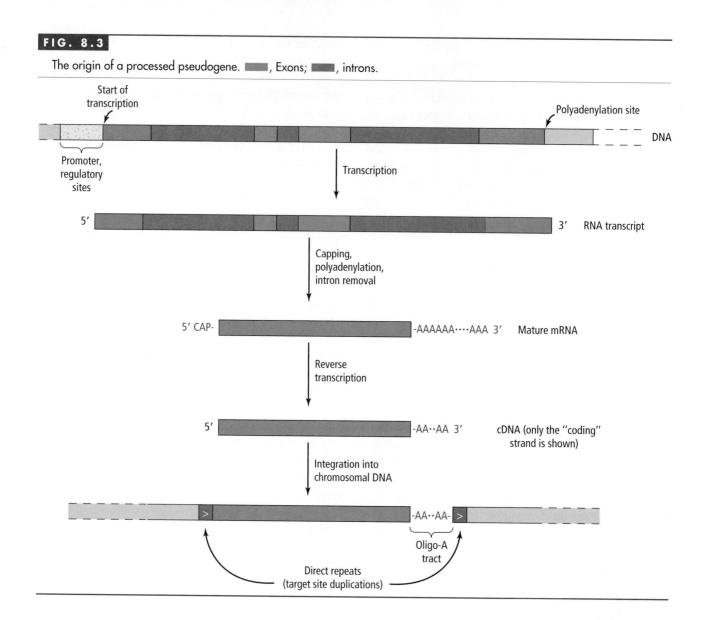

Start of transcription

Polyadenylation site

DNA

Promoter, regulatory sites

Transcription

5'   3'   RNA transcript

Capping, polyadenylation, intron removal

5' CAP-   -AAAAAA····AAA 3'   Mature mRNA

Reverse transcription

5'   -AA··AA 3'   cDNA (only the "coding" strand is shown)

Integration into chromosomal DNA

-AA··AA-

Oligo-A tract

Direct repeats (target site duplications)

The most populous tribe of SINEs are the **Alu sequences,** named after the presence of a cleavage site for the restriction endonuclease AluI in many of them. They occur in approximately 500,000 copies in the haploid genome. A full-length Alu sequence measures approximately 300 base pairs, contains an adenine-rich tract of anywhere between 7 and 50 base pairs at the 3' end, and is flanked by direct repeats of 7 to 21 base pairs. Different Alu sequences in the human genome differ in approximately 20% of their base pairs. Alu sequences are not translated, but perhaps one half of them can be transcribed by RNA polymerase III. The transcripts serve no recognized function and are degraded rapidly within the nucleus.

The Alu consensus sequence is more than 80% identical to the sequence of **7SL RNA,** a small cytoplasmic RNA that plays a role in the targeting of secreted proteins (see page 162). Because the 7SL RNA is present in all eukaryotes but Alu sequences are abundant only in vertebrates, the Alu sequences are thought to have originated from 7SL RNA, probably by reverse transcription.

At least some Alu sequences are mobile, and "jumping" Alu sequences have in a few instances been observed to cause mutations. Their mobility is thought to depend on reverse transcription (Fig. 8.4). Full-length Alu sequences constitute approximately 2% or 3% of the human genome, but truncated versions are not uncommon either, and altogeth-

FIG. 8.4

Hypothetical mechanism for the retroposition of Alu sequences. Transcription by RNA polymerase III typically starts at the first base of the Alu sequence and ends at a T-rich sequence downstream of the Alu sequence. Note that the direct repeats flanking the sequence arise as target site duplications during integration. Therefore they differ in different copies of the Alu sequence. LINE-1 sequences are thought to move by the same mechanism.

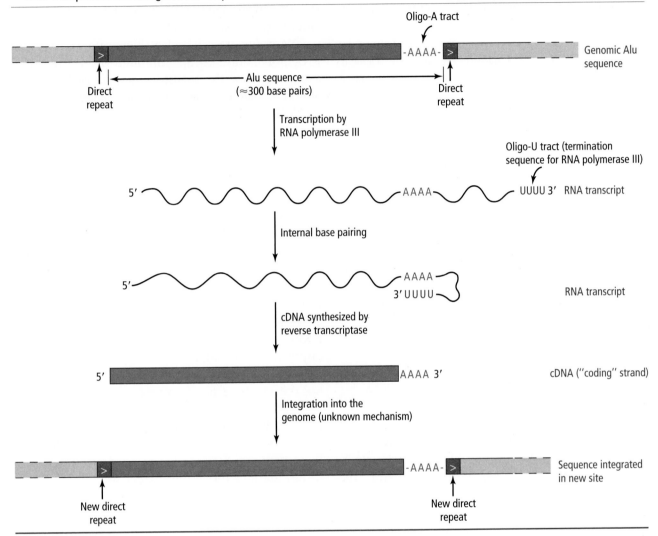

er the Alu-related sequences form perhaps 5% to 10% of our genome. Truncation of the sequence is a common accident during retroposition.

The most abundant LINEs in the human genome belong to the **LINE-1** family. Full-length LINE-1 sequences have approximately 5000 base pairs, and like the Alu sequences they have a poly-A tract at their 3′ end and are framed by direct repeats. *They encode a protein that resembles the retroviral reverse transcriptase.* On average, LINE-1 sequences differ from their consensus sequence by only 5%. The genome contains not more than approximately 3500 full-

length LINE-1 sequences, but there also are 50,000 to 100,000 partial sequences, most of them truncated at the 5′ end. Altogether approximately 5% of the human genome consists of LINE-1−related sequences.

Like Alu sequences, *LINE-1 sequences have been observed to jump on rare occasions,* and their mobility is thought to depend on reverse transcription and retroposition. Truncation of the sequence has been observed to occur during transposition. *LINE-1 sequences are endogenous sources of reverse transcriptase in vertebrate genomes.* This reverse transcriptase is thought to enable not only the LINEs themselves but also the Alu sequences to invade new positions in the genome. A useful function has not been demonstrated for SINEs and LINEs, and like other mobile elements (see Chapter 7), *they can cause mutations by jumping into a functional gene.* Therefore they have been vilified as "selfish DNA" or "molecular parasites." Unlike the bacterial insertion sequences and transposons (see Chapter 7), *the mobile elements of higher eukaryotes usually move through an RNA intermediate.*

TRANSCRIPTION AND TRANSLATION

In prokaryotes, transcription and translation occur in the same compartment. In eukaryotes, however, these two processes are separated both in space and in time: transcription takes place in the nucleus, translation in the cytoplasm. There is ample time for the posttranscriptional processing of the mRNA in the nucleus, and translation can start only after the fully processed mRNA has crossed from the nucleus into the cytoplasm. In the following sections, we trace the fate of eukaryotic mRNA from its synthesis by RNA polymerase to its translation by the ribosome.

Eukaryotes have three nuclear RNA polymerases

Although *E. coli* is content with a single RNA polymerase for the synthesis of all its cellular RNA, eukaryotes employ separate enzymes for the synthesis of rRNA, mRNA, and tRNA (Table 8.3). **RNA polymerase I** synthesizes the common precursor of the 5.8S, 18S, and 28S ribosomal RNA (see Chapter 6). *This enzyme is active in the nucleolus, where the ribosomal RNA is synthesized and ribosomal*

subunits are assembled from ribosomal RNA and proteins. The ribosomal subunits are exported from the nucleolus into the cytoplasm. **RNA polymerase II** is present in the nucleoplasm, where it synthesizes the mRNA precursors, and **RNA polymerase III**, also in the nucleoplasm, synthesizes the tRNAs and the 5S ribosomal RNA.

RNA polymerase II and, at higher concentrations, RNA polymerase III are inhibited by **α-amanitin**, a poison from the toadstool *Amanita phalloides. This toxin is the most common cause of fatal mushroom poisoning worldwide.*

Promoters, enhancers, and silencers are the regulatory elements of eukaryotic genes

As in prokaryotes (see Chapter 6), the promoters of different genes look quite different, with only one or a few areas of homology. Most protein-coding genes, which are transcribed by RNA polymerase II, contain the **TATA box** 25 to 30 base pairs upstream of the transcriptional initiation site. Other promoter elements, which are found less regularly, are poorly defined initiator (INR) elements at the transcriptional start site, as well as the CCAAT and GGGCG consensus sequences, which are between 60 and 120 base pairs upstream but occur in only 10% to 15% of eukaryotic promoters. Recombinant DNA studies have shown that most of the promoter elements promote transcription only if they are located in the correct $5' \rightarrow 3'$ orientation and only if they are located on the correct strand of the double helix. This suggests that the promoter elements are required for the correct positioning of RNA polymerase II on the transcriptional start site.

The eukaryotic RNA polymerases contain no functional equivalent of the bacterial σ subunit (see

---

TABLE 8.3

The eukaryotic RNA polymerases

Type	Location	Transcripts	Inhibition by α-amanitin
I	Nucleolus	Pre-rRNA	—
II	Nucleus	Pre-mRNA	+++
III	Nucleus	tRNA, 5S rRNA	+
Mitochondrial	Mitochondria	Mitochondrial RNAs	—

Chapter 6), but the promoter is recognized instead by a set of **general transcription factors.** The general transcription factors are DNA-binding proteins that are required for the transcription of *all* genes by a particular RNA polymerase, whereas **specific transcription factors** regulate the transcription of some, but not all, genes. *The RNA polymerase initiates transcription after binding to the promoter-associated transcription factors* (Fig. 8.5).

Enhancers and **silencers** are regulatory DNA sequences that mediate, respectively, an increase or a decrease in the transcription of neighboring genes. Positive control of transcription by enhancer sequences and their binding proteins is far more common than negative control. Some enhancer elements are attached to the promoter, but others are up to 5000 and occasionally up to 40,000 base pairs removed. They usually are upstream of the regulated gene, but they may be downstream or within an intron. In recombinant DNA experiments, they affect transcription even if they are on the "wrong" strand of the double helix or in the "wrong" $5' \rightarrow 3'$ orientation.

Enhancers and silencers affect gene transcription by the binding of regulatory proteins that act as specific transcription factors. *It is the DNA-bound proteins that increase or decrease the rate of transcription.* Most enhancers are organized as clusters of several binding sites for regulatory proteins, each approximately 15 to 20 base pairs long (see Fig. 8.6 for an example). The individual binding sites are called **response elements.**

Gene expression is regulated by DNA-binding proteins

Transcription is regulated by a vast number of DNA-binding proteins. *Most of them bind their response elements in a dimeric form,* either as homodimers of two identical subunits or as heterodimers of two slightly different subunits. The symmetry of these dimeric transcription factors is matched by their response elements, which frequently possess an incomplete dyad symmetry (see also Chapter 6, Fig. 6.35). Some recurrent structural motifs have been described in regulatory DNA-binding proteins. These are summarized in Table 8.4 and Figs. 8.7 and 8.8.

The dimeric transcription factors have a modular structure: a *DNA-binding module* provides both a non-

---

FIG. 8.5

Schematic model of the transcriptional initiation complex on RNA polymerase II promoters. Only the TATA binding protein (TBP) is required for transcription by all three nuclear RNA polymerases. The other "general" transcription factors shown here are involved only with transcriptional initiation by RNA polymerase II. In many genes the binding of TBP to the minor groove of the DNA induces a bend in the double helix and initiates strand separation. TAF, TBP-associated factors; TF IIA, TF IIB, TF IIF, TF IIH, transcription factors IIA, IIB, IIF, and IIH.

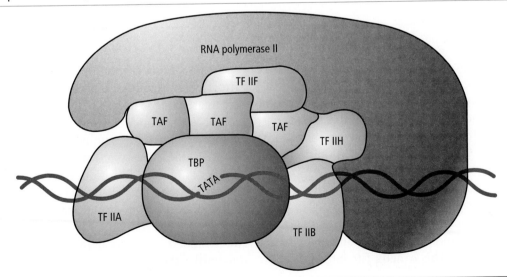

FIG. 8.6

The gene for the liver protein transthyretin (prealbumin), with its regulatory sites. The gene is drawn to scale to show its intron-exon structure and the multiple upstream binding sites for regulatory proteins. Note that in this gene, as in most others, the introns are far longer than the exons. Sites for the binding of regulatory proteins are clustered in the promoter and a distal enhancer. With the exception of AP1, which is present in all nucleated cells, the regulatory proteins are present in hepatocytes but not in most other cell types. ■, AP1; ●, C/EBP; ①, ③, ④, hepatocyte nuclear factors 1, 3, and 4.

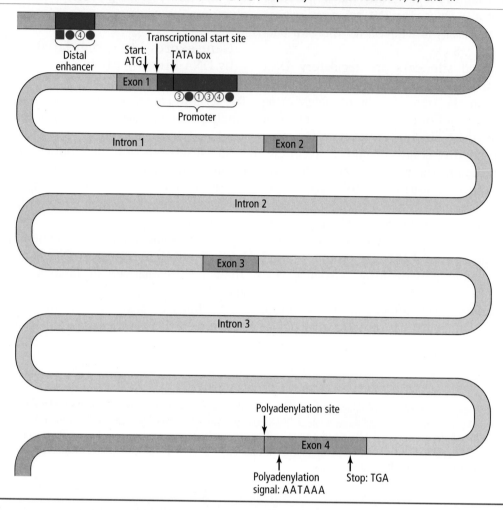

selective affinity for DNA and the ability to recognize the specific base sequence of the response element; a *dimerization module* allows the protein to assume the active dimeric state; and a *transcriptional activation (or inhibition) region* is required for the stimulation—or sometimes the inhibition—of transcription.

The DNA-binding module of the **helix-turn-helix, leucine zipper,** and **helix-loop-helix proteins** (Table 8.4) consists of an α-helix, 20 to 40 amino acids long, and has a high content of basic amino acid residues. This α-helix fits into the major

groove of the DNA double helix (Fig. 8.7, C). The **zinc finger proteins** contain between 2 and approximately 12 zinc ions in their DNA-binding region, each complexed to four amino acid side chains—either four cysteines or two cysteines and two histidines. The zinc finger is a loop of approximately 12 amino acid residues between two pairs of zinc-complexed amino acids (Fig. 8.8).

The dimerization of the transcription factors is effected by an amphipathic α-helix that forms a two-stranded coiled-coil in the dimeric protein—not unlike the α-helical coiled-coils in such struc-

TABLE 8.4

The major types of DNA-binding proteins in eukaryotes

Structural motif	Structural features	Examples
Helix-turn-helix proteins	Two α-helices separated by a β-turn. "Recognition helix" fitting in major groove of DNA.	"Homeodomain" proteins (proteins regulating embryonic development). Also most prokaryotic repressors.
Zinc finger proteins	Contain zinc bound to Cys and His side chains.	Receptors for steroid and thyroid hormones.
Leucine zipper proteins	Two α-helices, one with basic residues for DNA binding, one with regularly spaced Leu for dimerization.	C/EBP (gene activator in liver). c-Myc, c-Fos, c-Jun (growth regulators, protooncogene products).
Helix-loop-helix proteins	DNA-binding α-helix, and two dimerization helices separated by a nonhelical hoop.	Myo D-1, myogenin (proteins that induce muscle differentiation).

tural proteins as myosin, tropomyosin, and keratin (Chapter 12). The leucine zipper proteins, for example, display several leucine residues, spaced exactly seven amino acids apart, on the hydrophobic edge of the amphipathic helix. Because the α-helix has approximately 3.6 amino acids per turn (Chapter 2), these leucine residues are all on the same side of the helix.

To a large extent, *the transcription factors are regulated at the level of their own synthesis.* A different, and faster, level of control is effected by *protein-protein interactions,* which interfere with DNA binding or transcriptional activation. *Covalent modification by phosphorylation/dephosphorylation* is important, too: many transcription factors are phosphoproteins that are regulated by protein kinases and protein phosphatases. Finally, like the transcriptional regulators of prokaryotes (see Chapter 6), *some DNA-binding proteins of eukaryotes are regulated by small molecules that bind the transcription factors reversibly and act as positive or negative allosteric effectors.*

Specific transcription factors are important in several contexts:

1. *The specific transcription factors are responsible for tissue-specific gene expression.* The gene for transthyretin (prealbumin), for example, a plasma protein that is synthesized only in the liver and the choroid plexus (see Chapter 25), has at least 10 upstream binding sites for at least five different proteins (Fig. 8.6). With the exception of AP1, which is abundant in all nucleated cells, these transcription factors are present in much higher concentrations in hepatocytes than in other cells.

2. *Cell growth and differentiation are controlled by specific transcription factors.* Some transcriptional regulators stimulate, and others inhibit, cell proliferation. Also, the differentiation of stem cells into fully differentiated cells is controlled at the level of transcription, and embryogenesis can be understood as a sequence of developmental switches involving the appearance or disappearance of specific transcription factors.

3. *Some lipid-soluble hormones regulate transcription factors in their target cells.* The receptors for steroid hormones, thyroid hormones, retinoic acid, and calcitriol are zinc-finger proteins that have to form a complex with the hormone before they can bind to their response elements and stimulate transcription (see Chapter 27). The second messengers of water-soluble hormones, however, regulate transcription by inducing the phosphorylation of the transcription factors (see Chapter 27).

4. *Many viral genes can be expressed only in the presence of cellular transcription factors that have to bind to the promoters or enhancers of the viral genes.* Many viruses can infect only specific cell types because they depend on tissue-specific transcription factors in their host cell.

The design of agents that act on DNA-binding proteins and thereby affect gene transcription is a long-term objective in drug development. Agents of this kind could be useful in cancer therapy, in the treat-

FIG. 8.7

Binding of dimeric transcription factors to their response elements. The base sequences of the response elements show a dyad symmetry that matches the symmetry of the transcription factors. **A,** The schematic binding of a leucine zipper protein. The "zipper" is required for dimerization while the basic region binds to DNA. **B,** DNA binding by a helix-loop-helix protein. **C,** A computer graphics model of the binding of the carboxy-terminal portion ("basic region") of the leucine zipper protein C/EBF to its cognate binding site. (**C,** Elsevier Trends Journals, 1991.)

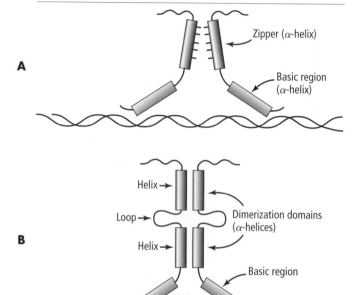

A

Zipper (α-helix)

Basic region (α-helix)

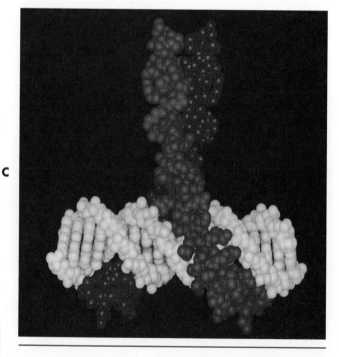

B

Helix →

Loop →

Helix →

Dimerization domains (α-helices)

Basic region

C

FIG. 8.8

The zinc finger. This structural motif occurs in 2 to 12 copies in the DNA-binding region of the zinc finger proteins. The amino acid residues on each side of the zinc are separated by approximately 3 or 4 amino acid residues, and the intervening loop contains approximately 12 residues.

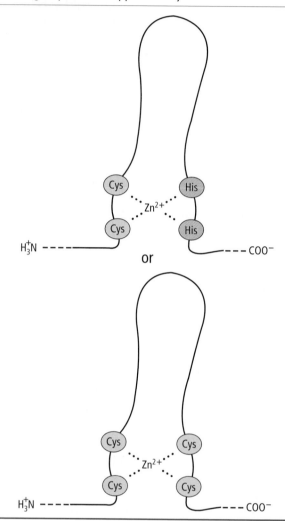

ment of some viral infections, and in the treatment of some genetic diseases.

Transcription is inhibited by histones and DNA methylation

Most of the sequence-specific DNA-binding proteins in eukaryotes (but not in prokaryotes; see Chapter 6) stimulate transcription, but *the histones inhibit transcription.* In the test tube, naked DNA is a far better template for transcription than the nucleosome-associated DNA of native chromatin. Once

FIG. 8.9

Structure of 5-methylcytosine in DNA. The methyl group does not interfere with the normal base pairing of cytosine.

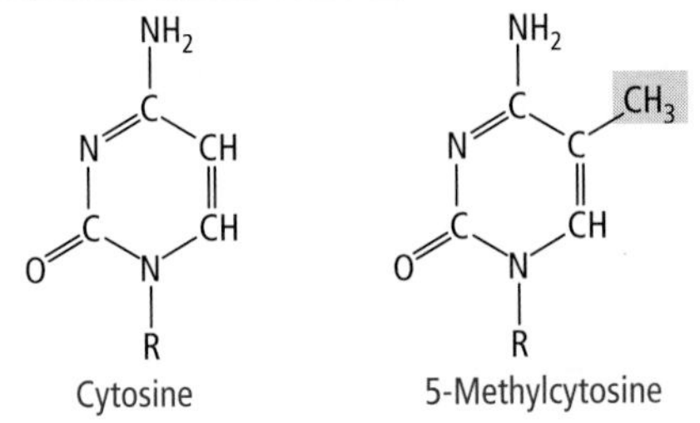

Cytosine   5-Methylcytosine

Eukaryotic mRNA is processed extensively by nuclear enzyme systems

Because most eukaryotic genes are patchworks of coding and noncoding sequences, the **primary transcripts** of protein-coding genes are much longer than the mature mRNAs. *These transcripts are processed in the nucleus, and the fully processed mature mRNA translocates to the cytoplasm, where it is translated.* Three processing steps occur almost uniformly with eukaryotic mRNA (Fig. 8.10):

1. *The 5′ end of the mRNA receives a cap.* The cap is a methylguanosine residue that is linked to the first nucleotide of the RNA through an unusual 5′-5′-triphosphate linkage (Fig. 8.11). Capping is the only definitely cotranscriptional event during mRNA processing. The cap is thought to protect the mRNA from the action of 5′-exonucleases and to assist in its binding to the ribosome.

2. *The 3′ end of the mRNA receives a poly-A tail.* Near its 3′ end, the primary transcript possesses a highly conserved AAUAAA consensus sequence as a **polyadenylation signal.** This sequence is recognized by a specific endonuclease that cleaves the RNA approximately 20 nucleotides downstream. Transcription may proceed for several hundred nucleotides beyond the polyadenylation site, but the 3′ end of the transcript is discarded. The newly created 3′ terminus, however, serves as a primer for the enzymatic addition of up to 250 adenine nucleotides. Although the poly-A tail associates with proteins that retard the action of 3′-exonucleases, it becomes progressively shorter during the lifetime of the mRNA. The only known eukaryotic mRNAs without poly-A tails are the histone mRNAs, whose half-lives are only a few minutes to an hour.

3. *The introns are removed from the primary transcript.* The intron-exon junctions of protein-coding nuclear genes, as well as a "branch site" within the intron, approximately 30 bases from the 3′ end, are marked by more-or-less-conserved consensus sequences (Fig. 8.12). The introns are removed by nuclear enzyme complexes called **spliceosomes.** The spliceosome contains five small RNAs (U1, U2, U4, U5, and U6), each between 106 and 185 nucleotides long. These are associated with proteins to form small nuclear ribonucleoprotein particles (**snRNPs,** or **"snurps"**). The mech-

started, RNA polymerase II can transcribe through a string of nucleosomes, although at a reduced rate. Transcriptional initiation, however, is reduced greatly or prevented altogether, especially when a nucleosome is bound over the promoter or enhancer of a gene. The structure of the nucleosome loosens during transcription, and possibly the histones are removed from the DNA altogether. Apparently, *the histones have to be displaced from promoters and enhancers by the competitive binding of sequence-specific transcription factors.* Transcriptional regulation in eukaryotes can be understood, in large part, as a competition between nonspecifically bound histones and sequence-specific transcription factors for relevant binding sites on the DNA.

Another more-or-less-nonspecific level of control is the methylation of cytosine residues to 5-methylcytosine (Fig. 8.9). Most of the methylcytosine is present in the sequence 5′-CG-3′ throughout the genome, and approximately 70% of the eligible sites are methylated. *Highly methylated areas of DNA are not transcribed.* For example, the transcriptionally inactive second X chromosome, which forms the Barr body in females, has a far higher 5-methylcytosine content than the active X chromosome.

The methylated CG sequence is a palindrome. The methylating enzyme systems act preferentially on hemimethylated CG sequences, and therefore both of the cytosines in a CG sequence usually are methylated. Thus *the methylation pattern of the DNA is potentially heritable through the cell generations,* even through the germline. This phenomenon, known as **genomic imprinting,** is a paradigm for the "inheritance of acquired traits."

FIG. 8.10

Posttranscriptional processing of mRNA in eukaryotes. All processing steps occur in the nucleus. The mature mRNA is transported into the cytoplasm, where it is translated by the ribosomes. Steps ④ and ⑤ take place on the spliceosome. ▭▬▭ , Exon.

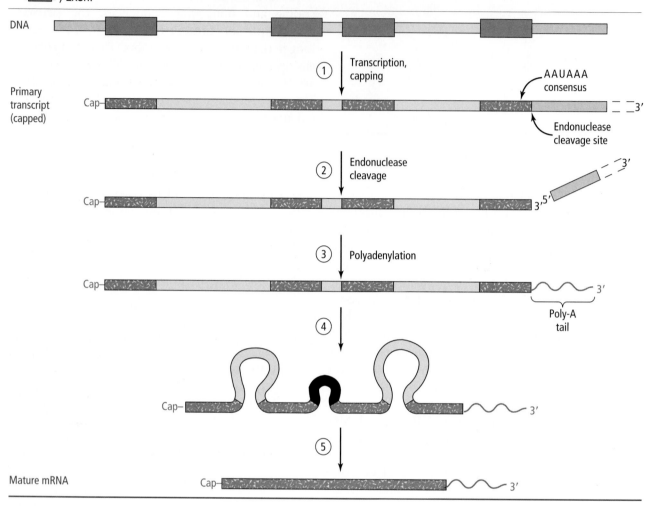

Translation is similar in prokaryotes and eukaryotes

The translational machinery of eukaryotes resembles the prokaryotic system in most respects, but there are two noteworthy differences:

1. *Eukaryotic polypeptides do not start with N-formylmethionine but rather with ordinary methionine.*
2. *Eukaryotic mRNA has no Shine-Delgarno sequence. It binds to proteins in the small ribosomal subunit* rather than the ribosomal RNA. This difference is important in genetic engineering: eukaryotic mRNAs are not translated by bacterial ribosomes unless their coding sequence is fused artificially with a bacterial ribosome-binding sequence in the 5′-untranslated region (see Chapter 10).

anism of the spliceosomal reactions is shown in Fig. 8.13.

Posttranscriptional processing and translation often are regulated

The regulation of transcription by DNA-binding proteins is the most important mechanism for the control of gene expression, both in prokaryotes and in eukaryotes.

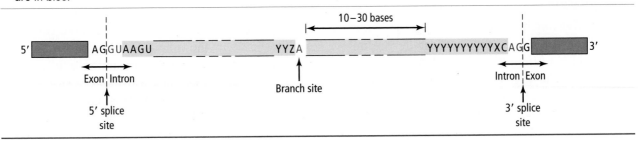

Eukaryotes use several additional mechanisms that operate at the posttranscriptional level.

Intranuclear degradation of primary transcriptor mRNA

A majority of all nuclear RNAs fall prey to nucleases before they can ever emerge into the cytoplasm as mature, translatable mRNAs. This extensive RNA degradation may prevent the inappropriate expression of genes. It also may protect the cell from viruses whose mRNAs are degraded in the nucleus. It is not known whether differences in nuclear RNAse activities participate in the tissue-specific regulation of gene expression.

Tissue-specific initiation and termination of transcription

Some genes can be transcribed from alternative promoters, yielding transcripts with different 5'-terminal portions. In other genes, alternative polyadenylation sites can be used, and this produces transcripts with different 3' ends. An example for the tissue-specific initiation of transcription is the use of alternative promoters in the gene for glucokinase (Fig. 8.14), an enzyme that is expressed only in the liver and in the insulin-producing β-cells of the pancreas (see Chapter 17). The significance, if any, of this tissue-specific transcriptional initiation is unknown.

Tissue-specific splicing

In some primary transcripts, sequences that are treated as introns by some cells are treated as exons by others. This leads to the formation of different mRNAs and different proteins from a single gene.

FIG. 8.12

Consensus sequences of mammalian introns. These sequences are recognized by the small nuclear ribonucleoprotein particles ("snurps") during the assembly of the spliceosome. They base-pair with the RNA molecules in the snurps. Mutations in the consensus sequences result in faulty splicing ("splice site mutation"). Y, pyrimidine; Z, purine; X, any base. Highly conserved bases are in blue.

FIG. 8.13

Splicing of introns from the transcripts of protein-coding genes in eukaryotes. The lariat intermediate has a $2' \rightarrow 5'$ (A $\rightarrow$ G) phosphodiester bond. Z, Purine; Y, pyrimidine; ψ, pseudouridine; A_m and U_m, 2-O-methylated adenosine and uridine.

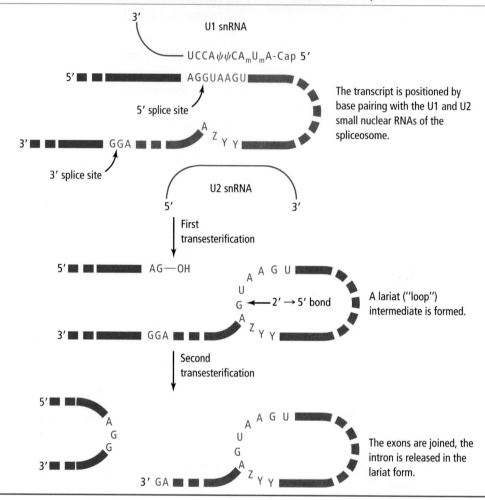

The molecular basis for these differences in the splicing machineries of different cells is not known at present, but differential splicing is a relatively common phenomenon. Figure 8.15 shows the tissue-specific splicing of the muscle protein tropomyosin.

Regulation of mRNA stability

The survival time of mature mRNA in the cytoplasm is regulated by nucleases that degrade the mRNA, and by mRNA-binding proteins that prevent nuclease attack. The regulation of transferrin receptor synthesis, described in Chapter 24, is a well-studied example for the regulation of mRNA stability by an mRNA-binding protein.

Regulation of translation

Ribosomal protein synthesis also can be regulated. The translation of ferritin mRNA in the liver, for example (see Chapter 24), is inhibited by the binding of a regulatory protein to the mRNA.

mRNA editing

This is a relatively uncommon mechanism in which a base in the mRNA is chemically altered posttranscriptionally. In the mRNA for apolipoprotein B in the intestine, for example, an amino acid–coding codon is changed enzymatically into a stop codon. The translation product of this edited mRNA is therefore shorter than that of the unedited mRNA (see Chapter 20).

FIG. 8.14

Tissue-specific transcription of the glucokinase gene in hepatocytes and pancreatic β-cells. Alternative promoters are used in the two cell types. The resulting polypeptides differ in the N-terminal region, which is encoded by exon 1 in the pancreas and by exon 1L or by exons 1L + 2A in the liver. ▬, Exon; ▭, intron.

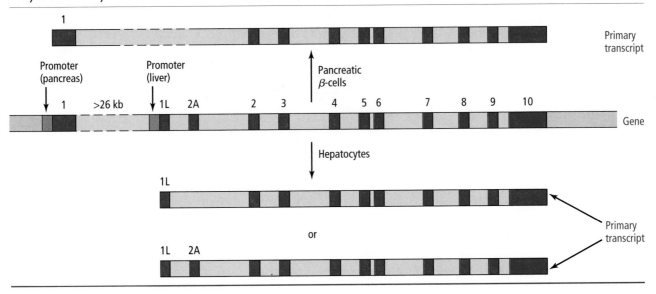

FIG. 8.15

The tropomyosin gene is a good example for tissue-specific splicing. Only 10 of the 13 exons are used in striated muscle, and 9 in smooth muscle. In this case, alternative polyadenylation signals are used in striated muscle and smooth muscle [Poly A (str) and Poly A (sm)].

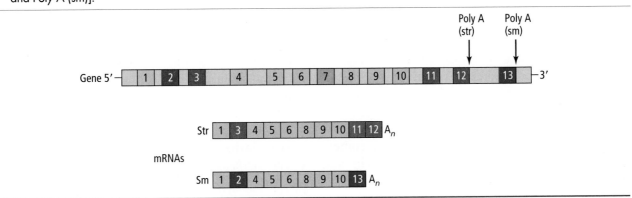

Diphtheria toxin inhibits protein synthesis

Diphtheria is a bacterial infection of the upper respiratory tract in which necrosis (death) of mucosal cells leads to severe pathologic changes and airway obstruction. The offending bacterium, *Corynebacterium diphtheriae*, causes this disease by secreting a toxic protein. After binding to a surface receptor on the mucosal cells, the toxin is cleaved proteolytically, and one of its fragments penetrates into the cell. *This active fragment is an enzyme that inactivates the elongation factor EF2* (Fig. 8.16). EF2 is the equivalent of the prokaryotic elongation factor EF-G (see Chapter 6), which catalyzes the GTP-driven movement of the ribosome along the mRNA. Because the toxin acts as an enzyme that inactivates the elongation factor irreversibly, a single toxin molecule is sufficient to inactivate thousands of EF2 molecules and to kill the cell by blocking its protein synthesis.

FIG. 8.16

Covalent modification of the eukaryotic elongation factor 2 (EF2, "translocase") by diphtheria toxin. The amino acid side chain in the elongation factor is diphthamide, a posttranslationally modified histidine.

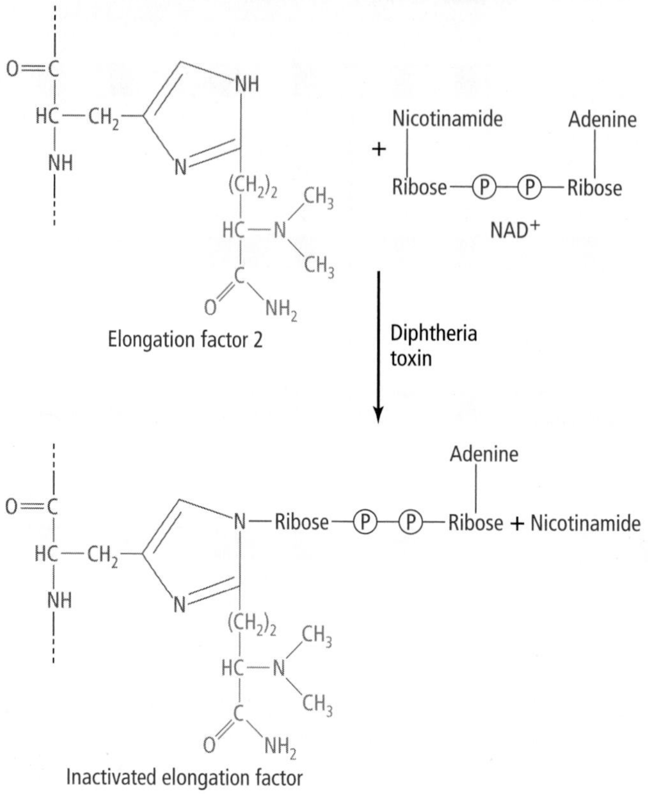

Interestingly, the gene for diphtheria toxin is not a regular denizen of the bacterial chromosome but belongs to a temperate phage (see Chapter 9) that is carried as a prophage in the bacterial genome. Only lysogenic strains of *C. diphtheriae* are pathogenic. Nonlysogenic strains are peaceful members of the normal bacterial flora on our skin and mucous membranes.

THE PROCESSING AND TARGETING OF EUKARYOTIC PROTEINS

Peptide bond formation by the ribosome is not the last step in protein synthesis. The remaining tasks are:

1. *The protein's higher-order structure has to be formed.* Most polypeptides fold spontaneously into their higher-order structure during translation, and this process is driven only by noncovalent interactions between different portions of the polypeptide. In some instances, however, helper proteins called **chaperones** assist in the folding process.
2. *Covalent modifications have to be introduced enzymatically.* These processes are collectively called **posttranslational processing**.
3. *The protein has to be transported to its proper destination.*

In the last part of this chapter, we trace the fate of eukaryotic proteins after their synthesis by the ribosome.

The secretory pathway starts at the rough endoplasmic reticulum

Some ribosomes are free-floating in the cytoplasm, whereas others are attached to the membrane of the rough endoplasmic reticulum. The ribosomes in these two locations have the same molecular structure, but they make different proteins: *free cytoplasmic ribosomes synthesize the proteins of cytoplasm, nucleus,*

TABLE 8.5

Use of the secretory pathway by different cell types

Cell	Secreted products	Reference page
Pancreatic acinar cells	Zymogens	Chapter 14
Pancreatic β-cells	Insulin, C-peptide	Chapter 26
Fibroblasts	Collagen, elastin, glycoproteins, proteoglycans	Chapter 13
Goblet cells	Glycoproteins ("mucins"), proteoglycans	Chapter 13
Intestinal mucosal cells	Chylomicrons	Chapter 18
Hepatocytes	Serum albumin, other plasma proteins, VLDL	Chapter 25

and mitochondria; the ER-bound ribosomes are in charge of secreted proteins (Table 8.5), plasma membrane proteins, and the proteins of ER, Golgi apparatus, and lysosomes.

The routing of secreted proteins through the **secretory pathway** is depicted in Fig. 8.17: during their synthesis by ribosomes on the rough ER, these proteins penetrate through the ER membrane into the lumen of the organelle. After moving through the ER, they are ferried to the Golgi by transfer vesicles that bud off from the ER and eventually fuse with the Golgi membrane. The Golgi packages the proteins into secretory vesicles, and these vesicles fuse with the plasma membrane to release their contents by **exocytosis**.

This road to the periphery also is an assembly line on which proteins are modified covalently by enzymes within ER, Golgi, or secretory vesicles. The most important types of covalent modification in the secretory pathway are listed in Table 8.6.

Plasma membrane proteins and the proteins of the ER and Golgi membranes also are processed in the secretory pathway. Unlike the secreted proteins, these proteins are not dissolved in the lumen of ER, transfer vesicles, Golgi, and secretory vesicles, but are part of their membranes.

O-linked oligosaccharides of glycoproteins are synthesized from nucleotide-activated sugars

The most complex type of posttranslational processing in the secretory pathway is the synthesis of the oligosaccharides in glycoproteins. Some oligosaccharides are bound covalently to the hydroxy groups of serine or threonine side chains in the polypeptides. These are called **O-linked oligosaccharides.** O-linked glycosylation takes place in the

Golgi apparatus, where the oligosaccharides are constructed by the stepwise addition of monosaccharides. *The precursors for these glycosylation reactions are nucleotide-activated monosaccharides* (see Fig. 8.18 and Fig. 8.19, A and Table 8.7).

The nucleotide is released when the sugar is transferred to the amino acid side chain or to the growing oligosaccharide chain, as shown in Fig. 8.19, B. The enzymes catalyzing these reactions are called **glycosyl transferases.** The synthesis of the activated sugars is discussed in Chapter 17.

N-linked oligosaccharides are synthesized through a lipid-linked intermediate

N-linked oligosaccharides are bound by an N-glycosidic bond to the amide group in the side chain of asparagine. N-linked glycosylation proceeds by a more complex route than O-linked glycosylation. *It starts with the construction of a mannose-rich oligosaccharide on **dolichol phosphate,** a lipid in the membrane of the rough ER. Like the O-linked oligosaccharides, the dolichol phosphate–bound oligosaccharide is synthesized by the stepwise addition of sugars from the activated precursors, namely UDP-GlcNAc, GDP-Man, and UDP-Glc. The whole oligosaccharide is then transferred to an asparagine side chain of a newly synthesized polypeptide (Fig. 8.20).

In the ER and Golgi, the glucose residues and one or more of the mannose residues are removed by exoglycosidases. The remaining core structure is again extended by the addition of monosaccharides from their activated precursors.

The oligosaccharides of glycoproteins show great structural diversity. They range in size from 2 sugar

FIG. 8.17

The secretory pathway. The proteins (⌇) are transported to the cell periphery through ER, transfer vesicles, Golgi apparatus, and secretory vesicles. The release from the cell is by exocytosis (fusion of the secretory vesicle membrane with the plasma membrane).

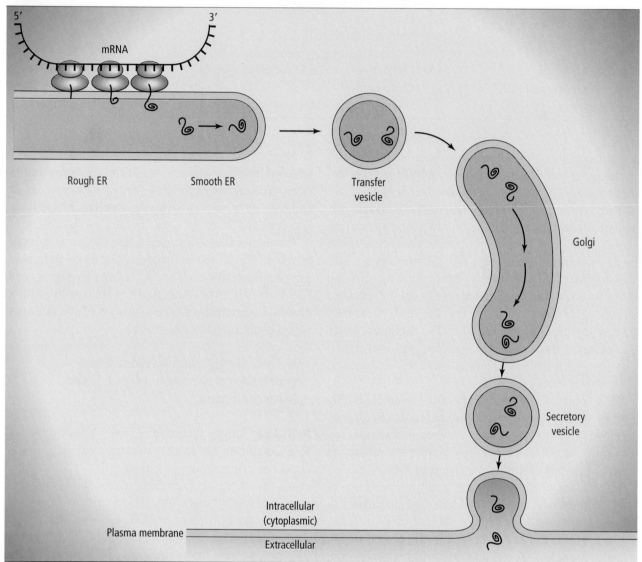

TABLE 8.6

Posttranslational processing in the secretory pathway

Type of processing	Examples
Removal of signal sequence	All proteins of the secretory pathway
Disulfide bond formation	Most proteins of the secretory pathway
Glycosylation	Collagen, other glycoproteins, proteoglycans
Amino acid modifications	Collagen, elastin
Partial proteolytic cleavage	Insulin, other peptide and protein hormones

FIG. 8.18

The structures of some monosaccharides commonly found in glycoproteins.

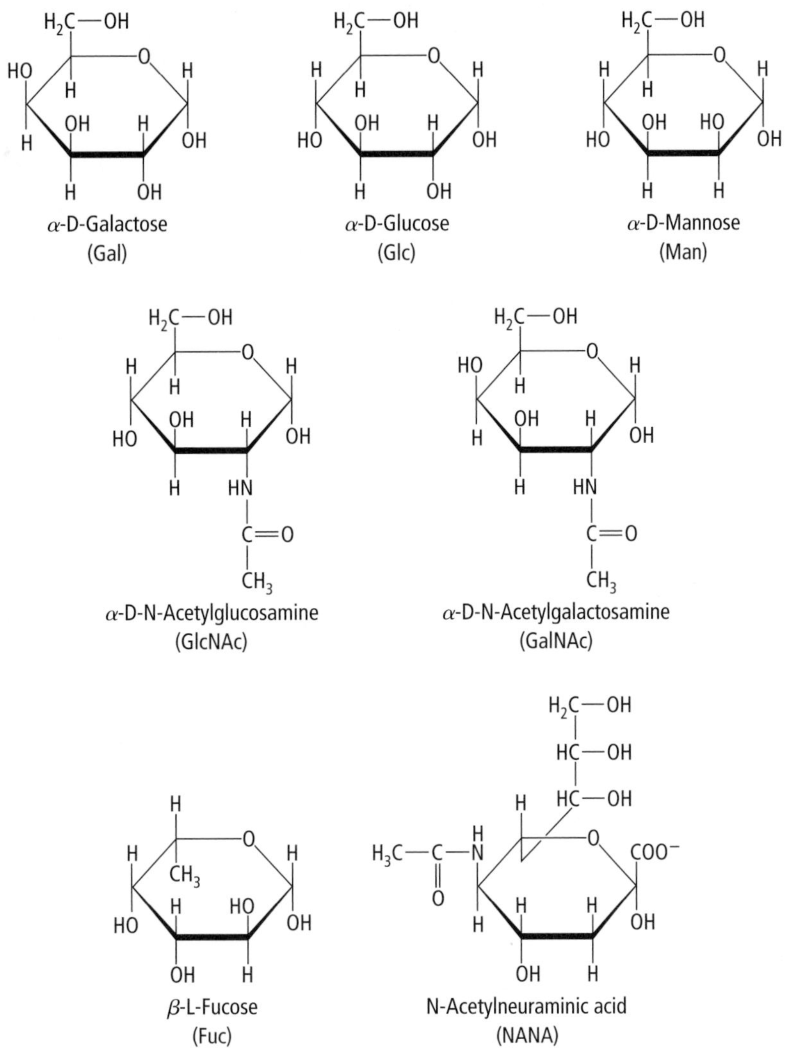

α-D-Galactose
(Gal)

α-D-Glucose
(Glc)

α-D-Mannose
(Man)

α-D-N-Acetylglucosamine
(GlcNAc)

α-D-N-Acetylgalactosamine
(GalNAc)

β-L-Fucose
(Fuc)

N-Acetylneuraminic acid
(NANA)

residues in the most simple O-linked oligosaccharides to more than 15 in some of the more complex N-linked oligosaccharides. Most are branched, and in many (but not all) cases, the terminal positions are occupied by the acidic amino sugar N-acetylneuraminic acid (NANA; see Fig. 8.18).

The oligosaccharides of glycoproteins are important for many of their biological functions, including the maintenance of their higher-order structure, water solubility, antigenicity, and the regulation of the protein's metabolic fate. The carbohydrate content of different glycoproteins varies from less than 10% to more than 50%.

Lysosomes are formed in a side branch of the secretory pathway

Lysosomal enzymes are directed to their proper destination by a molecular tag: they acquire a mannose 6-phosphate residue during the glycosylation reactions in the Golgi (Fig. 8.21). This molecular tag acts like a postal address, causing their sorting into the lysosomes. Like the secretory vesicles (Fig. 8.17), lysosomes are formed by budding from the Golgi.

In **I-cell disease,** a rare inherited disease that leads to mental deterioration and skeletal deformi-

FIG. 8.19

Synthesis of O-linked oligosaccharides in glycoproteins. **A,** Examples of activated monosaccharides used in the synthesis of oligosaccharides. The nucleotide is generally bound to the anomeric carbon (C-1 in the aldohexoses and their derivatives). The synthesis of the activated monosaccharides is described in Chapter 17). **B,** Two steps in the synthesis of an O-linked oligosaccharide in a glycoprotein. Each reaction requires a specific glycosyltransferase in the Golgi.

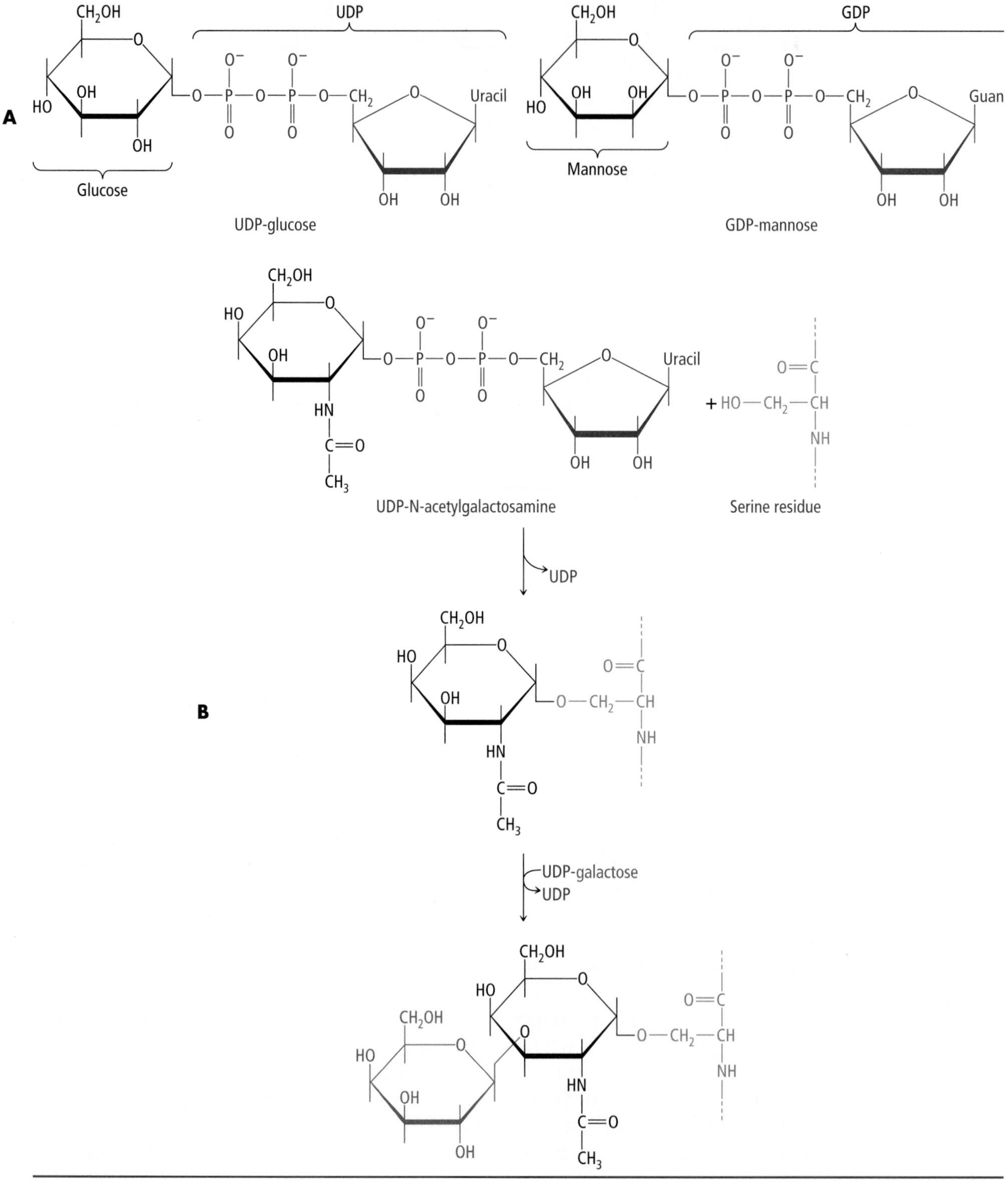

TABLE 8.7

Monosaccharides commonly found in glycoproteins

Monosaccharide	Type	Activated form	Comments
Galactose (Gal)	Aldohexose	UDP-Gal	Common
Glucose (Glc)	Aldohexose	UDP-Glc	Rare in mature glycoproteins
Mannose (Man)	Aldohexose	GDP-Man	Very common in N-linked oligosaccharides
Fucose (Fuc)	6-Deoxyhexose	GDP-Fuc	Both in O- and N-linked oligosaccharides
N-Acetylglucosamine (GlcNAc)	Amino sugar	UDP-GlcNAc	Linked to asparagine in N-linked oligosaccharides
N-Acetylgalactosamine (GalNAc)	Amino sugar	UDP-GalNAc	Common
N-Acetylneuraminic acid (NANA)	A sialic acid (acidic sugar derivative)	CMP-NANA	Often in terminal positions of both O- and N-linked oligosaccharides

FIG. 8.20

Synthesis of N-linked oligosaccharides in glycoproteins. **A,** Structure of dolichol phosphate. This lipid is present in the ER membrane, where it is used as a carrier of the core oligosaccharide. **B,** Structure of the dolichol-bound precursor oligosaccharide in N-linked glycosylation. This oligosaccharide is synthesized by the stepwise addition of the monosaccharides from activated precursors. The second phosphate residue in dolichol pyrophosphate is introduced by UDP-GlcNAc during the synthesis of the oligosaccharide. **C,** Transfer of the precursor oligosaccharide to an asparagine side chain of the polypeptide. This transfer reaction is cotranslational.

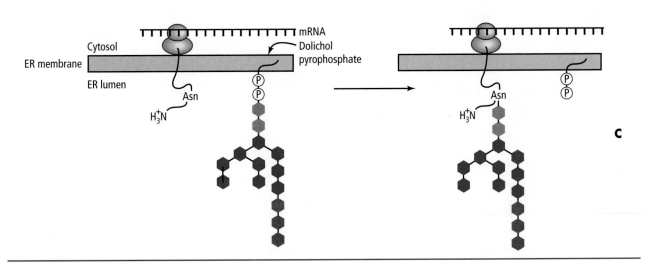

ties, one of the enzymes necessary for the attachment of mannose 6-phosphate to the lysosomal enzymes is absent. As a result, *the enzymes are not sorted into the lysosomes but rather are secreted.* Sphingolipids and glycosaminoglycans, which normally are degraded by lysosomal enzymes, accumulate in the lysosomes, whereas high levels of lysosomal enzymes are found in blood and other body fluids. I-cell disease is an example of a **lysosomal storage disease.** Other examples of lysosomal storage diseases are discussed in Chapters 13 and 19.

A signal sequence directs polypeptides to the endoplasmic reticulum

How does the cell "know" that a newly synthesized protein has to be processed through the secretory pathway? Polypeptides are synthesized from the amino to the carboxy terminus (see Chapter 6). In secreted proteins, as well as in proteins of plasma membrane, ER, Golgi, and lysosomes, the polypeptide starts with a **signal sequence** at the amino end. Signal sequences differ in different polypeptides, but usually they are 20 to 25 amino acids long and contain a high proportion of hydrophobic amino acids.

As soon as it emerges from the ribosome, the signal sequence binds to a cytoplasmic **signal recognition particle (SRP)** that contains a small RNA molecule of approximately 300 nucleotides (the **7SL RNA**) together with six protein subunits (Fig. 8.22). *Binding of the SRP halts translation* until the SRP–signal sequence–ribosome complex binds to a docking protein on the ER membrane. At this point, the SRP is released, translation resumes, and a pore forms in the ER membrane through which the polypeptide is passed. Soluble proteins enter the lumen of the ER, but membrane proteins "get

FIG. 8.22

Synthesis of a secreted protein by ribosomes on the rough ER. *SRP,* Signal recognition particle.

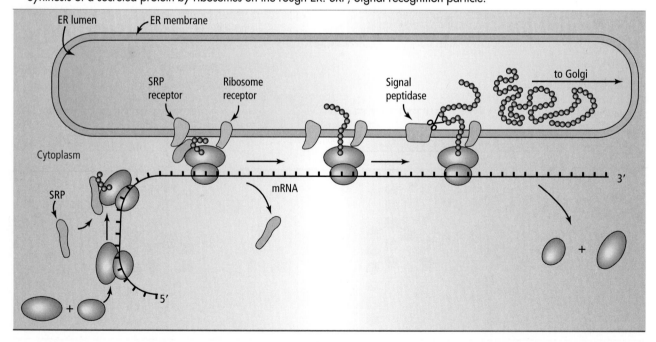

stuck" in the ER membrane. The signal sequence is no longer required beyond this stage. Even before translation is completed it is cleaved off by a **signal peptidase** in the ER.

The secreted proteins and membrane proteins of bacteria are synthesized similarly by ribosomes attached to the plasma membrane. Indeed, bacterial signal sequences can direct nascent polypeptides to the ER membranes of eukaryotic protein-synthesizing systems. Most likely, *the organelles of the secretory pathway have evolved from an infolding of the plasma membrane during eukaryotic evolution.*

Nuclear and mitochondrial proteins possess their own targeting sequences

Nuclear proteins and most mitochondrial proteins are synthesized by free cytoplasmic ribosomes. Nuclear proteins are directed through the nuclear pore complexes by short targeting sequences that are rich in the cationic amino acids lysine and arginine. These sequences often are in internal locations and are not cleaved off proteolytically. Most mitochondrial proteins are synthesized in the cytoplasm and have to be targeted to the outer membrane, the intermembranous space, the inner membrane, or the mitochondrial matrix. Initial targeting to the outer membrane requires an amino-terminal sequence rich in both the basic amino acids and serine and threonine. The subsequent partitioning between the different mitochondrial compartments is complex and frequently involves proteolytic cleavage events.

The endocytotic pathway brings proteins into the cell

Cells not only secrete proteins. They also are able to take up proteins, other macromolecules, and even large solid particles from their environment. This can be achieved by three processes (Fig. 8.23):

1. **Phagocytosis** (literally "cell eating") is the uptake of solid particles into the cell. The particle becomes surrounded by the plasma membrane and enclosed in a large membrane-bound vacuole. This phagocytic vacuole fuses with lysosomes or other intracellular vesicles, and its contents are digested within the cell. Unicellular eukary-

otes use phagocytosis for their own nutrition. In the human body, however, phagocytosis is limited mostly to granulocytes, monocytes, and macrophages, which participate in our immune defenses by eating up infectious microorganisms. These cells also engulf inanimate objects, such as dust particles in the lungs or urate crystals in the joints of gouty patients (see Chapter 23).

2. **Pinocytosis** ("cell drinking") is the nonselective uptake of fluid droplets into the cell. Pinocytotic vesicles contain dissolved substances at the same concentrations as the extracellular medium. Pinocytosis is used by secretory cells to retrieve the membrane material that is added to the plasma membrane during exocytosis.

3. **Receptor-mediated endocytosis** is a mechanism for the selective uptake of proteins or other high-molecular-weight materials. Its mechanism is similar to pinocytosis, but it requires a **receptor** for the endocytosed product. The receptor is a membrane protein to which the extracellular product binds selectively as a ligand. Binding is followed by the clustering of receptor-ligand complexes on the cell surface, and finally by the formation of an endocytotic vesicle. Endocytotic vesicles tend to fuse with each other and with intracellular vesicles to form larger structures called **endosomes,** which rapidly become acidified to a pH of approximately 5.0. In most cases, the endosome fuses with a lysosome to form a **secondary lysosome** in which the endocytosed material is digested by lysosomal enzymes. In most—but not all—cases, the receptor is recycled to the cell surface.

The most important uses of receptor-mediated endocytosis are:

1. *The uptake of nutritive substances.* The uptake of low-density lipoprotein (LDL, see Chapter 20) and of the iron-transferrin complex (see Chapter 24) are the most prominent examples of this.

2. *Waste disposal.* This function of receptor-mediated endocytosis is illustrated by the uptake of "worn-out" plasma proteins (see Chapter 25), hemoglobin-haptoglobin complexes, and heme-hemopexin complexes (Chapter 25) by hepatocytes or reticuloendothelial cells. The endocytosed products are digested by lysosomal enzymes.

FIG. 8.23

Cellular uptake of macromolecules and solid particles. **A,** Phagocytosis requires a cell surface protein (T) that acts as a receptor for the phagocytized particle, and it depends on the reversible assembly and disassembly of actin microfilaments (~) under the plasma membrane. Pseudopods are formed that flow round the particle. *L,* Lysosomes. **B,** Pinocytosis does not require a specific receptor. The cytoplasmic protein clathrin (/‾\ ) is required to form a coated pit, which subsequently forms a coated vesicle. Soluble extracellular molecules are taken up in proportion to their concentration in the extracellular medium. **C,** Receptor-mediated endocytosis is similar to pinocytosis but requires a receptor in the plasma membrane. **Y**, Receptor; ■, ligand.

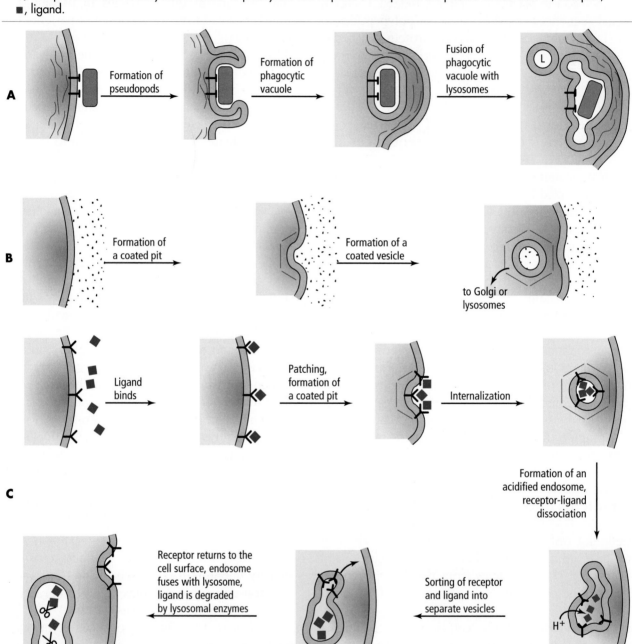

3. *Mucosal transfer.* In some cases, the endocytotic vesicle is not directed to the lysosomes but rather traverses the cell to fuse with the plasma membrane on the opposite side. The secretion of IgA across mucosal surfaces (see Chapter 25) is an example.

SUMMARY

Although the mechanisms of DNA replication and gene expression are similar in prokaryotes and eukaryotes, there are some noteworthy differences. Eukaryotes have far larger genomes than prokaryotes, and their DNA is packaged into chromosomes with the help of basic proteins called histones. Most of the DNA, dubbed "junk DNA," is noncoding, and most of this is of no obvious use for the organism. This junk DNA contains repetitive sequences, both in the form of simple-sequence DNA and in the form of moderately repetitive short and long interspersed elements. Some of these interspersed elements, most notably the Alu sequences and the LINE-1 sequences, are mobile. Their mobility depends on a LINE-encoded reverse transcriptase that allows them to move through an RNA intermediate in a process called retroposition.

The most remarkable feature of eukaryotic gene expression is the posttranscriptional processing of mRNA. Eukaryotic genes are patchworks of sequences called exons, which are represented in the mature mRNA, and introns, which do not appear in the mature mRNA because they are spliced out of the primary transcript. The removal of introns takes place in the nucleus and requires ribonucleoprotein particles called spliceosomes.

Most of the encoded proteins themselves are subject to extensive posttranslational processing. The cell also employs sophisticated mechanisms to direct its proteins to their proper destinations. Thus secreted proteins are channeled through the endoplasmic reticulum and the Golgi apparatus before they are released into the extracellular space by exocytosis.

Further Reading

Abel T, Maniatis T: Mechanism of eukaryotic gene regulation. In: Stamatoyannopoulos G, Nienhuis AW, Majerus PW,

Varmus H, editors: The molecular basis of blood diseases, pp. 33-70. W. B. Saunders, Philadelphia, 1994.

Allsopp RC et al.: Telomere length predicts replicative capacity of human fibroblasts. *Proc Natl Acad Sci USA* 89, 10114-10118, 1992.

Bernardi G: The human genome: organization and evolutionary history. *Annu Rev Genet* 29, 445-476, 1995.

Charlesworth B, Sniegowski P, Stephan W: The evolutionary dynamics of repetitive DNA in eukaryotes. *Nature* 371, 215-220, 1994.

Cowell IG: Repression versus activation in the control of gene transcription: *Trends Biochem Sci* 19, 38-42, 1994.

Dingwall C, Laskey RA: Nuclear targeting sequences—a consensus? *Trends Biochem Sci* 16, 478-481, 1991.

Drapkin R, Reinberg D: The multifunctional TF IIH complex and transcriptional control. *Trends Biochem Sci* 19, 504-508, 1994.

Glick BS, Beasley EM, Schatz G: Protein sorting in mitochondria. *Trends Biochem Sci* 17, 453-459, 1992.

Halban PA, Irminger J-C: Sorting and processing of secretory proteins. *Biochem J* 299, 1-18, 1994.

Holzman D: A "jumping gene" caught in the act. *Science* 254, 1728-1729, 1991.

Jennissen HP: Ubiquitin and the enigma of intracellular protein degradation. *Eur J Biochem* 231, 1-30, 1995.

Koleske AJ, Young RA: The RNA polymerase II holoenzyme and its implications for gene regulation. *Trends Biochem Sci* 20: 113-116, 1995.

Lingner J, Cooper JP, Cech TR: Telomerase and DNA end replication: no longer a lagging strand problem? *Science* 269, 1533-1534, 1995.

McCarthy JEG, Kollmus H: Cytoplasmic mRNA-protein interactions in eukaryotic gene expression. *Trends Biochem Sci* 20, 191-197, 1995.

Rippe K, Von Hippel PH, Langowski J: Action at a distance: DNA-looping and initiation of transcription. *Trends Biochem Sci* 20, 500-506, 1995.

Royle NJ: The proterminal regions and telomeres of human chromosomes. *Adv Genet* 32, 273-315, 1995.

Shay JW, Wright WE: The reactivation of telomerase activity in cancer progression: *Trends Genet* 12(4), 129-131, 1996.

Walter P, Johnson AE: Signal sequence recognition and protein targeting to the endoplasmic reticulum membrane. *Annu Rev Cell Biol* 10, 87-119, 1994.

Wek RC: eIF-2 Kinase: Regulators of general and gene-specific translation initiation. *Trends Biochem Sci* 19, 491-496, 1994.

Wolffe AP: Nucleosome positioning and modification: Chromatin structures that potentiate transcription. *Trends Biochem Sci* 19, 240-245, 1994.

QUESTIONS

1. The steroid hormone receptors can best be characterized as
   A. General transcription factors
   B. Zinc finger proteins
   C. Membrane proteins
   D. Histones
   E. Enhancers

2. Some pharmaceutical companies try frantically to find inhibitors of telomerase. A telomerase inhibitor could, in theory, be used to
   A. Boost the synthesis of muscle proteins
   B. Prevent viral infections
   C. Cure patients with cancer
   D. Cure patients with AIDS
   E. Make people immortal

3. Alu sequences can cause diseases by jumping into new genomic locations. Their mobility is thought to depend on the enzymes
   A. Transposase and RNA polymerase
   B. DNA polymerase and RNA replicase
   C. Peptidyl transferase and transposase
   D. Primase and integrase
   E. RNA polymerase and reverse transcriptase

4. Which is the best description of "enhancers" in eukaryotes?
   A. Regulatory DNA sequences within the coding sequences of genes that affect the rate of transcriptional elongation
   B. Binding sites for general transcription factors in the promoter
   C. Proteins that bind to regulatory base sequences in DNA
   D. DNA sequences outside the promoter region that contain multiple binding sites for regulatory proteins
   E. Proteins that enhance the rate of translational initiation by binding either to the ribosome or to the mRNA

5. A signal sequence has to be expected in the precursors of all the following proteins *except*
   A. Myoglobin, a cytoplasmic protein
   B. Acetylcholinesterase, a protein of the plasma membrane
   C. Collagen, a protein in the extracellular matrix of connective tissues
   D. Signal peptidase, a protein of the ER
   E. Acid maltase, a lysosomal hydrolase

Chapter 9

Introduction to Genetic Diseases

Genes encode proteins, and abnormal genes encode abnormal proteins. Abnormal proteins can cause disease. An abnormal gene arises by a **mutation**, a change in the DNA sequence. **Somatic mutations** occur in somatic cells and lead to an abnormal somatic cell clone. **Germline mutations,** however, are transmitted to the offspring and cause genetic diseases. The signs and symptoms of genetic diseases depend on the affected protein. If, for example, hemoglobin is affected, we have to expect a blood disease; if a structural protein of connective tissue is affected, a connective tissue disease results; and if a metabolic enzyme is affected, we will see a metabolic disease. Most mutations lead to an absent or nonfunctional protein product, but occasionally a mutation produces a protein with enhanced biological activity (for example, an enzyme with increased catalytic activity) or the protein is overproduced. In some cases, the mutant protein acquires new properties, either with or without the loss of its original function.

In this chapter, the various types of mutations are introduced, the importance of DNA repair is discussed, and the hemoglobinopathies are presented as examples of the relationship among the defective gene, its protein product, and the phenotypic expression of the disease.

| MUTATIONS AND DNA REPAIR |

Mutations either occur spontaneously or are induced by such external agents as radiation and chemicals. Although mutations provide the raw material for natural evolution, those that are of concern in medicine are undesirable: they lead to a genetic disease when they occur in the germline, and to a defective cell clone when they occur in a somatic cell. Somatic mutations can produce cells with reduced viability or impaired function, and *these mutations contribute to the normal aging process.* The most dangerous somatic mutations, however, are those that cause the cell to grow at an increased rate. *Mutations of this type lead to neoplastic diseases*, which are responsible for 20% of all deaths in industrialized countries. In the following sections, the molecular basis of mutagenesis and the DNA repair mechanisms that keep the mutation rate within tolerable limits are discussed.

The genes of somatic cells are present in two copies

All somatic cells of an organism are derived from a single ancestral cell, the fertilized ovum or the zygote. During repeated mitotic divisions, the replicated DNA is distributed equally to the daughter cells, and therefore *(almost) all somatic cells have the same genotype.* Moreover, the zygote contains two complete sets of genetic information, one from the sperm and one from the ovum. Therefore *the chromosomes, and the genes on them, are present in two copies in each somatic cell.* Somatic cells are said to be **diploid,** and the sperm and ovum are **haploid.** Most people have 46 chromosomes in their somatic cells, including 22 pairs of **autosomes** and two sex chromosomes—XX in females and XY in males.

The diploid state of somatic cells has an important implication for the expression of genetic diseases: an aberrant gene can be present in one copy, together with its normal counterpart. This condition is called **heterozygosity**. Worse, it can be present in two copies, without the normal counterpart. This condition is called **homozygosity**. In some cases, the heterozygous carriers of a disease gene are affected clinically. With respect to the disease gene, this pattern of inheritance is called **dominant**. In other cases, only individuals homozygous for the disease gene are ill. This inheritance pattern is called **recessive**.

At the biochemical level, *heterozygotes for a normal and a defective gene generally produce both the normal and the defective protein product*. Therefore it often is possible to identify asymptomatic heterozygous carriers of a recessive disease gene by quantitative biochemical determinations of the protein product.

A change in the base sequence of DNA can change the amino acid sequence of the encoded polypeptide

A **point mutation** is a change in a single base pair of the DNA. It is called **transition** if a purine is replaced by another purine or a pyrimidine by another pyrimidine, and **transversion** if a purine is replaced by a pyrimidine or a pyrimidine by a purine. If it occurs in the coding sequence of a gene, *the most common consequence of a point mutation is a single amino acid substitution in the polypeptide*. The effects on the biological properties of the polypeptide are variable: frequently the protein still is able to function normally, but in other cases its biological function is lost, either partially or completely.

Example:

$$
\begin{array}{ll}
\text{-ACA-TTA-CGC-} & \text{-ACA-TCA-CGC-} \\
\text{- Thr -Leu- Arg -} \longrightarrow & \text{- Thr - Ser - Arg -}
\end{array}
$$

Thanks to the degeneracy of the genetic code, some point mutations produce a codon that still codes for the same amino acid. **Silent mutations** of this kind are asymptomatic and can be identified only by DNA sequencing.

Example:

$$
\begin{array}{ll}
\text{-ACA-TTA-CGC-} & \text{-ACA-CTA-CGC-} \\
\text{- Thr -Leu- Arg -} \longrightarrow & \text{- Thr - Leu- Arg -}
\end{array}
$$

Point mutations in the untranscribed spacers between the genes or in the introns are silent unless they interfere with the initiation of transcription or RNA splicing.

A **nonsense mutation** is a point mutation that generates a stop codon. It causes the *premature termination of translation*, usually with the complete loss of function in the truncated protein.

Example:

$$
\begin{array}{ll}
\text{-ACA-TTA-CGC-} & \text{-ACA-TAA-CGC-} \\
\text{- Thr -Leu- Arg -} \longrightarrow & \text{- Thr -Stop . . . . .}
\end{array}
$$

Deletion and **insertion** are mutations in which bases are removed from the normal sequence or added to it. Some deletions and insertions are huge, affecting a large piece of the chromosome with dozens or hundreds of genes, but others affect only one or a few base pairs. The insertion or deletion of one or two base pairs in the coding sequence of a gene amounts to a **frameshift mutation**: beyond the site of the mutation, the mRNA is translated in the wrong reading frame and the amino acid sequence of the polypeptide is completely abnormal. The protein product most likely is devoid of any normal biological activity. The insertion or deletion of three base pairs, or any multiple of three, does not result in a frameshift, and the resulting protein is more likely to retain part or all of its biological activity.

Example:

$$
\begin{array}{ll}
\text{-CTC-ATC-GGA-CTT-} & \text{-CTC-TCG-GAC-TT--} \\
\text{- Leu - Ile - Gly -Leu-} \longrightarrow & \text{- Leu - Ser - Asp -----}
\end{array}
$$

or

$$
\begin{array}{ll}
\text{-CTC-ATC-GGA-CTT-} & \text{-CTC-GGA-CTT-----} \\
\text{- Leu - Ile - Gly -Leu-} \longrightarrow & \text{- Leu - Gly - Leu-----}
\end{array}
$$

Gene duplication is not a common cause of genetic disease, but it is important during evolution. A whole gene can duplicate as a result of homologous recombination between misaligned chromosomes during prophase of meiosis I. Gene families, such as the α- and β-like globin genes (see Section 2 of this chapter), originate by this mechanism.

A **translocation** is the transfer of genetic material from one chromosomal location to another. Translocations often involve large chunks of chromatin, sometimes a whole chromosome arm. A translocation does not necessarily cause disease unless the translocation breakpoint disrupts an important gene. *Translocated genes still are expressed normally*, provided they have not been severed from their regulatory sites.

A mutation in an intron-exon junction or at the branch site within the intron (see Fig. 8.12, Chapter 8) results in abnormal splicing and, in all likelihood, a nonfunctional protein product. Mutations in a promoter or enhancer leave the structure of the polypeptide intact but can increase or, more likely, decrease its rate of synthesis.

Repetitive DNA sequences sometimes can give rise to mutations. Some genetic diseases are caused by the amplification of a trinucleotide repeat within the confines of an important gene (Table 9.1). The mechanism by which these repeats become amplified is unknown.

Mutations can be induced by radiation and chemicals

The **basal mutation rate**, which is observed in the absence of environmental mutagens, is caused largely by errors during DNA replication. Spontaneous **tautomeric shifts** in the bases contribute to these errors: thymine, for example, normally is present in the keto form, which pairs with adenine. Very rarely, however, it shifts spontaneously to the enol form, which pairs with guanine. If a thymine in the template strand happens to be in the rare enol form at the moment of DNA replication, G instead of A is incorporated in the new strand. Similarly, adenine has a rare imino form that pairs with cytosine rather than thymine (Fig. 9.1). Fortunately these bases spend very little time in their less stable forms, so mutations caused by a tautomeric shift are rare.

Radiation is an important environmental cause of mutations. **Ionizing radiation**, including **X-rays**

and **radioactive radiation**, is sufficiently energy rich to displace electrons from their orbitals, creating short-lived, highly reactive intermediates that react with the DNA bases. *Ionizing radiation penetrates the whole body and therefore can cause both somatic and germline mutations.*

Ultraviolet (UV) radiation is a normal component of sunlight. It is nonionizing and cannot penetrate beyond the outer layers of the skin, but it nevertheless can form **pyrimidine dimers** from adjacent pyrimidine bases (Fig. 9.2). Therefore *sunlight is mutagenic*, causing both sunburn and skin cancer.

FIG. 9.1

Spontaneous tautomeric shifts of DNA bases as a cause of point mutations. **A,** Alternative structures of thymine and adenine. **B,** A base pair between guanine and the enol form of thymine.

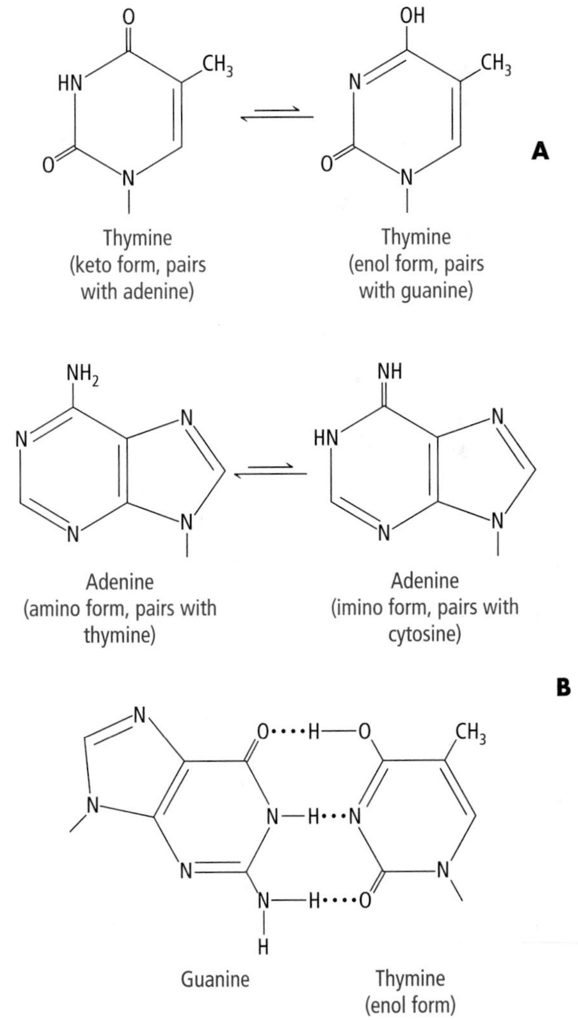

Thymine
(keto form, pairs with adenine)

Thymine
(enol form, pairs with guanine)

A

Adenine
(amino form, pairs with thymine)

Adenine
(imino form, pairs with cytosine)

B

Guanine

Thymine
(enol form)

Many chemicals can induce mutations as well:

1. **Base analogs** can cause mutations because *they are erroneously incorporated into DNA*. **Bromouracil** (Fig. 9.3) is incorporated into DNA in place of thymine. Although it usually pairs with adenine, the equilibrium between the keto and enol forms is more favorable for the enol form than in thymine, and mutations are caused by spontaneous tautomeric shifts.
2. **Alkylating agents** alkylate nitrogen or oxygen atoms in the bases (Fig. 9.4).
3. **Deaminating agents** turn the bases adenine, guanine, and cytosine into hypoxanthine, xanthine, and uracil, respectively. These abnormal bases lead to errors during DNA replication (Fig. 9.5).
4. **Intercalating agents** are planar, fused-ring structures that insert themselves between the stacked DNA bases (Fig. 9.6), causing frameshift mutations during DNA replication.

Fortunately most types of DNA damage can be repaired before the DNA is replicated. For this reason *mutagenic agents are most effective during the S phase of the cell cycle, when the new DNA is synthesized* (see Fig. 28.1, Chapter 28): there is less time available for repair before the replication event. The use of radiation therapy for cancer is based on this principle: because the cancer cells are the most rapidly divid-

TABLE 9.1

Genetic diseases caused by the amplification of a trinucleotide repeat sequence

Disease	*Amplified repeat*	*Location of repeat in gene*	*Copy number* Normal	*Copy number* Disease	*Signs and symptoms*
Fragile X	CGG	5′-Untranslated region	6-50	>100	Mental retardation in males
Myotonic dystrophy	CTG	3′-Untranslated region*	5-30	>60	Myotonia, muscle weakness
Spinal and bulbar muscular atrophy	CAG	Translated region†	17-26	40-52	Neurodegenerative disorders, with motor impairment‡
Huntington's disease	CAG	Translated region	11-34	37-86	Neurodegenerative disorders, with motor impairment‡
Spinocerebellar ataxia type 1	CAG	Translated region	19-36	43-81	Neurodegenerative disorders, with motor impairment‡
Dentatorubral-pallidoluysian atrophy	CAG	Translated region	7-23	49-75	Neurodegenerative disorders, with motor impairment‡
Machado-Joseph disease	CAG	Translated region	13-36	68-79	Neurodegenerative disorders, with motor impairment‡
Friedreich's ataxia	GAA	Intron	7-22	120-1700	Ataxia

* The gene codes for a protein kinase.
† The gene codes for the androgen receptor, a DNA-binding protein.
‡ In all of these disorders the amplified CAG repeat codes for a polyglutamine tract in the polypeptide. The functions of most of the gene products are unknown.

FIG. 9.2

Formation of a thymine dimer by ultraviolet UV radiation. Note that the two thymine residues are in the same strand of the double helix.

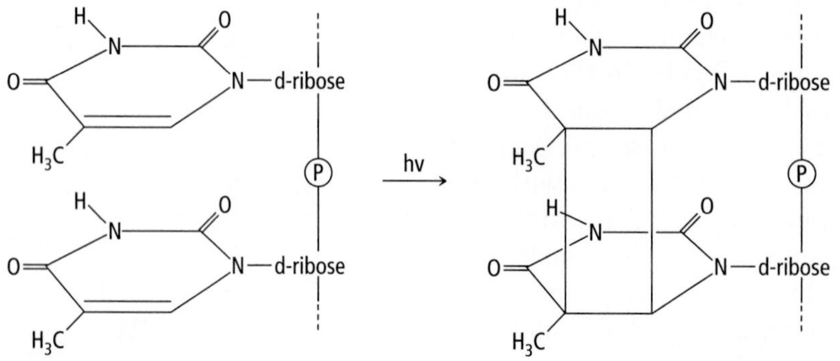

ing cells in the irradiated area, they are most likely to be in S phase and most likely to sustain fatal mutations. However, radiation actually can induce cancer by causing somatic mutations.

Damaged DNA can be repaired

Most types of DNA damage can be repaired by specialized enzyme systems. This is possible because *usually only one strand of the double helix is damaged, and the*

repair enzymes can receive their instructions from the undamaged complementary strand.

Direct repair by specialized enzyme systems is possible for some lesions. In *E. coli*, for example, thymine dimers can be repaired directly by a pho-

FIG. 9.3

The structure of bromouracil. The atomic radius of bromine is similar to that of a methyl group. Therefore bromouracil is incorporated into nucleotides and DNA in place of thymine.

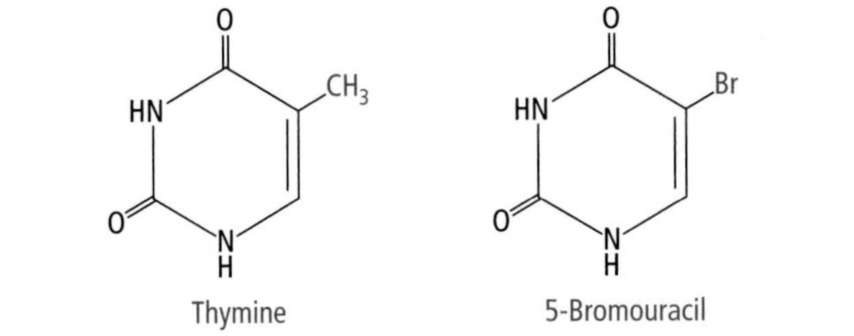

Thymine   5-Bromouracil

FIG. 9.4

Reactions of two alkylating agents with amino groups in DNA bases. Methyl bromide had been used as a grain fumigant but was banned for this use because of carcinogenic properties. Ethylene oxide is used for the sterilization of surgical instruments.

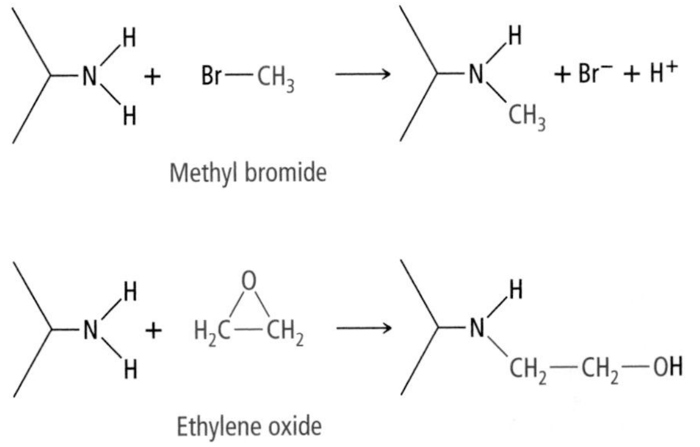

Methyl bromide

Ethylene oxide

FIG. 9.5

The action of a deaminating agent. HNO_2 can be formed from dietary nitrates in the intestine. **A,** The reaction of nitrous acid with adenine. **B,** Hypoxanthine pairs with cytosine instead of thymine.

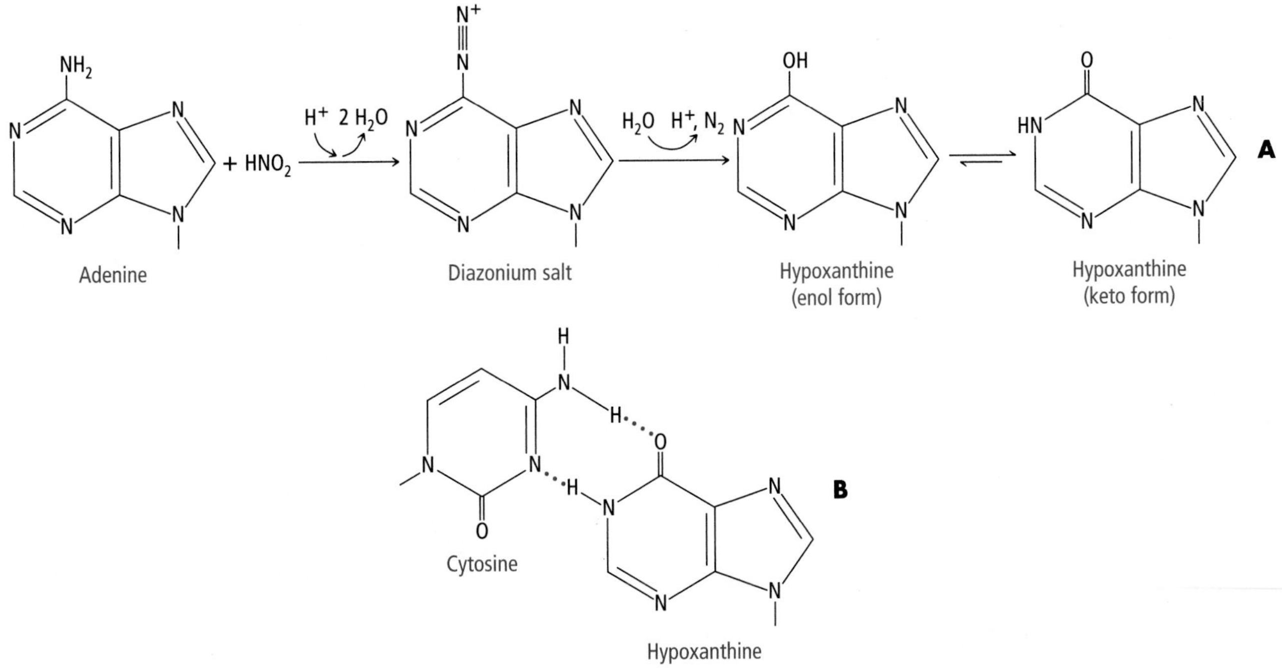

Adenine   Diazonium salt   Hypoxanthine   Hypoxanthine
                                                        (enol form)   (keto form)   **A**

Cytosine

Hypoxanthine   **B**

FIG. 9.6

Structures of intercalating agents. These planar ring systems cause frameshift mutations by inserting themselves between the DNA bases.

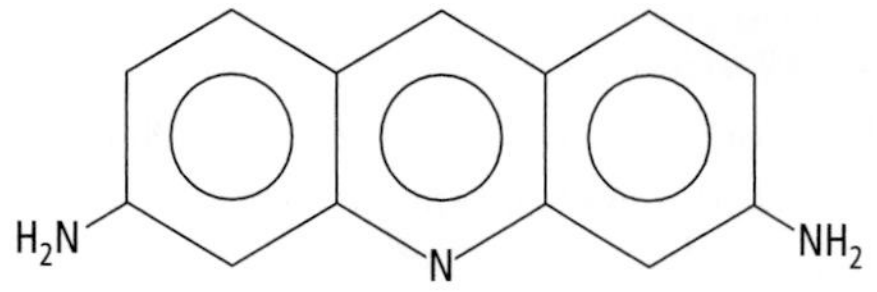

Proflavin
(= 2,8-Diaminoacridine)

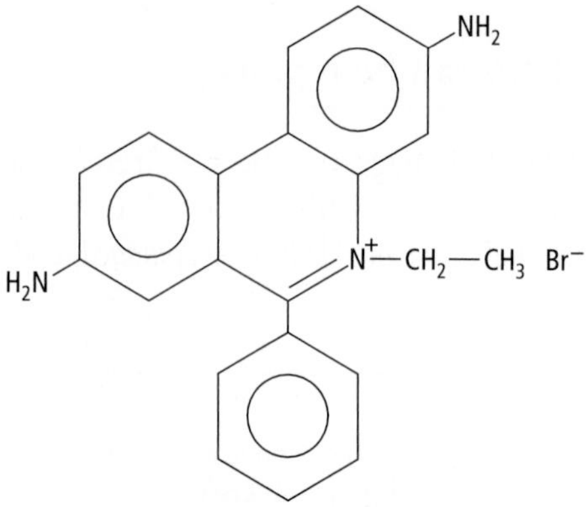

Ethidium bromide

toreactivating enzyme that binds to the dimer and cleaves it after exposure to visible light. Humans can repair O^6-alkyl derivatives of guanine by the direct transfer of the alkyl group to a cysteine side chain of the repair protein.

Depurination, the loss of a purine base by the spontaneous hydrolysis of its N-glycosidic bond with 2-deoxyribose, is a rather common type of DNA damage. It is repaired by the successive action of an **AP (apurinic) endonuclease,** DNA polymerase, and DNA ligase, as shown in Fig. 9.7.

In **base excision repair,** abnormal bases are removed from the DNA by specific **DNA glycosylases.** The deamination of adenine, guanine, and cytosine, for example, creates hypoxanthine, xanthine, and uracil. These bases are removed by the selective cleavage of the N-glycosidic bond between the base and 2-deoxyribose. This is followed by the action of AP endonuclease, DNA polymerase, and DNA ligase (Fig. 9.7). We see here the advantage of having thymine rather than uracil in DNA: if DNA contained uracil, the deamination of cytosine could not be recognized by the repair enzymes, and the mutation rate would be unpleasantly high.

Nucleotide excision repair removes bulky lesions including pyrimidine dimers and other photoproducts, adducts formed by the covalent binding of large foreign molecules to DNA, and some alkylated bases. Excision repair requires approximately 10 different proteins. These proteins form a "repair crew" that scans the DNA, recognizes the lesion, and

removes a portion of the damaged strand. The resulting gap is filled by DNA polymerase and DNA ligase (Fig. 9.8). Some lesions are recognized equally well and repaired in all forms of chromatin, but others are repaired preferentially if they occur in the template strand of a transcribed gene. It is believed that some variants of excision repair require the help of RNA polymerase or some other component of the transcriptional machinery to locate the damage.

Postreplication mismatch repair removes base mismatches and small insertions and deletions that arise from errors during DNA replication. This system has been described in *E. coli,* but it is equally important in eukaryotes. The repair enzymes can distinguish between the old strand and the newly synthesized strand because the old bacterial DNA is methylated at the palindrome GATC. The repair enzymes recognize hemimethylated GATC in newly replicated DNA and cleave the not-yet-methylated new strand either 5' or 3' of a mismatch. The damaged portion is removed by exonucleases, followed by the synthesis of new DNA and ligation. This system can eliminate base mismatches that are more than 1000 base pairs removed from the hemimethylated GATC sequence.

Defective DNA repair can cause disease

Xeroderma pigmentosum (XP) is a group of recessively inherited diseases in which numerous freckles and ulcerative lesions appear on sun-

FIG. 9.7

Repair of apurinic sites and of deaminated cytosine (uracil).

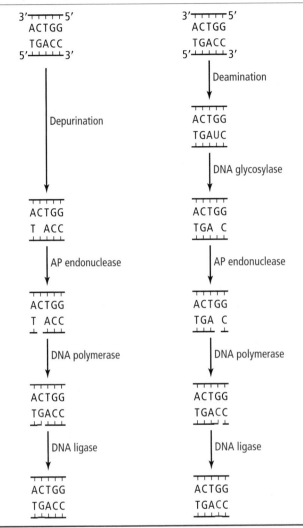

exposed skin. Skin cancer almost invariably develops at multiple sites, usually during the first and second decades of life. In some types of XP, the patients also show growth retardation and neurological degeneration. The only effective treatment for this otherwise fatal disease is the complete avoidance of sunlight.

The disease is caused by defects of nucleotide excision repair. This system is responsible for the repair of bulky DNA lesions, including the pyrimidine dimers that are formed by UV radiation in sun-exposed skin. At least seven subtypes have been identified in different patients, each caused by the deficiency of a different polypeptide in the repair system. Some of the XP mutations cripple both the genome-wide repair system and the preferential repair of transcribed DNA. They cause photosensitivity, skin cancer, and neurological symptoms. Others prevent only overall repair but permit the preferential repair of the transcribed strand. They cause only photosensitivity and skin cancer, but no neurological problems.

Cockayne's syndrome (CS) is a rare, recessively inherited disease characterized by growth retardation, neurological degeneration, and a wizened appearance, but without much photosensitivity and without an increased cancer risk. In these patients the overall excision repair is normal, but the preferential repair of the transcribed strand is deficient. Like XP, CS is genetically heterogeneous, with at least two types that are caused by deficiencies of two different gene products.

Xeroderma pigmentosum and CS demonstrate the different roles of the genome-wide excision repair system and the preferential repair of the transcribed strand: *the genome-wide system is required to protect dividing cells from DNA damage caused by external agents,* particularly UV radiation. The neurological degeneration and signs of early senility in CS, however, suggest that *the preferential repair of transcribed genes is important for the maintenance of nondividing end-stage cells that cannot be replaced once they are fatally injured by a mutation in an important gene.*

Bloom's syndrome, Fanconi's anemia, and **ataxia-telangiectasia** are associated with an increased incidence of chromosome breakage in cultured white blood cells, and there is an increased risk of leukemias and lymphomas. *These syndromes are thought to be caused by defects in the repair of double-strand DNA breaks.* The reduced activity of a DNA ligase has been demonstrated in patients with Bloom's syndrome. Patients with chromosome breakage syndromes are exquisitely sensitive to radiation, and their exposure to diagnostic X-rays therefore should be kept to a minimum.

Hereditary nonpolyposis colon cancer, finally, is an inherited cancer susceptibility syndrome that is caused by a defect of postreplication mismatch repair. This syndrome is discussed in Chapter 28.

THE HEMOGLOBINOPATHIES

Any gene can suffer mutations that cause the synthesis of a defective protein or prevent the synthesis

FIG. 9.8

The hypothetical sequence of events during the excision repair of a thymine dimer in humans. The repair complex may contain more than a dozen different polypeptides. Some of them *(XPB, XPD)* have helicase activity; others *(XPA, XPE)* recognize the damage or act as endonucleases *(XPG, ERCCI/XPF)*. The "XP" in the names of many of the repair proteins stands for "xero-derma pigmentosum," a disease that is caused by defects of excision repair proteins. Each XP protein is related to a different subtype ("complementation group") of this disease.

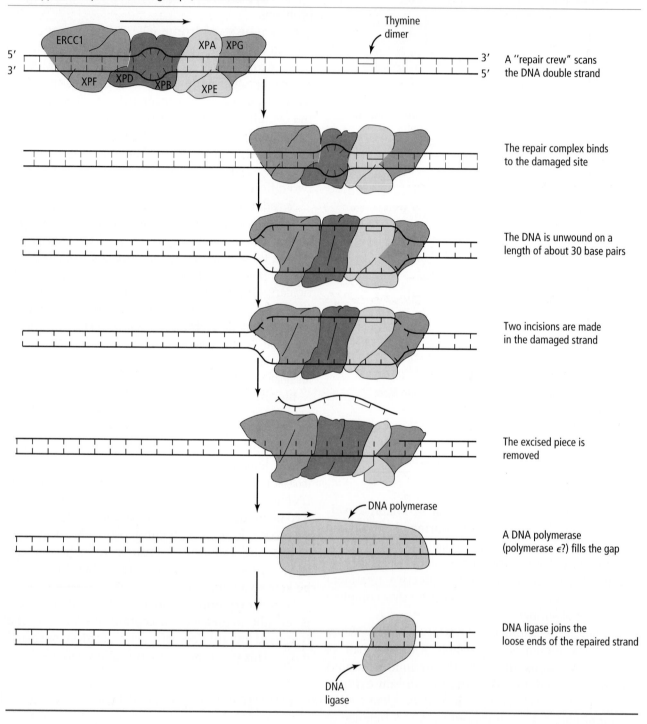

A "repair crew" scans the DNA double strand

The repair complex binds to the damaged site

The DNA is unwound on a length of about 30 base pairs

Two incisions are made in the damaged strand

The excised piece is removed

A DNA polymerase (polymerase ϵ?) fills the gap

DNA ligase joins the loose ends of the repaired strand

of the protein altogether. With 50,000 to 100,000 genes in the human genome, the number of genetic diseases is therefore impressive. Because mutations are rare events and serious genetic defects are removed from the population by selection, most of these diseases are rare. The **hemoglobinopathies,** however, are relatively common in many parts of the world. Also, our detailed knowledge of the structure and function of hemoglobin enables us to trace the mechanisms by which small molecular defects of a single polypeptide can lead to a clinical syndrome.

The hemoglobin genes are present in two gene clusters

The hemoglobins consist of two pairs of nonidentical polypeptides, and different hemoglobins can be formed by different combinations of these polypeptides (see Chapter 3). The genes for the hemoglobin chains are found on two chromosomes: the α-like genes are clustered on chromosome 16, and the β-like genes on chromosome 11 (Fig. 9.9). These gene clusters show some interesting features:

1. *Structurally related genes are placed close together on the chromosome.* Presumably, these genes arose from a single ancestral gene by **gene duplication.** Over time, the duplicated genes have mutated to produce the diversity we see today.
2. *The gene clusters contain **pseudogenes** (see Chapter 8),* which are related structurally to the "real" genes but cannot be transcribed and/or translated.
3. *The cluster on chromosome 16 contains two α-chain genes of identical structure.* This is unusual because most

protein-coding genes are present in only one copy in the haploid genome.

Not all of the α- and β-like globin genes are expressed at the same time. Figure 9.10 shows the expression of the genes during pre- and postnatal development: ϵ and ζ chains are limited to the early embryonic stage, and α and γ chains prevail during fetal development. *The newborn has approximately 75% HbF ($\alpha_2\gamma_2$) and 25% HbA ($\alpha_2\beta_2$), but HbF is replaced almost completely by HbA within 4 months after birth.*

More than 400 different point mutations have been described in the globin genes

More than 400 structural variants of hemoglobin α or β chains have been described in humans. Most of them are single amino acid substitutions that can be traced to a single base substitution in the gene. At least half of these mutations do not affect the function of the molecule sufficiently to cause disease. In those cases in which oxygen transport is affected, the change varies according to the site and the kind of the amino acid substitution:

1. *Mutations in the heme-binding pocket can cause methemoglobinemia.* A mutation replacing the proximal histidine by tyrosine, for example, makes the heme group inaccessible to methemoglobin reductase. Heterozygotes with this condition are cyanosed but otherwise in good health.
2. *Some mutations that affect the interface between the subunits lead to hemoglobins with abnormal oxygen-binding*

FIG. 9.9

Structures of the α- and β-like gene clusters. ψ, Pseudogene. The two α-chain genes are identical, and the two γ-chain genes ($^G\gamma$ and $^A\gamma$) code for polypeptides with a single Glycine $\leftrightarrow$ Alanine substitution.

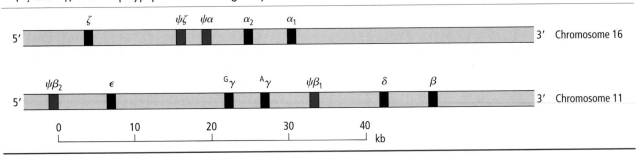

FIG. 9.10

Synthesis of globin chains during different stages of development.

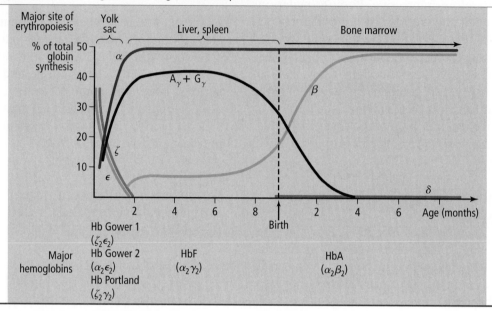

FIG. 9.11

The mutation in the β-chain gene leading to sickle cell hemoglobin (HbS).

$$H_3^+N — Val — His — Leu — Thr — Pro — Glu — Glu — \cdots$$
$$\cdots — CCT \quad GAG \quad GAG — \cdots$$
$$H_3^+N — Val — His — Leu — Thr — Pro — Val — Glu — \cdots$$
$$\cdots — CCT \quad GTG \quad GAG — \cdots$$

affinity. Hemoglobins with increased O_2 affinity lead to poor tissue oxygenation and a compensatory increase in erythropoiesis with polycythemia (increased number of red blood cells [RBCs]). Hemoglobins with low oxygen-binding affinity cause cyanosis.

3. *Some point mutations lead to abnormal processing of mRNA, premature degradation of mRNA, or increased proteolytic degradation of the α or β chain. These mutations cause thalassemia-like diseases.*

4. *Some abnormal hemoglobins cause hemolytic anemia because they have abnormal physical properties.* The most important example of this type of point mutation is hemoglobin S.

Sickle cell disease is caused by a point mutation in the β-chain gene

Sickle cell disease is a severe hemolytic disease that is common in people of African origin but also occurs in those from India, Saudi Arabia, and the Mediterranean region. *It is caused by the replacement of a glutamate residue in position 6 of the β chain by valine.* This can be traced to an A → T transversion in the β-chain gene (Fig. 9.11). The resultant **hemoglobin S (HbS)**, which can be characterized by the subunit structure $\alpha_2\beta_2^S$, is synthesized at a normal rate and

has a normal oxygen-binding affinity, but *it has a reduced water solubility in the deoxygenated form.* Deoxygenated but not oxygenated HbS forms an insoluble fibrous precipitate in the erythrocyte.

Because the mutation replaces a negatively charged amino acid residue with an uncharged one, *HbS can be separated from HbA by electrophoresis* (Fig. 9.12): because of its additional negative charge, HbA has a higher anodal mobility than HbS.

Only the homozygotes have sickle cell disease, so the mode of inheritance is characterized as autosomal recessive. The patient's erythrocytes tend to assume bizarre, often sickle-like shapes in the capillary beds and the veins, and the premature destruction of the sickled cells leads to a hemolytic type of anemia. Newborns still are healthy because most of their hemoglobin is HbF, but the first signs of the disease are likely to

FIG. 9.12

Electrophoresis of hemoglobin A and hemoglobin S at pH 8.6. Electrophoretic separation is possible because the sickle cell mutation (Glu → Val) removes a negative charge from the β chain.

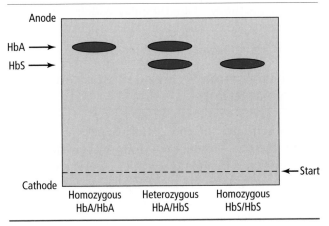

FIG. 9.13

Reaction of the terminal amino groups in hemoglobin with cyanate. Unlike carbamino hemoglobin, which is a normal product (see Chapter 3), carbamoyl hemoglobin has a relatively high oxygen-binding affinity.

$$\text{Polypeptide}-NH_2 + CO_2 \longrightarrow \text{Polypeptide}-NH-\overset{\overset{\displaystyle O}{\|}}{C}-O^- + H^+$$

Carbamino hemoglobin
(low O_2-affinity)

$$\text{Polypeptide}-NH_2 + O{=}C{=}NH \longrightarrow \text{Polypeptide}-NH-\overset{\overset{\displaystyle O}{\|}}{C}-NH_2$$

Carbamoyl hemoglobin
(high O_2-affinity)

appear 4 to 6 months after birth. Hemoglobin levels in the 6 to 11 g/dL range are usual in older children and adults with the disease.

The most insidious aspect of sickle cell disease is not the anemia but the tendency of the sickled cells to block capillary beds and thereby cause infarctions. Painful bone and joint infarctions are common. Multiple renal infarcts can lead to kidney failure, and many patients are crippled by recurrent central nervous system (CNS) infarctions. Some patients develop poorly healing leg ulcers. Recurrent attacks of severe pain in the extremities, bones, or abdomen, known as **painful crisis** or **sickling crisis,** are experienced by most patients. Episodes of **aplastic crisis** (bone marrow failure) may occur, and the sudden trapping of erythrocytes in the enlarged spleen, known as a **sequestration crisis,** is an important cause of death in children with the disease. At all ages, but particularly in early childhood, patients suffer increased mortality from infections. Other important causes of death are renal failure, cerebrovascular accidents, cardiac failure, and liver disease.

The treatment of sickle cell disease is based on the *strict avoidance of hypoxia and dehydration* (each of which temporarily increases the concentration of deoxy-HbS in RBCs) and the prompt treatment of any complications. Manipulations that increase the oxygen affinity of hemoglobin have been attempted. Thus **cyanate,** which increases the oxygen affinity by

covalent modification of the amino termini of the α and β chains (Fig. 9.13), has been found to be beneficial. However, cyanate is rarely used because of toxic side effects. Cyanate reacts not only with hemoglobin but also with the terminal amino groups of other proteins. An alternative approach involves manipulations that increase the synthesis of fetal hemoglobin.

Sickle cell heterozygotes are protected from tropical malaria

Heterozygotes with a normal β chain gene and the β^S gene have approximately 70% HbA and 30% HbS in their RBCs. Although these RBCs can sickle under conditions of extreme hypoxia, this does not occur in ordinary situations and therefore *the heterozygotes are healthy.* The heterozygous carrier state, also known as **sickle cell trait,** can be detected in the laboratory by exposing hemolyzed RBCs to anoxic conditions in vitro: if HbS is present, the solution becomes turbid.

Persons with the sickle cell trait not only are healthy, *they even enjoy a partial resistance to tropical malaria.* This has been shown in experiments in which normal homozygotes and sickle cell heterozygotes were deliberately infected with the malaria parasite. In areas with endemic malaria, young children with the sickle cell trait are as likely as others to get infected, but their disease is milder and less likely to be fatal. The connection between hemoglobin S and malaria is not altogether surprising: the malaria parasite, *Plasmodium falciparum,* spends part of its life cycle within the erythrocytes, where it is protected from immune attack. The presence of HbS appears to create a less hospitable environment for the parasite, perhaps even causing the premature destruction of the parasitized cells (Fig. 9.14).

The thalassemias are caused by reduced α or β chain production

The *thalassemias* are caused by the insufficient synthesis of structurally normal α or β chains. *They all result in anemia.* Also, the polypeptide that is present in excess amounts forms insoluble aggregates that are damaging to the cell and reduce its lifespan. The different types of thalassemia can be defined as follows:

α-**thalassemia**: Relative or absolute deficiency of α chains.

β-**thalassemia**: Relative or absolute deficiency of β chains.

Thalassemia minor: Heterozygous α or β thalassemia. Anemia may be present but is very mild.

Thalassemia major: Homozygous α or β thalassemia. Severe anemia.

The thalassemias are common in the Mediterranean countries, Africa, the Middle East, India, and Southeast Asia. Although experimental evidence is scarce, the heterozygous conditions are thought to provide some protection against malaria.

α-Thalassemia is caused most often by large deletions

The inheritance of the α-thalassemias is complicated by the presence of four rather than two α-chain genes in diploid somatic cells (Fig. 9.9). *Most patients with α-thalassemia have large deletions that remove one or both of the α-chain genes.* Figure 9.15 shows the possible deletion types.

Because α chains are required both before and after birth, the fetus is affected as well, and *a complete lack of α chains is fatal before or at birth.* Under these conditions, an abnormal hemoglobin of subunit structure γ_4 (**hemoglobin Barth's**) is formed that has a tenfold-higher oxygen affinity than hemoglo-

---

FIG. 9.14

The prevalence of heterozygosity for hemoglobin S ("sickle cell trait") in the Old World. In the United States, 8% of African Americans have the sickle cell trait, and approximately 1 in 600 has the disease.

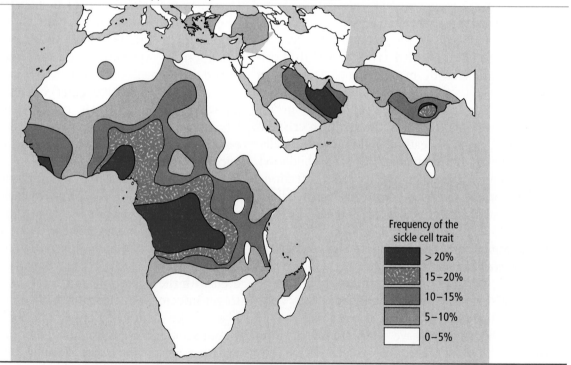

Frequency of the sickle cell trait

> 20%

15–20%

10–15%

5–10%

0–5%

Introduction to Genetic Diseases Genetic Information

bin A and cannot function as an effective oxygen carrier. A β_4 tetramer (**hemoglobin H**) is the predominant hemoglobin in patients with deletions of three α-chain genes. This aberrant hemoglobin is

FIG. 9.15

The deletion types in patients with α-thalassemia. **A,** One gene deleted ("silent carrier"): asymptomatic. **B,** Two genes deleted on different chromosomes: α-thalassemia minor, very mild anemia. **C,** Two genes deleted on the same chromosome: α-thalassemia minor, very mild anemia. **D,** Three genes deleted: hemoglobin H disease, moderately severe anemia. **E,** All four genes deleted: hemoglobin Barth's disease, hydrops fetalis.

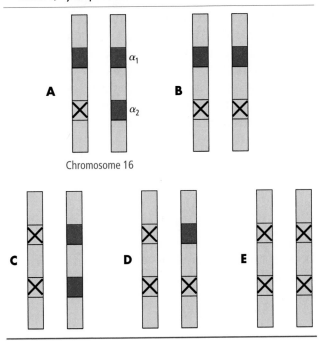

Chromosome 16

unstable. It denatures gradually and forms inclusion bodies in the cells. In most areas of the "thalassemia belt," only the deletion type depicted in Fig. 9.15, *A* and *B,* is prevalent. Approximately 2% of African Americans, for example, have the thalassemia minor phenotype of Fig. 9.15, *B.* In parts of India and Melanesia, a majority of individuals either are silent carriers (Fig. 9.15, *A*) or have the α-thalassemia minor phenotype (Fig. 9.15, *B*). The deletion type of Fig. 9.15, *C* and *E,* is common in Southeast Asia and occurs occasionally in the Mediterranean region. The severe homozygous deletion type has been identified as an important cause of stillbirth in Thailand.

Many different mutations can cause β-thalassemia

Some cases of β-thalassemia are caused by large deletions (Fig. 9.16), but most patients have single-base substitutions. More than 90 of these have been identified. Promoter mutations, splice site mutations, nonsense and frameshift mutations, and a mutation in the polyadenylation signal all have been observed in different patients. Splice site mutations, in particular, are very common.

Some β-thalassemia mutations result in a complete absence of β chains in the homozygous state (**β°-thalassemia**). Others cause a decrease in β-chain synthesis, and homozygotes have a small number of β chains (**β^+-thalassemia**). Because of the large number of different mutations, most β-thalassemia "homozygotes" actually are compound heterozygotes, with two different mutations in their two β-

FIG. 9.16

Deletions in the β-globin gene cluster. The deletions in the hereditary persistence of fetal hemoglobin (HPFH) group suggest that DNA sequences between the $^A\gamma$ and δ genes are important for the developmental switchoff of γ-chain synthesis.

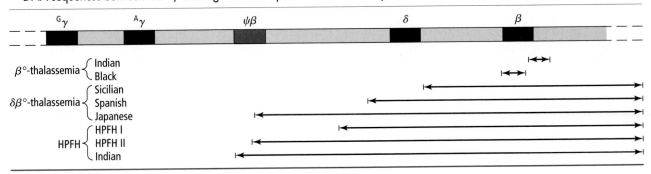

chain genes. "Homozygous" β^+-thalassemia shows a wide range of residual β-chain production and clinical severity. The milder forms, with clinical expression intermediate between the classical minor and major forms, are called **thalassemia intermedia.**

The heterozygous state (β-thalassemia minor) is a benign condition that requires no treatment. However, the homozygous state, known as **Cooley's anemia,** is a severe disease. *It is the most common type of severe thalassemia in the Mediterranean region and in many other countries.* The patients are healthy at birth because of the abundance of fetal hemoglobin, but *a severe anemia develops during the first year of life,* and most patients cannot maintain hemoglobin levels greater than 5 g/dL. The anemia is caused, in large part, by **abortive erythropoiesis:** the RBC precursors, which contain aggregates of excess α chains, are recognized as abnormal by phagocytic cells in the bone marrow and are destroyed before they can ever mature. The bone marrow responds to the anemia by working overtime, and a massive expansion of the red bone marrow leads to facial deformities ("chipmunk facies") and radiologic abnormalities. Also, most patients show extramedullary erythropoiesis in the liver and spleen.

Untreated patients with homozygous β^0-thalassemia are likely to die of severe anemia and intercurrent infections during infancy or childhood. They can survive to approximately 20 years of age if they are treated with regular transfusions of blood or packed erythrocytes, but they are likely to die at this time of iron overload. Severe anemia by itself increases intestinal iron absorption, and repeated blood transfusions introduce additional iron that cannot be excreted (see Chapter 24). For this reason, the patients are treated not only with regular blood transfusions but also with **desferrioxamine,** an iron chelator that must be administered chronically through a subcutaneous infusion pump. Desferrioxamine forms a soluble iron complex that can be excreted by the kidneys.

High levels of fetal hemoglobin protect the patient from the effects of β-thalassemia and sickle cell disease

Patients with homozygous β^0-thalassemia can survive (although with difficulty), but a complete absence of α chains leads to intrauterine death. One reason for this difference is that β^0 homozygotes still possess small amounts of HbA_2 and HbF. HbF accounts for less than 2% of the hemoglobin in most normal adults, and it occurs in only a small fraction of the RBCs. In homozygous β^0-thalassemia, however, it is the major hemoglobin, and *in these patients, the severity of the disease is inversely related to the HbF level.*

In some patients, including some of the deletion types (Fig. 9.16), the symptoms of β or $\delta\beta$ thalassemia remain mild because of high levels of HbF expression. These conditions are called **hereditary persistence of fetal hemoglobin (HPFH).** Not all cases of HPFH are caused by a deletion, and high levels of HbF have been found in some nonthalassemic subjects with near-normal levels of HbA. In some cases of nondeletion HPFH, the condition could be traced to a point mutation in the promoter region of one of the γ-chain genes.

A high level of HbF in adults is protective in all β-chain abnormalities, including sickle cell disease. Very little is known about the normal regulation of HbF synthesis, but several agents have been found to induce increased levels of γ-chain expression in adults. These include hydroxyurea, several derivatives of butyric acid, and the antitumor drug azacytidine. Unfortunately these agents are effective only at high doses and at the cost of many undesirable side effects. Azacytidine induces at least part of its effect by preventing the methylation of newly synthesized DNA in regulatory regions of the γ-chain genes. As in other genes (see Chapter 8), methylation inhibits the transcription of the γ-chain genes.

SUMMARY

Mutations are changes in DNA structure that either occur spontaneously or are induced by external agents. Somatic cells can become defective by mutations, and some mutations can transform a somatic cell into a tumor cell. Somatic mutations are the principal cause of cancer, and therefore essentially all mutagens also are carcinogens. Germline mutations, however, can lead to genetic diseases. Mutations can prevent the normal expression of a gene or cause the synthesis of a defective, nonfunctional protein, or the synthesis of a protein with abnormal biological properties. Cells use a variety of DNA repair systems to keep the mutation rate at a tolerable level. Most inherited defects of DNA repair (which are themselves the result of germline mutations) cause an increased cancer risk.

The hemoglobinopathies are classic examples of genetic diseases. Sickle cell disease is caused by a point mutation that leads to a Glu → Val substitution in the hemoglobin β chain. The erythrocytes of affected homozygotes sickle because deoxy-HbS has an abnormally low solubility, and the patient develops a hemolytic anemia and multiple tissue infarctions. The thalassemias are diseases in which either the hemoglobin α chains or β chains are underproduced. For this reason, hemoglobinopathies are the most common genetic diseases in malaria-infested parts of the world. Heterozygous carriers of the offending mutations have an increased resistance to the malaria parasite.

Further Reading

Bootsma D et al: Nucleotide excision repair syndromes: molecular basis and clinical symptoms. *Phil Trans R Soc London B*, 347, 75–81, 1995.

Chu G, Mayne L: Xeroderma pigmentosum, Cockayne syndrome and trichothiodystrophy: do the genes explain the diseases? *Trends Genet* 12 (5), 187–192, 1996.

Cooper DL, Lahue RS, Modrich P: Methyl-directed mismatch repair is bidirectional. *J Biol Chem* 268 (16), 11823–11829, 1993.

Handin RI, Lux SE, Stossel TP, editors: *Blood*. J. B. Lippincott, Philadelphia, 1995, pp. 1525–1700.

Hoeijmakers JHJ: Nucleotide excision repair. II: from yeast to mammals. *Trends Genet* 9 (16), 211–217, 1993.

Hoeijmakers JHJ, Bootsma D: incisions for excision. *Nature* 371, 654–655, 1994.

Huang JC, Hsu DS, Kazantsev A, Sancar A: Substrate spectrum of human excinuclease: repair of abasic sites, methylated bases, mismatches, and bulky adducts. *Proc Natl Acad Sci USA* 91, 12213–12217, 1994.

Morgan AR: Base mismatches and mutagenesis: how important is tautomerism? *Trends Biochem Sci* 18, 160–161, 1993.

Sancar A: DNA excision repair. *Annu Rev Biochem* 65, 43–81, 1996.

Scriver CR, Beaudet AL, Sly WS, Valle D, editors: *The metabolic basis of inherited disease*, 6th ed., Vol. 2. McGraw-Hill, New York, 1989, pp. 2281–2340, 2949–2971.

Seeberg E, Eide L, Bjoras M: The base excision repair pathway. *Trends Biochem Sci* 20 (10), 391–396, 1995.

Stamatoyannopoulos G, Nienhuis AW, Majerus PW, Varmus H, editors: *The molecular basis of blood diseases*. W. B. Saunders, Philadelphia, 1994, pp. 101–256.

Vos J-MH: *DNA repair mechanisms: impact on human diseases and cancer*. R. G. Landes, Austin, TX, 1995.

Williamson D, Carrell RW, Lehmann H: Haemoglobinopathies. In: Williams D, Marks V, editors: *Scientific foundations of biochemistry in clinical practice*, 2nd ed., Butterworth Heinemann, Oxford, 1994, pp. 420–445.

Wood RD: Proteins that participate in nucleotide excision repair of DNA in mammalian cells. *Phil Trans R Soc London B*, 347, 69–74, 1995.

Wood RD: DNA repair in eukaryotes. *Annu Rev Biochem* 65, 135–167, 1996.

QUESTIONS

1. You examine a 10-month-old infant who has numerous scaly and ulcerative skin lesions, as well as areas of hyperpigmentation. These lesions are present only on sun-exposed skin. You should consider the possibility that the child has a defect in
   A. Postreplication mismatch repair
   B. The repair of double-strand DNA breaks
   C. Removal of deaminated bases
   D. Base excision repair
   E. Nucleotide excision repair

2. The most important type of DNA damage in the child described in Question 1 is
   A. Double-strand DNA breaks
   B. Pyrimidine dimers
   C. Replication errors
   D. Insertions and deletions
   E. Base methylations

3. An 18-month-old girl of Middle Eastern ancestry who was treated initially for recurrent lung infections is found to have a blood hemoglobin concentration of 4.6%. The erythrocytes are smaller than normal and of somewhat irregular shape, and the mean intracorpuscular hemoglobin content is only 55% of normal. The levels of HbF and

HbA$_2$ are elevated mildly. This is most likely a case of
A. Sickle cell disease
B. A DNA repair defect
C. α-Thalassemia major
D. β-Thalassemia major
E. β-Thalassemia minor

4. Some patients with sickle cell disease have relatively mild symptoms because they also have
A. Bone marrow depression
B. Hemoglobin H
C. Increased α-chain synthesis
D. Increased γ-chain synthesis

Chapter 10

DNA Technology

Researchers have amassed a vast amount of information about the human genome during the past two decades. Far from being merely an intellectual pastime, this knowledge of our genes and their expression is revolutionizing medicine. The genes for most of the more important genetic diseases have been mapped and sequenced already, and molecular methods for the diagnosis of these diseases are available. Treatments based on the manipulation of gene expression or even the transfer of intact genes into the cells of patients with genetic diseases are in the experimental stage. Patients with a variety of diseases already are treated with proteins that have been produced by genetically engineered microorganisms. This chapter introduces the most important techniques of genetic engineering as they relate to medical practice.

| THE TOOLS |

The genetic engineer is a craftsman working in DNA, and like any other craftsman he needs a toolkit to work his material. There are several operations that occur in many applications: in many cases, for example, DNA has to be cut into handy fragments; DNA fragments must be separated by size; DNA of a specific, known sequence must be identified; and, of course, methods are required to determine the base sequence of DNA. In the first part of this chapter, we introduce the most important tools and procedures of genetic engineering.

Restriction endonucleases are used to cut large DNA molecules into smaller fragments

The DNA molecules in human chromosomes are huge, with lengths on the order of 100 million base pairs. To isolate, probe, clone, or sequence human DNA, these unwieldy molecules must be broken into smaller fragments.

The most useful DNA-cleaving reagents are the **restriction endonucleases.** These bacterial enzymes are useful because *they cleave double-stranded DNA very selectively at specific palindromic sequences.* These sequences do not occur very often in natural DNA molecules, and therefore the products of restriction endonuclease cleavage, the **restriction fragments,** are quite large, on the order of a few hundred to many thousand base pairs. Most restriction endonucleases do not cut in the center of their recognition sequence but rather one or two base pairs away from the symmetry axis in both strands. *This type of cleavage produces a double-stranded DNA molecule with short, single-stranded ends* (Fig. 10.1).

A large number of restriction endonucleases are known (Table 10.1), and more than a hundred of them are available commercially. Bacteria use restriction endonucleases as a defense against DNA viruses whose DNA they cleave. The bacteria protect susceptible sites in their own DNA by the methylation of bases within the recognition sequence: only the unmethylated viral DNA—not the methylated

FIG. 10.1

Generation of restriction fragments by the restriction endonuclease *Eco*RI. Both strands are cut. Note that the double-stranded DNA fragments have single-stranded ends.

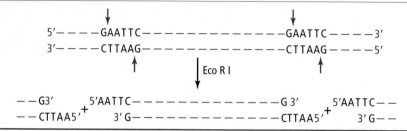

TABLE 10.1

Examples of restriction endonucleases*

Enzyme	Source	Cleavage specificity	No. of cleavage sites on λ phage DNA†
*Eco*RI	*Escherichia coli* RY 13	5′ G↓A A T T C 3′ 3′ C T T A A↑G 5′	5
*Eco*RII	*Escherichia coli* R 245	5′ ↓C C T G G 3′ 3′ G G A C C↑ 5′	>35
*Hind*III	*Haemophilus influenzae* R$_d$	5′ A↓A G C T T 3′ 3′ T T C G A↑A 5′	6
*Hae*III	*Haemophilus aegypticus*	5′ G G↓C C 3′ 3′ C C↑G G 5′	>50
*Bam*HI	*Bacillus amyloliquefaciens*	5′ G↓G A T C C 3′ 3′ C C T A G↑G 5′	5

* The first three letters in the name of each enzyme indicates the bacterium from which it is derived. Enzymes with a short recognition sequence, such as *Hae*III, cleave at many sites in natural DNA molecules and generate restriction fragments of small average size; those with a long recognition sequence cleave fewer sites and generate longer fragments.
† The λ phage DNA (see Chapter 7) consists of 48,513 base pairs.

bacterial DNA—is cleaved. This system is not absolutely reliable, of course, because occasionally the intruding viral DNA encounters the methyltransferase first, and once methylated, it is resistant to the restriction endonuclease.

Southern blotting is the standard procedure for the identification of restriction fragments

A restriction digest of DNA from a natural source, such as human genomic DNA, is likely to contain thousands of different restriction fragments. Let us assume that we want to identify a restriction fragment that carries a particular DNA sequence, for example, an exon of a protein-coding gene. In this situation we can use **Southern blotting** (named after Ed Southern, who developed the method in the 1970s). In this procedure (Fig. 10.2), the restriction digest is separated by electrophoresis in a cross-linked agarose or polyacrylamide gel. *This method separates the restriction fragments by size:* the smallest fragments move fastest, whereas the larger ones are retarded by the gel. Even restriction fragments differing in length by only one or a few nucleotides can be separated.

To recognize the desired fragment after electrophoresis, we need a specific reagent that reacts only with the correct fragment while ignoring everything else. This type of reagent is called a **molecular probe.** *A probe is a single-stranded oligonucleotide that is complementary to a sequence on the restriction*

FIG. 10.2

Identification of restriction fragments by Southern blotting. Only those restriction fragments with sequence complementarity to the probe are seen in the last step. This method provides two important pieces of information: it shows whether or not DNA sequences with complementarity to the probe are present in the genomic DNA, and it shows the approximate length of the restriction fragment carrying these sequences.

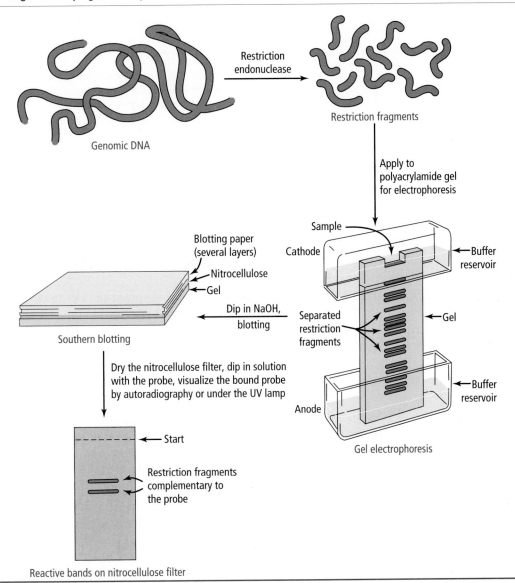

fragment. An mRNA, for example, can be used as a probe: it will bind to all restriction fragments that contain exon sequences of its gene. More commonly, however, a synthetic oligonucleotide is used. *The probe has to be at least 17 or 18 nucleotides long* because shorter sequences may be present, by chance, at multiple sites in the genome. Oligonucleotides of this size can be synthesized by chemical methods. To be recognizable, *the probe has to be labeled.* Probes can be constructed that contain a radioactive isotope such as tritium or phosphorus-32. These probes can be detected by autoradiography. Alternatively, a fluorescent group visible under the UV lamp can be attached to the probe.

The separated restriction fragments are double stranded, but *the probe can detect only single-stranded DNA.* Also, the restriction fragments are not bound tightly to the gel in which they were separated and

FIG. 10.3

Synthesis of molecular probes based on the partial amino acid sequence of a protein. The sequence is selected to consist of amino acids having only one or two codons in the genetic code (see Fig. 6.25). The possible DNA sequences shown here, when synthesized chemically and used as probes, will detect the template ("non-coding") strand in the protein-coding gene. "X" signifies any base.

Protein sequence	H_3^+N —·····— Met — Ser — Gln — Met — Trp — Thr —·····— COO^-
Possible codons	AUG AGU CAA AUG UGG ACX AGC CAG
Possible DNA sequences	5'A T G A G T C A A A T G T G G A C 3' 5'A T G A G T C A G A T G T G G A C 3' 5'A T G A G C C A A A T G T G G A C 3' 5'A T G A G C C A G A T G T G G A C 3'

therefore are easily leached out of the gel slab. In Southern blotting, the DNA is denatured by dipping the gel into a dilute sodium hydroxide solution and transferring ("blotting") the denatured, single-stranded DNA to a nitrocellulose filter. Effectively, *a replica of the gel slab with its separated restriction fragments is made on the nitrocellulose filter.* The nitrocellulose binds single-stranded DNA tightly, and the desired DNA fragment can be identified simply by dipping the nitrocellulose filter into a neutral solution of the probe and washing off the excess, unbound probe. The position of the probe, base-paired with the matching DNA fragment, now can be determined by autoradiography or fluorescence scanning.

Southern blotting can be used whenever at least a small part of the base sequence on the desired restriction fragment is already known. Can we also use this method to identify a gene of unknown base sequence if only the amino acid sequence of the encoded protein is known? Indeed, we cannot predict the exact base sequence of the gene because of the degeneracy of the genetic code: with the exception of methionine and tryptophan, all amino acids have between two and six codons (see Fig. 6.24, Chapter 8). A probe still can be made, however, if a sequence rich in methionine and/or tryptophan is selected and all possible complementary oligonucleotides are synthesized, as shown in Fig. 10.3.

Whereas Southern blotting identifies DNA fragments, **Northern blotting** is used similarly for the identification of RNAs with known base sequences. **Western blotting** is a method for the separation of polypeptides that are then analyzed by a monoclonal antibody.

DNA sequencing is a thriving industry

DNA can be sequenced by two methods. The **Maxam-Gilbert method** employs the partial chemical degradation of single-stranded DNA according to the procedure outlined in Fig. 10.4: the 5' terminus of the strand is labeled with radioactive phosphorus. The DNA is then divided into four batches and subjected to selective chemical cleavage at specific bases. The conditions are chosen to effect, on average, only one cleavage per chain. Methods are available for the selective cleavage of phosphodiester bonds on the 5' side of purines (A + G), pyrimidines (C + T), guanine, and cytosine. The fragments are separated according to size by polyacrylamide gel electrophoresis, and the gel is analyzed by autoradiography. *Only the radiolabeled 5' terminal fragments are detected.* This method can separate fragments differing in length by only one nucleotide, and the sequence can be deduced directly from the positions of fragments in the gel. DNAs of up to 250 nucleotides can be sequenced by this procedure.

The **Sanger dideoxy method** is an alternative method of DNA sequencing. It is based on the controlled interruption of enzymatic DNA synthesis by the inclusion of a dideoxyribonucleoside triphosphate in the in vitro system. *The dideoxyribonucleotide can be incorporated in the new strand by the DNA polymerase, but it leads to chain termination (Figs. 10.5 and 10.6).*

FIG. 10.4

Sequencing of the oligonucleotide 5' A G C A T T C G 3' by selective chemical cleavage (Maxam-Gilbert method). The conditions for the cleavage reactions are adjusted to produce, on average, one cleavage. ① The 5' end is labeled with radioactive phosphate. ② Four batches are cleaved separately on the 5' sides of G, A + G, C, and C + T, respectively. Only the radioactive fragments that are detected in the next step are shown here. ③ The fragments of step 2 are separated by polyacrylamide gel electrophoresis. The smallest fragments move fastest to the anode. Radioactive fragments are identified by autoradiography. The 5' → 3' sequence can be read from bottom to top, except for the first base.

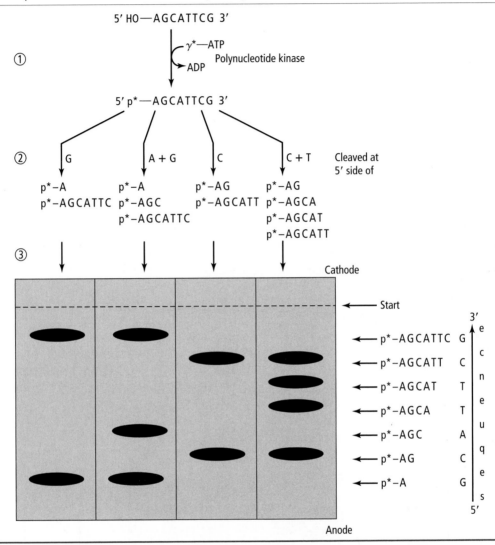

The pieces of newly synthesized DNA are separated by gel electrophoresis, and the sequence can be deduced from their sizes. Like the Maxam-Gilbert method, the Sanger dideoxy method can sequence up to approximately 250 nucleotides at a time.

DNA sequencing is technically easier and faster than protein sequencing (see Chapter 2), and *the amino acid sequences of many polypeptides have been deduced from the base sequences of their genes.* The complete genomes of some microorganisms have been sequenced already, including *Haemophilus influenzae*, *Mycoplasma genitalium* (an archaeal prokaryote), and even the 14-million-base-pair genome of baker's yeast, *Saccharomyces cerevisiae. It is expected that the entire human genome, with its 3.9 billion base pairs, will be sequenced by the year 2005,* at a cost of approximately 30 cents per base pair. A few thousand human genes have been sequenced already, and for many genetic diseases the molecular defect has been identified at the level of the DNA sequence. Sequencing the

FIG. 10.5

Structure of a dideoxy nucleoside triphosphate. DNA polymerases can incorporate a dideoxy nucleotide into a new DNA strand, but further chain growth is prevented for lack of a free 3'-hydroxy group.

FIG. 10.6

Sequencing of DNA by the controlled interruption of DNA synthesis (Sanger dideoxy method). A single-stranded DNA is required, and the primer is labeled with radioactive phosphorus (alternatively, it can be labeled with a fluorescent tag). Enzymatic DNA synthesis is performed in four separate test tubes. Each test tube contains all four deoxyribonucleoside triphosphates and one of the four dideoxyribonucleoside triphosphates. DNA synthesis is interrupted whenever a dideoxyribonucleotide is incorporated into the strand.

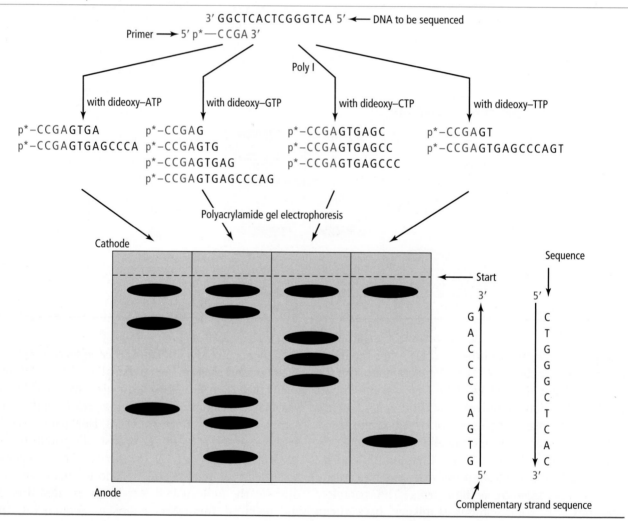

entire genome is expected to facilitate the identification of disease genes and the diagnosis of genetic defects, and to give us a better understanding of those genetic variations that are responsible for many of the normal differences among individuals.

THE DIAGNOSIS OF GENETIC DEFECTS

DNA-based diagnostic procedures represent the most rapidly expanding field in modern medical technology. These techniques can be used for the diagnosis of genetic defects, for example, in unaffected carriers of a recessively inherited disease gene or in the context of prenatal diagnosis. They also can be used to identify common polymorphisms, for example, in the blood group systems or the HLA system. Disease risks can be estimated by probing the DNA of healthy people, and even infectious diseases can be diagnosed by identifying the DNA of the pathogen. The following sections describe some representative procedures and applications of DNA-based diagnosis.

The sickle cell mutation obliterates the cleavage site of a restriction endonuclease

Sickle cell disease is caused by an A → T transversion in the hemoglobin β-chain gene (see Chapter 9). Fortuitously, this base substitution is within a palindrome that is cleaved by the restriction endonuclease MstII: *although the normal sequence is cleaved by the restriction enzyme, the mutated sequence is not* (Fig. 10.7, A). This unusual feature of the sickle cell mutation can be exploited for the molecular diagnosis of the disease and the heterozygous carrier state by Southern blotting, using a probe for a sequence 5′ of the mutation (Fig. 10.7, B): in the absence of the sickle cell mutation, this probe identifies a 1.15-kilobase (kb) fragment. If the mutation is present, however, MstII is unable to cleave the mutated site and the probed sequence is present on a 1.35-kb fragment. *This method can distinguish among the homozygous normal, homozygous affected, and heterozygous genotypes.*

Why should we diagnose the sickle cell mutation by Southern blotting rather than by hematologic methods or hemoglobin electrophoresis? One ad-

vantage is that the direct determination of the mutation permits an unambiguous diagnosis: hematologic abnormalities resembling sickle cell disease also can be caused by some other hemoglobinopathies, and some other abnormal hemoglobins can be confused with hemoglobin S during electrophoresis. Therefore *Southern blotting is preferred when a definitive diagnosis is required.* Also, nucleated cells suitable for DNA-based diagnostic tests are sometimes more readily available than a blood sample, particularly in prenatal diagnosis. Obtaining a sample of fetal blood (from the umbilical blood vessels) is a difficult and risky procedure. Cells derived from the fetal membranes, on the other hand, can be obtained readily by amniocentesis or chorionic villus sampling. *These fetal cells, which can be grown in culture, supply the DNA for the diagnostic test even though they do not express the hemoglobin genes.*

Sickle cell disease also can be diagnosed by Southern blotting with allele-specific oligonucleotide probes

Although the sickle cell mutation affects a restriction site, most other base substitutions do not. Therefore the method shown in Fig. 10.7 cannot be used for the diagnosis of other genetic diseases. A more generally applicable diagnostic procedure is the use of Southern blotting with **allele-specific oligonucleotide probes.** This procedure requires two synthetic oligonucleotide probes for the two sequence variants (**alleles**) of the gene, one complementary to the normal ("wild-type") allele and the other complementary to the mutant allele.

The use of allele-specific oligonucleotide probes requires a rigorous adjustment of the conditions during annealing. Annealing (base-pairing) is favored by low temperature and moderately high salt concentration. Under these conditions the probe binds not only to the exactly complementary sequence but also to related sequences. These assay conditions are said to be of **low stringency.** For the diagnosis of the sickle cell mutation, however, the probes have to distinguish between sequences that differ in only a single base, so the assay has to be performed at **high stringency,** for example, at elevated temperature or low ionic strength.

Figure 10.8 shows the use of Southern blotting with allele-specific oligonucleotide probes for the

FIG. 10.7

Molecular diagnosis of the sickle cell mutation by Southern blotting of an *MstII* restriction digest. **A,** The sickle cell mutation is within a palindromic sequence that is recognized by the restriction endonuclease *MstII*. The sickle cell mutation obliterates the *MstII* cleavage site. **B,** The sickle cell mutation generates a restriction fragment length polymorphism. ▬, Exons of the β-chain gene; ←, cleavage sites for *MstII*; ⊔, probe.

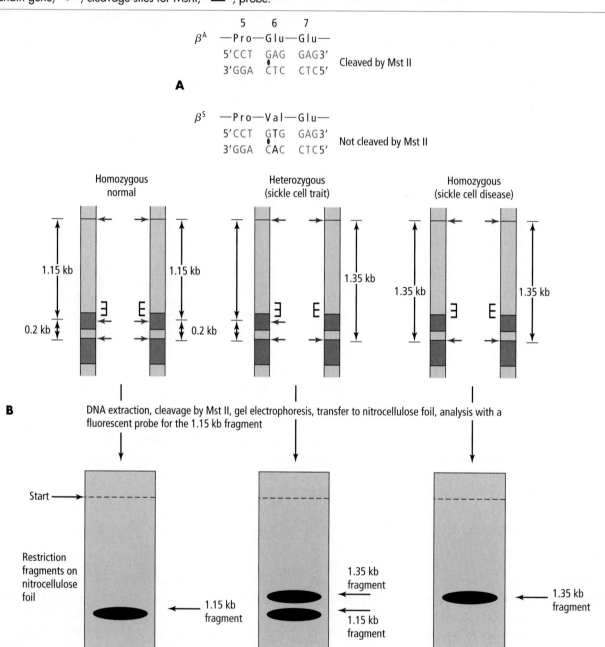

prenatal diagnosis of the sickle cell mutation: genomic DNA extracted from cultured amniotic cells is digested with a restriction endonuclease. The restriction digest is divided into two aliquots that are separated electrophoretically according to their size (lanes 1 and 2 in Fig. 10.8, *B*). After denaturation and transfer to a nitrocellulose filter, one aliquot is probed with the oligonucleotide for the normal sequence and the other is probed with the oligonucleotide for the mutated sequence. If the

FIG. 10.8

Prenatal diagnosis of sickle cell disease by Southern blotting with allele-specific oligonucleotide probes. Fetal cells are obtained either by chorionic villus sampling at 9 weeks or by amniocentesis at 15 weeks of gestation. **A,** The coding strand sequences of the normal β chain gene and the β^S gene in the area of the sickle cell mutation, and the structures of allele-specific oligonucleotide probes suitable for distinguishing between the normal and the mutated sequence. **B,** The procedure. ① Fetal cells are cultured. ② The DNA of the cultured cells is extracted. ③ The extracted DNA is treated with a restriction endonuclease. ④ Two aliquots of the restriction digest are separated on an agarose gel under identical conditions. ⑤ The DNA in the agarose gel is denatured with NaOH, then blotted to a nitrocellulose filter. ⑥ Lane 1 is treated with a probe for the normal DNA sequence; lane 2 with a probe for the sickle cell mutation.

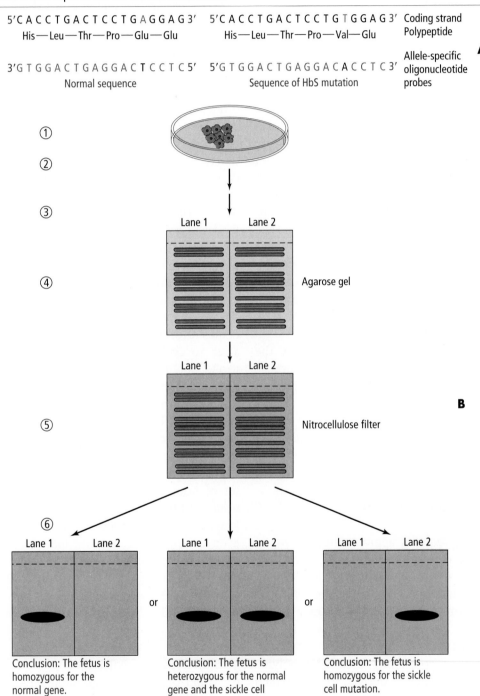

5′C A C C T G A C T C C T G A G G A G 3′   5′C A C C T G A C T C C T G T G G A G 3′   Coding strand

His—Leu—Thr—Pro—Glu—Glu   His—Leu—Thr—Pro—Val—Glu   Polypeptide

3′G T G G A C T G A G G A C T C C T C 5′   5′G T G G A C T G A G G A C A C C T C 3′   Allele-specific oligonucleotide probes

Normal sequence   Sequence of HbS mutation

A

B

Lane 1   Lane 2 — Agarose gel

Lane 1   Lane 2 — Nitrocellulose filter

Lane 1   Lane 2   or   Lane 1   Lane 2   or   Lane 1   Lane 2

Conclusion: The fetus is homozygous for the normal gene.

Conclusion: The fetus is heterozygous for the normal gene and the sickle cell mutation.

Conclusion: The fetus is homozygous for the sickle cell mutation.

fetus is homozygous for the normal β-chain gene, only the probe for the normal sequence binds. If the fetus has sickle cell disease, only the probe for the mutated sequence binds. If it is heterozygous, both probes bind. Unlike the method shown in Fig. 10.7, *this procedure discriminates between normal and mutated DNA not by identifying restriction fragments of different lengths, but rather by identifying a sequence variation between two fragments of equal length.*

There is one important limitation to the use of allele-specific oligonucleotide probes: *the method is applicable only when the molecular nature of the mutation is known.* In addition, *it requires that different patients with the disease all have the same mutation.* The latter requirement is fulfilled in the case of sickle cell disease: all patients have the same A $\rightarrow$ T substitution. However, in β-thalassemia, for example (see Chapter 9), we know of approximately 100 different mutations in the β-chain gene that all lead to the same disease. In this case, each individual mutation requires its own pair of allele-specific oligonucleotide probes. Diagnostic laboratories often deal with this problem by using probes only for those mutations that are most common in the patient population. This strategy can identify many carriers of a disease-causing mutation, but a negative result does not exclude the possibility that one of the less-common mutations is present.

This phenomenon—different mutations in the same gene all leading to the same disease because they all disrupt the normal function of the protein product—is called **allelic heterogeneity.** It is observed in most single-gene disorders, and *it is the most serious obstacle to the development of DNA-based diagnostic tests.*

DNA can be amplified by the polymerase chain reaction

Southern blotting requires approximately 10 μg of DNA, an amount that can be obtained from 1 mL of blood or from 10 mg of chorionic villus biopsy. If less than this amount is available, the DNA has to be amplified first, using the **polymerase chain reaction (PCR)**. The procedure, shown in Fig. 10.9, is based on the use of a heat-stable DNA polymerase. The most commonly used DNA polymerase, **Taq polymerase,** is derived from *Thermus aquaticus*, a thermophilic bacterium that was isolated originally from a hot spring in Yellowstone National Park. This enzyme functions best at temperatures close to 60°C and can survive repeated heating to 90°C.

Like other DNA polymerases, *Taq polymerase requires a base-paired primer with a free 3'-hydroxy group.* To amplify a specific section of genomic DNA, *two oligonucleotide primers are required that are complementary to sequences on the two strands of the double-stranded DNA. These primers form the ends of the amplified sequence.* Obviously the method can be used only if the sequences to the left and right of the interesting DNA are known.

PCR can be performed with a few nanograms of crude DNA. The primers are added to the DNA in very large ($>10^8$-fold) molar excess, together with a generous amount of Taq polymerase and the four deoxyribonucleoside triphosphates (dATP, dGTP, dCTP, and dTTP). The only additional requirement for the amplification reaction is a thermal cycling device. *The sample is alternately heated to 90°C to denature the double-stranded DNA, and cooled to 60°C for annealing of the primers and the polymerization reaction.* Each cycle takes a few minutes, and a total of 20 to 30 cycles commonly are employed. During each amplification cycle, the target DNA is doubled: theoretically, a single DNA molecule is copied into 2^{20} ($>10^6$) molecules after 20 cycles and into 2^{30} ($>10^9$) molecules after 30 cycles. Actually the efficiency is less than 100%, but it still is possible to produce 10^6 to 10^8 copies of the target DNA in a few hours. In classical PCR, the amplification product is electrophoresed on a cross-linked agarose or polyacrylamide gel and identified after staining without the use of probes.

PCR is convenient because *it is relatively fast* (a matter of hours) and, especially, because *it requires only small quantities of DNA* (1–10 ng). Diagnostic tests no longer require a blood sample: a buccal smear or even a single hair sent by mail is sufficient. One important limitation concerns the length of the amplified target DNA: it is difficult to reliably amplify DNA sequences longer than 3 kilobases. Although individual exons can be amplified readily, most genes are too large to be amplified in one piece. Also, the Taq polymerase has no proofreading 3'-exonuclease activity, so it has an error rate on the order of one base mismatch every few thousand base pairs.

FIG. 10.9

The polymerase chain reaction (PCR). The sequence to be amplified is defined by the 5′ ends of the oligonucleotide primers. The primers base-pair with the heat-denatured DNA strands by Watson-Crick base pairing. The Taq polymerase catalyzes DNA polymerization at 60°C and survives a temperature of 90°C during heat denaturation of the DNA. Neither primer nor Taq polymerase has to be added during repeated amplification cycles. Note that the amount of DNA between the primers increases geometrically: it doubles during each cycle of heating and cooling. ⊔⊔⊔ , Oligonucleotide primer.

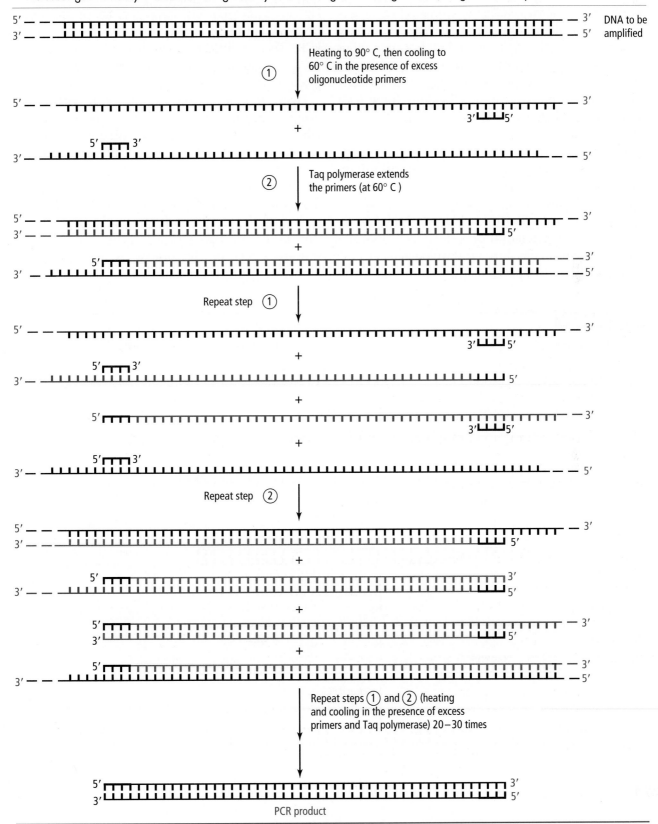

PCR with nested primers can be used for preimplantation diagnosis

DNA-based diagnostic procedures are employed in the **prenatal diagnosis** (antenatal diagnosis) of severe genetic diseases. *The aim of prenatal diagnosis is the detection of severe, debilitating genetic defects early in pregnancy, with the subsequent abortion of any affected fetus.* Fetal cells are obtained either by chorionic villus sampling at approximately 9 weeks of gestation or by amniocentesis at approximately 15 weeks. Usually these cells are propagated in cell culture for at least 1 or 2 weeks before the DNA is extracted for the diagnostic test.

The ethical problems associated with this approach can be mitigated by **preimplantation diagnosis:** the embryo is produced in the test tube and allowed to grow to the 8- or 16-cell stage. At this point, *a single cell is removed and its DNA is used for the diagnostic test.* The removal of a single cell does not seem to impair the further development of the embryo. Typically, approximately half a dozen ova

are fertilized in vitro at the same time, and all developing embryos are subjected to the test. Only the disease-free embryos are implanted.

Even "standard" PCR is not sufficiently powerful to amplify DNA reliably from a single cell. This feat requires **PCR with nested primers,** as shown in Fig. 10.10: a relatively large section of the target DNA is amplified initially through a 20- to 30-cycle PCR. The amplification product is then subjected to a second round of PCR with a new pair of primers.

Figure 10.11 shows the use of a PCR with nested primers for the preimplantation diagnosis of **cystic fibrosis (CF)**, a recessively inherited disease that is caused by the malfunction of a chloride channel in secretory cells. The patients have abnormally thick, viscous mucus secretions. The exocrine pancreas degenerates during the first years of life, with a pattern of cystic dilatation of intrapancreatic ducts and fibrosis of the parenchymal tissue, but the most serious aspect of the disease is a tendency for bronchial obstruction and, worst of all, recurrent

---

FIG. 10.10

The PCR with nested primers. This is the most sensitive method for DNA-based diagnosis. ⊔⊔⊔ , Primer.

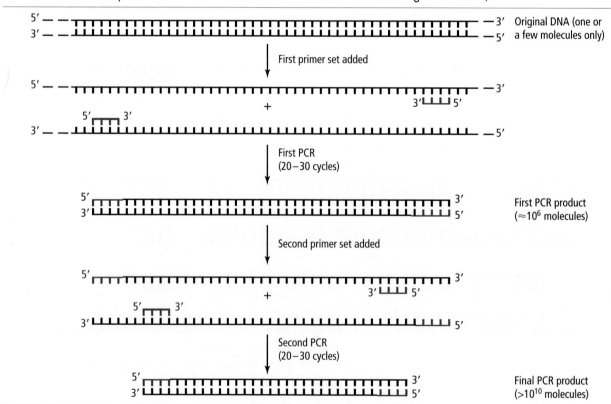

5′ — — ▯▯▯▯▯▯▯▯▯▯▯▯▯▯▯▯▯▯▯▯▯▯▯▯▯▯▯ — 3′ Original DNA (one or
3′ — — ▯▯▯▯▯▯▯▯▯▯▯▯▯▯▯▯▯▯▯▯▯▯▯▯▯▯▯ — 5′ a few molecules only)

First primer set added

First PCR (20–30 cycles)

First PCR product (≈10^6 molecules)

Second primer set added

Second PCR (20–30 cycles)

Final PCR product (>10^{10} molecules)

FIG. 10.11

Preimplantation diagnosis of cystic fibrosis, using PCR with nested primers. The most common cystic fibrosis mutation, the ΔPhe[508] mutation, is a three-base-pair deletion that results in a PCR product three nucleotides shorter than normal. The two PCR products can be separated by gel electrophoresis.

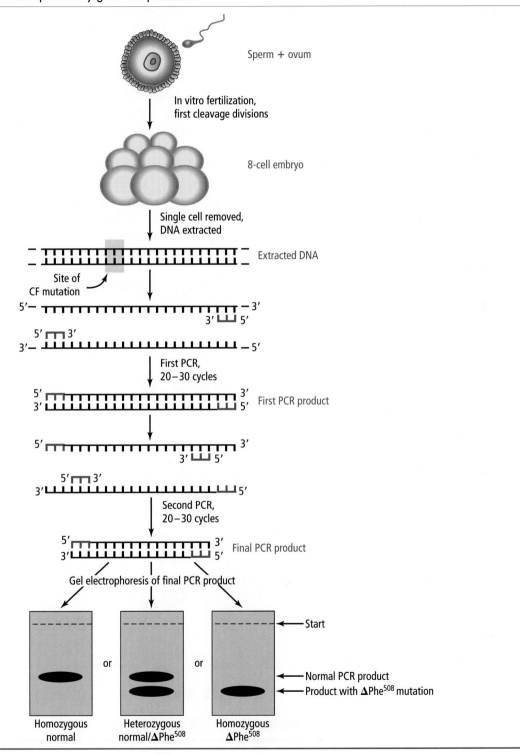

lung infections. The patients can be kept alive, often for three or four decades, by the liberal use of pancreatic enzyme supplements, antibiotics, and bronchodilators, but the quality of life is severely impaired and the treatment costs are staggering. CF is one of the most common genetic diseases, with an incidence of approximately 1 in 2000 in the white population. If both parents are heterozygous carriers of a CF mutation, the probability of an affected (homozygous) child is 25%, and prenatal or preimplantation diagnosis is indicated.

Any mutation that disrupts the normal function of the CF chloride channel can cause the disease, but in 70% of cases the mutation consists of a deletion of three successive base pairs that code for the amino acid phenylalanine in position 508 of the polypeptide (ΔPhe^{508} mutation). This mutation can be identified by PCR: using the same primer pair to amplify a short section of DNA around the site of the mutation, *the mutated sequence yields a PCR product three nucleotides shorter than normal*. This difference is sufficient to separate the two products by polyacrylamide gel electrophoresis. *The method shown in Fig. 10.11 for the CF mutation can be employed for all small insertions and deletions*. It is particularly useful for detecting such conditions as Huntington's disease and the fragile X syndrome, which are caused by the amplification of a trinucleotide repeat within the gene (Table 9.1, Chapter 9). In these cases, not only the presence of a mutation but also the exact copy number of the repeat sequence can be determined by the electrophoretic separation of the PCR products.

A variation of this procedure can be used for the diagnosis of single-base substitutions. In these cases, the PCR products have the same length and cannot be separated by electrophoresis, but the mutation nevertheless can be identified by allele-specific oligonucleotide probes. For this purpose, the electrophoresed PCR product is denatured and transferred to a nitrocellulose filter, as in classical Southern blotting (Fig. 10.2).

FIG. 10.12

The principle of deletion scanning with the PCR. Note that the primer pairs are designed to generate PCR products of different lengths that can be separated from each other by polyacrylamide gel electrophoresis. This method has been employed to amplify deletion-prone exons in patients with Duchenne muscular dystrophy. ▬, Exons; ⊔⊔, primer.

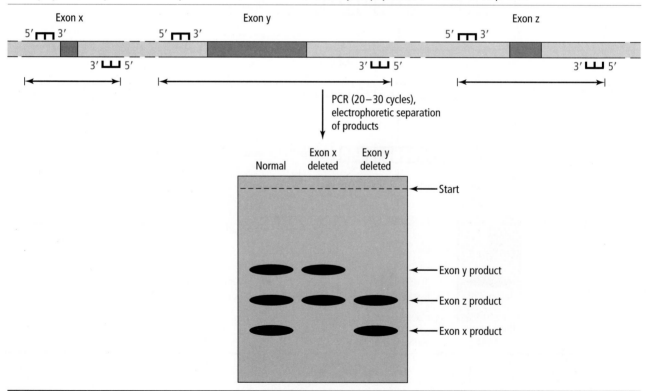

PCR can be used for deletion scanning

Some genetic diseases are caused by large deletions that remove either individual exons or the whole gene. **Duchenne muscular dystrophy (DMD)** is a severe, X-linked recessive muscle disease that is caused by mutations in the gene for the muscle protein dystrophin (see Chapter 12). The gene is unusually large, with 79 exons scattered over a total length of more than 2 million base pairs. More than half of the patients have large deletions that remove one or several exons from the gene.

Although different patients with DMD have different deletions, some exons are more likely to be deleted than others. The identification of deletions can be attempted by the method outlined in Fig. 10.12, using primer pairs for the PCR amplification of several deletion-prone exons. *Between 6 and 10 exons can be amplified simultaneously to yield PCR products of different sizes, and the deletion of one of the target exons can be recognized by the absence of its PCR product.*

A more complex application of PCR has been described for the diagnosis of α-thalassemia deletions in Southeast Asia and China (Fig. 10.13). The

---

FIG. 10.13

The use of PCR for the diagnosis of α-thalassemia deletions. **A,** The three most common α-thalassemia deletions in Southeast Asia and China. **B,** The use of two primer pairs for the amplification of two 156-base-pair segments at the 3′ ends of the α_1 and α_2 genes. The 5′ primers of the two amplifications are identical. They are complementary to a shared sequence near the 3′ ends of the two α-chain genes. The 3′ primers are different. They are complementary to sequences immediately 3′ of the two genes. The amplifications of the two segments are performed in different test tubes. ⊔⊔, Primer. The sizes of the primers and amplification products are not to scale. **C,** Identification of the PCR products from the α_2 and α_1 genes by polyacrylamide gel electrophoresis. This method can identify the lethal hydrops fetalis genotype during prenatal diagnosis. It also can distinguish between heterozygosity for the —^{SEA} deletion and homozygosity for one of the two smaller deletions in patients with clinical signs of α-thalassemia minor.

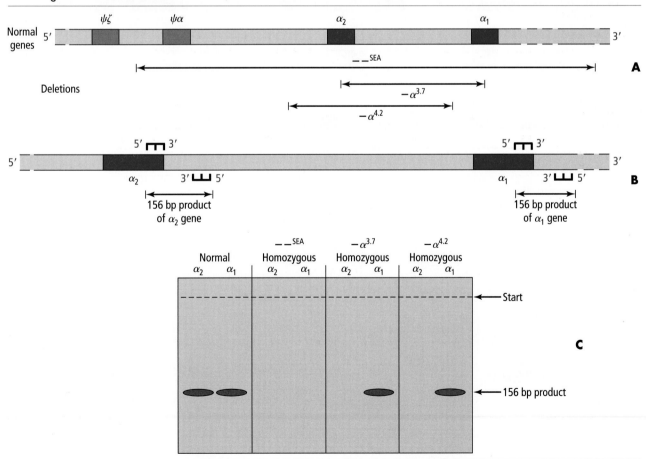

deletions can be identified readily if they are in the homozygous state, but the heterozygous carrier state is difficult to diagnose by PCR. The carrier state is diagnosed more easily by restriction endonuclease digestion and Southern blotting with a probe for a sequence within the α-like globin gene cluster (Fig. 10.14).

PCR is most suitable for the rapid detection of the lethal homozygous α-thalassemia major genotype during prenatal diagnosis: because very small amounts of DNA are sufficient, *the time-consuming culturing of fetal cells is not required.* Also, PCR does not require the time-consuming operations of blotting and probing; the PCR product can be identified directly in the stained gel. Therefore *PCR is intrinsically faster than Southern blotting.* Southern blotting, however, is the preferred procedure for carrier detection because it allows an unequivocal distinction between the different homozygous and heterozygous genotypes.

FIG. 10.14

The use of Southern blotting for the diagnosis of the most common α-thalassemia deletions (compare Fig. 10.13). The genomic DNA, extracted from leukocytes, cultured fibroblasts, or cultured amniotic cells, is cleaved with the restriction endonuclease *Bgl*II (↓). The probe that is used to detect the fragments hybridizes to a sequence in the 3′ portion of the zeta pseudogene ($\psi\zeta$). **A,** Fragments generated in three different deletion types. **B,** The appearance of restriction fragments after Southern blotting.

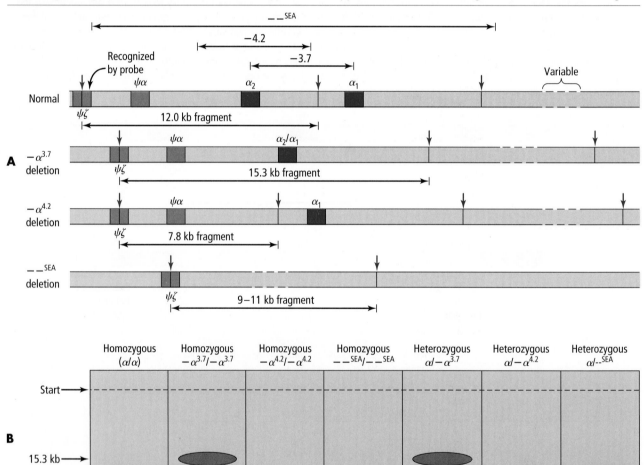

Allele-specific PCR can be used for the rapid diagnosis of point mutations

A synthetic oligonucleotide can prime DNA synthesis in PCR only if it is properly base-paired to the genomic DNA. If, in particular, the base at the 3′ end of the primer does not match the base in its target strand, the initiation of DNA synthesis is severely impaired.

In the case of single base substitutions, primers can be constructed whose 3′ ends correspond to the site of the mutation. *One of these allele-specific primers will amplify only the DNA of the normal gene, the other only that of the mutated gene.* In these assays, the allele-specific primers are used in conjunction with a second primer that recognizes a sequence common to the normal and the mutated gene. An example is shown in Fig. 10.15.

Dot-blot analysis permits rapid screening for mutations and genetic polymorphisms

Diagnostic procedures based on restriction endonuclease cleavage and Southern blotting require up to a few days, and even PCR-based procedures take many hours. However, there are situations that require a rapid, inexpensive screening test. For ex-

FIG. 10.15

The use of allele-specific PCR for the diagnosis of the sickle cell mutation. The 3′-terminal base of the allele-specific primer corresponds to the site of the mutation: one of the primers *(a)* amplifies only the normal allele; the other one *(s)* amplifies only the sickle cell allele. The "nonspecific" primer recognizes a sequence common to the HbA and HbS alleles. The DNA is amplified in two separate test tubes. The first test tube contains the *a* primer and the nonspecific primer, and the second contains the *s* primer and the nonspecific primer.

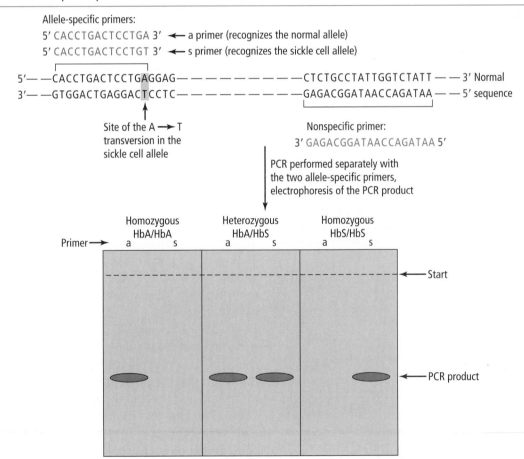

ample, 4% to 5% of the white population are unaffected heterozygous carriers of a mutation for cystic fibrosis (CF), a severe, recessively inherited disease that we encountered in the section on PCR with nested primers. Traditionally, diagnostic procedures for carrier detection are employed only in family members *after* the birth of an affected child. Is it possible, we may ask, to identify CF carriers in the general population and to alert couples at risk *before* an affected child is born? *If both prospective parents are identified as carriers, the birth of affected children can be prevented altogether,* either by prenatal diagnosis and selective abortion or by preimplantation diagnosis as shown in Fig. 10.11.

In approximately 70% of CF cases, the mutation consists of a three-base-pair deletion (ΔPhe^{508} mutation). This deletion can be identified by Southern blotting or PCR, but these procedures are too time consuming and expensive to be applied to large numbers of people. This situation requires the use of **dot-blotting** (Fig. 10.16): the extracted DNA is denatured and applied directly to a nitrocellulose filter without prior amplification or electrophoresis. This dot of denatured crude DNA is probed with allele-specific oligonucleotides for the presence of the ΔPhe^{508} mutation.

This method is simple, rapid, and inexpensive and therefore suitable for testing large numbers of people, thus making population screening possible. Of course, it cannot identify those 30% of CF carriers who have a mutation other than ΔPhe^{508}. Dot-blotting also can be employed to screen for the sickle cell mutation and other single-base substitutions. Dot-blotting can be used not only for the detection of disease-producing mutations, but also for the analysis of common polymorphisms. A polymorphism is defined as *the common occurrence of two or more DNA sequence variants in the population.* Blood group genes, for example, and the genes of the major histocompatibility complex are polymorphic. Traditionally these polymorphisms are identified by the use of antisera to the protein products (as in blood typing), or by electrophoresis (as in the case of hemoglobin A and hemoglobin S) (see Fig. 9.12, Chapter 9). Dot-blotting provides an alternative and more accurate approach to the analysis of these polymorphisms.

In addition to screening populations for a single mutation or polymorphism, *dot-blotting can even be used to test for different mutations or polymorphisms at the same time.* If this is desired, the DNA of a single individual can be dotted on several different filters, and each of these filters is analyzed with a different probe. It is even possible to analyze the same dot with more than one probe—for example, by probing one sequence variation with a fluorescent probe and another one with a radioactive probe, or by using probes fluorescing at different wavelengths. This approach, sometimes referred to as **multiplex genetic testing,** may become important in future efforts to prevent genetic diseases by identifying the unaffected carriers of recessive disease genes. It also may become important in identifying individuals who carry "susceptibility genes" for such multifactorial diseases as Alzheimer's disease or osteoporosis.

We have to realize at this point that *many recessively inherited diseases are preventable:* if all carriers in the population are identified, couples at risk can be directed either to remain childless or to use prenatal diagnosis or preimplantation diagnosis. Thus, all couples at risk for a child with sickle cell disease and most of those at risk for a child with cystic fibrosis can be identified readily with existing diagnostic methods.

FIG. 10.16

The use of dot-blotting for the diagnosis of a mutation with fluorescent-labeled probes for the normal and the mutated sequence. Denatured DNA from five different individuals is applied to two different nitrocellulose filters, each in a single dot. One filter is dipped into a solution with a probe for the normal sequence, the other into a solution with a probe for the mutant sequence. Excess probe is washed off and the bound probe is visualized under the UV lamp.

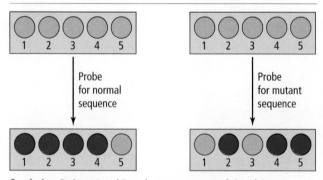

Conclusion: Patients 1 and 3 are homozygous normal, 2 and 4 are heterozygous, and 5 is homozygous for the mutation.

Scanning methods can be used to detect any mutation in a gene

Some genetic diseases show so much allelic heterogeneity that the use of allele-specific methods is an exercise in futility. In the bleeding disorder **hemophilia A**, for example (see Chapter 25), patients from different families usually have different mutations in the gene for clotting factor VIII. Therefore *an allele-specific probe that detects a hemophilia mutation in one family is useless in other families.*

One possible approach to this problem is to amplify the whole gene by PCR and to sequence the PCR products. This strategy may be possible for

The principle of mutation scanning by chemical mismatch detection. If the amplified gene segment from the patient did not contain a mutation, gel electrophoresis would show only the full-length product. The presence of a smaller fragment indicates a base mismatch, and the size of this fragment reveals how far the mutation is away from the end of the amplified sequence. ⊔⊔⊔ , Primer.

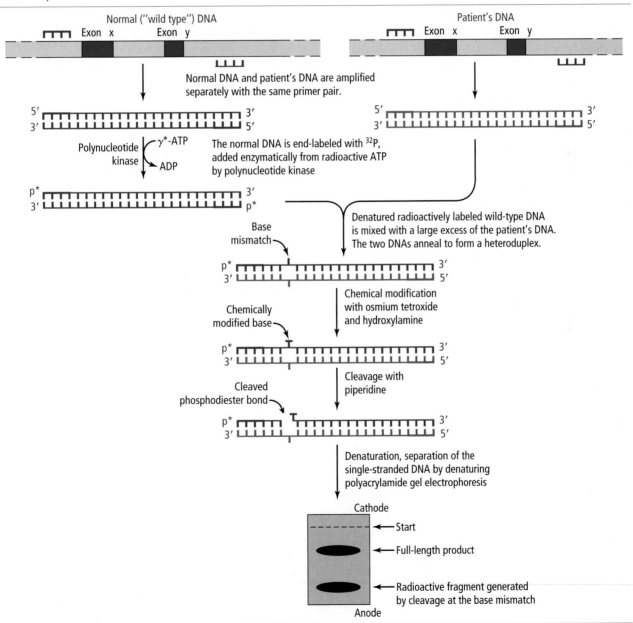

small genes, but it is too tedious for such large genes as the factor VIII gene (26 exons) or the dystrophin gene (79 exons).

Alternatively, we can use a **scanning method,** which can detect *any* mutation along the length of the gene. Several scanning methods have been developed; the most useful is **chemical mismatch detection.** In this method (Fig. 10.17), the important portions of the gene are amplified independently from the patient's DNA and from the normal, unmutated wild-type DNA. The PCR product of the wild-type DNA is end-labeled with ^{32}P and hybridized with a large excess of the unlabeled amplification product from the patient, to form a heteroduplex. Wild-type DNA and the patient's DNA are now base-paired *except at the site of the mutation.*

A mismatched base is more sensitive than the paired bases to certain chemical reagents. Specifically, an unmatched thymine can be modified chemically by osmium tetroxide and an unmatched cytosine by hydroxylamine, without affecting the base-paired thymines and cytosines in the molecule. The phosphodiester bonds at the modified bases then can be cleaved chemically by piperidine, and the products are separated by polyacrylamide gel electrophoresis under denaturing conditions. *If the patient's DNA contains a base substitution, gel electrophoresis will reveal the products of the chemical cleavage together with the full-length PCR product.* Once the approximate location of the mutation has been identified, the mismatch-containing PCR product can be sequenced.

Restriction fragment length polymorphisms are useful genetic markers

We saw before (Figs. 10.7 and 10.14) that some disease-producing mutations can be recognized because they change the length of a restriction fragment. Far more common than these disease-related variations are **restriction fragment length polymorphisms (RFLPs),** which are caused by sequence variations outside the genes. As shown in Figs. 10.7 and 10.18, an RFLP can be caused by a single-base change in a cleavage site for a restriction endonuclease. In other cases, it is caused by differences in the length of the DNA sequence between two restriction sites.

The most useful RFLPs are generated by tandemly repeated sequences with between two and two dozen nucleotides in the repeat unit (Fig. 10.18, C; see also Chapter 8). These repeats, commonly referred to as **variable number of tandem repeats (VNTRs),** occur in different repeat numbers in different people. For example, a sequence may be repeated only 5 or 6 times in some people and more than 20 times in others. Indeed, *we can expect different repeat numbers not only in different people but also on the two homologous chromosomes that carry the repeat in the diploid cell.*

Most RFLPs do not cause disease, but they still can be used for the diagnosis of genetic defects: if an RFLP is located close to a mutated gene, the two are transmitted together from one generation to the next simply because they are on the same DNA molecule. Therefore *the inheritance of the defective gene can be traced by tracing the inheritance of the associated restriction fragment.* The linkage pattern is, of course, different in different families: in some families the disease gene may be inherited together with a shorter fragment; in others it segregates with a longer fragment. For this reason, linkage studies are not suitable for population screening—only for studies in individual families.

The advantage of RFLPs is that *they can be used even if the sequence of the disease gene is unknown.* All we have to know is that the RFLP is located close to the disease gene on the same chromosome. Also, *the use of RFLPs is not affected by the vexing problem of allelic heterogeneity, which limits the usefulness of allele-specific methods.*

However, *RFLPs are useful only if they are very close to the affected gene,* ideally not more than 1 or 2 million base pairs removed. With greater distances, homologous recombination ("crossing-over") between the two locations is increasingly likely during prophase of meiosis I. This possibility of a crossing-over between the disease gene and the RFLP limits the accuracy of any prediction derived from linkage studies. Also, *linkage analysis requires the sampling of DNA from several family members,* not just from the patient, and a particular RFLP is useful ("informative") in some but not all families.

Tandem repeats are used for DNA fingerprinting

Polymorphic DNA sequences can be used not only to trace the inheritance of disease genes but also

FIG. 10.18

The origin of restriction fragment length polymorphisms. **A,** The polymorphism is caused by a base substitution in the recognition site of a restriction endonuclease. In this example the normal ("wild-type") allele is linked to the shorter fragment, and the mutant allele is linked to the longer fragment. ↓, Cleavage by the restriction endonuclease; ⊓⊓, probe used to detect the polymorphism. **B,** The polymorphism is caused by a variation in the length of the DNA between two restriction sites. In this example the mutant allele is linked to the shorter fragment. **C,** Tandemly repeated sequences (variable numbers of tandem repeats, VNTRs) provide the most useful RFLPs.

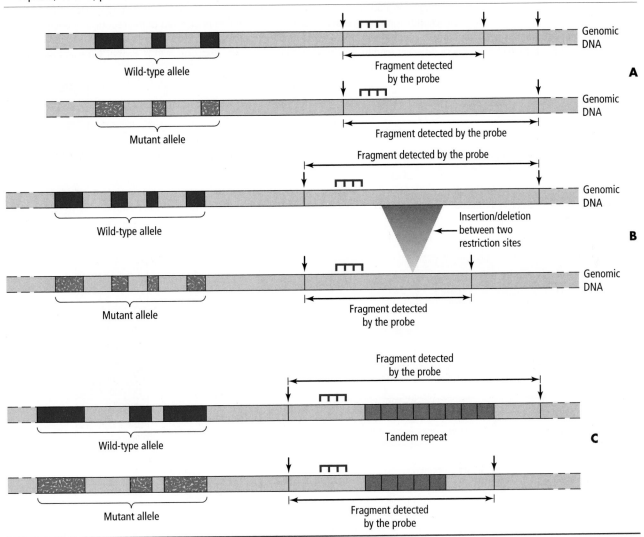

to identify persons in criminal cases. This use of DNA sequence variations is known as **DNA fingerprinting.**

Any detectable DNA sequence variation can be used for DNA fingerprinting, but the variable tandem repeats shown in Fig. 10.18, C are by far the most useful. **Microsatellites** are short tandem repeats, usually with two to four nucleotides in the repeat unit and a total length well below 1000 nucleotides. **Minisatellites** are longer, with a total repeat length of more than 1000 nucleotides.

DNA fingerprinting can be performed either with classical Southern blotting or with PCR (Fig. 10.19). Southern blotting is suitable when a large amount of DNA is available, for example, a drop of seminal fluid from a sexual offender. PCR is more sensitive and can be used when only a small amount of DNA

FIG. 10.19

Variable numbers of tandem repeats (VNTRs) used for DNA fingerprinting. **A,** Microsatellites consist of di-, tri-, or tetranucleotide repeats. They are used for single-locus DNA fingerprinting using PCR. Even if the repeat is present in many places throughout the genome, the use of the primers assures that only one of them is amplified. The two homologous chromosomes in each individual will produce two PCR products, and in most cases these will be of different lengths. This method does not require a probe because the PCR products can be identified directly by staining the gel after electrophoresis. ⊓⊓⊓, Primer. **B,** Minisatellites consist of longer repeat units, for example, $(AGGGCTGGAGG)_n$ or $(AGAGGTGGGCAGGTGG)_n$. They can be used for multilocus DNA fingerprinting, using Southern blotting with a frequently cutting restriction endonuclease (for example, HaeIII; see Table 10.1). The restriction fragments are detected with a probe that is directed at the repeat sequence itself, and therefore any fragment containing the repeat will be detected. If, for example, the repeat is present in 20 locations ("loci") in the genome, up to 40 fragments of different lengths will be seen after gel electrophoresis. ⊓⊓⊓, Probe; ↓, restriction site.

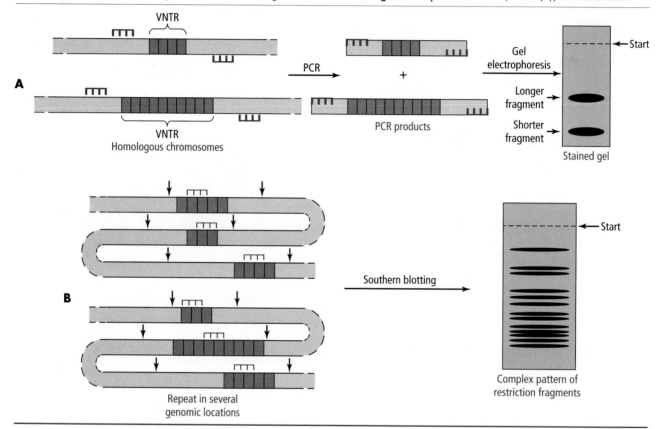

is available, for example, a single hair of a murderer stuck under a victim's fingernail. However, PCR requires more technical skill because it is sensitive to contamination.

Because variable numbers of tandem repeats are inherited as simple Mendelian traits, *DNA fingerprinting can be used for paternity testing.* DNA-based methods are supplementing and even replacing the time-honored immunologic methods of blood group typing and HLA typing for this purpose because they allow an almost 100% accurate determination of paternity—unless the alternative fathers are identical twins.

CLONING

DNA not only can be amplified in vitro by PCR; it also can be propagated in vivo after introduction into a bacterium or some other suitable host cell (for example, baker's yeast, frog oocytes, or cultured Chinese hamster ovary cells). *Cloning enables us to obtain large amounts of the cloned DNA.* This cloned DNA can be used for many purposes. The human genome project, for example, uses cloned DNA to sequence the human genome. In the following sections, we introduce the most important cloning techniques.

FIG. 10.20

The use of plasmid pBR322. This plasmid has been constructed specifically as a cloning vector. Several restriction endonucleases (*Bam*HI in this example) cleave the plasmid at unique sites within either the ampicillin-resistance (*amp-R*) gene or the tetracycline-resistance (*tet-R*) gene. In the application shown here, the *tet-R* gene is destroyed during cloning while the *amp-R* gene remains intact. Bacteria transformed by a recombinant plasmid can be selected because they can grow in the presence of ampicillin but not of tetracycline.

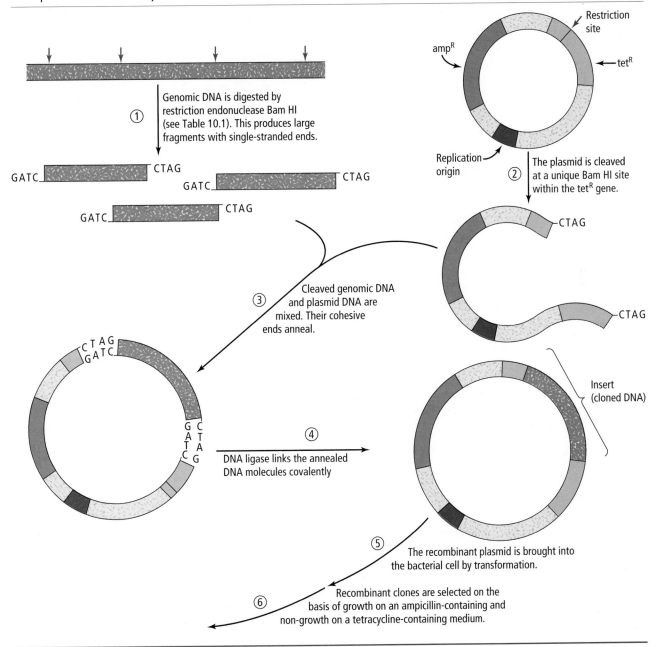

① Genomic DNA is digested by restriction endonuclease Bam HI (see Table 10.1). This produces large fragments with single-stranded ends.

② The plasmid is cleaved at a unique Bam HI site within the tet^R gene.

③ Cleaved genomic DNA and plasmid DNA are mixed. Their cohesive ends anneal.

④ DNA ligase links the annealed DNA molecules covalently

⑤ The recombinant plasmid is brought into the bacterial cell by transformation.

⑥ Recombinant clones are selected on the basis of growth on an ampicillin-containing and non-growth on a tetracycline-containing medium.

Genomic DNA fragments can be propagated in bacterial plasmids

Genetic engineers who want to propagate fragments of human DNA in a bacterial cell do not attempt to integrate this DNA in the bacterial chromosome, but the foreign DNA is inserted in a self-replicating entity called a **cloning vector**. A cloning vector can be a plasmid or a bacteriophage. Therefore *cloning requires the covalent joining of the foreign DNA with the vec-*

tor DNA. This joining has to be done in the test tube, not in the living cell.

Figure 10.20 shows the procedure for the cloning of a human DNA fragment with an R-factor plasmid carrying resistance genes for tetracycline and ampicillin. The method is based on the use of a highly selective restriction endonuclease that cleaves the circular plasmid DNA at only one site. The human DNA is cleaved with the same restriction endonuclease, generating large fragments with an average size of a few thousand base pairs. These restriction fragments end in short, single-stranded overhangs ("cohesive ends"); and when the cleaved plasmid is mixed with the fragments of human DNA, the two DNAs anneal (base-pair) spontaneously. When DNA ligase is added to the mixed DNAs, *plasmid DNA and human DNA are linked covalently into a single circular molecule.* This recombinant plasmid has to be brought into the bacterial cell by **transformation** (see Chapter 7). Transformation is rather inefficient, but it can proceed with reasonable yield if the recombinant plasmid is mixed with the bacteria in the presence of a high calcium concentration.

The recovery of a cloned DNA requires the two operations of selection and screening. **Selection** makes use of the antibiotic resistance gene(s) of the cloning vector. In the example of Fig. 10.20, the tetracycline-resistance gene has been disrupted by the insertion of the foreign DNA, whereas the ampicillin-resistance gene is still intact. Therefore properly transformed bacteria can grow in the presence of ampicillin but not of tetracycline. After the selection procedure, the transformed bacteria are plated on an agar plate, where each bacterium grows into a **clone** that forms a visible colony. *A large collection of bacterial clones, each containing a random piece of human genomic DNA, is called a* **genomic library.**

The **screening** of a genomic library is performed with a probe for the desired DNA sequence, according to the procedure outlined in Fig. 10.21. This requires prior knowledge of at least part of the base sequence. Once a clone with the desired sequence has been identified, the vector can be recovered from the bacterial clone and the insert can be excised with the same restriction endonuclease that had been used for the construction of the recombinant plasmid.

These procedures for the recovery of cloned DNA imply that *genomic libraries are useful only if they are very*

FIG. 10.21

Screening of bacterial clones in a genomic library with a radiolabeled probe. Only those clones (colonies) that contain the matching insert bind the probe and are identified by autoradiography. As an alternative to radioactive probes, fluorescent probes can be used to screen genomic libraries. Fluorescent probes can be detected directly under the UV lamp, without the need for autoradiography.

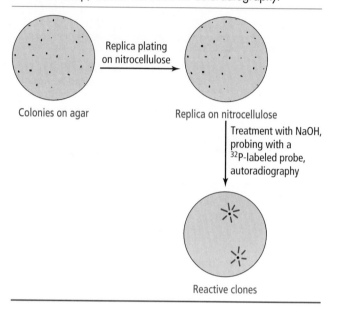

large. Each genomic DNA sequence should be represented in at least one of the clones.

Long stretches of DNA can be sequenced by chromosome walking

Genomic libraries can be used to find new genes. As we saw before (see, for example, Chapter 9), there are families of genes in the genome whose members are related structurally. If we know the partial or complete sequence of a protein-coding gene, we can construct probes that detect the gene in a genomic library. Sometimes, however, the probe hybridizes not only with the gene for which it was constructed but also with a different gene that encodes a structurally related protein. In one example, a probe was constructed for the gene of a receptor for substance K, a peptide neurotransmitter. When used to screen a genomic library, this probe identified the gene for the substance K receptor and also that for a different but structurally related receptor. This newly discovered receptor did

FIG. 10.22

Sequencing of a complete gene by chromosome walking. The method is based on the generation of overlapping restriction fragments and their cloning in a genomic library. The first clone is identified by the original probe. Its cloned fragment ("insert") is sequenced, and a new probe is synthesized that recognizes a sequence near the end of the insert. This new probe recognizes a new clone with an overlapping insert. This procedure can be repeated until the whole gene is sequenced. ▬▬ , Exons of the gene; ⊓ , probe.

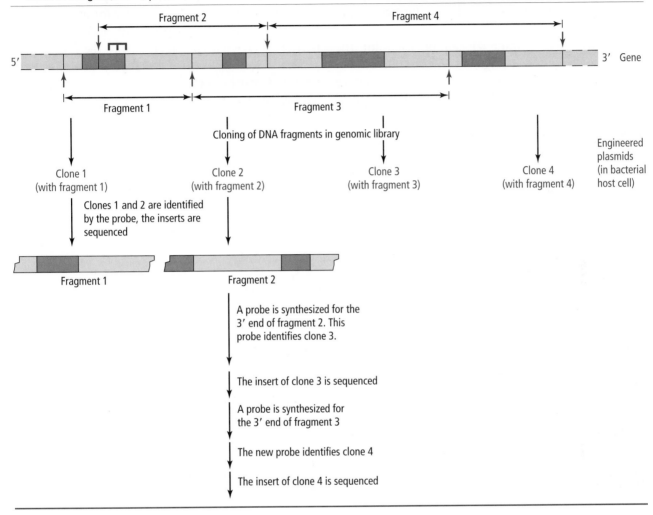

not bind substance K or related neuropeptides, but Δ¹-THC, the active constituent of marijuana. In all likelihood, an endogenous ligand exists for this "marijuana receptor," but the nature of this ligand still is unknown.

One limitation we encounter is the small size of the DNA inserts in genomic libraries: only a small fraction of the complete gene is present in an individual clone—typically a few thousand base pairs—but some eukaryotic genes are several hundred thousand base pairs long. To sequence a whole gene,

we have to resort to **chromosome walking**, as shown in Fig. 10.22: as soon as a reactive clone is identified with the original probe, a new probe is synthesized for an end sequence of the cloned fragment. *This new probe is used to screen the library for fragments that overlap the first one.*

Once a new clone is identified, its insert is sequenced as well and a new probe is synthesized for an end sequence of this fragment. By repeating these steps, long stretches of DNA can be sequenced from the cloned fragments in a genomic library.

Many different cloning vectors are available

Plasmid vectors suffer from a serious disadvantage: they can accommodate only small pieces of DNA, up to approximately 5 kb (5000 base pairs). Larger inserts tend to be deleted randomly during plasmid replication.

λ Phage (see Chapter 7) can be used for the cloning of larger DNA fragments. During its normal infective cycle, the linear double-stranded phage DNA of 48,513 base pairs is packaged into the capsid within the host cell. A stretch of approximately 15 kb in this DNA is not required for productive infection or integration into the host-cell chromosome. *This nonessential DNA can be replaced by an insert DNA* (Fig. 10.23). The recombinant phage DNA is mixed with the capsid proteins, and infective phage particles are assembled by **in vitro packaging**. *This step selects for the recombinant DNA because only DNA of the correct length can be packaged into the phage particle.*

λ Phage accommodates larger DNA inserts (10 to 15 kb) than the commonly used plasmid vectors. Also, the inefficient step of transformation is not required because the recombinant DNA in the phage particle is efficiently "injected" into the host cell.

Some cloning vectors are highly artificial constructs. **Cosmid vectors,** for example, contain the packaging signals of λ phage, an origin of replication, and an antibiotic-resistance gene. Pieces of foreign DNA 35 to 45 kb long can be inserted into this vector. With an insert of this size, it can be incorporated into a λ-phage particle by in vitro packaging. Although it enters the host cell like a

---

FIG. 10.23

The use of λ phage as a cloning vector. ■, Packaging signals ("cos sites"); ▨, phage genes essential for lytic or lysogenic infection; ▢, "nonessential" phage genes; ▢, insert DNA (human genomic DNA fragment or cDNA); ↓, cleavage site for restriction endonuclease. For proper packaging, the size of the insert DNA has to be similar to that of the nonessential phage genes that it replaces (≈ 15 kb).

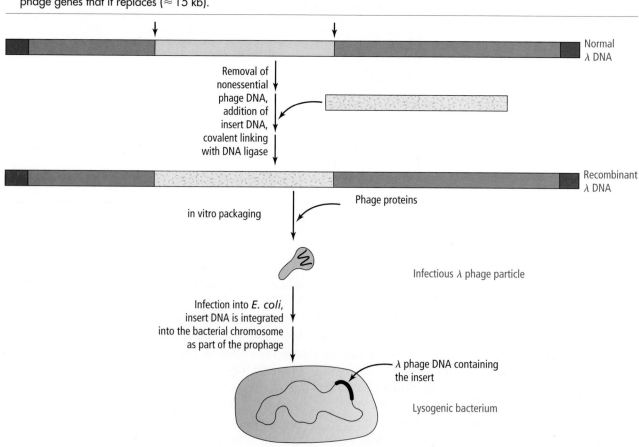

phage DNA, the cosmid DNA can neither make productive infection nor integrate itself into the host-cell DNA; rather, it replicates as a large plasmid.

cDNA libraries contain only expressed DNA

Only approximately 3% of the cloned DNA in genomic libraries codes for proteins. If we are interested specifically in the coding sequences, *we have to use mRNA rather than genomic DNA as a starting point*. The mRNA is extracted from a specific tissue or cell type such as brain, liver, or cultured fibroblasts. With the help of the retroviral enzyme **reverse transcriptase** (see Chapter 6), this extracted mRNA is used as a template for the synthesis of a double-stranded **complementary DNA (cDNA)**, as outlined in Fig. 10.24. The requirement of reverse transcrip-

FIG. 10.24

Procedure for the synthesis of cDNA for cloning in a plasmid or bacteriophage vector.

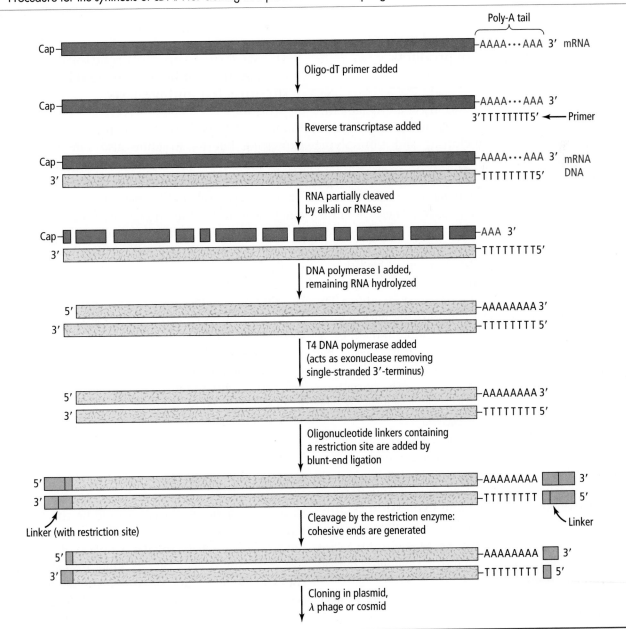

tase for a base-paired primer is fulfilled by the use of a synthetic oligo-dT, which base-pairs with the poly-A tails of the mRNA molecules.

A **cDNA library** is a collection of all the *expressed* DNA of a particular cell type or tissue. A cDNA library from bone marrow cells, for example, contains many clones with the cDNAs for hemoglobin α and β chains. A cDNA library from an insulinoma (an insulin-secreting tumor of pancreatic β cells), on the other hand, is rich in clones with the cDNA for proinsulin. For a genomic library, however, the cell type or tissue of origin is unimportant because the genomic DNA is the same in all cells of the organism.

Expression vectors are used to synthesize the protein products of cloned genes

Many human proteins can be used as therapeutic agents. They include hormones such as insulin and growth hormone; blood-clotting and fibrinolytic proteins such as clotting factors VIII and IX and tissue-type plasminogen activator (see Chapter 25); and humoral mediators of immune responses such as the interferons and interleukins. These proteins can be prepared from human tissues, but the yields are often unimpressive and the prices of the products may be staggering. Also, human-derived therapeutics can transmit deadly diseases. Many hemophiliacs, for example, were infected by the AIDS virus with the factor VIII concentrates with which they were treated, and some children died of a scrapie-like spongiform encephalopathy (caused by an infectious protein) after treatment with contaminated batches of human growth hormone. Therefore *many therapeutic proteins are now produced with the help of genetically engineered bacteria.*

The cloning strategies we have described are not useful for the production of proteins because the cloned DNA is propagated but its genes are not expressed. The effective transcription and translation of cloned DNA requires an **expression vector,** and the following conditions have to be met:

1. *Only cDNA, not genomic DNA, can be expressed in bacteria.* Bacteria cannot splice intron sequences out of a primary transcript.
2. *The coding sequence (cDNA) has to be joined to a strong bacterial promoter.*

3. *The 5'-untranslated region of the transcript must contain a bacterial ribosome-binding sequence (the Shine-Delgarno sequence; see Chapter 6).*

The expression vector has to provide a strong promoter together with the 5'-terminal part of the transcribed sequence. After ligating the insert DNA into the cloning vector, a transcript can be formed that contains the bacterial ribosome-binding sequence, the start codon, and the codons for the first few amino acids of a bacterial protein. This is followed by the sequence of the cloned cDNA. Expression vectors can be constructed with a bacterial signal sequence (see Chapter 8) that directs the secretion of the engineered protein.

The structure-function relationships of proteins can be determined by site-directed mutagenesis

Cloned DNA not only can be propagated and expressed, but its structure also can be changed deliberately by **site-directed mutagenesis.** *This approach is used to determine the structural requirements for the protein's biological functions.* If, for example, an amino acid residue in an enzyme is essential for its catalytic mechanism, then the substitution or deletion of this amino acid will abolish the enzyme's catalytic activity.

Figure 10.25 shows two technical approaches to site-directed mutagenesis. These manipulations are performed in vitro. After mutagenesis, the mutated insert DNA can be excised by a restriction endonuclease and inserted into an expression vector. After introduction into a host cell, the structurally altered protein is synthesized from the mutated DNA, and its properties can be studied.

GENE THERAPY

Most genetic diseases are caused by the mutational inactivation of an important gene. The most direct treatment for these diseases would be the artificial repair of the defective gene or the introduction of a functional gene that can take the place of the defective one. Approaches of this kind are called **gene therapy.** Gene therapy, as well as the related methods of **antisense technology,** are still in the experimental stage. We therefore can offer only a brief

FIG. 10.25

Site-directed mutagenesis of cloned DNA in vitro. **A,** A small piece of the cloned DNA is removed by a restriction endonuclease and replaced by a synthetic DNA containing the desired change. ↓, Restriction endonuclease cleavage. **B,** The DNA, inserted into a single-stranded cloning vector, is replicated with a DNA polymerase. The primer is a synthetic oligonucleotide that differs slightly from the original sequence. This primer becomes part of the new DNA strand. In this example, we achieve a G → C transversion.

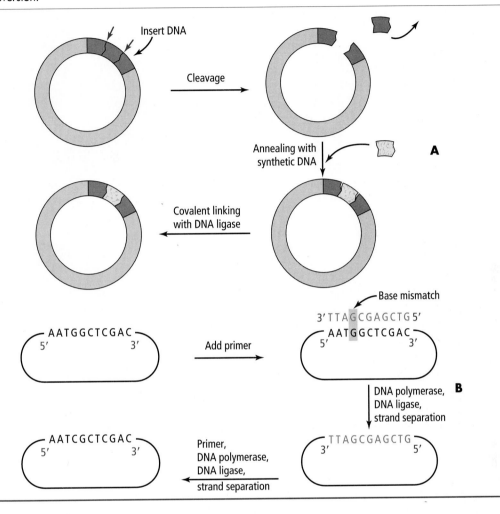

update of the most promising procedures and point to possible developments in the near future.

Foreign genes can be introduced into somatic cells

Somatic gene therapy is being developed for the treatment of genetic diseases and also for some nongenetic conditions. *This strategy does not target the germline but only the patient's somatic cells.* It does not even attempt to change all somatic cells, but the gene is delivered only to the affected tissue, if possible. In patients with Duchenne muscular dystrophy

(see Chapter 12), for example, an intact dystrophin gene is targeted specifically to muscle tissue, and in cystic fibrosis the intact gene for the CF chloride channel is targeted to the lung epithelium.

The delivery of the therapeutic gene to its target cells requires specialized techniques. Large DNA molecules do not easily cross biological membranes, and foreign DNAs are rarely integrated into the genome. In the most simple approaches, the foreign gene is delivered by physical methods (Fig. 10.26). To facilitate cell uptake, the gene can be enclosed in liposomes, artificial vesicles in which an aqueous core is surrounded by a lipid bilayer.

FIG. 10.26

Physical methods of gene delivery. **A,** The foreign gene is enclosed in a liposome. To facilitate the fusion of the liposome with the plasma membrane, the liposome is constructed in large part from cationic lipids. **B,** The foreign gene is covalently linked to a ligand that is taken up by receptor-mediated endocytosis. Only cells possessing the receptor for the ligand are transformed. Unless the endosome is disrupted, however, most of the foreign DNA is degraded by lysosomal enzymes. *L,* Ligand; *T*, receptor.

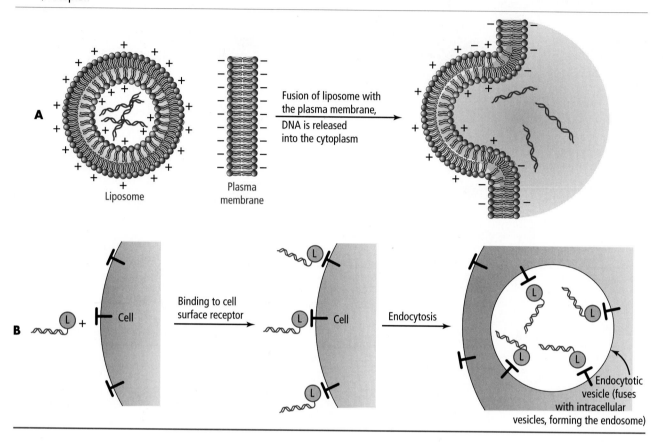

After fusion of the liposome with the plasma membrane of the target cell, the enclosed gene is released into the cytoplasm. *Liposome-mediated gene transfer is not cell type specific.* Injected liposomes may be taken up by any cell in the body, but they are most likely to end up in the endothelial cells lining the blood vessels.

Foreign genes also can be taken up by receptor-mediated endocytosis (see Chapter 8) if they are covalently bound to a suitable ligand. Hepatocytes, for example, possess a receptor that mediates the uptake of asialoglycoproteins (see Chapter 25). A foreign gene that is covalently bound to an asialoglycoprotein therefore is taken up by hepatocytes but not by other cells. Unfortunately the endocytosed gene-asialoglycoprotein conjugate usually is directed to the lysosomes, where it is degraded.

To avoid this undesirable outcome, the cells can be infected with an adenovirus at the same time. Adenoviruses disrupt the endosome and allow the endocytosed DNA to reach the cytoplasm.

The major disadvantage of both liposome-mediated and endocytotic delivery is the lack of stable integration of the foreign gene into the cellular genome. *The foreign DNA remains extrachromosomal, does not replicate, and is degraded rapidly by nucleases or diluted out of the cell with successive mitotic divisions.*

Retroviruses and DNA viruses are used as vectors for gene therapy

More promising than the physical methods of gene transfer is the use of viral vectors. Retroviruses are

FIG. 10.27

Construction of a retroviral vector for gene therapy. Both the retroviral provirus and the retroviral vector DNA are integrated in the producer cell genome. The vector RNA is packaged with the proteins produced by the retroviral provirus. The provirus RNA cannot be packaged because it lacks the packaging signal. ▬, Long terminal repeat; ▭, foreign gene to be transferred; ψ, packaging signal; gag, pol, env, normal retroviral genes.

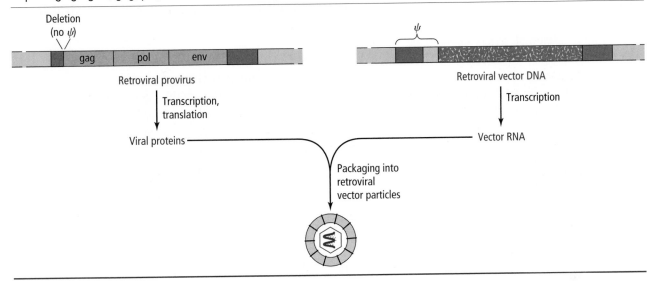

the most widely used vectors because they integrate their own cDNA into the host-cell genome during their normal reproductive cycle (see Chapter 7). Therefore *a foreign gene, incorporated into a retroviral genome, is targeted specifically to the chromosomes of the treated cell.*

The retroviral vectors that are used for gene therapy are highly artificial constructs. They contain the long terminal repeats of a "real" retrovirus, but *their pol, gag, and env genes are replaced by the foreign gene.* Retroviral vectors can carry inserts of approximately 7000 base pairs, enough to code for a large protein. The genes that are transferred by the retroviral vectors are not the natural genes with their intron-exon structure, but intronless constructs that either are produced from a cDNA or are synthesized chemically.

Retroviral vectors are produced in a cultured cell line ("producer cell") that contains the genome of a defective retrovirus. This defective retrovirus has all the retroviral genes but is lacking the packaging signal. Conversely, the retroviral vector cannot synthesize viral proteins but has the packaging signal. When the vector is introduced into the producer cell line, therefore, it is the vector RNA that is packaged into the virus particles, together with the

retroviral reverse transcriptase and integrase (Fig. 10.27).

When the vector enters its target cell, it can produce a cDNA copy of its RNA "genome" and integrate this cDNA with the aid of the reverse transcriptase and the integrase in the virus particle. Once in the host-cell chromosome, however, the vector cannot produce viral proteins for the formation of new virus particles. Instead, the insert gene is expressed to produce the desired protein product. Because of their inability to synthesize viral proteins and produce infectious virus particles, *retroviruses are "clean" vectors, with little or no cytotoxicity.*

Although retroviral vectors insert themselves specifically into the host-cell genome, retroviral gene transfer (known technically as **transfection**) is not particularly efficient. Even in cell cultures, less than 10% of the cells are transfected in most experiments. Also, with the sole exception of the AIDS virus, *retroviruses are not able to infect nondividing cells, and this is also true for the retroviral vectors.* Therefore these vectors are poorly suited for gene therapy of nondividing end-stage cells such as neurons and muscle fibers.

DNA viruses also are being explored as possible vectors for somatic gene therapy. Adenoviruses, for example, which are minor respiratory pathogens in humans, have been used to deliver the gene for the CF chloride channel to the respiratory epithelium of CF patients. In these adenoviral vectors, one of the viral genes is replaced by the transferred gene. Regrettably, *adenoviral vectors normally do not integrate their DNA into the host-cell DNA*, so the therapeutic benefits, if any, are transient. Also, viral proteins still are produced by the vector, and this gives rise both to cytotoxicity and to immunologic responses that may preclude the long-term use of the vector. However, these vectors can be produced more easily, and applied in higher titers, than the retroviral vectors, and they can infect nondividing cells.

Gene therapy has been attempted for various genetic diseases. Thus, the gene for adenosine deaminase (ADA) has been transfected successfully into lymphocytes of patients with ADA deficiency, an inherited immunodeficiency disease with severe malfunction of both B and T lymphocytes (see Chapter 23). Patients' lymphocytes are removed from the body, treated with the retroviral vector in vitro, and then injected back into the body.

The response to gene therapy depends, in large part, on the rate of gene expression that is required to cure the disease. The clotting disorder of dogs with hemophilia B (deficiency of clotting factor IX; see Chapter 25), for example, could be mitigated by the retroviral transfer of a factor IX gene into hepatocytes, although the factor IX level after this treatment was only 0.1% of normal. In the case of hemoglobin, however, a balanced synthesis of hemoglobin α and β chains is required, and the normal regulation of hemoglobin synthesis is poorly understood. Therefore the thalassemias may prove difficult to treat with gene therapy.

Some nongenetic conditions also are candidates for gene therapy. Cancer cells, for example, have been transfected with such cytokines as tumor necrosis factor (TNF) and interleukin-2 (IL-2) in attempts to stimulate the immune response against the tumor cells. Gene therapies for rheumatoid arthritis also are under investigation. This common disease is marked by an inflammatory process that is mediated by the cytokine interleukin-1 (IL-1). In this case, the transfected gene encodes either a soluble form of the IL-1 receptor or a receptor-blocking protein that prevents the action of IL-1. The vector carrying the gene is injected directly into the inflamed joint.

Antisense technology is aimed at blocking the expression of undesirable genes

Some diseases are caused not by the lack of a normal gene but rather by the expression or overexpression of an undesirable gene. In many cancers, for example, the malignant cells grow out of control because growth-stimulating genes are either overexpressed or mutated to produce superactive proteins. These genes are called **oncogenes** (see Chapter 28). Cancer growth can be blocked, theoretically, by inhibiting the expression of oncogenes in the tumor cells. Also, viral diseases can be treated by agents that inhibit selectively the expression of an essential viral gene.

Antisense technology is based on the use of oligonucleotides that are complementary to the base sequence of an undesirable mRNA. *By hybridizing with the mRNA, the antisense oligonucleotide blocks translation*. The antisense agent has to have a length of at least 16 to 18 nucleotides to prevent nonspecific hybridization with nontarget sequences. Both DNA and RNA oligonucleotides have been used experimentally, but problems are encountered because the antisense oligonucleotides are not taken up easily by their target cells and are degraded rapidly by cellular nucleases. Therefore *synthetic oligonucleotides commonly are used, in which the phosphodiester bonds are replaced by nuclease-resistant linkages* (Fig. 10.28). Even these nuclease-resistant analogs, however, show

FIG. 10.28

Structural modifications of the phosphodiester bonds in currently used antisense oligonucleotides.

d-ribose   d-ribose   d-ribose

$H_3C-P=O$ $^-O-P=O$ $^-S-P=O$

d-ribose   d-ribose   d-ribose

Methylphosphonate   Phosphodiester bond in DNA   Phosphorothioate

poor cell uptake and therefore have to be used at high concentrations. This is regrettable because the chemical synthesis of bulk quantities of antisense agents is quite expensive.

Like gene therapy, antisense technology still is in the experimental stage. Its most attractive feature is that, in theory, *the expression of any undesirable gene can be blocked by a complementary oligonucleotide analog.* It currently is expected that severe viral diseases such as AIDS will be the first diseases for which antisense therapies will be used.

The use of **antisense genes** combines the principles of gene therapy and antisense technology: a synthetic gene is introduced into the cell whose RNA transcript is complementary to the mRNA of an undesirable gene. The RNA transcript of the antisense gene is not translated.

Selective germline mutations can be produced

Germline cells, as well as somatic cells, can be manipulated genetically. In animal experiments, this can be achieved either by *the injection of foreign DNA into the zygote* or by *the manipulation of cultured embryonic stem cells.* Embryonic stem cells are early embryonic cells that are propagated in cell culture. Specific culturing conditions are required to maintain the cells in an undifferentiated state that can, in subsequent cell generations, give rise to any specialized cell type of the body: the cells have to remain **totipotent.**

Cultured embryonic stem cells can be treated with foreign DNA and implanted in an early embryo at the blastocyst stage. These blastocysts are implanted in foster animals, where they develop into chimeric animals. Some of the engineered stem cells in these animals enter the germline and transmit their genes to the next generation. Although the genetic change is present in the heterozygous state in these animals, it can be made homozygous by classical breeding.

Alternatively, genetically manipulated animals can be produced by **cloning:** *an oocyte is enucleated either by radiation treatment or by mechanical removal of the nucleus, and the nucleus of a genetically manipulated embryonic stem cell is introduced in vitro.* The cell is allowed to undergo the first cleavage divisions in the test tube before it is implanted into the uterus of a foster animal. Cloning can be used to produce large numbers of genetically identical animals, all descended from the same cultured cell line.

Gene disruptions can be achieved with the aid of DNA constructs that have partial sequence homology with the targeted gene. This foreign DNA is introduced into the target cells by microinjection or electroporation. In most cases, the artificially introduced DNA is degraded before it can be integrated into the genome, but *occasionally it becomes integrated into the chromosome by homologous recombination with the targeted gene* (Fig. 10.29).

Gene disruptions frequently have been induced in mice to create what is known as **knockout mice.** Knockout mice can be used as animal models of human genetic diseases. Also, the biological significance of proteins can be ascertained by observing the abnormalities (if any) when the functional protein is missing.

FIG. 10.29

Gene disruption in vivo by an artificial double-stranded DNA construct with sequence homology to the targeted gene. Gene disruption depends on homologous recombination between the exogenous DNA and the targeted gene. This principle is used for the production of "knockout mice." ▇, Normal cellular gene; ▇, exogenous DNA.

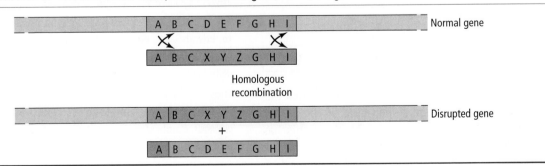

The same general procedures that are used for the production of knockout mice also have been used for the repair of defective genes or the introduction of new genes into the germline. In several instances, for example, the artificially induced gene defects in knockout mice have been corrected by the introduction of a new functional gene into the germline. In another example, giant mice were produced by introducing a gene for rat growth hormone, linked to the promoter of the metallothionein gene (see Chapter 24). When fed with heavy metals (metallothionein normally is induced by heavy metals), the livers of these animals produced large amounts of rat growth hormone.

Cloning, either with or without genetic manipulations of the cultured embryonic cells, has been performed in mice and sheep but not in humans, although *the cloning of human beings may become possible in the near future.* Sheep have been cloned not only from embryonic cells, but also from the cells of mature animals. Therefore, it may actually be possible to copy individuals with particular properties (for example, Mother Teresa or Idi Amin).

In theory, germline gene manipulations can be used to change permanently the genetic makeup of our species. For example, we are not able to synthesize ascorbic acid (vitamin C) because our fruit-eating ancestors lost the gene for the biosynthetic enzyme gulonolactone oxidase some 40 million years ago (see Chapters 17 and 24). The transfer of a gene for gulonolactone oxidase into the germline would restore our ability for vitamin C synthesis and eliminate any danger of scurvy—perhaps for the next 40 million years. This is not an example of gene therapy but rather of **enhancement engineering**. In contrast to gene therapy, which attempts to repair genetic defects, *enhancement engineering is aimed at improvements on a "normal" genetic constitution.* Needless to say, opinions about enhancement engineering are divided.

SUMMARY

A large amount of information about our genes has accumulated, and even the sequencing of the whole human genome is in full progress. Much of this has been possible because DNA can be cloned in bacterial cells. Either genomic DNA or cDNA, obtained by the reverse transcription of mRNA, can be cloned. Some cloning systems even permit the expression of the cloned genes, and many valuable proteins are produced commercially in genetically engineered bacteria.

The practicing physician is most likely to encounter DNA-directed techniques in the context of diagnostic tests for genetic diseases. These techniques require only the patient's DNA, not the encoded protein. If the sequences of both the normal gene and the mutated gene are known, allele-specific methods can be employed. Southern blotting with allele-specific oligonucleotide probes, in particular, is popular for these cases. If only small amounts of DNA are available, for example, in prenatal and preimplantation diagnosis, the DNA of interest has to be amplified by the polymerase chain reaction (PCR) first, before it can be analyzed by gel electrophoresis or the use of allele-specific probes. If the sequence of the gene and the nature of the mutation are unknown, however, neither PCR nor allele-specific oligonucleotides can be used. In many of these cases, however, it still is possible to trace the inheritance of the mutation by tracing closely linked restriction fragment length polymorphisms (RFLPs).

Various approaches to gene therapy also are under investigation. In the most advanced techniques, genes are targeted to somatic cells of the patient with the help of retroviral vectors. None of the currently available methods for gene delivery is particularly efficient, however, and gene therapy still is in the experimental stage.

Further Reading

Askari FK, McDonnell WM: Antisense oligonucleotide therapy. *N Engl J Med* 334 (5), 316–318, 1996.

Bentley DR: The direct diagnosis of genetic defects. In: Edwards RG, editor: *Preconception and preimplantation diagnosis.* Cambridge University Press, Cambridge, 1993, pp. 183–199.

Bentley DR, et al: Analysis of genetic variation in the single cell. In: Edwards RG, editor: *Preconception and preimplantation diagnosis.* Cambridge University Press, Cambridge, 1993, pp. 161–181.

Bronson SK, Smithies O: Altering mice by homologous

recombination using embryonic stem cells. *J Biol Chem* 269, 27155–27158, 1994.

Crystal RG: Transfer of genes to humans: early lessons and obstacles to success. *Science* 270, 404–410, 1995.

Fritsch EF, Wozney JM: Methods of molecular genetics. In: Stamatoyannopoulos G, Nienhuis AW, Majerus PW, Varmus H, editors: *The molecular basis of blood diseases.* W. B. Saunders, Philadelphia, 1994, pp. 3–32.

Korf B: Molecular diagnosis. *N Engl J Med* 332 (22), 1499–1502, 1995.

Lebo RV, et al.: Prenatal diagnosis of α-thalassemia by polymerase chain reaction and dual restriction enzyme analysis. *Hum Genet* 85, 293–299, 1990.

Malcolm S: Molecular genetics. In: Brock DJH, Rodeck CH, Ferguson-Smith MA, editors: *Prenatal diagnosis and screening.* Churchill Livingstone, New York, 1992, pp. 147–157.

Marx J: Marijuana receptor gene cloned. *Science* 249, 624–626, 1990.

Mueller RF: Molecular biology in relation to medical genetics. In: Emery AEH, Rimoin DL, editors: *Principles and practice of medical genetics*, 2nd ed., vol. 1. Churchill Livingstone, New York, 1990, pp. 33–51.

Mullis KB, Ferre F, Gibbs RA, editors: *PCR.* Birkhauser, Boston, 1994.

Sokol DL, Gewirtz AM: Gene therapy: basic concepts and recent advances. *Crit Rev Eukaryot Gene Expr* 6 (1), 29–57, 1996.

Southern EM: DNA chips: analyzing sequence by hybridization to oligonucleotides on a large scale. *Trends Genet* 12 (3), 110–115, 1996.

Trent RJ: *Molecular medicine.* Churchill-Livingstone, New York, 1993.

van de Woude S, van de Woude GF: Introduction to methods in molecular biology. In: De Vita VT, Hellman S, Rosenberg SA, editors: *Cancer: principles and practice of oncology*, 4th ed., vol. 1. J. B. Lippincott, Philadelphia, 1993, pp. 3–33.

Wilmut I, Schnieke AE, McWhir J, Kind AJ, Campbell KHS. Viable offspring derived from fetal and adult mammalian cells. *Nature* 385, 810–813, 1997.

Wilson JM: Adenoviruses as gene delivery vehicles. *N Engl J Med* 334 (18), 1185–1187, 1996.

Wu DY, Uggozoli L, Pal BK, Wallace RB: Allele-specific enzymatic amplification of β-globin genomic DNA for diagnosis of sickle cell anemia. *Proc Natl Acad Sci USA* 86, 2757–2760, 1989.

QUESTIONS

1. Large-scale DNA sequencing costs approximately 30 cents per base pair. How much money is required to sequence the whole human genome?
   - A. $100 million
   - B. $1 billion
   - C. $10 billion
   - D. $100 billion
   - E. $1 trillion

2. You have been instructed by the U.S. Department of Health to screen the whole population of New York City for the presence of the sickle cell mutation. Which method would be best for this project?
   - A. Southern blotting with allele-specific probes
   - B. PCR, with electrophoretic separation of the products
   - C. Linkage analysis with closely linked RFLPs
   - D. Chromosome walking
   - E. Dot blotting

3. Retroviral vectors are more popular than other viral vectors for somatic gene therapy because
   - A. They replicate faster than most other viruses.
   - B. They contain several copies of their DNA genome in the virus particle.
   - C. They can integrate themselves into the host-cell DNA.
   - D. Their replication is more accurate than that of most other viruses.
   - E. Their DNA has extensive sequence homology with normal cellular DNA.

4. The steps of classical Southern blotting include (1) denaturation of DNA with alkali; (2) electrophoresis in a cross-linked agarose or polyacrylamide gel; (3) application of a probe; (4) treatment of DNA with a restriction endonuclease, and (5) blotting of DNA to a nitrocellulose foil. The correct sequence of these steps is
   - A. $1 \rightarrow 4 \rightarrow 2 \rightarrow 5 \rightarrow 3$
   - B. $4 \rightarrow 3 \rightarrow 1 \rightarrow 2 \rightarrow 5$
   - C. $1 \rightarrow 5 \rightarrow 2 \rightarrow 3 \rightarrow 4$
   - D. $4 \rightarrow 2 \rightarrow 1 \rightarrow 5 \rightarrow 3$
   - E. $2 \rightarrow 1 \rightarrow 5 \rightarrow 4 \rightarrow 3$

5. If you want to use genetically engineered bacteria for the production of human growth hor-

mone, you need all of the following ingredients except

    A. A cDNA obtained by the reverse transcription of growth hormone mRNA

    B. A bacterial promoter sequence

    C. A sequence that codes for a bacterial ribosome-binding sequence

    D. Genomic DNA of the growth hormone gene

    E. Restriction endonucleases

6. PCR-based procedures often are preferred over Southern blotting for the prenatal diagnosis of genetic diseases after amniocentesis or chorionic villus sampling. Why?

    A. PCR requires less DNA, so lengthy cell culturing may not be necessary.

    B. PCR requires less technical skill than Southern blotting and is therefore less costly.

    C. PCR is less sensitive to contamination by extraneous DNA and therefore is less prone to false-positive results.

    D. Unlike Southern blotting, PCR does not require DNA from many family members.

    E. Unlike Southern blotting, PCR does not require any knowledge of the DNA sequence in and around the affected gene.

7. The classical PCR procedure (without allele-specific primers and without probes) can be used to

    A. Amplify the whole dystrophin gene with its 79 exons and 78 introns in one piece.

    B. Diagnose the sickle cell mutation after amniocentesis.

    C. Diagnose HIV infection in people with "at risk" lifestyles.

    D. Detect point mutations in a gene with an unknown sequence.

    E. All of the above can be done with PCR.

8. If you want to know whether the pharaoh Tutankhamen was a carrier of the sickle cell mutation, you should study the traces of DNA recovered from his mummy with

    A. Classical Southern blotting with allele-specific probes.

    B. Classical PCR (not allele-specific PCR), without the use of probes.

    C. PCR with blotting of the electrophoresed products to nitrocellulose and use of allele-specific probes.

    D. Dot-blotting with allele-specific probes.

    E. Linkage with closely linked VNTR polymorphisms.

9. Linkage studies with closely linked VNTR polymorphisms are the preferred diagnostic method for the detection of heterozygous carriers of recessive disease genes when

    A. There is allelic heterogeneity: you do not know which mutation is present in a known disease gene.

    B. There is locus heterogeneity: you do not know which gene is mutated.

    C. No case of the disease has so far occurred in the family.

    D. The disease is caused by a small deletion of a few base pairs.

    E. The exact molecular nature of the mutation is known.

10. To compare gene expression in rhabdomyosarcoma cells with gene expression in normal skeletal muscle, you have isolated mRNA from the two sources by affinity chromatography on an oligo-dT column. The *most direct* method for comparing the two mRNA patterns would be

    A. PCR with nested primers

    B. Dot-blotting

    C. Cloning

    D. Southern blotting

    E. Northern blotting

PART THREE

CELL AND TISSUE STRUCTURE

Chapter 11

Biological Membranes

Membranes are the only structural elements common to all cellular organisms. Each cell is surrounded by a **plasma membrane,** which forms the boundary between the cell and its environment. Eukaryotic but not prokaryotic cells possess intracellular membranes as well, which delineate their organelles. Acting as diffusion barriers, membranes effect a compartmentalization of biochemical processes.

The terms *plasma membrane* and *cell wall,* so often confused by students, should be strictly distinguished: the plasma membrane is a thin, flimsy structure that forms a diffusion barrier. The cell wall, however, is strong and stiff and maintains the shape of the cell. Plants and bacteria have a cell wall on top of their plasma membrane that contains the polysaccharides cellulose and peptidoglycan, respectively. We do not have cell walls: our cells are kept in shape by the **cytoskeleton** (discussed in Chapter 12), and the mechanical properties of our tissues depend in large part on the **extracellular matrix** (discussed in Chapter 13). In this chapter, we introduce the important properties of cellular membranes.

THE LIPID BILAYER

Under the electron microscope, biological membranes look like railroad tracks: in cross-section, a central electrolucent layer is sandwiched between two electron-dense layers. The total diameter of this trilaminar structure is approximately 8 nm. This appearance is common to essentially all biological membranes.

The chemical composition of membranes is, within limits, rather uniform as well: *they all consist of lipid and protein*. The protein/lipid ratio is high in membranes with high metabolic activity and low in metabolically more inert membranes. The inner mitochondrial membrane, for example, which contains the proteins of the respiratory chain and oxidative phosphorylation (see Chapter 16), is approximately 75% protein and 25% lipid. The myelin membrane, however, which forms an insulating layer around axons, is approximately 80% lipid and 20% protein. Carbohydrate is present only as a constituent of glycoproteins and glycolipids. In general, *lipids form the structural backbone of the membrane, whereas proteins are in charge of such specific functions as enzymatic activities, regulated transport, ion permeability and excitability, contact with structural proteins, and the transmission of physiological signals*. In the first part of this chapter, we introduce the structures of the major membrane lipids and the lipid bilayer, which forms the core of all biological membranes.

Membrane lipids are amphipathic

Unlike the triglycerides, which have very little affinity for water, membrane lipids are characterized as **amphiphilic** or **amphipathic**. These terms imply that *hydrophilic and hydrophobic parts are combined in the same molecule*. In the **phospholipids**, the hydrophilic part contains a phosphate group, and in the **glycolipids** it contains covalently attached carbohydrate. Based on their chemical building blocks, however, we can distinguish three classes of membrane lipids: the **phosphoglycerides**, the **sphingolipids**, and **cholesterol**.

The phosphoglycerides are the most abundant membrane lipids

The phosphoglycerides easily are the most abundant membrane lipids, accounting for more than half of the total lipids in most membranes. As their name

FIG. 11.1

Structures of the most common phosphoglycerides.

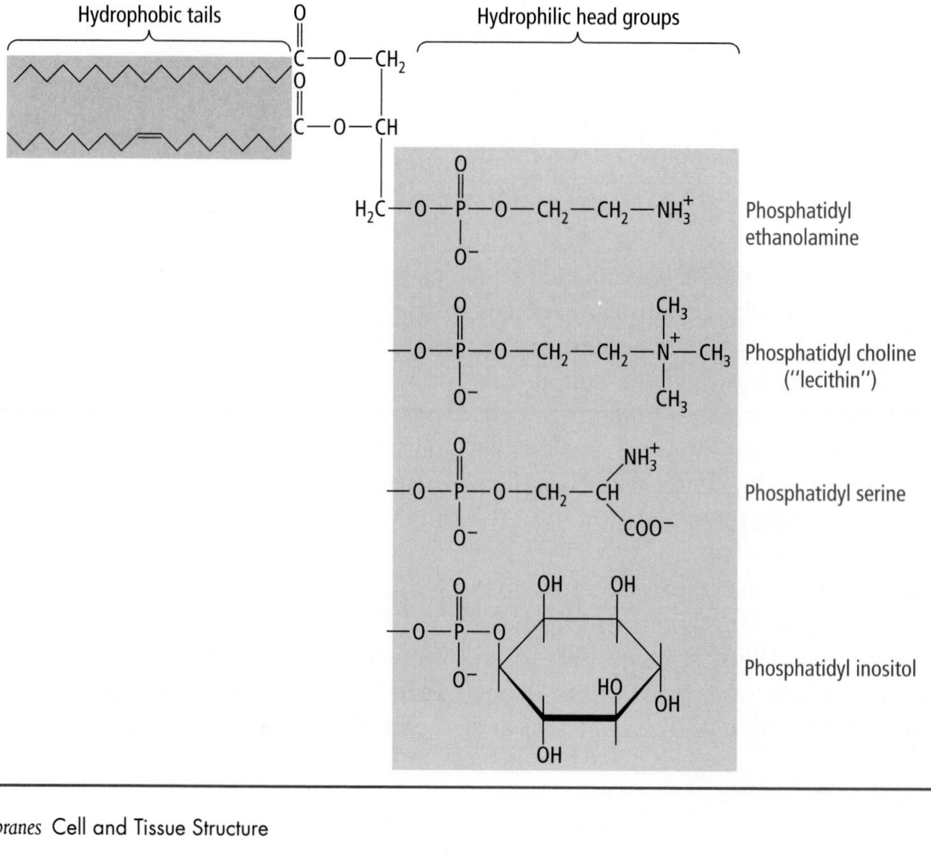

implies, they contain both phosphate and glycerol. If the third fatty acid residue of a triglyceride is replaced by a phosphate group, we obtain **phosphatidic acid** or **phosphatidate** as shown in Box 11.1. Phosphatidate is not a major membrane lipid itself but rather the parent compound and biosynthetic precursor of the phosphoglycerides (see Chapter 19).

The major membrane phosphoglycerides possess an alcohol, linked to the phosphate group in phosphatidic acid by a phosphodiester bond (Fig. 11.1). The phosphate is negatively charged at physiologic pH values, and also, the variable alcohol bound to the phosphate either is charged or has a high hydrogen-bonding potential. *Together with the phosphate, it forms*

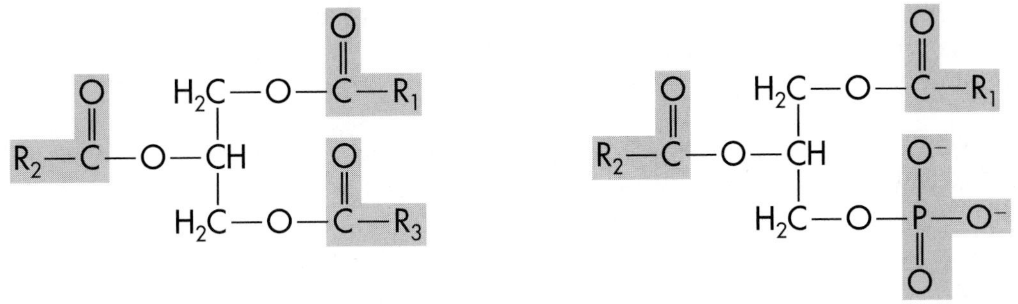

Triglyceride

Phosphatidate

Structures of cardiolipin and plasmalogen. **A,** Cardiolipin, a major lipid of the inner mitochondrial membrane. **B,** Ethanolamine plasmalogen. Plasmalogens account for up to 10% of the phospholipid in muscle and nervous tissue and are present in most other tissues as well.

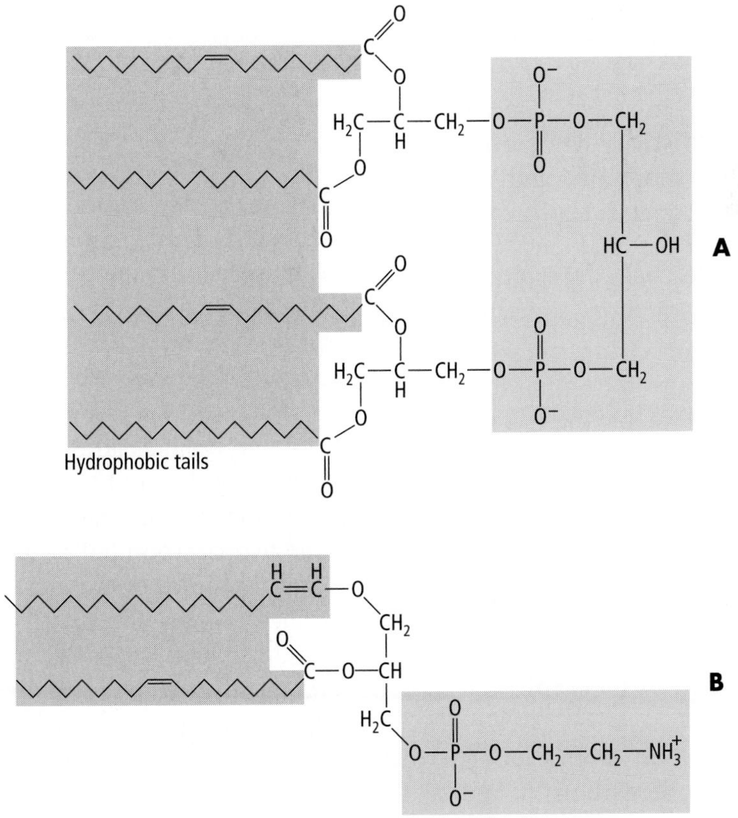

Hydrophobic tails

A

B

the hydrophilic head group of the molecule, and the two fatty acids form two hydrophobic tails. In the common phosphoglycerides, the fatty acid in position 1 usually is saturated (either palmitic or stearic acid), whereas that in position 2 is unsaturated.

Two less-common phosphoglycerides are shown in Fig. 11.2 (page 221). **Cardiolipin** (diphosphatidyl glycerol) is common only in the inner mitochondrial membrane. The widespread **plasmalogens**, usually with ethanolamine in their hydrophilic head group, are distinguished by the presence of an α-β-unsaturated fatty alcohol, rather than a fatty acid residue, in position 1.

Dipalmitoyl-phosphatidylcholine is the most important component of lung surfactant

Most phosphoglycerides function only as structural components of biological membranes. One phosphoglyceride, however, **dipalmitoyl phosphatidylcholine (dipalmitoyl lecithin)**, serves a special function as the major constituent of **lung surfactant**, a lipid and protein mixture that is secreted by type II pneumocytes in the alveolar walls. *Lung surfactant reduces the surface tension of the thin fluid film that lines the alveolar walls.* In its absence, the alveoli collapse, and the resulting respiratory impairment is immediately life threatening.

The deficiency of lung surfactant in preterm infants causes **respiratory distress syndrome**. This is a major cause of infant morbidity and mortality, causing 15% to 20% of neonatal deaths in Western countries. The maturity of the fetal lungs can be determined by assaying the lecithin/sphingomyelin (L/S) ratio in amniotic fluid. This ratio is low until 30 to 32 weeks of gestation. An infant born before this time is likely to suffer from respiratory distress syndrome. From 30 to 34 weeks, the L/S ratio rises to approximately 2.0 or above, indicating a sufficient amount of lung surfactant. *The L/S ratio is routinely determined for the timing of elective deliveries.*

Exogenous surfactant, administered by inhaler, has been found to be effective in the treatment of respiratory distress syndrome.

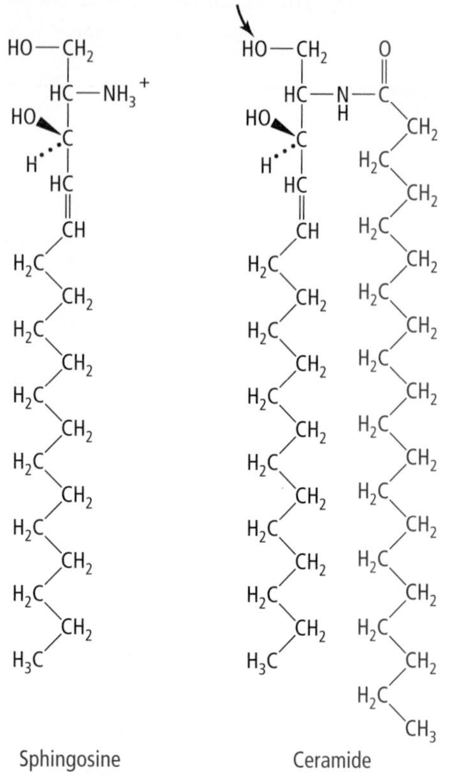

Most sphingolipids are glycolipids

Sphingosine is an 18-carbon amino alcohol that contains hydroxy groups at carbons 1 and 3, an

FIG. 11.3

Structures of sphingosine and ceramide. The fatty acid residues in ceramide often are very long (C-20 to C-24). The hydroxy group of ceramide that is substituted in the sphingolipids is marked by an arrow.

Sphingosine   Ceramide

amino group at carbon 2, and a long hydrocarbon tail. In the sphingolipids, the amino group of sphingosine forms an amide bond with a long-chain (C-18 to C-24) fatty acid. This structure is called **ceramide** (Fig. 11.3). Of the two hydroxy groups in ceramide, the one at C-3 remains unsubstituted, and the one at C-1 carries a variable substituent that forms the polar head group. *Like the phosphoglycerides, the sphingolipids have two hydrophobic tails.* Only one of these, however, is a fatty acid residue; the other one is the hydrocarbon tail of sphingosine itself.

The structures of the most important sphingolipids are shown in Fig. 11.4. Only sphingomyelin, which has the same head group as phosphatidylcholine (Fig. 11.1), qualifies as a phospholipid. The other sphingolipids are glycolipids. The most complex glycosphingolipids are the **gangliosides.** They contain complex oligosaccharides with between one and four

FIG. 11.4

The major types of sphingolipids.

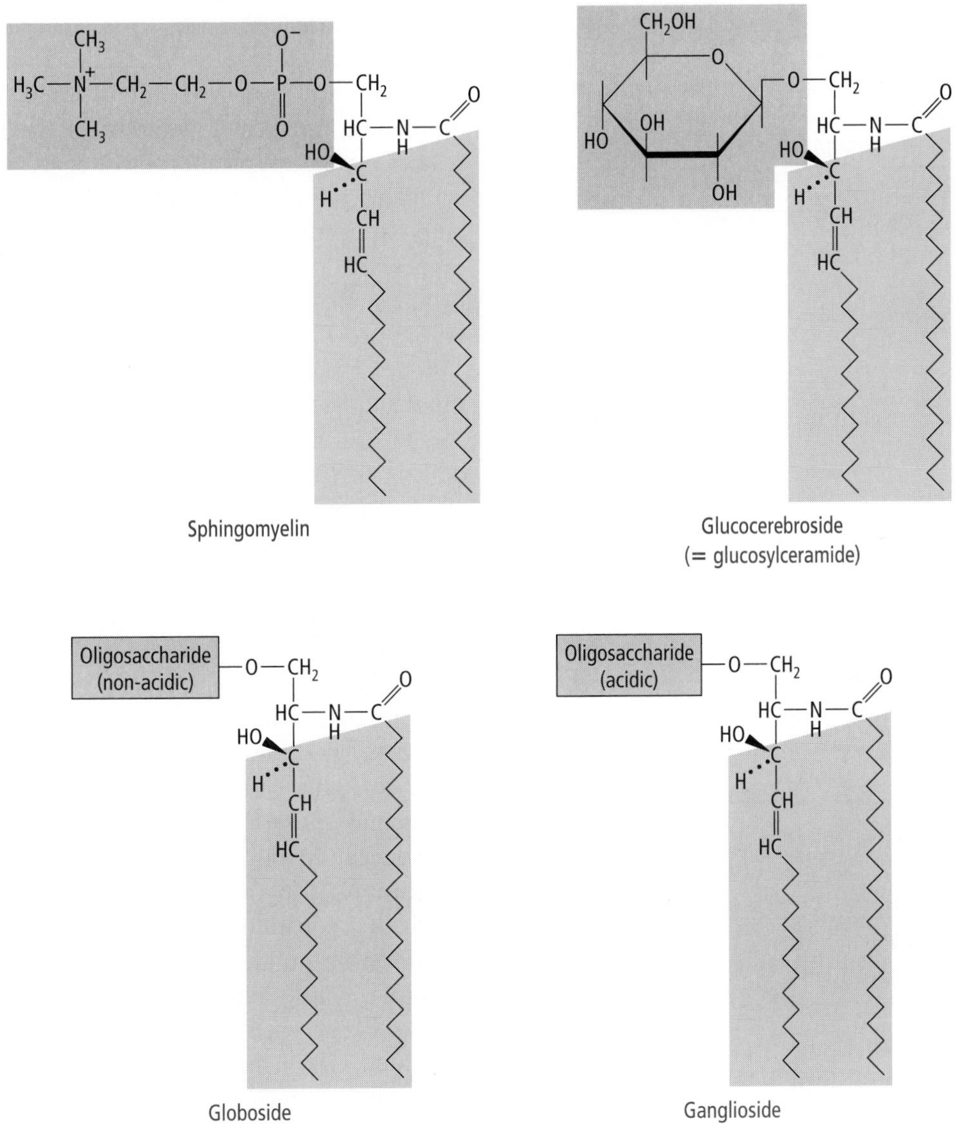

Sphingomyelin

Glucocerebroside
(= glucosylceramide)

Globoside

Ganglioside

residues of **N-acetylneuraminic acid (NANA)**, an acidic sugar derivative that occupies terminal positions in the oligosaccharide chain (Fig. 11.5, page 224).

The sphingolipids are less abundant than the phosphoglycerides, with the highest concentrations in the plasma membrane. The glycosphingolipids of the plasma membrane are concentrated in the exoplasmic leaflet, with their carbohydrate chains facing the extracellular space. Sphingomyelin and galactocerebroside (the latter partly in a sulfated form) are important components of myelin, and gangliosides and galactocerebroside are abundant in the gray matter of the brain.

Cholesterol is the most hydrophobic membrane lipid

Cholesterol (Fig. 11.6, page 224) is quite different from the other membrane lipids: instead of two long, wriggly hydrocarbon tails, it has a stiff carbocyclic ring structure, the **steroid ring system.** Moreover, instead of a stately hydrophilic head group, there is only a solitary hydroxy group at one end of the molecule. With this structure, *cholesterol is by far the least water-soluble membrane lipid.*

Cholesterol accounts for 10% or more of the

FIG. 11.5

Structures of complex glycosphingolipids. **A,** Ganglioside G_{M2}, a typical acidic glycosphingolipid. Some other gangliosides have two, three, or four residues of N-acetylneuraminic acid (NANA). **B,** The structure of N-acetylneuraminate (NANA), a sialic acid. This acidic sugar derivative is found in terminal positions of the oligosaccharides in gangliosides (and some glycoproteins).

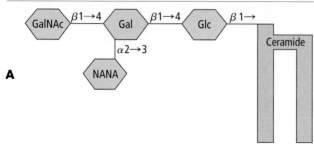

N-Acetylneuraminic acid
(NANA)

FIG. 11.6

The structure of cholesterol.

total lipid in the plasma membrane and the Golgi membrane but is less abundant in more internal membranes. It is prominent only in animals, including humans. Plants have different membrane steroids, the **phytosterols,** and most bacteria have no steroids at all.

Membrane lipids form a bilayer

In an aqueous environment, *the hydrophilic head groups of the membrane lipids always try to surround themselves with water, whereas the hydrophobic tails avoid water.* Membrane lipids do not dissolve well in water as individual molecules, but heavy agitation of the lipid in water results in some typical types of aggregates (Fig. 11.7). **Micelles** are globular structures that are formed by all polar lipids, including ordinary detergents. **Monolayers** are formed only at aqueous/nonaqueous interfaces—for example, between water and air; **bilayers** are formed within an aqueous environment. *All known biological membranes contain a lipid bilayer as their structural backbone.* Bilayers do not exist as flat, spread-out sheets in nature because the exposed edges do not like water, but they form small vesicles, 20 nm to 1 μm in diameter, that are known as liposomes.

The bilayer is held together by hydrophobic interactions. In addition, hydrophilic interactions exist between the head groups of neighboring lipid molecules, and between the head groups and the surrounding water. The geometry of the lipid molecules is important, too: *a bilayer can be formed only if the cross-sectional area of the head groups matches that of the hydrophobic tails.* If, for example, one of the fatty acids is removed from phosphatidylcholine (lecithin), the resulting lysolecithin no longer forms a bilayer. With its less-spacious hydrophobic end, lysolecithin feels more comfortable in a micelle than in a bilayer. For example, biological membranes are destabilized by treatment with phospholipase A_2. This enzyme, which occurs in many biological sources, including some snake venoms, hydrolyzes phosphoglycerides to the corresponding lysophosphoglycerides.

The lipid bilayer is a two-dimensional fluid

Because of its noncovalent character, the lipid bilayer lacks structural strength. Its mechanical properties are not unlike those of an ordinary soap bubble (Fig. 11.7, *E*). For example, it is easily deformed by even slight forces. Also, the hydrophobic tails of the lipids can merrily wriggle around, and each individual molecule is free to diffuse laterally in the plane of the bilayer. This lateral diffusion proceeds

FIG. 11.7

Behavior of polar lipids in water. **A,** A *micelle* is a small, spherical structure with a hydrophilic surface and a hydrophobic core. **B,** A *bilayer* is the prototype of a biological membrane. As in the micelle, the hydrophilic head groups are on the surface and the hydrophobic tails are buried in the center. **C,** A *liposome* is the prototype of a membrane-bound vesicle. It forms spontaneously from a lipid bilayer. **D,** A *monolayer* forms at the interface between water and air. **E,** A *soap bubble* consists of two monolayers enclosing a thin water film.

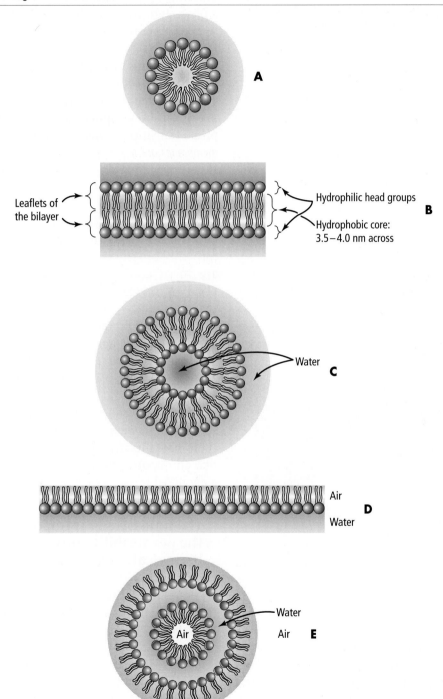

A

Leaflets of the bilayer

Hydrophilic head groups

Hydrophobic core: 3.5–4.0 nm across

B

Water

C

Air

Water

D

Water

Air

E

FIG. 11.8

Effect of a *cis* double bond on the array of fatty acid chains in the hydrophobic core of the lipid bilayer. **A,** The geometry of *cis* and *trans* double bonds. There is no free rotation around the C=C bond, and all four substituents of the double-bonded carbons are in the same plane. The double bonds in natural fatty acids are always in *cis* configuration. **B,** An unsaturated fatty acid in the lipid bilayer.

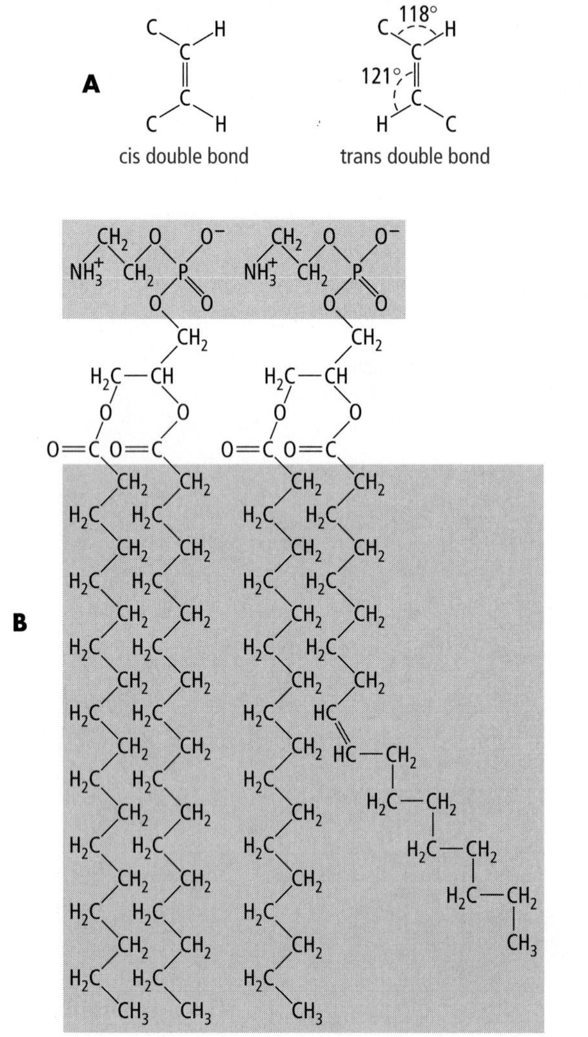

cis double bond   trans double bond

verse diffusion of the more polar membrane lipids, known as flip-flop, is essentially impossible in artificial lipid bilayers. It is observed occasionally in "real" membranes, where proteins can assist the flip-flopping lipids.

When a synthetic lipid bilayer that contains only one lipid (e.g., lecithin or sphingomyelin) is cooled, a phase transition can be observed at a well-defined temperature: the membrane "freezes." The lipids no longer move relative to each other, and their hydrophobic tails are aligned in parallel like a platoon of soldiers standing at attention.

In real membranes, which contain a mixture of many different lipids together with proteins, the phase transition is gradual. *At ordinary body temperature, membranes are in a more-or-less fluid state.* Their fluidity is determined by their lipid composition: long, saturated fatty acid chains in the membrane lipids make the membrane more rigid because they align themselves parallel to each other, forming multiple van der Waals interactions. Unsaturated fatty acids disturb this orderly array because their double bonds are in *cis* configuration (Fig. 11.8). The *cis* double bond introduces a kink in the hydrocarbon chain that destabilizes the regular parallel alignment of the hydrophobic tails. Therefore *a high content of unsaturated fatty acid residues in the membrane lipids makes the membrane more fluid.*

Cholesterol also is important for membrane fluidity. With its rigid ring system (Fig. 11.6), *it decreases the fluidity of most membranes.* It can, however, also insert itself between the fatty acid chains and prevent their crystallization. In this respect, cholesterol acts like an impurity that decreases the melting point of a chemical.

The lipid bilayer is important for the permeability properties of biological membranes

To penetrate a lipid bilayer, a substance has to pass from the aqueous solution through the region of the hydrophilic head groups, then across the hydrophobic core and out between the head groups on the opposite side. Figure 11.9 summarizes the permeability properties of lipid bilayers. Lipid-soluble molecules, blood gases (which are both small and nonpolar), and, to a limited extent, very small water-soluble molecules—including water itself—pene-

at speeds of approximately 1 μm/sec in artificial bilayers. Transverse diffusion, however, presents a problem: to switch from one leaflet of the bilayer to the other, the polar head group has to abandon its interactions with water molecules and neighboring head groups to dive across the hydrophobic core. This is energetically so unfavorable that *trans-*

FIG. 11.9

Permeability properties of a typical lipid bilayer.

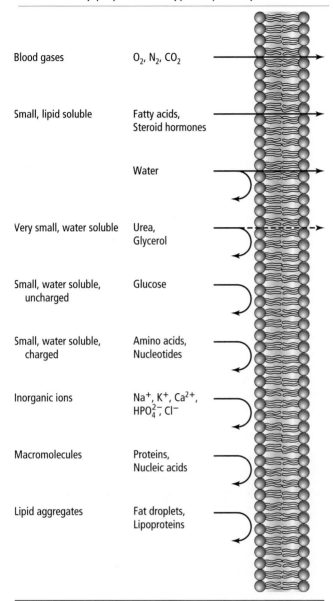

Blood gases	O_2, N_2, CO_2
Small, lipid soluble	Fatty acids, Steroid hormones
	Water
Very small, water soluble	Urea, Glycerol
Small, water soluble, uncharged	Glucose
Small, water soluble, charged	Amino acids, Nucleotides
Inorganic ions	Na^+, K^+, Ca^{2+}, HPO_4^{2-}, Cl^-
Macromolecules	Proteins, Nucleic acids
Lipid aggregates	Fat droplets, Lipoproteins

brane potentials. In real membranes, the resting membrane potential and the excitability properties are regulated by specific ion channels that are formed by membrane proteins.

Not only water-soluble molecules but also very insoluble ones experience problems penetrating biological membranes. Triglycerides, in particular, form droplets in aqueous environments that are jected by the hydrophilic head groups of the membrane lipids. This property is important for the intestinal absorption of triglycerides (see Chapter 14).

The permeability properties of biological membranes are important for the distribution of drugs in the body. Unlike physiologic metabolites, *most drugs are not transported by specific membrane carriers but have to rely on passive diffusion across the lipid bilayer.* Only lipid-soluble drugs are free to diffuse throughout the body, whereas most water-soluble drugs are not able to enter cells or to penetrate the blood-brain barrier. Many drugs possess ionizable groups. *These drugs can cross membranes only in the uncharged form.* Some very small lipophilic substances, however, can dissolve in the lipid bilayer, resulting in an increase of membrane fluidity. Inhalation anesthetics such as ether, chloroform, halothane, and possibly ethanol, are thought to act by this mechanism.

MEMBRANE PROTEINS AND SPECIALIZED MEMBRANE FUNCTIONS

The continuity of biological membranes, their flexibility, and their barrier function for water-soluble molecules can be explained by the properties of the lipid bilayer. However, membranes have many specific functions that depend on membrane proteins. These functions include:

- *Interactions with the cytoskeleton and the extracellular matrix.* These interactions are essential for the integrity of the cell and of the tissue as a whole.
- *Enzymatic activities.* Many important biochemical reactions are catalyzed by membrane-bound enzymes.
- *Regulated transport.* Many water-soluble nutrients, metabolic intermediates, and waste products have to be transported across membranes,

trate. Other water-soluble molecules, as well as macromolecules such as proteins and nucleic acids, are rejected. *Most of the important nutrients, metabolic intermediates, and coenzymes are water soluble and therefore cannot cross the lipid bilayer.* Lipid bilayers also are impermeable to such inorganic ions as sodium, potassium, and even protons. Therefore *the electrical conductivity of lipid bilayers is very low.* This property is a prerequisite for the maintenance of electrical mem-

although they cannot diffuse across a simple lipid bilayer.

- *Regulated permeability for inorganic ions.* This is the basis for the excitability properties of biological membranes.
- *Signal transduction.* Cells must be able to respond to hormones, neurotransmitters, and other extracellular signals, and these messages have to be relayed across the plasma membrane.

Most of the specialized membrane functions will be discussed in later chapters. In the following sections, we introduce the principles of protein-lipid interactions in biological membranes and the properties of carrier-mediated membrane transport.

Membranes contain integral and peripheral membrane proteins

Proteins account for 50% to 65% of the total mass in most membranes. *These proteins are globular proteins,* and most of them have a high content of α-helical structure. According to the **fluid-mosaic model** of membrane structure (Fig. 11.10), the membrane proteins associate with the lipid bilayer in different ways:

1. **Integral membrane proteins** are embedded in the lipid bilayer. In the most common type of integral membrane protein, the polypeptide traverses the lipid bilayer by means of a **transmembrane helix.** This is a stretch of α helix, approximately 25 amino acids long, that consists mostly of hydrophobic amino acid residues. *The nonpolar side chains of these amino acids interact with the membrane lipids, and the peptide bonds form hydrogen bonds with each other.* In the α helix, the rise per amino acid is approximately 0.15 nm (see Chapter 2), and therefore a 25-amino-acid helix measures approximately 3.75 nm, corresponding to the diameter of the hydrophobic core of the lipid bilayer (Fig. 11.7, B). Some integral membrane pro-

FIG. 11.10

The fluid-mosaic model of membrane structure. *1, 2, 3,* Integral membrane proteins traversing the lipid bilayer; *4,* protein anchored by a covalently bound lipid (myristyl, farnesyl, or geranylgeranyl); *5, 6,* peripheral membrane proteins bound to integral membrane proteins; *7,* peripheral membrane protein adsorbed to the head groups of membrane lipids; *8,* cytoskeletal protein attached to an integral membrane protein.

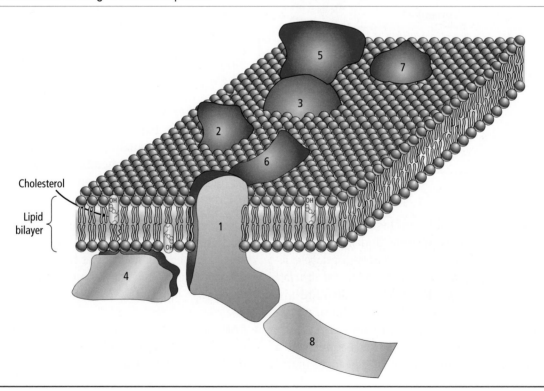

Cholesterol

Lipid bilayer

teins traverse the lipid bilayer only once; others criss-cross many times (Fig. 11.11). The solubilization of integral membrane proteins requires the use of mild nonionic detergents, which dissolve the lipid bilayer without denaturing the proteins.

2. **Peripheral membrane proteins** do not traverse the bilayer. They are attached to the membrane surface by noncovalent interactions with integral membrane proteins or the hydrophilic head groups of the membrane lipids. Experimentally, peripheral membrane proteins can be detached from the membrane by treatment with high salt concentrations or by pH changes.

Some proteins are attached to the membrane by covalently bound lipids (Fig. 11.12). On the outer surface of the plasma membrane, we find proteins that are covalently bound to phosphatidylinositol by means of an oligosaccharide chain. Trehalase on intestinal microvilli (see Chapter 14), alkaline phosphatase on osteoblasts (see Chapter 25), and carcinoembryonic antigen (a tumor marker) are attached to the membrane in this way. Other lipid tags are used by proteins on the inner surface of the plasma membrane or on organellar membranes: a myristic acid chain (saturated C-14 fatty acid) is attached by an amide bond to the N-terminal glycine of some proteins. Others have palmitic acid (saturated C-16 fatty acid) bound to the side chain of an internal serine, threonine, or cysteine residue. Also a farnesyl (C-15 isoprenoid) or geranylgeranyl (C-20 isoprenoid) group is sometimes present, bound to the

FIG. 11.11

Examples of membrane-spanning integral membrane proteins. The membrane-spanning segments are formed by nonpolar α helices. **A,** Glycophorin A, a major protein of the erythrocyte membrane. ◆ and ⬟, Carbohydrate; 0, nonpolar residues; c, charged residues. **B,** Band 3 protein, another major protein of the RBC membrane. The polypeptide consists of 929 amino acid residues and traverses the membrane approximately a dozen times. It is present in a dimeric form, functioning as an anion channel and as an attachment point for cytoskeletal proteins.

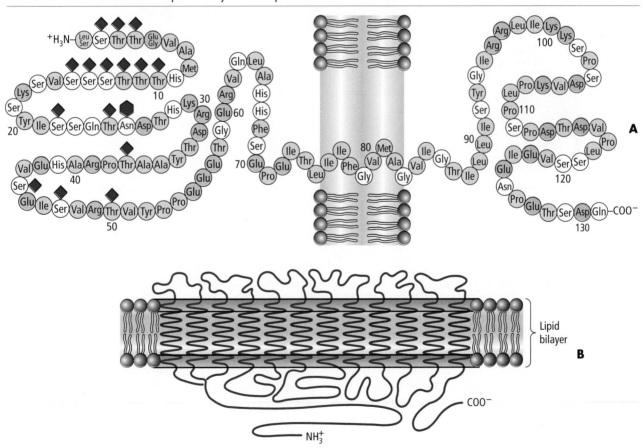

FIG. 11.12

Attachment of proteins to the plasma membrane by covalently bound lipids. *EA*, Ethanolamine; *Man*, D-mannose; *GlcNH₂*, non-acetylated glucosamine. The structure of the glycoinositol phospholipid anchor shown on the right varies somewhat in different membrane proteins.

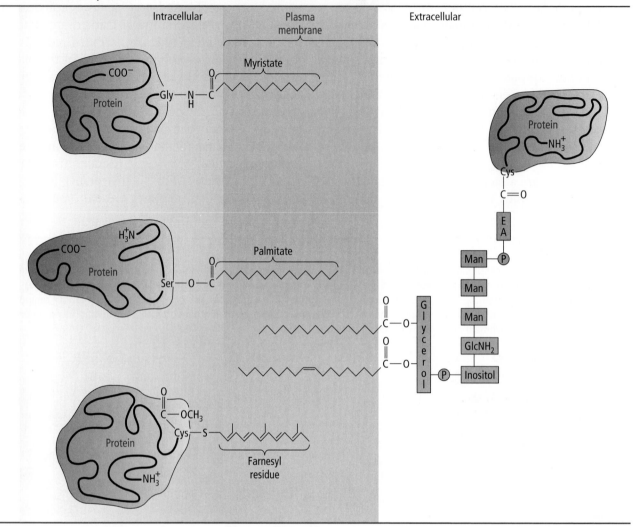

side chain of a methylated C-terminal cysteine residue.

Membranes are asymmetric

Although membrane proteins can, in principle, diffuse laterally in the plane of the membrane, lateral diffusion often is restricted by binding to other membrane proteins, cytoskeletal proteins, or proteins of the extracellular matrix. The transverse diffusion ("flip-flop") of membrane proteins has never been observed. This is not surprising because the water-exposed portions of the membrane proteins interact extensively with the surrounding water molecules. In erythrocytes, for example, the asymmetric orientation of the membrane proteins does not change during the 120-day lifespan of the cell.

Even membrane lipids flip-flop so rarely that their distribution in the membrane is asymmetric. The plasma membrane of most cells, for example, contains most of its phosphatidyl ethanolamine, phosphatidyl serine, and phosphoinositides in the cytoplasmic leaflet and most of its glycolipids, phosphatidyl choline, and sphingomyelin in the exoplasmic leaflet (Fig. 11.13).

FIG. 11.13

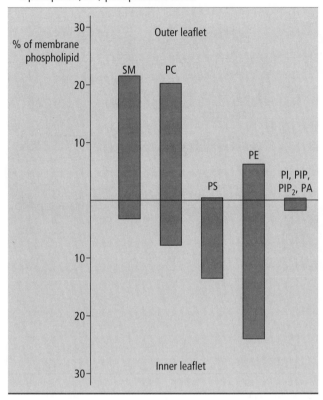

Distribution of phospholipids in the outer and inner leaflets of the erythrocyte membrane. *SM*, Sphingomyelin; *PC*, phosphatidylcholine; *PS*, phosphatidylserine; *PE*, phosphatidylethanolamine; *PI*, phosphatidylinositol; *PIP*, phosphatidylinositol 4-phosphate; *PIP₂*, phosphatidylinositol 4,5-isphosphate; *PA*, phosphatidic acid.

Cell surfaces have a fluffy carbohydrate coat

Unlike many intracellular membranes, *the plasma membrane has a high content of glycolipids and glycoproteins.* In essentially all cases, *these glycolipids and glycoproteins are oriented with their carbohydrate tails facing the extracellular space* (see Fig. 11.11, *A* for an example). These carbohydrate tails, which make up 3% to 10% of the total mass of the plasma membrane, surround the cell with a smooth hydrophilic coat, the **glycocalyx.**

The carbohydrate portions of membrane glycoproteins and glycolipids are constructed on their protein or lipid core by enzymes in the ER and Golgi (see Chapters 8 and 19). Being located in the lumen of these organelles, *the enzymes form the carbohydrates only on the lumenal surface.* When Golgi-derived vesicles fuse with the plasma membrane,

these carbohydrates are placed on the exoplasmic face (Fig. 11.14).

Membranes are sensitive to chemical and mechanical injury

Being noncovalent structures, biological membranes can be destroyed by even mild chemical or physical insults. Any agent that disrupts hydrophobic interactions is likely to damage the lipid bilayer. *Exposed membranes tolerate neither nonpolar organic solvents nor detergents.* Some commonly used disinfectants and antiseptics, including phenol, ethanol, and the cationic detergents, act in part by disrupting the membranes of microorganisms.

Mechanical insults by crystalline materials are injurious as well. In sickle cell disease, for example (see Chapter 9), precipitates of deoxyhemoglobin S are thought to damage the erythrocyte membrane. In patients with gouty arthritis, the lysosomal membrane in phagocytic cells suffers mechanical damage from the needle-sharp sodium urate crystals that these cells ingest. This leads to the death of the phagocytic cell and an inflammatory response (see Chapter 23). Also, *slow freezing is not tolerated by animal and human cells,* in part because of osmotic stress and in part because the relentlessly growing ice crystals damage the cellular membranes irreversibly.

Quick-freezing of dispersed cells or small tissue samples avoids the formation of large ice crystals, and structural membrane damage is minimized. In sperm banking, the samples are frozen quickly in the presence of 10% glycerol or some other antifreeze that further reduces the formation of large ice crystals. The preservation of viable human bodies by freezing, so popular with science-fiction writers, will not be possible anytime soon, because the large heat capacity of the body makes rapid freezing impossible.

Membrane carriers form channels across the lipid bilayer

Although most lipid-soluble substances can diffuse across biological membranes by **passive diffusion,** water-soluble substances require specific transport mechanisms. A few membranes, most notably the outer mitochondrial membrane, are riddled with pores that allow the nonselective passage of small,

FIG. 11.14

Placement of a glycoprotein in the plasma membrane. Note that the lumenal surface of the organelles corresponds to the exoplasmic face of the plasma membrane. Glycolipids are synthesized the same way, with their carbohydrate initially facing the lumen of the ER and Golgi.

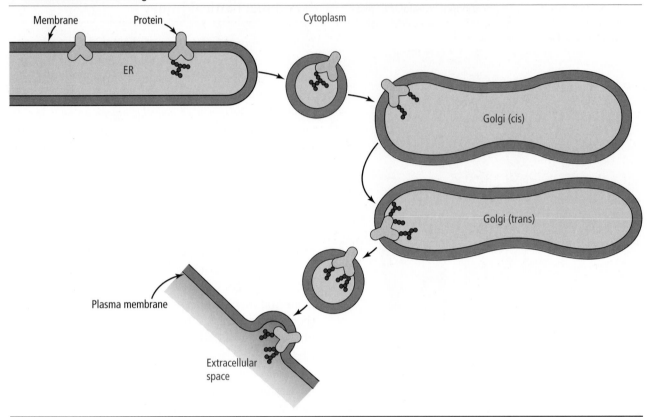

water-soluble molecules. In most membranes, however, *water-soluble molecules have to be transported by carrier-mediated transport* (Table 11.1). Carriers are membrane-spanning proteins or glycoproteins that form a **gated channel** across the lipid bilayer. Unlike a simple pore, *the gated channel has a specific binding site for the transported molecule*. The channel undergoes conformational changes that allow the substrate to bind on one side and to be released on the opposite side of the membrane (Fig. 11.15).

Facilitated diffusion is a type of carrier-mediated transport that does not use an external energy source. Therefore the net transport of the substrate is always down its electrochemical gradient. The uptake of glucose into erythrocytes is effected by facilitated diffusion (Fig. 11.15). Not only RBCs but also most other cells take up glucose by this cost-efficient mechanism. The transport of a single substrate by a membrane carrier, as in the facilitated diffusion of glucose, is called **uniport**.

Carrier-mediated transport is substrate specific and saturable, and it can be selectively inhibited

Carrier-mediated transport, even if it is passive, can be distinguished from simple diffusion by three important features:

1. *Substrate specificity.* Carrier-mediated transport requires the specific, noncovalent binding of the substrate to the carrier. This is similar to the formation of the enzyme-substrate complex in enzymatic reactions (see Chapter 4). Therefore, *transport depends on the proper fit between substrate and*

TABLE 11.1

Transport of small molecules and inorganic ions across biological membranes

Type of transport	Carrier required	Transport against gradient	Metabolic energy required	ATP hydrolysis	Example
Passive diffusion	−	−	−	−	Steroid hormones, many drugs
Facilitated diffusion	+	−	−	−	Glucose in RBCs and blood-brain barrier
Active transport	+	+	+	+	Na^+, K^+-ATPase, Ca^{2+}-ATPase
Secondary active transport	+	+	+	−	Sodium cotransport of glucose in kidney and intestine

FIG. 11.15

Facilitated diffusion of glucose across the erythrocyte membrane. There is no external energy source, so the net transport is down the concentration gradient. Actually, all steps in this cycle are reversible, and a net transport of glucose into the cell takes place only because glucose is consumed in the cell, thereby maintaining a concentration gradient.

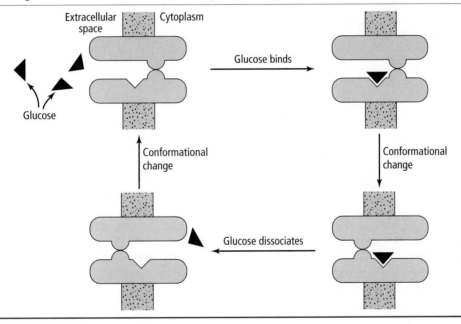

carrier. The glucose transporter in RBCs, for example, transports D-glucose but not L-glucose, and it has markedly reduced affinities for other hexoses such as D-mannose and D-galactose.

2. *Saturability.* The rate of passive diffusion is directly proportional to the concentration gradient, but *carrier-mediated transport shows the same saturation kinetics as enzymatic reactions* (Fig. 11.16). The V_{max} of carrier-mediated transport is directly proportional to the number of carriers in the membrane.

3. *Specific inhibition and physiologic regulation.* Like enzymes, membrane carriers can be specifically inhibited. Glucose transport into erythrocytes, for example, is competitively inhibited by various glucose analogs. Carrier-mediated transport also can be a rate-limiting and regulated step in meta-

FIG. 11.16

Saturability of carrier-mediated transport. We assume that the substrate moves from a compartment with variable concentration (concentration on the x axis) to a compartment where its concentration is zero. This corresponds to the assumption of negligible product concentration in Michaelis-Menten kinetics (see Chapter 4). Compare this graph with Fig. 4.6 (Chapter 4). On the other hand, in carrier-independent passive diffusion, the rate of transport is directly proportional to the concentration gradient.

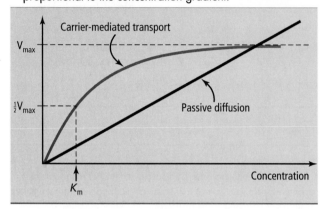

1

$$\Delta G = R \times T \times \ln \frac{c_2}{c_1}$$
$$= 2.303 \times R \times T \times \lg \frac{c_2}{c_1}$$

where R is the gas constant

$$\left(1.987 \times 10^{-3} \frac{kcal}{mol \times K}\right)$$

and T is the absolute temperature. We now can calculate the energy required to pump 1 mol of an uncharged molecule against a tenfold concentration gradient

$$\left(\frac{c_2}{c_1} = 10\right)$$

at 25°C (298 K):

$$\Delta G = 2.303 \times 1.987 \times 10^{-3} \frac{kcal}{mol \times K}$$
$$\times 298\ K \times \lg 10$$
$$= +1.36\ kcal/mol$$

If an ion is transported from a compartment with the concentration c1 to a compartment with the concentration c2, the energy requirement is determined not only by the concentration gradient but also by the interaction of the ion's charge with the membrane potential:

2

$$\Delta G = [2.303 \times R \times T \times \lg \frac{c_2}{c_1}]$$
$$+ [Z \times F \times \Delta V]$$

where Z is the charge of the ion, F is the Faraday constant

$$\left(23.062 \frac{kcal}{V \times mol}\right),$$

and ΔV is the membrane potential in volts.

Substituting the values of Fig. 11.17 into equation 2, we can, for example, calculate the energy required to pump a sodium ion out of the cell:

bolic pathways. Although, for example, glucose uptake by RBCs is not regulated, the facilitated diffusion of glucose into adipose tissue and muscle is stimulated by insulin. Insulin increases the V_{max} of glucose transport into these tissues by increasing the number of glucose carriers in the plasma membrane.

Transport up an electrochemical gradient requires metabolic energy

The cost-conscious mechanism of facilitated diffusion is sufficient for the transport of many substrates. In other cases, however, the cell has to accumulate a molecule or ion actively against a concentration gradient or electrochemical gradient. This type of transport, known as **active transport,** requires metabolic energy.

Like chemical reactions, *membrane transport is driven by the free energy change ΔG (see Chapter 4, Equation 5). Fortunately the situation is less complex because there is no enthalpy change ($\Delta H = 0$), and the process is purely entropy driven.* For an uncharged molecule, the driving force ΔG for the transfer of a molecule from a compartment with the concentration c_1 to a compartment with the concentration c_2 is given by the equation

FIG. 11.17

Typical ion distributions across the plasma membrane. All concentrations are in mM (mmol/liter). ΔV, Membrane potential.

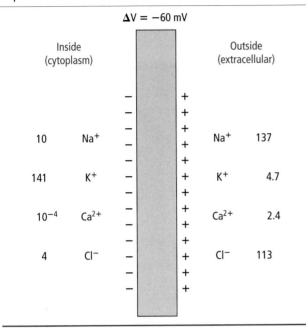

$$\Delta V = -60 \text{ mV}$$

Inside (cytoplasm) / Outside (extracellular)

Inside			Outside	
10	Na$^+$		Na$^+$	137
141	K$^+$		K$^+$	4.7
10^{-4}	Ca^{2+}		Ca^{2+}	2.4
4	Cl$^-$		Cl$^-$	113

$$\Delta G = 2.303 \times 1.987 \times 10^{-3} \frac{\text{kcal}}{\text{mol} \times \text{K}}$$

$$\times\ 298\ \text{K} \times \lg \frac{137}{10}$$

$$+\ 1 \times 23.062 \frac{\text{kcal}}{\text{V} \times \text{mol}} \times 0.06\ \text{V}$$

$$=\ 1.545 \frac{\text{kcal}}{\text{mol}} + 1.384 \frac{\text{kcal}}{\text{mol}}$$

$$=\ +2.929\ \text{kcal/mol}$$

Equation 2 defines the **electrochemical gradient** for ions. The electrochemical gradient is large for such ions as Na$^+$ and Ca^{2+}, for which the two components of equation 2 have the same sign, and small for such ions as K$^+$ and Cl$^-$ where they have opposite signs. The pumping of ions against their electrochemical gradient requires metabolic energy, which is supplied by the hydrolysis of ATP, either directly or indirectly.

The sodium-potassium ATPase is an ATP-driven membrane pump

The classical example for an ATP-driven membrane pump is the **sodium-potassium ATPase**. *This pump is located in the plasma membrane of all cells,* with highest activity in nervous tissue and muscle. It maintains the normal gradients of sodium and potassium across the plasma membrane by pumping sodium out of the cell and potassium into the cell.

The Na$^+$,K$^+$-ATPase is a tetrameric glycoprotein with two α subunits (molecular weight [MW] 112,000) and two β subunits (MW 55,000). Both subunits span the membrane several times, and the two α subunits are thought to form the gated channel. This channel has binding sites for sodium and potassium. A tentative model for the functioning of the pump is shown in Fig. 11.18. In this model, the phosphorylation of an aspartate side chain in one of the α subunits stabilizes an "outside-open" conformation that has a high affinity for K$^+$. Its dephosphorylation stabilizes an "inside-open" conformation with a high Na$^+$ affinity. During each transport cycle, three Na$^+$ are transported out of the cell, two K$^+$ are transported into the cell, and one ATP is consumed. Because of the net transport of an electrical charge, this transport is called **electrogenic**.

Although ATP hydrolysis and ion transport are tightly coupled, *the sodium-potassium ATPase is a major consumer of metabolic energy,* accounting for perhaps 20% or 25% of the basal metabolic rate. The brain allots at least half of its energy to sodium-potassium pumping.

Protons and calcium also are often transported by ATP-driven membrane pumps. The sarcoplasmic reticulum of muscle fibers and the plasma membrane of most cells contain a **Ca^{2+}-ATPase** that pumps calcium out of the cytoplasm. It constitutes approximately 80% of the total membrane protein in the sarcoplasmic reticulum of skeletal muscle and consumes close to 10% of the total metabolic energy in resting muscle. Like the Na$^+$,K$^+$-ATPase, the Ca^{2+}-ATPase is phosphorylated reversibly during the transport cycle.

Sodium cotransport is used for the cellular uptake of many molecules

The coupled transport of two different substrates by the same carrier is called **cotransport**. If, as in the case of the Na$^+$,K$^+$-ATPase, the two substrates are transported in opposite directions, the mechanism is called **antiport**; if they are transported in the same direction, it is called **symport**. Antiports that are not coupled to ATP hydrolysis occur, for example, in the inner mitochondrial membrane, where they exchange metabolites between the intermembranous space and the mitochondrial matrix (see Chapter 16).

The best-known example for symport is **sodium cotransport**, which often is used for the cellular uptake of small molecules. In the intestinal mucosa,

FIG. 11.18

A model for the functioning of the Na$^+$,K$^+$-ATPase.

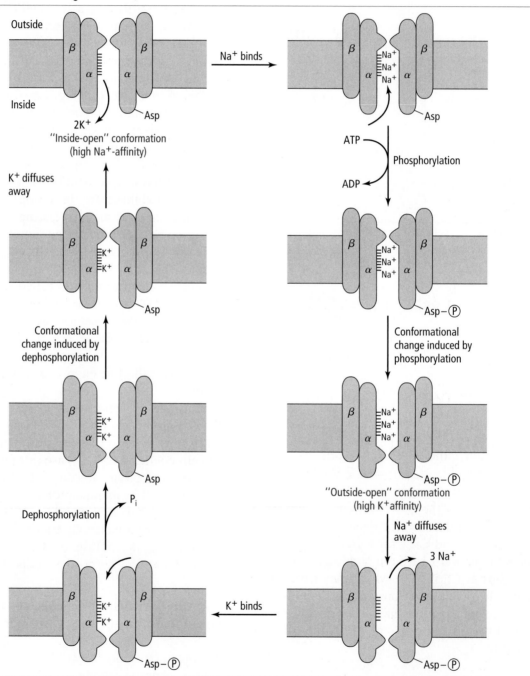

for example, glucose and amino acids are absorbed into the cell by sodium cotransport (Fig. 11.19). The same type of transport is used in the proximal renal tubules for the reabsorption of glucose and amino acids from the primary filtrate. Indeed, kidney and intestine often use the same sodium cotransporter, and therefore many transport defects are expressed in both organs (see Chapter 21).

FIG. 11.19

Absorption of glucose in the brush border of the small intestine. The apical (lumenal) membrane and the basolateral (serosal) membrane of the epithelial cells are physiologically different. The tight junctions between adjacent cells prevent not only the diffusion of solutes around the cells but also the lateral diffusion of membrane proteins. Therefore different sets of carriers are present in the two parts of the plasma membrane.

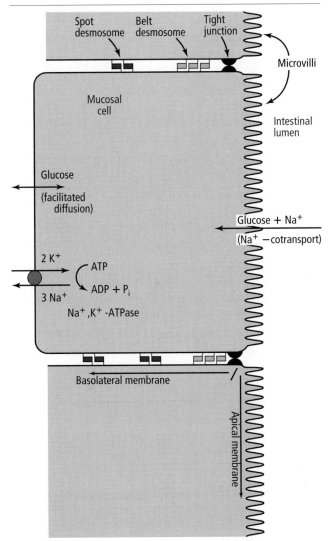

Sodium cotransport can accumulate a substrate against a concentration gradient because the substrate is transported only together with a sodium ion, and the transport of the sodium ion into the cell is down a steep electrochemical gradient (see Fig. 11.17). *Although the carrier does not hydrolyze ATP, sodium cotransport consumes energy by dissipating the actively maintained sodium gradient.* This type of transport, which depends on the continued activity of the sodium-potassium ATPase, is characterized as **secondary active transport**.

The sodium-potassium ATPase is inhibited by cardiotonic steroids

Steroidal glycosides from the plant *Digitalis purpurea* L. are a time-honored treatment for congestive heart failure. *They increase the force of myocardial contraction by blocking the Na^+,K^+-ATPase.* The force of contraction depends directly on the calcium concentration in the cytoplasm, where the contractile elements are located. The cardiotonic steroids increase the cytoplasmic Ca^{2+} concentration because the major mechanism for the removal of Ca^{2+} out of the myocardial cell is a Ca^{2+}/Na^+ antiporter in the plasma membrane (Fig. 11.20). *This antiporter depends on a sodium gradient for effective calcium transport.* With

FIG. 11.20

Regulation of the intracellular calcium concentration in myocardial cells. Cardiotonic steroids (digitalis) reduce the sodium gradient and therefore the effectiveness of the Ca^{2+}/Na^+ antiporter in the plasma membrane.

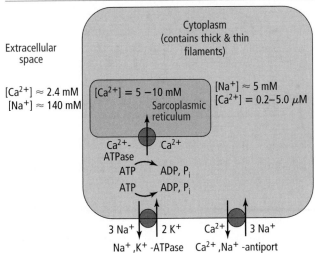

decreased activity of the Na^+,K^+-ATPase, the sodium gradient diminishes, and more calcium remains in the cytoplasm. This provides more Ca^{2+} for uptake into the sarcoplasmic reticulum by the Ca^{2+}-ATPase. The sarcoplasmic Ca^{2+}, in turn, is released during contraction in response to membrane depolarization. *Cardiotonic steroids are very toxic*, and overdosage results in fatal arrhythmias because a near-normal Na^+ gradient is required for the normal excitability of the myocardial cells and the conducting system.

Zachowski A: Phospholipids in animal eukaryotic membranes: transverse asymmetry and movement. *Biochem J* 294, 1-14, 1993.

SUMMARY

Biological membranes are a universal element of cell structure. They are diffusion barriers and sites of specific, regulated transport. All biological membranes consist of lipids and proteins. The membrane lipids include the phosphoglycerides, sphingolipids, and cholesterol. These lipids are amphipathic, with hydrophilic and hydrophobic parts combined in the same molecule. In the form of a lipid bilayer, they form the structural backbone of all biological membranes. Integral membrane proteins are embedded in the lipid bilayer, whereas peripheral membrane proteins are attached to its surface. Most integral membrane proteins traverse the lipid bilayer in the form of a transmembrane α-helix.

The lipid bilayer is responsible for the barrier function of the membrane, particularly its impermeability to hydrophilic solutes. Membrane proteins are in charge of specialized functions. Membrane proteins can act as enzymes, as structural links between the cytoskeleton and the extracellular matrix, as components of signaling pathways, and as carriers that transport hydrophilic substrates across the membrane. Some types of carrier-mediated transport are passive; others are driven by the hydrolysis of ATP, either directly or indirectly.

Further Reading

Hanin I, Pepeu G, editors: *Phospholipids*. Plenum Press, New York, 1990.

Kuroki Y, Voelker DR: Pulmonary surfactant proteins. *J Biol Chem* 269 (42), 25943-25946, 1994.

QUESTIONS

1. An almost ubiquitous structural feature of *integral* membrane proteins is
   A. Several segments of antiparallel β-pleated sheet structure.
   B. A covalent bond with a fatty acid residue in a phosphoglyceride.
   C. An extended fibrous structure that forms multiple salt bonds with the head groups of membrane phospholipids.
   D. Several amphipathic α helices.
   E. At least one nonpolar membrane-crossing α helix.

2. Which is true concerning the prevalence of lipids in biological membranes?
   A. Triglycerides and phosphoglycerides are the most abundant lipids in most membranes.
   B. Most membrane sphingolipids are phospholipids.
   C. Cholesterol is common in the nuclear and inner mitochondrial membranes but not in the plasma membrane of most cells.
   D. The glycolipids of the plasma membrane are found in the outer leaflet of the bilayer.
   E. Membranes in the brain have a high phosphoglyceride content but only very small amounts of sphingolipids.

3. The transport of glucose across the capillary endothelium of cerebral blood vessels ("blood-brain barrier") is effected by facilitated diffusion. This means that
   A. Specific inhibition of cerebral glucose uptake is not possible.
   B. The cerebral glucose uptake is always directly proportional to the concentration gradient for glucose across the endothelium.
   C. The inhibition of ATP synthesis in the endothelial cells will prevent glucose uptake into the brain.

D. As long as glucose is only consumed but not produced in the brain, the cerebrospinal fluid glucose concentration is always less than the blood glucose concentration.

E. There is no upper limit to the amount of glucose that can be taken up by the brain.

4. Many properties of biological membranes depend on the structure of the lipid bilayer. Typical features of lipid bilayers include

A. Impermeability for small inorganic ions such as sodium and protons

B. Rapid exchange of phospholipids between the two leaflets of the bilayer

C. High electrical conductivity

D. Lack of lateral mobility of membrane lipids at normal body temperature

E. Permeability for proteins

Chapter 12

The Cytoskeleton

Membranes are suitable as diffusion barriers, but they lack mechanical strength. They cannot maintain the shape of the cell or make it resistant to external forces. Mechanical strength requires intracellular fibers that are collectively known as the **cytoskeleton.** The most important cytoskeletal elements are:

1. The **membrane skeleton** is a fibrous meshwork that reinforces the plasma membrane. It is linked to integral membrane proteins.
2. **Microfilaments,** with a diameter of approximately 7 nm, consist mainly of the protein actin. They are important for the physical consistency of the cytoplasm and for cell motility.
3. **Intermediate filaments** are somewhat thicker than the microfilaments (8–12 nm). They provide mechanical support for the cell.
4. **Microtubules** are polymers of the protein tubulin. With a diameter of 24 nm, they are the thickest and strongest elements of the cytoskeleton. They are important for the maintenance of cell shape, for intracellular transport processes, and as the structural backbone of cilia and flagella.

The erythrocyte membrane is reinforced by a spectrin network

During their 120-day lifespan, erythrocytes travel approximately 300 miles, part of this through tortuous capillary channels where they are exposed to mechanical insults. Under these conditions, the cells can maintain their structural integrity, charac-teristic shape, and resilience only because *they possess a meshwork of long, thin fibers right under their plasma membrane.*

These fibers are formed from two long polypep-tides, **α-spectrin** and **β-spectrin.** The most impor-tant structural motif in these polypeptides is the **spectrin repeat,** a sequence of 106 amino acids that is repeated (with variations) 20 times in the α chain and 17 times in the β chain. Each of these repeats consists of three α-helical segments that form a coiled-coil structure (Fig. 12.1).

Spectrin forms an antiparallel dimer, with an α chain and a β chain lying side by side. These α-β dimers condense head to head to form a tetramer — a long, flexible, wormlike molecule with a contour length of 200 nm and a diameter of 5 nm. The ends of the spectrin tetramer are noncovalently bound to short (35-nm) actin filaments. This interaction is facilitated by two other proteins, **band 4.1 protein** (so named after its migration in gel electrophoresis) and **adducin.** By binding several spectrin tetramers, *the actin filaments form the nodes of a two-dimensional net-work* that can be likened to a fishing net or a piece of very thin, flexible chicken wire (Fig. 12.2, B).

The spectrin network is attached to the mem-brane by the peripheral membrane protein **ankyrin,** which is itself bound to the integral membrane pro-tein **band 3 protein.** This binding is stabilized by **band 4.2 protein** (pallidin). The actin microfila-ments interact with the membrane through band 4.1 protein, which binds weakly to the integral mem-brane proteins **glycophorin A and C,** and to the head groups of phosphatidyl serine.

FIG. 12.1

Structure of a spectrin dimer. The spectrin repeat consists of three α-helical coiled coils with a total of 106 amino acid residues.

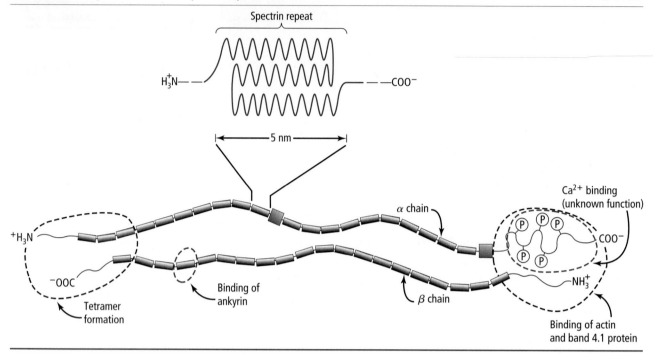

Defects of the erythrocyte membrane skeleton cause hemolytic diseases

Hereditary spherocytosis (HS) is the most common type of inherited hemolytic anemia in northwestern Europe, with a prevalence of approximately 1 in 5000. The disease is marked by an abundance of *small erythrocytes with a round rather than biconcave disc-like shape.* These abnormal cells are fragile, and they rupture easily during their passage through the splenic cords. HS is a heterogeneous group of disorders with various clinical severities, inherited as an autosomal dominant trait in approximately 75% of cases. Different components of the membrane skeleton, including spectrin and ankyrin, are defunct in different patients. A reduced amount of spectrin is a general finding, probably because any spectrin that is not tightly bound in the membrane skeleton falls prey to proteolytic enzymes during RBC maturation. The severity of the disease is proportional to the spectrin deficiency. Causal treatments are not possible at present, but splenectomy cures the anemia in most patients.

Hereditary elliptocytosis (HE) is a related group of inherited diseases in which the erythrocytes are ellipsoidal rather than spherical. Like HS, HE is a heterogeneous group of disorders. The mode of inheritance and clinical expression are variable, and several molecular defects of the membrane skeleton have been described in different patients. These include abnormalities in the structure of spectrin, protein 4.1, protein 4.2, and ankyrin.

Dystrophin forms a membrane skeleton in muscle fibers

The membrane skeletons of cells other than erythrocytes are not known in molecular detail. There are at least two different genes for spectrin α chains and five for spectrin β chains, and spectrin seems to be present in most nucleated cells. Different variants of a protein with distinct tissue distributions are called **isoforms.** In the case of spectrin, the different isoforms are encoded by different genes, but in some other cases they are produced by the alternative splicing of a single transcript.

Dystrophin is a distant relative of spectrin; it is found in skeletal, cardiac, and smooth muscle, and to a lesser extent in the brain. It is a very large protein, with 3685 amino acids in the polypeptide. Besides an

FIG. 12.2

Hypothetical model of the membrane skeleton in RBCs. **A,** In transverse section. **B,** In tangential section.

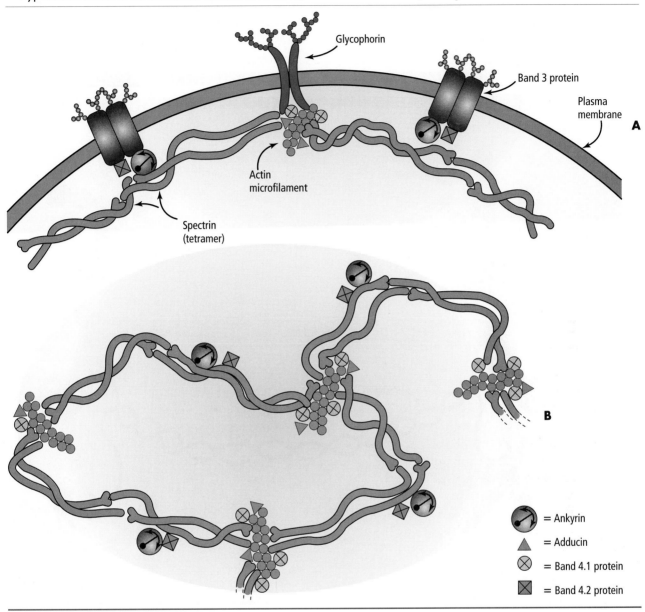

Glycophorin

Band 3 protein

Plasma membrane

A

Actin microfilament

Spectrin (tetramer)

B

= Ankyrin

= Adducin

= Band 4.1 protein

= Band 4.2 protein

actin-binding domain and 24 spectrin repeats, it has a calcium-binding domain and a unique carboxy terminus that is required for membrane attachment (Fig. 12.3). Like spectrin, dystrophin is thought to form antiparallel dimers. *Dystrophin is bound to a complex of membrane proteins, and these membrane proteins, in turn, are bound to extracellular matrix proteins.* These matrix proteins include the ubiquitous laminins of the basement membrane.

Duchenne muscular dystrophy is caused by the absence of dystrophin

Dystrophin constitutes only 0.002% of the total muscle protein in humans, but its absence is the cause of Duchenne muscular dystrophy (DMD), the most common (1 in every 3500 males) and most deadly form of inherited muscle disease. This X-linked recessive disease causes progressive muscle

FIG. 12.3

Structure of dystrophin, the major component of the membrane skeleton in muscle fibers. **A,** The domain structure of dystrophin. ▭, Actin-binding domain; ▬, calcium-binding domain; ▨, membrane attachment; ▪, spectrin repeat. Dystrophin is thought to form an antiparallel dimer. **B,** The dystrophin-associated proteins in the sarcolemma. These proteins link the cytoskeleton to the extracellular matrix. α-D, α-Dystroglycan; β-D, β-dystroglycan; *Sar*, sarcoglycan complex; *Syn*, syntrophin; A0, A0 protein.

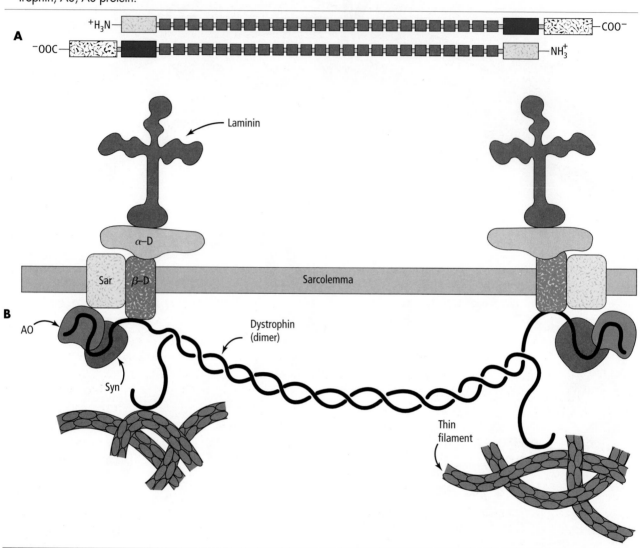

weakness and muscle wasting, which starts at 1 or 2 years of age and progresses relentlessly until the patient dies of heart failure or weakness of the respiratory muscles, usually at approximately 20 years of age.

Most patients with DMD have deletions that eliminate large portions of the dystrophin gene. The mutation rate is very high, and approximately one third of the patients did not inherit the defective gene but have a new mutation. This high mutation rate is not altogether surprising because *the dystrophin gene is the largest gene ever identified in humans.* With its 79 exons, the gene straddles 2.5 million base pairs of DNA!

Dystrophin is thought to stabilize the sarcolemma during the deformations that accompany muscle contraction. Also, unlike the RBC, the muscle fiber is surrounded by an extracellular matrix, and *interactions between the cytoskeleton and the extracellular matrix proteins are important for the structural integrity of the tissue.*

There is no effective treatment for DMD, but the

FIG. 12.4

Structure of keratin, the major intermediate filament protein of epithelial tissues. **A,** The domain structure of a single polypeptide (type I keratin). The central, mostly α-helical part consists of approximately 310 amino acids. **B,** A parallel heterodimer formed from a type I and a type II keratin polypeptide.

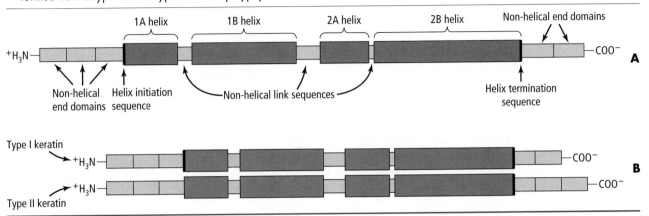

disease is a prime candidate for gene therapy (see Chapter 10). Gene therapy is facilitated by the multinucleated nature of muscle fibers—the fiber may be saved if only one of its many nuclei acquires the foreign gene—and by the fact that a tight regulation of dystrophin expression does not seem to be required. However, the large size of the gene makes the construction of vectors difficult, and the commonly used retroviral vectors require dividing cells and therefore are not particularly good at transfecting muscle fibers.

The keratins are the most important structural proteins of epithelial tissues

The **intermediate filaments** are structural elements in the cytoplasm of most cells. All intermediate filament proteins have the same general structure, with a central α-helical portion that is interrupted by short, nonhelical linker sequences. This portion is framed by end domains that are thought to aid in fiber formation (Fig. 12.4, *A*).

The most conspicuous intermediate filament proteins are the **keratins,** which form the horny layer of the skin as well as such skin appendages as hair and fingernails. There are two different types of keratin, the acidic (type I) and the basic (type II) keratins. Approximately 15 different variants of each exist. *They form obligatory heterodimers, with a type I polypeptide always arranged in parallel with a type II polypeptide* (Fig. 12.4, *B*). The heterodimer is a **coiled-coil,** with the two α-helical polypeptides wound around each other. The contacts between the two α helices are formed by hydrophobic amino acid side chains on one edge of each helix. Cross-sections show that the keratin fibril contains between 12 and 24 of these heterodimers, probably in a staggered array.

The two-stranded coiled-coil structure is not unique to the keratins but occurs in many other proteins as well, including myosin (see Fig. 12.8), tropomyosin (see Fig. 12.7), and the dimerization domains of many DNA-binding proteins (see Chapter 8). Spectrin (see Fig. 12.1) and the long arm of laminin (see Fig. 13.15, Chapter 13), however, contain not a two-stranded but rather a three-stranded α-helical coiled coil.

Different keratins are expressed in different cell types. In the basal layer of the epidermis, for example, K14 is the major type I keratin and K5 is the major type II keratin. In the more mature cells of the spinous and granular layers, keratins K10 and K1 are the major type I and type II keratins, respectively (Fig. 12.5). Single-layered epithelia express keratins 18, 19, and/or 20 (type I) and keratins 7 and 8 (type II), and various other keratin pairs are expressed in hair and nails.

Many types of intermediate filament proteins other than the keratins are expressed in various cell types (Table 12.1). *All of them are dynamic structures that can be assembled and disassembled rapidly.* In many cases, the phosphorylation of intermediate filament proteins by various protein kinases causes disassembly

TABLE 12.1

The major types of intermediate filament proteins*

Protein	Tissue or cell type
Keratin	Epithelial cells, hair, nails
Vimentin	Embryonic tissues, mesenchymal cells, most cultured cells
Desmin	Muscle tissue, at Z disk in skeletal muscle
Glial fibrillary acidic protein	Astrocytes, Schwann cells
Peripherin	Neurons of the peripheral nervous system (PNS)
α-Internexin	Neurons of the central nervous system (CNS)
Neurofilament proteins (NF-L, NF-M, NF-H)	Neurons of CNS and PNS
Lamin	Nucleus in all nucleated cells, under the nuclear membrane. This is the only noncytoplasmic intermediate filament protein.

* All of these proteins have the general structure depicted in Fig. 12.4, A for keratin.

FIG. 12.5

The layers of human skin. The epidermal cells are held together by numerous spot desmosomes. These spot desmosomes are attachment points for the intracellular keratin filaments.

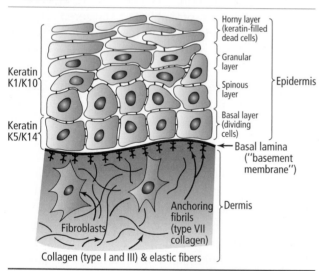

of the filaments; their dephosphorylation by specific protein phosphatases causes filament formation.

Abnormalities of keratin structure cause skin diseases

Epidermolysis bullosa (EB) is a group of inherited skin diseases in which even mild mechanical stress causes damage at the dermis-epidermis junction, with painful blistering. Approximately 1 in 5000 individuals has some form of EB. In most cases the disease is inherited as an autosomal dominant trait.

In some patients with EB, the molecular defect has been traced to point mutations in the genes of either keratin K14 or keratin K5. Various point mutations at the ends of the central helical domains (helix initiation and termination sequences in Fig. 12.4, A), in particular, have been found in different affected families.

The clinical presentation of EB can be explained by the expression patterns of K5 and K14: only the basal cells of the epidermis form these polypeptides. Therefore *shear forces easily destroy the basal cell layer while the overlying cells are left intact.* The base of the epidermis fills with extracellular fluid, and a blister forms.

Point mutations in the genes for K1 and K10, the major keratins of the spinous and granular cell layers, have been identified as causes of **epidermolytic hyperkeratosis,** a dominantly inherited type of skin disease with scaling, hyperkeratosis, and blistering.

Striated muscle contains thick and thin filaments

We already have encountered actin microfilaments as anchoring points for proteins of the membrane skeleton (Figs. 12.2 and 12.3). In muscle tissue, they are essential elements of the contractile apparatus, together with the thicker myosin filaments.

The skeletal muscle fiber, with a typical diameter of 20 to 50 μm and a length of 1 to 40 mm, is divided functionally into **myofibrils,** which run lengthwise along the muscle fiber (Fig. 12.6, A). The myofibrils are cylindrical in shape, approximately 0.6 μm in diameter, and surrounded by cisternae of the sarcoplasmic reticulum. They are organized into **sarcomeres** by transverse partitions known as **Z disks.** Invaginations of the plasma membrane form the **T-tubules** (T for transverse), which reach each sarcomere at the level of the Z disk. The T-tubules are in close apposition to the cisternae of the sarcoplasmic reticulum, which in turn envelop the sides of the sarcomere.

Attached to the Z disk are the **thin filaments** (7 nm in diameter), which consist of the protein **actin** together with **tropomyosin** and **troponin.** Suspended in the center of the sarcomere are the thick filaments (16 nm in diameter) that are formed by the protein **myosin.** Thick and thin filaments overlap considerably. Based on the light microscopic appearance, the area near the Z disk that contains only thin filaments is called the I band (I for isotropic), and the area of the thick filaments is called the A band (A for anisotropic). In the center of the A band is the somewhat lighter H zone, which contains only thick filaments (Fig. 12.6, B and C).

The length of the filaments does not change during contraction, but the thick and thin filaments slide along each other until the ends of the thin filaments touch or almost touch each other in the center of the sarcomere. The H band and the I zone shrink, and the sarcomere shortens to approximately 70% of its original length.

Actin is a globular protein that polymerizes into a fibrous structure

Actin, the major protein of the thin filaments, consists of globular subunits called **G-actin** (MW 42,000). Under conditions of physiologic ionic strength and magnesium concentration, *these globular units polymerize head to tail* to form a fibrous structure called **F-actin.** The resulting microfilament consists of two strands of F-actin coiled around each other (Fig. 12.7, A).

Actin microfilaments also contain troponin and tropomyosin. Tropomyosin is a long, thin, coiled-coil of two α-helical polypeptides with a length of 40 nm. These tropomyosin molecules spiral along the microfilament near the groove between the two actin strands. Troponin consists of the three subunits Tn-T (tropomyosin binding), Tn-I (inhibitory, actin binding), and Tn-C (calcium binding). This heterotrimeric complex is spaced at regular intervals of 38.5 nm along the thin filament, corresponding to the length of the spiraling tropomyosin dimer. *Troponin is a regulatory protein that makes the thin filament sensitive to calcium.*

Myosin is a two-headed molecule with ATPase activity

Myosin, which forms the thick filaments, consists of one pair of heavy chains (MW 230,000 each) and two pairs of nonidentical light chains (MW 16,000 and 20,000). The carboxy-terminal 60% of the two heavy chains forms an α-helical coiled-coil with a length of 130 nm and a diameter of 2 nm. It is interrupted by a hinge region that acts as a joint, allowing the molecule to bend at different angles. The amino-terminal ends of the two heavy chains form two globular heads, and each of these heads is associated with two nonidentical light chains (Fig. 12.8, A).

The myosin heads possess an ATPase activity, but this activity is minimal in the absence of actin. Although ATP is hydrolyzed quickly, ADP and inorganic phosphate remain tightly bound to the catalytic site and prevent the access of further ATP molecules. The myosin heads can interact with actin, too, and in the presence of pure actin filaments the ATPase activity of the myosin heads is stimulated 200-fold. *The myosin heads interact with the actin of the thin filament and hydrolyze ATP during contraction while the fibrous tails bundle the molecules together in the thick filament.* Approximately 300 to 400 myosin molecules aggregate laterally in the thick filament, with their globular heads protruding on all sides. In the middle of the filament the molecules are bundled tail to tail; therefore this central portion has no heads (Fig. 12.8, B).

Calcium and ATP are required for muscle contraction

The myosin heads of the thick filament have to bind the actin of the thin filament during muscle con-

FIG. 12.6

Structure of the skeletal muscle fiber. **A,** Section through a muscle fiber. The fiber has a diameter of 20 to 50 μm and is surrounded by the plasma membrane (sarcolemma). Its nuclei (*N*, up to 100 per fiber) are located peripherally, and the mitochondria are interspersed between the myofibrils. More than 100 myofibrils (0.6 to 1.0 μm diameter) run the length of the muscle fiber. **B,** The sarcomere structure of the myofibril in the relaxed state. **C,** The sarcomere in the contracted state. **D,** A cross section through the overlap zone of thick and thin filaments: the filaments are neatly packed, with each thick filament surrounded by six thin filaments and each thin filament surrounded by three thick filaments.

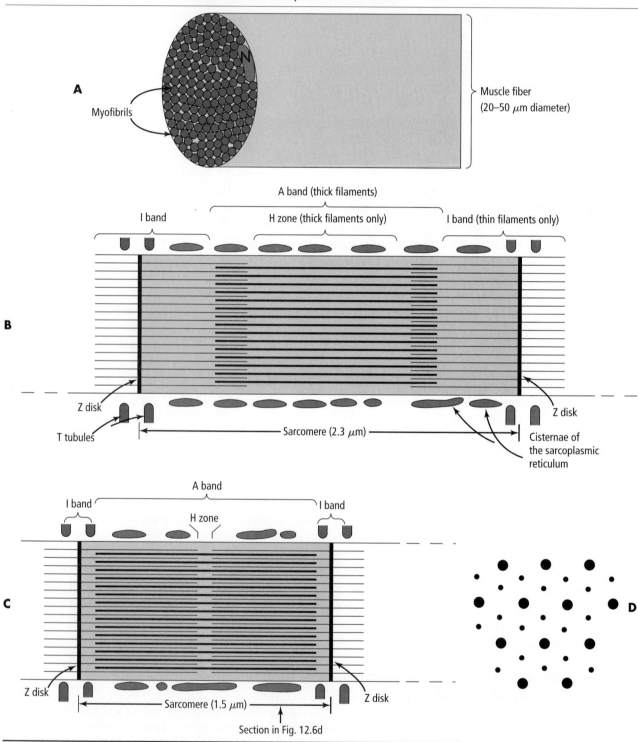

FIG. 12.7

The thin filaments of skeletal muscle. **A,** A simplified model of thin filament structure. The troponin complex (*TN-C, TN-I,* and *TN-T*) binds to a specific site on the dimeric tropomyosin (*TM*) molecule. **B,** The position of tropomyosin (*T*) in the relaxed state (low [Ca^{2+}]) and the contracted state high ([Ca^{2+}]). When tropomyosin moves into the groove between the actin monomers, the myosin-binding sites on actin become exposed.

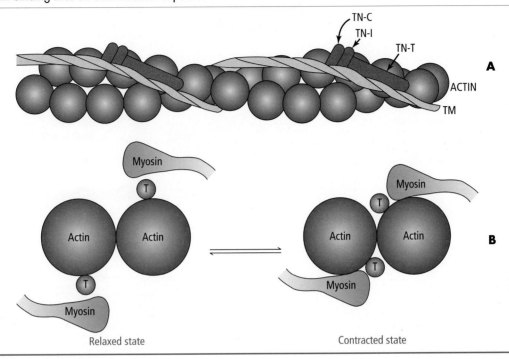

FIG. 12.8

Structure of myosin and the thick filaments. **A,** Structure of a single myosin molecule. **B,** Structure of the thick filaments in skeletal muscle. The globular heads of myosin are on the surface of the filament. Its center consists only of the fibrous tails and is therefore without globular heads. The packed tails have a diameter of 10.7 nm.

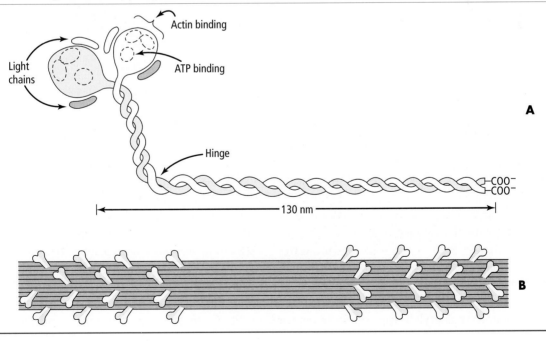

FIG. 12.9

The mechanism of muscle contraction. In this model, the conformational change of the myosin molecule ("power stroke") is induced by the binding of the myosin head to the thin filament and the subsequent release of ADP and inorganic phosphate. ATP is required to detach the myosin head from the thin filament.

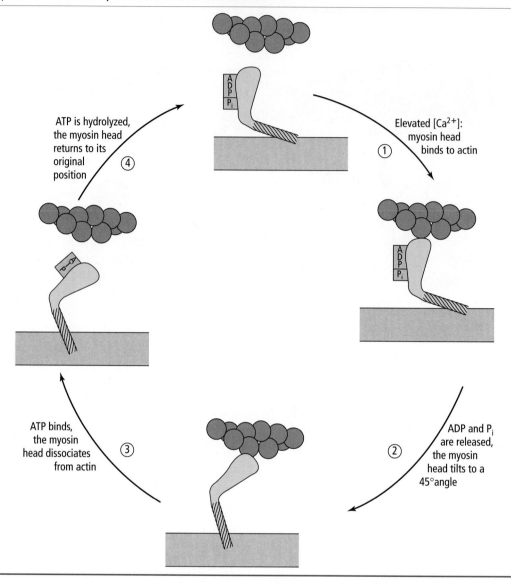

ATP is hydrolyzed, the myosin head returns to its original position ④

Elevated [Ca²⁺]: myosin head binds to actin ①

ATP binds, the myosin head dissociates from actin ③

ADP and Pᵢ are released, the myosin head tilts to a 45°angle ②

traction, but *this interaction can take place only when calcium is bound to the troponin complex on the thin filament.* In the resting muscle fiber, the calcium concentration is maintained at a level of only 10^{-7} M—10,000 times lower than in the extracellular space—by the action of the Ca^{2+}-ATPase in the sarcoplasmic reticulum (see Chapter 11). This calcium concentration is not sufficient to engage the troponin complex.

Muscle contraction is triggered by the action of the neurotransmitter acetylcholine on its receptor in the neuromuscular junction (see Chapter 26). Acetylcholine depolarizes the membrane of the muscle fiber, and this depolarization is relayed into the interior through the T-tubules. Through the contacts between T-tubules and the sarcoplasmic reticulum, *membrane depolarization triggers the release of calcium from the sarcoplasmic reticulum,* and the cytoplasmic calcium level increases up to 100-fold, to approximately 10^{-5} M. Four Ca^{2+} ions bind to troponin C on the thin filaments, and *this results in a* conformational change in the troponin complex that pulls tropomyosin from the myosin-binding sites of actin (Fig. 12.7, B). The myosin heads now are able to bind to actin.

The resulting interaction is depicted in Fig. 12.9: in the resting state, ADP and inorganic phosphate are tightly bound to the myosin heads. In this form, the myosin heads bind to the exposed actin of the thin filaments as soon as the cytoplasmic calcium level rises and tropomyosin is removed from the myosin-binding sites on the thin filament. *Actin binding causes the release of the bound ADP and phosphate; this, in turn, induces a conformational change in the myosin that pulls the thick filament approximately 7 nm along the thin filament.* ATP is required to detach the myosin head from actin but is then rapidly hydrolyzed to ADP and phosphate.

In death, the cytoplasmic Ca^{2+} concentration rises and ATP is depleted. Therefore the myosin heads bind to the thin filaments, their dissociation is no longer possible in the absence of ATP, and the muscle becomes stiff. This phenomenon is called **rigor mortis.**

Non-muscle cells also contain actin and myosin

Non-muscle cells contain rather large amounts of actin together with much smaller amounts of myosin. Six different isoforms of actin in human tissues are known. They are very similar and can even copolymerize in the same filament. The actin of non-muscle cells forms long filaments similar to those in muscle, but the non-muscle myosin (there are several isoforms that differ widely in their structures and properties) forms only very short, thin, inconspicuous fibrils.

The actin microfilaments of non-muscle cells spread and sprawl throughout the cytoplasm, without the highly ordered array typical of muscle cells. They are most abundant right under the plasma membrane, where they are known as **stress fibers.** Non-muscle actin polymerizes and depolymerizes rapidly, and *this polymerization/depolymerization is responsible for gel-sol transitions in the cytoplasmic matrix.* The aggregation state of actin is regulated by a large number of actin-binding proteins (Table 12.2). Many specialized cellular functions also depend on actin microfilaments, including

TABLE 12.2

Some actin-binding proteins of non-muscle cells

Protein	Properties
Tropomyosin	Strengthens actin filaments; may determine their length in some systems
α-Actinin	Crosslinks actin filaments
Gelsolin	Depolymerizes actin filaments at high ($>1\ \mu M$) calcium concentration
Fodrin	Spectrin-like; connects actin filaments
Fimbrin	Crosslinks neighboring actin filaments
Caldesmon	Binds to actin/tropomyosin filaments and prevents myosin binding at low ($<1\ \mu M$) calcium concentration
Vinculin	Binds both to α-actinin and to membrane proteins; thereby anchors actin filaments to the plasma membrane

1. Ameboid motility of macrophages and neutrophils;
2. Phagocytosis;
3. Contraction of intestinal microvilli;
4. Formation of the cleavage furrow during mitosis;
5. Shape change of activated platelets (see Chapter 25);
6. Outgrowth of dendrites and axons in developing neuroblasts.

Actin-dependent processes are inhibited by **cytochalasin B,** a fungal metabolite that prevents actin polymerization by capping one of the ends of the growing microfilament. **Phalloidin,** another fungal toxin, prevents the depolymerization of actin filaments. These agents change the shapes of many cells, inhibit cell motility, and prevent the outgrowth of axons from ganglia.

Microtubules consist of tubulin

Microtubules are thick, stiff, hollow tubes with an outer diameter of 24 nm and an inner diameter of 14 nm. *Like the actin microfilaments, they are formed by the*

FIG. 12.10

Structure of microtubules. **A,** Side view. **B,** Cross-sectional view. The ring of 13 tubulin subunits is actually arranged helically along the axis of the microtubule so that the two α-tubulin units separated by a dash are on different cross-sectional planes.

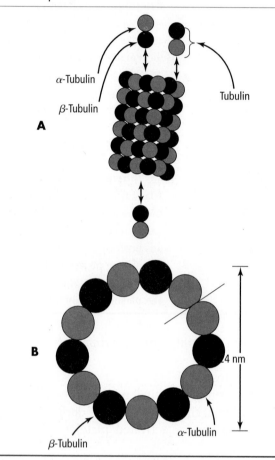

Microtubules occur in all nucleated cells. They often extend into cell processes and therefore are thought to be important for the *maintenance of cell shape.* They also are required for many *intracellular transport processes.* During mitosis, for example, the chromosomes are pulled to opposite poles of the cell by the microtubules ("spindle fibers") of the mitotic spindle. Microtubules also are used to bring vesicular organelles from the perikaryon of neurons to the nerve terminals, a process known as *fast axoplasmic transport.*

Like the actin filaments, microtubules are regulated by numerous associated proteins (microtubule-associated proteins, or MAPs). During fast axoplasmic transport, for example, proteins with ATPase activity (MAP 1c and kinesin) pull vesicles actively along the microtubules, at a speed of approximately 25 cm/day (3 μm/sec).

Colchicine, the poison of autumn crocus, blocks the polymerization of tubulin and inhibits microtubule-dependent cellular processes. It acts, for example, as a mitosis inhibitor because it prevents the formation of microtubules in the mitotic spindle.

All eukaryotic cilia and flagella contain a 9 + 2 array of microtubules

Cilia and flagella are hairlike cell appendages that are capable of beating or swirling motions (Fig. 12.11). Ciliated cells are found in many epithelia, including those of the bronchial tree, nasal sinuses, and Fallopian tubes. The only flagellated cell in humans is the sperm cell. Eukaryotic cilia and flagella are surrounded by a membrane that is continuous with the plasma membrane. In cross-section, two single microtubules are seen in the center, and nine double microtubules in the periphery. The double microtubules consist of a circular A fiber and a crescent-shaped B fiber. Unlike the cytoplasmic microtubules, which appear to be assembled and disassembled continuously, *the microtubules of cilia and flagella are permanent structures,* held in place by various structural proteins: the central microtubules are surrounded by a central sheath; radial spoke proteins connect this sheath with the outer doublet microtubules; and the doublet microtubules are connected by elastic bands formed by the protein nexin (Fig. 12.12).

The A subfiber of the doublet microtubules extends two arms that consist of the protein **dynein.**

polymerization of a soluble globular protein. This protein is called **tubulin** and consists of two subunits, α-tubulin and β-tubulin, with molecular weights of 53,000 each.

These building blocks polymerize in a helical array, with 13 protein subunits per turn (Fig. 12.10). Microtubules may reach lengths of several micrometers, containing thousands of tubulin molecules. Approximately one half of the tubulin in the cell is polymerized into microtubules at any time, and *the microtubules can be assembled and disassembled rapidly as required.* In this respect, they resemble the actin microfilaments of non-muscle cells. Like the actin and myosin filaments, microtubules have a distinct polarity. They tend to assemble at one end (the A end) and disassemble at the other end (the D end).

FIG. 12.11

The motile patterns of cilia and flagella. **A,** Cilium. **B,** Flagellum. Sperm flagella beat 30 to 40 times per second.

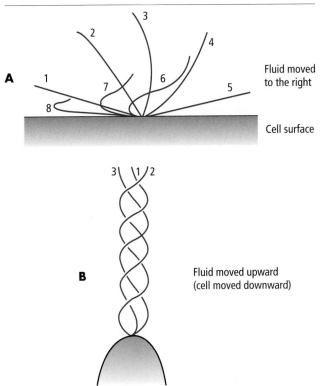

FIG. 12.12

Cross section through a cilium or flagellum. All eukaryotic (but not prokaryotic) cilia and flagella have this general structure.

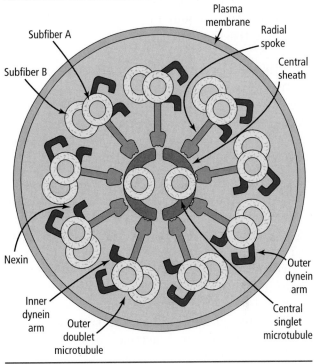

The outer dynein arms have three globular heads; the inner arms have either two or three. Each of these heads is formed by a separate large polypeptide. Like the myosin heads, *the dynein heads have ATPase activity, and they can walk along the B subfiber of a neighboring doublet microtubule* in the same way that the globular heads of myosin walk along the actin filaments in muscle cells (Fig. 12.9). Even the role of ATP is similar in the two systems: ATP is required to dissociate the dynein heads from the neighboring B subfiber as it is required to dissociate the myosin heads from the thin filament.

Structural defects of cilia and flagella cause bronchitis, sinusitis, and infertility

Recessively inherited defects in the microtubule-associated proteins of cilia and flagella result in the **immotile cilia syndrome** (population incidence = 1 in 20,000 to 1 in 50,000). This disorder is genetically and biochemically heterogeneous: in some patients, the dynein arms are either absent or abnormally short. In others, the radial spokes or the central sheath are absent or abnormal, and some patients are lacking the two central microtubules. Cilia and flagella are completely immotile, feebly motile, or show erratic movements.

Patients with this syndrome suffer from chronic or recurrent infections of the bronchial tree and the nasal sinuses. In these locations, epithelial cells have to move mucus by coordinated beatings of their cilia. In the lower respiratory tract, the epithelium is covered by a mucus blanket with a thickness of approximately 5 μm. Most inhaled particles and microorganisms get caught on this glue trap and are moved up the bronchi and the trachea by coordinated ciliary motion. This "mucus elevator" removes approximately 30 to 40 g of mucus from the bronchial system every day.

Men with this syndrome are infertile because their sperm cells are paralyzed, and even in vitro fertilization is not possible. Women also have reduced fertility, presumably from lack of ciliary movement in their Fallopian tubes. The most surprising observation, however, is that 50% of all patients with immotile cilia syndrome have a complete situs inversus (left-right inversion of the internal organs). Possibly the beating of cilia on embryonic epithelia is required for the development of a normal left-right asymmetry.

Cells are connected by specialized intercellular junctions

In epithelia and in other tissues with high cell density, the structural integrity and the function of the tissue depend on specialized cell-cell contacts (Fig. 12.13):

1. **Adherent junctions** glue the cells in a tissue together. They occur in two varieties: the **spot desmosome** or **macula adherens** can be understood as a spot weld between neighboring cells. These junctions are most conspicuous in stratified epithelia such as the epidermis, but they also are common in other tissues, including the myocardium. The **belt desmosome** or **zonula adherens** occurs only in single-layered epithelia such as the intestinal mucosa. The cells of these epithelia are encircled completely by a belt desmosome close to the border between their apical and basolateral surfaces.

   Cell-cell contact in the adherens junctions is established by adhesive transmembrane glycoproteins that include the **cadherins** in the belt desmosome and the related **desmogleins** and **desmocollins** in the spot desmosome. *These cell surface glycoproteins form homotypic interactions:* they bind specifically to the same type of glycoprotein on the neighboring cell surface. These adhesive plasma membrane glycoproteins are bound to a set of peripheral membrane proteins on the cytoplasmic side of the membrane, which include β-catenin, α-catenin, and plakoglobin in the belt desmosome. *These proteins are bound to the actin stress fibers underlying the plasma membrane.* The peripheral membrane proteins in the spot desmosome differ from those in the belt desmosome, with the exception of plakoglobin, which is present in both. Most importantly, *the spot desmosome interacts not with actin microfilaments but with intermediate filaments.* In epithelial tissues, these intermediate filaments consist of keratin. Structural defects of desmosomal proteins are not common, but a

FIG. 12.13

The three major types of cell-cell junction. **A,** The belt desmosome ("adherens junction"). The major adhesive membrane protein is E-cadherin (⬛). E-cadherin is bound to β-catenin or plakoglobin (⬭) on the cytoplasmic side of the membrane, and these are bound to α-catenin (⬤), which interacts with actin microfilaments ("stress fibers"). Spot desmosomes have a similar molecular architecture, but they are linked to intermediate filaments, not to microfilaments. **B,** The tight junction of an epithelial cell. Unlike the adhesive proteins of the desmosome, the proteins of the tight junction are space-filling and do not allow the diffusion of extracellular solutes or of membrane components. **C,** The gap junction. In the "open" state, the central pore allows the passage of solutes with molecular weights up to about 1200 daltons.

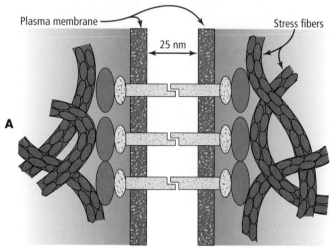

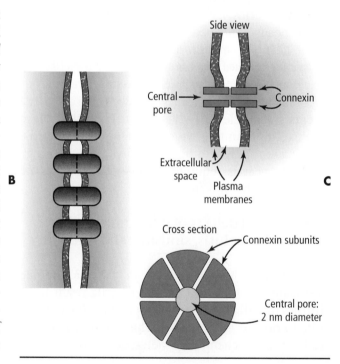

family of autoimmune dermatoses known as **pemphigus** are caused by autoantibodies to desmosomal proteins in the skin.

2. **Tight junctions** are beltlike adhesions between neighboring cells in single-layered epithelia. *They form a watertight seal around the cell that prevents the diffusion of solutes through the extracellular clefts.* Typical examples for epithelia with tight junctions include the intestinal mucosa, the renal tubules, and the cerebral capillaries, where tight junctions between the endothelial cells form the blood-brain barrier. *Tight junctions also prevent the lateral diffusion of membrane lipids and membrane proteins,* thereby compartmentalizing the plasma membrane into physiologically distinct areas. In the intestinal mucosal cells, for example, the tight junction forms the boundary between the apical (lumenal) and basolateral surfaces. The apical membrane of this cell type is distinguished by an abundance of glycolipids and a paucity of phospholipids in its outer leaflet, and by the presence of membrane-bound digestive enzymes (see Fig. 14.5). The intestinal mucosal cells also possess a belt desmosome encircling the cell in parallel with the tight junction (Fig. 11.19), and spot desmosomes on the lateral surface. Tight junctions are formed by a protein lattice whose components have not been characterized biochemically.

3. **Gap junctions** are small channels that interconnect the cytoplasm of neighboring cells. With a diameter of 2 nm, *they allow the passage of molecules up to a molecular weight of approximately 1200.* Each half-channel is formed by six subunits of the transmembrane protein **connexin**. Gap junctions respond to the level of cytosolic calcium: an increase in the calcium concentration closes the channel. This mechanism is important during cell death, when the cytosolic calcium concentration increases. In this situation, the surrounding cells have to sever their trade relations with the dead neighbor to maintain their own ion gradients and to prevent a unidirectional drain of their metabolites.

SUMMARY

The cytoskeleton consists of intracellular fibers that participate in the maintenance of cell shape, cell motility, and intracellular transport processes. There are several types of cytoskeletal fibers that are formed either from fibrous proteins or by the polymerization of globular protein subunits. Some cytoskeletal proteins, such as spectrin in erythrocytes and dystrophin in muscle fibers, reinforce the plasma membrane. The intermediate filaments, however, like the keratins of epithelial tissues, extend throughout the cytoplasm. Actin-based microfilaments are present in all human cells. They consist of globular actin subunits and can be assembled and disassembled rapidly, thereby regulating the physical consistency of the cytoplasm. They also are required for various kinds of cell motility, including ameboid motility and muscle contraction. Muscle cells contain a highly specialized contractile cytoskeleton based on actin microfilaments ("thin filaments") and myosin filaments ("thick filaments"). Microtubules are large cytoskeletal elements that are formed by the polymerization of the protein tubulin. They participate in various intracellular transport processes, and they reinforce cilia and flagella. Several genetic diseases, including hereditary spherocytosis, Duchenne muscular dystrophy, immotile cilia syndrome, and various skin diseases are caused by abnormalities of cytoskeletal proteins.

Further Reading

Campbell KP: Three muscular dystrophies: loss of cytoskeleton-extracellular matrix linkage. *Cell* 80, 675–679, 1995.

Cohen C, Parry DAD: α-Helical coiled coils: more facts and better predictions. *Science* 263, 488–489, 1994.

Cowin P: Unraveling the cytoplasmic interactions of the cadherin superfamily. *Proc Natl Acad Sci USA* 91, 10759–10761, 1994.

Fuchs E: Intermediate filaments: structure, dynamics, function, and disease. *Annu Rev Biochem* 63, 345–382, 1994.

Hemler ME, Mihich E, editors: *Cell adhesion molecules.* Plenum Press, New York, 1993.

Kreis T, Vale R, editors: *Guidebook to the cytoskeletal and motor proteins.* Oxford University Press, Oxford, 1993.

Lux SE, Palek J: Disorders of the red cell membrane. In: Handin RI, Lux SE, Stossel TP, editors: *Blood.* J. B. Lippincott, Philadelphia, 1995, pp. 1701–1818.

Scriver CR, Beaudet AL, Sly WS, Valle D, editors: *The metabolic basis of inherited disease*, 6th ed., vol. 2. McGraw-Hill, New York, 1989, pp. 2367–2408, 2869–2902, 2739–2750.

Steinert PM, Bale SJ: Genetic skin diseases caused by mutations in keratin intermediate filaments. *Trends Genet* 9 (8), 280–284, 1993.

Stossel TP: The machinery of cell crawling. *Sci Am* Sept. 1994, 54–63.

Tinsley JM, Blake DJ, Zuellig RA, Davies KE: Increasing complexity of the dystrophin-associated protein complex. *Proc Natl Acad Sci USA* 91, 8307–8313, 1994.

Trinick J: Titin and nebulin: protein rulers in muscle? *Trends Biochem Sci* 19, 405–408, 1994.

van de Klundert FAJM, Raats JMH, Bloemendal H.

Intermediate filaments: regulation of gene expression and assembly. *Eur J Biochem* 214, 351–366, 1993.

Walker RA, Sheetz MP: Cytoplasmic microtubule-associated motors. *Annu Rev Biochem* 62, 429–451, 1993.

QUESTIONS

1. Some cytoskeletal fibers can be assembled and disassembled rapidly as needed because they are formed from globular protein subunits. This type of fiber includes the
   A. Intermediate filaments and actin microfilaments
   B. Thick and thin filaments of skeletal muscle
   C. Proteins of the membrane skeleton (spectrin, dystrophin) and the microtubules
   D. Intermediate filaments and the thick filaments of skeletal muscle
   E. Actin microfilaments and microtubules

2. Colchicine is a plant alkaloid that prevents the formation of microtubules. This drug is most likely to inhibit
   A. The mechanical integrity of the horny layer of the skin
   B. Mitosis
   C. Muscle contraction
   D. The electrical coupling between myocardial cells
   E. The contraction of intestinal microvilli

3. The structural integrity of the epidermis depends critically on the presence of
   A. Keratin filaments and belt desmosomes
   B. Actin microfilaments and tight junctions
   C. Keratin filaments and spot desmosomes
   D. Thick (myosin) filaments and gap junctions
   E. Keratin filaments and tight junctions

4. Recurrent respiratory infections in children can be caused by a great variety of abnormalities. One possibility to consider in a child who presents with repeated bouts of bronchitis and sinusitis is an inherited defect in the protein
   A. Dynein
   B. Tropomyosin
   C. Connexin
   D. Keratin
   E. Dystrophin

Chapter 13

The Extracellular Matrix

In soft tissues such as liver, brain, and epithelial tissues, most of the available space is filled by the cells. The cells in these tissues are separated by narrow clefts, approximately 20 nm wide, that contain glycoproteins in an aqueous medium. *The consistency and mechanical properties of these tissues are determined by the cytoskeletal proteins and by specialized cell-cell adhesions.*

The cells of connective tissues, however, are separated by vast expanses of extracellular matrix. This extracellular matrix contains various types of proteinaceous fibers embedded in an amorphous ground substance of hydrated glycoproteins and proteoglycans. *The mechanical properties of these tissues are determined by the composition of the extracellular matrix,* and in particular by the amount, kind, and spatial orientation of its fibers. In this chapter, we examine the constituents of the extracellular matrix in such tissues as the dermis, cartilage, tendon, and bones.

FIBROUS PROTEINS OF THE EXTRACELLULAR MATRIX

The functions of the extracellular matrix (Fig. 13.1) vary with the tissue. In bone and cartilage, it has to provide structural rigidity; in tendons, tensile strength; in skin and blood vessels, elasticity. The **amorphous ground substance,** consisting of highly hydrated polysaccharides, proteoglycans, and glycoproteins, acts as a *flexible space filler and molecular glue* that holds the cells and fibers of the tissue together. The **fibers** that are embedded in this ground substance provide *tensile strength and elasticity.* We will introduce the molecular building blocks of the fibers before turning to the components of the amorphous ground substance.

The collagens are the most abundant proteins in the body

The collagens account for approximately 25% of the body protein in adults and 15% to 20% in children. As shown in Table 13.1, *collagen is most abundant in strong, tough, connective tissues,* including tendon, bone, cartilage, and the dermis. Soft parenchymatous tissues such as liver and brain have very little collagen.

TABLE 13.1

Approximate collagen contents of different tissues, expressed as percentage of the dry weight

Tissue	Collagen content (%)
Demineralized bone*	90
Tendons	80–90
Skin†	50–70
Cartilage	50–70
Arteries	10–25
Lung	10
Liver	4

* Bone from which the inorganic components (mostly calcium phosphates) have been removed by acid treatment.
† Mostly in the dermis. The major structural proteins of the epidermis are the keratins (see Chapter 12).

FIG. 13.1

Major constituents of the extracellular matrix. Collagen fibers and elastic fibers are required for tensile strength and elasticity, respectively. The amorphous ground substance is formed from proteoglycans, adhesive glycoproteins, and the polysaccharide hyaluronic acid. The extracellular matrix is linked to the cytoskeleton through proteins in the plasma membrane.

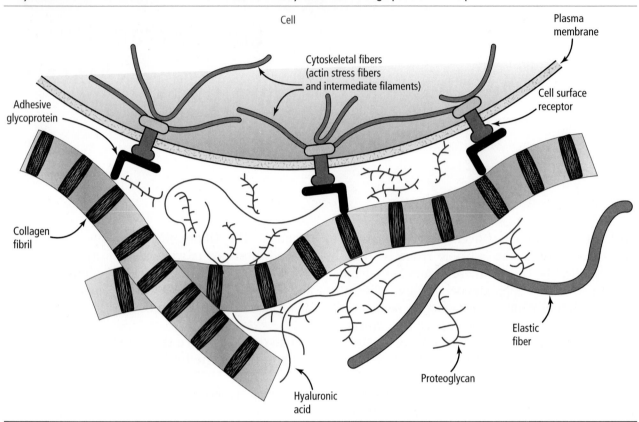

The collagens are a large protein family with close to 20 members (Table 13.2). They all consist of three polypeptides that form a characteristic triple helix, but their supermolecular structures differ. Only types I, II, III, V, VI, and XI form fibrils. Type IV collagen, a major constituent of basement membranes, is the most important nonfibrillar collagen.

The tropocollagen molecule forms a long triple helix

A typical collagen such as type I collagen has a very unusual amino acid composition. Glycine accounts for not less than 33% of the amino acid residues, and proline contributes another 10%. Most remarkably, collagen contains 3-hydroxyproline ($\leq 0.5\%$), 4-hydroxyproline ($\approx 10\%$), and 5-hydroxylysine ($\approx 1\%$) (Fig. 13.2). These hydroxylated amino acids are not represented in the genetic code, and therefore *they have to be synthesized posttranslationally from prolyl and lysyl residues in the polypeptide.* Collagen also has a small amount of carbohydrate, most of it linked to the hydroxy group of hydroxylysine in the form of a Glu-Gal disaccharide. The carbohydrate content of the fibrillar collagens is low ($0.5-1\%$ in types I and III), but it is higher in some of the nonfibrillar types (14% in type IV). Nutritionally, collagen is an inferior protein because some of the essential amino acids, including isoleucine, phenylalanine/tyrosine, and the sulfur amino acids are present in insufficient amounts. Therefore Jell-O (**gelatin** is denatured collagen) is not a good source of dietary protein.

The basic structural unit of collagen fibers, the **tropocollagen** molecule, consists of *three intertwined polypeptides* (Fig. 13.3). The most abundant type, type I collagen, consists of two different polypeptides,

TABLE 13.2

The collagens

Type	Most common composition	Structural features	Tissue distribution
I	$[\alpha 1(I)]_2$, $\alpha 2(I)$	67-nm-banded fibrils	Most abundant type, in most connective tissues
II	$[\alpha 1(II)]_3$	67-nm-banded fibrils	Cartilage, vitreous humor
III	$[\alpha 1(III)]_3$	67-nm-banded fibrils	Fetal tissues, skin, blood vessels, lungs, uterus, intestine, tendons, fresh scars
IV	$[\alpha 1(IV)]_2$, $\alpha 2(IV)$*	Globular C-terminal end domain; forms a branched network	All basement membranes
V	$[\alpha 1(V)]_2$, $\alpha 2(V)$†	67-nm-banded fibrils	Most tissues, minor component associated with type I collagen
VI	$\alpha 1(VI)$, $\alpha 2(VI)$, $\alpha 3(VI)$	C- and N-terminal globular domains; forms atypical fibrils	Most tissues, including cartilage
VII	$[\alpha 1(VII)]_3$	Dimer	Anchoring fibrils under basement membranes
VIII	$[\alpha 1(VIII)]_2$, $\alpha 2(VIII)$	Short helix, globular end domains, no fibril formation	Formed by endothelial cells, in Descemet's membrane
IX	$\alpha 1(IX)$, $\alpha 2(IX)$, $\alpha 3(IX)$	With bound dermatan sulfate	On surface of type II collagen fibrils in cartilage
X	$[\alpha 1(X)]_3$	Similar to type VIII	Calcifying cartilage
XI	$\alpha 1(XI)$, $\alpha 2(XI)$, $\alpha 1(III)$	67-nm-banded fibrils	Cartilage
XII	$[\alpha 1(XII)]_3$	Many globular domains	On surface of type I collagen fibrils
XIII	$[\alpha 1(XIII)]_3$ (?)	With transmembrane domain	Minor collagen in skin, intestine
XIV	$[\alpha 1(XIV)]_3$ (?)	Nonfibrillar	Like type XII
XV	$[\alpha 1(XV)]_3$ (?)	Nonfibrillar	Many tissues
XVI	$[\alpha 1(XVI)]_3$ (?)	Nonfibrillar	On surface of collagen fibrils
XVII	$[\alpha 1(XVII)]_3$ (?)	With transmembrane domain	Hemidesmosomes of skin
XVIII	$[\alpha 1(XVIII)]_3$ (?)	Nonfibrillar	Liver, kidney, skeletal muscle
XIX	$[\alpha 1(XIX)]_3$ (?)	Nonfibrillar	On surface of collagen fibrils, in rhabdomyosarcomas

* Tissue-specific $\alpha 3(IV)$, $\alpha 4(IV)$, $\alpha 5(IV)$, and $\alpha 6(IV)$ chains also occur.
† A less abundant $\alpha 3(V)$ chain is also often present.

each with approximately 1050 amino acids: an $\alpha 1(I)$ chain that is present in two copies and an $\alpha 2(I)$ chain in one copy, yielding the structural formula $[\alpha 1(I)]_2 \alpha 2(I)$ (see Table 13.2). *These polypeptides have very unusual amino acid sequences, with glycine in every third position.*

Each of the three polypeptides in tropocollagen forms a helical structure. This helix is called a **polyproline type II helix** because it resembles a helix type that is formed by the synthetic polypeptide polyproline. It is quite unlike the familiar α helix: the α helix is a tightly packed, right-handed helix with 3.6 amino acids per turn and a rise per amino acid of 0.15 nm (see Chapter 2); the polyproline helix is an extended, left-handed helix with 3 amino acids per turn and a rise per amino acid of 0.30 nm. This means that *the polyproline helix is twice as extended as the α helix.* It also means that *all the glycine residues are on the same side of the helix.* Unlike the α helix, the polyproline helix is not stabilized by hydrogen bonds between peptide bonds but by steric repulsion of the bulky proline and hydroxyproline side chains.

The three helical polypeptides of the tropocollagen molecule are wound around each other in a right-handed triple helix. Like the β-pleated sheet (see Chapter 2), the triple helix is stabilized by hydrogen bonds between the peptide bonds of the different polypeptides. Now we understand why one edge of each polyproline helix has to be lined with glycine residues: only the glycine side chain is small enough to permit close contact between the main chains of the polypeptides. It is the peptide bonds of the glycine residues that form the interchain hydrogen bonds. *The whole molecule looks like a three-stranded rope,* with a total length of 300 nm and a diameter of 1.5 nm.

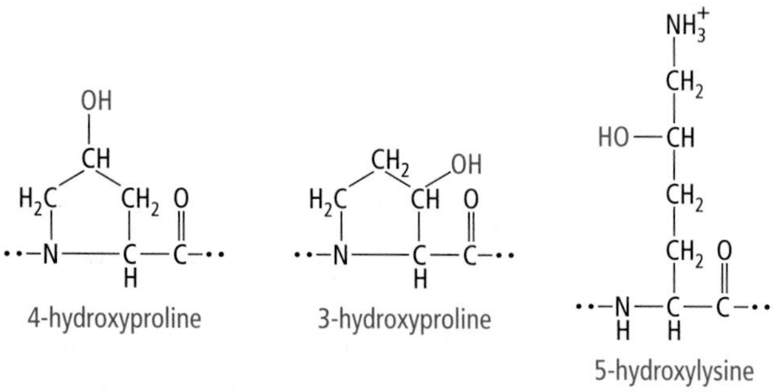

Collagen fibrils consist of a staggered array of tropocollagen molecules

As might be expected, *the long, ropelike tropocollagen molecules form fibrils by aligning themselves in parallel.* This alignment is rather precise, with a characteristic staggered array in which the end of one molecule extends 67 nm beyond that of its neighbor and with gaps of approximately 35 nm between the end of one molecule and the beginning of the next (Fig. 13.4). Fibril formation depends on interactions

---

FIG. 13.2

Hydroxylated amino acids in collagen.

4-hydroxyproline   3-hydroxyproline   5-hydroxylysine

FIG. 13.3

The triple-helical structure of collagen. The tropocollagen molecule has a length of approximately 300 nm and a diameter close to 1.5 nm. In the typical fibrillar collagens, only short terminal portions of the polypeptides (the "telopeptides") are not triple helical.

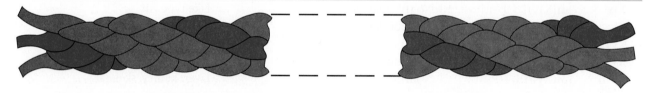

FIG. 13.4

The typical staggered array of tropocollagen molecules in the collagen fibril. The telopeptides participate in covalent cross-linking.

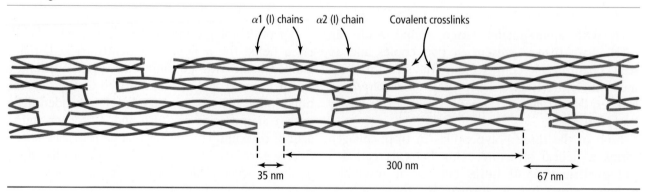

α1 (I) chains   α2 (I) chain   Covalent crosslinks

35 nm   300 nm   67 nm

between amino acid side chains in neighboring molecules. Collagen types I, II, III, V, and XI form typical cross-striated fibrils with diameters anywhere between 10 and 300 nm that contain hundreds or even thousands of tropocollagen molecules in cross-section. More often than not, a single fibril contains more than one type of collagen.

Collagen fibrils have great tensile strength, and a fibril of 1 mm diameter would be able to carry a weight of approximately 10 kg. This tensile strength is exploited fully in tendons, where the fibrils are arranged in parallel. Collagen also is durable, with lifespans ranging from some weeks (blood vessels, fresh scars) to many years (bone). Collagen degradation is initiated by an extracellular collagenase that cleaves the polypeptide at a single site approximately three quarters down the length of the triple helix. The resulting fragments unravel spontaneously and are degraded further by other proteases. Intact, triple-helical collagen is very resistant to common proteases such as pepsin and trypsin.

Collagen synthesis requires extensive posttranslational processing

Like all other extracellular proteins, *collagen is processed through the secretory pathway* (see Chapter 8). The polypeptides that are synthesized by ribosomes on the rough endoplasmic reticulum are called **preprocollagen.** They contain not only the 1050 amino acids of mature tropocollagen but also additional sequences at the amino and carboxy ends. In the $\alpha 1(I)$ chain of type I collagen, these sequences, called **propeptides,** measure approximately 170 and 220 amino acid residues at their N-terminal and C-terminal ends, respectively. The propeptides are globular and have neither the unusual amino acid composition and sequence nor the triple-helical structure of mature collagen. The processing of type I collagen is shown in Fig. 13.5:

1. *Approximately 25 amino acids are removed from the amino ends of pro-$\alpha 1(I)$ and pro-$\alpha 2(I)$ chains by* **signal peptidase.** This cotranslational reaction (see Chapter 8) converts preprocollagen to **procollagen.**
2. *Intrachain disulfide bonds are formed in the N-terminal propeptides of the $\alpha 1(I)$ chain; interchain disulfide bonds are formed between the C-terminal propeptides.*
3. *Some of the prolyl and lysyl side chains become hydrox-*

ylated. 4-Hydroxyproline, 3-hydroxyproline, and 5-hydroxylysine are formed by three different enzymes.

4. *Some of the 5-hydroxylysyl residues become glycosylated.* The glycosyl transferases that catalyze these reactions use UDP-galactose and UDP-glucose as precursors (see Chapter 8).
5. *The triple helix forms in the C $\rightarrow$ N terminal direction.* The interchain disulfide bonds in the C-terminal propeptides are required for initiation of triple helix formation. Because the amino acid hydroxylating enzymes and the glycosyl transferases act only on the non–triple-helical polypeptides, any delay in triple helix formation and any imperfection of the triple-helical structure is likely to cause overhydroxylation and overglycosylation.
6. *Procollagen is secreted.* Only triple-helical procollagen can be secreted; improperly coiled molecules are degraded.
7. *The N- and C-terminal propeptides are removed by extracellular proteases.* The resulting tropocollagen molecules are triple-helical, with the exception of a few amino acids at the N- and C-terminal ends, the **telopeptides.** In the $\alpha 1(I)$ chains, for example, the helical sequence consists of 1014 amino acids (338 Gly-X-Y repeats), the N-terminal telopeptide has 16, and the C-terminal telopeptide has 26.
8. *The tropocollagen molecules assemble into fibrils.* We realize at this point that the propeptides have two different functions:

- They initiate the formation of the triple helix in the ER, and
- They prevent premature fibril formation.

9. *The molecules in the fibril become cross-linked covalently.* Cross-linking is initiated by **lysyl oxidase.** This oxygen-dependent, copper-containing enzyme acts in the gaps between the ends of the tropocollagen molecules during fibril formation, oxidizing some of the lysyl residues in the telopeptides to allysine and some of the hydroxylysyl residues to hydroxy-allysine. The aldehyde groups created in these reactions react nonenzymatically with other allysyl residues, unmodified lysyl and hydroxylysyl residues, and sometimes histidyl residues to form a variety of covalent cross-links (Fig. 13.6). Cross-linking is essential for the formation of a strong collagen fibril.

FIG. 13.5

Posttranslational processing of type I collagen, the most abundant fibrillar collagen.

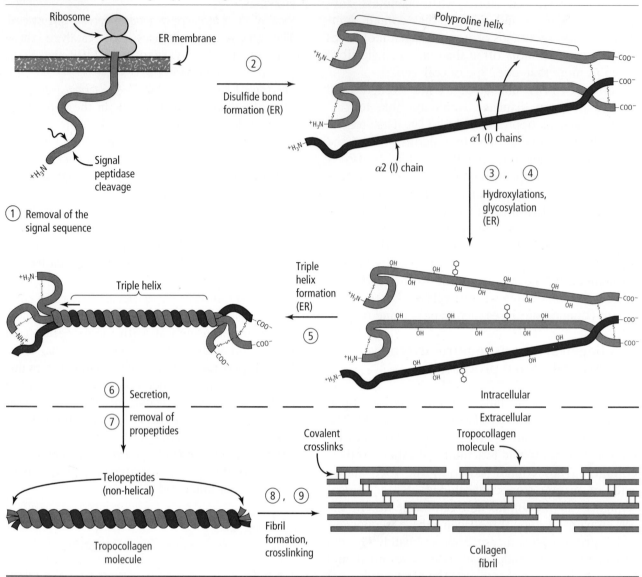

Collagen genes have unusual structures

Unlike the genes for the hemoglobin chains (see Chapter 9), the genes for different collagen chains are not clustered but are scattered throughout the genome. They typically consist of approximately 50 exons, but the exons account for only some 20% of their length. The exons coding for the triple-helical portions of the collagens are quite remarkable: *they generally start with a codon for glycine and encode a fixed number of Gly-X-Y units*. As shown in Table 13.3 for the $\alpha 1(I)$ chain of type I collagen, most exons consist of 54 base pairs (bp) encoding six Gly-X-Y units. These exons were most likely generated by **exon duplication** during the evolution of the collagen genes, whereas the 108- and 162-bp exons may be the result of **exon fusion.** The 45-bp exons probably arose by a 9-bp deletion from the primordial 54-bp exon, and the 99-bp exons may have originated by the fusion of a 45-bp exon with a 54-bp exon.

FIG. 13.6

Covalent cross-linking of collagen. **A,** The lysyl oxidase reaction. **B,** An aldol cross-link in collagen. **C,** An "advanced" type of covalent cross-link in collagen formed from allysine (①), hydroxyallysine (②), and hydroxylysine (③).

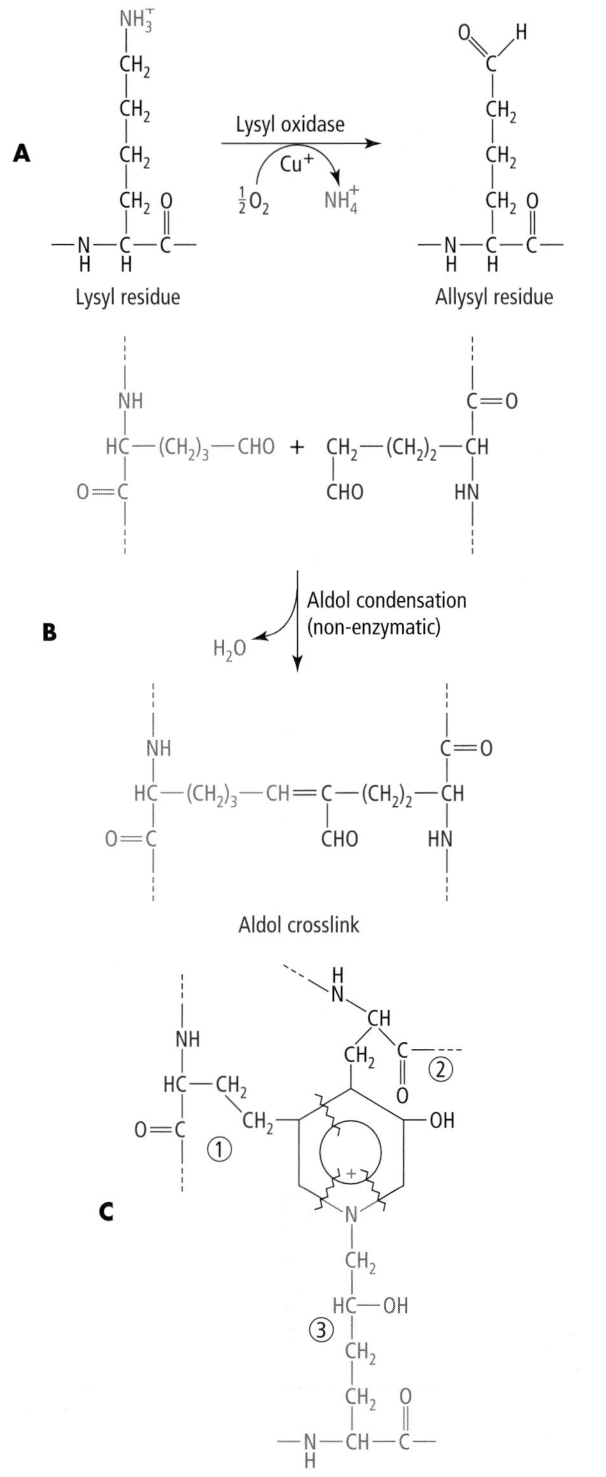

TABLE 13.3

Sizes of the 41 exons coding for the triple-helical part of the $\alpha(1)(I)$ chain in type I collagen*

Exon length	Encoded sequence	No. of exons
54	$(Gly\text{-}X\text{-}Y)_6$	21
108	$(Gly\text{-}X\text{-}Y)_{12}$	9
162	$(Gly\text{-}X\text{-}Y)_{18}$	1
45	$(Gly\text{-}X\text{-}Y)_5$	5
99	$(Gly\text{-}X\text{-}Y)_{11}$	5

* Each exon begins with a codon for glycine and encodes a fixed number of Gly-X-Y repeats.

Collagen metabolism is altered in aging and disease

The meat of young animals is soft and tender, whereas that of old animals is tough and unpalatable; according to experts, the same is true for human flesh. The reason for this age-related change is that *the collagen of old animals and humans has more covalent cross-links than that of the young.* Also, the amount of collagen, relative to the proteins of parenchymal cells, increases with age. The gourmet knows, of course, that actin and myosin taste much better than collagen!

Collagen synthesis also is stimulated by injury. During wound healing, fibroblasts migrate to the site of the lesion to form abundant collagen. Scar tissue consists mostly of collagen. The death of parenchymal cells in such tissues as liver, spleen, and kidney also is followed by the proliferation of fibroblasts and the deposition of a collagen-rich extracellular matrix. In **liver cirrhosis,** for example, which is the common outcome of a variety of liver diseases, most of the parenchymal cells are replaced by fibrous connective tissue (a cirrhotic liver would taste awful!).

In bacterial tissue infections, collagen synthesis is stimulated around the infected site, and the infection is walled off in a localized **abscess.** Abscess formation is not always successful, however: *some pathogenic bacteria secrete collagenases that cleave tropocollagen proteolytically.* These bacteria can spread far and wide through the tissues. Typical examples are the anaerobic bacteria (*Clostridium histolyticum, Clostridium perfringens*) that cause **gas gangrene,** a severe form of wound infection.

One step in collagen synthesis—the hydroxylation of prolyl and lysyl side chains in procollagen—requires ascorbic acid (vitamin C). These reactions therefore are blocked in vitamin C deficiency (**scurvy**). Hydroxyproline, in particular, is required to stabilize the triple helix. *Without hydroxyproline, the triple helix denatures spontaneously at body temperature,* and most of the abnormal collagen is degraded intracellularly because it fails to form the secretable triple-helical structure. The result is a generalized hemorrhagic tendency, loose teeth, poor wound healing, rupture of scar tissue, and other signs of connective tissue weakness.

Many genetic defects of collagen structure and biosynthesis are known

Connective tissue diseases can result from inherited abnormalities in the procollagen chains themselves, or from deficiencies of enzymes for their posttranslational processing. These diseases are classified according to their phenotypic expression.

Osteogenesis imperfecta (OI) is a group of diseases in which *brittle bones ("glass bones") are the most prominent feature.* It includes very mild forms with occasional pathological fractures, but also severe forms that cause skeletal deformities and dwarfism or even perinatal death. Extraskeletal manifestations include a blue discoloration of the sclera, hearing loss, and poor tooth development. The incidence of OI is approximately 1 in 10,000, and the inheritance is autosomal dominant in most cases.

OI is caused by mutations in the genes for the α1 and α2 chains of type I collagen. Approximately 100 different mutations have been identified in different patients, many of them point mutations that replace a glycine residue with another amino acid. Interestingly, these point mutations, which impair the formation of the triple helix in the endoplasmic reticulum (ER), are most damaging when they occur near the carboxy end of the triple helix. This is because the triple helix forms in the C → N terminal direction in the ER (Fig. 13.5). The amino acid substitution arrests the coiling process, and this results in

---

FIG. 13.7

Single amino acid substitutions in the α1 chain of type I collagen are "included" mutations. The abnormal polypeptide initially is included in the molecule, but molecules with at least one abnormal chain are degraded or nonfunctional. Heterozygotes form 50% normal and 50% abnormal α1 chains, but 75% of the triple-stranded molecules contain at least one abnormal chain and therefore are useless. A similar heterozygous mutation in the gene for the α2 chain would disrupt only 50% of the molecules and cause a milder disease.

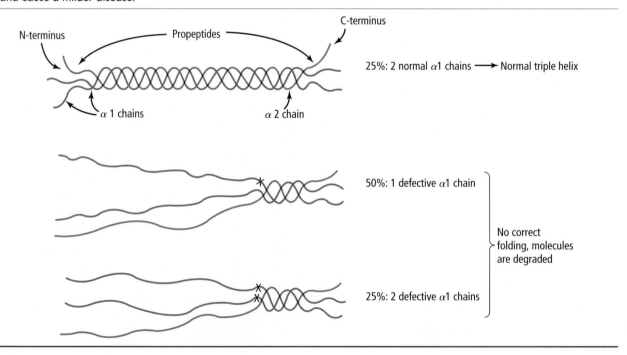

overhydroxylation and overglycosylation of amino acid residues N-terminal to the site of the mutation. This prevents the completion of the triple helix, and the uncoiled polypeptides fall prey to intracellular proteases. Point mutations of this kind are most damaging when they appear in the gene for the $\alpha 1$ chain, which is present in two copies in the triple helix. In this case, three quarters of the molecules formed by a heterozygous patient contain at least one defective $\alpha 1$ chain and are degraded (Fig. 13.7). Why are the bones affected so badly by mutations in the type I collagen genes? The likely reason is that almost all of the collagen in bone is type I collagen. In most other tissues, type I collagen occurs together with type II (cartilage) or type III collagen (skin, blood vessels, hollow viscera).

Ehlers-Danlos syndrome is a heterogeneous group of diseases characterized by *stretchy skin and loose joints*. The "indiarubber man" who could bend and twist himself into incredible shapes and package himself into tiny boxes had Ehlers-Danlos syndrome. The price for this virtuosity is fragile skin that bruises easily. Even small wounds heal poorly, with the formation of characteristic "cigarette paper" scars. Some forms of Ehlers-Danlos syndrome can be traced to defects in collagen synthesis, including deficiencies of lysyl hydroxylase or lysyl oxidase, or the incomplete removal of the propeptides (Table 13.4).

Structural defects of type III collagen result in Ehlers-Danlos syndrome type IV. This disease often is complicated by the rupture of large blood vessels, the colon, or the gravid uterus. These tissues are rich in type III collagen.

Abnormalities of type II collagen, the "cartilage collagen," affect endochondral bone formation and cause skeletal deformities and dwarfism. **Spondylo-epiphyseal dysplasia**, a dominantly inherited form

---

TABLE 13.4

Diseases affecting connective tissue proteins

Disease	Inheritance*	Cause	Signs and symptoms
Scurvy	—	Deficiency of dietary vitamin C	Hemorrhages, easy bruising
Osteogenesis imperfecta	AD (most)	Mutations in genes for type I collagen	Brittle bones, blue sclera, deafness
Ehlers-Danlos syndrome			
Type I (gravis)	AD	Not known	Hyperextensible skin, easy bruising, "cigarette paper" scars, hypermobile joints
Type II (mitis)	AD	Not known	Like type I, but milder
Type III	AD	Not known	Joint hypermobility, no scarring
Type IV	AD	Mutations in gene for type III collagen	Rupture of arteries, bowel, and gravid uterus
Type VI	AR	Deficiency of lysyl hydroxylase	Extensible skin, joint hypermotility, ocular fragility
Type VII	AD	Failure to remove the N-terminal propeptides in a type I collagen chain	Joint hypermobility, hip dislocation
Spondyloepiphyseal dysplasia	AD	Mutations in gene for type II collagen	Short-limbed dwarfism
Epidermolysis bullosa dystrophica	AD or AR	Mutations in gene for type VII collagen	Abnormal skin blistering
Marfan syndrome	AD	Mutations in gene for fibrillin	Tall stature, lens dislocation, aortic aneurysm

* AD, Autosomal dominant; AR, autosomal recessive.

of dwarfism, is caused by structural defects of type II collagen.

Type VII collagen forms anchoring fibrils at the dermis-epidermis junction that anchor the basement membrane to the underlying dermis (see Chapter 12, Fig. 12.5). The absence of this collagen causes the dystrophic variety of **epidermolysis bullosa.** As mentioned in Chapter 12, most other forms of these skin-blistering diseases are caused by abnormalities not of collagen but rather of keratin, the major structural protein of the epidermis.

Elastin is the most important constituent of elastic fibers

Elastic fibers guarantee the elasticity of such tissues as the skin, arteries, lungs, and ligaments. These "rubber band" fibers consist of the protein **elastin.** Like collagen, elastin has an aberrant amino acid composition, with high proportions of glycine (31%), alanine (22%), and proline (11%). Some 4-hydroxyproline (1%) also is present, but there is no hydroxylysine. *Like collagen, elastin contains covalent cross-links that are derived from allysine.* Therefore lysyl oxidase is required for the synthesis of elastin as well as that of collagen. **Desmosine** (Fig. 13.8) is an unusual allysine-derived cross-link in elastin (but not collagen) that connects four sites in two different polypeptides (Fig. 13.9).

In the elastic fibers, amorphous elastin is associated with microfibrils. One of the glycoproteins in these microfibrils, **fibrillin,** is defective in patients with **Marfan syndrome.** Patients with this dominantly inherited condition are unusually tall, with long, spidery fingers (arachnodactyly); the lens is displaced (ectopia lentis); and the media of the large arteries is abnormally weak. Many patients die suddenly in midlife after rupture of the dilated aorta.

THE AMORPHOUS GROUND SUBSTANCE

The collagen fibers and elastic fibers are embedded in an amorphous ground substance of nonfibrous glycoproteins, proteoglycans, and the polysaccharide hyaluronic acid. The components of the amorphous ground substance are not required for tensile strength, but they are important for the deformability and resilience of the tissue, and they participate

FIG. 13.8

FIG. 13.8

The structure of desmosine. This covalent cross-link occurs in elastin but not in collagen. Besides desmosine, elastin also contains some of the cross-links typical for collagen.

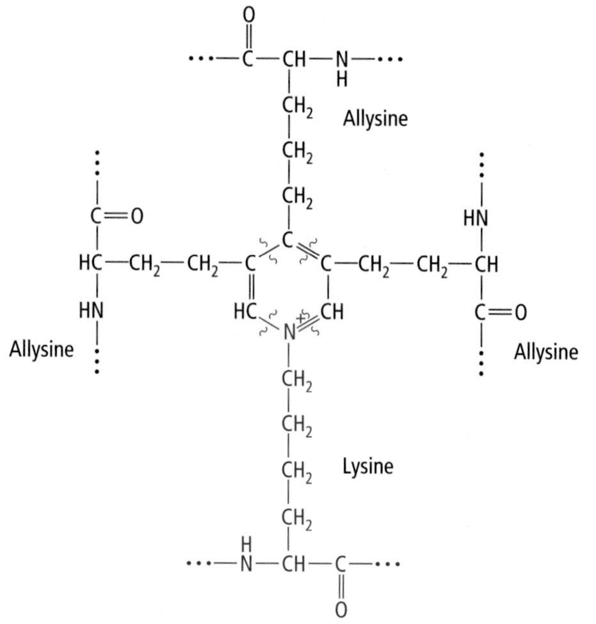

in tissue cohesion by binding to cell surfaces and fibers.

Hyaluronic acid is a huge polysaccharide in the extracellular matrix

Major components of the ground substance are the **glycosaminoglycans (GAGs),** unbranched acidic polysaccharides that consist of repeating disaccharide units. One of their building blocks always is an acetylated or, less commonly, a sulfated amino sugar; the second component usually—but not always—is a uronic acid. Uronic acids are hexose derivatives in which C-6 of a hexose is oxidized to a carboxy group (Fig. 13.10).

Hyaluronic acid is a GAG that consists of repeating disaccharide units of glucuronic acid and N-acetylglucosamine in $\beta 1,3$ and $\beta 1,4$ glycosidic linkage (Fig. 13.11). More than 10,000 disaccharide units form a huge, unbranched molecule with a molecular weight up to 10^7 daltons and a length of up to 10 μm. The negative charges of hyaluronic acid bind water and cations, and the β-glycosidic bonds favor an extended conformation. *At low concentrations, hyaluronic*

FIG. 13.9

A model for the structure of elastin. Elastic recoil during relaxation is thought to depend on hydrophobic interactions between amino acid side chains in the polypeptide.

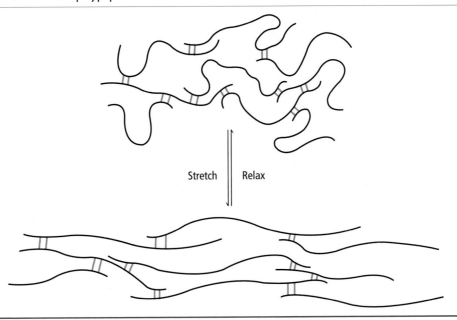

Stretch | Relax

acid forms viscous solutions, and at higher concentrations it forms a hydrated gel. **Wharton's jelly** in the umbilical cord is a hyaluronate-based gel. The **vitreous body** of the eye is a gel of sodium hyaluronate with an interspersed network of type II collagen fibrils. **Synovial fluid** is a lubricant that contains 0.3% hyaluronic acid together with a glycoprotein.

In the tissues, the long, extended hyaluronate molecules tend to push cells and fibers apart. Migrating cells in embryonic tissues are surrounded by a hyaluronate-rich matrix, but the hyaluronic acid content of the extracellular matrix declines as the cells settle to form coherent tissues.

Sulfated GAGs are covalently bound to core proteins

GAGs other than hyaluronic acid carry sulfate groups in the form of sulfate esters and, sometimes, in amide bond with the nitrogen of the amino sugar. These sulfate groups contribute additional negative charges. *The sulfated GAGs are much shorter than hyaluronic acid, and they are covalently bound to amino acid side chains in a core protein,* much as oligosaccharides are bound to amino acid side chains in "ordinary" glycoproteins.

The core protein with its covalently attached

GAGs is called a **proteoglycan.** *Different proteoglycans have different core proteins, and an individual core protein can carry more than one kind of GAG.* Also, the linkage to the core protein differs in different proteoglycans. Even the GAGs themselves differ somewhat in different proteoglycans and in different tissues. The chain length and the degree of sulfation, for example, vary considerably for any given GAG. Proteoglycans are found in many places:

1. *Proteoglycans are major components of the amorphous ground substance of connective tissues* (see Fig. 13.13).
2. *Some proteoglycans reside in the plasma membrane,* many of them as integral membrane proteins (Fig. 13.12). Heparan sulfate and, less commonly, chondroitin sulfate are present in these cell surface proteoglycans. Together with glycolipids and glycoproteins, they contribute to the **glycocalyx** (see Chapter 11).
3. *Mucus contains proteoglycans.* Proteoglycans and **mucins** (glycoproteins with abundant O-linked oligosaccharides) are responsible for the slimy consistency of mucous secretions.
4. *Heparin is formed by mast cells and basophils,* as is histamine (see Chapter 26). Heparin has anticoagulant and lipid-clearing properties. When it is released

FIG. 13.10

Amino sugars and uronic acids are the most common building blocks of the glycosaminoglycans. In the amino sugars the hydroxy group at C-2 of the hexose is replaced by an amino group. This amino group is most often acetylated and sometimes sulfated. In the uronic acids, C-6 of the hexose is oxidized to a carboxy group. *N*-Acetylglucosamine and *N*-Acetylgalactosamine are the most common amino sugars, and glucuronic acid and iduronic acid (a C-5 epimer of glucuronic acid) are the most common uronic acids. The amino sugars but not the uronic acids are also common in glycoproteins and glycolipids. The D and L series of monosaccharides are designated according to the absolute configuration at the asymmetrical carbon farthest away from the carbonyl carbon. Therefore the C-5 epimer of D-glucuronic acid belongs to the "L" series.

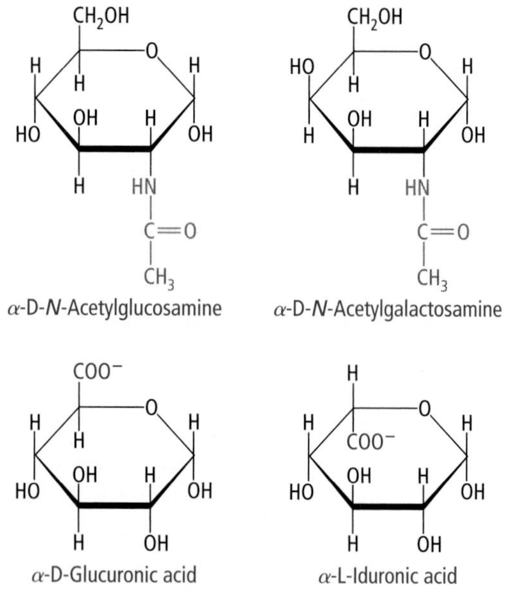

α-D-*N*-Acetylglucosamine

α-D-*N*-Acetylgalactosamine

α-D-Glucuronic acid

α-L-Iduronic acid

together with histamine during inflammatory and allergic reactions, histamine increases vascular permeability and heparin prevents excessive fibrin formation in the interstitial space.

Cartilage contains large proteoglycan aggregates

Approximately two thirds of the dry weight of cartilage consists of type I and type II collagen; most of the rest is contributed by a large proteoglycan called **aggrecan**. Aggrecan has a core protein of 2316 amino acids, which can be divided into different structural and functional domains (Fig. 13.13): the N-terminal part forms two globular domains that do not carry GAGs and that bind to hyaluronic acid.

These are followed by a keratan sulfate–containing domain and a large chondroitin sulfate–containing domain. The carboxy end forms another globular domain without attached GAGs.

The aggrecan molecule looks like a test tube brush, with approximately 100 chondroitin sulfate chains and 50 to 80 keratan sulfate chains extending from the core protein in all directions. Like hyaluronic acid, the sulfated GAGs of aggrecan are sprawling, hydrated polysaccharide chains that fill a large volume. In all, the aggrecan molecule has a molecular weight of approximately 2×10^6 and a length of 400 nm (0.4 μm).

Aggrecan molecules, as their name implies, are gregarious. They form large **proteoglycan aggregates** in which the GAG-free N-terminal domains of the core protein are noncovalently bound to hyaluronic acid. This binding is reinforced by a small, noncovalently bound link protein (Fig. 13.14). The proteoglycan aggregates are very large. At intervals of 40 nm, a single hyaluronic acid molecule binds up to a few hundred aggrecan molecules. The resulting aggregate has a molecular weight of 1 to 5×10^8 daltons and a length of a few micrometers. The volume occupied by a single proteoglycan aggregate is larger than a bacterial cell!

The proteoglycan aggregates of cartilage are responsible for the elasticity, resilience, and gel-like properties of this tissue, whereas the collagen fibers that are embedded in the proteoglycan matrix prevent tearing of the tissue in response to stretch and shear forces.

Bone consists of calcium phosphates in a collagenous matrix

Bone consists of approximately 10% water, 20% organic materials, and 70% inorganic salts. *The organic matrix is mostly type I collagen; the inorganic salts are derived from calcium phosphate* $(Ca_3(PO_4)_2)$. **Hydroxyapatite,** $3 Ca_3(PO_4)_2 \cdot Ca(OH)_2$, is the major inorganic component. There also are considerable amounts of Mg^{2+}, Na^+, CO_3^{2-}, fluoride, and citrate. Other metal ions also can be incorporated into this "bone salt." Sr^{2+}, for example, can take the place of Ca^{2+} in the crystal lattice. Radioactive ^{90}Sr, formed during nuclear blasts, can stay in bone for many years, causing damage to the rapidly dividing cells of the neighboring bone marrow.

FIG. 13.11

The most important glycosaminoglycans (GAGs). The structures of the GAGs are quite variable. Thus, chondroitin 4-sulfate has sulfur on C-4 rather than C-6 of the amino sugar; dermatan sulfate contains some glucuronic acid besides iduronic acid, and the sulfate of the amino sugar may be either on C-4 or on C-6; heparan sulfate contains some iduronic acid besides glucuronic acid; and heparin contains both glucuronic acid and iduronic acid.

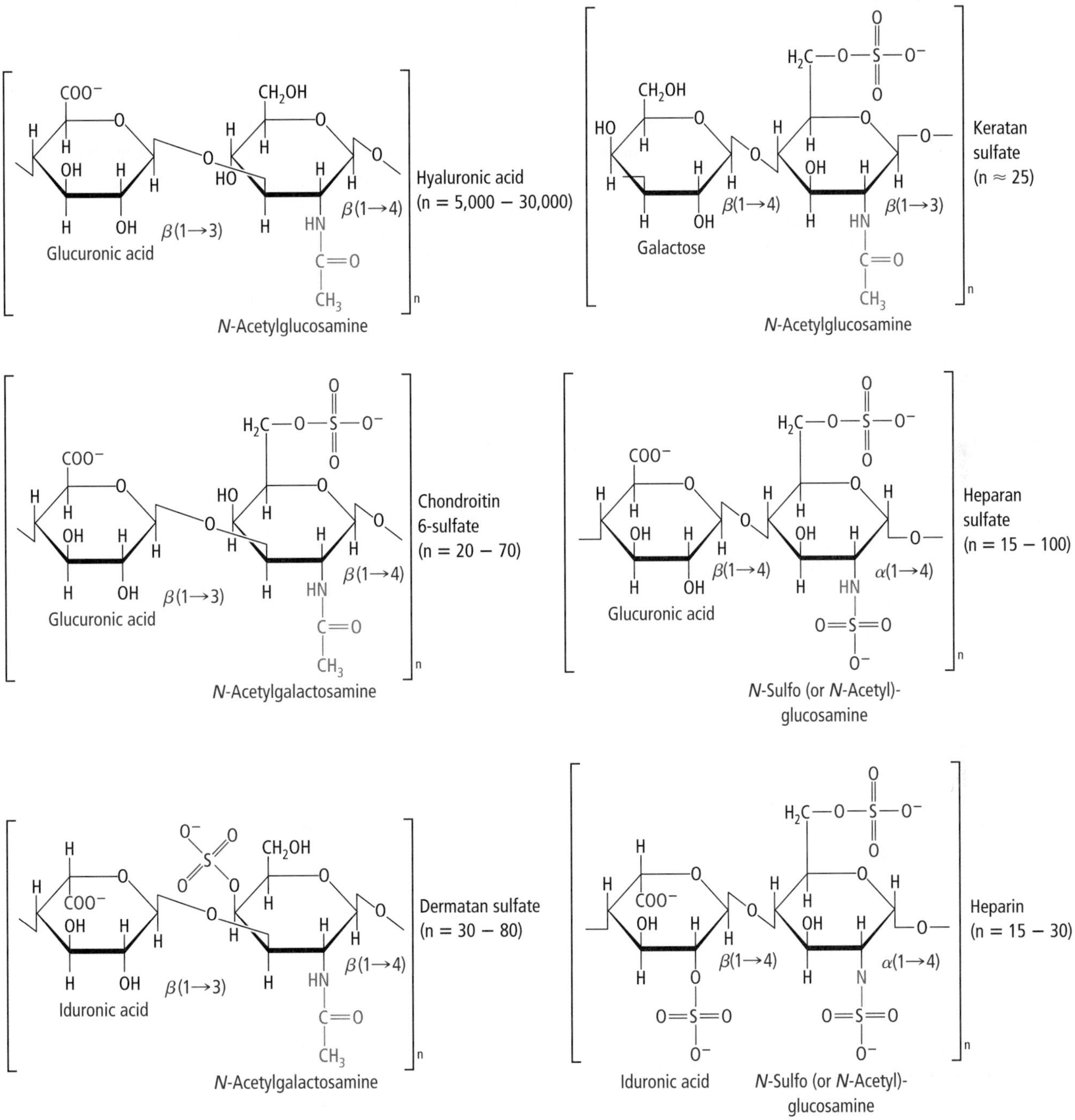

FIG. 13.12

Structure of a surface proteoglycan that is present in the plasma membrane of many epithelial cells. Note that more than one GAG may be present, and that N- or O-linked oligosaccharides may be present as well.

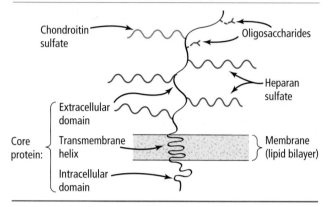

During bone formation, the collagenous organic matrix is deposited first. Mineralization is initiated by the formation of insoluble $CaHPO_4 \cdot 2H_2O$ in the gaps between the ends of tropocollagen molecules in the collagen fibrils (see Fig. 13.4). This salt, which is more soluble than the bone salt, is converted spontaneously to hydroxyapatite. Plasma and extracellular fluid are supersaturated with the components of bone salt, but the mineralization of soft tissues is prevented by inorganic pyrophosphate, which prevents the growth of hydroxyapatite crystals. In bone, pyrophosphate is destroyed by **alkaline phosphatase,** an enzyme on the surface of osteoblasts and in the extracellular medium (see Chapter 25). Patients who are deficient in alkaline phosphatase suffer from **hypophosphatasia.** This recessively inherited disease is characterized by

FIG. 13.13

Structure of aggrecan, the major proteoglycan of cartilage. **A,** Overall structure (schematic). **B,** Covalent attachment of chondroitin sulfate to serine side chains in aggrecan. The xylose-galactose-galactose linker sequence has been found in several other proteoglycans as well. **C,** Covalent attachment of keratan sulfate to serine (sometimes threonine) side chains in aggrecan. In some other proteoglycans, keratan sulfate is bound N-glycosidically to asparagine rather than O-glycosidically to serine. NANA, N-acetylneuraminic acid.

Oligosaccharides (N-linked)

Oligosaccharides (O-linked)

Core protein

^+H_3N —

— COO^-

A

N-terminal globular (binds hyaluronic acid)

C-terminal globular (unknown function)

Keratan sulfate containing

Chondroitin sulfate containing

B Ser — O — Xyl — Gal — Gal — [GlcUA — GalNAc]$_n$

with SO_4^- on GalNAc

Ser — O — GalNAc — [Gal — GlcNAc]$_n$ **C**

with SO_4^- on GlcNAc

Gal — NANA

poor bone mineralization similar to that seen in patients with rickets or osteomalacia.

In pathological situations, *bones become demineralized whenever either the calcium or the phosphate concentration in the plasma and the extracellular medium is reduced.* This mechanism contributes to the impaired mineralization in **rickets** and **osteomalacia** (vitamin D deficiency; see Chapter 24). **Hypophosphatemia,** also known as **vitamin D–resistant rickets,** is an inherited defect of renal phosphate reabsorption that leads to decreased serum phosphate levels and impaired bone mineralization. Also, *the solubility of the bone salt increases profoundly at decreased pH values. Chronic acidosis therefore leads to bone demineralization.* In patients with renal failure, bone demineralization results from a combination of impaired vitamin D metabolism (see Chapter 24) and an incompletely compensated metabolic acidosis. *Poorly mineralized bones have a soft consistency, much like cartilage, and they bend rather than break under stress.*

Impaired formation of the organic matrix leads to brittle bones that break easily. Osteogenesis imperfecta and the far more common **osteoporosis** are caused by impaired synthesis of type I collagen. Both the calcium content and the collagen content are reduced in osteoporotic bone.

Metastatic calcification is the inappropriate deposition of insoluble calcium salts in soft tissues. It is

---

FIG. 13.14

Structure of the proteoglycan aggregate in cartilage.

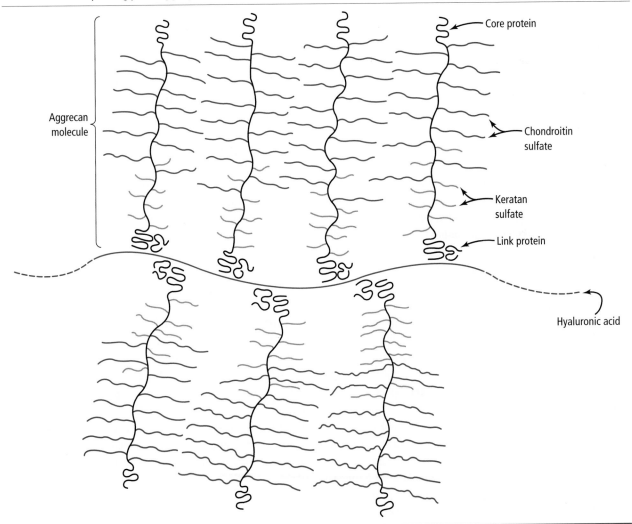

Core protein

Aggrecan molecule

Chondroitin sulfate

Keratan sulfate

Link protein

Hyaluronic acid

caused by prolonged periods of hypercalcemia or hyperphosphatemia when the solubility product for the formation of $CaHPO_4 \cdot 2H_2O$ is exceeded.

Basement membranes contain type IV collagen, laminin, and heparan sulfate proteoglycans

The basal lamina, commonly called "basement membrane" although it is structurally unrelated to biological membranes, is a specialized structure of the extracellular matrix. With a thickness of only 60 to 100 nm, it underlies layers of epithelial cells and surrounds such cells as muscle fibers and adipocytes. The nonfibrillar **type IV collagen** is a major component of the basal lamina. This collagen contains a triple helix, just like the fibrillar collagens, but the triple helix is interrupted at approximately 20 sites. These imperfections make a streamlined fibrillar structure impossible. In addition, the C terminus of the polypeptide forms a globular, nonhelical domain. *Instead of fibrils, type IV collagen forms an irregular, two-dimensional network in the basal lamina.*

Besides type IV collagen, basement membranes contain **laminin,** a large, cross-shaped glycoprotein consisting of three polypeptides (Fig. 13.15). Laminin is remarkable for its multiple binding affinities: it contains binding sites for cell surface receptors, type IV collagen, heparan sulfate proteoglycans, and the basement membrane glycoprotein entactin (nidogen). *It acts as a molecular glue that attaches the other components of the basement membrane to the overlying cells.* Laminin is an example of a **multiadhesive protein.**

Laminin binds to the cell surface through a specific transmembrane protein that functions as a laminin receptor. The major laminin receptor belongs to the **integrin** class of receptors, which consist of two transmembrane polypeptides. Integrin receptors include not only various laminin receptors but also receptors for fibronectin, fibrillar collagens, and other extracellular matrix proteins. Far from acting only as a glue, *laminin induces physiologic responses in the cells.* Some cell types proliferate or change their shape in response to laminin binding, and epithelial cells spread on laminin-coated surfaces. In this respect, *laminin acts similarly to hormones and growth factors, which also act on their target cells through cell surface receptors* (see Chapters 27 and 28).

Besides laminin and type IV collagen, basement membranes contain smaller amounts of heparan sulfate proteoglycans. These proteoglycans may be important in endothelial basement membranes that serve as filters for plasma proteins. This filter function is most evident in the double-thickness basement membrane of the renal glomerulus. *This "membrane" retains the negatively charged plasma proteins while cationic proteins of equal size can pass through.* Almost all plasma proteins have isoelectric points well below the normal blood pH of 7.4 and therefore are negatively charged. The heparan sulfate content of the glomerular basement membrane is decreased in patients with proteinuria from diabetes mellitus or other causes. This suggests that heparan sulfate proteoglycans help to form pores in the basement membrane that are lined by negative charges and therefore are less permeable to anionic than to cationic macromolecules.

Fibronectin glues cells and collagen fibers together

Fibronectin is the most abundant multiadhesive protein in connective tissues, and it even occurs as a circulating plasma protein in a concentration of approximately 30 mg/100 mL. Like laminin, it is a very large protein. It is formed from two similar polypeptides, each with a length of some 2500 amino acids, which are linked by disulfide bonds near their carboxy termini (Fig. 13.16). Many structurally different fibronectins are formed by differential splicing of the transcript from a single gene, and by the combination of the different polypeptides in the dimeric protein. Plasma fibronectin is a soluble dimer; tissue fibronectin forms disulfidebonded fibrils.

Fibronectin is formed from three different types of sequences called modules. These modules are, with considerable variations, repeated many times, forming a total of six globular domains. Not surprisingly, *most of these modules are encoded by separate exons.* Sequences homologous to the type I and type II modules also are present in some other, unrelated proteins. Apparently *both exon shuffling and exon duplication (see Chapter 8) occurred during the evolution of the fibronectin gene.*

Different parts of the molecule bind to cell surface receptors, heparan sulfate proteoglycans, fibril-

FIG. 13.15

Laminin and the structure of the basal lamina. **A,** Structure of laminin. **B,** Hypothetical position of laminin on the cell surface.

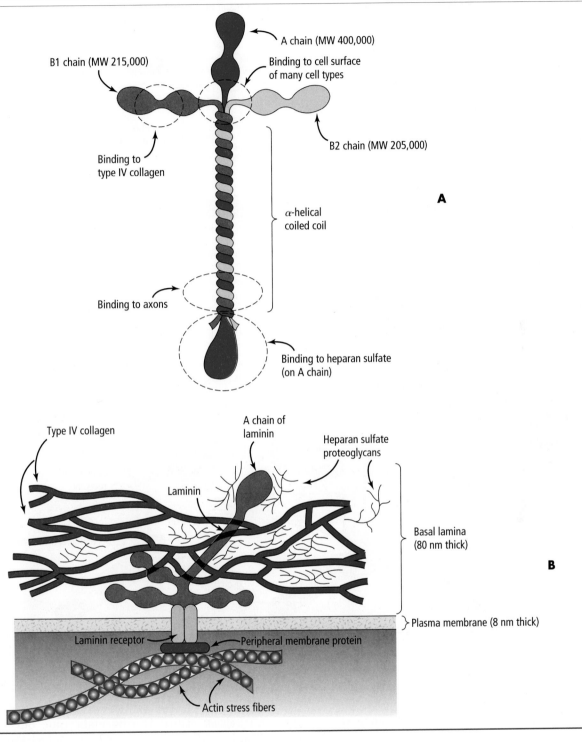

FIG. 13.16

Fibronectin and cell-to-fiber adhesion. **A,** Domain structure of fibronectin. The cell-binding site is surprisingly small, with the sequence Arg-Gly-Asp-Ser as the minimal required structure. As a result of alternative splicing, the binding site for lymphoid cells is present in some but not all fibronectins. **B,** Hypothetical position of fibronectin on the cell surface.

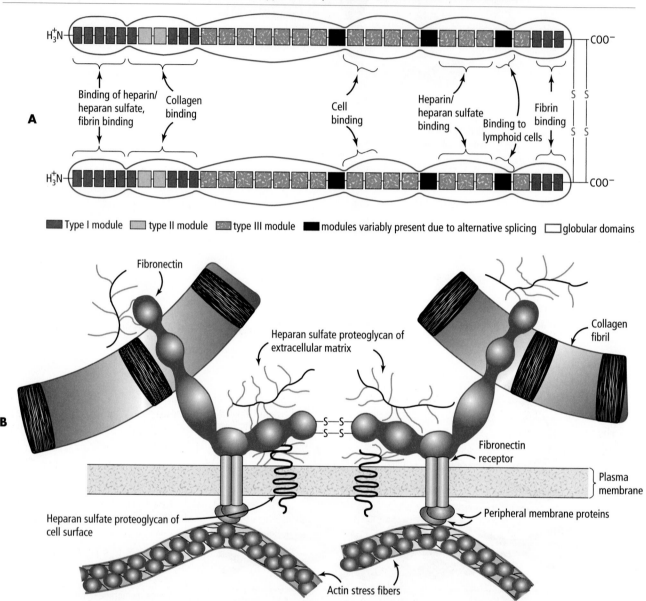

lar collagens, and fibrin. The binding to cell surface receptors of the integrin type is mediated by the surprisingly short sequence Arg-Gly-Asp-Ser in the ninth and tenth type III modules. *Fibronectin glues the cells to the fibrous meshwork of the* *extracellular matrix.* During embryonic development, fibronectin is necessary for the migration of cells along fibrous tracks. During wound healing, it is incorporated into the fibrin clot and even becomes covalently cross-linked to fibrin by transglutami-

FIG. 13.17

Synthesis of chondroitin sulfate.

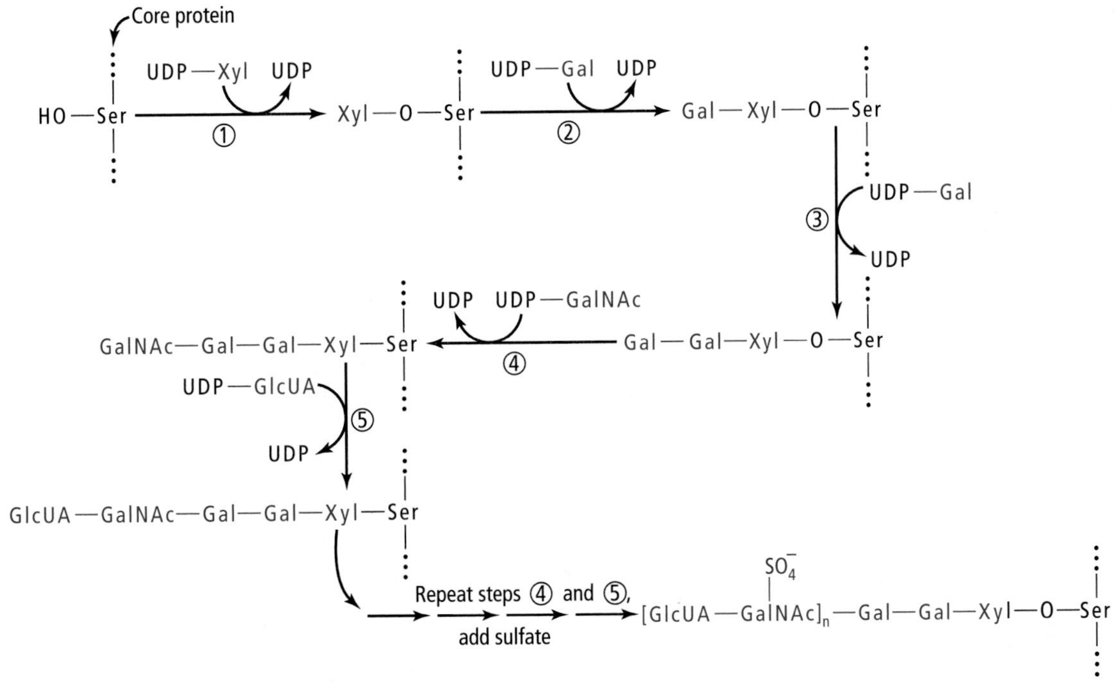

nase (factor XIII, see Chapter 25). This enmeshed fibronectin is thought to attract fibroblasts and, perhaps, endothelial cells, which play key roles in wound healing.

Malignant cells, unlike their normal counterparts, often are devoid of surface-bound fibronectin. They do, however, possess fibronectin receptors, and *the binding of these receptors to tissue fibronectin is thought to be an important event in metastasis.* In many cases, the treatment of cancerous animals with synthetic peptide analogs of the Arg-Gly-Asp-Ser recognition sequence has resulted in an inhibition of tumor metastasis, presumably because the synthetic peptide competes with tissue fibronectin for surface receptors on itinerant tumor cells.

Proteoglycans are synthesized in the ER and degraded in lysosomes

Like procollagen, the proteoglycans of the extracellular matrix are processed through the secretory pathway. *The core protein is made by ribosomes on the rough ER, and the polysaccharides are constructed in the ER and Golgi.* The precursors of the GAG chains are nucleotide-activated sugars, including UDP-N-acetylglucosamine, UDP-N-acetylgalactosamine, UDP-glucuronic acid, UDP-galactose, and UDP-xylose (Fig. 13.17, see also Chapter 8).

Some modifications are introduced in the polysaccharide after the formation of the glycosidic bonds: iduronic acid is formed by the epimerization of glucuronic acid, and sulfate groups are introduced during or after the synthesis of the polysaccharide by the transfer of sulfate from **phosphoadenosine phosphosulfate (PAPS)** (Fig. 13.18). *PAPS provides an activated sulfate for sulfation reactions much as ATP provides an activated phosphate for phosphorylation reactions.*

Unlike collagen, the proteoglycans have to be taken up into the cell by endocytosis before they can be degraded. The endocytotic vesicle becomes acidified and fuses with a lysosome, and *the GAGs are degraded by lysosomal enzymes.* Many different enzymes have to cooperate in the degradation of GAGs. The complete degradation of heparan sulfate, for example,

FIG. 13.18

Structure of phosphoadenosine phosphosulfate (PAPS), which is used as an "activated sulfate" in sulfation reactions. PAPS is biosynthetically derived from ATP. Note that the phosphate-sulfate bond is an energy-rich, mixed anhydride bond. It is cleaved when the sulfate is transferred to the acceptor.

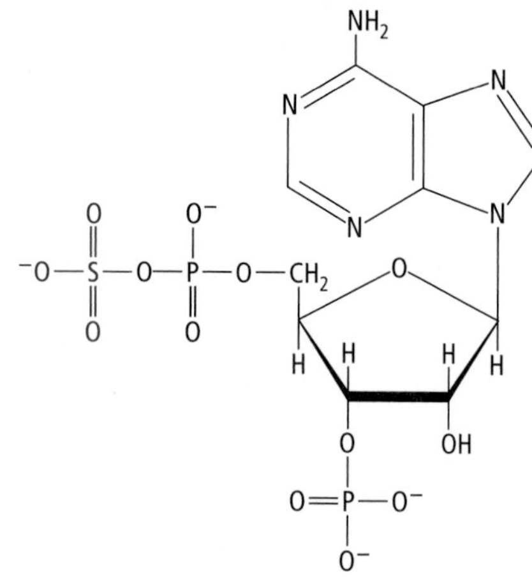

requires three different exoglycosidases, four sulfatases, and an acetyltransferase.

The major pathways for the lysosomal degradation of sulfated GAGs proceed by the *stepwise removal of monosaccharides from the nonreducing end* by exoglycosidases, together with the removal of sulfate residues by sulfatases. Only hyaluronic acid and chondroitin sulfate can be degraded by a lysosomal endoglycosidase ("hyaluronidase").

Mucopolysaccharidoses are caused by the deficiency of GAG-degrading lysosomal enzymes

The deficiency of only one of the required lysosomal enzymes can interrupt the ordered sequence of GAG degradation. As a result, *the undegraded GAGs accumulate in the lysosomes*. Some of the accumulating polysaccharide is processed to smaller fragments by endoglycosidases, and these fragments often appear in blood and urine, where they can be detected in diagnostic tests. This type of disease is called a **mucopolysaccharidosis**. Mucopolysaccharide is an obsolete name for GAG, but "glycosaminoglycanosis" does not seem to sound right. The mucopolysaccharidoses are examples of **lysosomal storage diseases.** Another group of lysosomal storage diseases,

the lipid storage diseases, will be encountered in Chapter 19.

Some features of the mucopolysaccharidoses (Table 13.5) should be emphasized:

1. *The enzyme deficiency is generalized, affecting all organ systems.* This is a feature of all lysosomal storage diseases. It applies also to the lipid storage diseases (see Chapter 19) and Pompe's disease (see Chapter 17).

2. *The diseases are inherited as autosomal recessive or (type II) X-linked recessive traits.* This means that heterozygotes, who typically have one half of the normal enzyme activity, are healthy. Heterozygotes can be identified (with difficulty) by determination of the enzyme activity in cultured leukocytes, fibroblasts, or other cells.

3. *Many mucopolysaccharidoses are known in both severe and mild forms.* Patients with severe disease have no detectable enzyme activity, whereas those with less severe disease have an enzyme with abnormally low activity. The difference between types IH and IS in Table 13.5 is an example.

4. *Most mucopolysaccharidoses are not apparent at birth,* but signs and symptoms develop gradually as more and more mucopolysaccharide accumulates.

5. *Defects in the degradation of keratan sulfate and dermatan sulfate cause skeletal deformities and other connective tissue abnormalities.* Common manifestations include coarse facial features ("gargoylism"), short stature, corneal clouding, hearing loss, joint stiffness, valvular heart disease, obstructive lung disease, and hepatosplenomegaly. All of these problems are caused by the excessive deposition of GAGs in the tissues.

6. *Only defects in heparan sulfate degradation cause mental retardation and neurological degeneration.* Heparan sulfate is the only important GAG in the central nervous system.

7. *Chondroitin sulfate and hyaluronic acid do not accumulate* because they can be alternatively degraded by lysosomal hyaluronidase, an endoglycosidase.

The mucopolysaccharidoses are rare diseases, with a combined incidence of perhaps 1 in 10,000 to 1 in 20,000 live births. Specific treatment in the form of enzyme replacement has been attempted, but success has been limited because of poor tissue uptake of the injected enzymes and because of immunological responses.

TABLE 13.5

The mucopolysaccharidoses

Systematic name	*Common name*	*Inheritance**	*Enzyme deficiency*	*GAG(s) affected*	*Clinical features*
IH	Hurler	AR	α-L-Iduronidase (complete deficiency)	Dermatan sulfate, heparan sulfate	Skeletal deformities, dwarfism, corneal clouding, hepatosplenomegaly, valvular heart disease, mental retardation, death at ≤10 years
IS	Scheie	AR	α-L-Iduronidase (partial deficiency)	Dermatan sulfate, heparan sulfate	Corneal clouding, stiff joints, normal intelligence and life span
II	Hunter	XR	Iduronate sulfatase	Dermatan sulfate, heparan sulfate	Similar to Hurler, but no corneal clouding, death at 10-15 years
IIIA	Sanfilippo A	AR	Heparan-*N*-sulfatase	Heparan sulfate	Severe to profound mental retardation, mild physical abnormalities
IIIB	Sanfilippo B	AR	α-*N*-Acetyl-glucosaminidase	Heparan sulfate	Severe to profound mental retardation, mild physical abnormalities
IIIC	Sanfilippo C	AR	Acetyl-CoA: α-glucosaminide acetyltransferase	Heparan sulfate	Severe to profound mental retardation, mild physical abnormalities
IIID	Sanfilippo D	AR	*N*-Acetylglucosamine 6-sulfatase	Heparan sulfate	Severe to profound mental retardation, mild physical abnormalities
IVA	Morquio A	AR	Galactose 6-sulfatase	Keratan sulfate	Severe skeletal deformities, corneal clouding, normal intelligence
IVB	Morquio B	AR	β-Galactosidase	Keratan sulfate	Severe skeletal deformities, corneal clouding, normal intelligence
VI	Maroteaux-Lamy	AR	*N*-Acetylgalactosamine 4-sulfatase	Dermatan sulfate	Severe skeletal deformities, corneal clouding, normal intelligence
VII	Sly	AR	β-Glucuronidase	Dermatan sulfate, heparan sulfate	Skeletal deformities, hepatosplenomegaly

* AR, Autosomal recessive; XR, X-linked recessive.

SUMMARY

The extracellular matrix of connective tissue consists of an amorphous ground substance and fibers. The most abundant fiber type is formed from collagen, a long, ropelike molecule that consists of three intertwined polypeptides. There are many types of collagen; they differ in structure, properties, and tissue distribution. Collagen is synthesized from a larger precursor called procollagen, which is processed in the organelles of the secretory pathway and extracellularly. Several inherited connective tissue diseases, including osteogenesis imperfecta and Ehlers-Danlos syndrome, are caused by abnormalities of collagen structure or biosynthesis.

The amorphous ground substance consists of proteoglycans, hyaluronic acid, and multiadhesive glycoproteins. Hyaluronic acid and the sulfated glycosaminoglycan chains of the proteoglycans are highly hydrated, with a mucilaginous or gel-like consistency. Multiadhesive glycoproteins such as laminin and fibronectin bind both to cell surfaces and to fibrous matrix proteins and thereby glue these components together. Through cell surface receptors in the plasma membrane of connective tissue cells, laminin and fibronectin establish a connection between the extracellular matrix and the cytoskeleton and regulate the growth and behavior of the cells. The mucopolysaccharidoses are lysosomal storage diseases caused by deficiencies of lysosomal enzymes for glycosaminoglycan degradation. These diseases result in connective tissue abnormalities and/or mental impairment.

Further Reading

Arnaout MA: Structure, function and regulation of cell adhesion molecules. In: Frank MM, Austen KF, Claman HN, Unanue ER: *Samter's immunologic diseases*, 5th ed., vol. 1. Little, Brown, Boston, 1995, pp. 161–182.

Loftus JC, Smith JW, Ginsberg MH: Integrin-mediated cell adhesion: the extracellular face. *J Biol Chem* 269 (41), 25235–25238, 1994.

Muir H: The chondrocyte, architect of cartilage. *BioEssays* 17 (12), 1039–1048, 1995.

Nicholls AC: Collagen disorders. In: Holton JB, editor: *The inherited metabolic diseases*, 2nd ed., Churchill Livingstone, New York, 1994, pp. 379–420.1

Roberts DD, Mecham RP, editors: *Cell surface and extracellular glycoconjugates*. Academic Press, San Diego, 1993.

Rowe DW, Shapiro JR: Heritable disorders of structural proteins. In: Kelly N, Harris ED, Ruddy S, Sledge CB: *Textbook of rheumatology*, 4th ed., vol. 2. W. B. Saunders, Philadelphia, 1993, pp. 1567–1592.

Scriver CR, Beaudet AL, Sly WS, Valle D, editors: *The metabolic basis of inherited disease*, 6th ed., vol. 2. McGraw-Hill, New York, 1989, pp. 1565–1622, pp. 2805–2842.

QUESTIONS

1. In a home for handicapped children you see an 11-year-old girl who is only 90 cm tall, wheelchair bound, and with multiple limb deformities. The nurse tells you that the girl has "glass bones" and has suffered many severe fractures. Most likely, this girl has a mutation in a gene for
   A. Type I collagen
   B. Type III collagen
   C. Elastin
   D. Fibronectin
   E. Fibrillin

2. Besides the ubiquitous type I collagen, cartilage contains large quantities of
   A. Type III collagen and fibronectin
   B. Type VII collagen and elastin
   C. Elastin and hyaluronic acid
   D. Type III collagen and laminin
   E. Type II collagen and proteoglycans

3. A first-semester medical student presents with follicular hyperkeratosis (gooseflesh), numerous small subcutaneous hemorrhages, and loose teeth. He reports that for the last 4 months he has been living only on canned foods, spaghetti, and soft drinks. The process that is most likely impaired in this student is
   A. The removal of propeptides from procollagen
   B. The hydroxylation of prolyl and lysyl residues in procollagen
   C. The formation of allysine residues in collagen
   D. The formation of covalent cross-links between allysine and lysine residues in collagen
   E. The formation of desmosine in elastin

4. Some mucopolysaccharidoses cause only connective tissue problems such as skeletal deformities, corneal clouding, or valvular heart disease. In some forms, however, the patients suffer from mental deficiency. The degradation of which glycosaminoglycan is impaired in those diseases in which mental deficiency is a prominent sign?
   A. Hyaluronic acid
   B. Chondroitin sulfate
   C. Dermatan sulfate
   D. Heparan sulfate
   E. Keratan sulfate

5. Poor mineralization leads to soft bones that bend easily. Conditions that can be expected to cause poor bone mineralization include all of the following except
   A. Increased intestinal absorption of dietary calcium
   B. Increased renal excretion of inorganic phosphate
   C. A deficiency of alkaline phosphatase in bone
   D. Chronic acidosis

PART FOUR

Metabolism

Chapter 14

Digestive Enzymes

The major dietary nutrients—most notably the polysaccharides, proteins, and nucleic acids—are large, polymeric structures. These nutrients cannot be absorbed in the intact state. They have to be hydrolyzed into their building blocks, which in turn are absorbed by the intestinal mucosa. *The whole process of digestion consists of hydrolytic cleavage reactions*, performed by digestive enzymes in the lumen of the gastrointestinal tract. Approximately 30 g of digestive enzymes are secreted per day. Most of these enzymes have narrow substrate specificities, hydrolyzing only specific bonds in their substrates. Therefore several enzymes have to cooperate in the digestion of more complex nutrients such as proteins and polysaccharides (Table 14.1).

Saliva contains α-amylase and lysozyme

The major function of saliva is not the digestion of nutrients but the conversion of food into a homogeneous mass during mastication. The only noteworthy enzymes in saliva are **α-amylase** and **lysozyme.** α-Amylase cleaves α-1,4 glycosidic bonds in starch. Starch occurs in two forms. **Amylose** (see Fig. 1.5, *A*, Chapter 1) is a polymer of glucose, linked by α-1,4 glycosidic bonds. **Amylopectin**, which usually forms the larger part of the starch in plants,

TABLE 14.1

Dietary nutrients and their fates in the gastrointestinal tract

Nutrient	Products generated	Enzymes	Sites of digestion
Starch, glycogen	Glucose	α-Amylase, di- and oligosaccharidases	Saliva, intestinal lumen, brush border
Maltose	Glucose	Glucoamylase, sucrase	}
Sucrose	Glucose + fructose	Sucrase	Brush border
Lactose	Glucose + galactose	Lactase	
Proteins	Amino acids, di- and tripeptides	Pepsin, pancreatic enzymes, brush border enzymes	Stomach, intestinal lumen, brush border
Triglycerides	Fatty acids, 2-mono-acylglycerol	Pancreatic lipase	Intestinal lumen
Nucleic acids	Nucleosides, bases	DNAses, RNAses	Intestinal lumen
"Fiber": cellulose, hemicelluloses, lignin, etc.	Acetate, propionate, lactate, H_2, CH_4, CO_2	Only very limited fermentation by colon bacteria	

FIG. 14.1

The pattern of starch digestion by α-amylase. This enzyme acts strictly as an endoglycosidase. It is unable to cleave the bonds in maltose, maltotriose, and the α-limit dextrins. ↓, Cleavage sites.

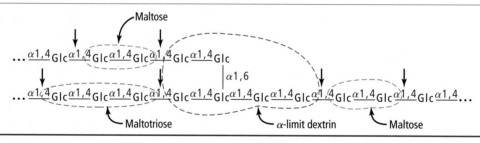

is a branched molecule with a variable number of α-1,6 glycosidic bonds in addition to the α-1,4 bonds.

α-Amylase is an **endoglycosidase.** In contrast to **exoglycosidases,** which remove monosaccharides from the ends of an oligo- or polysaccharide, endoglycosidases cleave internal bonds. Indeed, α-amylase does not act on di- and trisaccharides, and therefore it produces **maltose, maltotriose,** and **α-limit dextrins** rather than free glucose (Fig. 14.1). Maltose is a disaccharide; maltotriose is a trisaccharide of glucose residues in α-1,4 glycosidic linkage, and α-limit dextrins are oligosaccharides containing an α-1,6 glycosidic bond. α-Amylase is active at the normal salivary pH of 6.5 to 7.0, but it is rapidly denatured in the acidic environment of the stomach. Therefore it makes only a minor contribu-

tion to starch digestion. It does, however, keep the teeth clean by dissolving starchy bits of food that remain lodged between the teeth after a meal. Cancer patients whose salivary glands have been destroyed by radiation therapy develop rapid tooth decay.

The other salivary enzyme, **lysozyme** (see Chapter 4), is also an endoglycosidase. Its substrate specificity, however, is radically different from that of α-amylase. It hydrolyzes β-1,4 glycosidic bonds in **peptidoglycan,** a cross-linked polysaccharide in bacterial cell walls (Fig. 4.16, Chapter 4). Although *lysozyme can kill some types of bacteria,* others are resistant because their peptidoglycan is protected from the enzyme by other cell wall components or (in gram-negative bacteria) by an overlying outer membrane. Indeed, saliva contains a lush bacterial flora that is harmless and that even helps in the suppression of pathogenic bacteria and yeasts. Nevertheless, many other bacteria are killed by lysozyme, and wounded animals make use of this effect by licking their wounds.

Protein digestion starts in the stomach

With a pH close to 2.0, the stomach provides an extremely acidic environment. The proton gradient between gastric juice and the blood—an almost millionfold concentration difference—is the steepest ion gradient anywhere in the body. This acidic environment is functionally very important:

1. *It is fatal for most microorganisms,* so bacterial counts are extremely low in the stomach. Many food-acquired intestinal infections are aided by achlorhydria (lack of gastric acid) or gastrectomy (surgical removal of the stomach). Also, pathogens are more likely to establish an intestinal infection when ingested in water or other fluids than in solid food because solid foods remain in the stomach far longer than do fluids.
2. *Dietary proteins become denatured by gastric acid.* This is important for protein digestion because proteins in their native conformation often are poor substrates for proteases.
3. *The acidic environment is required for the action of* **pepsin.** Pepsin is a protease that works optimally at pH values close to 2.0. Pepsin is a *carboxyl protease* (see Chapter 4). Its catalytic mechanism requires two aspartate side chains in the active site, one in the protonated form and the other in the deprotonated form.

Pepsin acts mostly as an **endopeptidase.** Endopeptidases cleave peptide bonds in the interior of a poly- or oligopeptide. **Exopeptidases,** on the other hand, remove amino acids from the end of the peptide. **Aminopeptidases** are exopeptidases that attack the amino terminus of the peptide; **carboxypeptidases** act on the carboxy terminus.

Pepsin does not cleave at random. It prefers peptide bonds formed by the amino groups of aromatic and other large hydrophobic amino acids. Therefore the major breakdown products are not free amino acids but rather a mixture of oligopeptides, known as **peptones.** Neither gastric acid nor pepsin is essential for life, and protein digestion still is possible after total gastrectomy.

Most digestive enzymes in the small intestine are derived from the pancreas

As the acidic stomach contents reach the duodenum, they are rapidly neutralized by bicarbonate in the pancreatic secretions. The exocrine pancreas is a factory for a large number of digestive enzymes that attack all major kinds of nutrients. Copious amounts of α-amylase are secreted by the pancreas. This pancreatic α-amylase differs chemically from the salivary enzyme, but it has essentially the same cleavage specificity. *Closely related enzymes that catalyze the same reaction but differ in their molecular structure, kinetic parameters, electrophoretic mobility, or other properties are called* **isoenzymes.**

Proteolytic enzymes from the pancreas include the endopeptidases **trypsin, chymotrypsin,** and **elastase.** *All three are serine proteases* (see Chapter 4), but they differ in their cleavage specificities (Table 14.2). They degrade the peptones to ever smaller peptide fragments. Their action is complemented by **carboxypeptidases A and B,** which act on the carboxy termini of the peptides to remove nonpolar and basic amino acids, respectively. Several other enzymes are contributed by the pancreas, including **pancreatic lipase,** various **phospholipases,** and **nucleases.**

Fat digestion requires bile salts

The digestion of dietary triglycerides is complicated by their insolubility. Triglycerides tend to form large droplets in water that provide only a small surface area for enzymatic attack. A small fraction of dietary triglycerides are digested by an acid-stable **lingual lipase,** which is secreted by glands at the base of the tongue and which can function in the acidic environment of the stomach. Together with phospholipids and other emulsifiers already present in the food, the free (unesterified) fatty acids produced by the lingual lipase disperse the dietary fat into small emulsion droplets.

Pancreatic lipase binds to these emulsion droplets with the aid of a **colipase.** This colipase is a small protein, secreted by the pancreas as an inactive pre-

TABLE 14.2

Enzymes of protein digestion

Enzyme	Source	Type	Catalytic mechanism	Cleavage specificity
Pepsin	Stomach	Endopeptidase	Carboxyl protease	NH-side of hydrophobic amino acids
Trypsin	Pancreas	Endopeptidase	Serine protease	CO-side of basic amino acids
Chymotrypsin	Pancreas	Endopeptidase	Serine protease	CO-side of hydrophobic amino acids
Elastase	Pancreas	Endopeptidase	Serine protease	CO-side of small amino acids
Carboxypeptidase A	Pancreas	Carboxypeptidase	Metalloprotease (Zn^{2+})	Hydrophobic amino acids at C terminus
Carboxypeptidase B	Pancreas	Carboxypeptidase	Metalloprotease (Zn^{2+})	Basic amino acids at C terminus

FIG. 14.2

The action of pancreatic lipase on dietary triglycerides: only two of the three fatty acids are released. Fatty acids and 2-monoacylglycerol are sufficiently water soluble to diffuse from the mixed bile salt micelles to the mucosal cell surface. They are also sufficiently lipid soluble to diffuse through the plasma membrane of the mucosal cells.

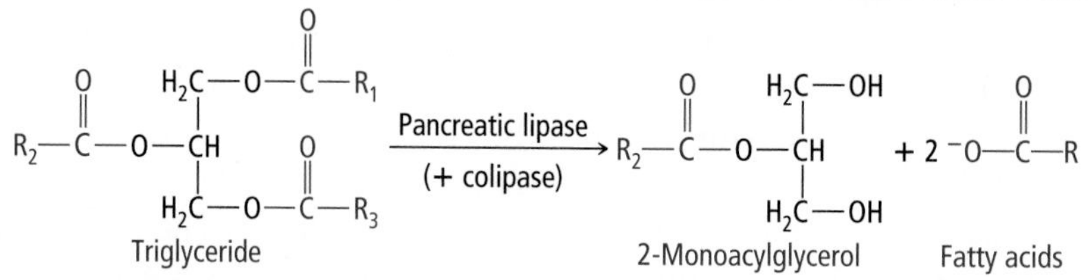

cursor that is activated by trypsin in the duodenum. *Pancreatic lipase hydrolyzes dietary triglycerides to free fatty acids and 2-monoacylglycerol* (Fig. 14.2). Unlike the triglycerides, which are essentially insoluble, *the products of fat digestion are slightly soluble in water.*

The effective absorption of fatty acids and 2-monoacylglycerol requires the presence of **bile salts,** amphipathic products that act as emulsifiers in the small intestine (Fig. 14.3). Between 20 and 50 g of bile salts reaches the intestine every day. The bile salts form **micelles** in which their hydrophilic surface faces the aqueous surroundings while the hydrophobic surface associates with lipids (Fig. 14.4). In their natural habitat in the small intestine, the micelles acquire fatty acids, 2-monoacylglycerol, and other lipids. The resulting **mixed micelles** are lamellar structures. With diameters between 4 and 60 nm, they are much smaller than emulsion droplets. Being small and diffusible, *they ferry the lipids rapidly through the unstirred layer overlying the intestinal mucosa.* From the mixed micelles, fatty acids and 2-monoacylglycerol diffuse to the brush border and

enter the mucosal cells, probably by passive diffusion across the microvillar membrane. Bile salts facilitate the absorption not only of fatty acids and 2-monoacylglycerol but also of other dietary lipids, including cholesterol and the fat-soluble vitamins. In general, *those lipids with the lowest water solubility are most dependent on bile salts for their absorption.*

Fat malabsorption can result from pancreatic failure, lack of bile salts, or extensive intestinal diseases. Patients with pancreatic failure have bulky, fatty stools that contain undigested triglycerides. This condition is called **steatorrhea.** Because of impaired micelle formation, patients with pancreatic failure also are unable to absorb other dietary lipids, exposing them to deficiencies of fat-soluble vitamins. A lack of bile salts has similar consequences: although most of the dietary fat still is digested, the breakdown products are absorbed incompletely, and approximately one third of the dietary fat appears in the stools in the form of free fatty acids, mono-, di-, and triglycerides.

Fat malabsorption can be treated effectively by

FIG. 14.3

Structure of glycocholate, the most abundant bile salt in humans. The protonated forms of the bile salts are called "bile acids." **A,** Structure. **B,** Stereochemistry. Note that the molecule has a hydrophilic surface and a hydrophobic surface.

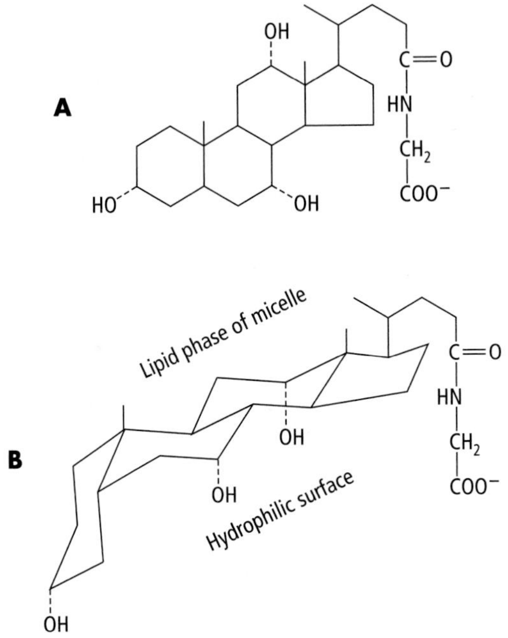

TABLE 14.3

Disaccharidases and oligosaccharidases of the intestinal brush border

Enzyme	Cleavage specificity
Glucoamylase	Maltose, maltotriose, acts as exo-glycosidase on α-1,4 bonds at the nonreducing end of starch and starch-derived oligosaccharides
Sucrase	Sucrose, maltose, maltotriose
Isomaltase	α-1,6 Bonds in isomaltose and α-limit dextrins
Lactase*	Lactose; also cellobiose†
Cerebrosidase*	Gluco- and galactocerebroside
Trehalase	Trehalose‡

* The lactase and cerebrosidase activities reside in two different globular domains of the same polypeptide (see Fig. 14.5).
† Cellobiose is a disaccharide of two glucose residues in β-1,4 glycosidic linkage.
‡ Trehalose is a disaccharide of two glucose residues in α,α'-1,1 glycosidic linkage; common only in mushrooms and insects.

replacement therapy. Both pancreatic enzymes and bile salts are available in tablet form and are used routinely in patients with pancreatic insufficiency or biliary disease.

The digestion of proteins and carbohydrates is completed in the intestinal brush border

Although the crypts of Lieberkühn in the small intestine secrete between 1 and 2 L of a watery fluid every day, this secretion is almost devoid of digestive enzymes. Digestive enzymes are, however, present on the lumenal surface of the intestinal mucosal cells. This surface, known as the **brush border,** may measure more than 200 m² because of the extensive folding of the villi and the innumerable microvilli. Various endopeptidases, aminopeptidases, carboxypeptidases, and **dipeptidases** of the brush border act on the small oligopeptides formed by pepsin and the pancreatic enzymes. Nevertheless, a sizable portion of the di-

etary protein is absorbed not in the form of free amino acids but rather as di- and tripeptides. These are further hydrolyzed to free amino acids by cytoplasmic enzymes in the mucosal cells.

Disaccharidases and **oligosaccharidases** (Table 14.3) hydrolyze the dietary disaccharides sucrose and lactose, as well as the maltose, maltotriose, and α-limit dextrins that are formed by the action of α-amylase on starch.

The brush border enzymes are firmly attached to the cell surface, with their catalytic domains protruding into the intestinal lumen (Fig. 14.5).

Not everything can be digested

The digestion of most nutrients is incomplete: approximately 95% of the dietary fat and variable proportions of other dietary lipids are utilized. Starch is digested with an efficiency of 70% to 90%, depending on the dietary source. Protein digestion is somewhat variable. Keratins and some plant proteins are incompletely digested, but overall no more than 5 to 20 g of protein is excreted in the stools every day. The digested protein includes not only dietary protein but also considerable amounts from secreted digestive enzymes and desquamated mucosal cells.

FIG. 14.4

Sequence of events in fat digestion. Other dietary lipids (cholesterol, phospholipids, fat-soluble vitamins, etc.) are absorbed by the same mechanism, requiring mixed bile salt micelles for their diffusion to the brush border.

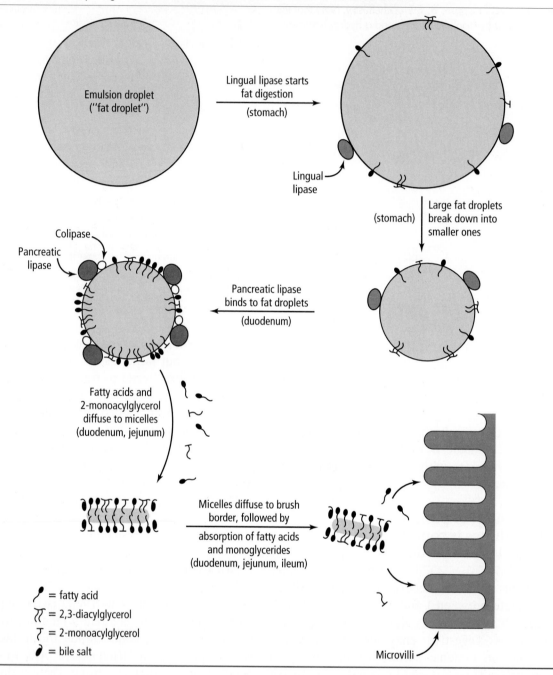

Emulsion droplet ("fat droplet")

Lingual lipase starts fat digestion (stomach)

Lingual lipase

(stomach) Large fat droplets break down into smaller ones

Colipase

Pancreatic lipase

Pancreatic lipase binds to fat droplets (duodenum)

Fatty acids and 2-monoacylglycerol diffuse to micelles (duodenum, jejunum)

Micelles diffuse to brush border, followed by absorption of fatty acids and monoglycerides (duodenum, jejunum, ileum)

Microvilli

= fatty acid

= 2,3-diacylglycerol

= 2-monoacylglycerol

= bile salt

Some polymers in vegetables, including cellulose, hemicelluloses, inulin, pectin, lignin, and suberin, are not attacked by our digestive enzymes at all. A small percentage of this undigestible "dietary fiber" is hydrolyzed and anaerobically fermented by the lush bacterial flora of the colon. Important products of this bacterial fermentation include the gases **hydrogen, methane,** and **carbon dioxide** (a potentially flammable mixture) and the organic acids **acetate, propionate, butyrate,** and **lactate.** Both the gases and the acids are for the most part absorbed through the colonic mucosa.

FIG. 14.5

Anchoring of disaccharidases to the surface of the microvilli in the intestinal brush border. The sucrase-isomaltase complex is biosynthetically derived from a single polypeptide that is cleaved by pancreatic proteases. Isomaltase and lactase/cerebrosidase have transmembrane α-helices; trehalase is anchored by glycosyl phosphatidylinositol (see Fig. 11.12, Chapter 11). All of these enzymes are glycoproteins.

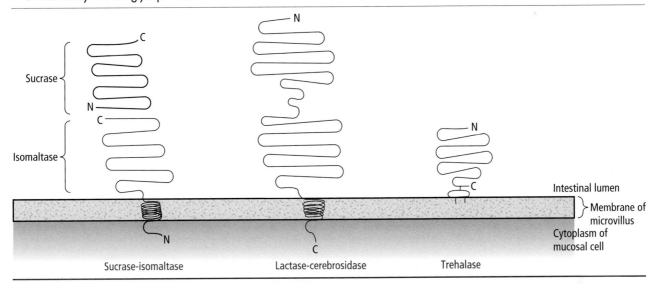

Some vegetables contain undigestible carbohydrates that nevertheless are consumed avidly by colon bacteria. Beans and peas, for example, contain raffinose (galactose-glucose-fructose), stachyose (galactose-galactose-glucose-fructose), and other oligosaccharides with galactose residues in α-1,6-glycosidic linkage. Upon entering the colon, these oligosaccharides are rapidly fermented to acids and gas. The result is harmless but distressing: in addition to flatulence, abdominal discomfort can occur because of the irritant effect of the acids on the intestinal mucosa and the osmotic activity of the deprotonated acids.

Also, any gastrointestinal condition that impairs the digestion of otherwise well-digested carbohydrates or proteins is likely to cause flatulence. These conditions often can be treated with orally administered digestive enzymes.

Many adults cannot digest large amounts of lactose

The disaccharide **lactose** is abundant only in milk and milk products. It therefore is not surprising that the activity of intestinal lactase is maximal in infants and tends to decline in later life. In some people, a high lactase activity is maintained throughout life. Individuals with this phenotype, called **lactase persistence,** can digest almost any amount of lactose. In others, the lactase activity declines to only 5% to 10% of the original level. In this situation, called **lactase restriction,** the consumption of more than 200 to 800 ml of milk results in intestinal discomfort with flatulence, abdominal pain, and diarrhea. These effects are caused by the osmotic activity of the undigested lactose and by the excessive formation of gas and acids by intestinal bacteria (including our old friend *Escherichia coli;* see the *lac* operon, Chapter 6), for whom lactose is a welcome treat. Individuals with lactase restriction therefore show **lactose intolerance.** Lactose intolerance is not an important clinical problem because most people have enough common sense to adjust their milk intake to their digestive capacity. It should be routinely considered, however, in patients with ill-defined abdominal complaints ("irritable bowel syndrome").

Various lactase preparations are commercially available. They are taken in tablet form or are mixed with the milk. These pharmaceutical products contain lactases of microbial origin.

Lactase persistence is a simple Mendelian trait that is dominant over lactase restriction. In most parts of the world, the majority of the population

TABLE 14.4

Approximate prevalence of lactase restriction (nonpersistent lactase) in various populations

Population/country	% With low lactose-digesting capacity
Sweden	1
Britain	6
Germany	15
Greece	53
Morocco	78
Tuareg (Niger)	13
Fulani (Nigeria, Senegal)	0-22
Ibo, Yoruba (Nigeria)	89
Saudi Arabia: Bedouins	23
Other Arabs	56
India (different areas)	27-67
Thailand	98
China	93-100
North American Indians	63-95

has the lactase-restricted phenotype. Lactase persistence prevails only in Europeans and in some desert nomads of Arabia and Africa (Table 14.4). Most other mammalian species have a nonpersistent lactase, and lactase persistence is thought to have evolved quite recently in populations where adults have developed the habit of consuming the milk of such domestic animals as cattle, horses, camels, or reindeer. This may very well be the case for the natives of northern Europe: according to an early anthropologist, "They [the Germans] do not eat much cereal food, but live chiefly on milk and meat. . . ." *

Biochemically, lactase restriction can be demonstrated in two ways. In the **lactose tolerance test,** which closely resembles the procedure of the glucose tolerance test (see Chapter 29), the blood glucose level is determined before and after the ingestion of 50 g of lactose. A rise in blood glucose of less than 20 mg/100 ml indicates lactase restriction. Alternatively, the hydrogen content of breath can be determined before and after an oral lactose load. An increased hydrogen content indicates that undigested lactose has been fermented by colon bacteria.

Many digestive enzymes are released as inactive precursors

Like other extracellular proteins, *digestive enzymes are produced by the secretory pathway* (see Chapter 8), with an N-terminal signal sequence that is removed in the endoplasmic reticulum (ER) during or shortly after translation. Among the digestive enzymes, the proteases and phospholipases are dangerous fellows because *they can potentially attack proteins and membrane lipids in the cells in which they are synthesized.* Self-digestion is prevented by an elegant mechanism: the dangerous enzymes (but not lipases and glycosidases) are synthesized and secreted as inactive precursors called **zymogens.** The zymogens are stored in the synthesizing cells within membrane-bound vesicles called **zymogen granules.** The zymogens are released by exocytosis and activated by selective proteolytic cleavage in the lumen of the GI tract.

Pepsinogen, after its secretion from the chief cells of the stomach, is converted to active pepsin by the proteolytic removal of a 44-amino-acid peptide from its amino terminus. This reaction occurs by autoactivation at pH values below 5. At pH values above 2.0, the cleaved peptide remains bound to pepsin, masking its active site and thereby acting as a pepsin inhibitor. With or without the bound peptide, *pepsin is essentially inactive at pH values close to 7.0.*

The pancreatic zymogens include **trypsinogen, chymotrypsinogen** (Fig. 14.6), **proelastase, procarboxypeptidases,** and **prophospholipases.** *All of these zymogens are activated by trypsin in the intestinal lumen.* Trypsinogen itself is activated to trypsin either by trypsin or by the duodenal enzyme **enteropeptidase.**

The pancreas protects itself not only by synthesizing the more dangerous enzymes as inactive zymogens, but also by a **trypsin inhibitor.** The pancreatic trypsin inhibitor is a small (6-kDa) polypeptide that binds very tightly (but noncovalently) to trypsin. It is present in the cytoplasm of the acinar cells and in the ductal system, where it inactivates any trypsin that is erroneously activated within the organ.

Despite these protective mechanisms, the premature activation of pancreatic zymogens does occur

---

* Caesar, *Gallic War* 4,1. Archeological evidence shows that the traditional staple food in northern Europe actually consisted of a porridge prepared from crushed grains and cow's milk.

FIG. 14.6

Activation of chymotrypsinogen to chymotrypsin. These reactions take place in the duodenum. Although π-chymotrypsin is fully active, α-chymotrypsin is the predominant form in the small intestine.

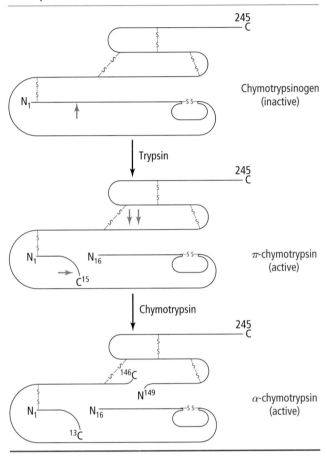

but the "brush border enzymes" of the small intestine are membrane proteins on the surface of the mucosal cells.

Proteins first are denatured by gastric acid and then are digested by pepsin in the stomach and by the pancreatic enzymes trypsin, chymotrypsin, elastase, carboxypeptidase A, and carboxypeptidase B in the lumen of the small intestine. Their digestion is completed by aminopeptidases and dipeptidases on the surface of the intestinal mucosal cells. Starch is digested to maltose, maltotriose, and α-limit dextrins by the pancreatic α-amylase, and these products are hydrolyzed to free glucose by brush border enzymes. Also, the dietary disaccharides sucrose and lactose are hydrolyzed by brush border enzymes. Dietary triglycerides are digested to free fatty acids and 2-monoacylglycerol by pancreatic lipase, and these breakdown products are absorbed with the aid of bile salts.

The digestive enzymes are products of the "secretory pathway." Proteases and phospholipases generally are synthesized as inactive zymogens that are activated by partial proteolysis in the lumen of the GI tract.

Further Reading

Berk JE: Gas. In: Haubrich WS, Schaffner F, Berk JE, editors: *Gastroenterology*, 5th ed., vol. 1. W. B. Saunders, Philadelphia, 1995, pp. 113-128.

Haubrich WS, Schaffner F, Berk JE, editors: *Gastroenterology*, 5th ed., vol. 2. W. B. Saunders, Philadelphia, 1995, pp. 955-975, 1087-1100.

Johnson LR, et al, editors: *Physiology of the gastrointestinal tract*, 3rd ed., vol. 2. Raven Press, New York, 1994, pp. 1723-1934.

Scriver CR, Beaudet AL, Sly WS, Valle D, editors: *The metabolic basis of inherited disease*, 6th ed., vol. 2. McGraw-Hill, New York, 1989, pp. 2975-3006.

in **acute pancreatitis**, an often life-threatening condition in which the pancreas digests itself. The enzymes not only wreak havoc within the pancreas, they also spill over into the abdominal cavity, where the pancreatic lipase finds ample substrate in the intraabdominal adipose tissue. Acute pancreatitis is diagnosed by the determination of lipase or amylase in the blood (see Chapter 25).

SUMMARY

Digestion consists of hydrolytic cleavage reactions in which macromolecular nutrients are hydrolyzed to their monomeric building blocks. Most digestive enzymes are secreted into the lumen of the GI tract,

QUESTIONS

1. A Chinese student complains to the school physician at the U.S. medical school where he is studying that he suffers from bouts of flatulence and diarrhea shortly after each breakfast. His usual breakfast consists of two candy bars, a small bag of potato chips, and three glasses of fresh milk.

He never had digestive problems in his home country, where his diet consisted only of rice and vegetables. He most likely has a low level of

A. Pepsin
B. Pancreatic lipase
C. Lactase
D. Trypsin
E. α-Amylase

2. Patients who have had a pancreatectomy (surgical removal of the pancreas) should take supplements of digestive enzymes with each meal. These enzyme supplements need not contain

A. α-Amylase
B. Proteases
C. Lipase
D. Disaccharidases

Chapter 15

Introduction to Metabolic Pathways

The metabolic activities of cells are dictated by two major concerns:

1. *The cell has to synthesize the macromolecules that are required for its structure and function.* Proteins have to be synthesized from amino acids, complex carbohydrates from monosaccharides, membrane lipids from fatty acids and other building blocks, and nucleic acids from nucleotides.

2. *Energy is required* for biosynthetic activity, for the active transport of inorganic ions and other substrates across membranes, and for various specialized functions. This energy has to be generated by the degradation of dietary nutrients to simple-structured metabolic intermediates and their eventual oxidation to carbon dioxide and water.

An unsuspecting nutrient molecule entering a cell therefore has two possible fates: it can be used as a building block for the synthesis of a cellular macromolecule, or it can be degraded and eventually oxidized to carbon dioxide and water. These degradative processes are coupled with the generation of metabolic energy in the form of ATP.

The accumulation of a protein, polysaccharide, lipid, or other biosynthetic product would be injurious to the cell, so these macromolecules have to be degraded again by hydrolytic cleavage reactions (pathway ② in Fig. 15.1). A **steady state** has to be maintained in which the rates of synthesis and degradation are balanced and the amount of the biosynthetic product remains constant.

Different nutrients also can be interconverted through metabolic intermediates (pathways ③ and ④ in Fig. 15.1). Most amino acids, for example, can be converted to glucose, and glucose can be converted to fatty acids.

Those processes in which a larger or more elaborate molecule is produced from simple-structured precursors are called **anabolic**, and those that de-

FIG. 15.1

The major types of metabolic activity in the cell.

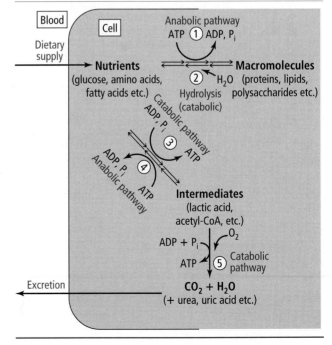

FIG. 15.2

The metabolic functions of the major organelles.

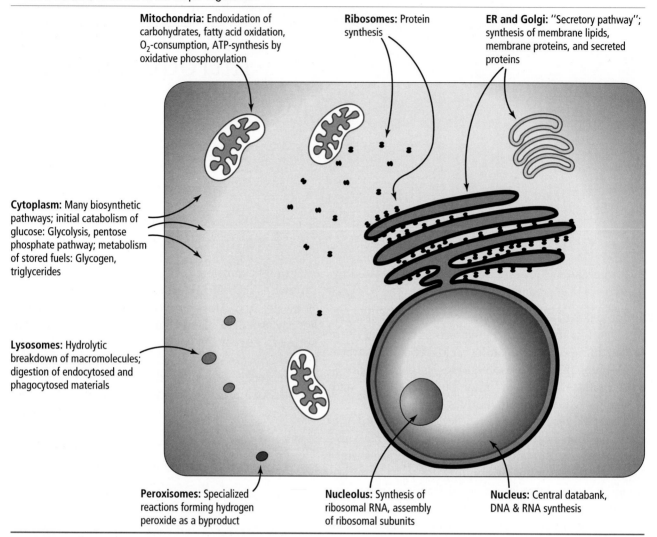

Mitochondria: Endoxidation of carbohydrates, fatty acid oxidation, O_2-consumption, ATP-synthesis by oxidative phosphorylation

Ribosomes: Protein synthesis

ER and Golgi: "Secretory pathway"; synthesis of membrane lipids, membrane proteins, and secreted proteins

Cytoplasm: Many biosynthetic pathways; initial catabolism of glucose: Glycolysis, pentose phosphate pathway; metabolism of stored fuels: Glycogen, triglycerides

Lysosomes: Hydrolytic breakdown of macromolecules; digestion of endocytosed and phagocytosed materials

Peroxisomes: Specialized reactions forming hydrogen peroxide as a byproduct

Nucleolus: Synthesis of ribosomal RNA, assembly of ribosomal subunits

Nucleus: Central databank, DNA & RNA synthesis

grade a complex molecule to simple products are called catabolic. As a general rule, *anabolic processes require metabolic energy* in the form of ATP or some other "energy-rich" metabolite, whereas *catabolic processes are exergonic and often are coupled to ATP synthesis*. Most of the ATP is produced during the endoxidation of metabolic intermediates by oxidative reactions in the mitochondria (pathway ⑤ in Fig. 15.1).

Metabolic processes are compartmentalized

The eukaryotic cell is partitioned by membranous structures that form organelles. Each organelle has

its own enzymatic outfit and is in charge of distinctive metabolic activities. As shown in Fig. 15.2, the cytoplasm, the endoplasmic reticulum (ER), and the Golgi apparatus are concerned mainly with biosynthetic reactions. The cytoplasm also performs tasks in the initial, anaerobic degradation of nutrients, particularly carbohydrates.

The mitochondria are the powerhouses of the cell. They use molecular oxygen to oxidize nutrients and metabolic intermediates to carbon dioxide and water. The lysosomes are "catabolic" organelles, but their task is limited to the hydrolysis of cellular macromolecules and of endo- or phagocytosed materials. They do not produce ATP.

BOX 15.1

Ethanol $\xrightarrow[\Delta G^{0'} = +5.5 \text{ kcal/mol}]{\text{NAD}^+ \quad ① \quad \text{NADH, H}^+}$ Acetaldehyde $\xrightarrow[\Delta G^{01} = -12.9 \text{ kcal/mol}]{\text{NAD}^+, \text{H}_2\text{O} \quad ② \quad \text{NADH, H}^+}$ Acetic acid

$$\Delta G^{0'} = +0.7 \text{ kcal/mol} \quad ③$$

GTP, CoA-SH

GMP, PP$_i$

Acetyl-CoA

Both the organellar membranes and the plasma membrane contain numerous carriers that permit the exchange of metabolites among the different compartments.

The free energy changes in metabolic pathways are additive

Most metabolic processes, such as the synthesis of glucose from lactic acid, the synthesis of cholesterol from acetyl-CoA, and the oxidation of acetyl-CoA to carbon dioxide and water, do not consist of a single reaction. They require a whole sequence of reactions that form a **metabolic pathway**. *The direction in which the pathway proceeds depends on the sum of the free energy changes of the individual reactions.* Let us consider the simple pathway shown in Box 15.1. Under standard conditions this pathway will proceed to the right, although two of the three reactions are endergonic: the sum of the standard free energy changes is -6.7 kcal/mol. The actual free energy changes, however, may be quite different from the standard free energy changes. Reaction ①, for example, has a very unfavorable equilibrium. With equal concentrations of NAD$^+$ and NADH, there would be only one molecule of acetaldehyde at equilibrium for every 10,000 molecules of ethanol (see Table 4.2 in Chapter 4). Under aerobic conditions, however, [NAD$^+$] is always far higher than [NADH]. If [NAD$^+$] is 100 times higher than [NADH], for example, we have to expect one molecule of acetaldehyde in equilibrium with 100 molecules of ethanol, and with an [NAD$^+$]/[NADH]

ratio of 1000, the [ethanol]/[acetaldehyde] ratio is 10. Therefore this seemingly "irreversible" reaction is actually "reversible" under normal cellular conditions.

Reaction ③ appears freely reversible with its $\Delta G^{0'}$ of $+0.7$ kcal/mol. Under "real cell" conditions, however, the GTP concentration is some 100 times higher than the GMP concentration, and the level of inorganic pyrophosphate (PP$_i$) is extremely low because this product is rapidly cleaved to inorganic phosphate by various pyrophosphatases. Therefore this reaction actually proceeds only in the direction of acetyl-CoA formation.

The terms **"freely reversible"** and **"(physiologically) irreversible"** are used to indicate whether or not a reaction can proceed in both directions under ordinary cellular conditions.

Most metabolic pathways are regulated

The activities of metabolic pathways have to be adjusted to the physiological needs of both the cell and the organism. Three major possibilities exist for the regulation of enzymes in a pathway:

1. *The amount of the enzyme can be adjusted by a change in its rate of synthesis or degradation.* In Chapter 6 we encountered an example of this type of regulation, which is called **adaptive control**, in the lactose operon of the bacterium *Escherichia coli*. Similar mechanisms are at work in our cells, too. Metabolic enzymes have lifespans ranging from 1 hour to several days, so this is a long-term type of regulation.

2. *Some enzymes can be modified covalently, most often by the phosphorylation and dephosphorylation of specific amino acid side chains.* Either the phosphorylated or the dephosphorylated enzyme may be the catalytically active form. This regulatory mechanism requires a **protein kinase** (phosphorylating enzyme) and a **protein phosphatase** (dephosphorylating enzyme):

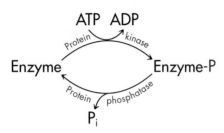

Protein kinases and protein phosphatases are regulated enzymes themselves. They respond to either metabolites or hormones.

3. *Some metabolic enzymes are regulated directly by allosteric effectors.* In most cases the allosteric effector is a substrate, intermediate, or product of the pathway. Some enzymes are regulated both by phosphorylation/dephosphorylation and by allosteric effectors. In these cases the equilibrium between an active and an inactive conformation is affected both by covalent modification and by the reversible, noncovalent binding of allosteric effectors (see Fig. 17.16, Chapter 17 for two examples).

4. Competitive inhibition is most important in the form of **product inhibition:** the product of the reaction competes with the substrate by forming an enzyme-product complex.

Feedback inhibition and feedforward stimulation are the most important regulatory principles

Let us consider a simple anabolic pathway in which a biosynthetic product such as heme, cholesterol, or a purine is synthesized from a simple precursor:

$$\text{Substrate A} \xrightarrow{(1)} \text{B} \xrightarrow{(2)} \text{C} \xrightarrow{(3)} \text{D} \xrightarrow{(4)} \text{Product E}$$

This pathway has to be active when the end product E is needed. When there is already an oversupply of product E, on the other hand, the pathway has to be inhibited. In fact, *anabolic pathways generally are inhibited by high concentrations of the end product.* This principle of regulation is called **feedback inhibition** (Fig. 15.3, *A*).

Not all enzymes in a pathway are regulated. Short-term regulation, in particular, affects only one or a few enzymes in the pathway. Which enzyme is most suitable for regulation?

1. *A regulated enzyme has to be present in lower activity in vivo than the other enzymes in the pathway:* it has to catalyze the rate-limiting step.
2. *It should serve an essential function in only one metabolic pathway.*
3. *It should catalyze the first irreversible reaction of the pathway.* This reaction is called the **committed step.** Regulation of the committed step ensures that only the substrate of the pathway accumulates when the regulated enzyme is inhibited. If a later reaction were regulated, one or more metabolic intermediates would accumulate and possibly cause toxic effects. The inhibition of enzyme ④ in the pathway shown earlier, for example, would inevitably result in an undesirable buildup of intermediate D, and possibly C and B as well.

FIG. 15.3

Regulation of metabolic pathways. The indicated regulatory influences (−−−$\pm$→, stimulation; −−−−→, inhibition) may work through changes in the enzyme concentration (regulation of enzyme synthesis or degradation), by direct allosteric effects, or by effects on protein kinases and protein phosphatases that regulate the phosphorylation state of the enzyme. **A,** Anabolic pathway: feedback inhibition. **B,** Catabolic pathway: regulation by ATP and ADP. **C,** Catabolic pathway: regulation by feedforward stimulation.

A A → B → C → D → E

B A → B → C → D → E → → → $CO_2 + H_2O$, ADP + P_i → ATP

C A → B → C → D → E → → → $CO_2 + H_2O$

In energy-producing catabolic pathways (Fig. 15.3, B), the important product is ATP. Therefore *ATP is used as a feedback inhibitor*: when ATP is in short supply, the catabolic pathways are stimulated, and when it is abundant they are inhibited. The ATP level is inversely related to the concentrations of ADP and AMP. Indeed, *ADP and AMP often act opposite to ATP in the regulation of metabolic pathways.*

In **feedforward stimulation,** a substrate stimulates the pathway by which it is utilized (Fig. 15.3, C). The induction of the *lac* operon of *E. coli* in the presence of lactose (see Chapter 6) is an example of feedforward stimulation.

Hormones can regulate the synthesis or, sometimes, the degradation of metabolic enzymes, or they change the phosphorylation state of the rate-limiting enzyme. Hormones are released in response to physiological stimuli, including carbohydrate feeding (insulin), fasting (glucagon), stress (epinephrine, cortisol), and physical exercise (epinephrine). They coordinate the activities of different tissues in these situations.

Inborn errors of metabolism are diseases in which a metabolic pathway is interrupted by an enzyme deficiency

What is expected when one of the enzymes in a metabolic pathway is deficient as a result of a mutation in the enzyme-coding gene (Fig. 15.4)? The immediate effects of the enzyme deficiency are always the *accumulation of the substrate* and the *lack of the product.*

If an anabolic pathway is affected (Fig. 15.4, A), *clinical signs and symptoms can be caused by the lack of the end product.* An example of this situation is **oculocutaneous albinism.** The "classical" albino has an inherited deficiency of tyrosinase, an enzyme that

FIG. 15.4

Consequences of an enzyme deficiency. **A,** Anabolic pathway: metabolite C accumulates, product E is deficient. C is either excreted or diverted into alternative pathways. Clinical signs and symptoms may be caused either by the deficiency of the product or by the accumulation of C. **B,** Catabolic pathway: a nutrient or one of its metabolites accumulates. Unless the pathway is essential for ATP synthesis (glycolysis, TCA cycle, etc.), the clinical signs are caused not by ATP deficiency but by the accumulation of the nutrient and/or its metabolites. **C,** Degradation of a macromolecule: the undegraded molecule C accumulates, mostly within the cells. The result is a "storage disease."

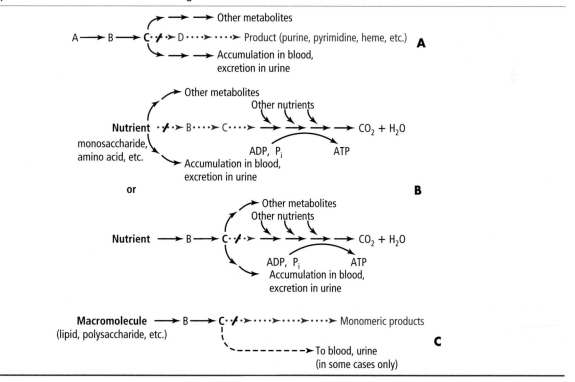

is required for the synthesis of the dark pigment melanin (see Chapter 21). In other metabolic disorders, however (see the porphyrias in Chapter 22 for an example), it is not the lack of the end product but rather the accumulation of a toxic metabolic intermediate that causes signs of disease.

The deficiency of an enzyme in a major catabolic, ATP-producing pathway such as glycolysis or the TCA cycle (see Chapter 16) is likely to cause serious problems for those cells that depend on the pathway for the generation of their metabolic energy. More commonly, however, an enzyme deficiency affects only the catabolism of a specialized substrate such as fructose (see Chapter 17), galactose (see Chapter 17), or phenylalanine (see Chapter 21). In these cases (Fig. 15.4, B), problems are caused not by a lack of ATP, which still can be synthesized from other substrates, but by *the abnormal accumulation of the nutrient or its immediate metabolites*. Some of these diseases can be treated very effectively simply by avoiding the offending nutrient.

If the intracellular degradation of a macromolecule by hydrolytic enzymes is blocked (pathway ② in Fig. 15.1), problems arise through the *abnormal accumulation ("storage") of the nondegradable macromolecule* (Fig. 15.4, C). This pattern of metabolic disease is called a **storage disease.** The mucopolysaccharidoses (see Chapter 13), glycogen storage diseases (see Chapter 17), and lipid storage diseases (see Chapter 19) are the most prominent examples. Many but not all storage diseases are caused by the deficiency of a lysosomal enzyme.

Isoenzymes are enzymes that catalyze the same reaction but differ in their molecular structures. In most cases the isoenzymes are encoded by different genes, and the expression of these genes is tissue specific. Therefore *an inherited enzyme deficiency may block a pathway only in certain tissues or cell types but not in others.*

Hundreds of different enzyme deficiencies have been recognized in inherited metabolic diseases. Most of these are rare, with frequencies of less than 1 in 10,000 in the population. However, they give valuable information about the normal roles of the affected pathways. Most of these diseases, which are collectively called **inborn errors of metabolism,** are recessively inherited: the heterozygotes, who typically have one half of the normal enzyme activity, are healthy. In many cases a near-total deficiency of the enzyme is required to cause signs of disease.

Vitamin deficiencies, toxins, and hormonal abnormalities also can disrupt metabolic pathways

Most metabolic pathways require not only enzymes but also coenzymes. Many coenzymes, in turn, are derived from dietary **vitamins** (see Chapter 24). *A vitamin deficiency can interrupt a metabolic pathway by depriving it of an essential coenzyme.* Most vitamin-derived coenzymes (such as NAD, FAD, and coenzyme A) participate in many different metabolic pathways, and all of these are affected by the vitamin deficiency.

Some toxins are enzyme inhibitors and therefore can produce effects resembling those of an inherited enzyme deficiency. Lead (see Chapter 21), arsenic (see Chapter 16), and cyanide (see Chapter 16) are examples of toxins that produce their effects by inhibiting metabolic enzymes.

Endocrine disorders such as diabetes mellitus and Cushing's syndrome are the most complex metabolic diseases, because the affected hormones act simultaneously on many metabolic pathways in a variety of tissues. The most important example, diabetes mellitus, will be discussed in Chapter 29.

SUMMARY

Biosynthetic processes can be characterized as either anabolic or catabolic. Anabolic, or biosynthetic, processes produce a complex biosynthetic product from simple precursors, whereas catabolic processes degrade complex molecules to more simple ones. Anabolic processes consume metabolic energy, and this energy has to be supplied by catabolic processes.

Metabolic interconversions take the form of metabolic pathways. The direction of the pathway is determined by the sum of the standard free energy changes of the individual reactions and by the cellular concentrations of substrates and products. Enzymes in metabolic pathways can be regulated by adjustments of their own synthesis or degradation, by covalent modifications, or by reversibly binding ligands. The regulated enzymes often are inhibited by a product of the pathway (feedback inhibition) or are stimulated by a substrate (feedforward stimulation).

Metabolic pathways can be interrupted as a result of an inherited enzyme deficiency, a vitamin deficiency, or toxic inhibition of one of the enzymes in the pathway. Signs of disease may be caused by a missing product of the pathway or by the accumulation of a nutrient or metabolic intermediate.

QUESTIONS

1. The generation of metabolic energy from glucose requires a pathway known as glycolysis. Based on the principles of metabolic regulation that you know, the most likely mechanism of regulation for this pathway is

   A. Inhibition of the first irreversible step by glucose
   B. Inhibition of the first irreversible step by ADP
   C. Inhibition of the last irreversible step by ADP
   D. Inhibition of the first irreversible step by ATP

2. Under physiological conditions, the "reversibility" of a metabolic reaction is affected by all of the following except
   A. Concentration of the substrate
   B. Concentration of the enzyme
   C. The energy charge if ATP and ADP participate in the reaction
   D. The standard free energy change of the reaction

Chapter 16

The Oxidation of Glucose

Glycolysis, the TCA Cycle, and

Oxidative Phosphorylation

Each cell has to generate metabolic energy. To this end, it has to degrade exogenous nutrients such as glucose, fatty acids, and amino acids, or stored reserves such as triglycerides or glycogen. Under aerobic conditions these substrates are oxidized to carbon dioxide and water. Carbohydrates yield approximately 4 kcal/g, triglycerides 9.3 kcal/g, and proteins 5.5 kcal/g. Molecular oxygen is consumed stoichiometrically during oxidative metabolism, as exemplified by the oxidation of the carbohydrate glucose and the triglyceride tripalmitate:

$$C_6H_{12}O_6 + 6\,O_2 \longrightarrow 6\,CO_2 + 6\,H_2O$$
Glucose

$$C_{51}H_{98}O_6 + 72^1/_2\,O_2 \longrightarrow$$
Tripalmitate
$$51\,CO_2 + 49\,H_2O$$

The **respiratory quotient (RQ)** is the molar ratio of CO_2 produced per unit of O_2 consumed. The RQ for the oxidation of carbohydrates is 1.0, for fat approximately 0.7, and for protein approximately 0.8.

Most cells can generate metabolic energy from various alternative substrates including glucose, fatty acids, and amino acids. Others are more specialized. A few cell types—for example, neurons and red blood cells—depend mostly or exclusively on glucose for their energy needs. In this chapter,

we trace the fate of glucose through its major catabolic pathways.

GLYCOLYSIS: FROM GLUCOSE TO PYRUVATE

All cells in the human body can generate metabolic energy from glucose. Despite its simple stoichiometry, glucose oxidation is a complex process that requires reactions both in the cytoplasm and in the mitochondria. The initial reaction sequence, known as *glycolysis*, takes place in the cytoplasm and converts one molecule of the six-carbon sugar glucose into two molecules of the three-carbon acid pyruvate.

Glucose is the principal transported carbohydrate in humans

All major dietary carbohydrates contain glucose, either as their only building block, as in starch and glycogen, or together with another monosaccharide, as in sucrose and lactose. Therefore the largest portion of the dietary carbohydrate reaches the consuming tissues in the form of glucose. Fructose and galactose, obtained from dietary sucrose and lactose, respectively, can be converted to glucose in the liver (Fig. 16.1).

FIG. 16.1

The role of glucose as the principal transported carbohydrate in the human body. Note the important role of the liver in glucose metabolism.

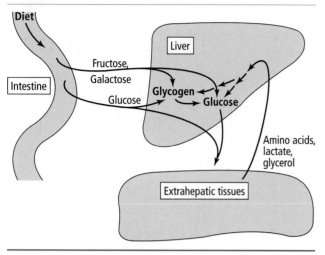

Being water soluble, glucose can be transported easily by the blood. However, it cannot be stored effectively because of its osmotic activity. For storage it has to be converted to the polysaccharide **glycogen,** which is present in many cells, being most plentiful in liver and muscle tissue.

The **blood glucose level** is tightly regulated: in the fasting state it is maintained at 4.0 to 5.5 mM (70 to 100 mg/dL), and even after a carbohydrate-rich meal it rarely rises above 8.5 mM (150 mg/dL). *In the fasting state the blood glucose level is maintained by the liver,* which produces glucose initially from its stored glycogen and later from such noncarbohydrates as amino acids, lactate, and glycerol. The maintenance of a more-or-less-constant blood glucose level is essential for those tissues that depend on glucose as their principal energy source, most notably the brain.

Glucose degradation begins in the cytoplasm and ends in the mitochondria

The steps in glucose oxidation are summarized in Fig. 16.2: after entering the cell by facilitated diffusion across the plasma membrane (see Chapter 11), *glucose is processed to two molecules of the three-carbon compound* **pyruvate.** This pathway is called **glycolysis.**

Under aerobic conditions, pyruvate enters the mitochondrion, where it is oxidatively decarboxylated

to the two-carbon compound **acetyl-CoA.** Acetyl-CoA then enters the **tricarboxylic acid cycle (TCA cycle)** by reacting with the four-carbon compound oxaloacetate to form the six-carbon compound citrate. Citrate is converted back to oxaloacetate in the reactions of the TCA cycle while two carbons are released as CO_2.

In these pathways *the hydrogen of the substrate does not directly form water but is transferred initially to the coenzymes NAD and FAD (see Chapter 5). The reduced coenzymes are then reoxidized by molecular oxygen in the* **respiratory chain** *of the inner mitochondrial membrane. The reoxidation of the reduced coenzymes is coupled to ATP synthesis in the process of* **oxidative phosphorylation.** This is the major energy source for most cells. A small amount of useful energy in the form of ATP or GTP also is produced directly in glycolysis and the TCA cycle by **substrate-level phosphorylation.**

Glycolysis participates only in carbohydrate metabolism, but acetyl-CoA also is formed in the degradation of fatty acids and amino acids. *The TCA cycle and oxidative phosphorylation therefore are the final common pathway for the oxidation of all major nutrients.*

Glycolysis begins with ATP-dependent phosphorylations

All cells in the human body can metabolize glucose by glycolysis. After entering the cell, glucose initially is phosphorylated by **hexokinase.** This enzyme produces **glucose 6-phosphate** by the transfer of the terminal phosphate of ATP to the hydroxy group at C-6 of glucose (Fig. 16.3). This reaction is exergonic ($\Delta G^{o'} = -4.0$ kcal/mol; Table 16.1) because an energy-rich phosphoanhydride bond in ATP is cleaved while a "low-energy" phosphate ester bond is formed. Therefore, and because the ATP concentration in the cell is usually far higher than the ADP concentration, the hexokinase reaction is irreversible under ordinary conditions.

The hexokinase reaction is not specific for glycolysis: *glucose always is phosphorylated to glucose 6-phosphate before it is converted to other products in the major metabolic pathways.* This reaction commits glucose to intracellular metabolism because, unlike glucose, which can leave the cell on the same carrier on which it entered, *glucose 6-phosphate is not transported across the plasma membrane.*

FIG. 16.2

The steps in glucose oxidation. The cytoplasmic reaction sequence from glucose to pyruvate is known as glycolysis. The catabolic pathways convert the carbon of the substrate to carbon dioxide. The hydrogen initially is transferred to the coenzymes NAD^+ and FAD. The reduced coenzymes then are reoxidized by the respiratory chain. Most of the ATP is produced in the process of oxidative phosphorylation, which couples the oxidation of the reduced coenzymes to ATP synthesis.

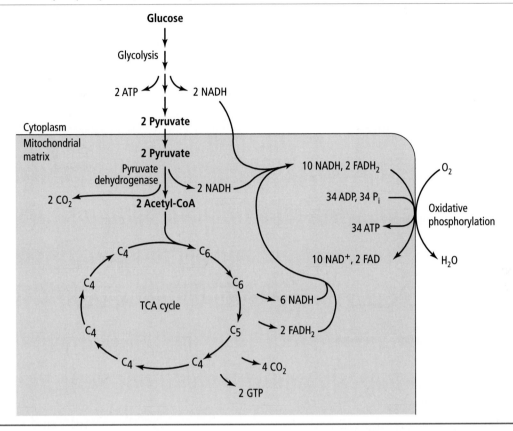

In glycolysis, glucose 6-phosphate is converted to fructose 6-phosphate in the freely reversible **phosphohexose isomerase** reaction. Fructose 6-phosphate then is phosphorylated to fructose 1,6-bisphosphate by **phosphofructokinase (PFK)**. This is the first irreversible reaction specific for glycolysis: it is its **committed step.**

The reactions from glucose to fructose 1,6-bisphosphate require two high-energy phosphate bonds in ATP. This initial investment has to be recovered in later reactions of the pathway.

Most glycolytic intermediates have three carbons

The six-carbon intermediate fructose 1,6-bisphosphate is cleaved into two triose phosphates by the enzyme **aldolase**: carbons 1, 2, and 3 form dihydroxyacetone phosphate, and carbons 4, 5, and 6 form glyceraldehyde 3-phosphate. The two triose phosphates are interconverted in the reversible **triose phosphate isomerase** reaction. Aldolase and triose phosphate isomerase establish an equilibrium among fructose 1,6-bisphosphate, dihydroxyacetone phosphate, and glyceraldehyde 3-phosphate. Although only glyceraldehyde 3-phosphate is a substrate for the next glycolytic reaction, triose phosphate isomerase ensures that all six glucose-derived carbons can proceed through the pathway.

The next reactions produce ATP while glyceraldehyde 3-phosphate is oxidized to 3-phosphoglycerate. First, glyceraldehyde 3-phosphate is converted to the energy-rich intermediate 1,3-bisphosphoglycerate by **glyceraldehyde 3-phosphate dehydrogenase**. In this reaction the aldehyde group of the substrate is oxidized to a carboxy group, which

FIG. 16.3

The reactions of glycolysis, the major catabolic pathway for glucose. It is active in the cytoplasm of all cells in the human body.

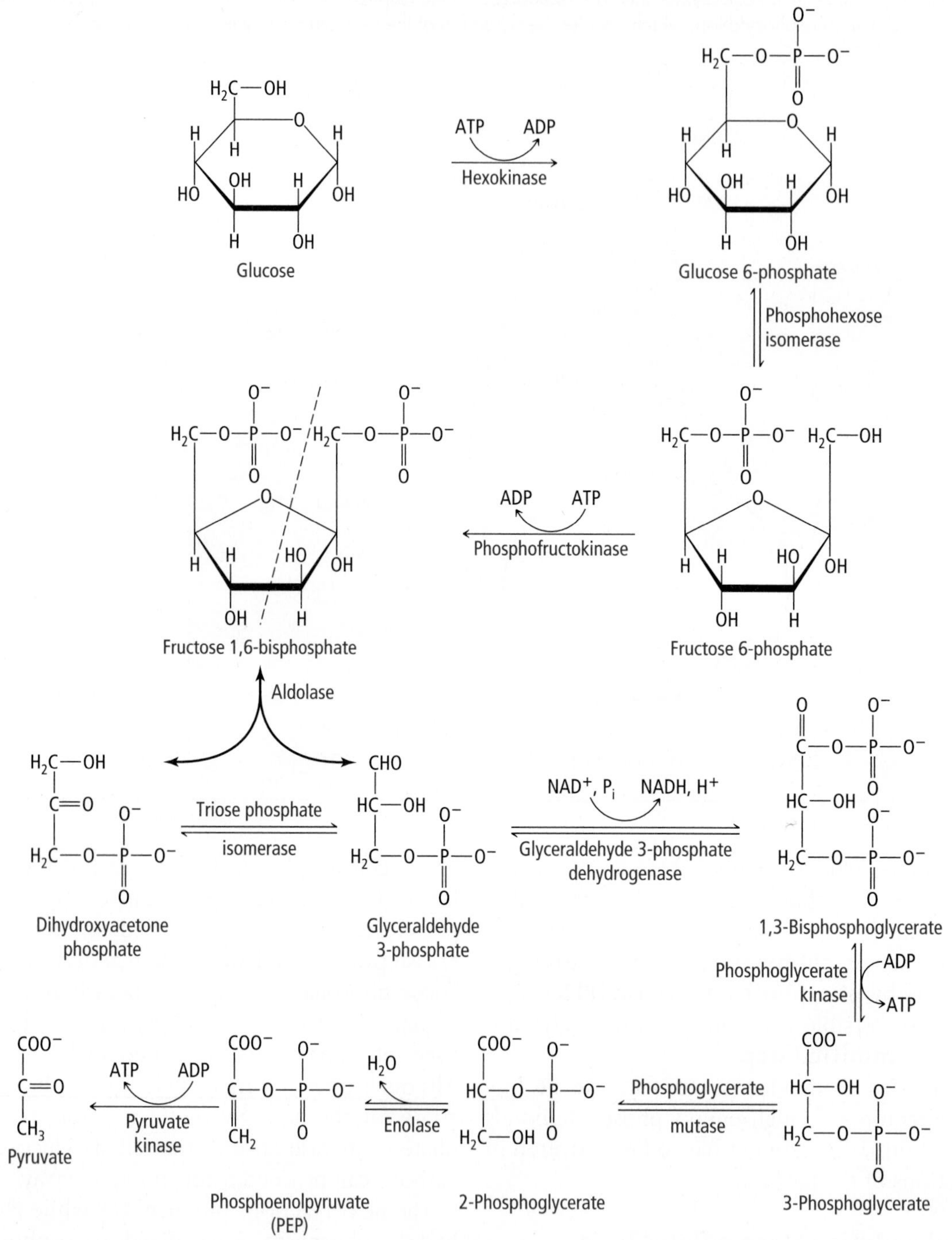

Glucose
ATP
ADP
Hexokinase
Glucose 6-phosphate
Phosphohexose isomerase
Fructose 6-phosphate
ADP
ATP
Phosphofructokinase
Fructose 1,6-bisphosphate
Aldolase
Dihydroxyacetone phosphate
Triose phosphate isomerase
Glyceraldehyde 3-phosphate
NAD+, Pi
NADH, H+
Glyceraldehyde 3-phosphate dehydrogenase
1,3-Bisphosphoglycerate
Phosphoglycerate kinase
ADP
ATP
3-Phosphoglycerate
Phosphoglycerate mutase
2-Phosphoglycerate
H2O
Enolase
Phosphoenolpyruvate (PEP)
ATP
ADP
Pyruvate kinase
Pyruvate

TABLE 16.1

Standard free energy changes of glycolytic reactions

Reaction	Enzyme	$\Delta G^{0\prime}$ (kcal/mol)
Glucose $\xrightarrow{\text{ATP}\quad\text{ADP}}$ Glucose 6-phosphate	Hexokinase	−4.0
Glucose 6-phosphate $\rightleftharpoons$ Fructose 6-phosphate	Phosphohexose isomerase	+0.4
Fructose 6-phosphate $\xrightarrow{\text{ATP}\quad\text{ADP}}$ Fructose 1,6-bisphosphate	Phosphofructokinase	−3.4
Fructose 1,6-bisphosphate $\rightleftharpoons$ Dihydroxyacetone phosphate + Glyceraldehyde 3-phosphate	Aldolase	+5.7
Dihydroxyacetone phosphate $\rightleftharpoons$ Glyceraldehyde 3-phosphate	Triose phosphate isomerase	+1.8
Glyceraldehyde 3-phosphate $\underset{}{\overset{\text{NADH}^+,\ P_i \quad\quad \text{NAD}^+,\ H^+}{\rightleftharpoons}}$ 1,3-bisphosphoglycerate	Glyceraldehyde 3-phosphate dehydrogenase	+1.5
1,3-Bisphosphoglycerate $\underset{}{\overset{\text{ADP}\quad\text{ATP}}{\rightleftharpoons}}$ 3-Phosphoglycerate	Phosphoglycerate kinase	−4.5
3-Phosphoglycerate $\rightleftharpoons$ 2-Phosphoglycerate	Phosphoglycerate mutase	+1.1
2-Phosphoglycerate $\underset{}{\overset{\text{H}_2\text{O}}{\rightleftharpoons}}$ Phosphoenolpyruvate (PEP)	Enolase	+0.4
Phosphoenolpyruvate $\xrightarrow{\text{ADP}\quad\text{ATP}}$ Pyruvate	Pyruvate kinase	−7.5

in turn forms an energy-rich mixed anhydride bond with phosphate. The enzyme couples the exergonic oxidation with the endergonic formation of a mixed anhydride bond. Note that in this reaction the phosphate group is derived not from ATP but from inorganic phosphate. Also, NADH is formed, which is a valuable product because its oxidation in the respiratory chain is a source of ATP (Fig. 16.2).

Simple hydrolysis of the mixed anhydride bond would release not less than 11.8 kcal/mol in the form of heat. Instead of hydrolyzing the bond, however, the energy-conscious cell uses this energy by transferring the phosphate to ADP, forming ATP. This reaction is catalyzed by **phosphoglycerate kinase.** The principle of ATP synthesis that we encounter here is known as **substrate-level phosphorylation:** *an energy-rich intermediate (in this case 1,3-bisphosphoglycerate) is formed in the pathway. This energy-rich intermediate then is used for the synthesis of an energy-rich nucleotide (in this case ATP).* We shall encounter other examples of substrate-level phosphorylation in the last reaction of glycolysis and in the TCA cycle.

3-Phosphoglycerate is isomerized to 2-phosphoglycerate by **phosphoglycerate mutase** ("mutase" is an old-fashioned name for isomerases that shift

the position of a phosphate group within the molecule). 2-Phosphoglycerate, in turn, is dehydrated to phosphoenolpyruvate (PEP) by **enolase.**

In the last reaction of glycolysis, catalyzed by **pyruvate kinase,** the phosphate group of PEP is transferred to ADP. Although ATP is synthesized, this reaction is highly exergonic, with a $\Delta G^{o\prime}$ of −7.5 kcal/mol. This implies a free energy content of 14.8 kcal/mol for the phosphate ester bond in PEP. Why is this phosphate ester so unusually energy rich? The initial transfer of phosphate from PEP to ADP is indeed endergonic. However, the enolpyruvate formed in this reaction rearranges almost immediately to pyruvate, and enolpyruvate effectively is removed from the equilibrium (Fig. 16.4).

Only the hexokinase, PFK, and pyruvate kinase reactions are "irreversible." All other glycolytic reactions can proceed in either direction under physiological conditions. The equilibria of the aldolase and triose phosphate isomerase reactions are very unfavorable (Table 16.1). Fructose 1,6-bisphosphate, however, is formed in the irreversible PFK reaction, and glyceraldehyde 3-phosphate is consumed rapidly in the next reactions of the pathway. The actual equilibrium of the glyceraldehyde 3-phosphate dehydrogenase reaction is far more favorable than sug-

FIG. 16.4

The pyruvate kinase reaction. Pyruvate shows keto-enol tautomerism, the keto form being energetically far more stable than the enol form.

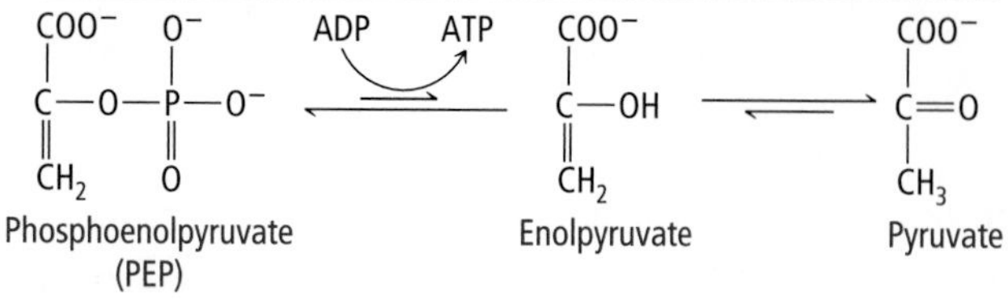

Phosphoenolpyruvate (PEP)   Enolpyruvate   Pyruvate

TABLE 16.2

Products formed during the conversion of one molecule of glucose to two molecules of pyruvate in aerobic glycolysis*

Enzyme	Product
Hexokinase	− 1 ATP
Phosphofructokinase	− 1 ATP
Glyceraldehyde 3-phosphate dehydrogenase	+ 2 NADH
Phosphoglycerate kinase	+ 2 ATP
Pyruvate kinase	+ 2 ATP
	2 ATP + 2 NADH

* Note that all reactions beyond the aldolase reaction occur twice for each glucose molecule.

---

gested by its $\Delta G^{o\prime}$ value of + 1.5 kcal/mol because the concentration of NAD^+ far exceeds that of NADH in the aerobic cell.

Besides two molecules of pyruvate, glycolysis produces two molecules of ATP and two molecules of NADH from each molecule of glucose (Table 16.2).

PFK is the most important regulated enzyme of glycolysis

The requirement for glycolytic activity varies in different physiological states. Most tissues glycolyze heavily after a carbohydrate-rich meal, when excess dietary glucose has to be metabolized. During fasting, most tissues reduce their glycolytic activity markedly while covering their energy needs by the oxidation of fatty acids and other alternative substrates.

The *long-term control* of glycolysis, particularly in the liver, is effected by changes in the amounts of several glycolytic enzymes. These changes reflect alterations in the rates of enzyme synthesis and, possibly, degradation.

The most important enzyme for the *short-term control* of glycolysis is PFK. This enzyme, which catalyzes the committed step of glycolysis, is

- *inhibited by ATP and stimulated by AMP and ADP*
- *inhibited by low pH*
- *inhibited by citrate*
- *stimulated by insulin and inhibited by glucagon (in the liver)*

The response to ATP and AMP adjusts the activity of the enzyme to the immediate energy needs of the cell. It *increases glycolytic activity when the ATP consumption is increased*, as in contracting muscle, and in metabolic emergencies when the oxygen-dependent system of oxidative phosphorylation in the mitochondria fails.

Citrate is a mitochondrial metabolite that signals an abundance of energy and metabolic intermediates. An increased acidity dampens glycolytic activity when pyruvic and lactic acid, the end products of glycolysis, accumulate to dangerous levels.

Of the important hormones, *insulin is released in response to elevated blood glucose after a carbohydrate-rich meal, whereas the glucagon level is increased in the fasting state.* The effects of these hormones on PFK are part of their overall role in the regulation of the blood glucose level (see Chapter 17). The hormonal effects are tissue specific: in humans, glucagon is important only in the liver, having little effect on other tissues. Epinephrine is a powerful activator of PFK in muscle but not in most other tissues. In the brain, which depends on glucose metabolism at all times, PFK responds neither to insulin nor to other hormones.

Besides PFK, hexokinase and pyruvate kinase frequently are regulated. Like PFK, these enzymes catalyze physiologically irreversible reactions. In most tissues (but not in the liver), hexokinase is competitively inhibited by its own product glucose 6-phosphate. This product inhibition prevents an accumulation of glucose 6-phosphate when the supply of glucose exceeds the capacity of the metabolizing pathways. Otherwise the excessive formation of glucose 6-phosphate would deplete the cell of inorganic phosphate and thereby impair ATP synthesis. Pyruvate kinase, finally, is inhibited by ATP in many tissues. This effect is most important in the liver, where it participates in the reciprocal regulation of glycolysis and gluconeogenesis (see Chapter 17).

FIG. 16.5

Anaerobic glycolysis: lactate dehydrogenase regenerates NAD$^+$ for the glyceraldehyde 3-phosphate dehydrogenase reaction. The conversion of glucose to lactic acid can proceed smoothly with a net synthesis of two ATP molecules.

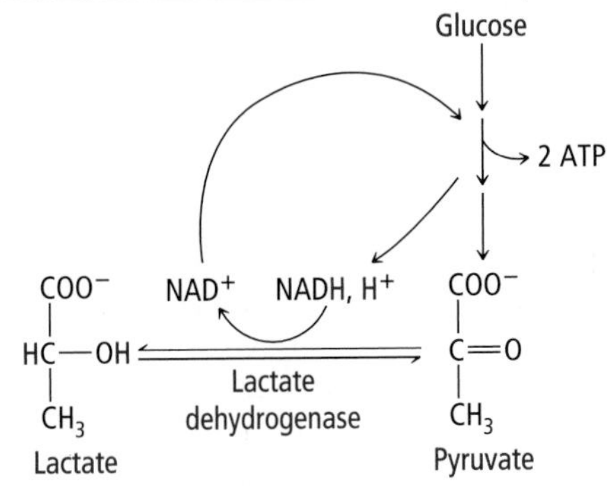

Lactate is produced by glycolysis under anaerobic conditions

Although the mitochondrial oxidation of pyruvate and NADH requires molecular oxygen, the reactions of glycolysis do not. Therefore *glycolysis should be able to supply ATP under anaerobic conditions*. With pyruvate as end product, however, this is not possible because NAD$^+$ is converted to NADH, and the pathway would soon grind to a halt for lack of NAD$^+$.

The solution to this problem is elegantly simple: the hydrogen of NADH is transferred to the keto group of pyruvate, forming lactate. This reaction, catalyzed by **lactate dehydrogenase (LDH)**, regenerates NAD$^+$ for the glyceraldehyde 3-phosphate dehydrogenase reaction of glycolysis:

$$\text{Pyruvate} + \text{NADH} + \text{H}^+ \longrightarrow$$
$$\text{Lactate} + \text{NAD}^+ \quad \Delta G^{0\prime} = -6.0 \text{ kcal/mol}$$

The overall balance of anaerobic glycolysis (Fig. 16.5) is:

$$\text{Glucose} + 2 \text{ ADP} + 2 \text{ P}_i \longrightarrow$$
$$2 \text{ Lactate} + 2 \text{ ATP} + 2 \text{ H}_2\text{O}$$

Despite its unbalanced equilibrium, the LDH reaction is physiologically reversible because NAD$^+$ is always far more abundant than NADH under aerobic conditions. In fact, *lactate is a metabolic dead end*, and the LDH reaction is the only way to channel lactate back into the metabolic pathways. Being an acid,

lactic acid tends to acidify the cell in which it is formed. Therefore it has to be released through an anion channel in the plasma membrane and transported to aerobic tissues, where it is converted to pyruvate first, before it can be oxidized to CO$_2$ and H$_2$O or converted back to glucose (by gluconeogenesis; see Chapter 17).

The two ATPs formed in glycolysis amount to only 14.6 kcal of useful energy, whereas the complete oxidation of glucose produces approximately 270 kcal (see Table 16.6, page 323). Therefore anaerobic glycolysis is suitable only for cells with low energy requirements and as a temporary device to survive episodes of hypoxia or to cope with increased energy demands:

1. *Mature erythrocytes do not have mitochondria.* They do not engage in biosynthetic activity, and they require ATP only for the maintenance of ion gradients across their membranes. Their modest energy requirements are met by the anaerobic glycolysis of 15 to 20 g of glucose per day.

2. *Skeletal muscle* has to increase its ATP production more than twentyfold during bouts of vigorous contraction, for example, a 100-m sprint. In this situation the supply of oxygen from the blood becomes a limiting factor, and the tissue depends to a large extent on the anaerobic glycolysis of glucose and, more importantly, of stored glycogen. The lactate concentration in the blood rises five- to tenfold in this situation.

3. *Hypoxia* resulting from vascular obstruction or other causes—for example, in the myocardium during acute myocardial infarction—stimulates glycolysis at the level of PFK while preventing the mitochondrial oxidation of pyruvate and NADH. *Anaerobic glycolysis helps the cells to survive brief episodes of hypoxia.* It is a mixed blessing, however, because lactic acid acidifies the tissue and actually can contribute to cell death and tissue necrosis.

Anaerobic glycolysis is important because *carbohydrates are the only metabolic substrates that can produce ATP under anaerobic conditions.*

Lactic acid accumulates in many metabolic disorders

The acidity of the blood is tightly regulated at a pH of 7.35 to 7.40. A decrease of the blood pH below

TABLE 16.3

Conditions resulting in lactic acidosis

Condition	Mechanism	Reference
Physical exercise	Anaerobic glycolysis in muscle	
Severe lung disease		
High altitude	Impaired respiration	
Drowning		
Severe anemia		
Carbon monoxide poisoning	Impaired oxygen delivery	Chapter 3
Sickling crisis		Chapter 9
Cyanide poisoning	Inhibition of oxidative phosphorylation	Chapter 16 (p. 324)
Alcohol intoxication	Impaired gluconeogenesis	Chapter 29
von Gierke's disease	Impaired gluconeogenesis	Chapter 17
Pyruvate dehydrogenase deficiency	Impaired pyruvate oxidation	Chapter 16 (p. 307)
Leukemia	Anaerobic glycolysis by neoplastic cells	
Metastatic carcinoma		

this range is called **acidosis;** an increase is **alkalosis.** Hypoventilation can cause acidosis because carbon dioxide and carbonic acid accumulate:

$$CO_2 + H_2O \underset{\text{carbonic anhydrase}}{\overset{\text{Spontaneous, or}}{\rightleftharpoons}} H_2CO_3$$

$$\updownarrow \text{Spontaneous}$$

$$HCO_3^- + H^+$$

This type of acidosis is called **respiratory acidosis.** *Metabolic acidosis, on the other hand, is caused either by an overproduction of organic acids or by renal disease.*

Lactic acidosis is the most common type of metabolic acidosis. It is caused either by increased production or by decreased utilization of lactic acid. The most common cause is an impairment of oxidative metabolism, resulting from respiratory failure, impaired oxygen transport, or direct inhibition of oxidative phosphorylation. The cellular energy charge decreases, PFK becomes activated, and a large amount of pyruvate is formed at a time when its mitochondrial oxidation is impaired. The excess is converted to lactate. The mitochondria are unable to oxidize NADH to NAD^+ under anaerobic conditions, and because of the resulting increase in the $[NADH]/[NAD^+]$ ratio the LDH reaction becomes essentially irreversible in the direction of lactate formation. Other conditions that result in an increased $[NADH]/[NAD^+]$ ratio also increase lactic acid formation. This occurs, for example, in alcohol intoxication, when rapid ethanol oxidation produces a large amount of NADH in the liver (see Chapter 29). Finally, any enzymatic defect that prevents the utilization of pyruvate, either by mitochondrial oxidation or by gluconeogenesis, is likely to cause lactic acidosis. Some causes of lactic acidosis are listed in Table 16.3.

Genetic defects and toxins can inhibit glycolysis

A complete deficiency of any glycolytic enzyme would be fatal, at least if such cells as neurons or erythrocytes, which depend on glucose as their principal energy source, were affected. Partial deficiencies of glycolytic enzymes in RBCs, however, are seen as rare causes of hemolytic anemia. **Pyruvate kinase deficiency** occurs with a frequency of approximately 1 in 10,000. In this recessively inherited condition, the erythrocytes have anywhere between 5% and 25% of the normal pyruvate kinase activity. The severity of the hemolytic anemia depends on the residual enzyme activity.

Glycolysis can be inhibited by **fluoride ions,** which inhibit enolase. Sodium fluoride is used in the clinical laboratory to inhibit glycolysis in blood

FIG. 16.6

Uncoupling of substrate-level phosphorylation in glycolysis by arsenate. An unstable mixed anhydride is formed between arsenate and 3-phosphoglycerate. This anhydride hydrolyzes spontaneously. The pathway can proceed because the product of this hydrolysis, 3-phosphoglycerate, is a normal glycolytic intermediate.

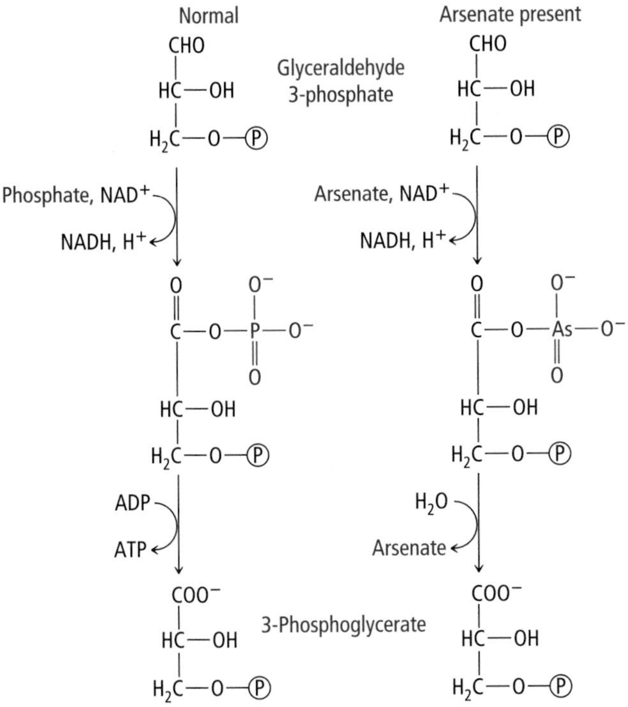

samples that are used for the determination of the blood glucose level.

Arsenate uncouples substrate-level phosphorylation with glyceraldehyde 3-phosphate dehydrogenase and phosphoglycerate kinase, by competing with phosphate as a substrate of the glyceraldehyde 3-phosphate dehydrogenase reaction (Fig. 16.6). The term "uncoupling" implies that *the pathway can proceed, but the ATP synthesis normally coupled to the enzymatic reactions no longer takes place*. Indeed, the net ATP yield of glycolysis is zero in the presence of arsenate.

PYRUVATE DEHYDROGENASE AND THE TCA CYCLE: FROM PYRUVATE TO CARBON DIOXIDE AND REDUCED COENZYMES

Under anaerobic conditions, pyruvate is reduced to lactate. Under aerobic conditions, however, it is transported into the mitochondrion, where it is oxi-dized to carbon dioxide and water. The mitochondrial pathways of pyruvate oxidation include the pyruvate dehydrogenase reaction and the tricarboxylic acid (TCA) cycle. These pathways convert the carbon skeleton of pyruvate to carbon dioxide while electrons (and protons) are transferred to the coenzymes NAD^+ and FAD.

Pyruvate is decarboxylated to acetyl-CoA in the mitochondria

After entering the mitochondrial matrix, pyruvate is oxidatively decarboxylated to acetyl-CoA:

$$\text{Pyruvate} + NAD^+ + \text{CoA-SH} \longrightarrow \text{Acetyl-CoA} + NADH + CO_2$$

This irreversible reaction is catalyzed by **pyruvate dehydrogenase**, an aggregate of three distinct enzymes:

1. *The pyruvate dehydrogenase component* (E_1), which contains **thiamine pyrophosphate** as a prosthetic group
2. *The dihydrolipoyl transacetylase component* (E_2), containing **lipoic acid** covalently bound to a lysine side chain
3. *The dihydrolipoyl dehydrogenase component* (E_3), an FAD-containing flavoprotein

The enzyme complex contains multiple copies of each component in an orderly array. Besides the tightly bound prosthetic groups, coenzyme A and NAD^+ are required for the reaction.

The structures of thiamine pyrophosphate and lipoic acid are shown in Fig. 16.7. Thiamine pyrophosphate acts as a carrier of pyruvate and of the hydroxyethyl group that is formed by its decarboxylation. Lipoic acid participates as an oxidation-reduction (redox) system and as a carrier of the acetyl group before it is transferred to coenzyme A.

The reaction sequence is shown in Fig. 16.8. Note that pyruvate is decarboxylated while it is bound to thiamine pyrophosphate. The resulting hydroxyethyl residue, which is at the oxidation state of acetaldehyde ("activated acetaldehyde"), is oxidized to an acetyl residue during its transfer to lipoic acid, with lipoic acid itself acting as the oxidant. After the transfer of the acetyl residue to coenzyme A, the free dihydrolipoic acid thus formed is oxidized by the dihydrolipoyl dehydrogenase component of the enzyme complex in an NAD^+-dependent reaction.

Acetyl-CoA is formed from carbohydrates, fatty acids, and amino acids

Acetyl-CoA is formed not only from carbohydrates through glycolysis and the pyruvate dehydrogenase reaction, but also from fatty acids in the pathway of β-oxidation (see Chapter 18). Amino acids also are degraded to acetyl-CoA, either directly ("ketogenic" amino acids) or via pyruvate ("glucogenic" amino acids).

The major fate of acetyl-CoA in most cells is oxidation in the TCA cycle, but acetyl-CoA is also a substrate for biosynthetic processes, most notably the synthesis of fatty acids, cholesterol, and ketone bodies

---

FIG. 16.7

Structures of thiamine pyrophosphate and lipoic acid. In the pyruvate dehydrogenase complex, thiamine pyrophosphate is bound noncovalently to the apoprotein while lipoic acid is covalently bound by an amide bond with a lysine side chain.

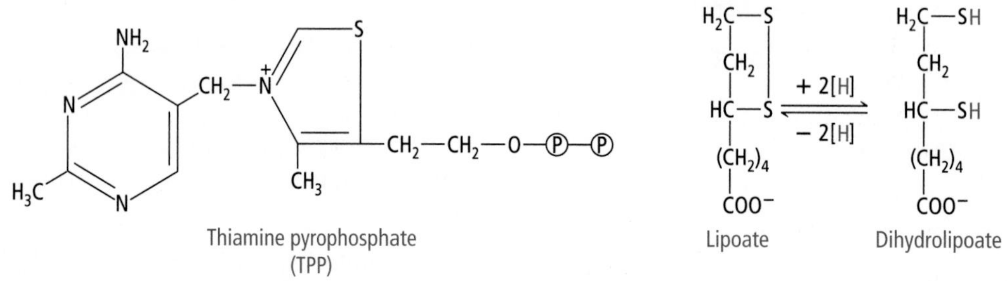

Thiamine pyrophosphate (TPP)

Lipoate   Dihydrolipoate

FIG. 16.8

The pyruvate dehydrogenase reaction.

The Oxidation of Glucose Metabolism

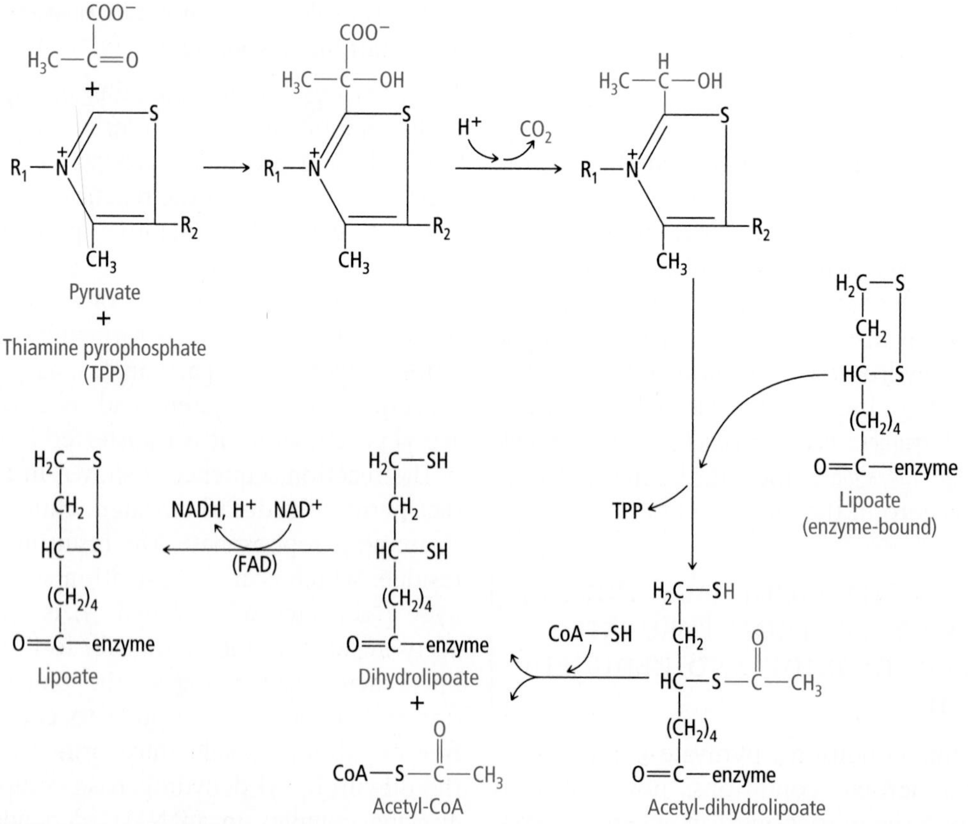

(Fig. 16.9). After a carbohydrate-rich meal, for example, acetyl-CoA is formed from glucose and then is converted to fatty acids and triglycerides. In **acetylation reactions**, acetyl-CoA is used as an activated form of acetate for the synthesis of acetic acid esters and amides (Fig. 16.10).

The pyruvate dehydrogenase reaction is impaired in several diseases

With the exception of lipoic acid, the coenzymes of pyruvate dehydrogenase require vitamins for their synthesis: pantothenic acid (coenzyme A), niacin (NAD), riboflavin (FAD), and thiamine (TPP). A deficiency of any of these vitamins can impair the pyruvate dehydrogenase reaction. This is most clearly demonstrated by **thiamine deficiency (beriberi** and **Wernicke-Korsakoff syndrome**; see Chapter 24). In this condition the blood levels of pyruvate, lactate, and alanine are elevated, espe-cially after a carbohydrate-rich meal. Pyruvate accu-mulates because its major reaction is inhibited, and most of the excess either is reduced to lactate or is transaminated to alanine.

Inherited partial deficiencies of pyruvate dehy-drogenase occasionally are seen. The nervous sys-tem is affected most seriously, and lactic acidosis is present. The clinical expression and the prognosis depend on the residual enzyme activity. With severe deficiencies ($< 40\%$ of normal enzyme activity), symptoms appear in early infancy and often include mental retardation, microcephaly, optical atrophy, and severe motor dysfunction. In less severe cases, the major manifestation is a slowly progressive spinocerebellar ataxia (motor incoordination) that begins to develop later during childhood. Fibroblast cultures obtained from the patient's skin are useful for enzymatic diagnosis. Treatment can be attempted by placing the patient on a low-carbohydrate diet. Therapeutic trials with megadoses of thiamine or other required vitamins also are indicated.

Arsenite, the most toxic form of arsenic, poi-sons pyruvate dehydrogenase by binding to the sulfhydryl groups in dihydrolipoic acid (Fig. 16.11). A similar reaction of arsenite with closely spaced sulfhydryl groups in immature keratin leads to its incorporation in hair and fingernails. Its determi-nation in hair has been used forensically in cases of alleged arsenic poisoning.

FIG. 16.9

The sources and fates of acetyl-CoA.

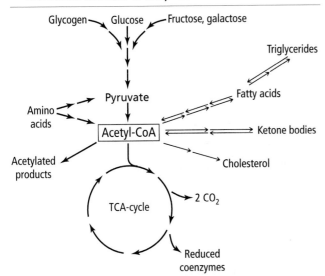

FIG. 16.11

Reaction of arsenite with dihydrolipoic acid.

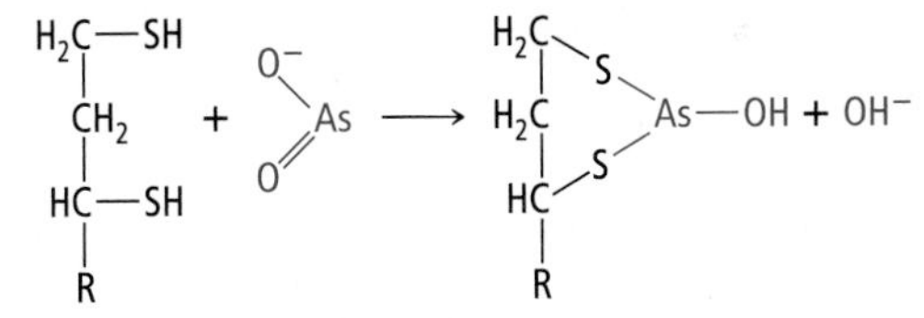

Lipoic acid   Arsenite

FIG. 16.10

Synthesis of acetylcholine in cholinergic neurons. This is an example of an acetylation reaction.

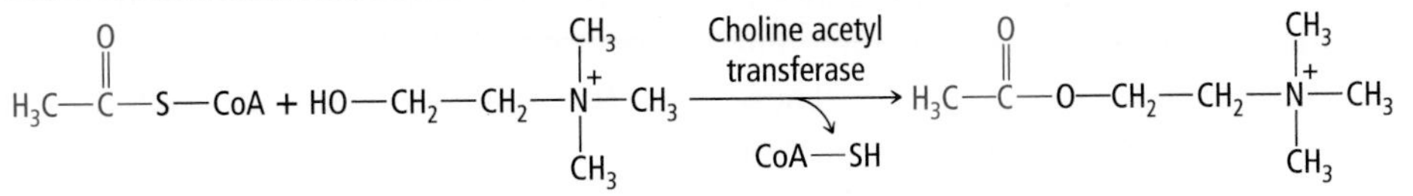

FIG. 16.12

Reactions of the tricarboxylic acid (TCA) cycle.

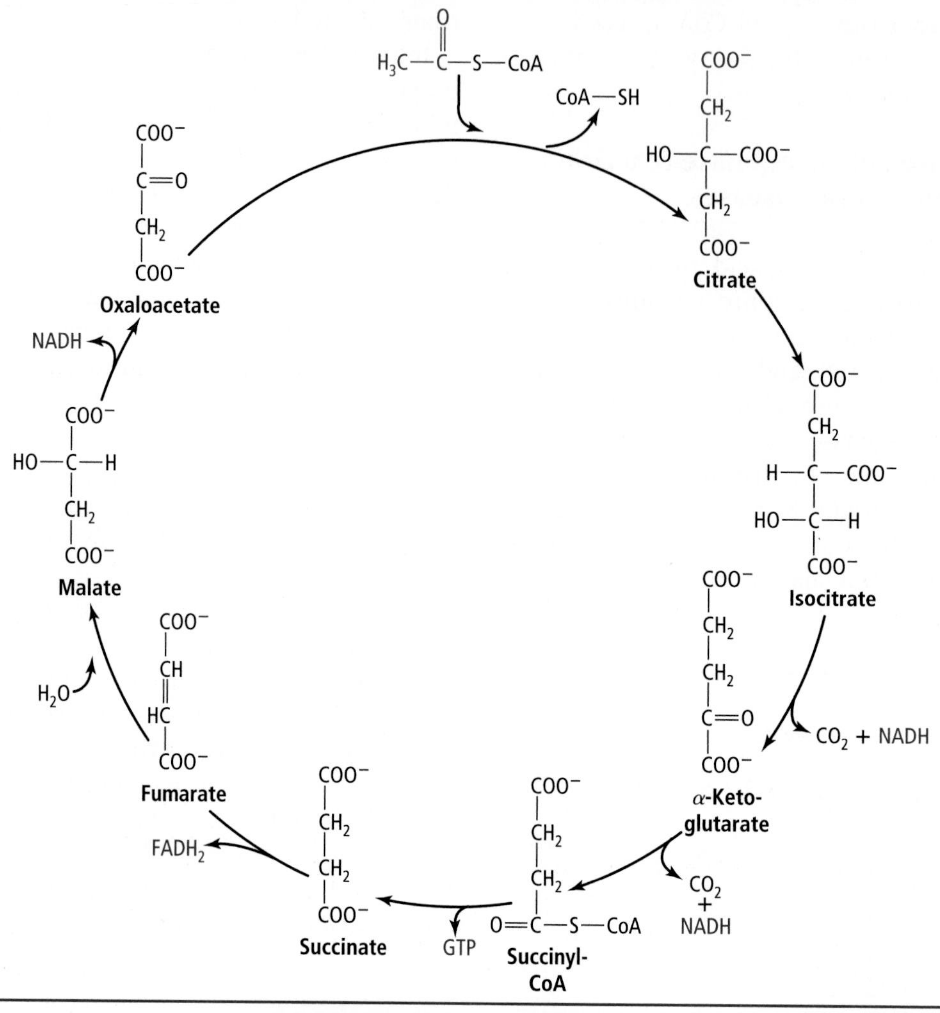

The TCA cycle produces two molecules of carbon dioxide for each acetyl residue

The TCA cycle, also known as the **citric acid cycle** *or* **Krebs cycle,** *is the final common pathway for the oxidation of all major nutrients.* Most of its enzymes are present in soluble form in the mitochondrial matrix, and *it is active in all cells that possess mitochondria.*

The first intermediate of the cycle is citrate, a six-carbon compound formed by a reaction between acetyl-CoA and the four-carbon compound oxaloacetate. The remaining reactions of the cycle (Fig. 16.12) regenerate oxaloacetate from citrate. These reactions release two carbons in the form of carbon dioxide.

Citrate synthase is an exclusively mitochondrial enzyme in mammalian tissues. It forms a bond between the methyl group of the acetyl residue in acetyl-CoA and the keto carbon of oxaloacetate. The CoA-thioester of citrate that is formed initially hydrolyzes subsequently, thereby making the reaction irreversible (Table 16.4).

In the next reaction, citrate is isomerized to isocitrate by the enzyme **aconitase**. First citrate is dehydrated to aconitate, and then aconitate is hydrated to isocitrate (Fig. 16.13). The enzyme establishes an equilibrium containing 90% citrate, 3% aconitate, and 7% isocitrate.

Fluoroacetate, a toxin that has been used as a rodenticide and that can cause fatal poisoning in humans, is metabolically converted to fluorocitrate

Reaction equilibria of the pyruvate dehydrogenase reaction and the TCA-cycle reactions

Enzyme	$\Delta G^{o'}$ (kcal/mol)	Products
Pyruvate dehydrogenase	−8.0	CO_2, NADH
Citrate synthase	−8.5	
Aconitase	+1.6	
Isocitrate dehydrogenase	−2.0	CO_2, NADH
α-Ketoglutarate dehydrogenase	−8.0	CO_2, NADH
Succinyl-CoA synthetase	−0.7	GTP
Succinate dehydrogenase	≈0	$FADH_2$
Fumarase	−0.9	
Malate dehydrogenase	+7.1	NADH

The aconitase reaction.

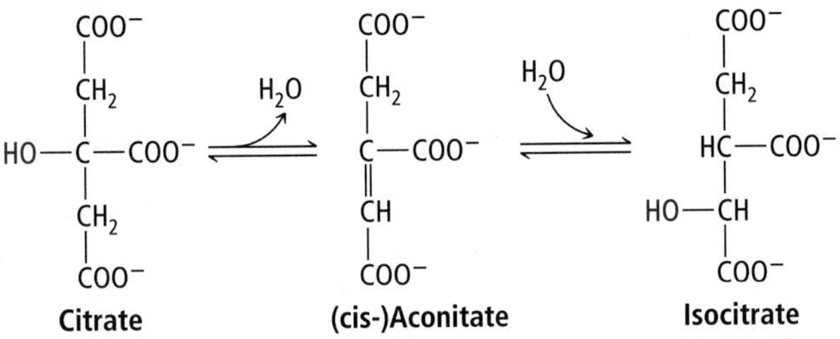

Citrate   **(cis-)Aconitate**   **Isocitrate**

by the same enzymes that normally metabolize acetate (Fig. 16.14). The resulting fluorocitrate is a potent inhibitor of aconitase.

Isocitrate is oxidatively decarboxylated to α-ketoglutarate (2-oxoglutarate) by **isocitrate dehydrogenase** (Fig. 16.15). Oxalosuccinate is an enzyme-bound intermediate in this reaction. The isocitrate dehydrogenase of the TCA cycle is an NAD-linked enzyme. NADP-linked isocitrate dehydrogenases of unknown function are also present in both the cytoplasm and the mitochondria of many tissues.

The next reaction of the cycle, catalyzed by α-**ketoglutarate dehydrogenase,** also is an oxidative decarboxylation. Its mechanism is different from that of the isocitrate dehydrogenase reaction and resembles that of pyruvate dehydrogenase: the substrate is an α-ketoacid, its carboxy carbon is released as CO_2, and the original keto carbon is oxidized to the level of a carboxy group, which is bound to coenzyme A. Like pyruvate dehydrogenase, α-ketoglutarate dehydrogenase is a multienzyme complex with three components: the α-ketoglutarate dehydrogenase component (E_1'), the transsuccinylase component (E_2'), and the dihydrolipoyl dehydrogenase component (E_3'). The first two components are different from those in the pyruvate dehydrogenase complex, but E_3' is identical to E_3. This implies that genetic defects of the dihydrolipoyl dehydrogenase impair the oxidative decarboxylation of both pyruvate and α-ketoglutarate. The coenzyme requirements of the two multienzyme complexes are identical.

In the next reaction, catalyzed by **succinyl-CoA synthetase** (also known as **succinyl thiokinase**), the hydrolysis of the energy-rich thioester bond in succinyl-CoA is coupled to the synthesis of GTP from GDP and inorganic phosphate. This is another example of substrate-level phosphorylation: an energy-rich bond in a metabolic intermediate is used for the synthesis of a phosphoanhydride bond in a nucleotide. GTP is equivalent to ATP, with which it is in equilibrium through the nucleoside diphosphate kinase reaction:

$$GTP + ADP \rightleftharpoons GDP + ATP$$

Succinate is a four-carbon dicarboxylic acid. In the remaining reactions, two hydrogens of succinate have to be replaced by oxygen to complete the cycle with the formation of oxaloacetate.

Succinate first is oxidized to fumarate by the transfer of two carbon-bound hydrogens to the FAD prosthetic group of the enzyme **succinate dehydrogenase (SDH).** Unlike the other TCA-cycle enzymes, which are soluble in the mitochondrial

FIG. 16.14

Metabolic activation of fluoroacetate to fluorocitrate. Fluorocitrate is an inhibitor of aconitase.

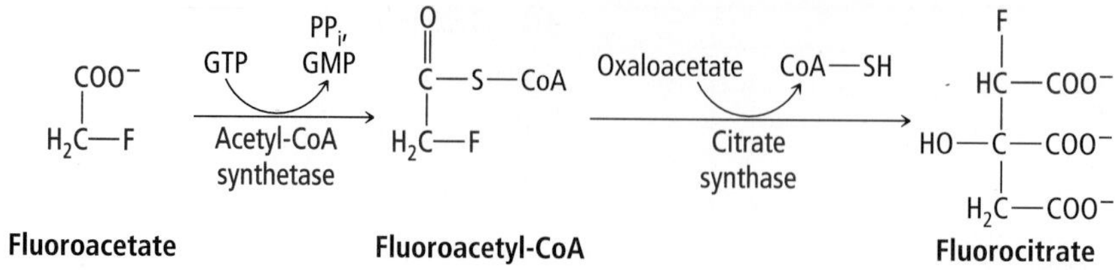

Fluoroacetate — Fluoroacetyl-CoA — Fluorocitrate

FIG. 16.15

The isocitrate dehydrogenase reaction.

Isocitrate — Oxalosuccinate — α-Ketoglutarate

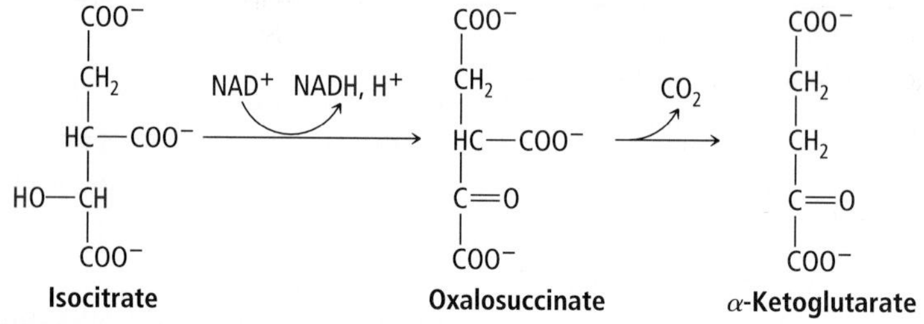

matrix, SDH is an integral protein of the inner mitochondrial membrane. This is a strategic location for the regeneration of its prosthetic group: unlike NADH, $FADH_2$ is a tightly bound prosthetic group that cannot simply diffuse away to be reoxidized in a different enzymatic reaction. It has to transfer its hydrogen to ubiquinone, a component of the respiratory chain in the inner mitochondrial membrane (see Fig. 16.25). SDH contains non-heme iron, which channels electrons from $FADH_2$ to ubiquinone.

Why does SDH use enzyme-bound FAD rather than soluble NAD^+ to abstract hydrogen from its substrate? The reason is that the FAD in SDH has a higher standard redox potential than does NAD. This means that FAD has a higher affinity for hydrogen than does NAD^+. Indeed, if NAD^+ were used, the reaction would be irreversible in the direction of succinate formation.

Fumarate is hydrated to L-malate by **fumarase**. Like the enolase reaction of glycolysis, this is a freely reversible lyase reaction.

Malate finally is oxidized to oxaloacetate in the NAD^+-dependent **malate dehydrogenase** reaction. Like lactate dehydrogenase, malate dehydrogenase interconverts an α-hydroxy acid and an α-keto acid.

As in the lactate dehydrogenase reaction, the equilibrium favors the hydroxy acid (Table 16.4). The reaction nevertheless can proceed in the right direction because the $[NAD^+]/[NADH]$ ratio in the mitochondrion is very high under aerobic conditions, and because oxaloacetate is consumed in the irreversible citrate synthase reaction.

Reduced coenzymes are the most important products of the TCA cycle

The important products of the TCA cycle are listed in Table 16.4. While two carbons (in the form of the acetyl residue in acetyl-CoA) enter the cycle, two carbons are released as carbon dioxide. The other product of oxidative metabolism, water, is not formed: instead, *hydrogen is transferred from the substrate to the coenzymes NAD^+ and FAD.* Not less than three molecules of NADH and one molecule of $FADH_2$ are formed in each turn of the cycle. *These reduced coenzymes, together with those formed in glycolysis, the pyruvate dehydrogenase reaction, and other catabolic pathways, are the fuel for the respiratory chain, where they are reoxidized by molecular oxygen.* Oxidative phosphorylation produces *three ATPs from each NADH and two ATPs from each $FADH_2$* that is oxidized in the respiratory chain.

BOX 16.1

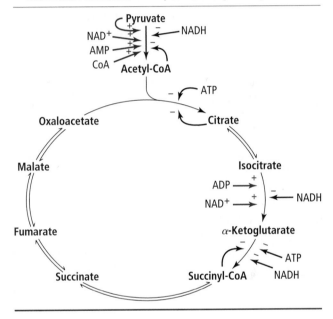

Enzyme—Ser—OH (active)

Protein kinase (ATP → ADP)

Protein phosphatase (P$_i$)

Enzyme—Ser—O—P—O$^-$ (inactive)

The overall energy yield from the oxidation of one acetyl residue is therefore 12 high-energy phosphate bonds. Only one of them is derived from substrate-level phosphorylation. The others are produced during the reoxidation of the reduced coenzymes.

There is no alternative to the respiratory chain for the oxidation of the reduced coenzymes in the mitochondrion. Therefore, unlike glycolysis, *the TCA cycle cannot function under anaerobic conditions.* Without molecular oxygen the cycle soon would grind to a halt for lack of NAD$^+$ and FAD.

Energy charge and [NADH]/[NAD$^+$] ratio are most important for the regulation of pyruvate dehydrogenase and the TCA cycle

The important product of mitochondrial oxidation is ATP. Therefore the rates of the pyruvate dehydrogenase reaction and the TCA cycle have to be adjusted to the cell's need for ATP: *the rate-limiting enzymes should be stimulated by low energy charge and inhibited by high energy charge.*

NADH is an important product, too. The activity of the respiratory chain increases when the energy demand is increased, and the immediate result of this is a decreased [NADH]/[NAD$^+$] ratio. In this situation the catabolic pathways have to produce more NADH as a substrate for the respiratory chain: they should be *stimulated by NAD$^+$ and inhibited by NADH.*

Evidently the catabolic mitochondrial pathways have to work in full gear when ATP is in short supply and the respiratory chain needs more fuel in the form of NADH and FADH$_2$. However, there should also be a more direct feedback inhibition of the irreversible reactions, to avoid an undesirable accumulation of metabolic intermediates (Fig. 16.16).

Pyruvate dehydrogenase, which is outside the

FIG. 16.16

Regulatory effects on pyruvate dehydrogenase and the TCA cycle. Note the importance of energy charge and the [NADH]/[NAD$^+$] ratio, and the product inhibition of the irreversible reactions. ——$^+$→, Stimulation; ——→, inhibition.

TCA cycle, is important because *it channels carbohydrate-derived carbons irreversibly into the metabolic pool of acetyl-CoA* and thereby into the TCA cycle. Pyruvate dehydrogenase is inhibited by its products NADH and acetyl-CoA and is stimulated by AMP. It also is inactivated by the phosphorylation of a single serine side chain, and reactivated by dephosphorylation as shown in Box 16.1. The protein kinase that phosphorylates the enzyme complex is allosterically activated by high energy charge, high [NADH]/[NAD$^+$] ratio, and high [acetyl-CoA]/[CoA] ratio, and is inhibited by pyruvate. The action of the protein kinase is opposed by a protein phosphatase that removes the bound phosphate by a hydrolytic cleavage reaction.

Some of the TCA-cycle enzymes are regulated, too. **Citrate synthase** is inhibited by ATP. More important, however, is the availability of oxaloacetate. The K_m of citrate synthase for this substrate is on the same order of magnitude as its intramitochondrial concentration ($\approx 10\ \mu M$). Citrate also acts as a competitive inhibitor with respect to oxaloacetate.

Isocitrate dehydrogenase is inhibited by high energy charge and high [NADH]/[NAD$^+$] ratio. Citrate, which accumulates in addition to isocitrate when isocitrate dehydrogenase is inhibited, can leave the mitochondrion and act as an allosteric effector in the pathways of glycolysis, gluconeogenesis (see Fig. 17.6, *B*, Chapter 17), and fatty acid biosynthesis (see Fig. 18.14, Chapter 18). Therefore elevations of mitochondrial energy charge and [NADH]/[NAD$^+$] ratio can affect these cytoplasmic pathways via inhibition of isocitrate dehydrogenase.

α-Ketoglutarate dehydrogenase, like pyruvate dehydrogenase, is inhibited by its own products (succinyl-CoA and NADH) and by high energy charge, but unlike pyruvate dehydrogenase it is not regulated by phosphorylation/dephosphorylation.

Except in anoxia, the mitochondrial [NAD$^+$]/[NADH] ratio is so high that NAD$^+$, as a substrate of the dehydrogenase reactions, is rarely a limiting factor. The equilibrium of the NAD-dependent malate dehydrogenase reaction, however, is very unfavorable (see Table 16.4). With an elevated [NADH]/[NAD$^+$] ratio, the [malate]/[oxaloacetate] ratio also is increased and citrate synthase suffers from a shortage of oxaloacetate.

The TCA cycle provides an important pool of metabolic intermediates

The TCA cycle not only is the final common pathway for the oxidation of metabolic fuels, it also provides a variety of metabolites as starting materials for biosynthetic reactions. Figure 16.17 summarizes some of the important reactions. One problem, however, arises when TCA-cycle intermediates are removed for biosynthesis: the mitochondrion soon is depleted of oxaloacetate, and the citrate synthase

FIG. 16.17

Some reactions of TCA-cycle intermediates.

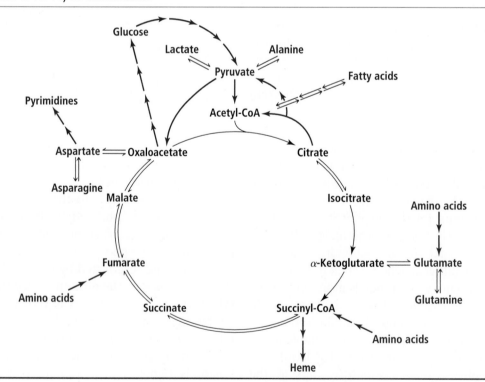

reaction is deprived of one of its substrates. *Therefore biosynthetic reactions that consume TCA-cycle intermediates have to be balanced by reactions that produce them.* This latter type of reaction is called **anaplerotic** (from the Greek word for "to fill up").

Some of the biosynthetic reactions are quite tissue specific: the use of oxaloacetate for the synthesis of glucose in the gluconeogenic pathway (see Chapter 17) is important in the liver during fasting, and the use of succinyl-CoA for heme biosynthesis (see Chapter 22) is most important in the erythropoietic cells of the bone marrow.

The three α-ketoacids—pyruvate, α-ketoglutarate, and oxaloacetate—are structurally related to the amino acids alanine, glutamate, and aspartate (Fig. 16.18). When the amino acids are in short sup-

ply they can be synthesized from the α-ketoacids. Under most conditions, however, excess dietary amino acids are metabolized to their corresponding α-ketoacids. Most other amino acids also are degraded to TCA-cycle intermediates.

Another important anaplerotic reaction is the carboxylation of pyruvate to oxaloacetate. This reaction, catalyzed by **pyruvate carboxylase**, is a typical *ATP-dependent carboxylation*: a carbon, derived from inorganic bicarbonate, is introduced into the substrate in the form of a carboxy group. The reaction requires **biotin**, a prosthetic group covalently bound to the apoenzyme by an amide bond with a lysine side chain.

The reaction proceeds in two steps (Fig. 16.19). First, CO_2 is bound to a nitrogen in biotin to pro-

---

FIG. 16.18

Alpha-keto acids and their corresponding alpha-amino acids.

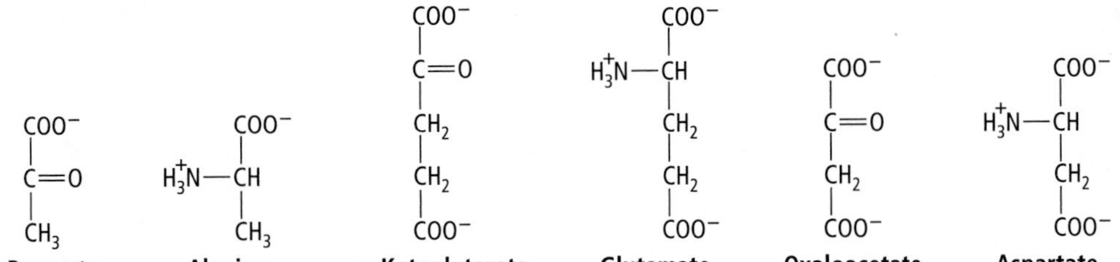

Pyruvate   Alanine α-Ketoglutarate   Glutamate   Oxaloacetate   Aspartate

---

FIG. 16.19

The pyruvate carboxylase reaction. This general mechanism applies to all biotin- and ATP-dependent carboxylations.

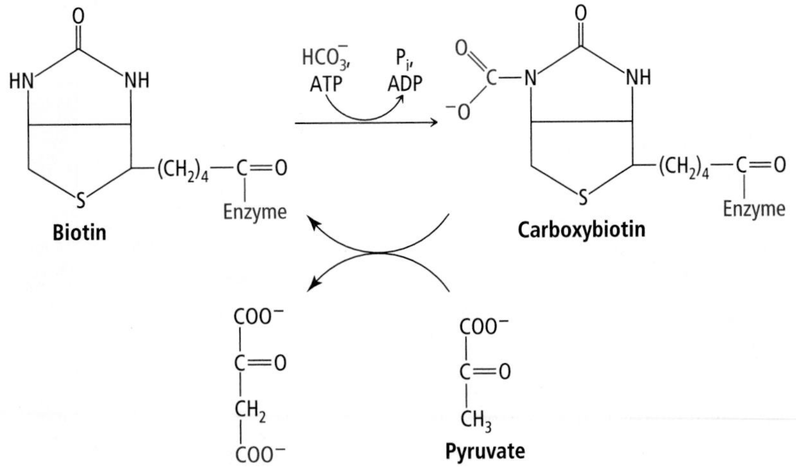

duce **carboxy-biotin.** This endergonic reaction $\Delta G^{0\prime} = +4.7$ kcal/mol) is made possible by the concomitant hydrolysis of ATP to ADP + phosphate ($\Delta G^{0\prime} = -7.3$ kcal/mol), resulting in an overall free energy change of -2.6 kcal/mol ($4.7 - 7.3$ kcal/mol). Carboxy-biotin can be considered an activated form of carbon dioxide. In the next step, the carboxy group of carboxy-biotin is transferred to pyruvate to form oxaloacetate.

Pyruvate carboxylase is a strictly mitochondrial enzyme. It requires manganese or magnesium for its activity, and acetyl-CoA is a positive allosteric effector. Indeed, the enzyme has an absolute requirement for acetyl-CoA. Patients with a genetic deficiency of pyruvate carboxylase (a rare, recessively inherited condition) suffer from lactic acidosis and CNS dysfunction.

Most intermediates of mitochondrial metabolism can be transported across the inner mitochondrial membrane

Mitochondrial metabolism depends on a continuous exchange of metabolites between the cytoplasm and the mitochondrial matrix. Pyruvate, for example, has to be transported into the mitochondrion. TCA-cycle intermediates or their products have to be transported to the cytoplasm for use in biosynthetic reactions. ADP and inorganic phosphate have to enter the mitochondrion as substrates for oxidative phosphorylation, and ATP has to pass from the mitochondrion to the cytoplasm, where it is used for energy-dependent processes.

The transfer of small, water-soluble molecules across the outer mitochondrial membrane is unproblematic because this membrane contains numerous pores formed by the protein porin. The inner membrane, however, which has to support a steep proton gradient during oxidative phosphorylation (see Fig. 16.26), is impermeable to hydrophilic solutes. Metabolites have to be transported across this membrane by specific carriers. Of the important intermediates, acetyl-CoA, oxaloacetate, fumarate, NAD+, and NADH are not transported. Of the nucleotides, only ADP and ATP are transported. The other TCA-cycle intermediates, however, are translocated, as are pyruvate and phosphate. Those amino acids that are directly derived from pyruvate, α-ketoglutarate, and oxaloacetate are transported as well.

The mitochondrial translocases, summarized in Fig. 16.20, are antiporters that, within limits, *maintain electroneutrality by transporting like charges in opposite directions*. They do not hydrolyze ATP but may consume energy by dissipating actively maintained ion gradients or reducing the membrane potential, which normally is positive outside and negative inside. For example, the transport of hydroxyl ions out of the mitochondrion by the phosphate carrier consumes energy indirectly by dissipating an actively maintained proton gradient (see Fig. 16.26). The ATP/ADP exchange, on the other hand, is electrogenic: ADP

FIG. 16.20

Translocases that transport metabolites across the inner mitochondrial membrane.

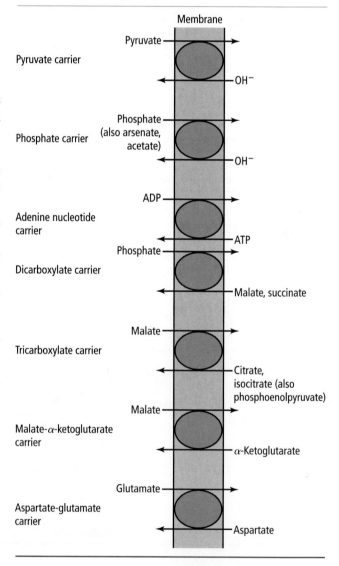

has approximately three negative charges at physiological pH; ATP has approximately four. This net transport of approximately one negative charge out of the mitochondrion weakens the membrane potential, which is an essential component of the proton gradient.

The transport of hydrogen from cytoplasmic NADH into the mitochondrion poses a special problem: for oxidation by the respiratory chain, NADH has to be in the mitochondrial matrix, but neither NADH nor NAD$^+$ is transported across the inner mitochondrial membrane. This necessitates the use of shuttle systems to transfer the hydrogen of cytoplasmic NADH (derived from glycolysis) to the respiratory chain in the inner mitochondrial membrane. The two principal shuttles, the **glycerol phosphate shuttle** and the **malate-aspartate shuttle,** are shown in Fig. 16.21.

The glycerol phosphate shuttle transfers the hydrogen first to dihydroxyacetone phosphate, forming glycerol phosphate, and then to the FAD prosthetic group of the mitochondrial glycerol

---

FIG. 16.21

The glycerol phosphate shuttle **(A)** and the malate-aspartate shuttle **(B).** Both of these shuttles are active in most cell types.
A, The mitochondrial glycerol phosphate dehydrogenase is an integral protein of the inner mitochondrial membrane, whose glycerol phosphate-binding site is on the cytoplasmic surface. Therefore glycerol phosphate need not cross the membrane. The FAD prosthetic group of the enzyme is regenerated by transfer of its hydrogen to ubiquinone (Q), a component of the respiratory chain. **B,** The arrows indicate the direction in which the shuttle proceeds during the transport of cytoplasmic hydrogen into the mitochondrion. Actually, the shuttle is freely reversible and can transport hydrogen out of the mitochondrion in some situations.

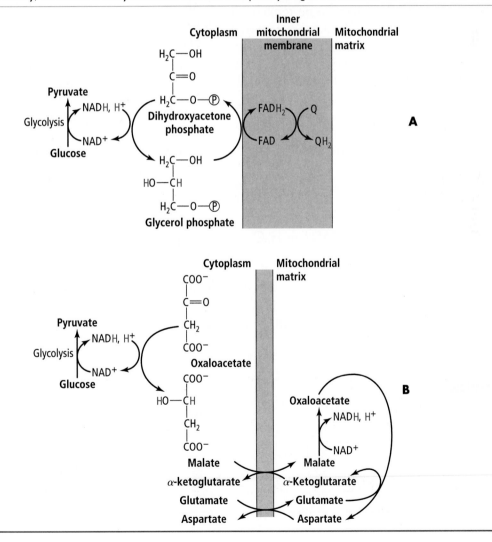

phosphate dehydrogenase, an integral protein of the inner mitochondrial membrane. Like succinate dehydrogenase, this enzyme regenerates its FAD by the direct transfer of electrons to the respiratory chain. *Only two ATPs are produced.*

The malate-aspartate shuttle transfers hydrogen from cytoplasmic NADH to oxaloacetate, forming malate. After its transport into the mitochondrion, malate forms NADH in the malate dehydrogenase reaction of the TCA cycle. This NADH can be oxidized by the respiratory chain, *producing three ATPs.*

THE RESPIRATORY CHAIN AND OXIDATIVE PHOSPHORYLATION

During all of the catabolic processes encountered so far, hydrogen was transferred from the substrate to NAD^+ or FAD. Indeed, *the formation of reduced coenzymes is a common feature of all major catabolic pathways.* Obviously, NADH and $FADH_2$ have to be reoxidized to NAD^+ and FAD, respectively, which are required as substrates of the pathways. In the mitochondrion, the coenzymes are oxidized by molecular oxygen in the **respiratory chain,** which is located in the inner mitochondrial membrane.

The respiratory chain uses molecular oxygen to oxidize NADH and $FADH_2$

The overall reactions in the respiratory chain are simple enough:

$$NADH + H^+ + \tfrac{1}{2} O_2 \longrightarrow NAD^+ + H_2O$$

$$FADH_2 + \tfrac{1}{2} O_2 \longrightarrow FAD + H_2O$$

The free energy changes of these reactions, however, are remarkable: the oxidation of $NADH + H^+$

releases 52.6 kcal/mol under standard conditions. This corresponds to the free energy content of not less than seven phosphoanhydride bonds in ATP. The energy yield from the oxidation of the $FADH_2$ in mitochondrial flavoproteins is variable. It is on the order of 40 kcal/mol.

During the oxidation of the reduced coenzymes, part of this energy is harvested as ATP in the process of **oxidative phosphorylation.** To achieve this, *the oxidations are broken down into several sequential reactions with smaller free energy changes.* In these reactions the components of the respiratory chain accept and donate electrons, either with or without accompanying protons. Schematically, a simple hydrogen transport chain can be described as shown in Box 16.2. The individual reactions in this chain are:

1. $NADH + H^+ + A \longrightarrow NAD^+ + AH_2$
2. $AH_2 + B \qquad \longrightarrow A + BH_2$
3. $BH_2 + C \qquad \longrightarrow B + CH_2$
4. $CH_2 + \tfrac{1}{2} O_2 \qquad \longrightarrow C + H_2O$

The sum of the free energy changes in these four reactions equals that of the overall reaction:

$$NADH + H^+ + \tfrac{1}{2} O_2 \longrightarrow NAD^+ + H_2O$$

Electron carriers can react with "hydrogen" carriers because a hydrogen atom consists of one electron and one proton. Protons can be exchanged readily with the solvent during redox reactions. Iron, for example, which is a component of many electron carriers, can accept an electron from a hydrogen carrier such as FAD while a proton is released:

$$FADH_2 + 2 Fe^{3+} \longrightarrow FAD + 2 Fe^{2+} + 2 H^+$$

Fe^{2+}, in turn, can donate an electron to a hydrogen

BOX 16.2

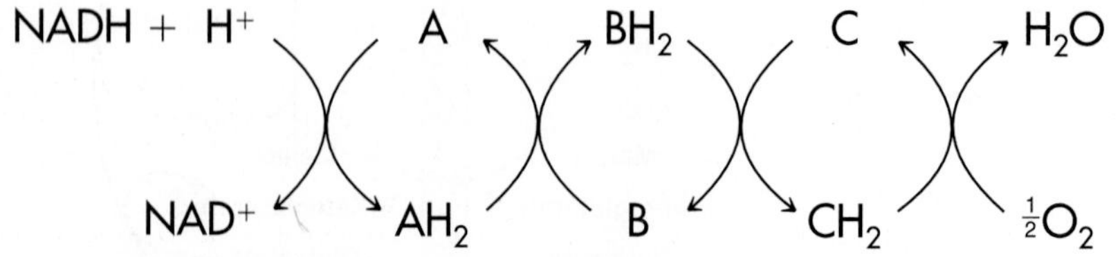

carrier while a proton enters from the aqueous solvent, for example:

$$2 \, Fe^{2+} + \tfrac{1}{2} \, O_2 + 2 \, H^+ \longrightarrow 2 \, Fe^{3+} + H_2O$$

The standard reduction potential is the most useful property of redox couples

Redox reactions are defined as electron-transfer reactions. This implies the participation of two substrates: a reduced substrate, or **reductant,** which donates electrons and becomes oxidized, and an oxidized substrate, or **oxidant,** which accepts electrons and becomes reduced during the reaction.

A substance that can exist in either an oxidized or a reduced form is called a **redox couple.** $FAD/FADH_2$, Fe^{3+}/Fe^{2+}, and $\tfrac{1}{2} \, O_2/H_2O$ are examples of redox couples. During a redox reaction, each redox couple undergoes a "half-reaction."

Examples:

$$FAD + 2 \, H^+ + 2 \, e^- \Longleftrightarrow FADH_2$$

$$Fe^{3+} + e^- \Longleftrightarrow Fe^{2+}$$

$$\tfrac{1}{2} \, O_2 + 2 \, H^+ + 2 \, e^- \Longleftrightarrow H_2O$$

For the equilibrium of redox reactions, *the important property of a redox couple is its tendency to accept or donate electrons.* This tendency can be determined experimentally by allowing the two half-reactions of a redox reaction to proceed in separate compartments and measuring the resulting electron motive force (in volts).

The **reduction potential,** also called the **redox potential,** commonly is determined under standard conditions, with a temperature of 25°C and reactant concentrations of 1 M. The reference system, whose reduction potential is arbitrarily set as 0 volt, is the hydrogen electrode, with a half-reaction of $2H^+ + 2e^- \longleftrightarrow H_2$. A **standard reduction potential** $E°$ of less than zero means that a redox couple has a greater tendency to donate electrons, or a greater "reducing power," than the hydrogen molecule. A standard reduction potential above zero means a greater tendency to accept electrons. $E°$ is

the property not of a reaction, but of a redox couple (Table 16.5).

For biological systems, the standard conditions are modified: the concentrations of reactants other than H^+ are kept at 1 M, but the proton concentration is fixed at 10^{-7} M (pH = 7.0). Reduction potentials determined under these conditions are designated as $E°'$. These are the same "biological" standard conditions that are used for the definition of standard free energy changes (see Chapter 4).

Under standard conditions, the driving force for a redox reaction can be expressed as the difference between the standard reduction potentials of the participating redox couples ($\Delta E°'$):

$$\Delta E^{0'} = E^{0'}_{oxidant} - E^{0'}_{reductant}$$

For the reaction

$$NADH + H^+ + \tfrac{1}{2} \, O_2 \longrightarrow NAD^+ + H_2O$$

TABLE 16.5

Standard reduction potentials of some biologically important redox couples

Oxidant/reductant	$E°'$ (volt)
Acetate/acetaldehyde	− 0.60
$2 \, H^+/H_2$	− 0.42*
$NAD^+/NADH + H^+$	− 0.32
$NADP^+/NADPH + H^+$	− 0.32
Lipoate/Dihydrolipoate	− 0.29
Acetoacetate/β-Hydroxybutyrate	− 0.27
Glutathione oxidized/reduced	− 0.23
Acetaldehyde/Ethanol	− 0.20
Pyruvate/Lactate	− 0.19
Oxaloacetate/Malate	− 0.17
Fumarate/Succinate	+ 0.03
Cytochrome b Fe^{3+}/Fe^{2+}	+ 0.08
Dehydroascorbate/Ascorbate	+ 0.08
Ubiquinone/Ubiquinol	+ 0.10
Cytochrome c Fe^{3+}/Fe^{2+}	+ 0.22
Fe^{3+}/Fe^{2+}	+ 0.77†
$\tfrac{1}{2} \, O_2/H_2O$	+ 0.82

* The reduction potential of the hydrogen electrode is set at zero for "chemical" standard conditions, with a proton concentration of 1 M. The shift into the negative range is caused by the far lower proton concentration under "biological" standard conditions (at a pH of 7.0).
† Standard reduction potential of inorganic iron. The reduction potentials of the iron in heme proteins and iron-sulfur proteins may be markedly different.

the standard reduction potentials are:

$$NAD^+/NADH + H^+: E^{0\prime} = -0.32 \text{ volt}$$

$$\tfrac{1}{2}O_2 + 2H^+/H_2O: E^{0\prime} = +0.82 \text{ volt}$$

$$\begin{aligned}
\Delta E^{0\prime} &= E^{0\prime}_{\tfrac{1}{2}O_2 + 2H^+/H_2O} - E^{0\prime}_{NAD^+/NADH+H^+} \\
&= 0.82 \text{ volt} - (-0.32 \text{ volt}) \\
&= +1.14 \text{ volt}
\end{aligned}$$

As in the case of free energy changes, the actual driving force of the reaction under nonstandard conditions (ΔE) depends also on the relative reactant concentrations. There is, indeed, a simple relationship between $\Delta G^{0\prime}$ and $\Delta E^{0\prime}$:

$$\Delta G^{0\prime} = -n \times F \times \Delta E^{0\prime}$$

in which n is the number of electrons transferred and F is the Faraday constant (23.06 kcal V^{-1} mol^{-1}).

A positive $\Delta E^{0\prime}$, like a negative $\Delta G^{0\prime}$, signifies an exergonic reaction. In the earlier example of NADH oxidation by molecular oxygen, $\Delta G^{0\prime}$ can be calculated as

$$\begin{aligned}
\Delta G^{0\prime} &= -n \times F \times \Delta E^{0\prime} \\
&= -2 \times 23.06 \times 1.14 \\
&= -52.6 \text{ kcal/mol}
\end{aligned}$$

In redox reactions, electrons are transferred from a redox couple with a lower reduction potential to one with a higher reduction potential.

The respiratory chain contains flavoproteins, iron-sulfur proteins, cytochromes, ubiquinone, and protein-bound copper

The components of the respiratory chain act as either "hydrogen" carriers or electron carriers. The **flavoproteins** are important hydrogen carriers. Two electrons and two protons are transferred to the FAD or FMN prosthetic group during the transition from the oxidized to the reduced state. Single-electron transfers are possible, too. In this case an unstable free radical is generated (Fig. 16.22). Flavoproteins often are associated with iron-sulfur proteins, and one-electron transfers are thought to occur between the flavin and the non-heme iron. Typically, the standard reduction potentials of the flavoproteins are higher than that of NAD$^+$/NADH but lower than those of the cytochromes. The flavoproteins of the respiratory chain are integral membrane proteins.

The **iron-sulfur proteins**, also known as **non-heme iron proteins**, are electron carriers in which iron is complexed to cysteine side chains. Many iron-sulfur proteins contain inorganic sulfide as well (Fig. 16.23). In these cases, hydrogen sulfide is released when the protein is treated with acid in vitro. *The protein-bound iron participates in electron transfers by changing its oxidation state between the ferrous (Fe^{2+}) and ferric (Fe^{3+}) forms.* The standard reduction potentials are variable, depending on the polypeptide environment of the non-heme iron. Like the flavoproteins, the iron-sulfur proteins of the respiratory chain are integral membrane proteins.

FIG. 16.22

Structures of oxidized and reduced flavins.

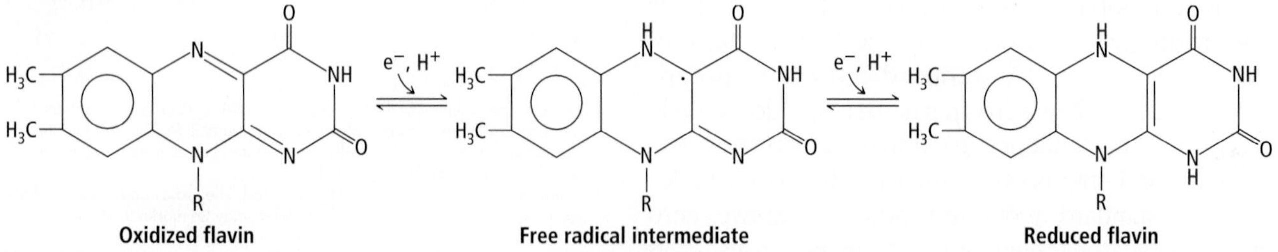

Oxidized flavin — Free radical intermediate — Reduced flavin

The **cytochromes** are electron carriers that contain an iron-porphyrin as a prosthetic group. In most cases, this iron-porphyrin is the heme group. In contrast to hemoglobin and myoglobin, *the heme iron of the cytochromes undergoes valence changes between* Fe^{2+} *and* Fe^{3+} *during its normal functioning,* thereby acting as a reversible electron carrier. Also, in most cytochromes (but not cytochrome a/a_3), the heme iron is bound to two amino acid side chains, thereby preventing the binding of molecular oxygen, carbon monoxide, and other potential ligands. Though the heme group of cytochrome b is bound to the apoprotein by noncovalent interactions, it is covalently bound in cytochromes c and c_1. Cytochromes a and a_3 contain **heme a** rather than

"ordinary" heme. In this iron porphyrin, a methyl group of heme is oxidized to a formyl group, and a hydrophobic isoprenoid chain is attached to one of the vinyl groups. With the exception of cytochrome c, the cytochromes of the respiratory chain are integral membrane proteins.

Ubiquinone, also known as **coenzyme Q**, is a mobile, diffusible hydrogen carrier, not permanently associated with an apoprotein. It has a hydrocarbon tail of (usually) 10 isoprene (branched 5-carbon) units, which makes it strongly hydrophobic and confines it to the lipid bilayer of the inner mitochondrial membrane. Like the flavin coenzymes, ubiquinone carries two hydrogens but can act in one-electron transfers by forming a free-radical intermediate (Fig. 16.24).

Protein-bound **copper** participates in the last reaction of the respiratory chain, the transfer of electrons to molecular oxygen. It acts as an electron carrier by a valence change between the Cu^{1+} and Cu^{2+} forms.

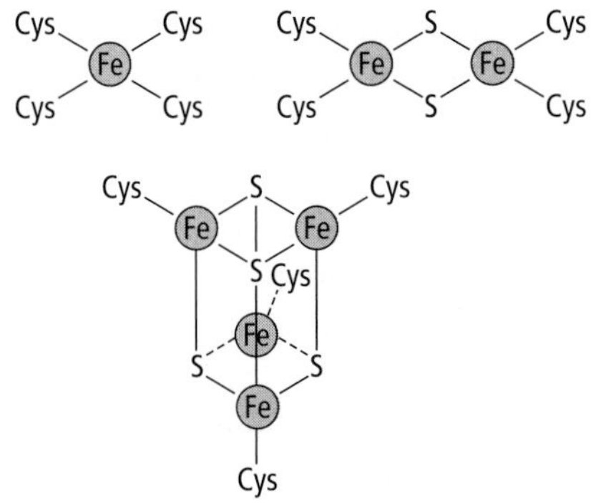

The respiratory chain contains three large multiprotein complexes

Four members of the respiratory chain are freely diffusible: NADH, ubiquinone, cytochrome c, and molecular oxygen. NADH has to be present in the mitochondrial matrix. Ubiquinone is mobile within the lipid bilayer. Cytochrome c is a peripheral membrane protein on the outer membrane surface. Mo-

---

FIG. 16.23

Iron-sulfur complexes in proteins. The iron in these complexes can change its oxidation state reversibly between the ferrous (Fe^{2+}) and ferric (Fe^{3+}) forms.

FIG. 16.24

Structure of ubiquinone (coenzyme Q).

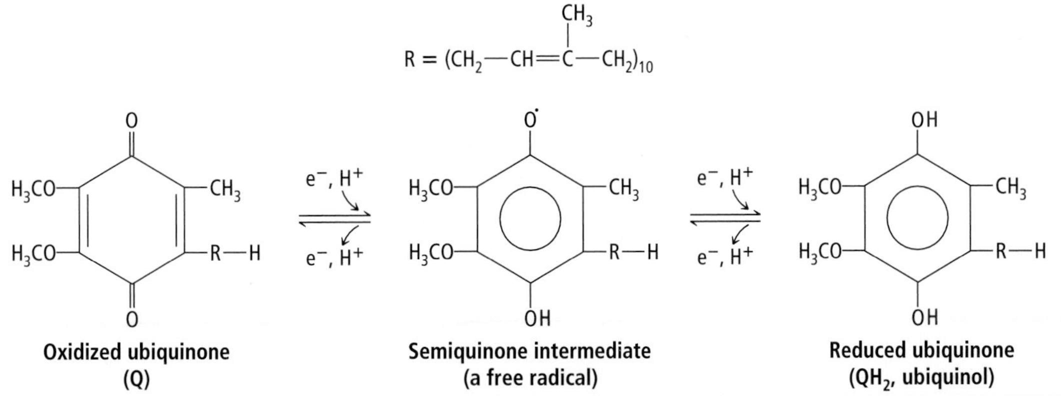

$$R = (CH_2 - CH = \overset{\overset{\textstyle CH_3}{|}}{C} - CH_2)_{10}$$

Oxidized ubiquinone (Q)   Semiquinone intermediate (a free radical)   Reduced ubiquinone (QH$_2$, ubiquinol)

lecular oxygen, freely diffusible across membranes, receives electrons and protons on the matrix side of the inner mitochondrial membrane.

The other components of the respiratory chain are constituents of three large protein complexes, which are arranged asymmetrically in the membrane (Fig. 16.25).

1. The **NADH-Q reductase complex**, also called **NADH dehydrogenase**, transfers electrons from NADH to ubiquinone. It contains FMN and several iron-sulfur centers. Electrons are transferred from NADH to FMN, then through a succession of iron-sulfur centers to ubiquinone.
2. The **QH$_2$-cytochrome c reductase complex**, also called **cytochrome reductase**, contains cytochrome b, an iron-sulfur protein, and cytochrome c$_1$.
3. The **cytochrome oxidase complex** consists of 13 different polypeptides, two heme a groups, and two copper ions. Each of the two heme a groups, known as heme a and heme a$_3$, is located near a copper ion. O$_2$ is tightly bound between heme a$_3$ and copper during its reduction, to be released only after its complete reduction to H$_2$O. The reduction of oxygen is thought to occur by the sequential transfer of four electrons. Cytochrome oxidase has a very high affinity for molecular oxygen. Therefore oxidative phosphorylation is near maximal even at very low oxygen partial pressure.

Mitochondrial flavoproteins, including succinate dehydrogenase and the mitochondrial glycerol phosphate dehydrogenase, bypass the NADH-Q reductase complex. They transfer their electrons directly to ubiquinone.

Electron transport and ATP synthesis are coupled through a proton gradient

In oxidative phosphorylation, *the exergonic redox reactions of the respiratory chain are coupled to the endergonic synthesis of ATP from ADP and inorganic phosphate.* Which of these redox reactions are actually used to synthesize ATP? Early observations showed that three sites in the respiratory chain are important, one in each of the three protein complexes (Fig. 16.25). Each of these "phosphorylation sites" is responsible for the synthesis of approximately one ATP for each pair of electrons. Therefore *the respiratory chain oxidation of one NADH yields three ATPs.* The **P/O ratio** is defined as the number of high-energy phosphate bonds formed for each oxygen atom consumed. The P/O ratio for NADH oxidation is 3. The transfer of electrons from mitochondrial flavoproteins toubiquinone is not

---

FIG. 16.25

The respiratory chain. The shaded structures are multiprotein complexes in the inner mitochondrial membrane. NADH and succinate are in the matrix space, ubiquinone (Q) is in the lipid bilayer of the membrane, and cytochrome c is a peripheral membrane protein, bound to the outer surface of the inner mitochondrial membrane. The standard redox potentials are shown for some components. →, Sites of proton pumping ("phosphorylation sites").

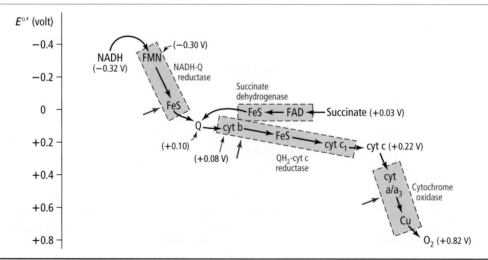

accompanied by ATP synthesis. Therefore *the P/O ratio for the oxidation of FADH₂ is only 2.*

According to the **chemiosmotic hypothesis,** oxidative phosphorylation proceeds in two steps (Fig. 16.26). In the first step, *protons are translocated from the mitochondrial matrix to the intermembranous space.* This proton pumping is fueled by the redox reactions in the respiratory chain. The three "phosphorylation sites" actually are sites of proton pumping. The mechanism by which proton translocation is coupled to redox reactions in the respiratory chain is not known. Proton pumping by the respiratory chain creates a proton gradient of approximately one pH unit across the inner mitochondrial membrane, inside alkaline. It also helps to maintain a membrane potential of 100 to 200 mV, inside negative. Concentration gradient and electrical potential add up to a steep electrochemical gradient for protons, amounting to approximately 4 to 6 kcal/mol.

The impermeability of the inner mitochondrial membrane both to protons and to other inorganic ions (which would dissipate the membrane potential) is an absolute requirement for oxidative phosphorylation. We saw before (see Fig. 16.20) that most translocases of the inner mitochondrial membrane are antiporters that effect electroneutral exchanges, thereby minimizing the effects of substrate transport on the membrane potential.

FIG. 16.26

The two steps in oxidative phosphorylation. The inner mitochondrial membrane acts like a storage battery that is charged by the proton pumps of the respiratory chain. **A,** Protons are pumped out of the mitochondrial matrix. Proton pumping is fueled by the exergonic redox reactions in the respiratory chain. **B,** Protons move back into the matrix space through a specific proton channel. This proton channel is coupled to an ATP-synthesizing enzyme (the F_1 ATPase). ATP synthesis is fueled by the flow of protons down their electrochemical gradient.

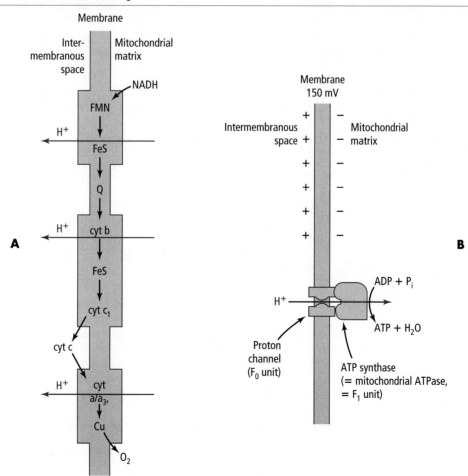

In the second step of oxidative phosphorylation, *the proton gradient is utilized for ATP synthesis*: protons are allowed to move back into the mitochondrion through a specific proton channel. This proton channel is coupled to an ATP-synthesizing enzyme, the **mitochondrial ATP synthase.**

The mitochondrial ATP synthase, also known as the F_1 unit (F_1 stands for "coupling factor 1"), is a protein complex of subunit structure $\alpha_3\beta_3\gamma\delta$ and a molecular weight of 380 kDa. It can be visualized in the electron microscope as small buttons on the inner surface of the inner mitochondrial membrane. The F_1 unit is attached to the **F_0 unit** (oligomycin-sensitive factor), an integral membrane protein that contains the proton channel.

Proton flow through the F_0 unit and ATP synthesis by the F_1 unit are tightly coupled: *ATP is synthesized only when protons flow, and protons can flow only when ATP*

FIG. 16.27

Isolation of the F_1 ATPase. Note that the isolated ATP synthase does not synthesize but rather hydrolyzes ATP. This enzyme therefore is often called the "mitochondrial ATPase" or "F_1 ATPase." An intact membrane with a steep proton gradient is an absolute requirement for ATP synthesis.

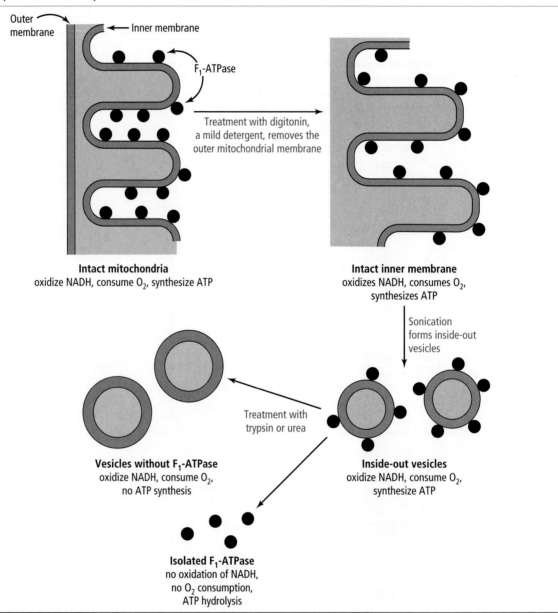

Outer membrane

Inner membrane

F_1-ATPase

Treatment with digitonin, a mild detergent, removes the outer mitochondrial membrane

Intact mitochondria
oxidize NADH, consume O_2, synthesize ATP

Intact inner membrane
oxidizes NADH, consumes O_2, synthesizes ATP

Sonication forms inside-out vesicles

Treatment with trypsin or urea

Vesicles without F_1-ATPase
oxidize NADH, consume O_2, no ATP synthesis

Inside-out vesicles
oxidize NADH, consume O_2, synthesize ATP

Isolated F_1-ATPase
no oxidation of NADH, no O_2 consumption, ATP hydrolysis

is synthesized. Neither the mechanism nor the stoichiometry of ATP synthesis is known in any detail, but for energetic reasons the translocation of at least two protons is required for the synthesis of one ATP.

In the absence of a sufficient proton gradient, the ATP synthase hydrolyzes, rather than synthesizes ATP, as shown in Fig. 16.27. Therefore the term **mitochondrial ATPase** is sometimes applied to the ATP-synthesizing complex. Energetically, *mitochondrial ATP synthesis is the reversal of an ATP-dependent membrane transport.*

The efficiency of glucose oxidation is close to 40%

We are now in a position to examine the efficiency of ATP synthesis from the oxidation of glucose. As shown in Table 16.6, 36 to 38 high-energy phosphate bonds are generated. Only four of these are produced by substrate-level phosphorylation in glycolysis and TCA cycle; the rest are from oxidative phosphorylation.

Anaerobic glycolysis, on the other hand, yields not more than two molecules of ATP. Evidently, *only aerobic metabolism can supply sufficient energy for such tissues as the brain and the myocardium, which have to maintain a high metabolic rate at all times.*

Under standard conditions, the free energy of hydrolysis for a phosphoanhydride bond in ATP is approximately -7.3 kcal/mol. The total yield of chemical energy during glucose oxidation, assuming 37 ATP formed, is therefore

$$37 \times 7.3 = 270.1 \text{ kcal/mol}$$

TABLE 16.6

Energy yield from glucose oxidation

Pathway	Yield	
Glycolysis		2 ATP
	2 NADH $\rightarrow$	4 or 6 ATP*
Pyruvate dehydrogenase	2 NADH $\rightarrow$	6 ATP
TCA cycle	2 GTP $\rightarrow$	2 ATP
	6 NADH $\rightarrow$	18 ATP
	2 FADH$_2$ $\rightarrow$	4 ATP
		36 or 38 ATP

* The energy yield from cytoplasmic NADH depends on the shuttle system used.

The total heat released by glucose oxidation in the bomb calorimeter is 686 kcal/mol. Therefore the efficiency of ATP synthesis in glucose oxidation is $270.1/686 = 0.396 = 39.6\%$. The balance is released as heat.

Even with ATP synthesis, the overall equilibrium of the oxidative pathways is so overwhelmingly in favor of substrate oxidation that *the cells are able to maintain a high [ATP]/[ADP] ratio.* In resting muscle, for example, the [ATP]/[ADP] ratio is on the order of 100:1.

Under most conditions, the rate of oxidative phosphorylation is limited by the availability of ADP

Respiratory control is based on a tight coupling between electron flow in the respiratory chain and ATP synthesis: *in the absence of electron flow, ATP cannot be synthesized, and when ATP synthesis is not possible for lack of ADP or phosphate, electrons cannot flow.* Unless the proton gradient is dissipated through the F_o/F_1 ATPase, it will build up to such proportions that the redox reactions in the respiratory chain grind to a halt, unable to pump against the overwhelming gradient.

There is no specific physiological control point, or "rate-limiting step," in oxidative phosphorylation, but its rate depends on the availability of its substrates. Possible limiting factors include

NADH
Oxygen
ADP
Phosphate
The capacity of the respiratory chain itself when all substrates are freely available (its V_{max})

Under most conditions, *the rate-limiting factor is the supply of ADP.* Phosphate and (except in starvation) NADH are not often limiting. With increased metabolic activity, as in contracting muscle, the rate of oxidative phosphorylation increases initially in proportion to the increased ADP concentration, until either the oxygen supply or the capacity of the respiratory chain becomes limiting.

An increased rate of oxidative phosphorylation increases the mitochondrial [NAD$^+$]/[NADH] ratio. This, together with the decreased energy charge that induced the increased rate of oxidative phosphorylation in the first place, stimulates pyruvate dehydrogenase and the regulated enzymes of the TCA cycle (see Fig. 16.16). NADH production thereby is adjusted to the requirements for oxidative phosphorylation.

Oxidative phosphorylation is inhibited by many poisons

Electron flow through the respiratory chain can be blocked by *site-specific inhibitors* (Table 16.7). **Rotenone,** obtained from the roots of some tropical plants, inhibits electron flow from the iron-sulfur complexes in the NADH-Q reductase complex to ubiquinone. It is a very effective poison for fish, which take it up through their gills, but it is not very toxic to humans because of its poor intestinal absorption. Humans therefore can eat the poisoned fish with impunity. Rotenone is also in favor asa "natural" insecticide. Besides rotenone, some **barbiturates** inhibit electron flow through the NADH-Q reductase complex. This action is unrelated to the useful sedative-hypnotic properties of barbiturates, but it may play a role in barbiturate poisoning.

Antimycin A, an antibiotic produced by a streptomycete, blocks electron flow through the QH_2-cytochrome c reductase complex.

In the cytochrome oxidase complex, several inhibitors bind to the heme iron in cytochrome a/a_3 whose sixth coordination position is not occupied by an amino acid side chain but is reserved for oxygen. **Cyanide** and **azide** bind to the ferric form of the iron; carbon monoxide binds to the ferrous form. **Hydrogen sulfide** also is a potent inhibitor. Carbon monoxide has a higher affinity for hemoglobin than for cytochrome oxidase, but the other agents induce their clinically important toxicity by inhibiting electron flow.

Uncouplers of oxidative phosphorylation prevent ATP synthesis without inhibiting electron flow. Most uncouplers interfere with the proton gradient across the inner mitochondrial membrane. **2,4-Dinitrophenol** and **pentachlorophenol** (Fig. 16.28) are diffusible, lipophilic organic acids. *They dissipate the proton gradient by transporting protons across the inner mitochondrial membrane.* Without a sufficient proton gradient, ATP synthesis is no longer possible. Electron flow, however, is not blocked but actually increases because the respiratory chain no longer has to pump protons against a steep gradient.

Some endogenous compounds, including free fatty acids, bilirubin, and possibly thyroxine, also can act as uncouplers at concentrations well above the physiological range. In the case of bilirubin, which deposits in the basal ganglia of infants with severe hyperbilirubinemia (see Chapter 22), a role of the uncoupling effect in the resulting brain damage is possible.

Valinomycin is a transport antibiotic that makes

TABLE 16.7

Inhibitors of oxidative phosphorylation

Inhibitor	Mechanism
Inhibitors of electron flow	
Rotenone, amytal	Inhibits NADH-Q reductase
Antimycin A	Inhibits QH_2-cytochrome c reductase
Cyanide, azide, hydrogen sulfide, carbon monoxide	Inhibits cytochrome oxidase
Oligomycin	Inhibits the F_1/F_o ATPase
Uncouplers	
2,4-Dinitrophenol, pentachlorophenol	Transports protons across the inner mitochondrial membrane
Valinomycin	Transports potassium across the inner mitochondrial membrane
Arsenate	Substitutes for phosphate during ATP synthesis
Atractyloside	Inhibits ATP-ADP translocation

the inner mitochondrial membrane permeable for potassium. It acts as an uncoupler because the translocation of potassium ions dissipates the membrane potential, which is an essential component of the proton-motive force.

Arsenate uncouples oxidative phosphorylation by an entirely different mechanism: after getting a free ride into the mitochondrion on the phosphate transporter, it competes with phosphate for ATP synthesis. The resulting γ-arsenate analogue of ATP hydrolyzes spontaneously back to ADP and arsenate.

Oligomycin is an antibiotic that inhibits oxidative phosphorylation by blocking proton flow through the F_o/F_1 ATPase. It prevents ATP synthesis and leads to the buildup of a very steep proton gradient that inhibits electron flow through the respiratory chain.

The plant product **atractyloside** prevents ATP synthesis by blocking the ATP/ADP antiporter in the inner mitochondrial membrane (see Fig. 16.20). The resulting lack of ADP in the mitochondrial matrix stops both ATP synthesis and electron flow.

Oxygen deficiency is rapidly fatal

Although the ATP concentration in various tissues is only 1 to 5 g/kg, approximately 70 kg of ATP is synthesized in the human body every day, the vast majority of it by oxidative phosphorylation. This means that the average ATP molecule has a lifespan of only 1 to 5 minutes and that most cells will be depleted of ATP very soon after the cessation of oxidative phosphorylation.

FIG. 16.28

Structures of 2,4-dinitrophenol and pentachlorophenol. These chemicals are highly diffusible, acidic substances that can penetrate the inner mitochondrial membrane, even in the negatively charged deprotonated form. They uncouple oxidative phosphorylation by transporting protons across the membrane.

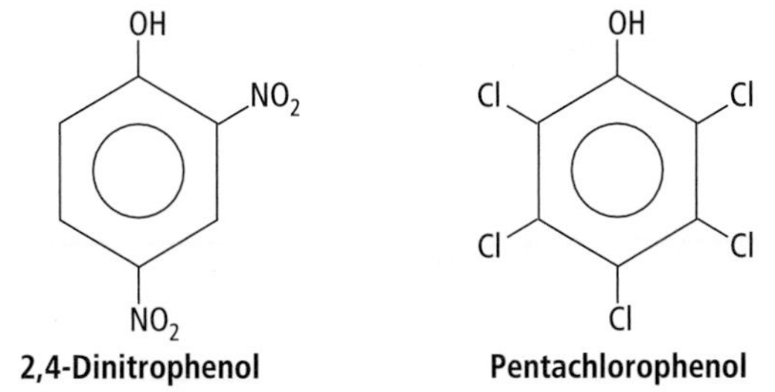

2,4-Dinitrophenol   **Pentachlorophenol**

The most common cause for a failure of oxidative phosphorylation is **hypoxia** (insufficient oxygen) or **anoxia** (complete lack of oxygen). Oxygen deficiency is caused most commonly by **ischemia** (interruption of the blood supply). Ischemic anoxia causes cell death within a few minutes (neurons), half an hour to 2 hours (myocardium, liver, kidney), or several hours (fibroblasts, epidermis, skeletal muscle). In ischemic cell injury and cell death (Fig. 16.29), some of the events are

- *All energy-dependent processes, including active membrane transport, are no longer possible.*
- *Osmotic imbalances are caused by the failure to maintain normal ion gradients.* Cellular edema (swelling) develops, and similar abnormalities afflict membrane-bounded organelles, including lysosomes and mitochondria.
- *Glycolysis is stimulated by low energy charge* at the level of PFK, with the resultant accumulation of lactic acid. This stimulation of glycolysis under anaerobic conditions is known as the **Pasteur effect**. Glycolysis is fueled by stored glycogen, whose breakdown also is stimulated by low energy charge (see Chapter 17). Lactic acid decreases the pH of the ischemic tissue.
- *Both the plasma membrane and the organellar membranes become leaky* because of osmotic stress and increased acidity. Cellular enzymes leak into the interstitial space and finally appear in the blood. Lysosomal enzymes are released, and in their acidified environment, they attack cellular proteins, glycoproteins, glycolipids, phosphate esters, and other substrates. Some of these hydrolytic cleavages, especially those of carboxylic esters and phosphate esters, further acidify the environment.

Ischemic tissue injury is not entirely the result of oxygen deficiency. In animal experiments, cells have survived "pure" anoxia, without interruption of the blood flow, longer than ischemic anoxia. This fact points to the importance of accumulating metabolic products, such as lactic acid, in ischemic cell injury.

In ischemia, *loss of function always precedes cell death.* Ischemic myocardial tissue, for example, can survive for 30 to 60 minutes, but its contractility is lost within less than 1 minute. Similarly, although neurons survive for some minutes, consciousness is lost almost immediately after a sudden interruption of the blood supply to the brain. This is likely to take place, for example, after decapitation on the guillotine.

Inhibitors of oxidative phosphorylation also can be rapidly fatal

Cyanide (HCN) blocks the respiratory chain by binding to the ferric iron in cytochrome a/a_3. Although not particularly potent (the lethal dose of HCN in humans is approximately 1 mg/kg), cyanide is absorbed rapidly from the gastrointestinal tract, and the effect of inhaled HCN gas is almost instantaneous, forestalling any effective measures of treatment. Cyanides are popular for suicide as well as homicide. They also are used for the extermination of rodents and insects—and, in some states, of murderers: in the gas chamber, HCN gas is used to block the condemned felon's respiratory chain.

The metabolic derangements of cyanide poisoning resemble those of hypoxia (Fig. 16.29). Hyperventilation develops rapidly. This hyperventilation is caused not by hypoxia or hypercapnia (elevated CO_2)—the oxygen saturation of hemoglobin actually is increased and the carbon dioxide concentration of the blood is decreased—but by a massive lactic acidosis. Unable to synthesize ATP by oxidative phosphorylation, *all tissues switch to anaerobic glycolysis and release lactic acid into the blood*. Metabolic acidosis of any cause is a powerful stimulus for the

FIG. 16.29

The metabolic consequences of hypoxia. A decreased energy charge and decreased [NAD$^+$]/[NADH] ratio are the initial results of oxygen deficiency. The mitochondrial oxidative pathways are arrested for lack of NAD$^+$. The regulated enzymes of glycolysis and glycogen degradation (phosphofructokinase and glycogen phosphorylase) are stimulated by low energy charge. The accumulation of lactic acid acidifies the cell. Both the plasma membrane and the organellar membranes are damaged by the increased acidity and by osmotic imbalances that result from the failure of ATP-dependent ion pumps. Lysosomal enzymes, which are active at low pH, initiate autolysis.

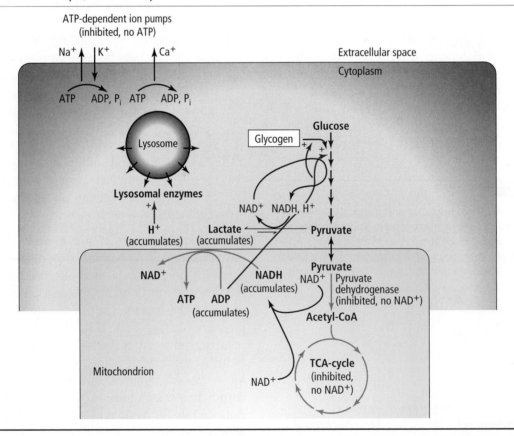

respiratory center. Hyperventilation tends to increase the pH of blood and tissues because *the removal of respiratory carbon dioxide reduces the proton concentration* according to the equilibrium

$$HCO_3^- + H^+ \rightleftharpoons H_2CO_3 \rightleftharpoons CO_2 + H_2O$$

The treatment of cyanide poisoning is aimed at the removal of the poison from cytochrome oxidase. Sodium nitrite, in moderate doses, is given to induce methemoglobin formation. The ferric iron in methemoglobin binds cyanide avidly, thereby removing it from the ferric iron in cytochrome a/a_3. Sodium thiosulfate also is given; it reacts with cyanide to form the far-less-toxic thiocyanate. This reaction is catalyzed by the enzyme rhodanase in the liver and, to a lesser extent, in other tissues.

Pentachlorophenol (Fig. 16.28) is a popular wood preservative that kills termites, fungi, bacteria, and, occasionally, humans by uncoupling their oxidative phosphorylation. Like cyanide poisoning, pentachlorophenol poisoning leads to a failure of oxidative phosphorylation and to lactic acidosis. In contrast to cyanide poisoning, however, *oxygen consumption and NADH oxidation are not decreased but increased.* A high $[NAD^+]/[NADH]$ ratio and low energy charge stimulate the oxidative pathways. With impaired ATP synthesis, however, *the energy of fuel oxidation is released as heat.* Hyperthermia therefore is a prominent sign in pentachlorophenol poisoning.

Mutations in mitochondrial DNA can cause disease

Any complete malfunction of mitochondrial oxidative metabolism is fatal. Genetic diseases in which mitochondrial oxidation is impaired are indeed rare. Most of these mitochondrial diseases are caused by mutations in the mitochondrial DNA.

The mitochondrial genome (see Chapter 8) consists of a circular DNA molecule of 16,569 base pairs, which encodes 13 polypeptides, 22 tRNAs, and the 2 RNAs of the mitochondrial ribosomes (12S and 16S). The mitochondrially encoded polypeptides include seven subunits of NADH-Q reductase, one subunit of QH_2-cytochrome c reductase, three subunits of cytochrome oxidase, and two subunits of ATP synthase. All other mitochondrial proteins are encoded by nuclear genes and synthesized by cytoplasmic ribosomes.

Leber's hereditary optic neuropathy (LHON) is characterized by the sudden onset of blindness in adults, associated with a degeneration of the optic nerve. The most common mutation in patients with this disease is a single-base substitution at base pair 11,778 of the mitochondrial DNA, in the gene for one of the subunits of NADH-Q reductase. Other patients have point mutations in genes for other respiratory chain components, including subunits of NADH-Q reductase, QH_2-cytochrome c reductase, and cytochrome oxidase. All of these mutations impair electron flow through the respiratory chain and reduce ATP synthesis. They lead to blindness because the optic nerve has a high energy demand and depends almost entirely on oxidative phosphorylation for its ATP supply. LHON is transmitted from an affected mother to all of her children, but not from an affected father. The reason for this unusual inheritance pattern is that almost all mitochondria in the zygote are derived from the ovum rather than from the sperm.

Mutations in the genes for ATP synthase subunits and for mitochondrial tRNAs are known as well. These mutations lead to diseases that are characterized by neurological abnormalities, abnormalities of red muscle fibers, cardiomyopathy, retinal degeneration, and/or lactic acidosis. All affected tissues rely heavily on oxidative metabolism and therefore are vulnerable to mitochondrial diseases. In some cases the disease-producing mutation is present in all mitochondria, but in other cases some mitochondria are unaffected while others bear the mutation, even in the same cell. The latter case is called **heteroplasmy.** Most cells have hundreds of mitochondria, and each mitochondrion has several copies of the mitochondrial genome.

Mitochondrial DNA has a higher mutation rate than does nuclear DNA. For this reason mutations in the mitochondrial DNA accumulate during our lifetime, and the oxidative capacity declines with advancing age. Deletions in the mitochondrial DNA, in particular, accumulate with age in such tissues as the heart, muscles, and the brain. It is thought that these deletions gradually spread in the mitochondrial population because the shortened DNA replicates faster than the full-length mitochondrial DNA, provided that the origin of replication is spared. The gradual decline of mitochondrial function with age explains why many inherited mitochondrial mutations become symptomatic only at an advanced age, when the combined effects of the inherited mutation and of acquired somatic mutations decrease oxidative phosphorylation below a critical threshold.

Reactive oxygen derivatives are formed during oxidative metabolism

The reduction of one molecule of oxygen to two molecules of water requires four electrons (and four protons). A partial reduction of molecular oxygen by fewer than four electrons is possible, but the products are very reactive. The reduction of molecular oxygen by a single electron produces **superoxide**:

$$O_2 + e^- \longrightarrow O_2^-$$

Superoxide

Superoxide is both an anion and a free radical. A free radical is not a terrorist at large but rather *a highly reactive substance with an unpaired electron*. Like other free radicals, superoxide is very short lived. It initiates chain reactions in which another molecule is converted to a free radical, which in turn reacts with a third molecule, and so on (see lipid peroxidation, Chapter 18). It also forms other reactive oxygen species as shown in Box 16.3. The superoxide radical is thought to be formed in small quantities by many oxygenases, but the most important source probably is cytochrome oxidase.

Hydrogen peroxide also is formed by many flavoproteins. Unlike NADH and NADPH, $FADH_2$ and $FMNH_2$ are tightly bound prosthetic groups. Therefore, after being reduced in a dehydrogenase reaction, the flavin coenzyme cannot be reoxidized by diffusing to a different enzyme and participating in a different reaction.

Flavoproteins of the inner mitochondrial membrane, such as succinate dehydrogenase and the mitochondrial glycerol phosphate dehydrogenase, can donate their hydrogen to ubiquinone:

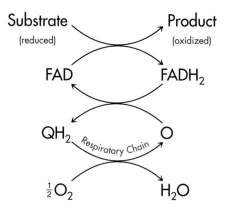

Flavoproteins in other locations transfer their hydrogen directly to molecular oxygen, with the formation of hydrogen peroxide:

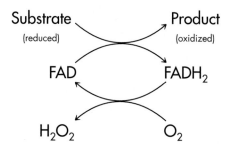

Xanthine oxidase (see Chapter 23) and monoamine oxidase (MAO, Chapter 26) are prominent examples of H_2O_2-forming flavoproteins.

Several enzymes have evolved to destroy the reactive oxygen derivatives. **Superoxide dismutase** eliminates the superoxide radical:

$$2\,O_2^- + 2\,H^+ \xrightarrow[\text{dismutase}]{\text{Superoxide}} H_2O_2 + O_2$$

It is present in all tissues, both in the cytoplasm and in the mitochondria. The mitochondrial enzyme is activated by manganese, and the cytoplasmic enzyme contains copper and zinc. *Superoxide dismutase is*

BOX 16.3

$$O_2^- \underset{}{\overset{H^+}{\rightleftharpoons}} HO_2^- \xrightarrow[\text{}]{HO_2^-\quad O_2} H_2O_2 \overset{}{\rightleftharpoons} 2\,{}^{\cdot}OH$$

| Superoxide radical | Hydroperoxide radical | Hydrogen peroxide | Hydroxy radical |

required for aerobic life. It is present in all aerobic organisms, but not in obligate anaerobes.

Hydrogen peroxide is destroyed by the heme-containing enzyme **catalase:**

$$2 H_2O_2 \xrightarrow{\text{Catalase}} 2 H_2O + O_2$$

This enzyme is present in blood and tissues (which is why hydrogen peroxide bubbles when it is applied to wounds), with the highest concentrations (up to 40% of the total protein) in peroxisomes.

Peroxidases are enzymes that react hydrogen peroxide with organic substrates. For purposes of detoxification, **glutathione peroxidase** is probably most important in human tissues. The enzyme uses glutathione, a tripeptide with a sulfhydryl group (see Chapter 17), as a substrate:

$$2 \text{ Glutathione-SH} + H_2O_2 \longrightarrow$$
$$\text{Glutathione-S-S-enoihtatulG} + 2 H_2O$$

Some vitamins and metabolites can terminate free-radical–mediated oxidative reactions by acting as scavengers of free radicals. Important protective agents are vitamin E and the retinoids (see Chapter 24), which are lipophilic and are thought to act in biological membranes, and the water-soluble agents ascorbic acid, bilirubin, and uric acid.

The medical importance of reactive oxygen derivatives is not entirely clear. They probably are important for the nonenzymatic oxidation of polyunsaturated fatty acid residues in membrane lipids and triglycerides (see Chapter 18). They also may cause other types of cellular damage rather nonselectively, including somatic mutations. Some investigators consider oxygen the most important (and least avoidable) environmental mutagen. Oxidative enzymes are conspicuously absent from the nucleus, and the high mutation rate of mitochondrial DNA may well be caused by the dangerous proximity of cytochrome oxidase and other oxidative enzymes, which pollute the environment with reactive oxygen derivatives.

Oxygen derivatives also may play specific roles in some diseases. The formation of toxic H_2O_2 by MAO has been indicted as a contributing factor for the neuronal degeneration in patients with Parkinson's disease (see Chapter 26). The dopaminergic nigrostriatal neurons that gradually are destroyed in this disease have a high MAO activity, and treatment with MAO inhibitors has been claimed not only to relieve the symptoms in the short term, but also to delay the progression of the disease.

Besides the possibility for chronic damage, reactive oxygen derivatives are a likely factor in acute oxygen toxicity. The administration of pure oxygen is beneficial in some situations, but it is accompanied by the danger of serious toxicity. Laboratory animals die in an atmosphere of pure oxygen, and premature infants have developed retrolental fibroplasia, with resulting blindness, after oxygen treatment.

SUMMARY

The catabolism of glucose is initiated in the cytoplasm and completed in the mitochondria. The cytoplasmic reaction sequence, known as glycolysis, produces two molecules of the three-carbon compound pyruvate from the six-carbon substrate glucose. It also produces two molecules of ATP and two molecules of NADH.

Under aerobic conditions, pyruvate enters the mitochondrion, where it is oxidatively decarboxylated to the two-carbon acetyl residue in acetyl-CoA. This reaction also forms carbon dioxide and NADH. Acetyl-CoA is formed not only from carbohydrates through glycolysis and the pyruvate dehydrogenase reaction, but also from fatty acids and amino acids.

The tricarboxylic acid cycle (TCA cycle) is the final common pathway for the oxidation of the acetyl-CoA formed from carbohydrates, fatty acids, and amino acids. In the first reaction of the cycle, acetyl-CoA reacts with the four-carbon compound oxaloacetate to form the six-carbon compound citrate. Citrate then is converted back to oxaloacetate in the remaining reactions of the TCA cycle. Each round of the cycle produces two molecules of carbon dioxide, one GTP, three NADHs, and one $FADH_2$ from the acetyl residue.

The reduced coenzymes are reoxidized by molecular oxygen in the respiratory chain. The redox reactions of the respiratory chain create a proton gradient across the inner mitochondrial membrane, and this proton gradient is used for ATP synthesis by the mitochondrial ATP synthase. The efficiency of ATP synthesis during glucose oxidation is close to

40%. Oxidative phosphorylation is the principal energy source for most tissues.

Oxidative phosphorylation is controlled directly by the level of cellular ADP; glycolysis, pyruvate dehydrogenase, and the TCA cycle are inhibited by high energy charge and stimulated by low energy charge. The regulated mitochondrial reactions also are stimulated by a high [NAD$^+$]/[NADH] ratio. These regulatory mechanisms ensure that an adequate cellular ATP pool is maintained at all times.

Under anaerobic conditions, the pyruvate formed in glycolysis is reduced to lactate in the lactate dehydrogenase (LDH) reaction. Anaerobic glycolysis produces two molecules of ATP for each glucose molecule; it therefore can tide the cell over during brief periods of hypoxia, but the accumulating lactic acid tends to acidify the tissue. Red blood cells depend on anaerobic glycolysis at all times; skeletal muscle forms lactate during periods of vigorous contraction; ischemic tissues switch to anaerobic glycolysis when ATP no longer is produced by oxidative phosphorylation.

Further Reading

Babcock GT, Wikstrom M: Oxygen activation and the conservation of energy in cell respiration. *Nature* 356, 301-309, 1992.

Behal RH, Buxton DB, Robertson JG, Olson MS: Regulation of the pyruvate dehydrogenase multienzyme complex. *Annu Rev Nutr* 13, 497-520, 1993.

Massey V: Activation of molecular oxygen by flavins and flavoproteins. *J Biol Chem* 269 (36), 22459-22462, 1994.

Pedersen PL, Amzel LM: ATP synthases. *J Biol Chem* 268 (14), 9937-9940, 1993.

Scriver CR, Beaudet AL, Sly WS, Valle D, editors: *The metabolic basis of inherited disease*, 6th ed., vol. 1. McGraw-Hill, New York, 1989. pp. 869-888, 2341-2366.

Sies H: Strategies of antioxidant defense. *Eur J Biochem* 215, 213-219, 1993.

Wallace DC: Mitochondrial diseases: genotype versus phenotype. *Trends Genet* 9 (4), 128-133, 1993.

QUESTIONS

1. Some enzymes of the TCA cycle are physiologically regulated. The most common regulatory effect on these enzymes is
   A. Inhibition by ATP
   B. Inhibition by ADP
   C. Inhibition by NAD$^+$
   D. Stimulation by citrate
   E. Inhibition by acetyl-CoA

2. Some individuals are born with a partial deficiency of pyruvate dehydrogenase in all tissues. Which tissue suffers most from this abnormality?
   A. Liver
   B. Muscle
   C. Erythrocytes
   D. Adipose tissue
   E. Brain

3. Which biochemical changes take place in brain cells shortly after decapitation on the guillotine?
   A. The rate of glycolysis is reduced.
   B. TCA-cycle activity is increased.
   C. The [Lactate]/[Pyruvate] concentration ratio is increased.
   D. All electron carriers in the respiratory chain are converted to the oxidized state.
   E. The potassium concentration in the cells increases, and the sodium concentration decreases.

4. Assume that the concentration of one of the glycolytic enzymes is reduced to 50% of normal as a result of a heterozygous mutation. The reduced activity of which enzyme would decrease overall glycolytic activity to the greatest extent?
   A. Hexokinase
   B. Phosphofructokinase
   C. Aldolase
   D. Enolase
   E. Pyruvate kinase

5. Assume that the NADH-Q reductase complex is inhibited by the fish poison rotenone. A likely result of this inhibition will be that
   A. The mitochondria can no longer oxidize glycerol phosphate to dihydroxyacetone phosphate.
   B. Most or all of the mitochondrial NAD will be in the oxidized state.
   C. Most or all of the mitochondrial ubiquinone will be in the oxidized state.
   D. The proton gradient across the inner mitochondrial membrane will be very steep.
   E. Phosphofructokinase will be inhibited.

6. Following the advice of her biochemistry profes-

sor, an overweight medical student goes on a sawdust diet (it fills the stomach but cannot be digested). She should make sure that the sawdust is not from wood that has been treated with the uncoupler pentachlorophenol. Pentachlorophenol would cause

A. Weight gain
B. Reduced oxygen consumption (while she is still alive)
C. Reduced TCA-cycle activity
D. Hyperthermia
E. An increased $[NADH]/[NAD^+]$ ratio

7. Muscle contraction causes an immediate increase in the rate of oxidative phosphorylation because contraction

A. Decreases the pH
B. Increases the NAD^+ concentration
C. Increases the activity of phosphofructokinase
D. Decreases the activity of pyruvate dehydrogenase
E. Increases the ADP concentration

Chapter 17

Carbohydrate Metabolism

Carbohydrates are important both for the generation of metabolic energy and for biosynthetic purposes. The most important functions of carbohydrate metabolism are:

1. *The generation of metabolic energy by the catabolism of glucose.* We encountered the glycolytic pathway and its mitochondrial sequels in Chapter 16.
2. *The maintenance of a normal blood glucose level.* Glucose is readily available after a carbohydrate-rich meal, but in the fasting state it has to be produced either by the degradation of stored glycogen or by synthesis from noncarbohydrates.
3. *The utilization of dietary monosaccharides other than glucose.* Fructose and galactose, in particular, have to be channeled into the major metabolic pathways of glucose.
4. *The provision of specialized monosaccharides as biosynthetic precursors:* ribose for the synthesis of nucleotides and nucleic acids, and amino sugars and acidic sugar derivatives for the synthesis of glycolipids, glycoproteins, and proteoglycans.

| GLUCONEOGENESIS |

Most cells in our body can generate metabolic energy from a variety of substrates, including glucose, fatty acids, amino acids and ketone bodies. Only some specialists, like the brain and the erythrocytes, depend on glucose. The brain alone consumes about 120 grams per day, and for optimal functioning it requires a blood glucose concentration of 4.0 to 5.5 mM (70 to 100 mg/dL).

Dietary carbohydrates maintain the blood glucose level only for a few hours after a meal. After this time, glucose has to be supplied by the liver, the "guardian of the milieu interieur." The liver can produce glucose by two pathways:

1. Stored glycogen is degraded. The glycogen reserves of the liver, however, rarely exceed 100 g and therefore are depleted within 24 hours.
2. Glucose is synthesized from such noncarbohydrate precursors as amino acids, lactic acid, and glycerol in the pathway of **gluconeogenesis.** This is the only source of glucose during prolonged fasting.

Only the liver and the renal cortex have a complete gluconeogenic pathway. On a weight basis, the gluconeogenic capacity of the renal cortex equals that of the liver, but because of the size difference between these tissues the gluconeogenic activity in the kidney amounts to only 10% of that in the liver.

Three irreversible reactions of glycolysis have to be bypassed in gluconeogenesis

The most obvious strategy for the synthesis of glucose from simple metabolic intermediates would be a reversal of glycolysis, with glucose being formed from pyruvate. A simple reversal of glycolysis, however, is not possible because three of the glycolytic reactions are physiologically irreversible: those catalyzed by **hexokinase, phosphofructo-**

kinase (PFK), and **pyruvate kinase.** *If these reactions can be bypassed, the synthesis of glucose from pyruvate should be possible* (Fig. 17.1).

The pyruvate kinase reaction of glycolysis is irreversible despite ATP synthesis. Without ATP involvement 14.8 kcal/mol would be required to convert pyruvate back to phosphoenolpyruvate (PEP). This

feat cannot be achieved in a single reaction. Instead, pyruvate first is carboxylated to oxaloacetate, which then is decarboxylated and phosphorylated to PEP (Fig. 17.2). We encountered the first reaction, catalyzed by pyruvate carboxylase, as an anaplerotic reaction of the TCA cycle (see Chapter 16). It requires ATP in addition to enzyme-bound biotin. The second reaction, catalyzed by **PEP-carboxykinase,** requires GTP. The consumption of two high-energy phosphate bonds in the synthesis of PEP from pyruvate results in a $\Delta G^{o\prime}$ value of + 0.2 kcal/mol. The reactions proceed from pyruvate to PEP because of the high cellular concentration ratios of [ATP]/[ADP], [GTP]/[GDP], and [Pyruvate]/[PEP].

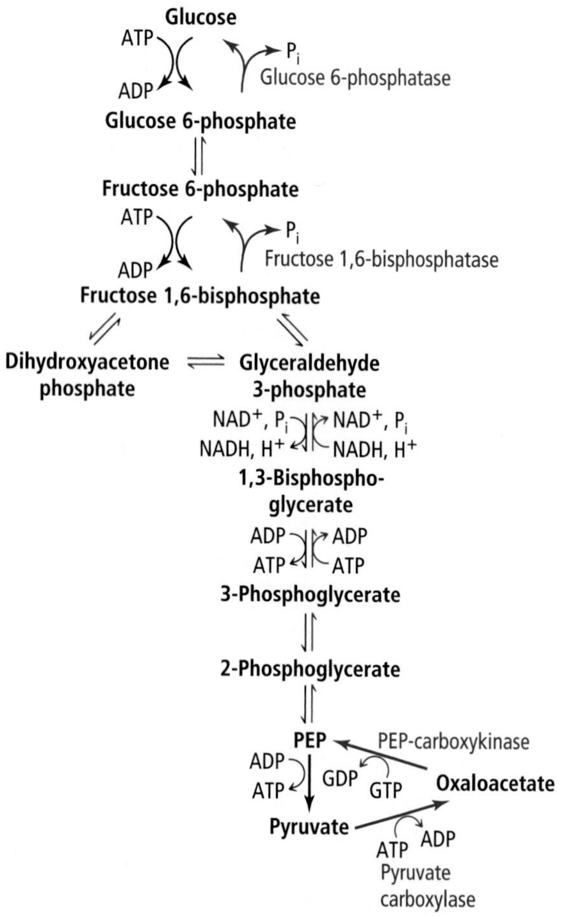

Pyruvate carboxylase is a strictly mitochondrial enzyme, but PEP-carboxykinase is both mitochondrial and cytoplasmic. PEP is transported across the inner mitochondrial membrane; oxaloacetate is shuttled into the cytoplasm after being reduced to malate or transaminated to aspartate.

PEP is processed to fructose 1,6-bisphosphate through the reversible reactions of glycolysis. The irreversible PFK reaction is bypassed by **fructose 1,6-bisphosphatase,** which hydrolyzes the phosphate from carbon 1 of its substrate.

The hexokinase reaction also is bypassed by the hydrolytic cleavage of the phosphate ester, catalyzed by **glucose 6-phosphatase.** Unlike the other gluconeogenic enzymes, which are cytoplasmic (except pyruvate carboxylase), this enzyme resides on the lumenal surface of the endoplasmic reticulum (ER) membrane. Both the fructose 1,6-bisphosphatase and the glucose 6-phosphatase reactions, being hydrolytic cleavages, are irreversible (Fig. 17.3).

Gluconeogenesis is expensive: six phosphoanhydride bonds are required for the synthesis of one

FIG. 17.1

The reactions of glycolysis and gluconeogenesis.

FIG. 17.2

The first bypass of gluconeogenesis: from pyruvate to phosphoenolpyruvate (PEP).

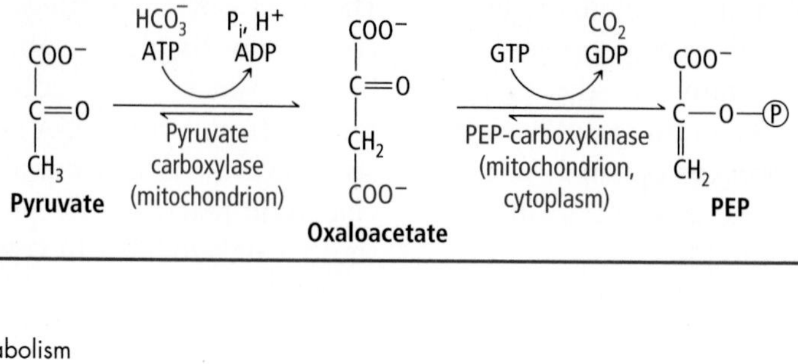

glucose molecule from two molecules of lactate. Pyruvate carboxylase consumes two ATPs, PEP-carboxykinase consumes two GTPs, and glyceraldehyde 3-phosphate dehydrogenase consumes two ATPs in the reversal of substrate-level phosphorylation.

Acetyl-CoA is not a precursor for gluconeogenesis

In addition to pyruvate, **lactate** and **alanine** are convenient substrates of gluconeogenesis (Fig. 17.4) because they can be converted to pyruvate by the lactate dehydrogenase reaction and by transamination (see Chapter 21), respectively. **Oxaloacetate** is not only a gluconeogenic intermediate but also a member of the TCA cycle. This is important because most amino acids are degraded to TCA-cycle intermediates such as α-ketoglutarate, succinyl-CoA, and fumarate. Through the reactions of the cycle and the gluconeogenic pathway, *the carbon skeletons of these "glucogenic" amino acids can be converted to glucose.*

Glycerol is another substrate of gluconeogenesis. It enters the pathway at the level of the triose phosphates (Fig. 17.5).

FIG. 17.3

The second and third bypasses of gluconeogenesis.

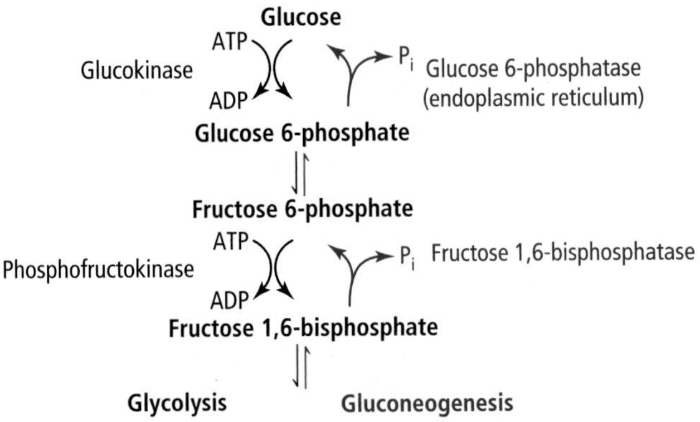

FIG. 17.4

The most important substrates of gluconeogenesis. Although acetyl-CoA enters the TCA cycle, it is not a substrate of gluconeogenesis because the citrate synthase reaction does not involve the net synthesis of a TCA-cycle intermediate.

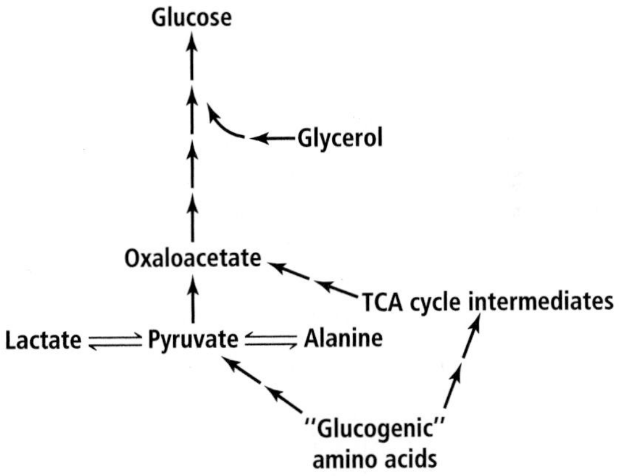

FIG. 17.5

Glycerol enters gluconeogenesis (and glycolysis) at the level of the triose phosphates. The glycerol for gluconeogenesis is derived from triglyceride hydrolysis in adipose tissue.

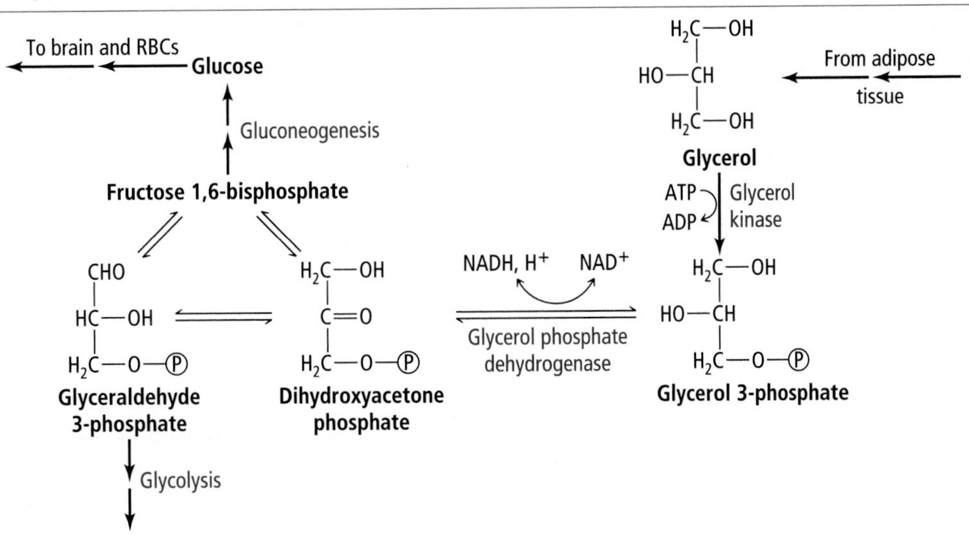

Acetyl-CoA cannot be converted to glucose. The pyruvate dehydrogenase reaction is irreversible, and there are no alternative reactions to channel acetyl-CoA into gluconeogenesis. *Also, substances that are degraded to acetyl-CoA, such as fatty acids (see Chapter 18), ketone bodies (see Chapter 18), and ethanol (see Chapter 29), are not substrates of gluconeogenesis.*

Glucogenic amino acids are the most important precursors for gluconeogenesis during fasting: *fatty acids from adipose tissue provide for the energy needs of most tissues, and protein breakdown in skeletal muscle and other tissues supplies amino acids for gluconeogenesis.* Additional substrates are lactate, derived from anaerobic cells such as the erythrocytes, and glycerol, which is released from adipose tissue together with fatty acids. The fatty acids themselves, however, which contain 95% of the energy value of triglycerides, are not substrates of gluconeogenesis.

The reciprocal regulation of glycolysis and gluconeogenesis in the liver is important for the maintenance of a normal blood glucose level

Only those enzymes that catalyze the irreversible reactions between pyruvate and PEP, between fructose 1,6-bisphosphate and fructose 6-phosphate, and between glucose 6-phosphate and glucose are suitable for regulation. A simultaneous activity of the opposing enzymes in each of these three substrate cycles would lead to a **futile cycle** that achieves little but ATP hydrolysis.

Both cellular metabolites and hormones participate in the reciprocal regulation of hepatic glycolysis and gluconeogenesis. Some metabolites act as reversibly binding allosteric effectors or competitive inhibitors of the regulated enzymes. Hormones, on the other hand, affect the enzymes in two ways:

1. *They regulate the amount of the enzyme in the cell* by altering the rate of enzyme synthesis and, sometimes, of enzyme degradation. This type of regulation requires a few days for a maximal effect.
2. *They trigger the phosphorylation or dephosphorylation of metabolic enzymes,* thereby changing enzyme activity without changing the number of enzyme molecules in the cell. These effects are important for the minute-to-minute regulation of enzyme activity.

Some hormones, most notably the steroid and thyroid hormones, enter their target cells and affect gene expression directly by binding to nuclear transcription factors. Others bind to a receptor on the cell surface and induce the formation of an intracellular **second messenger.** Second messengers can regulate metabolic enzymes in the short term by inducing their phosphorylation or dephosphorylation. They also can regulate the synthesis of the enzyme protein at the level of transcription.

Several hormones participate in the regulation of hepatic glycolysis and gluconeogenesis:

1. Glucagon is a peptide hormone, produced by the α-cells in the endocrine pancreas. It is released in response to a decreased blood glucose level, so its plasma level is somewhat higher in the fasting state than after a carbohydrate-containing meal. *It stimulates the glucose-producing pathways (including gluconeogenesis) and inhibits the glucose-consuming pathways in the liver, and thereby prevents the development of hypoglycemia.* The glucagon effects are mediated by the second messenger **cyclic AMP (cAMP).** cAMP stimulates **protein kinase A,** which phosphorylates several metabolic and regulatory enzymes. Phosphorylation either increases or decreases the activity of the enzyme. Protein kinase A phosphorylates some nuclear proteins as well, thereby regulating the synthesis of some metabolic enzymes at the level of transcription.
2. The catecholamines **epinephrine** and **norepinephrine** are "stress hormones" that are released during physical exercise and cold exposure, and in psychological emergencies such as during a difficult biochemistry examination. They induce slight increases in cAMP levels in the liver, so *they favor gluconeogenesis over glycolysis.*
3. **Glucocorticoids** are stress hormones that affect gene transcription directly, without the need for a second messenger (see Chapter 27). Acting at the level of gene transcription, *they stimulate gluconeogenesis.*
4. **Insulin** is released from pancreatic β-cells in response to an increased blood glucose level; its plasma concentration is up to 10 times higher after a carbohydrate-rich meal than during prolonged fasting. It reduces the cAMP level in the

FIG. 17.6

The reciprocal regulation of glycolysis and gluconeogenesis in the liver. ①, Glucokinase; ②, phosphofructokinase; ③, pyruvate kinase; ④, pyruvate carboxylase; ⑤, PEP-carboxykinase; ⑥, fructose 1,6-bisphosphatase; ⑦, glucose 6-phosphatase $\xrightarrow{+}$, Stimulation; $\longrightarrow$, inhibition. **A,** Substrate flow during fasting and in the well-fed state, and the effects of hormones on the amounts of glycolytic and gluconeogenic enzymes. Regulation of enzyme synthesis and degradation is the most important long-term (hours to days) control mechanism. In most cases, the hormone acts by changing the rate of transcription or by affecting the stability of the mRNA. Some of the insulin effects shown here require the presence of glucose. **B,** Short-term regulation of glycolysis and gluconeogenesis by reversibly binding effectors and by phosphorylation/dephosphorylation. $\dashrightarrow$, Allosteric and competitive effects; $\cdots\blacktriangleright$, phosphorylation. Only pyruvate kinase and phosphofructo-2-kinase/fructose-2,6-bisphosphatase are regulated by cAMP-dependent phosphorylation.

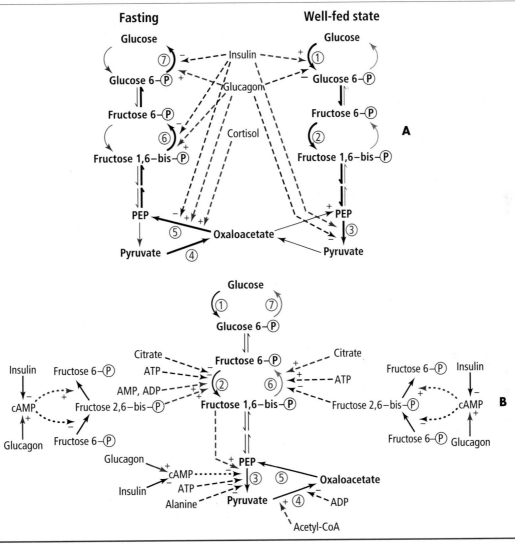

liver, probably by activating a cAMP-degrading phosphodiesterase, which means that *it opposes the effects of glucagon and the catecholamines.* It also affects gene expression independently of the cAMP system. *Insulin stimulates the glucose-consuming pathways and inhibits the glucose-producing pathways in the liver.*

The day-to-day regulation of glycolysis and gluconeogenesis is effected by an action of the hormones on the amount of the key enzymes (Fig. 17.6, *A*). Insulin represses the gluconeogenic enzymes and induces most of the glycolytic enzymes, and these effects are counteracted by glucagon and the other insulin antagonists. *Insulin causes the liver to metabolize excess glucose in the well-fed state, and the insulin-antagonistic hormones prevent hypoglycemia during fasting.*

Glycolysis and gluconeogenesis are fine-tuned by allosteric effectors and hormone-induced enzyme phosphorylations

The short-term control of glycolysis and gluconeogenesis is shown in Fig. 17.6, *B*.

Pyruvate kinase is the most important regulated enzyme in the PEP-pyruvate cycle. It is inhibited allosterically by ATP and alanine and activated by fructose 1,6-bisphosphate. The concentration of fructose 1,6-bisphosphate is increased whenever PFK is activated and fructose 1,6-bisphosphatase is inhibited. Its effect on pyruvate kinase is an example of *feedforward stimulation.* Pyruvate kinase also is inhibited by the cAMP-induced phosphorylation of a single serine side chain in the enzyme protein.

PEP-carboxykinase is not known to be subject to short-term regulation, but pyruvate carboxylase is activated allosterically by acetyl-CoA and competitively inhibited by its product ADP.

PFK and fructose 1,6-bisphosphatase in the liver are oppositely regulated by adenine nucleotides and citrate. Whereas AMP and ADP stimulate PFK, fructose 1,6-bisphosphatase is stimulated by ATP and citrate. Therefore *glycolysis prevails when energy and metabolic intermediates are in short supply, and gluconeogenesis is*
favored when they are plentiful. The most potent modulator of these two enzymes, however, is **fructose 2,6-bisphosphate.** This regulatory metabolite, not to be confused with the glycolytic intermediate fructose 1,6-bisphosphate, is an allosteric activator of PFK and a competitive inhibitor of fructose 1,6-bisphosphatase.

Fructose 2,6-bisphosphate is both synthesized from and degraded to fructose 6-phosphate by a unique bifunctional enzyme that combines the activities of a 6-phosphofructo-2-kinase (PFK-2) and a fructose 2,6-bisphosphatase on the same polypeptide. This bifunctional enzyme is regulated by phosphorylation/dephosphorylation: the dephosphorylated enzyme acts as a kinase, and the phosphorylated form acts as a phosphatase (Fig. 17.7).

The phosphorylation state of the bifunctional enzyme is under hormonal control: glucagon, acting through its second messenger cAMP and the cAMP-activated protein kinase A, phosphorylates the bifunctional enzyme. Insulin opposes glucagon by lowering the cellular cAMP concentration. In addition, it stimulates the protein phosphatase that dephosphorylates the bifunctional enzyme. *By adjusting the cellular concentration of fructose 2,6-bisphosphate, insulin and glucagon can affect glycolytic/gluconeogenic activity within minutes.* Fructose 6-phosphate also regulates the bifunctional enzyme: it stimulates the kinase activity and inhibits the phosphatase activity by an allosteric mechanism.

FIG. 17.7

Synthesis and degradation of fructose 2,6-bisphosphate, the most important regulator of phosphofructokinase and fructose 1,6-bisphosphatase. This regulatory metabolite is synthesized and degraded by a bifunctional enzyme that combines the kinase and phosphatase activities on the same polypeptide. cAMP-induced phosphorylation inhibits the kinase activity and stimulates the phosphatase activity of the bifunctional enzyme. ·····▸, Phosphorylation; ·····▸, dephosphorylation; – –▸, allosteric effect; ─+─▸, stimulation; ──▸, inhibition.

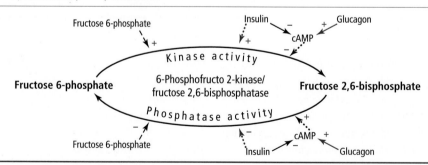

The enzymes of the glucose/glucose 6-phosphate cycle are regulated, in large part, by substrate availability. The phosphorylation of glucose in the liver is effected by hexokinase 4, an isoenzyme of hexokinase that is better known as **glucokinase**. The most important kinetic difference between glucokinase and the other isoenzymes of hexokinase is the Michaelis constant for glucose: the other forms of hexokinase have K_m values on the order of 0.1 mM (2 mg/dL), but glucokinase has a K_m of approximately 10 mM (200 mg/dL). Glucokinase also shows a sigmoidal rather than a hyperbolic relationship between glucose concentration and reaction rate (Fig. 17.8). The steep part of the curve is in the range of physiological glucose concentrations, so the reaction rate varies substantially with alterations of the glucose level. The glucose concentration in the portal circulation exceeds that in systemic blood after a carbohydrate-rich meal, and glucose readily equilibrates across the hepatocyte membrane by a high-capacity bidirectional transporter. Glucokinase also is regulated by a protein that inhibits its activity in the presence of fructose 6-phosphate. Therefore glucose phosphorylation is suppressed when a large amount of fructose 6-phosphate is formed by gluconeogenesis or glycogen degradation.

Glucose 6-phosphatase also is affected by substrate availability: with a K_m of 3 mM for glucose 6-phosphate, it is not saturated under ordinary conditions (see Table 17.2). Therefore an increased production of glucose 6-phosphate by gluconeogenesis (or glycogen degradation) is followed by an increased flow through the glucose 6-phosphatase reaction.

The stimulation of gluconeogenesis by high energy charge and by high concentrations of citrate and acetyl-CoA appears strange: gluconeogenesis is required during fasting, and we would expect decreased rather than increased levels of ATP and metabolites in a starving organism. Actually, however, the liver is not starved, even during prolonged fasting: under hormonal direction, triglycerides are degraded in adipose tissue during fasting. The fasting liver metabolizes fatty acids from adipose tissue much more avidly than it metabolizes dietary glucose after a meal, so high levels of ATP and acetyl-CoA indeed are maintained in the fasting state. Now we can appreciate the energy source for gluconeogenesis: *the six high-energy phosphate bonds needed for the synthesis of a glucose molecule are supplied by fatty acid oxidation.*

GLYCOGEN METABOLISM

Glucose cannot be stored because it is water soluble and osmotically active. For storage, it has to be converted to the insoluble polymer glycogen. The electron microscope reveals glycogen granules in many cell types, but the most important stores are in liver and skeletal muscle. In the well-fed state, the glycogen content of the liver is up to 8% of the fresh weight—100 to 120 g in an adult. The glycogen concentration in skeletal muscle approaches 1%, but because most people have more muscle than liver, the total amount of muscle glycogen exceeds that in the liver.

Liver and muscle store glycogen for different purposes: *the liver synthesizes glycogen after a carbohydrate-rich meal and degrades it to free glucose during fasting.* This glucose is released into the blood for use by needy tissues. *Skeletal muscle synthesizes glycogen at rest and degrades it during exercise.* Muscle glycogen does not contribute to the blood glucose but rather is used for

FIG. 17.8

Approximate reaction rates of hexokinase (isoenzymes 1, 2, and 3) and glucokinase at different substrate concentrations. The sigmoidal relationship between reaction rate and substrate concentration for glucokinase accentuates the increase of the reaction rate with increased glucose level.

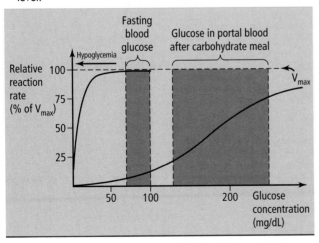

the generation of metabolic energy in the working muscles themselves.

Glycogen is a branched polymer of glucose residues

Glycogen is a polymer of approximately 10,000 to 40,000 glucose residues, held together by α-1,4 glycosidic bonds. With a molecular weight between 10^6 and 10^7 daltons, it is as big as a complete human ribosome (4.2×10^6 Da). The molecule is branched: approximately 1 in 12 glucose residues serves as a branch point by forming an α-1,6 glycosidic bond with another glucose residue (Fig. 17.9). Theoretically, the molecule has only one reducing end with a free hydroxy group at carbon 1 but a large number of nonreducing ends with a free hydroxy group at carbon 4. The enzymes of glycogen synthesis and glycogen degradation are nested between the outer branches of the molecule and act only on the nonreducing ends. Therefore *the many nonreducing end branches of glycogen facilitate its rapid synthesis and degradation.*

Glycogen is synthesized from glucose

The steps in the synthesis of glycogen from glucose are outlined in Figs. 17.10 and 17.11. Glucose-6-phosphate is synthesized from free glucose by hexokinase (glucokinase in the liver). **Phosphoglucomutase** then isomerizes glucose 6-phosphate to glucose 1-phosphate in a reversible reaction. At equilibrium, approximately 95% of the substrate is present as glucose 6-phosphate and 5% as glucose 1-phosphate. UDP-glucose finally is formed in a reaction between glucose 1-phosphate and UTP. This otherwise-reversible reaction is driven to completion by the subsequent hydrolysis of pyrophosphate. UDP-glucose is the activated form of glucose for glycogen synthesis.

The UDP residue in UDP-glucose is attached to carbon 1 of glucose, so it is this carbon that forms the glycosidic bond. UDP-glucose is used not only for glycogen synthesis, but also for the synthesis of glycolipids and glycoproteins (see Chapters 8 and 19). The bond between glucose and UDP is indeed energy rich, and with a free energy content of 7.3 kcal/mol it rivals the phosphoanhydride bonds in ATP. The free energy content of an α-1,4 glycosidic bond in glycogen is only 4.5 kcal/mol.

The principal actor in glycogen synthesis is **glycogen synthase.** This enzyme creates the α-1,4 glycosidic bonds in glycogen by transferring the glucose residue from UDP-glucose to the 4-hydroxy group at the nonreducing end of the glycogen molecule (Fig. 17.11). This reaction elongates the outer

---

FIG. 17.9

Structure of glycogen. *Left,* Overall structure. Note the large number of nonreducing ends, which are required as substrates for the enzymes of glycogen metabolism. *Right,* The structure around a branch point.

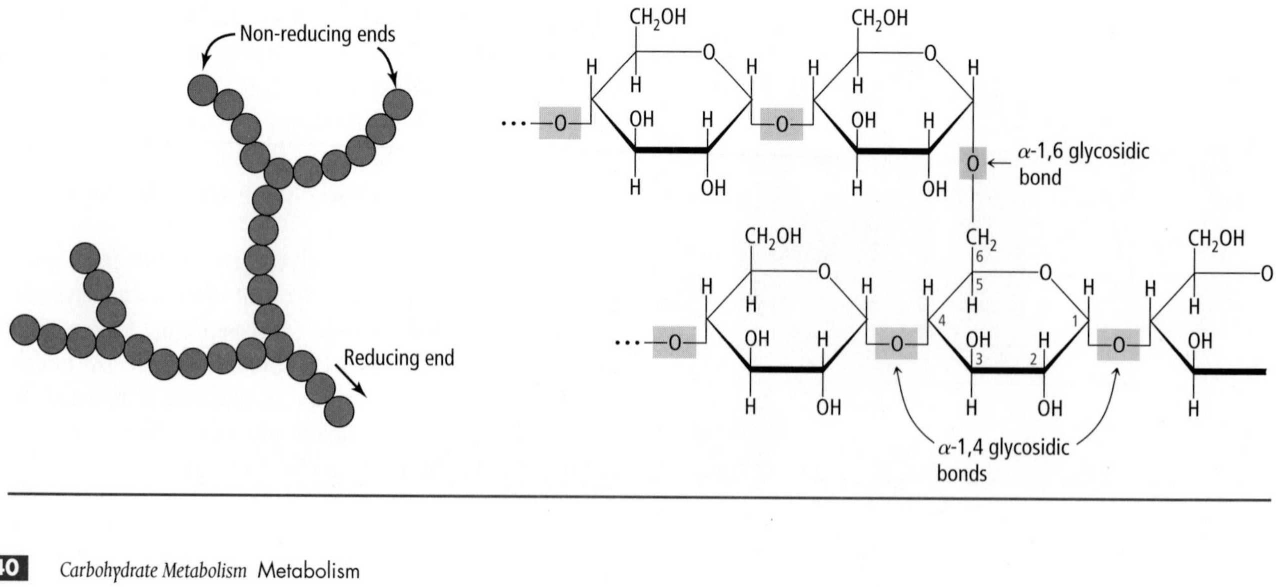

branches of the glycogen molecule by one glucose residue at a time.

Glycogen synthase cannot form the α-1,6 glycosidic bonds at the branch points. Branching requires a **branching enzyme**, which transfers a string of glucose residues, typically seven in length, from the end of an unbranched chain to carbon number 6 of a glucose residue in a more interior location (Fig. 17.12).

Glycogen synthesis from glucose consumes *two*

Synthesis of UDP-glucose. UDP-glucose is the activated form of glucose for glycogen synthesis, but also for the synthesis of other complex carbohydrates (see Table 8.7, Chapter 8).

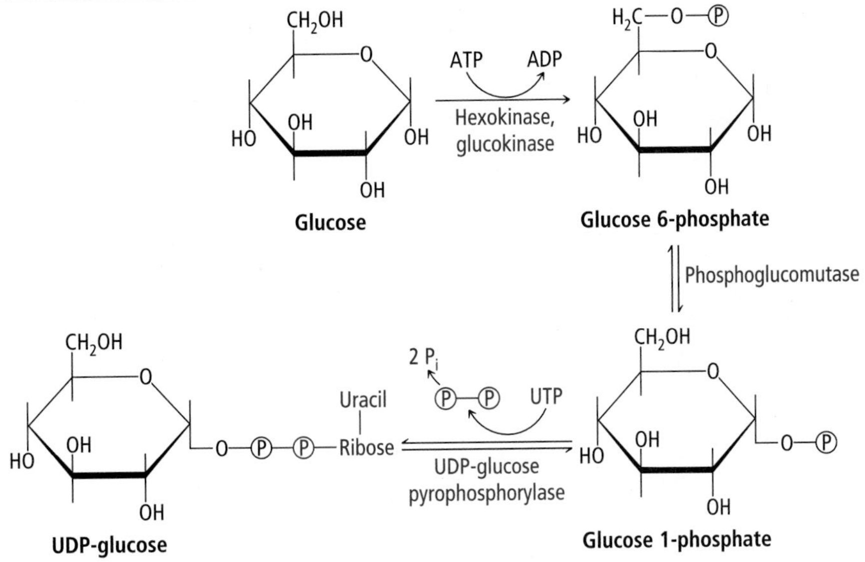

The glycogen synthase reaction.

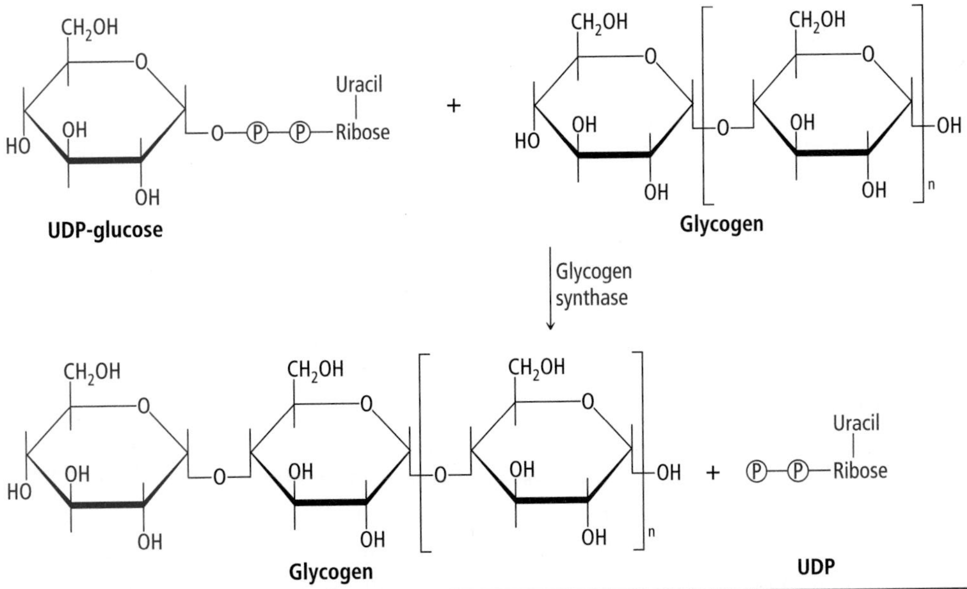

FIG. 17.12

The action of the branching enzyme.

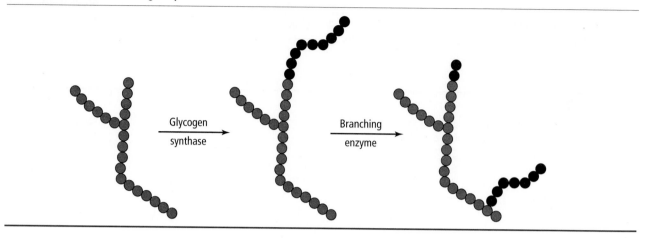

FIG. 17.13

The glycogen phosphorylase reaction.

Glucose 1-phosphate

phosphoanhydride bonds for each glucose residue: hexokinase consumes one ATP, and UTP is required for the formation of UDP-glucose.

Glycogen is degraded by phosphorolytic cleavage

Glycogen phosphorylase, the major enzyme of glycogen degradation, catalyzes the phosphorolytic cleavage of a glucose residue from the nonreducing end of the molecule. This cleavage produces not free glucose but glucose 1-phosphate (Fig. 17.13). The reaction is freely reversible, and at equilibrium the concentration of inorganic phosphate is 3.6 times higher than that of glucose 1-phosphate. Glycogen phosphorylase can be used for glycogen synthesis in vitro, but in the living cell it degrades glycogen because the cellular [Phosphate]/[Glucose 1-phosphate] ratio is at least 100.

Glycogen phosphorylase does not cleave the α-1,6 glycosidic bonds at the branch points. It does not

FIG. 17.14

The action of the debranching enzyme.

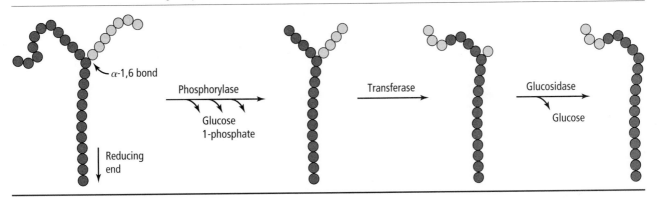

even go near the branch points, typically stopping four residues before. The branches have to be removed by a **debranching enzyme**, which combines transferase and α-1,6-glucosidase activities on the same polypeptide: the transferase activity, cleaving an α-1,4 glycosidic bond, removes a block of three glucose residues beyond the branch point and transfers these to carbon 4 at the nonreducing end of a chain. The glucose residue at the branch point itself is not transferred but cleaved hydrolytically by the α-1,6 glucosidase activity of the debranching enzyme (Fig. 17.14). Therefore the glucose residue at the branch point is released as free glucose rather than glucose 1-phosphate. Overall, *approximately 92% of the glucose residues in glycogen form glucose 1-phosphate, and 8% form free glucose.*

Glucose 1-phosphate is in equilibrium with glucose 6-phosphate through the phosphoglucomutase reaction. The further fate of glycogen-derived glucose differs in different tissues: *the liver cleaves glucose 6-phosphate to free glucose* in the glucose 6-phosphatase reaction, and being an altruistic organ, it releases this glucose into the blood for use by such needy tissues as the brain and the blood cells (Fig. 17.15). Muscles, in contrast, do not have glucose 6-phosphatase. Therefore *glucose 6-phosphate has to be metabolized within the muscle fiber,* mostly by glycolysis.

Anaerobic glycolysis from glycogen produces three rather than two molecules of ATP for each glucose residue: the ATP-consuming hexokinase reaction is not required because glucose 6-phosphate is generated by glycogen phosphorylase and phosphoglucomutase, which do not consume ATP.

Glycogen metabolism is regulated by hormones and metabolites

Glycogen synthesis and glycogen degradation should not be active at the same time, to avoid an ATP-consuming futile cycle. The important regulated enzymes are glycogen synthase and glycogen phosphorylase. Both of these can be phosphorylated and dephosphorylated on specific serine side chains by protein kinases and a protein phosphatase, respectively. In both cases the more active form of the enzyme is designated by the letter *a*, the less active form by *b* (Fig. 17.16).

Glycogen synthase is more active in the dephosphorylated form, and glycogen phosphorylase is more active in the phosphorylated form. Therefore *the simultaneous phosphorylation of both enzymes will switch the cell from glycogen synthesis to glycogen degradation.*

The phosphorylation state of the enzymes is regulated by hormones and their second messengers. Insulin stimulates glycogen synthesis both in the liver and in skeletal muscle. It ensures that excess carbohydrate is stored away as glycogen after a meal. Glucagon stimulates glycogen degradation in the liver, but not in muscle, when the blood glucose level is low—as, for example, in the fasting state. The catecholamines norepinephrine and epinephrine are powerful activators of glycogen breakdown in both muscle and liver. They mobilize glycogen when glucose is needed to fuel muscle contraction. *Both glycogen synthase and glycogen phosphorylase become dephosphorylated when insulin is abundant, and they become phosphorylated when glucagon or the catecholamines prevail.*

FIG. 17.15

Metabolic fates of glycogen in liver and muscle. Note that the liver possesses glucose 6-phosphatase, which forms free glucose both in gluconeogenesis (see Fig. 17.1, page 334) and from glycogen. This enzyme is not present in muscle tissue. **A,** Liver. **B,** Muscle.

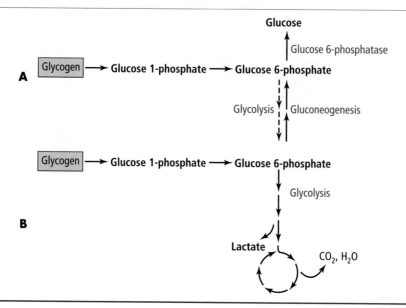

FIG. 17.16

Regulation of glycogen synthase and glycogen phosphorylase by covalent modification and allosteric effectors. Note that the simultaneous phosphorylation of the two enzymes leads to glycogen degradation, and their dephosphorylation leads to glycogen synthesis. $\xrightarrow{+}$, Allosteric activation; $\xrightarrow{}$, allosteric inhibition.

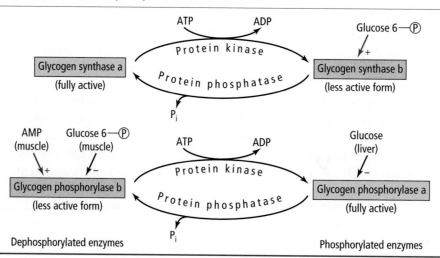

The hormones act both on the protein kinases that phosphorylate the enzymes—there are several of them—and on the dephosphorylating enzyme **protein phosphatase-1.** Superimposed on the hormonal actions are the effects of such allosteric effectors as glucose, glucose 6-phosphate, and AMP.

Figure 17.17 gives an impression of the great complexity of these regulatory mechanisms.

The actions of glucagon are initiated when the hormone binds to a receptor on the outer surface of the plasma membrane. This interaction leads to the activation of **adenylate cyclase,** an enzyme that

FIG. 17.17

Regulation of glycogen metabolism in the liver. Note that the hormones affect glycogen synthase and glycogen phosphorylase through the protein kinases and the protein phosphatase (phosphatase-1) that regulate their phosphorylation state. $--\blacktriangleright$, Allosteric effects; $\cdots\blacktriangleright$, phosphorylation; $\cdots\blacktriangleright$, dephosphorylation; $\longrightarrow$, activation; $\longrightarrow$, inhibition. **A,** Hormonal effects on the phosphorylation of the glycogen-metabolizing enzymes by protein kinases in the liver. MAP kinases, mitogen-activated protein kinases; GSK-3, glycogen synthase kinase-3. **B,** Hormonal effects on the dephosphorylation of the glycogen-metabolizing enzymes by protein phosphatase-1, and the effects of allosteric effectors.

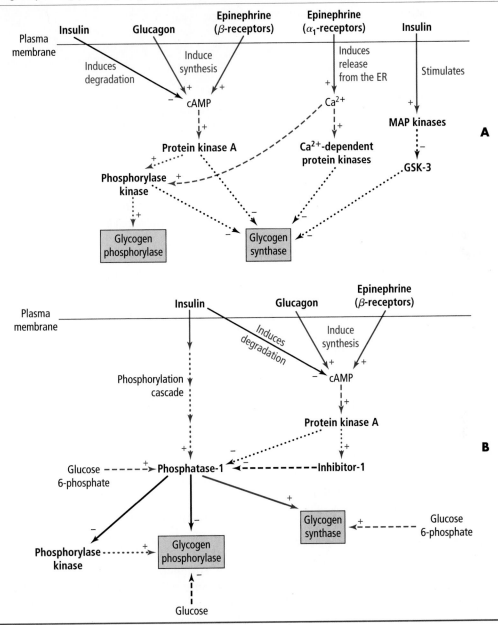

synthesizes the second messenger cAMP on the inner surface of the plasma membrane. cAMP is an allosteric activator of protein kinase A, and this protein kinase phosphorylates and thereby inactivates glycogen synthase. It also phosphorylates and thereby activates **phosphorylase kinase,** and phosphorylase kinase in turn phosphorylates both glycogen phosphorylase and glycogen synthase. *All regulated enzymes of glycogen metabolism become phosphorylated by the cAMP-induced phosphorylation cascade.* The catecholamines (norepinephrine and epinephrine) *stimulate cAMP synthesis* by an action on **β-adrenergic receptors**. Acting on **α₁-adrenergic receptors**, on the other hand, *they cause an increase in the cytoplasmic calcium concentration.* α₁-Receptors prevail in the liver; β-receptors are more important in muscle tissue. Calcium stimulates phosphorylase kinase synergistically with cAMP. It also stimulates several other protein kinases, and some of these are able to phosphorylate and thereby inactivate glycogen synthase.

Insulin is thought to mediate its effects through protein phosphorylation cascades, without the need for a second messenger. It affects glycogen metabolism by at least three mechanisms:

- *It reduces the level of cAMP,* probably by activating a cAMP-degrading phosphodiesterase.
- *It inhibits glycogen synthase kinase-3* (GSK-3), one of those enzymes that phosphorylate and inactivate glycogen synthase.
- *It stimulates protein phosphatase-1,* the enzyme that dephosphorylates glycogen synthase, glycogen phosphorylase, and phosphorylase kinase.

Phosphatase-1 is a key enzyme in the regulation of glycogen metabolism. Besides being activated by an insulin-triggered phosphorylation, it also can be phosphorylated at a different site by protein kinase A. By this latter phosphorylation, however, the enzyme is not activated but is removed from the glycogen granule to which it is otherwise bound through a glycogen-binding subunit. Like glycogen synthase and glycogen phosphorylase, phosphatase-1 normally is nested between the outer branches of the glycogen molecule. Phosphatase-1 also is inhibited allosterically by the cAMP-activated phosphoprotein **inhibitor-1**, and stimulated by glucose 6-phosphate (Fig. 17.17, *B*).

Superimposed on the hormonal regulation by phosphorylation/dephosphorylation are the actions of allosteric effectors. Glucose 6-phosphate stimulates glycogen deposition not only by stimulating phosphatase-1 but also by stimulating glycogen synthase b—and, in muscle tissue, by inhibiting glycogen phosphorylase. Glycogen phosphorylase in muscle and other extrahepatic tissues also is stimulated powerfully by AMP. This allosteric effect ensures that *glycogen is degraded rapidly in metabolic emergencies,* particularly in hypoxia, when it is required as a substrate of anaerobic glycolysis. Unlike other

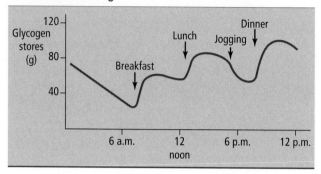

FIG. 17.18

Changes in the glycogen stores of the liver in the course of a day. Glycogen metabolism in the liver regulates the blood glucose level in the short term, and gluconeogenesis is important for the long-term regulation after more than 12 to 24 hours of fasting.

forms of stored energy, *glycogen can be used for ATP synthesis under anaerobic conditions.*

Glycogen phosphorylase in the liver, finally, is inhibited by glucose. Glucose not only inhibits the enzyme directly, but more importantly, it induces a conformational change that exposes the covalently bound phosphate to the action of the protein phosphatase. The intracellular glucose concentration in the liver approximates the blood glucose level, so *glycogen degradation in the liver is regulated directly by the blood glucose level.* The glycogen concentration in the liver varies widely with the nutritional state (Fig. 17.18).

The effects of the second messengers on glycogen metabolism are similar in muscle and liver, although the stimuli that regulate them are different. Epinephrine, but not glucagon, elevates the cAMP concentration in skeletal muscle, and although calcium levels in the liver are raised by epinephrine via α₁-adrenergic receptors, the cytoplasmic calcium concentration in the muscle fiber is regulated by neuronal stimulation. *The calcium that is released from the sarcoplasmic reticulum during excitation-contraction coupling (see Chapter 12) synchronizes glycogen degradation with muscle contraction.*

Glycogen accumulates in several enzyme deficiencies

Any deficiency of a glycogen-degrading enzyme will cause the abnormal accumulation of glycogen in the

TABLE 17.1

Glycogen storage diseases

Type	Enzyme deficiency	Organ(s) affected	Clinical course
I (von Gierke's disease)	Glucose 6-phosphatase	Liver, kidney	Severe hepatomegaly, severe hypoglycemia, lactic acidosis, ketosis, hyperuricemia
II (Pompe's disease)	α-1,4 Glucosidase ("acid maltase")	All organs	Death from cardiac failure in infants
III (Cori's disease)	Debranching enzyme	Muscle, liver	Like I, but much milder
IV (Andersen's disease)	Branching enzyme	Liver, myocardium	Death from liver cirrhosis usually before age 2
V (McArdle's disease)	Phosphorylase	Muscle	Muscle cramps and pain upon exertion, easy fatigability, normal life expectancy
VI (Hers' disease)	Phosphorylase	Liver	Like type I, but milder, with less severe hypoglycemia
VII (Tarui's disease)	Phosphofructokinase	Muscle, RBCs	Like type V
VIII	Phosphorylase kinase*	Liver	Mild hepatomegaly and hypoglycemia

* There is also an X-linked form of phosphorylase kinase deficiency affecting muscle, and several autosomal recessive forms affecting liver, muscle + liver, or muscle + heart. The enzyme contains four different subunits, and one of these is encoded by a gene on the X chromosome.

affected tissue. The resulting diseases, summarized in Table 17.1, are known collectively as the **glycogen storage diseases.** These rare diseases, with an overall incidence of approximately 1 in 40,000, are inherited as autosomal recessive traits (except for the X-linked forms of phosphorylase kinase deficiency). Because different isoenzymes are present in different tissues, a deficiency often is limited to one or a few organ systems. *Clinically, the glycogen storage diseases are distinguished as hepatic, myopathic, and generalized types* (Table 17.1).

Most of the hepatic types are severe diseases, with *hepatomegaly and fasting hypoglycemia.* The classical example is **von Gierke's disease,** which is caused by a deficiency of glucose 6-phosphatase. The patients have severe hepatomegaly, and they may die of severe hypoglycemia, which develops within 3 to 4 hours of fasting. This result is not surprising, because glucose 6-phosphatase is required for the formation of glucose both by glycogen breakdown and by gluconeogenesis: as soon as the supply of dietary glucose is exhausted, hypoglycemia is inevitable. The patients can be kept alive only by regular carbohydrate feeding, day and night.

von Gierke's disease illustrates the importance of endogenous glucose formation: *without the synthesis of glucose by glycogen degradation and gluconeogene-*

sis, we would die of hypoglycemia within hours after the last meal.

McArdle's disease, caused by a deficiency of glycogen phosphorylase in skeletal muscle, is a typical example of the myopathic type of glycogen storage disease. Although otherwise in good health, the patients complain about muscle weakness and painful cramps on exertion. Some patients experience acute episodes of myoglobinuria (excretion of myoglobin in the urine), and some develop persistent muscle weakness and muscle wasting as they grow older. This disease shows that *the utilization of muscle glycogen is not essential for life but is necessary for normal performance during physical exercise.*

One biochemical finding in McArdle's disease is of interest: after muscular activity, these patients do not show the expected increase in the blood level of lactic acid. This demonstrates that *the most important source of lactic acid during muscular activity is not free glucose from the blood but stored muscle glycogen.*

Pompe's disease is a generalized glycogen storage disease. The deficient enzyme, surprisingly, is lysosomal: in all tissues a small amount of glycogen normally is taken up by lysosomes, where it is degraded by a lysosomal α-glucosidase ("acid maltase"). Lysosomes are thought to ingest glycogen particles incidentally during the uptake of other cellular macromolecules. Pompe's disease is fatal: affected infants develop severe cardiomegaly and die of cardiac failure at an early age.

The metabolism of fructose and galactose

Dietary sources contain substantial amounts of fructose and galactose, besides glucose. Free fructose is present in honey and in many fruits, but most dietary fructose comes in the form of the disaccharide sucrose (table sugar). Galactose is a common com-

ponent of glycolipids and glycoproteins, but the most important dietary source is the disaccharide lactose in milk and milk products. These monosaccharides have to be channeled into the major pathways of glucose metabolism.

Fructose is channeled into glycolysis/gluconeogenesis

Fructose is less rapidly absorbed from the intestine than is glucose, but once in the blood it is metabolized more rapidly: its plasma half-life after IV injec-

FIG. 17.19

Metabolism of fructose in the liver. **A,** Pathways. **B,** Substrate flow after a good meal. **C,** Substrate flow when the blood glucose level is low.

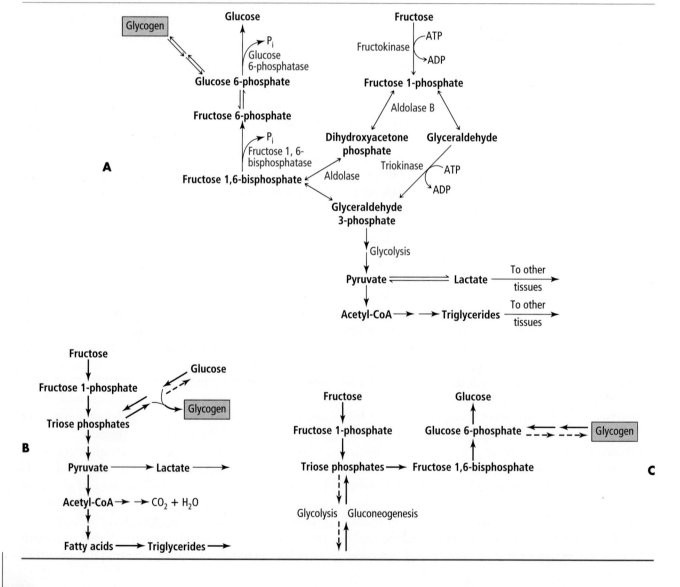

tion has been found to be only half that of glucose (18 min versus 43 min). Some of the fructose is phosphorylated to the glycolytic intermediate fructose 6-phosphate by hexokinase. The K_m of hexokinase for fructose, however, is approximately 20 times higher than that for glucose, so this pathway is important only when the fructose concentration is very high.

Most of the dietary fructose is phosphorylated by **fructokinase** *in the liver, kidney, and intestine.* The liver alone accounts for almost half of the total fructose metabolism. Fructokinase produces not fructose 6-phosphate but fructose 1-phosphate, which is not a glycolytic intermediate (Fig. 17.19). Fructose 1-phosphate is cleaved to dihydroxyacetone phosphate and glyceraldehyde by **aldolase B,** an isoenzyme of aldolase that can cleave both fructose 1,6-bisphosphate and fructose 1-phosphate. The products of aldolase B are metabolized further by glycolysis or gluconeogenesis.

Excess fructose is toxic

The metabolism of large amounts of fructose by the liver is not entirely unproblematic: the activity of fructokinase exceeds that of aldolase B (Table 17.2), and therefore *fructose 1-phosphate tends to accumulate.* This metabolite, in turn, is a potent allosteric effector of several enzymes of carbohydrate metabolism.

Also, because the tissue concentration of fructose 1-phosphate in the liver can reach 10 μmol/g, a substantial portion of the phosphate in the cell becomes tied up in fructose 1-phosphate. This can impair oxidative phosphorylation and cause liver damage.

Also, *the liver metabolizes fructose faster than glucose* (compare the activities of glucokinase and fructokinase in Table 17.2). The PFK reaction, in particular, which controls the rate of glycolysis from glucose and glycogen, is bypassed by fructose, and pyruvate kinase is stimulated by fructose 1-phosphate as it is by fructose 1,6-bisphosphate (Fig. 17.6, *B,* page 337).

Fructose has been used as a substitute for glucose in parenteral (intravenous) nutrition. Also, diabetic diets were formulated in which a large portion of the dietary carbohydrate was supplied as fructose, based on the reasoning that the insulin-dependent PFK reaction would be bypassed. It soon was found, however, that excess fructose can cause liver damage, increased lactate formation, hypertriglyceridemia, and hyperuricemia. Therefore fructose no longer is used in parenteral nutrition. It is also of doubtful value in diabetic diets because the diabetic liver metabolizes the triose phosphates not by glycolysis but by gluconeogenesis (see Chapter 29), effectively converting dietary fructose into blood glucose.

TABLE 17.2

Kinetic properties of fructose-metabolizing enzymes in the liver, and, for comparison, the glucose-metabolizing enzyme glucokinase

Enzyme	V_{max} (μmol/min per g of tissue)	K_m for the carbohydrate substrate (mM)
Glucokinase	1*	10
Fructose carrier (in plasma membrane)	30	67-200‡
Fructokinase	10	0.5
Aldolase B:		
Cleavage of fructose 1-phosphate	2-3	1
Cleavage of fructose 1,6-bisphosphate	2-3	0.004-0.012
Triokinase	2	0.01
Fructose 1,6-bisphosphatase	4*	1†
Glucose 6-phosphatase	10*	2.5-3‡

* Depends on the nutritional state.
† Depends on the allosteric effectors.
‡ After a sweet meal, the fructose concentration in the portal vein reaches approximately 2 to 3 mM. The usual glucose 6-phosphate concentration in the liver is approximately 0.2 mM (higher during fasting; lower after a meal).

Fructose leads to an increased formation of lactic acid because it is rapidly metabolized to pyruvate, and pyruvate is in equilibrium with lactate. The hypertriglyceridemia can be traced to the rapid synthesis of fatty acids and triglycerides from fructose in the liver. The liver releases these triglycerides into the blood in the form of very-low-density lipoprotein (VLDL; see Chapter 20).

Inborn errors of fructose metabolism cause hypoglycemia and liver damage

Deficiencies of fructose-metabolizing enzymes occasionally are seen. Fructokinase deficiency leads to **essential fructosuria,** with fructose appearing in the urine after a meal containing fructose (or sucrose). This rare condition is asymptomatic. It sometimes is detected incidentally during urinalysis when "reducing sugar" (fructose) is present while enzymatic glucose tests, such as the glucose oxidase method, are negative. Most of the fructose eventually is metabolized by hexokinase in muscle and adipose tissue.

Patients with aldolase B deficiency have **hereditary fructose intolerance.** They complain about nausea and vomiting after eating fructose or sucrose, and this is accompanied by signs of hypoglycemia (weakness, trembling, and sweating). Liver damage can develop in untreated cases, and the patient eventually may succumb to liver cirrhosis. Hypoglycemia and liver damage both are attributed to the intracellular accumulation of fructose 1-phosphate: besides tying up phosphate and thereby impairing ATP synthesis, fructose 1-phosphate inhibits aldolase, phosphohexose isomerase, and glycogen phosphorylase, and it stimulates glucokinase.

Fructose, like glucose, is transported across the plasma membrane, but *fructose 1-phosphate is a strictly intracellular metabolite.* Therefore fructose but not fructose 1-phosphate is elevated in the blood and urine of patients with fructose intolerance. Most monosaccharides, including glucose, fructose, and galactose, are transported, but *their phosphorylated derivatives cannot penetrate the plasma membrane.*

A deficiency of the gluconeogenic enzyme fructose 1,6-bisphosphatase results in fructose intolerance similar to aldolase B deficiency, but these patients also have fasting hypoglycemia. They can form glucose from stored glycogen, but gluconeo-genesis is blocked. Glycogen degradation can maintain a reasonably normal blood glucose level for many hours, but *the defect in gluconeogenesis results in dangerous hypoglycemia when the period of fasting exceeds 12 to 18 hours.* By that time, most of the liver glycogen is depleted.

Fructose intolerance is treated by excluding fructose from the diet. Indeed, most affected children spontaneously develop a strong aversion to sweets. The term *conditioned taste aversion* is applied to this situation, in which the experience of illness or malaise after eating leads to a strong aversion to the offending food. On the bright side, adults with fructose intolerance have excellent teeth!

Galactose is channeled into the pathways of glucose metabolism

Like fructose, dietary galactose is metabolized mostly in the liver. The main pathway is outlined in Fig. 17.20: galactose 1-phosphate is formed by **galactokinase,** and UDP-galactose then is formed from galactose 1-phosphate and UDP-glucose. UDP-galactose is epimerized to UDP-glucose, which is recycled in the galactose 1-phosphate-uridyl-transferase reaction. The net reaction of the pathway is *the ATP-dependent conversion of galactose to glucose 1-phosphate.* Because of its reversibility, the epimerase reaction is also useful as an endogenous source of UDP-galactose for the synthesis of glycolipids, glycoproteins, and proteoglycans.

FIG. 17.20

Galactose metabolism.

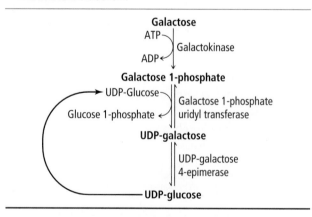

Galactosemia is an inborn error of galactose metabolism

In **classical galactosemia,** an autosomal recessive disease with an estimated population incidence of 1 in 40,000, a deficiency of galactose 1-phosphate-uridyl transferase leads to the accumulation of galactose and galactose 1-phosphate after the ingestion of milk or other galactose-containing foods. This disease is evident within weeks after birth: feeding difficulties and vomiting result in poor weight gain, and jaundice is present that often is misdiagnosed as a protracted physiological jaundice of the newborn (see Chapter 22). This jaundice is caused not by hemolysis, as evidenced by normal hemoglobin levels, but by liver dysfunction. The blood levels of alanine transaminase and aspartate transaminase are elevated, indicating hepatocellular damage (see Chapter 25). The central nervous system is affected as well, as evidenced by an abnormal lethargy or irritability. Mental deficiency, liver cirrhosis, and cataracts develop in untreated cases.

Whereas the liver damage in galactosemia is caused by the accumulation of galactose 1-phosphate and the concomitant depletion of inorganic phosphate, cataract formation is caused by free galactose: aldose reductase in the lens, the same enzyme that forms sorbitol from glucose in the polyol pathway (see Fig. 17.23, page 355), reduces galactose to galactitol, which accumulates in the lens and causes cataracts. Patients with a deficiency of galactokinase get cataracts even though they do not suffer from liver damage.

The diagnosis is suggested by the presence of reducing material (galactose) in the urine, with a negative glucose oxidase test. In addition, galactose 1-phosphate-uridyl transferase can be determined in RBCs: the patients are lacking the enzyme completely, and the unaffected heterozygotes have a reduced enzyme activity. All clinical signs of galactosemia can be avoided by placing the patient on a milk-free diet, so the diagnosis should be made as early as possible.

THE MINOR PATHWAYS OF CARBOHYDRATE METABOLISM

Carbohydrates not only are substrates for the generation of metabolic energy, they also are required for the synthesis of nucleotides, glycolipids, glycoproteins, and other specialized products. The principal task of the "minor pathways" of carbohydrate metabolism is the provision of metabolites for specialized biosynthetic purposes.

The pentose phosphate pathway supplies NADPH and ribose 5-phosphate

The important products of the cytoplasmic **pentose phosphate pathway,** also known as the **hexose monophosphate shunt,** are ribose 5-phosphate and NADPH. Although NADPH has the same redox potential as NADH, the functions of the two coenzymes are different: NAD^+ collects hydrogen from catabolic substrates for transfer to the respiratory chain, but *the hydrogen of NADPH is required for reductive biosynthesis.* The synthesis of fatty acids and cholesterol from acetyl-CoA, in particular, requires NADPH.

The **oxidative branch** of the pentose phosphate pathway, which is initiated by **glucose 6-phosphate dehydrogenase,** produces NADPH in a sequence of irreversible reactions (Fig. 17.21). The **nonoxidative branch** (Fig. 17.22) consists of reversible rearrangements of phosphorylated monosaccharides. It links ribulose 5-phosphate, the product of the oxidative branch, to the glycolytic and gluconeogenic pathways.

The nonequilibrium nature of the reactions in the oxidative branch enables the cell to maintain a high $[NADPH]/[NADP^+]$ ratio. Well-fed liver cells, for example, contain 50 to 100 times more NADPH than $NADP^+$. This is in marked contrast to NAD: under aerobic conditions, NAD^+ may be more than 100 times more abundant than NADH. For this reason, *the cells employ NADPH rather than NADH whenever a strong reducing agent is required.*

The most important enzymes of the nonoxidative branch are **transketolase** and **transaldolase.** Transketolase transfers a two-carbon unit; transaldolase transfers a three-carbon unit. Transketolase (but not transaldolase) contains enzyme-bound thiamine pyrophosphate, which acts as a transient carrier of the two-carbon unit.

The overall balance of the pentose phosphate pathway, as shown in Figs. 17.21 and 17.22, can be written as:

$$3 \text{ Glucose 6-phosphate } + 6 \text{ NADP}^+ \longrightarrow$$
$$2 \text{ Fructose 6-phosphate } + \text{ Glyceraldehyde}$$
$$\text{3-phosphate} + 6 \text{ NADPH} + 6 \text{ H}^+ + 3 \text{ CO}_2$$

Besides the glycolytic intermediates, *two molecules*

of NADPH *are formed for each carbon released as* CO_2. Actually, however, the pentose phosphate pathway can run in different modes according to the relative needs of the cell for NADPH and ribose 5-phosphate:

FIG. 17.21

The oxidative branch of the pentose phosphate pathway.

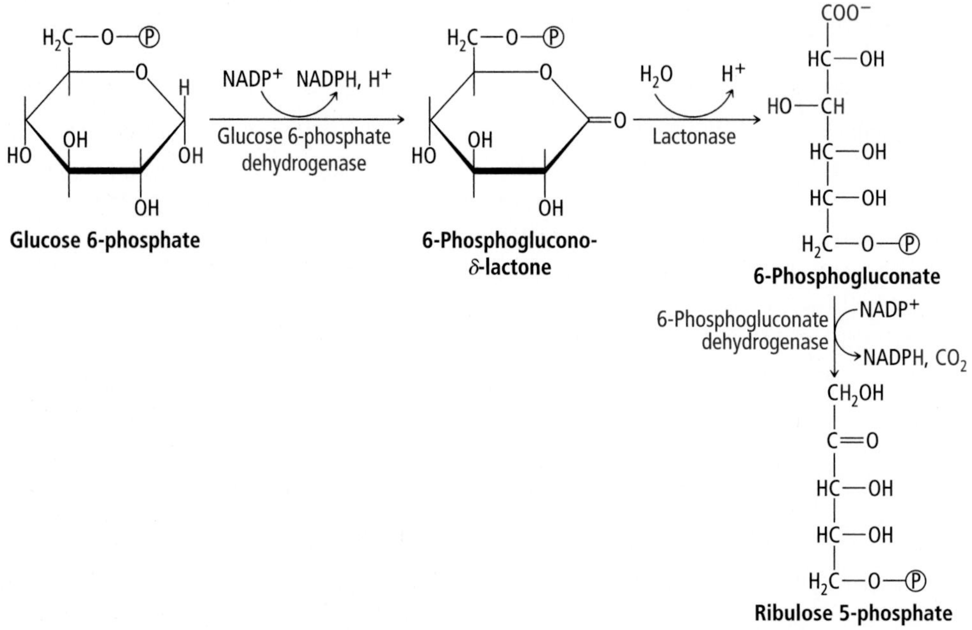

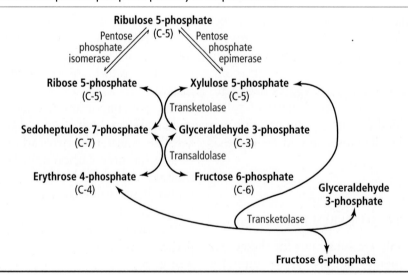

FIG. 17.22

The nonoxidative branch of the pentose phosphate pathway in adipose tissue.

1. If the cell needs more ribose 5-phosphate than NADPH, ribose 5-phosphate is formed not only through the oxidative branch but also by a reversal of the reactions in the nonoxidative branch. This may be important in muscle tissue, where the activity of glucose 6-phosphate dehydrogenase is very low and where an adequate nucleotide pool has to be maintained.

2. If the needs for ribose 5-phosphate and NADPH are balanced, the oxidative branch and the pentose phosphate isomerase reaction supply both products, with little substrate flow through the nonoxidative branch.

3. If the cell needs more NADPH than ribose 5-phosphate, the oxidative and the nonoxidative branch together form fructose 6-phosphate and glyceraldehyde 3-phosphate. These are converted back to glucose 6-phosphate in the gluconeogenic reactions. In this mode, the pathway runs a cyclic course, and theoretically, the whole glucose molecule can be oxidized to CO_2 and NADPH.

Pentose phosphate pathway activity is minimal in muscle and brain, where almost all of the glucose is degraded by glycolysis, but it accounts for a significant portion of the total glucose oxidation in tissues with active fatty acid or cholesterol synthesis, including liver, adrenal cortex, and the lactating (but not the nonlactating) mammary gland.

NADPH is also important for the antioxidant defenses of the body (see the next paragraph), so the pentose phosphate pathway is well developed in cells that are exposed to a high oxygen partial pressure. In the cornea of the eye, for example, it accounts for 60% of the total glucose consumption.

The amounts of glucose 6-phosphate dehydrogenase and phosphogluconate dehydrogenase are increased in the well-fed state, and this effect most likely is mediated by insulin. In the short term, glucose 6-phosphate dehydrogenase is inhibited by a high [NADPH]/[NADP$^+$] ratio. Therefore *any increase in the consumption of NADPH results in an increased activity of the oxidative branch.*

Glucose 6-phosphate dehydrogenase deficiency causes drug-induced hemolytic anemia

Erythrocytes require NADPH not for reductive biosynthesis but for the maintenance of a reducing environment: because the cell cannot replace defective proteins by new synthesis during its 120-day lifespan, any damage by peroxides or other oxidizing agents has to be avoided. NADPH plays a key role in the antioxidant defenses of the cell because it is required to maintain **glutathione** in the reduced state. Glutathione is the tripeptide γ-Glu-Cys-Gly. It functions as a reducing agent by forming a disulfide bond with a second glutathione molecule as shown in Box 17.1. For example, it can destroy hydrogen peroxide in a reaction that is catalyzed by **glutathione peroxidase** which appears in Box 17.2.

BOX 17.1

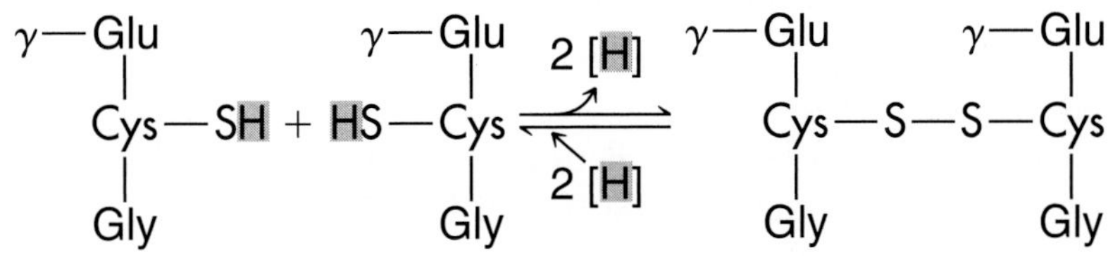

BOX 17.2

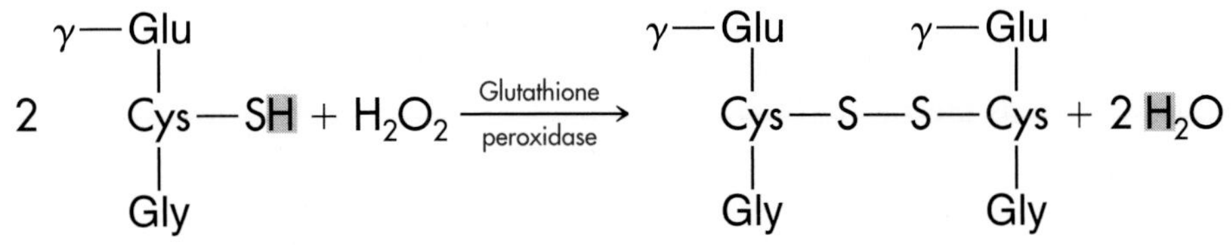

BOX 17.3

$$\underset{\text{Gly}}{\overset{\gamma\text{—Glu}}{|}}\underset{\text{Cys—S—S—Cys}}{\overset{}{|}}\underset{\text{Gly}}{\overset{\gamma\text{—Glu}}{|}} + \text{NADPH} + \text{H}^+ \xrightarrow[\text{reductase}]{\text{Glutathione}} 2 \underset{\text{Gly}}{\overset{\gamma\text{—Glu}}{|}}\overset{}{\underset{}{\text{Cys—SH}}} + \text{NADP}^+$$

Reduced glutathione is essential for protecting cellular proteins from oxidative damage. Therefore the dimeric, oxidized form has to be reduced back by the enzyme **glutathione reductase** shown in Box 17.3. We see now that *the antioxidant defenses of the cell would be seriously compromised in the absence of NADPH.*

Exactly this happens in the erythrocytes of individuals with a partial deficiency of glucose 6-phosphate dehydrogenase. This common, X-linked recessive trait is expressed in all tissues, but only the erythrocytes are seriously affected. Unlike other cells, RBCs do not possess alternative routes for NADPH synthesis (see malic enzyme, Chapter 18), and they cannot compensate for a low enzyme activity by synthesizing more enzyme. The abnormal enzymes found in patients with this deficiency are the result of missense mutations, which either reduce the catalytic activity of the enzyme (decreased V_{max} or increased K_m) or decrease its lifespan. Not less than 300 genetic variants of glucose 6-phosphate dehydrogenase are known so far, more than for any other human enzyme.

Glucose 6-phosphate dehydrogenase deficiency is harmless under ordinary conditions; problems arise only when the erythrocytes are exposed to oxidative stress. This is caused most commonly by drugs that either are oxidants themselves or give rise to oxidizing products during their metabolism. A large amount of glutathione becomes oxidized, and a large amount of NADPH is required for its reduction. In such situations, the abnormally sluggish glucose 6-phosphate dehydrogenase is not able to keep pace with the increased demand. Without sufficient NADPH and reduced glutathione, membrane proteins become covalently cross-linked, aggregates of oxidized hemoglobin (known as **Heinz bodies**) become visible in the cells, and a hemolytic crisis develops within 2 or 3 days after the initial exposure to the drug.

The offending drugs include the antimalarial primaquine, the sulfonamides sulfanilamide and sulfamethoxazole, acetanilid (a minor analgesic), nalidixic acid (an antimicrobial drug), nitrofurantoin (a urinary antiseptic), and many other drugs. Not only do these drugs have to be avoided, but even ordinary broad beans (*Vicia faba*) are dangerous. They cause **favism,** an often life-threatening attack of hemolysis with hemoglobinuria that occurs 24 to 48 hours after the consumption of broad beans. Even in the sixth century BC, Pythagoras strongly advised against the eating of beans, possibly because of the high prevalence of favism in Greece.*

Infectious diseases also are a fairly common cause of hemolysis in individuals with glucose 6-phosphate dehydrogenase deficiency. Viral hepatitis, pneumonia, and typhoid fever, for example, can lead to unexpected hemolytic complications.

Glucose 6-phosphate dehydrogenase deficiency is rare in northern Europe but very common in Africa, the Mediterranean region, the Middle East, India, and Southeast Asia. *It affects more than 100 million people (mostly males) worldwide,* including approximately 11% of males in the U.S. African American population. This high incidence is related to a partial protection of heterozygous females (but not hemizygous males) against malarial infection.

Fructose is the principal sugar in seminal fluid

Fructose serves some specialized functions in the human body. In seminal fluid, which contains up to 11 mM (200 mg/dL) free fructose, it replaces glucose as the principal monosaccharide. It is the major

---

* According to some scholars, however, Pythagoras' injunction against beans stems from the belief that beans contain the souls of dead people. Pythagoras was one of the first European philosophers to believe in the transmigration of the soul.

FIG. 17.23

The polyol pathway.

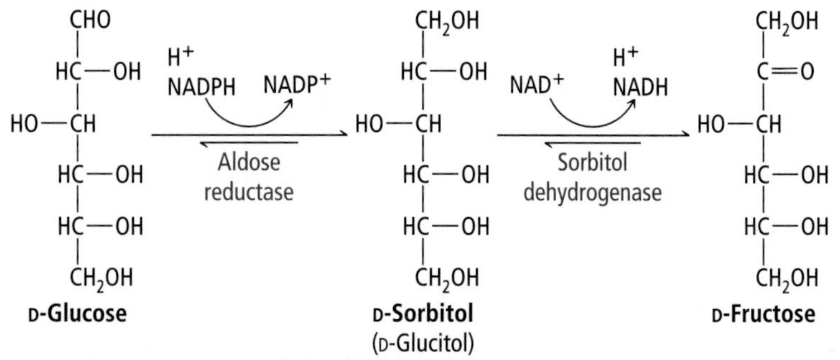

```
    CHO                              CH₂OH                            CH₂OH
  HC—OH       H⁺                   HC—OH                             C=O
HO—CH    NADPH  NADP⁺            HO—CH       NAD⁺  H⁺             HO—CH
  HC—OH    ⟶   Aldose             HC—OH         ⟶  NADH           HC—OH
  HC—OH         reductase          HC—OH            Sorbitol        HC—OH
  CH₂OH                            CH₂OH            dehydrogenase    CH₂OH
 D-Glucose                        D-Sorbitol                      D-Fructose
                                  (D-Glucitol)
```

TABLE 17.3

Sugars in glycolipids, glycoproteins, and proteoglycans

Sugar	Type	Activated form	Occurrence
Mannose	Hexose	GDP-Man	Glycoproteins (especially N linked)
Galactose	Hexose	UDP-Gal	Glycoproteins, glycolipids, proteoglycans
Glucose	Hexose	UDP-Glc	Glycoproteins (rare), glycolipids
Fucose	Deoxyhexose	GDP-Fuc	Glycoproteins, glycolipids
N-acetylglucosamine	Aminohexose	UDP-GlcNAc	Glycoproteins, proteoglycans
N-acetylgalactosamine	Aminohexose	UDP-GalNAc	Glycoproteins, glycolipids, proteoglycans
Glucuronic acid	Uronic acid	UDP-GlcUA	Proteoglycans
Iduronic acid	Uronic acid	None*	Proteoglycans
N-acetylneuraminic acid	Sialic acid	CMP-NANA	Glycoproteins, glycolipids

* Formed by the epimerization of glucuronic acid in the proteoglycan.

energy source for the sperm cells in their all-important race for the ovum. The advantage of fructose over glucose may be that bacteria, which compete with the sperm cells for the available nutrient, often prefer glucose over other energy sources (see Chapter 6).

The fructose is synthesized in the seminal vesicles by the **polyol pathway** (Fig. 17.23). This pathway is given its direction by the choice of cofactors: the cellular NADPH concentration far exceeds that of NADP⁺, and NAD⁺ is far more abundant than NADH. Therefore glucose is converted to fructose, not fructose to glucose. This pathway is active not only in seminal vesicles but in many other tissues as well, including the lens, retina, blood vessels, and peripheral nerves.

Amino sugars and sugar acids are made from glucose

Several monosaccharide derivatives are required specifically for the synthesis of glycolipids, glycoproteins, and proteoglycans. *These products, which are required as nucleotide-activated precursors (Table 17.3), can be made from glucose.* The synthesis of the activated **amino sugars** is shown in Fig. 17.24.

UDP-glucuronic acid is made by the NAD⁺-dependent oxidation of carbon 6 in UDP-glucose (Fig. 17.25). Free glucuronic acid, produced only by the degradation of proteoglycans and other glucuronic acid–containing products (reaction ③ in Fig. 17.25), is metabolized to an intermediate of the pentose phosphate pathway. Mammals other than

FIG. 17.24

Synthesis of amino sugars.

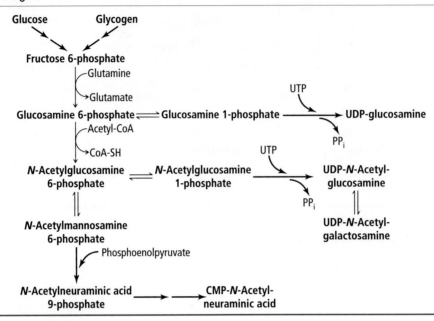

FIG. 17.25

The uronic acid pathway.

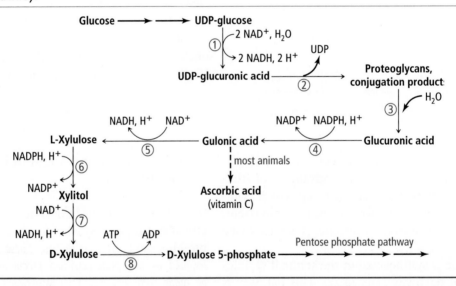

primates, guinea pigs, and fruit bats can convert the intermediate gulonic acid to **ascorbic acid (vitamin C;** see Chapter 24). Unlike us, these animals do not get scurvy on a vitamin C–deficient diet. Most likely, our ancestors subsisted on a fruit-based diet that contained a dependable supply of ascorbic acid, so they could afford to lose the ability for ascorbic acid biosynthesis.

A rare genetic condition, **essential pentosuria,** is caused by an enzymatic block in the conversion of L-xylulose to xylitol (reaction ⑥ in Fig. 17.25). Individuals with this otherwise-harmless condition excrete L-xylulose in the urine, and the presence of this "reducing sugar" may lead to a misdiagnosis of diabetes mellitus unless specific tests for glucose, such as the glucose oxidase method, are employed.

SUMMARY

Glucose is an important metabolic substrate for most tissues, and it is a required fuel for brain and erythrocytes. Therefore the normal blood glucose level of 70 to 100 mg/dL has to be maintained at all times. In the absence of a dietary supply, the liver produces glucose by two pathways: gluconeogenesis and glycogen degradation.

Gluconeogenesis uses amino acids, lactate, and glycerol as substrates for glucose synthesis. This pathway is based on a reversal of glycolysis, with specific gluconeogenic enzymes bypassing the three irreversible reactions of glycolysis. This pathway is the only source of glucose during long-term fasting.

Glycogen is the intracellular storage form of carbohydrate, and the degradation of liver glycogen is the major source of blood glucose during short-term fasting. Extrahepatic tissues use their glycogen not for blood glucose regulation but as an extra fuel for times of extra demand—especially in contracting muscle—and as a backup fuel for periods of hypoxia, when glycogen is fermented to lactic acid.

Glucose metabolism is regulated by hormones: insulin stimulates the glucose-consuming pathways of glycolysis and glycogen synthesis, and glucagon and epinephrine stimulate the glucose-producing pathways of gluconeogenesis and glycogen degradation.

Dietary monosaccharides other than glucose are channeled into glycolysis. *Galactose* is effectively converted to glucose 6-phosphate; *fructose* enters the main sequence at the level of the triose phosphates. These reactions take place mostly in the liver.

The "minor pathways" of carbohydrate metabolism supply specialized products: the *pentose phosphate pathway* provides ribose 5-phosphate and NADPH, and fructose, galactose, amino sugars, and sugar acids are produced from glucose in other specialized reaction sequences.

Further Reading

Cornish-Bowden A, Cardenas M: Hexokinase and "glucokinase" in liver metabolism. *Trends Biochem Sci* 16, 281-282, 1991.

Dent P et al.: The molecular mechanism by which insulin stimulates glycogen synthesis in mammalian skeletal muscle. *Nature* 348, 302-308, 1990.

Dunger DB, Holton JB: Disorders of carbohydrate metabolism. In: Holton JB, editor: *The inherited metabolic diseases*, 2nd ed. Churchill Livingstone, New York, 1994, pp. 21-65.

Henry RR, Crapo PA: Current issues in fructose metabolism. *Annu Rev Nutr* 11, 21-39, 1991.

Luzzato L: Glucose-6-phosphate dehydrogenase deficiency and the pentose phosphate pathway. In: Handin RI, Lux SE, Stossel TP, editors: *Blood*. J. B. Lippincott, Philadelphia, 1995, pp. 1897-1923.

Pilkis SJ: Molecular physiology of the regulation of hepatic gluconeogenesis and glycolysis. *Annu Rev Physiol* 54, 885-909, 1992.

Printz RL, Magnuson MA, Granner DK: Mammalian glucokinase. *Annu Rev Nutr* 13, 463-496, 1993.

Scriver CR, Beaudet AL, Sly WS, Valle D, editors: *The metabolic basis of inherited disease*, 6th ed. McGraw-Hill, New York, 1989, pp. 399-491, 2237-2266.

QUESTIONS

1. Ischemic tissues have an increased rate of glycolysis. Most of this is fueled not by glucose but by locally stored glycogen that is degraded in response to ischemia. This response depends on the activation of glycogen phosphorylase by
   A. ATP
   B. AMP
   C. Low pH
   D. Carbon dioxide
   E. Glucose 6-phosphate

2. Several inborn errors of carbohydrate metabolism can cause fasting hypoglycemia. The most severe fasting hypoglycemia is expected in deficiencies of
   A. Phosphofructokinase
   B. Aldolase
   C. Glycogen phosphorylase
   D. Fructose 1,6-bisphosphatase
   E. Glucose 6-phosphatase

3. A medical student of Middle Eastern ethnic background develops an episode of hemolysis and hemoglobinuria 24 hours after injecting himself with a street drug of unknown composition. He probably has a low activity of the RBC enzyme
    A. Glucose 6-phosphate dehydrogenase
    B. Hexokinase
    C. Phosphofructokinase
    D. Fructokinase
    E. Glucose 6-phosphatase

4. Liver glycogen normally is synthesized after a meal and is degraded during fasting. Which pharmacological manipulation would enhance glycogen degradation in the liver?
    A. An inhibitor of α-adrenergic receptors
    B. An inhibitor of β-adrenergic receptors
    C. The injection of insulin
    D. A drug that activates protein phosphatase 1
    E. A drug that inhibits the degradation of cAMP

5. Glycogen degradation is an important energy source for exercising muscle. How many high-energy phosphate bonds are synthesized by converting one glucose residue in glycogen to lactic acid?
    A. one
    B. two
    C. three
    D. four
    E. five

Chapter 18

The Metabolism of Fatty Acids and Triglycerides

Dietary triglycerides are a major source of metabolic energy, accounting for close to 40% of the total calories in typical Western diets. Approximately 95% of their energy content is contributed by their fatty acids, and only 5% by the glycerol. Triglycerides are also important as the principal storage form of energy in the body. Most people carry between 5 and 20 kg of triglycerides in their adipose tissue. These triglycerides are synthesized in the well-fed state and degraded during fasting. With an energy content of 9.3 kcal/g, a fat store of 12 kg of triglyceride contains 110,000 kcal—enough to keep us alive for almost 3 months without food.

This chapter describes those metabolic pathways of fatty acids and triglycerides that are related to their role as sources of metabolic energy.

THE GENERATION OF METABOLIC ENERGY FROM FATTY ACIDS

Fatty acids of dietary origin are oxidized by most tissues after a meal, and the excess is stored away in adipose tissue. The stored triglycerides are degraded in the fasting state, when the released fatty acids are the main energy source for the body. In the following sections we will trace the pathways for the utilization of dietary fat, fat storage in adipose tissue, and the mitochondrial oxidation of fatty acids.

Fatty acids differ in their chain length and in the number of carbon-carbon double bonds

A typical fatty acid consists of an unbranched hydrocarbon chain with a carboxy group at one end. Most naturally occurring fatty acids have an even number of carbons, with chain lengths of 16 and 18 being the most common. Structural modifications, including hydroxy groups or methyl groups attached to the hydrocarbon chain, occasionally are present but are not a common feature of most lipids.

In **saturated fatty acids,** the carbons are linked exclusively by single bonds. Of the fatty acids listed in Table 18.1, **acetic acid** does not occur in natural fats and oils, but vinegar contains approximately 5% acetic acid. **Butyric acid** is also uncommon in natural fats, except for milkfat. It is distinguished by its smell, which resembles that of malodorous feet. In the production of some types of cheese, butyric acid is released from milkfat by the action of microbial lipases and contributes to the flavor of the product. **Myristic acid** is a major fatty acid in nutmeg, coconut, and palm kernel oil; **palmitic acid** and **stearic acid** are the most abundant saturated fatty acids in animal and human fat, accounting for 30% to 40% of the fatty acids in our adipose tissue.

The carbons of the fatty acids are numbered, starting with the carboxy carbon. Alternatively, they are designated by Greek letters: as in the amino

TABLE 18.1

Structures of some naturally occurring saturated fatty acids

No. of carbons	Fatty acid	Structure	
2	Acetic acid	H_3C—COOH	╱COOH
4	Butyric acid	H_3C—$(CH_2)_2$—COOH	∧COOH
14	Myristic acid	H_3C—$(CH_2)_{12}$—COOH	∧∧∧∧∧∧∧COOH
16	Palmitic acid	H_3C—$(CH_2)_{14}$—COOH	∧∧∧∧∧∧∧∧COOH
18	Stearic acid	H_3C—$(CH_2)_{16}$—COOH	∧∧∧∧∧∧∧∧∧COOH
20	Arachidic acid	H_3C—$(CH_2)_{18}$—COOH	∧∧∧∧∧∧∧∧∧∧COOH
22	Behenic acid	H_3C—$(CH_2)_{20}$—COOH	∧∧∧∧∧∧∧∧∧∧∧COOH
24	Lignoceric acid	H_3C—$(CH_2)_{22}$—COOH	∧∧∧∧∧∧∧∧∧∧∧∧COOH

BOX 18.1

$$H_3C-(CH_2)_{16}-COOH =$$

chain with numbering: ω 18/17, 16/15, 14/13, 12/11, 10/9, 8/7, 6/5 (δ), 4/3 (γ/β), 2 (α) — COOH

acids, the α-carbon is the one next to the carboxy carbon, the β-carbon is carbon 3, etc. The last carbon in the chain is the ω (omega) carbon, as in the example of stearic acid which is shown in Box 18.1. **Monounsaturated fatty acids** have one carbon-carbon double bond, and **polyunsaturated fatty acids** have more than one. The double bonds of the polyunsaturated fatty acids are always three carbons apart, with a single methylene (—CH_2—) group in between. The positions of the double bonds are specified by their distance from the carboxy end: A Δ^9 double bond, for example, is between carbons 9 and 10. Alternatively, the distance from the omega carbon can be specified. The latter designation is useful because fatty acids can be elongated and shortened only at the carboxy end. If, for example, oleic acid (see Table 18.2) is elongated by two carbons, the product is no longer a Δ^9 fatty acid, but Δ^{11}; yet it is still an ω9 fatty acid. Also, *humans are not able to introduce new double bonds beyond Δ^9*. For this reason some of the polyunsaturated fatty acids, notably linoleic acid and possibly α-linolenic acid, are *nutritionally essential*. As shown in Table 18.2, the structures of unsaturated fatty acids can be described by a formula indicating the chain length, the number of double bonds, and their locations.

There is no free rotation around the carbon-carbon double bond, and the substituents are fixed in *cis* or *trans* configuration:

cis   or   *trans*

The *trans* configuration favors an extended shape of the hydrocarbon chain; a *cis* double bond forms an angle of 120°:

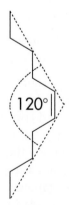

120°

Only fatty acids with cis double bonds are common in nature.

TABLE 18.2

Structures of some unsaturated fatty acids

Fatty acid	Biosynthetic class	Formula	Structure	Nutritionally essential
Palmitoleic acid	$\omega 7$	16:1;9	$H_3C—(CH_2)_5—CH{=}CH—(CH_2)_7—COOH$	No
Oleic acid	$\omega 9$	18:1;9	$H_3C—(CH_2)_7—CH{=}CH—(CH_2)_7—COOH$	No
Linoleic acid	$\omega 6$	18:2;9,12	$H_3C—(CH_2)_3—(CH_2—CH{=}CH)_2—(CH_2)_7—COOH$	Yes
α-Linolenic acid	$\omega 3$	18:3;9,12,15	$H_3C—(CH_2—CH{=}CH)_3—(CH_2)_7—COOH$	Yes
Arachidonic acid	$\omega 6$	20:4;5,8,11,14	$H_3C—(CH_2)_3—(CH_2—CH{=}CH)_4—(CH_2)_3—COOH$	No*

* Can be synthesized from dietary linoleic acid.

BOX 18.2

$$R—COO^- + HS—CoA \xrightarrow[\text{Acyl-CoA synthetase}]{ATP \quad AMP, PP_i} R—\overset{\overset{\displaystyle O}{\|}}{C}—S—CoA$$

The properties of the fatty acids can be predicted from their structures:

1. With a pK value close to 4.8, the carboxy group is approximately 99% deprotonated at physiological pH values.
2. *Long-chain fatty acids are slightly water soluble in the deprotonated state but not in the protonated state.*
3. *Double bonds decrease the melting point of the fatty acid.* Stearic acid, for example, has a melting point of 70°C; oleic acid 16°C; linoleic acid −5°C, and α-linolenic acid −11°C, even though these 18-carbon fatty acids all have approximately the same molecular weight. The same is true for fats and oils: the softer the margarine, the higher its content of unsaturated fatty acids.

Chylomicrons transport triglycerides from the intestine to other tissues

The main products of fat digestion are *2-monoacylglyc-erol and free fatty acids* (see Chapter 14). After their absorption, the fatty acids are activated to **acyl-CoA** in the endoplasmic reticulum (ER) of the intestinal mucosal cell (see Box 18.2). This reaction is made irreversible by the subsequent hydrolysis of inorganic pyrophosphate. The triglycerides then are resyn-thesized from 2-monoacylglycerol and acyl-CoA (Fig. 18.1).

Why are triglycerides first hydrolyzed in the intestinal lumen, only to be resynthesized in the mucosal cell? The reason is that free fatty acids and monoglycerides, being slightly water soluble, can diffuse to the cell surface for absorption. Triglycerides, on the other hand, cannot be absorbed.

The triglycerides are incorporated into **chylomi-crons,** a type of lipoprotein that consists of 98% to 99% lipid and 1% to 2% protein. Most of their lipid is triglyceride, but they also contain other dietary lipids such as cholesterol, cholesterol esters, phospholipids, and fat-soluble vitamins. The protein component of the chylomicrons is synthesized at the rough ER, and the lipids are added in the smooth ER and Golgi—following the familiar secretory pathway (see Chapter 8).

The chylomicrons are small fat droplets with a size of up to 1 µm. They are secreted into the extracellular space, collected by local lymph vessels, and transported to the left brachiocephalic vein by the thoracic duct.

The utilization of triglycerides requires **lipoprotein lipase (LPL)**. This enzyme is synthesized in adipose tissue, skeletal muscle, the myocardium, the lactating mammary gland, spleen, lung, kidney, and aorta, but not in liver and brain. LPL is attached

FIG. 18.1

Absorption and transport of dietary fat. *LPL*, Lipoprotein lipase.

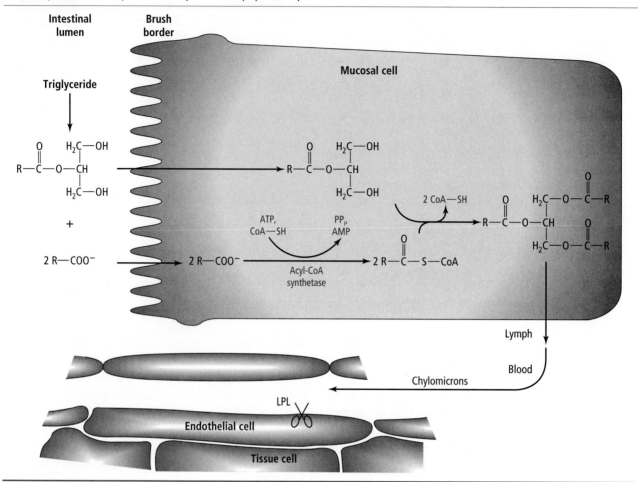

to heparan sulfate proteoglycans on the surface of the capillary endothelium. As the chylomicrons pass through the capillaries they bind to LPL, and their triglycerides are hydrolyzed to free fatty acids and 2-monoacylglycerol. Most of the fatty acids and monoglyceride diffuse directly into the tissue (Fig. 18.2).

Different tissues have different isoenzymes of LPL, which are subject to adaptive control: LPL activity in adipose tissue is increased in the well-fed state and decreased during fasting. In skeletal muscle and the myocardium, in contrast, LPL activity is moderately high both in the well-fed state and during fasting. Also, the K_m of the myocardial enzyme for chylomicrons is approximately 10 times lower than that of the enzyme in adipose tissue. Shortly after a fatty meal, when chylomicrons are abundant,

most of the triglycerides are used by adipose tissue. During the transition from the fed to the fasted state, however, *dietary triglycerides are rerouted from adipose tissue to skeletal muscle and the myocardium*.

LPL can be solubilized by injected heparin, which also increases its enzymatic activity. The evaluation of LPL activity in the laboratory is based on the determination of serum lipase activities before and after heparin injection.

Adipose tissue is specialized for the storage of triglycerides

Approximately 90% of the fresh weight of adipose tissue is triglyceride. With an energy value of 9.3 kcal/g, this triglyceride is a highly concentrated store of metabolic energy. Glycogen, on the other

FIG. 18.2

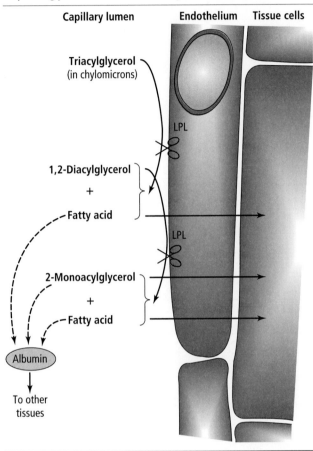

Hydrolysis of triglycerides in chylomicrons by lipoprotein lipase. The breakdown products diffuse mostly into the tissue cells. A smaller portion becomes noncovalently bound to serum albumin and is carried to distant sites. Lipoprotein lipase (LPL) is noncovalently bound to heparan sulfate proteoglycans of the endothelial plasma membrane.

Capillary lumen   **Endothelium**   **Tissue cells**

Triacylglycerol (in chylomicrons)

LPL

1,2-Diacylglycerol

+

Fatty acid

LPL

2-Monoacylglycerol

+

Fatty acid

Albumin

To other tissues

hand, has a caloric value of only 4.1 kcal/g. In addition, triglycerides are stored without accompanying water, whereas glycogen is hydrated: a glycogen granule contains approximately 2 g of water with every gram of glycogen. A fat store of 15 kg has an energy value of 140,000 kcal. This amount of energy in the form of hydrated glycogen would weigh 100 kg!

After a mixed meal, most of the fatty acids for triglyceride synthesis in adipose tissue are derived from the action of lipoprotein lipase on chylomicron triglycerides. These fatty acids have to be activated to their CoA-thioesters before they can be used for triglyceride synthesis. The glycerol moiety of the triglycerides is derived from **glycerol 3-phosphate.** The only important source of this precursor in adipose tissue is the **glycerol phosphate dehydrogenase** reaction, which reduces the glycolytic intermediate dihydroxyacetone phosphate in an NADH-dependent reaction. This is the same enzyme that participates in the glycerol phosphate shuttle (see Chapter 16) and in gluconeogenesis from glycerol (see Chapter 17). The reaction is freely reversible. An alternative reaction for the generation of glycerol phosphate, the phosphorylation of glycerol by glycerol kinase, is important in the liver but not in adipose tissue.

The reactions of triglyceride synthesis in adipose tissue are summarized in Fig. 18.3. This pathway operates in other tissues as well, including the liver and the lactating mammary gland. It differs, however, from triglyceride synthesis in the intestine, where 2-monoacylglycerol rather than glycerol phosphate is a precursor (see Fig. 18.1).

Triglyceride metabolism in adipose tissue is under hormonal control

Insulin stimulates fat synthesis by several mechanisms:

1. *It increases the rate of glycolysis,* and glycolysis is required for triglyceride synthesis because it supplies glycerol phosphate. In adipose tissue, the most important control site is probably not the PFK reaction but rather the tissue uptake of glucose. Insulin favors glycolysis in adipose tissue by increasing the number of functional glucose carriers in the plasma membrane.
2. *Lipoprotein lipase activity in adipose tissue is increased by insulin.* This increases the supply of fatty acid substrates.
3. *Insulin induces the glycerolphosphate-acyl transferase,* which adds the first fatty acid to glycerol phosphate in the biosynthetic pathway (see Fig. 18.3).

Lipolysis (triglyceride hydrolysis) requires the sequential removal of the three fatty acids from glycerol. The first cleavage, which is rate limiting, is catalyzed by the **hormone-sensitive adipose tissue lipase.** The hormonal influences on the lipase are summarized in Fig. 18.4. The enzyme is phosphorylated and activated by the cyclic AMP-dependent protein kinase A, the same enzyme that operates in the regulation of glycogen metabolism

FIG. 18.3

Triglyceride synthesis in adipose tissue and the liver. Note that this pathway differs from that in the intestine (Fig. 18.1).

Dihydroxyacetone phosphate ⟵ Glycolytic reactions ⟵ Glucose

NADH, H⁺ ⟶ | Glycerol phosphate dehydrogenase
NAD⁺ ⟵ |

H_2C-OH
$HO-CH$
$H_2C-O-P-O^-$
‖ O
O^-

ADP   ATP
Glycerol kinase (liver, not adipose tissue) ⟵ Glycerol

Glycerol 3-phosphate

| 2 Acyl-CoA
↓ 2 CoA-SH

Phosphatidate:
$R-C-O-CH$
$H_2C-O-C-R$
$H_2C-O-P-O^-$
O^-

P_i Acyl-CoA   CoA-SH ⟶

Triglyceride (= Triacylglycerol):
$R-C-O-CH$
$H_2C-O-C-R$
$H_2C-O-C-R$

Phosphatidate

Triglyceride (= Triacylglycerol)

FIG. 18.4

Hormonal regulation of lipolysis in adipose tissue.

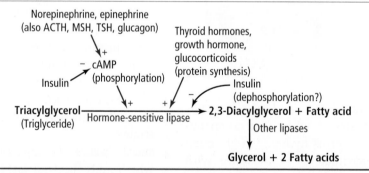

Norepinephrine, epinephrine (also ACTH, MSH, TSH, glucagon)

Thyroid hormones, growth hormone, glucocorticoids (protein synthesis)

− cAMP (phosphorylation)

Insulin

Insulin (dephosphorylation?)

Triacylglycerol (Triglyceride) ⟶ Hormone-sensitive lipase ⟶ 2,3-Diacylglycerol + Fatty acid

Other lipases ↓

Glycerol + 2 Fatty acids

(see Chapter 17). *The most important lipolytic agents in humans are the catecholamines,* which act through β-adrenergic receptors, cAMP, and protein kinase A. Norepinephrine, released from sympathetic nerve terminals in adipose tissue, is more important than circulating epinephrine: in animal experiments, sympathetic denervation has caused excessive fat accumulation in the denervated portions of adipose tissue, an effect that becomes most obvious under conditions of food deprivation or cold exposure, when fat is degraded in the surrounding innervated tissue.

Glucocorticoids, growth hormone, and the **thyroid hormones** facilitate lipolysis not by the direct stimulation of cAMP formation but by inducing the synthesis of lipolytic proteins. Thus, glucocorticoids induce the de novo synthesis of the hormone-sensitive lipase and thereby augment the lipolytic

BOX 18.3

Carnitine

Palmitoyl-carnitine

response to the catecholamines. This effect shows regional differences: in patients with Cushing's syndrome (excess glucocorticoids), adipose tissue is reduced in the extremities while truncal obesity and a "buffalo hump" develop. This shows that adipose tissue in the abdomen and neck does not respond well to the lipolytic action of these hormones.

The lipolytic hormones are antagonized by insulin, which inhibits the hormone-sensitive lipase by poorly known mechanisms, either by decreasing the level of cAMP in the cells or by inducing the dephosphorylation of the lipase. Adipose tissue is very sensitive to insulin, and even the moderately high levels of this hormone during the transition from the fed to the fasted state powerfully inhibit lipolysis.

Insulin ensures that *triglycerides are synthesized after a meal and degraded during fasting*. The sympathetic nervous system, on the other hand, ensures that *triglycerides are hydrolyzed during cold exposure, stress, and physical exercise*.

Unlike liver and intestine, *adipose tissue does not release particulate lipid in the form of lipoproteins, but releases "free" (unesterified) fatty acids*, which bind noncovalently and reversibly to serum albumin for their transport to distant sites. These albumin-bound fatty acids have a rapid turnover, with a plasma half-life of only 3 min. *The plasma levels of free fatty acids are minimal after a carbohydrate-rich meal and rise approximately fivefold within several days of fasting*. Fatty acids are the major fuel for most tissues during fasting, and glycerol, which is released from adipose tissue together with the fatty acids, is a convenient substrate for gluconeogenesis (see Fig. 18.8).

Fatty acids have to enter the mitochondrion before they can be oxidized

With the exception of some specialized cell types such as neurons and erythrocytes, all cells of the body can oxidize fatty acids. *The mitochondrion is the principal site of fatty acid oxidation*, so the fatty acids have to be transported into the mitochondrion first. Although protonated fatty acids can diffuse passively across membranes, the transport of long-chain fatty acids (those with 14 or more carbons) into the mitochondrion is not effected by passive diffusion. These fatty acids are activated rapidly to their CoA-thioesters by enzymes on the ER membrane and the outer mitochondrial membrane, so the concentrations of the free fatty acids in the cytoplasm are extremely low. In addition, long-chain fatty acids cannot be activated within the mitochondrial matrix. Because the CoA-thioesters of the fatty acids are the actual substrates of mitochondrial β-oxidation, free fatty acids diffusing passively into the mitochondrion cannot be oxidized.

The transport of long-chain fatty acids across the inner mitochondrial membrane requires the coenzyme **carnitine** as shown in Box 18.3. The fatty acid is transferred from coenzyme A to the hydroxy group of carnitine in the reversible **carnitine-palmitoyl transferase** reaction. Two carnitine-palmitoyl transferases, designated I and II, are present on the outer and the inner surface of the inner mitochondrial membrane, respectively. Carnitine and acyl-carnitine cross the membrane by facilitated exchange diffusion (Fig. 18.5).

FIG. 18.5

Transport of long-chain fatty acids into the mitochondrion. The carnitine-palmitoyl transferase reaction is freely reversible.

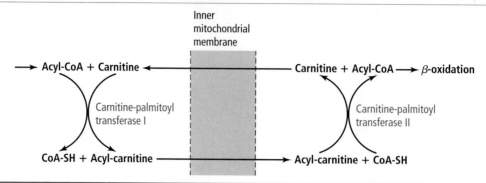

The mitochondrial uptake of short- and medium-chain fatty acids does not require carnitine: fatty acids with a chain length of up to approximately 12 carbons diffuse passively across the membrane and subsequently are activated in the mitochondrion.

β-Oxidation degrades fatty acids to acetyl-CoA

The principal fate of acyl-CoA in the mitochondrion is β-oxidation (Fig. 18.6). Each cycle of β-oxidation shortens the fatty acid by two carbons and produces an acetyl residue in acetyl-CoA. NADH and FADH$_2$ are formed in two oxidative reactions during each cycle. These reduced coenzymes are used as substrates for the respiratory chain. The reaction sequence is called β-oxidation because it is the β-carbon (carbon 3) that is oxidized.

The stoichiometry for the β-oxidation of palmitate is:

$$\text{Palmitoyl-CoA} + 7\ \text{FAD} + 7\ \text{NAD}^+ + 7\ \text{CoA} + 7\ \text{H}_2\text{O} \longrightarrow 8\ \text{Acetyl-CoA} + 7\ \text{FADH}_2 + 7\ \text{NADH} + 7\ \text{H}^+$$

The energy yield can be calculated as:

8 Acetyl-CoA ⟶	96 ATP
7 FADH$_2$ ⟶	14 ATP
7 NADH ⟶	21 ATP
	131 ATP
	− 2 ATP
	129 ATP

FIG. 18.6

Reaction sequence of β-oxidation. These reactions take place in the mitochondrial matrix of most cells.

$$R-CH_2-CH_2-\overset{\overset{\displaystyle O}{\|}}{C}-S-CoA$$
Acyl-CoA

FAD ⟶ FADH$_2$ — Acyl-CoA dehydrogenase

$$R-\overset{\overset{\displaystyle H}{|}}{C}=\overset{\underset{\displaystyle H}{|}}{C}-\overset{\overset{\displaystyle O}{\|}}{C}-S-CoA$$
***trans*-Δ2-Enoyl-CoA**

H$_2$O ⟶ — Enoyl-CoA hydratase

$$R-\overset{\overset{\displaystyle OH}{|}}{CH}-CH_2-\overset{\overset{\displaystyle O}{\|}}{C}-S-CoA$$
3-L-Hydroxyacyl-CoA

NAD$^+$ ⟶ NADH, H$^+$ — 3-L-Hydroxyacyl-CoA dehydrogenase

$$R-\overset{\overset{\displaystyle O}{\|}}{C}-CH_2-\overset{\overset{\displaystyle O}{\|}}{C}-S-CoA$$
3-Ketoacyl-CoA

CoA-SH ⟶ — β-Ketothiolase

$$R-\overset{\overset{\displaystyle O}{\|}}{C}-S-CoA + H_3C-\overset{\overset{\displaystyle O}{\|}}{C}-S-CoA$$
Acyl-CoA   **Acetyl-CoA**

BOX 18.4

$$\xrightarrow{\;\beta\text{-Oxidation}\;} R-\overset{H}{\underset{}{C}}=\overset{H}{\underset{}{C}}-CH_2-\overset{O}{\overset{\|}{C}}-S-CoA \xrightarrow[\text{isomerase}]{\text{Enoyl-CoA}} R-CH_2-\overset{H}{\underset{}{C}}=\overset{}{\underset{H}{C}}-\overset{O}{\overset{\|}{C}}-S-CoA$$

Two ATPs are subtracted because the initial activation of palmitate to palmitoyl-CoA requires two high-energy phosphate bonds in ATP. *The energy yield is close to 40%* — approximately the same as for glucose oxidation (see Chapter 16).

β-Oxidation is regulated by the supply of fatty acids

Those cells that oxidize fatty acids are able to obtain their energy from alternative fuels, such as glucose and amino acids, as well. Within rather wide limits, the use of fatty acids by the tissues is proportional to the plasma free fatty acid level, and therefore *fatty acid oxidation is for the most part regulated at the level of the hormone-sensitive adipose tissue lipase.*

An additional regulated step is the uptake of fatty acids into the mitochondrion: *carnitine-palmitoyl transferase is allosterically inhibited by malonyl-CoA.* Malonyl-CoA is formed in the regulated step of fatty acid synthesis (see Fig. 18.14, page 376), so its cytoplasmic concentration is high whenever fatty acid synthesis is stimulated. Therefore *fatty acid oxidation is inhibited when fatty acid synthesis is active.* Carnitine-acyl transferase I in the liver is also subject to long-term regulation: its activity is increased in prolonged fasting.

The oxidation of some fatty acids requires specialized reactions

Mitochondrial β-oxidation can smoothly oxidize unbranched saturated fatty acids with an even number of carbons and a chain length up to 18 or 20 carbons. Fatty acids that do not fit this description require additional enzymatic reactions.

1. **Unsaturated fatty acids** require modifications of their double bonds before β-oxidation: the enoyl-CoA intermediate of β-oxidation has a *trans*-Δ^2 double bond, but the double bonds in the natural fatty acids are in *cis* configuration and

may be encountered in either the Δ^2 or Δ^3 position. A *cis*-Δ^3 double bond can be isomerized to a *trans*-Δ^2 double bond as shown in Box 18.4. The product is an intermediate of β-oxidation. *cis*-Δ^4 double bonds also can be dealt with effectively as shown in Box 18.5. Also, fatty acids with *trans* double bonds, which occur in the hydrogenated fats of margarine, peanut butter, and many processed foods, are oxidized readily.

2. **α-Oxidation** is a minor pathway in the ER and mitochondria. It oxidizes carbon 2 (the α-carbon) and then releases carbon 1 as CO_2, thereby *shortening the fatty acid by one carbon at a time.* The function of α-oxidation is not the production of ATP but rather the degradation of methylated fatty acids. This is illustrated by **Refsum's disease,** a rare, recessively inherited defect of α-oxidation. The patients accumulate excessive quantities of **phytanic acid** in their body lipids. This unusual fatty acid is derived from the alcohol phytol, an isoprenoid that occurs as a constituent of chlorophyll in green vegetables as shown in Box 18.6. Phytanic acid cannot be β-oxidized without prior modification because the β-carbon is methylated. Its degradation normally is initiated by α-oxidation, followed by a round of β-oxidation, which yields propionyl-CoA rather than acetyl-CoA.

   Refsum's disease patients present with a variety of neurological disturbances, including cerebellar ataxia, peripheral neuropathy, nerve deafness, motor weakness, and retinitis pigmentosa. The patients respond to dietary restriction of green vegetables and of ruminant milk and meat, which contain large amounts of phytanic acid.

3. **ω-Oxidation** is a microsomal system that oxidizes the last carbon of the fatty acid (the ω-carbon) to a carboxy group, thereby producing a dicarboxylic acid. This process occurs mostly with medium-chain fatty acids. The dicarboxylic acids can be activated at either end, followed by β-oxidation.

BOX 18.5

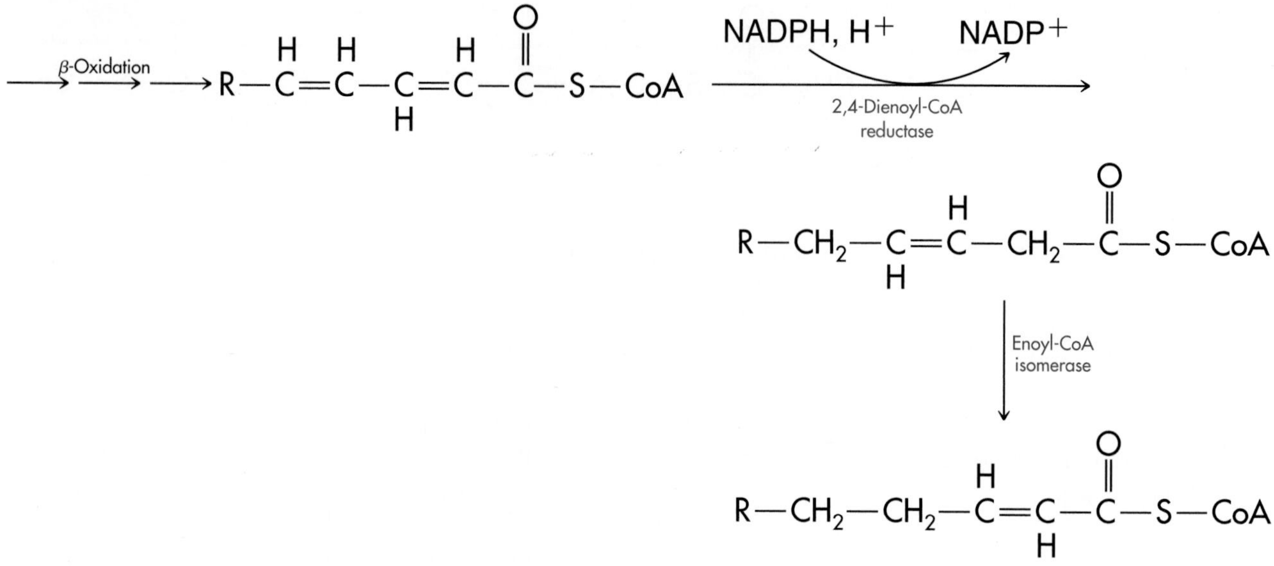

$$\xrightarrow{\beta\text{-Oxidation}} \quad R-\underset{H}{\overset{H}{C}}=\underset{H}{C}-\underset{H}{\overset{H}{C}}=C-\overset{O}{\overset{\|}{C}}-S-CoA \xrightarrow[\substack{2,4\text{-Dienoyl-CoA}\\\text{reductase}}]{\text{NADPH, H}^+ \qquad \text{NADP}^+}$$

$$R-CH_2-\underset{H}{C}=\overset{H}{C}-CH_2-\overset{O}{\overset{\|}{C}}-S-CoA$$

$$\Big\downarrow \substack{\text{Enoyl-CoA}\\\text{isomerase}}$$

$$R-CH_2-CH_2-\underset{H}{C}=\overset{H}{C}-\overset{O}{\overset{\|}{C}}-S-CoA$$

BOX 18.6

$$H_3C-\underset{\underset{CH_3}{|}}{CH}-(CH_2)_3-\underset{\underset{CH_3}{|}}{CH}-(CH_2)_3-\underset{\underset{CH_3}{|}}{CH}-(CH_2)_3-\underset{\underset{CH_3}{|}}{CH}-CH_2-COOH$$

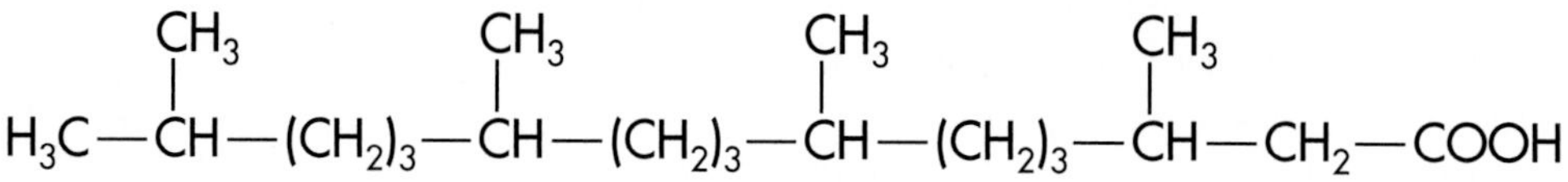

Phytanic acid

BOX 18.7

$$\underset{\underset{\text{Propionyl-CoA}}{}}{\underset{CH_2}{\overset{CH_3}{|}}-\overset{O}{\overset{\|}{C}}-S-CoA} \xrightarrow[\substack{\text{Propionyl-CoA carboxylase}\\\text{(biotin)}}]{\text{HCO}_3^-, \quad P_i \\ \text{ATP} \quad \text{ADP}} \underset{\text{D-Methylmalonyl-CoA}}{{}^-OOC-\underset{\underset{}{|}}{\overset{CH_3}{\overset{|}{CH}}}-\overset{O}{\overset{\|}{C}}-S-CoA}$$

$$\Big\updownarrow \substack{\text{Methylmalonyl-CoA}\\\text{racemase}}$$

$$\underset{\text{Succinyl-CoA}}{{}^-OOC-CH_2-CH_2-\overset{O}{\overset{\|}{C}}-S-CoA} \xleftarrow[\substack{\text{Methylmalonyl-CoA mutase}\\(B_{12})}]{} \underset{\text{L-Methylmalonyl-CoA}}{{}^-OOC-\underset{\underset{CH_3}{|}}{CH}-\overset{O}{\overset{\|}{C}}-S-CoA}$$

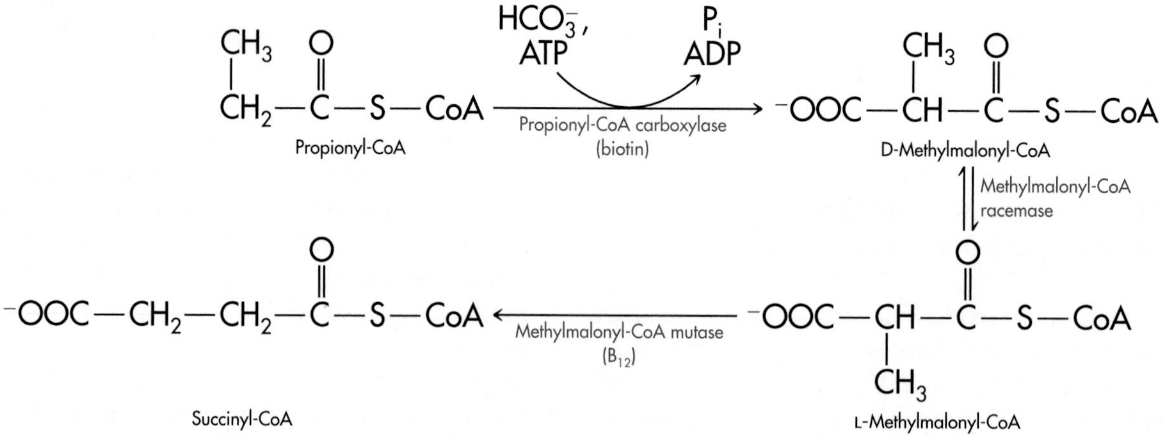

4. **Peroxisomal β-oxidation** uses essentially the same reaction sequence as the mitochondrial system, except for the very first reaction, which is catalyzed by an H₂O₂-producing flavoprotein. The peroxisomal system can handle very long fat-

ty acids (chain lengths of $\geqq$ 20 carbons), which are poor substrates for mitochondrial β-oxidation. Peroxisomal β-oxidation can proceed only to the stage of octanoyl-CoA.

5. **Odd-chain fatty acids** are β-oxidized normally,

FIG. 18.7

Formation of ketone bodies in liver mitochondria.

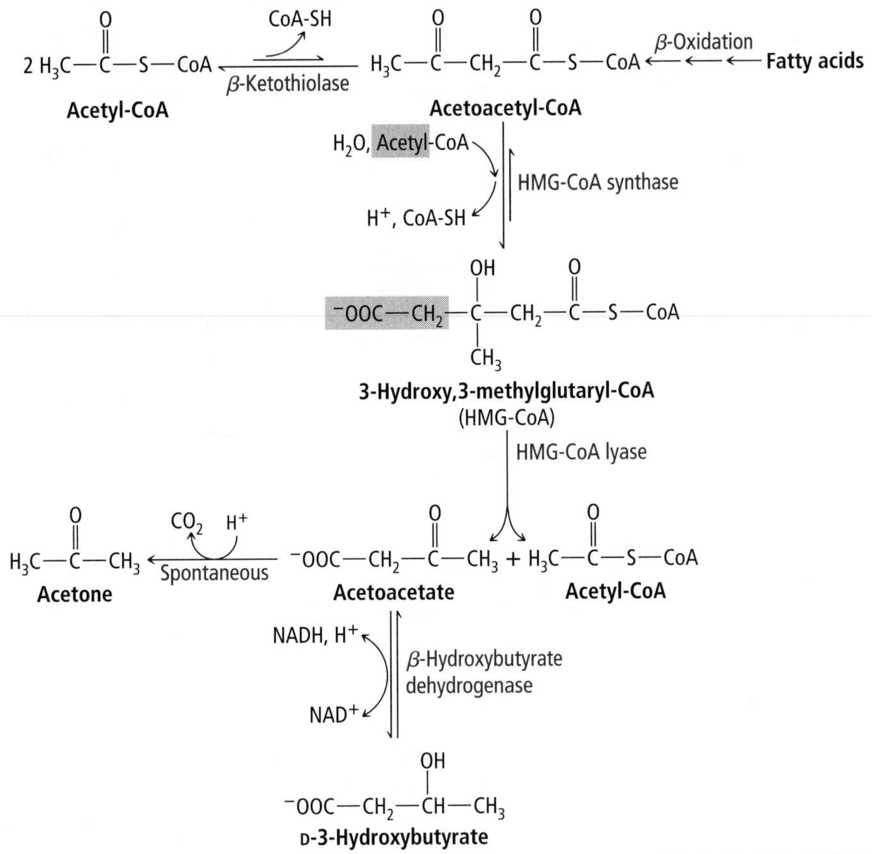

but the last step produces propionyl-CoA rather than acetyl-CoA. *Propionyl-CoA is converted to succinyl-CoA via methylmalonyl-CoA* as shown in Box 18.7. This reaction sequence requires both biotin and deoxyadenosylcobalamin, a coenzyme form of vitamin B_{12} (see Chapter 24). Unlike acetyl-CoA, propionyl-CoA is a substrate of gluconeogenesis.

The liver converts excess fatty acids to ketone bodies

The term **ketone bodies** is applied to the three biosynthetically related products **acetoacetate, β-hydroxybutyrate,** and **acetone.** Acetoacetate and β-hydroxybutyrate *are formed from acetyl-CoA in liver mitochondria.* The liver releases the ketone bodies into the blood for transport to other tissues, where they are used as an important source of metabolic energy. The pathway of **ketogenesis** is shown in Fig. 18.7.

A very small amount of acetone is formed by the nonenzymatic decarboxylation of acetoacetate. It serves no recognized biological function, and most is exhaled through the lungs. In diabetic ketoacidosis, however (see Chapter 29), it appears in significant quantity, and its smell in the patient's breath is a valuable aid in the diagnosis of this life-threatening condition.

The utilization of ketone bodies in the mitochondria of extrahepatic tissues requires the reaction of acetoacetate with succinyl-CoA as shown in Box 18.8. Although any substrate—including glucose—that is degraded to acetyl-CoA in the liver can be converted to ketone bodies, ketogenesis usually is associated with fatty acid oxidation. When dietary carbohydrate is plentiful, the liver channels only a moderate amount of glucose through the glycolytic

BOX 18.8

$$\longrightarrow \quad \longrightarrow \beta\text{-Hydroxybutyrate}$$

From blood

$\longrightarrow \quad \longrightarrow$ Acetoacetate $\quad +$ Succinyl-CoA $\rightleftharpoons$ Acetoacetyl-CoA $+$ Succinate

CoA-SH $\searrow$ | β-ketothiolase (β-oxidation)

2 Acetyl-CoA $\longrightarrow$ TCA cycle

FIG. 18.8

Effects of insulin, glucagon, and epinephrine on lipolysis in adipose tissue and on the utilization of fatty acids and glycerol by the liver. Hormones that stimulate lipolysis in adipose tissue also facilitate β-oxidation of fatty acids and gluconeogenesis in the liver. Of the insulin antagonists, glucagon is more effective in the liver and epinephrine is more effective in adipose tissue. ··⁺►, Stimulation ···►, inhibition.

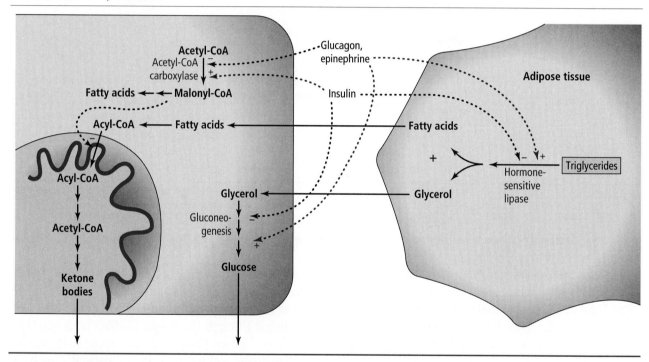

pathway, and most of this is released as lactate, used for fatty acid synthesis, or oxidized in the TCA cycle. During fasting, on the other hand, a large amount of free fatty acids from adipose tissue are β-oxidized to acetyl-CoA. The liver has a very high capacity for fatty acid oxidation, and *mitochondrial fatty acid uptake and β-oxidation are less tightly regulated than glycolysis and the pyruvate dehydrogenase reaction.* The acetyl-CoA formed by β-oxidation is not used for biosyn-

thetic activities during fasting, and its oxidation by the TCA cycle is reduced as well because the liver obtains most of its energy from the respiratory chain oxidation of the NADH and FADH$_2$ formed during β-oxidation (Figs. 18.8 and 18.9).

Besides substrate availability, *enzyme induction is important for ketogenesis.* The synthesis of HMG-CoA synthase—the rate-limiting enzyme of ketogenesis from acetyl-CoA—is stimulated powerfully by fast-

FIG. 18.9

The fates of fatty acids and acetyl-CoA in the liver when the plasma free fatty acid level is low (after a carbohydrate-rich meal) and during fasting. **A,** After a carbohydrate-rich meal. **B,** During fasting.

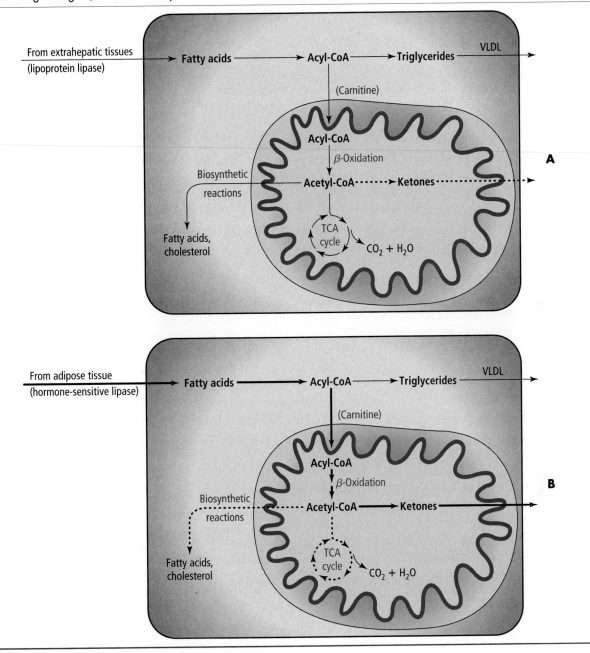

ing, fat feeding, and insulin deficiency. Fatty acids, in particular, are excellent inducers of this enzyme, acting at the level of transcription. The importance of ketogenesis during fasting and in diabetes mellitus will be discussed in Chapter 29.

Defects of β-oxidation cause muscle weakness and fasting hypoglycemia

Some tissues, including nervous tissue and RBCs, do not oxidize fatty acids. Other tissues, however, including muscle and liver, derive most of their energy from fatty acids, at least in the fasting state. It is these tissues that are compromised by defects of β-oxidation.

Carnitine deficiency can result from defects of carnitine biosynthesis, defective transport into the cells, or excessive renal excretion. Carnitine normally is synthesized from protein-bound lysine in the kidney and, to a far lesser extent, in the liver (see Chapter 21, page 443), and it has to be transported to other tissues by the blood.

Carnitine also is depleted in many organic acidurias, including methylmalonic aciduria (see Chapter 21, page 437) and medium-chain acyl-CoA dehydrogenase deficiency (to be discussed shortly), because the accumulating acids form carnitine esters, which are excreted in the urine. Carnitine esters of many organic acids can be formed from the CoA-thioesters of the acids in reactions analogous to the carnitine-palmitoyl transferase reaction. The formation of these water-soluble, excretable carnitine esters is a detoxification mechanism for the disposal of potentially hazardous organic acids.

If the liver is affected, carnitine deficiency leads to *hypoketotic hypoglycemia during periods of extended fasting*. Gluconeogenesis requires energy in the form of ATP and GTP, and fatty acid oxidation is the only important energy source for the fasting liver. Therefore *any defect in the main sequence of β-oxidation prevents gluconeogenesis*. Ketogenesis is impaired as well because the supply of acetyl-CoA from β-oxidation is curtailed. The lack of ketone bodies adds to the effect of the hypoglycemia because the brain depends entirely on a combination of glucose and ketone bodies during periods of fasting.

The muscles also suffer in carnitine deficiency. *Muscle weakness and muscle cramps on exertion* are the most typical complaints. Histologically, many patients show an unusual abundance of fat droplets in muscle tissue and liver, and some develop fatty degeneration of the liver. This is to be expected, because excess acyl-CoA that cannot be transported into the mitochondrion is diverted into triglyceride synthesis.

Carnitine deficiency can be treated with oral carnitine, but the intestinal absorption of carnitine is rather poor. Intestinal bacteria metabolize most of the ingested carnitine to inactive products, including trimethylamine (see Chapter 21, page 432). At high doses of oral carnitine (>200 mg/kg daily),

trimethylamine causes a harmless but embarrassing side effect: a body odor like rotten fish.

Understandably, carnitine supplements are also popular with athletes who try to boost their performance by increasing their β-oxidation.

Deficiencies of enzymes within the β-oxidation sequence are known as well. The most common of these is **medium-chain acyl-CoA dehydrogenase deficiency.** The affected enzyme catalyzes the first reaction in the β-oxidation of medium-chain (C_5 to C_{12}) fatty acids. (Two other acyl-CoA dehydrogenases take care of short-chain and long-chain fatty acids.) This fairly common condition often presents with *fasting hypoglycemia* during the first 2 years of life. Although many cases go undiagnosed, some patients develop severe and even fatal episodes of hypoglycemia, often in the context of an infection, when the child eats little and the brain depends on the liver for its nourishment. Many of those patients traditionally diagnosed with "Reye's syndrome" or "sudden infant death syndrome" have turned out to suffer from medium-chain acyl-CoA dehydrogenase deficiency. At autopsy, patients who have died of this disease show a typical fatty infiltration of the liver.

Most patients with medium-chain acyl-CoA dehydrogenase deficiency do well as long as they avoid excessive fasting. A low-fat diet is recommended, and the carnitine deficiency that is caused by the urinary excretion of carnitine esters should be corrected by oral carnitine supplements.

THE CARBOHYDRATE-TO-FAT PATHWAY

We already have observed (see Chapter 17) that fatty acids cannot be converted into carbohydrates. Carbohydrates, on the other hand, can be converted into triglycerides. This requires the synthesis of both fatty acids and glycerol from glucose. Carbohydrate-to-fat conversion is not very important under most conditions, but it occurs on a high-carbohydrate diet when excess energy from dietary carbohydrate is stored away as triglyceride in adipose tissue.

Fatty acids are synthesized from acetyl-CoA

In humans, endogenous fatty acid synthesis is important only in a few tissues, including the liver and the lactating mammary gland. *Acetyl-CoA is the precur-*

sor of the carbons in the fatty acid, and NADPH is required for the reductive reactions of the pathway. In a first step, acetyl-CoA is carboxylated to malonyl-CoA by **acetyl-CoA carboxylase** as shown in Box 18.9. This is a typical ATP-dependent carboxylation, with enzyme-bound biotin as a carrier of the carboxy group (see Chapter 16). Because its product malonyl-CoA is not used in other metabolic pathways, *this reaction is the committed step of fatty acid biosynthesis.*

The other reactions of fatty acid synthesis are catalyzed by the cytoplasmic **fatty acid synthase** **complex.** This complex is a dimer of two identical polypeptide chains (Fig. 18.10). Two sulfhydryl groups in each of the two polypeptides act as carriers of acyl groups during fatty acid synthesis. One of these belongs to a cysteine side chain, and the other to **phosphopantetheine** (Fig. 18.11), a prosthetic group that is covalently bound to a serine side chain. The phosphopantetheine-containing domain of the polypeptide is known as **acyl carrier protein (ACP).** The growing fatty acid is bound covalently to these sulfhydryl groups during its synthesis.

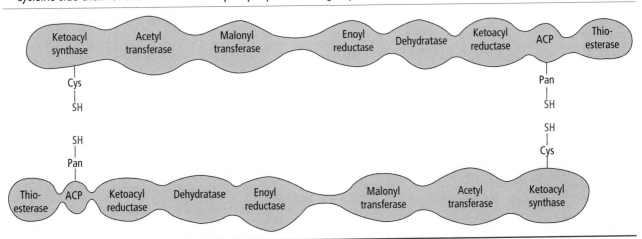

BOX 18.9

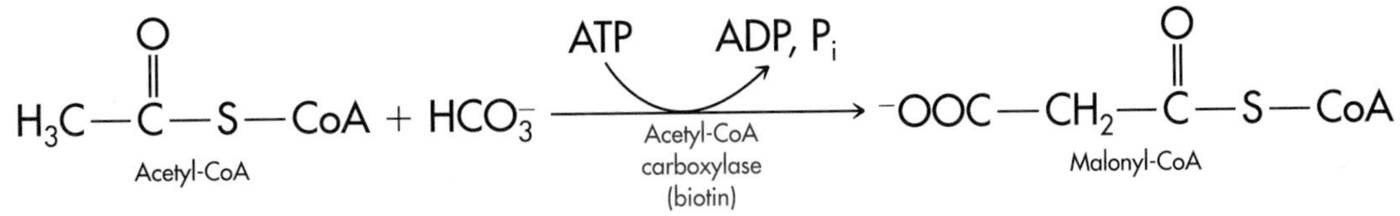

FIG. 18.10

Structure of the mammalian fatty acid synthase complex. During fatty acid synthesis, acyl groups are transferred between the cysteine side chain of one subunit and the phosphopantetheine group of the other subunit.

FIG. 18.11

The phosphopantetheine group in the fatty acid synthase complex. It resembles coenzyme A in its structure and in its ability to form a thioester bond with organic acids.

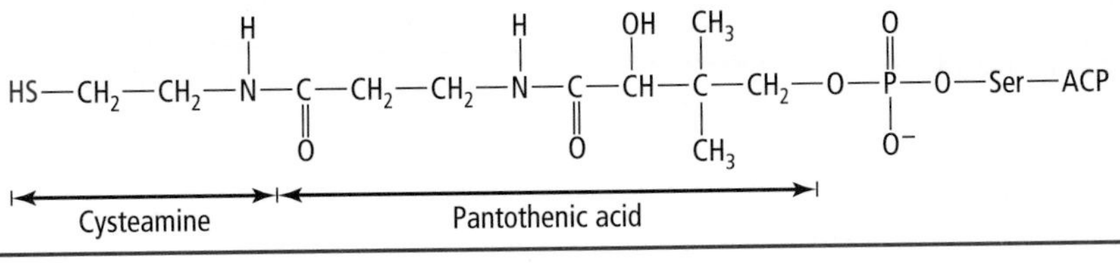

FIG. 18.12

Reactions of the first elongation cycle in fatty acid biosynthesis. The cysteine side chain and the phosphopantetheine group actually belong to two separate polypeptides in the fatty acid synthase complex.

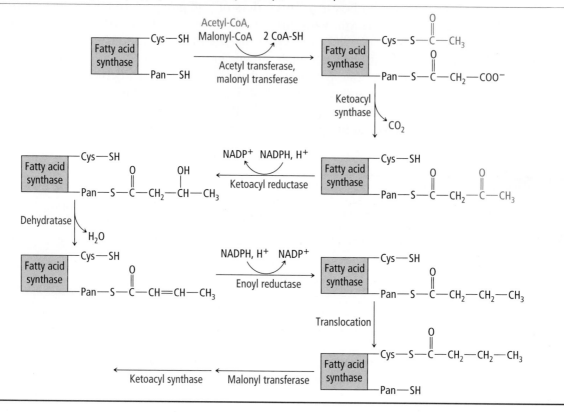

The first elongation cycle of fatty acid synthesis is shown in Fig. 18.12. It includes two reductive reactions in which NADPH is required as the reductant. In the second cycle, a malonyl residue again is transferred to the phosphopantetheine group, then the butyryl residue is transferred to C-2 of the malonyl residue with accompanying decarboxylation, followed by the ketoacyl reductase, dehydratase, and enoyl reductase reactions. This cycle is repeated until a chain length of 16 carbons is reached. At this point the product, palmitic acid, is released hydrolytically. This reaction is catalyzed by the thioesterase domain of the fatty acid synthase.

The stoichiometry for the synthesis of palmitic acid is

$$\text{Acetyl-CoA} + 7 \text{ Malonyl-CoA} + 14 \text{ NADPH} + 14 \text{ H}^+ \longrightarrow \text{Palmitate} + 7 \text{ CO}_2 + 14 \text{ NADP}^+ + 8 \text{ CoA-SH} + 6 \text{ H}_2\text{O}$$

Because malonyl-CoA is formed from acetyl-CoA in the reaction

$$\text{Acetyl-CoA} + \text{CO}_2 + \text{ATP} + \text{H}_2\text{O} \longrightarrow \text{Malonyl-CoA} + \text{ADP} + \text{P}_i + \text{H}^+$$

we can write the overall reaction as

$$8 \text{ Acetyl-CoA} + 7 \text{ ATP} + 14 \text{ NADPH} + 6 \text{ H}^+ + \text{H}_2\text{O} \longrightarrow \text{Palmitate} + 14 \text{ NADP}^+ + 8 \text{ CoA-SH} + 7 \text{ ADP} + 7 \text{ P}_i$$

Now we understand why most naturally occurring fatty acids have an even number of carbons: they are synthesized by the addition of a two-carbon unit during each cycle of fatty acid synthesis.

The acetyl-CoA for fatty acid biosynthesis is derived from mitochondrial citrate

Fatty acid synthesis takes place in the cytoplasm, but acetyl-CoA is produced in the mitochondrion.

FIG. 18.13

Transport of acetyl units from the mitochondrion to the cytoplasm. The inner mitochondrial membrane has carriers for citrate, pyruvate, and malate, but not for acetyl-CoA and oxaloacetate.

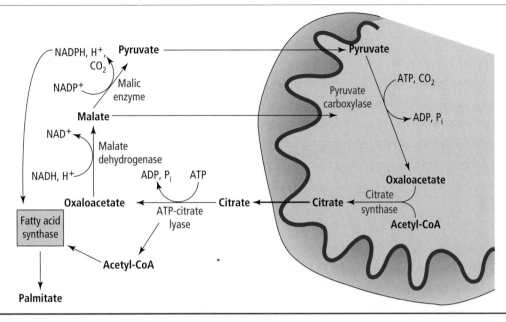

Unlike most other mitochondrial metabolites, *acetyl-CoA cannot cross the inner mitochondrial membrane*. It has to be converted to citrate first, using the citrate synthase reaction of the TCA cycle. Citrate leaves the mitochondrion on the tricarboxylate transporter and is cleaved back to acetyl-CoA and oxaloacetate in a reaction catalyzed by **ATP-citrate lyase** in the cytoplasm. While acetyl-CoA is used for fatty acid synthesis, oxaloacetate is shuttled back into the mitochondrion either as malate or as pyruvate (Fig. 18.13). During the formation of pyruvate, NADPH is produced by **malic enzyme**. This reaction theoretically can supply half of the NADPH required for fatty acid synthesis. The remaining NADPH has to come from the pentose phosphate pathway.

Excess carbohydrate is converted to triglycerides after a meal

Fatty acid synthesis is regulated in part by adaptive control: the levels of acetyl-CoA carboxylase, fatty acid synthase, ATP-citrate lyase, and glucose 6-phosphate dehydrogenase in the liver are increased by carbohydrate feeding and decreased during fasting. A fat-free, carbohydrate-based diet is the most po-

tent inducer of these enzymes. The dietary effects are mediated, in part, by insulin.

The short-term regulation of fatty acid synthesis takes place at the level of acetyl-CoA carboxylase. This enzyme can exist in an inactive monomeric form (MW 400 kDa) and an active polymeric form (MW 6000 to 8000 kDa). The most important allosteric regulators are citrate, which stabilizes the active polymeric form, and palmitoyl-CoA, which dissociates the complex into the inactive monomers. The well-fed liver has a higher citrate level and a lower acyl-CoA level than the fasting liver.

Hormones are important, too: *insulin stimulates, and glucagon and epinephrine inhibit, acetyl-CoA carboxylase.* These hormonal effects depend on two protein kinases that phosphorylate and inactivate acetyl-CoA carboxylase (Fig. 18.14): the cAMP-activated protein kinase A mediates the inhibitory effects of glucagon and β-adrenergic agonists, and the **AMP-activated protein kinase** not only is activated by AMP, it also is inhibited in the presence of insulin. It mediates most of the stimulatory effect of insulin on acetyl-CoA carboxylase. Metabolic emergencies with a decreased cellular energy charge (high AMP) also lead to a rapid switchoff of fatty acid synthesis via this protein kinase.

FIG. 18.14

Regulation of acetyl-CoA carboxylase by allosteric effectors and hormones. ——$^+$→, Stimulation; ——→, inhibition.

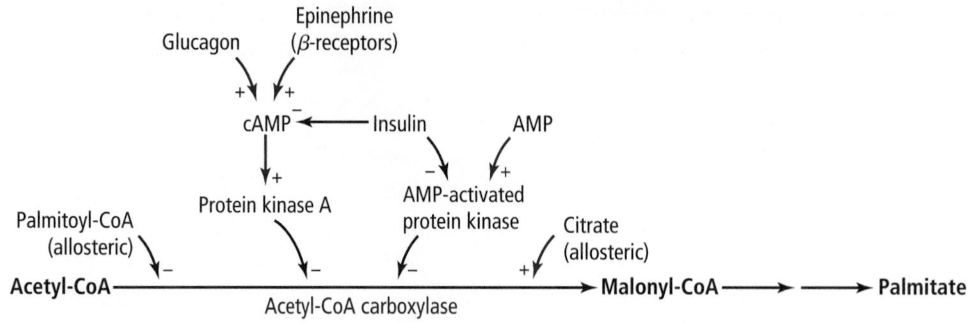

BOX 18.10

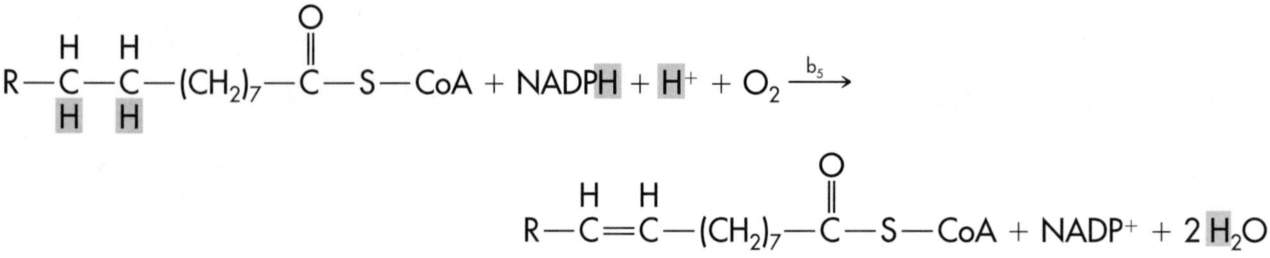

The regulatory mechanisms ensure that *the liver converts excess dietary carbohydrate into fatty acids.* These fatty acids are esterified to triglycerides, and the triglycerides are released as constituents of very-low-density lipoprotein (VLDL). Like the chylomicron triglycerides, VLDL triglycerides are hydrolyzed by lipoprotein lipase in extrahepatic tissues, including adipose tissue. This carbohydrate-to-fat pathway is important only on a high-carbohydrate diet when the regulated enzymes are stimulated by insulin (Fig. 18.15). Thus people, like geese, can be fattened on a carbohydrate-based diet.

Most fatty acids can be synthesized from palmitate by desaturation and chain elongation

The fatty acid synthase complex produces palmitate, a saturated, 16-carbon, fatty acid. The fatty acids in our triglycerides and membrane lipids, however, have chain lengths of up to 24 or 26 carbons, C-18 fatty acids being the most common. Also, only approximately 50% of our fatty acids are saturated; another 40% are monounsaturated, and perhaps 10%

are polyunsaturated. Most of these fatty acids can be synthesized in the human body.

Chain elongation is possible both in the ER (the **microsomes**) and in the mitochondrion. Like the fatty acid synthase complex, *the elongation systems add two carbons at a time.* The mitochondrial system prefers fatty acids with fewer than 16 carbons. Microsomal chain elongation, on the other hand, works best with palmitate. Chain elongation occurs with unsaturated as well as saturated fatty acids.

The **desaturation** of fatty acids is effected by membrane-bound desaturase systems in the ER of the liver and other organs. *The desaturases are monooxygenases:* molecular oxygen is the oxidant, and a reduced coenzyme, either NADH or NADPH, is oxidized together with the substrate. Cytochrome b_5 participates in the reaction by channeling electrons from NAD(P)H to oxygen as shown in Box 18.10. The first double bond is introduced in position Δ^9 of palmitic or stearic acid, producing palmitoleic acid or oleic acid, respectively. Oleic acid is the most abundant unsaturated fatty acid in our lipids. Additional double bonds can be introduced between the first double bond and the carboxy group, but not

FIG. 18.15

The carbohydrate-to-fat pathway that operates after a carbohydrate-rich meal. Unlike some animal species, humans synthesize fatty acids mostly in the liver, rather than in adipose tissue. Many reactions on this pathway are stimulated by insulin, including hepatic glucokinase and phosphofructokinase (①), acetyl-CoA carboxylase and fatty acid synthase (②), lipoprotein lipase in adipose tissue (③), glucose uptake into adipose tissue (④), and phosphofructokinase in adipose tissue (⑤).

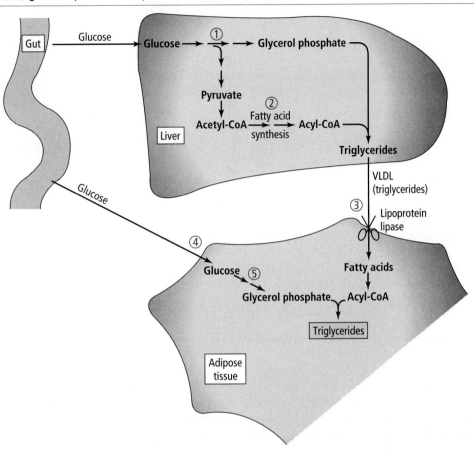

beyond Δ^9. Therefore many polyunsaturated fatty acids can be synthesized from dietary palmitic or stearic acid by a combination of desaturation and chain elongation. These belong to the ω^7 and ω^9 classes.

Some polyunsaturated fatty acids are nutritionally essential

Linoleic acid (18:2;9,12) and α-linolenic acid (18:3;9, 12,15), the parent compounds of the ω^6 and ω^3 classes of polyunsaturated fatty acids, respectively, cannot be synthesized in the human body and therefore are nutritionally essential. **Essential fatty acid deficiency** is characterized by *dermatitis and poor wound healing*. It has been observed in patients kept on total parenteral nutrition for long time pe-

riods, in patients suffering from severe fat malabsorption, and in infants fed on low-fat milk formulas. The symptoms are cured readily by dietary linoleic acid. A diet that supplies as little as 1% of the calories in the form of essential fatty acids is considered adequate. The requirement for linolenic acid is not well established, and attempts to induce a deficiency syndrome by selective omission of linolenic acid from the diet have been unsuccessful not only in humans but also in many animal species.

Polyunsaturated fatty acids can be oxidized nonenzymatically

In the presence of oxygen, polyunsaturated fatty acids are susceptible to a nonenzymatic process known as **autooxidation** or **peroxidation.** It oc-

FIG. 18.16

Autooxidation ("peroxidation") of polyunsaturated fatty acids.

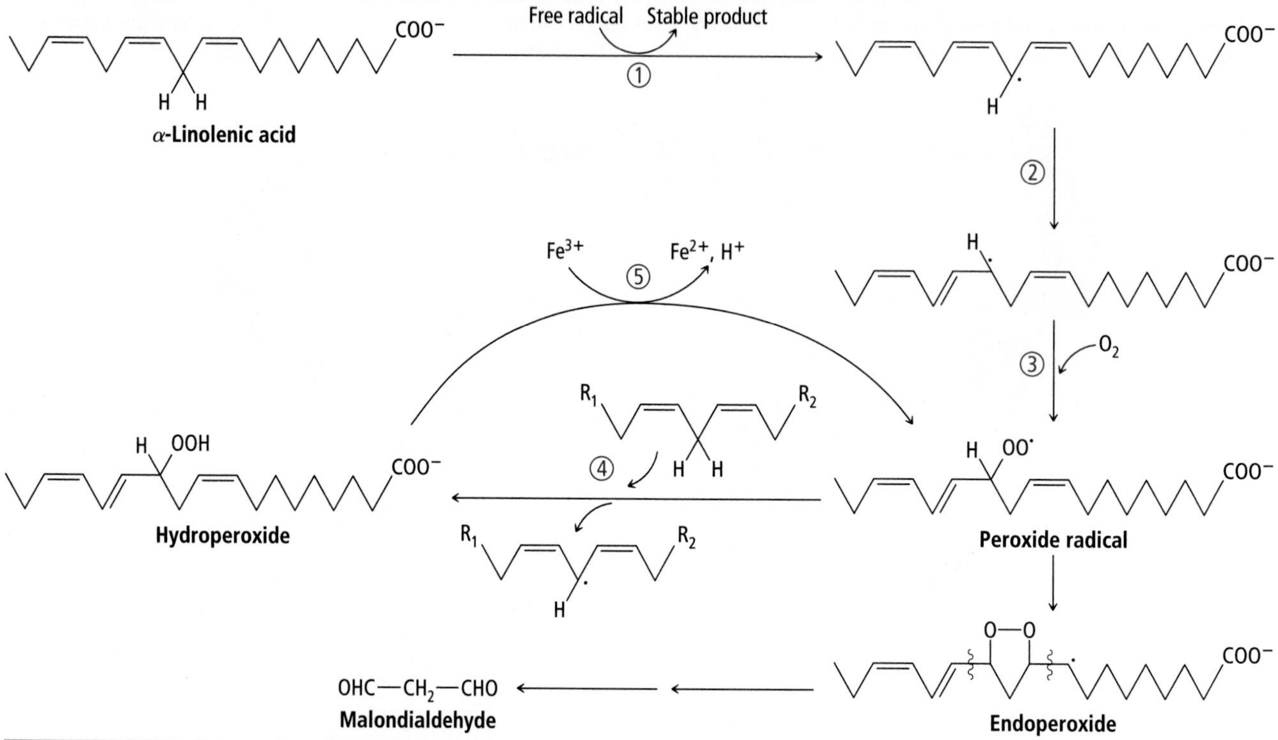

curs both outside the body, where it is responsible for rancidity, and in vivo. The basis for this susceptibility is the relative ease with which a hydrogen atom can be abstracted from the methylene group between two double bonds of a polyunsaturated fatty acid. This oxidative reaction (reaction ① in Fig. 18.16) is initiated by a free radical that may be derived from another polyunsaturated fatty acid (reaction ④ in Fig. 18.16) or from partially reduced oxygen generated during oxidative metabolism (see Chapter 16).

In the latter case, the initiator may be a superoxide radical:

$$\text{[H] from fatty acid}$$

$$O_2^{\cdot-} \xrightarrow[\text{Reaction ① (Fig. 18.16)}]{} O_2H^- \xrightarrow{H^+} H_2O_2$$

Or it may be a peroxide radical generated from hydrogen peroxide with the aid of a metal ion which is shown in Box 18.11. Similarly, hydroperoxide de-

rivatives of polyunsaturated fatty acids can be converted back into reactive peroxide radicals by the mechanism shown in Box 18.11 for hydrogen peroxide (reaction ⑤ in Fig. 18.16). This implies the possibility of *a branching chain reaction leading to an avalanche of free radicals.* The fatty acid itself finally may be degraded to smaller products. If at least three double bonds—always three carbons apart— are present in the fatty acid, **malondialdehyde** is a prominent product. Malondialdehyde is chemically reactive. It cross-links proteins and other molecules, resulting in membrane damage and the accumulation of **lipofuscin**, a poorly degradable polymeric product that contains partially decomposed polyunsaturated fatty acids and cross-linked, denatured proteins. It accumulates as "age pigment" in the lysosomes of older people. Lipofuscin accumulation is probably harmless, but there is also a potential for mutagenesis, either by malondialdehyde or by stray radicals formed during lipid peroxidation.

Experimentally, lipid peroxidation can be induced

$$H_2O_2 + Fe^{3+} \longrightarrow HOO\cdot + Fe^{2+} + H^+$$

$$HOO\cdot \xrightarrow[\text{Reaction } \textcircled{1} \text{ (Fig. 18.16)}]{\substack{[H] \text{ from} \\ \text{fatty acid}}} H_2O_2$$

by various enzymes, especially metalloenzymes such as xanthine oxidase or superoxide dismutase, but the mechanisms of lipid peroxidation in the living cell are not well understood.

Both enzymatic and nonenzymatic mechanisms limit the extent of lipid peroxidation: the enzymes **catalase, superoxide dismutase,** and **glutathione peroxidase** (see Chapters 16 and 17) destroy dangerous products of oxidative metabolism. Some vitamins and metabolites, including **vitamin E** and the **retinoids** (see Chapter 24), **uric acid** (see Chapter 23), and **ascorbate** (see Chapter 24) are protective because they react with free radicals or other oxidants, forming harmless, non−free radical products.

Lipid peroxidation has been implicated in ailments as diverse as cancer, atherosclerosis, and cell damage during inflammatory processes and aging, but its importance in these conditions is still controversial.

on the other hand, is stimulated by norepinephrine and epinephrine and is inhibited by insulin. These agents regulate the hormone-sensitive adipose tissue lipase, which catalyzes the first and rate-limiting step of triglyceride hydrolysis. Adipose-tissue-derived fatty acids are the most important energy source for the body during fasting.

Fatty acids are oxidized by the pathway of β-oxidation, which is active in the mitochondria of most cells. β-Oxidation produces acetyl-CoA, and this acetyl-CoA is oxidized in the TCA cycle. The fasting liver, however, converts adipose-tissue−derived fatty acids into ketone bodies. The ketone bodies are released into the blood and oxidized in extrahepatic tissues.

Fatty acids can be synthesized from acetyl-CoA. This pathway is most active in the liver, where it is used to convert excess dietary carbohydrate into fatty acids and triglycerides. These triglycerides are transported to other tissues as constituents of very-low-density lipoprotein.

SUMMARY

Dietary triglycerides are hydrolyzed to free fatty acids and 2-monoacylglycerol by the pancreatic lipase. After their absorption, these products are used for the resynthesis of triglycerides in the intestinal mucosa, and these triglycerides are transported to other tissues as constituents of chylomicrons. The chylomicron triglycerides are hydrolyzed by the endothelial enzyme lipoprotein lipase, and the breakdown products are utilized by the tissue.

Adipose tissue receives a large part of the dietary triglycerides. Under the stimulatory influence of insulin, the adipose cells use the fatty acids generated by lipoprotein lipase for the synthesis of storage triglycerides. The hydrolysis of stored triglycerides,

Further Reading

Bensadoun A: Lipoprotein lipase. *Annu Rev Nutr* 11, 217-237, 1991.

Bieber LL: Carnitine. *Annu Rev Biochem* 57, 261-283, 1988.

Rice-Evans C, Burdon R: Free radical-lipid interactions and their pathological consequences. *Prog Lipid Res* 32 (1), 71-110, 1993.

Roe CR, Coates PM: Acyl-CoA dehydrogenase deficiencies. In: Scriver CR, Beaudet AL, Sly WS, Valle D, editors: *The metabolic basis of inherited disease*, 6th ed., vol. 1. McGraw-Hill, New York, 1989, pp. 889-914.

Saloranta C, Groop L: Interactions between glucose and FFA metabolism in man. *Diabetes Metab Rev* 12 (1), 15-36, 1996.

QUESTIONS

1. Like many other tissues, the myocardium can use the triglycerides in chylomicrons for its own energy needs. The utilization of chylomicron triglycerides requires the enzyme
   A. Acetyl-CoA carboxylase
   B. Glucose 6-phosphate dehydrogenase
   C. Phospholipase A$_2$
   D. Lipoprotein lipase
   E. Hormone-sensitive lipase

2. The excessive formation of ketone bodies occurs in many disease states. The most important regulated step determining the rate of ketogenesis is catalyzed by
   A. Acyl-CoA dehydrogenase
   B. Pyruvate kinase
   C. Hormone-sensitive adipose tissue lipase
   D. Acetyl-CoA carboxylase
   E. Glucose 6-phosphate dehydrogenase

3. The ackee fruit, which grows in Jamaica, contains a toxin that inhibits the acyl-CoA dehydrogenase of β-oxidation. This toxin is dangerous because it can cause
   A. Impaired β-oxidation in the brain
   B. Fasting hypoglycemia
   C. Ketoacidosis
   D. Inhibition of lipolysis in adipose tissue
   E. Impaired formation of triglycerides in the liver

4. A pharmaceutical company wants to develop an anti-obesity drug that acts directly on adipose tissue metabolism. The most promising drug type would be agents that
   A. Stimulate β-adrenergic receptors
   B. Inhibit adenylate cyclase
   C. Stimulate glucose uptake into adipose cells
   D. Inhibit the hormone-sensitive adipose tissue lipase
   E. Stimulate insulin receptors in adipose tissue

Chapter 19

The Metabolism of Membrane Lipids

Whereas the triglycerides are used for the storage of metabolic energy, the membrane lipids are essential components of all biological membranes. There are three chemical classes of membrane lipids: the **phosphoglycerides**, the **sphingolipids**, and the **steroids**. Most cells are able to synthesize these lipids themselves, but a considerable interorgan exchange of membrane lipids also takes place in the form of plasma lipoproteins. This chapter is concerned with the major reactions for the biosynthesis and degradation of the three classes of membrane lipids.

THE METABOLISM OF PHOSPHOGLYCERIDES AND SPHINGOLIPIDS

Both phosphoglycerides and sphingolipids can be synthesized de novo ("from scratch") in all cells except erythrocytes. Although phospholipids are transported in the blood, most of the phosphoglycerides and sphingolipids are synthesized in the cells where they are needed. In the following sections we will introduce the most important reactions for the synthesis and degradation of these membrane lipids.

Phosphatidic acid is an intermediate in phosphoglyceride synthesis

The enzymes of phosphoglyceride synthesis either are cytoplasmic or are associated with the membrane of the ER. **Phosphatidic acid**, synthesized from glycerol phosphate, is a key intermediate as

shown in Box 19.1. This is the same reaction sequence that is used for the synthesis of triglycerides in tissues other than the intestine (see Chapter 18).

There are two pathways for the de novo synthesis of phosphoglycerides: in the **phosphatidic acid pathway**, phosphatidate is activated in the form of CDP-diacylglycerol; in the **salvage pathway** the alcohol that becomes bound to phosphatidate is activated. The two pathways are shown in Figs. 19.1 and 19.2 for the synthesis of phosphatidylinositol and phosphatidylcholine, respectively. In both cases, *CTP is used to activate one of the substrates*. These reactions are similar to the activation of glucose for glycogen synthesis (see Chapter 17). In the subsequent reaction, however, a phosphoanhydride bond in the CDP derivative is cleaved and one of the phosphate groups is incorporated in the product.

The phosphatidic acid pathway is used for the synthesis of phosphatidylinositol and cardiolipin, and the salvage pathway is the major source of phosphatidylethanolamine and phosphatidylcholine.

Phosphoglycerides are remodeled extensively after their initial synthesis

Phosphoglycerides are degraded by **phospholipases**. These enzymes, which are present in essentially all tissues, are classified according to their cleavage specificity as shown in Box 19.2. Phospholipases are used not only for the final degradation but also for the remodeling of phosphoglycerides. The fatty acids in positions 1 and 2, for example, can be exchanged by hydrolysis and re-acylation as shown

BOX 19.1

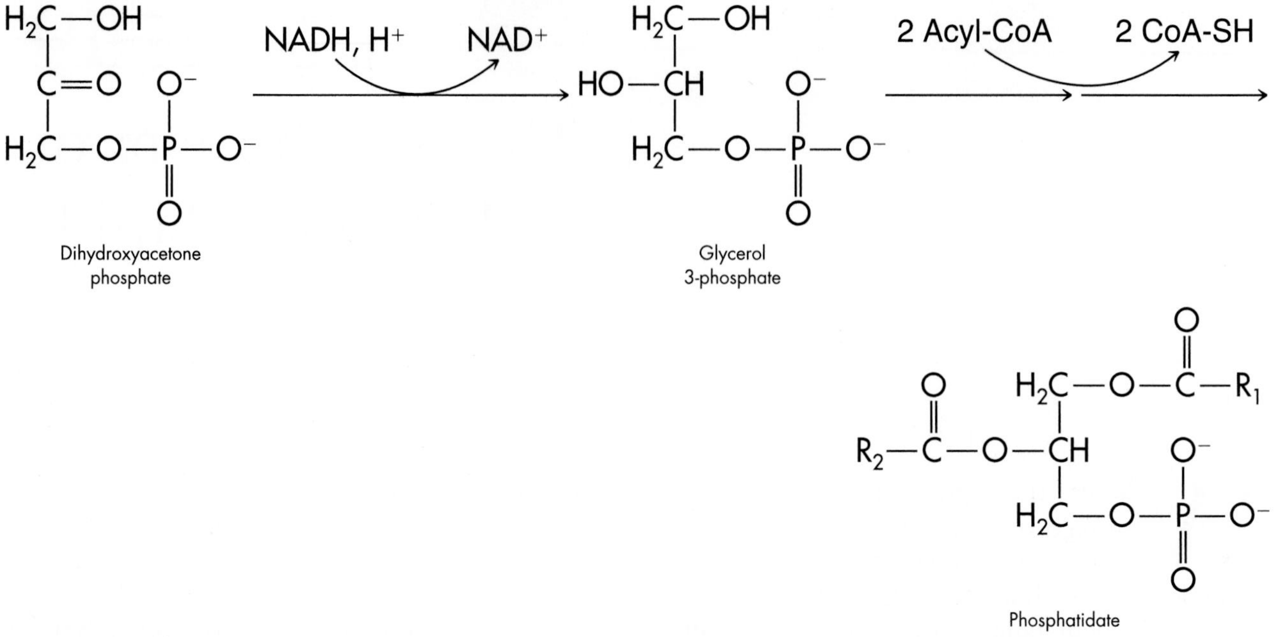

Dihydroxyacetone phosphate

Glycerol 3-phosphate

Phosphatidate

FIG. 19.1

Synthesis of phosphatidylinositol by the phosphatidic acid pathway.

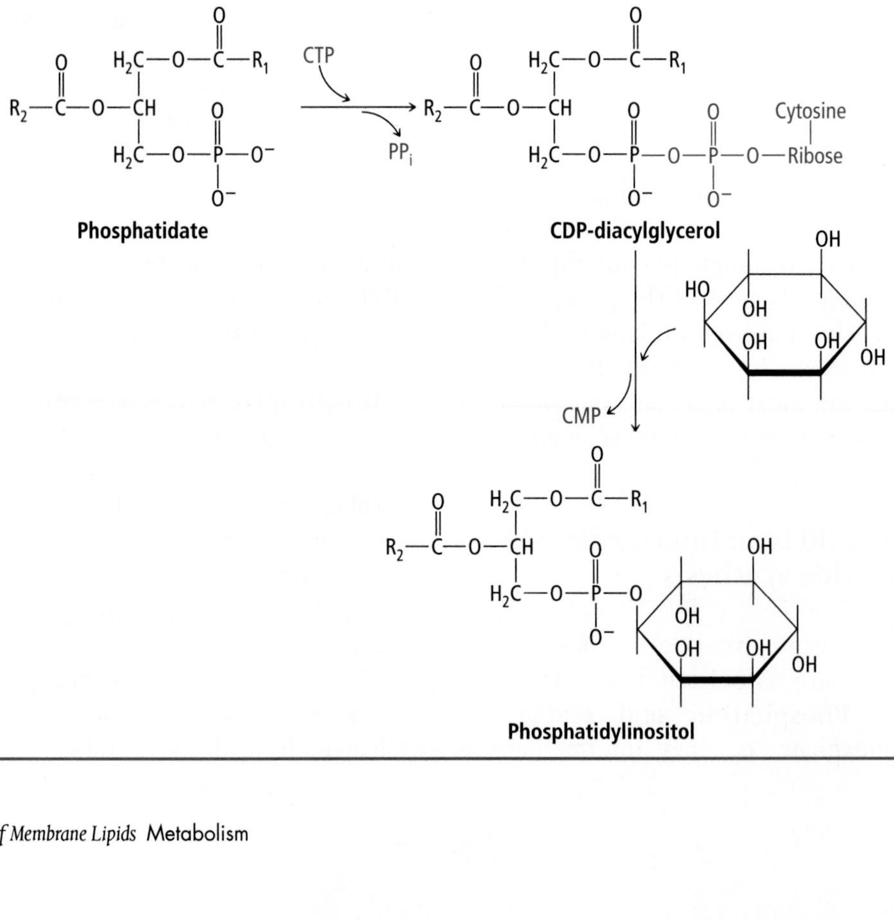

Phosphatidate

CDP-diacylglycerol

Phosphatidylinositol

FIG. 19.2

Synthesis of phosphatidylcholine by the salvage pathway.

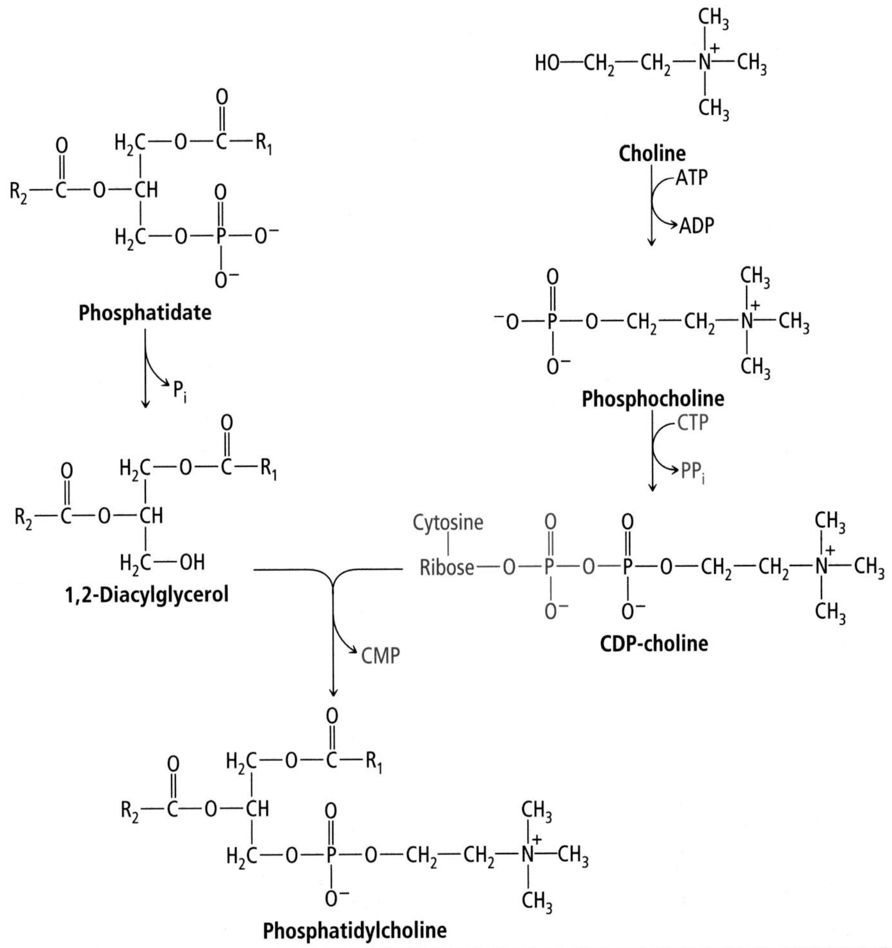

Phosphatidate

Choline

Phosphocholine

1,2-Diacylglycerol

CDP-choline

Phosphatidylcholine

BOX 19.2

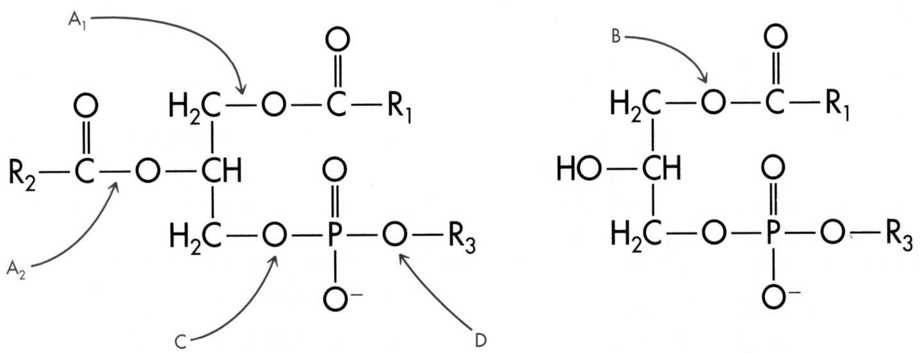

BOX 19.3

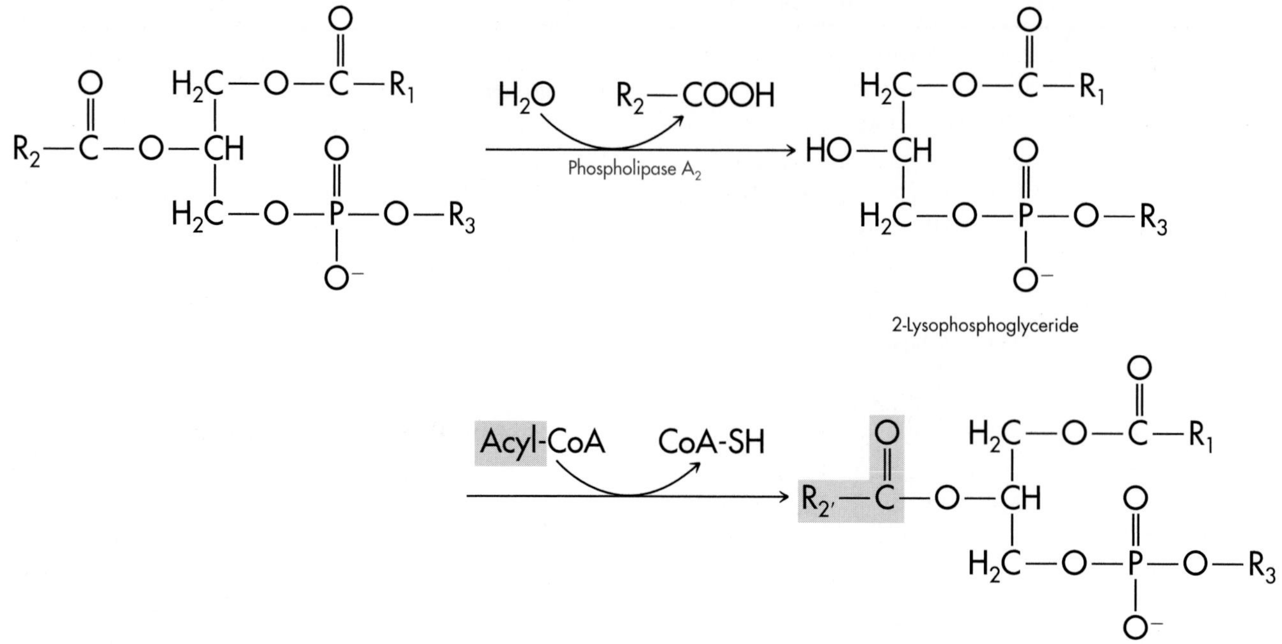

2-Lysophosphoglyceride

BOX 19.4

Phosphatidate—O—CH$_2$—CH—NH$_3^+$ with COO$^-$ branch
Phosphatidylserine

→ (Liver mitochondria, releasing CO$_2$) →

Phosphatidate—O—CH$_2$—CH$_2$—NH$_3^+$
Phosphatidylethanolamine

3 SAM → 3 SAH (Liver microsomes)

Phosphatidate—O—CH$_2$—CH$_2$—N$^+$ with three CH$_3$ groups
Phosphatidylcholine

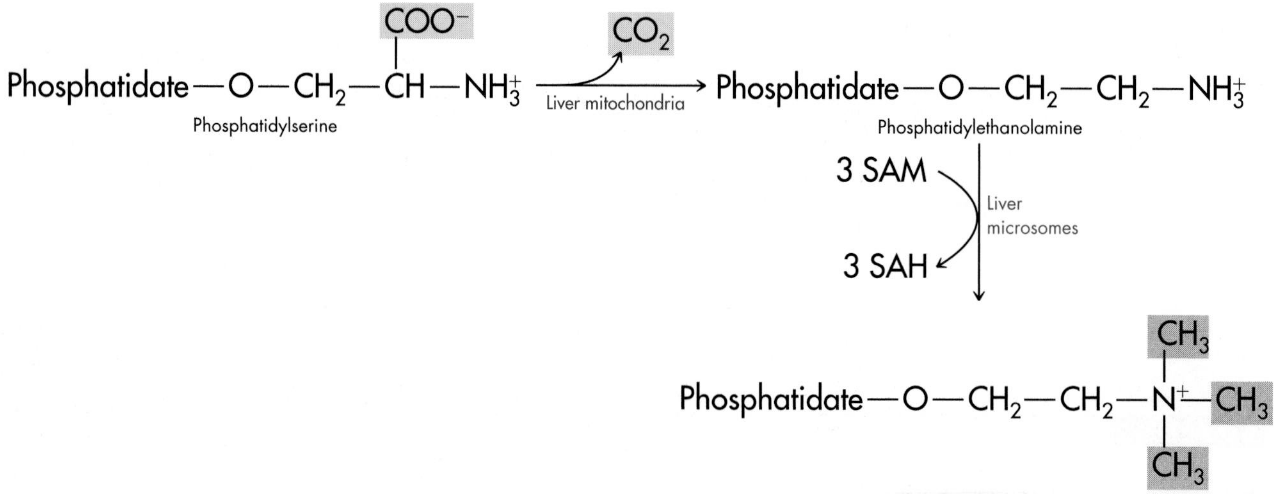

in Box 19.3. The acyltransferase catalyzing the last step in this sequence is specific for both the lysophosphoglyceride and the fatty acid. The specificities of these enzymes are largely responsible for the presence of specific fatty acids in positions 1 and 2 of the phosphoglycerides: C-1 usually is occupied by a saturated fatty acid, and the fatty acid in position 2 usually is unsaturated.

The alcoholic substituent of phosphatidic acid also is exchangeable. Thus, phosphatidylserine is synthesized mostly by base exchange with ethanolamine in human tissues:

Phosphatidylethanolamine + Serine $\rightleftharpoons$
Phosphatidylserine + Ethanolamine

Phosphatidylethanolamine can be made by the decarboxylation of phosphatidylserine, and phosphatidylcholine can be made by the methylation of phosphatidylethanolamine as shown in Box 19.4. **Plasmalogens,** which constitute up to 10% of the phosphoglycerides in muscle and brain, are synthesized from dihydroxyacetone phosphate (Fig. 19.3). Most plasmalogens contain ethanolamine, although choline, serine, or inositol is sometimes present instead.

Platelet activating factor (**PAF;** see Fig. 19.3) is formed by white blood cells and acts as a mediator of hypersensitivity reactions and acute inflammatory responses. In concentrations as low as 10^{-11} to 10^{-10} M it induces platelet adhesion, vasodilation, and chemotaxis of polymorphonuclear leukocytes. The presence of an acetyl group, instead of a long-chain acyl group, in position 2 makes PAF more water soluble than other phosphoglycerides, enabling it to diffuse through an aqueous medium.

Sphingolipids are synthesized from ceramide

Ceramide, consisting of sphingosine and a long-chain fatty acid, is the core structure of the sphingolipids:

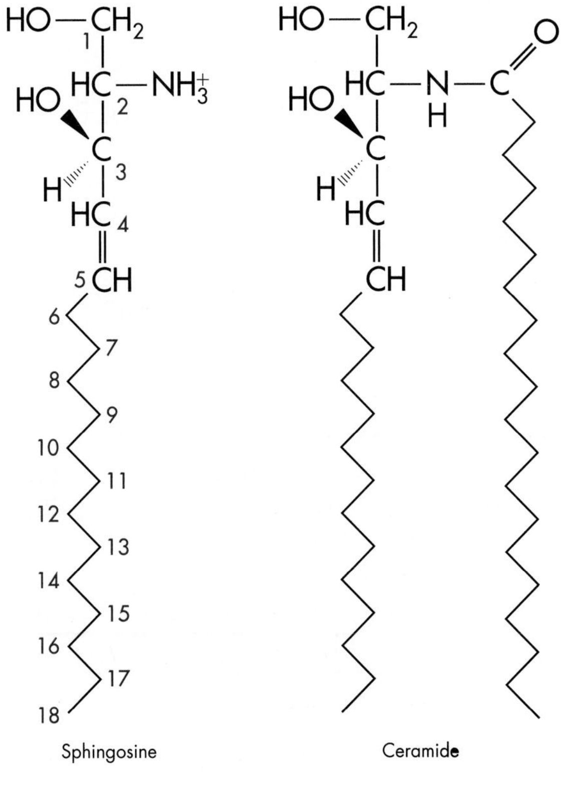

Sphingosine   Ceramide

The primary hydroxy group at C-1 of sphingosine is substituted by phosphocholine in sphingomyelin and by a mono- and or oligosaccharide in the glycosphingolipids (for structures, see Chapter 11). Sphingosine is synthesized in the ER of most cells from palmitoyl-CoA and serine, and the fatty acid is introduced from its CoA-thioester.

During the synthesis of the sphingolipids in the ER and Golgi, *the hydroxy group at C-1 of sphingosine is not activated, but its substituent is introduced from an activated precursor.* The most important source of phosphocholine for the synthesis of sphingomyelin is phosphatidylcholine:

Ceramide + Phosphatidylcholine $\longrightarrow$ Sphingomyelin + 1,2-Diacylglycerol

During the synthesis of the glycosphingolipids, the monosaccharide residues are introduced from their activated precursors (see Table 8.7, Chapter 8). The oligosaccharide chains of the complex glycosphingolipids (globosides and gangliosides) are constructed by the stepwise addition of monosaccharides as shown in Box 19.5.

The ABO blood group substances are oligosaccharides in glycosphingolipids

Blood group substances are components of the erythrocyte membrane that differ in different individuals because of genetic polymorphisms. Some two dozen blood group systems have been described. Of these, the ABO system is most important for blood transfusions. The blood group substances of this system have been isolated from erythrocyte membranes and identified as glycosphingolipids. Their antigenic specificities are caused by variations in the terminal sugar of the oligosaccharide as shown in Box 19.6. The GalNAc transferase and the Gal transferase are encoded by two allelic variants of the same gene, which are known as the A allele and the B allele, respectively. A third allele of this gene, the O allele, encodes an inactive form of the enzyme. Approximately 40% to 45% of Caucasians have two copies of the O allele. These persons have only the H substance and are classified as blood group O. Another 40% to 45% have the A allele, either in two copies or in one copy together with the O allele. They have blood group A. Another 10%

FIG. 19.3

Synthesis of plasmalogens and platelet activating factor *(PAF)*.

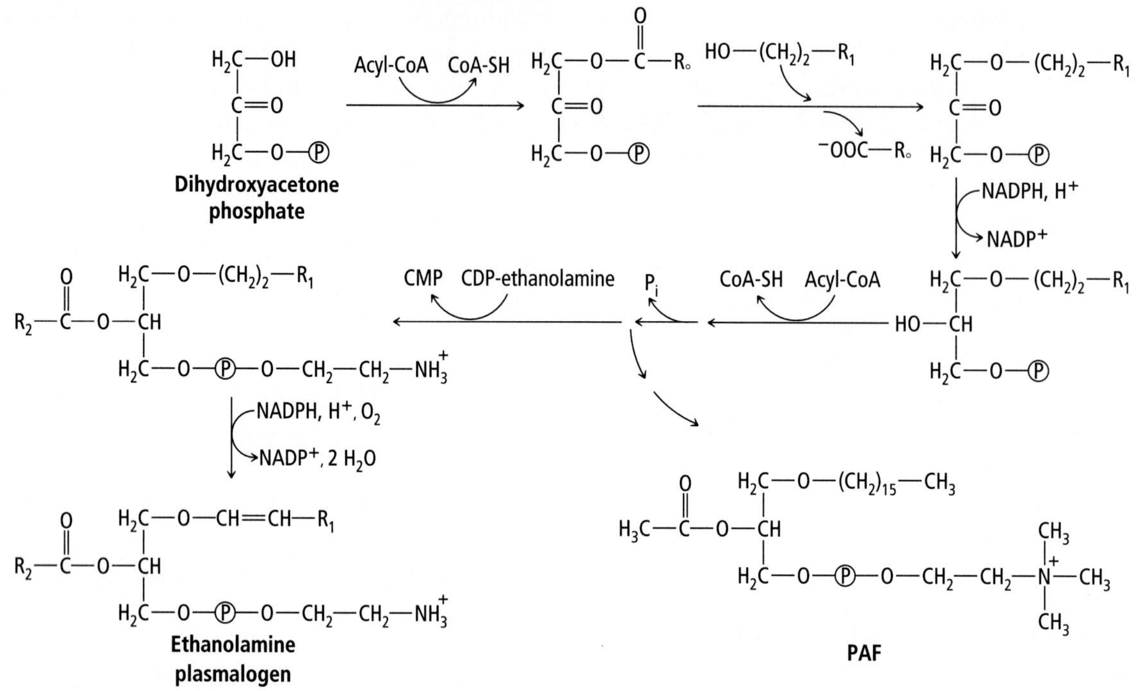

Ethanolamine plasmalogen

PAF

BOX 19.5

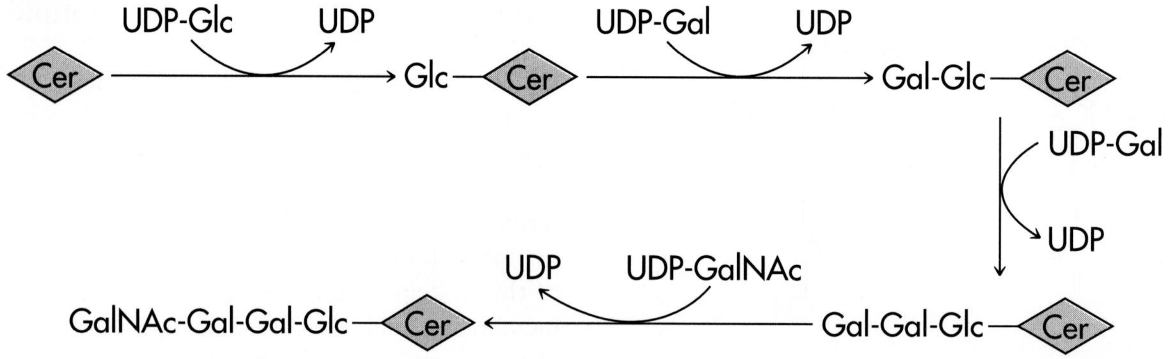

have the B allele, either in two copies or in one copy together with the O allele. They have blood group B. The remaining 5% have one copy of the A allele and one copy of the B allele. They have blood group AB.

The blood group substances of some other blood group systems, including the Lewis system, are oligosaccharides. In other cases, however, blood group substances arise from variations in the amino acid sequence of a membrane glycoprotein. The antigens of the MN blood group system, for example, are variants of the membrane protein glycophorin A (see Fig. 11.11, Chapter 11) that differ in the amino acid residues at positions 1 and 5.

Deficiencies of sphingolipid-degrading enzymes cause lipid storage diseases

Sphingolipids are degraded by lysosomal enzymes. In the case of the complex glycosphingolipids, these de-

BOX 19.6

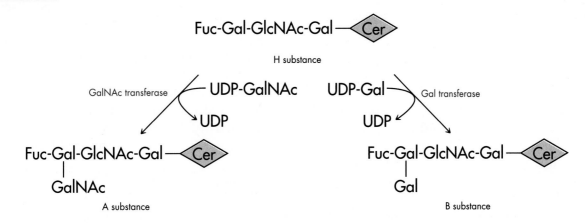

Fuc-Gal-GlcNAc-Gal — Cer

H substance

GalNAc transferase

UDP-GalNAc

UDP-Gal

Gal transferase

UDP

UDP

Fuc-Gal-GlcNAc-Gal — Cer
|
GalNAc

A substance

Fuc-Gal-GlcNAc-Gal — Cer
|
Gal

B substance

FIG. 19.4

Lysosomal degradation of sphingolipids. The numbered reactions refer to the storage diseases in Table 19.1. *There are two different β-galactosidases, one for ganglioside G_{m1} and the other for galactocerebroside. Lactosyl ceramide is degraded by both.

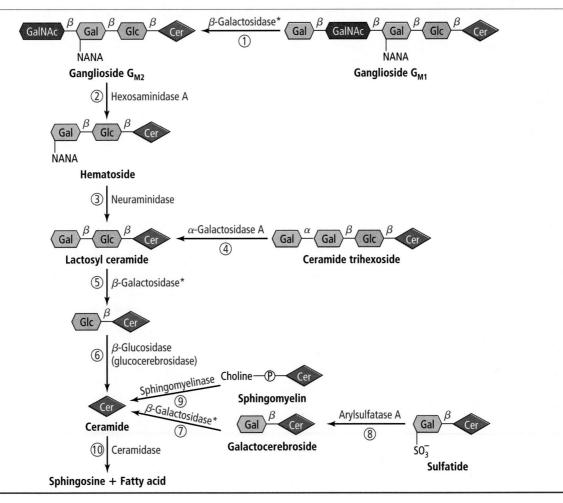

grading enzymes are exoglycosidases, which remove terminal sugars from the oligosaccharide. These exoglycosidases have narrow substrate specificities for the monosaccharide they remove and the type of bond they cleave. Figure 19.4 shows the degradation of some of the more important sphingolipids.

A deficiency of any of these enzymes leads to an accumulation of its substrate in the lysosomes. The resulting disease is called a **lipid storage disease** or **sphingolipidosis.** *The enzyme deficiency is expressed in all tissues.* If it is complete, the disease is severe, with the progressive accumulation of the insoluble, nondegradable, and nonexcretable lipid. The nervous system is seriously affected in essentially all cases because of its high sphingolipid content and turnover. Hepatosplenomegaly is also common because phagocytic cells in the spleen and liver remove erythrocytes from the circulation, and nondegradable lipid from the RBC membrane accumulates in these tissues.

The diagnosis of lipid storage diseases is performed in specialized laboratories by the determination of the enzyme activities in cultured leukocytes, cultured skin fibroblasts, or, for prenatal diagnosis, cultured amniotic cells. The inheritance is autosomal recessive, except for Fabry's disease, which is X-linked recessive. In the more severe diseases, affected homozygotes have near-zero enzyme activity. Heterozygotes can be identified because their enzyme activity is approximately one half of normal. Milder variants of lipid storage diseases also occur in which affected homozygotes have greatly decreased, but not completely absent, enzyme activity. The severity and prognosis of the disease depend largely on this residual enzyme activity.

Tay-Sachs disease is caused by a complete deficiency of hexosaminidase A (reaction ② in Fig. 19.4), leading to an accumulation of ganglioside G_{M2}. Although affected children appear normal at birth, they develop signs of mental and neurological deterioration within the first year of life. This is accompanied by hepatomegaly. The disease is relentlessly progressive, causing death before age 3. The old name "amaurotic idiocy" refers to the apparent blindness of the patients (Gr. ἀμαυρός, obscure). Ophthalmoscopy shows a cherry-red spot in the fovea centralis. This actually represents its normal color, which is accentuated by the gray appearance of the surrounding lipid-laden ganglion cells. It is

TABLE 19.1

Examples of lipid storage diseases

Disease	Enzyme deficiency*	Incidence	Clinical course
Generalized gangliosidosis	1	Unknown	Mental retardation, hepatomegaly, skeletal abnormalities
Tay-Sachs	2	1 in 3600 (Ashkenazi Jews)	Mental retardation, blindness, hepatosplenomegaly, death in infancy
Gaucher's	6	Infantile: rare; adult: 1 in 600 (Ashkenazi Jews)	Infantile form similar to Tay-Sachs; adult-onset form without mental retardation
Fabry's	4	1 in 40,000	Skin rash, renal failure
Krabbe's (globoid leukodystrophy)	7	1 in 50,000 (Sweden); lower elsewhere	Mental retardation, myelin nearly absent
Metachromatic leukodystrophy	8	1 in 100,000	Demyelination, mental deterioration; different degrees of severity
Niemann-Pick	9	Rare	Hepatosplenomegaly, mental retardation, early death
Farber's	10	Rare	Hoarse voice, mental retardation, dermatitis, skeletal abnormalities, early death

* The numbers refer to the numbered reactions of Fig. 19.4.

not diagnostic for Tay-Sachs disease, however, because it is seen in some other lipid storage diseases as well. Tay-Sachs disease is very rare in most populations, but in Ashkenazi Jews it occurs with a frequency of approximately 1 in 3600 births.

Table 19.1 shows some examples of lipid storage diseases. Of these diseases, the adult-onset form of Gaucher's disease is the most common in the United States. Like Tay-Sachs disease, it is most prevalent in Ashkenazi Jews. In this disease, in which patients typically possess a residual enzyme activity between 10% and 20% of normal, mental retardation is absent and the patients present in midlife with splenomegaly, thrombocytopenia, abdominal discomfort, and bone erosion.

CHOLESTEROL METABOLISM

Cholesterol is the only important membrane steroid in animals and humans. The human body contains approximately 140 g of cholesterol, the majority of which is "free" (unesterified) cholesterol in the cellular membranes. It is most abundant in those tissues that also contain large amounts of other membrane lipids, namely, the nervous system.

Cholesterol esters, in which the hydroxy group of cholesterol is esterified with a long-chain fatty acid, are used as an *intracellular storage form of cholesterol.* They are abundant in some steroid hormone–producing tissues, particularly the adrenal cortex, where they form conspicuous lipid droplets throughout the cytoplasm. They are also prominent in the plasma lipoproteins, where approximately 70% of the cholesterol is esterified.

Cholesterol is the least-soluble membrane lipid

Cholesterol contains a condensed four-ring system, known as the **cyclopentanoperhydrophenanthren,** or the **steroid** ring system. This ring system is decorated with a hydroxy group, two methyl groups, and a branched hydrocarbon chain. The molecule contains eight asymmetric carbons, but only 1 of the 256 possible stereoisomers occurs in nature. Substituents of the steroid nucleus can be in α or β configuration. Those in β configuration, indicated by bold lines, face upward from the plane of the steroid ring; those in α configuration, indicated

by broken lines, point behind the plane of the ring. The angular methyl groups (C-18 and C-19), as well as the hydroxy group at carbon 3, are in β configuration as shown in Box 19.7.

Cholesterol has a very low water solubility: approximately 0.2 mg will dissolve in 100 mL of water at 25°C. This is some 300 times less than the concentration of unesterified cholesterol actually circulating in the plasma in the form of lipoproteins. Cholesterol esters are even less soluble than cholesterol itself.

Only animals and humans form significant amounts of cholesterol. Plants contain other steroids, which are collectively called **phytosterols.** Ergosterol (mostly in fungi) and β-sitosterol (in higher plants) are examples of phytosterols. They are poorly absorbed from dietary sources and therefore are present only in small amounts in the human body. Bacteria do not produce steroids. Dietary cholesterol is derived from animals, and *a vegetarian diet is essentially cholesterol free.*

Both endogenous synthesis and the diet are important sources of cholesterol

Most people in Western countries eat close to 1 g of cholesterol per day. Its absorption depends on the presence of bile salts and is influenced by the amount of dietary cholesterol: it may be above 60% on a low-cholesterol diet, but an absorption of 30% is more typical for a high-cholesterol diet.

Endogenous cholesterol synthesis amounts to 0.5 to 1 g per day, depending on the dietary supply. All nucleated cells can synthesize cholesterol, but the liver is the most important site, accounting for at least 50% of the total. Some endocrine tissues, such as the adrenal cortex and the corpus luteum, which produce steroid hormones, have very high rates of cholesterol synthesis.

Dietary cholesterol is absorbed as free cholesterol. Most of this is converted to cholesterol esters by the microsomal enzyme **acyl-CoA-cholesterol acyl transferase (ACAT)** in the intestinal mucosa. Together with other dietary lipids, *the cholesterol esters are packaged into chylomicrons.* After the removal of most of the triglycerides by the extrahepatic lipoprotein lipase (see Chapter 18), the cholesterol-rich remnant particles are taken up by the liver. Thus, *most of the dietary cholesterol is directed to the liver.*

BOX 19.7

Cholesterol

A cholesterol ester
(Oleyl-cholesterol)

$H_3C-(CH_2)_7-C=C-(CH_2)_7-C-O-$

FIG. 19.5

Interorgan transport of cholesterol.

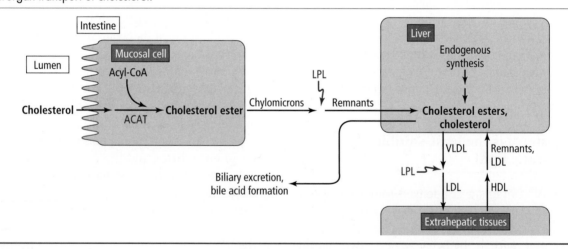

The liver, in turn, releases cholesterol and choles- terol esters as constituents of very-low-density lipoprotein (VLDL), together with triglycerides and phospholipids. VLDL is processed to low-density lipoprotein (LDL), which is taken up both by the liver and by extrahepatic tissues. *LDL is the principal external source of cholesterol for most cells.* The transport of cholesterol from the extrahepatic tissues to the liver requires high-density lipoprotein (HDL) to- gether with other lipoproteins (Fig. 19.5). Details of lipoprotein function and metabolism will be de- scribed in Chapter 20.

FIG. 19.6

The stages of cholesterol synthesis.

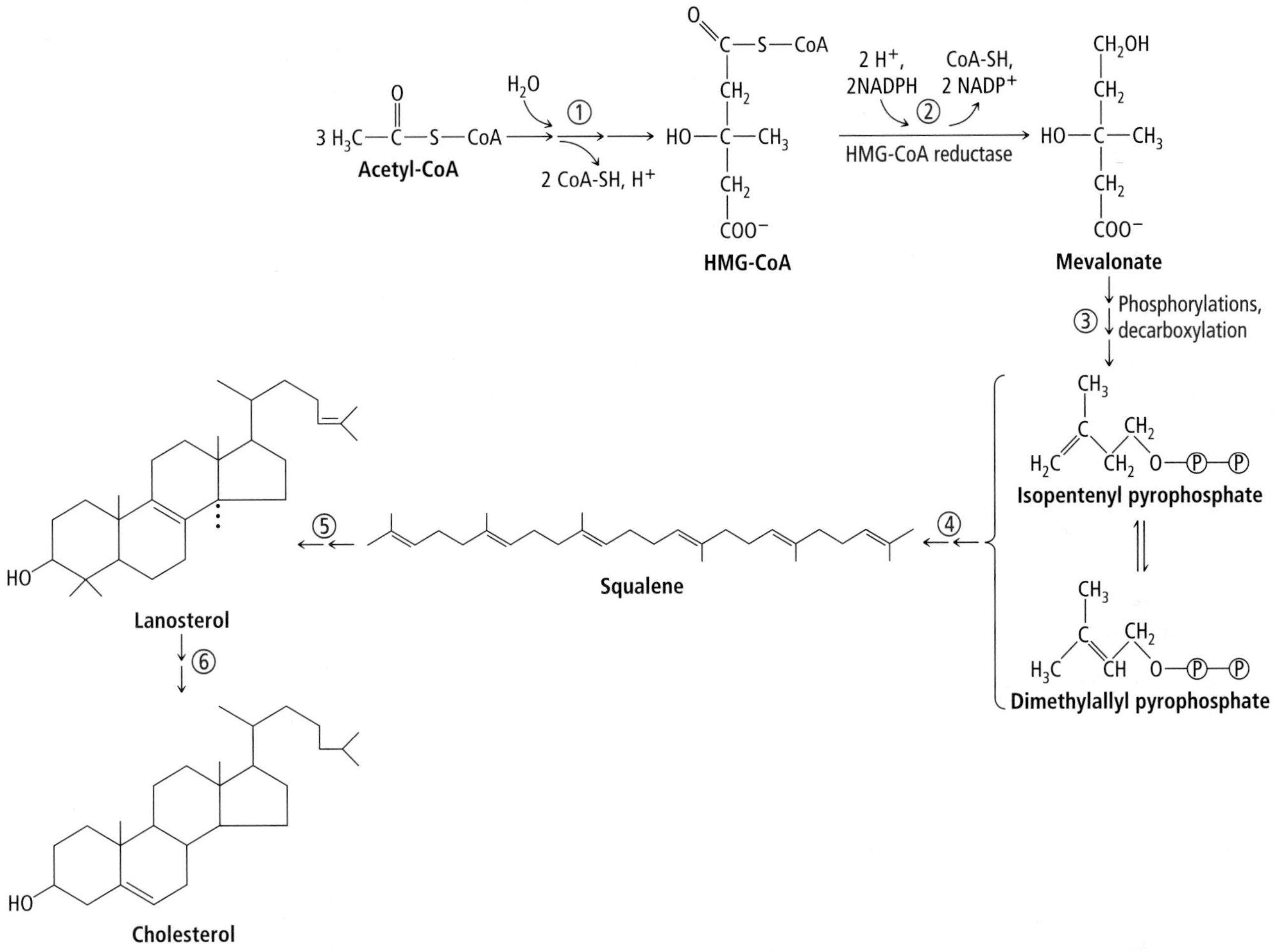

Cholesterol is synthesized from acetyl-CoA

All 27 carbons of cholesterol are biosynthetically derived from the acetyl residue in acetyl-CoA. The enzymes of the biosynthetic pathway, which number close to 30, are found in the cytosol and the ER. The pathway is shown in a very abbreviated form in Fig. 19.6. The first reactions, up to HMG-CoA, are shared with the synthesis of the ketone bodies (see Chapter 18). Whereas ketogenesis is mitochondrial, however, the HMG-CoA for cholesterol synthesis is formed by a cytoplasmic HMG-CoA synthase.

The NADPH-dependent formation of mevalonate from HMG-CoA (reaction ② in Fig. 19.6) is the committed step of cholesterol synthesis. The six-carbon compound mevalonate then is processed to the branched-chain five-carbon compounds **isopetenyl pyrophosphate** and **dimethylallyl pyrophosphate** (reaction sequence ③ in Fig. 19.6). Six of these five-carbon units form the 30-carbon compound **squalene** (reaction sequence ④ in Fig. 19.6), and squalene is cyclized to **lanosterol,** the first steroid product of the pathway. Lanosterol, finally, is processed to cholesterol.

HMG-CoA reductase is the most important regulated enzyme of cholesterol biosynthesis

Cholesterol biosynthesis is regulated by feedback inhibition: *the rate-limiting enzyme, HMG-CoA reductase, is inhibited by free cholesterol.* This effect is mediated at both the transcriptional and the posttranscriptional levels. HMG-CoA reductase has a lifespan of approximately 4 hours, so a change in its rate of synthesis or degradation can affect cholesterol synthesis rather rapidly.

Insulin stimulates HMG-CoA reductase, and this effect is thought to be mediated by the AMP-activated protein kinase: like acetyl-CoA carboxylase (see Chapter 18), HMG-CoA reductase is phosphorylated and inactivated by this insulin-inhibited enzyme.

The isoprenoids are derived from the pathway of cholesterol biosynthesis

The **isoprenoids** are biosynthetic products that are derived from the branched-chain five-carbon compounds isopentenyl pyrophosphate and dimethylallyl pyrophosphate. Besides cholesterol and the other steroids, relatively few isoprenoids are synthesized in the human body, including:

- the side chain of **ubiquinone** (see Fig. 16.24, Chapter 16)
- **dolichol,** which participates in the synthesis of the N-linked oligosaccharides in glycoproteins (see Fig. 8.21, Chapter 8)
- the side chain of **heme a,** the prosthetic group of cytochrome a/a$_3$
- **farnesyl** and **geranylgeranyl groups,** which are used to anchor proteins to membranes (see Fig. 11.12, Chapter 11)

Plants produce a far greater variety of isoprenoids. All fat-soluble vitamins, for example, are isoprenoids. Phytanic acid, which accumulates in patients with Refsum's disease (see page 368), also shows the typical isoprenoid structure.

Bile acids are synthesized from cholesterol

The steroid nucleus of cholesterol cannot be degraded in the human body. *Cholesterol has to be disposed of by the biliary system, either as itself or after its conversion to bile acids.*

Bladder bile contains approximately 400 mg/dL cholesterol. Because the intestinal absorption of biliary cholesterol, like that of dietary cholesterol, is on the order of only 50%, *as much as 500 mg of cholesterol may be eliminated from the body per day.* Cholesterol is metabolized to coprostanol, cholestanone, and other "neutral sterols" by the intestinal flora.

The **bile acids,** more properly called **bile salts** because they are present in the deprotonated form at pH 7, are formed from cholesterol in hepatocytes and are secreted actively into the bile canaliculi. They are not useless excretory products but rather serve a vital function in lipid absorption (see Chapter 14). *Approximately half of the cholesterol in the body eventually is metabolized to bile salts.* The **primary bile acids,** which are synthesized in the liver, include **cholic acid** and **chenodeoxycholic acid,** cholic acid being the more abundant. The liver releases the bile acids not in the free form but as conjugation products with glycine or taurine (Fig. 19.7). In humans the ratio of glycine conjugates to taurine conjugates is approximately 3:1.

The structural differences between cholesterol and the bile acids are:

1. The hydrocarbon chain at C-17 of the steroid nucleus is shortened by three carbons, and the terminal carbon is oxidized to a carboxy group.
2. One or two hydroxy groups are present in addition to the one inherited from cholesterol.
3. All hydroxy groups in the bile acids are in α configuration. Even the configuration at C-3, which is β in cholesterol, is inverted in the bile acids.
4. The fusion between the A and the B rings is in *cis* configuration because the angular methyl group C-19 and the hydrogen at C-5 are both in β configuration. The result is a bend between the planes of rings A and B.

The acidic groups in the glycine and taurine conjugates are almost fully deprotonated at physiological pH values. The hydroxy groups all point to the same side of the molecule and form a hydrophilic surface; the opposite surface is hydrophobic. This property is important for the formation of bile salt micelles.

7α-Hydroxylase catalyzes the regulated step of bile acid synthesis

The committed step in bile acid synthesis (Fig. 19.8) is the introduction of a hydroxy group in position 7 of cholesterol by the microsomal enzyme *7α-*

FIG. 19.7

Structures of the primary bile salts (bile acids), compared with cholesterol.

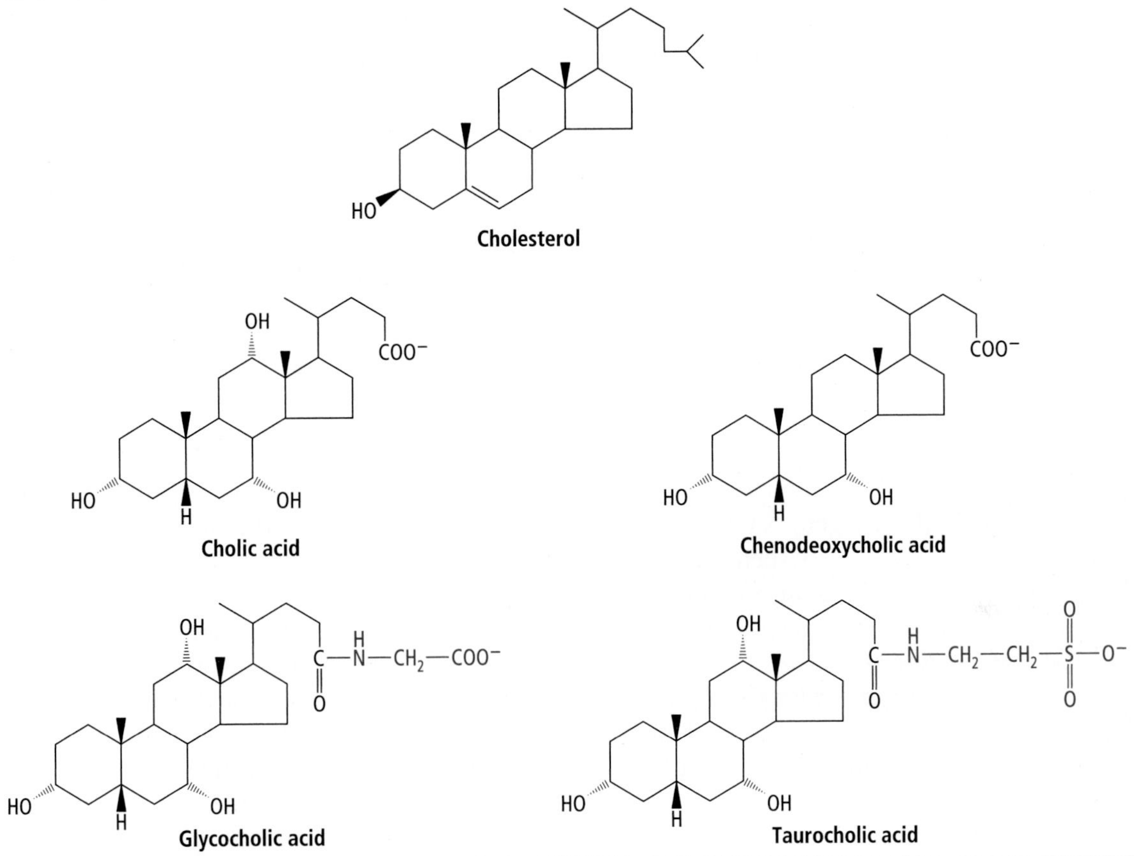
HO
Cholesterol
OH
COO⁻
HO
H
OH
Cholic acid
COO⁻
HO
H
OH
Chenodeoxycholic acid
OH
C—N—CH₂—COO⁻
H
O
HO
H
OH
Glycocholic acid
OH
C—N—CH₂—CH₂—S—O⁻
H
O
O
O
HO
H
OH
Taurocholic acid

FIG. 19.8

Synthesis of the primary bile acids by ER-associated enzymes in hepatocytes.

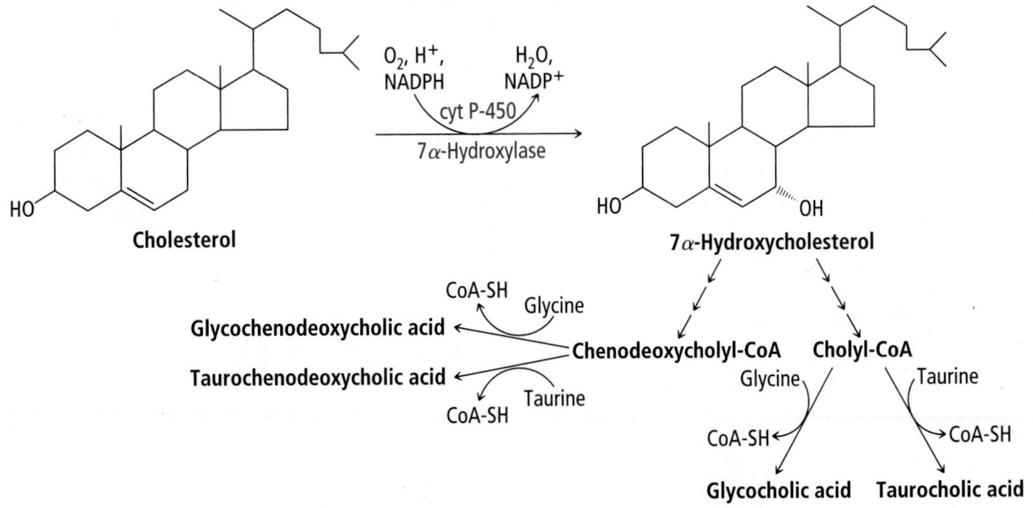
HO
Cholesterol
O₂, H⁺,
NADPH
H₂O,
NADP⁺
cyt P-450
7α-Hydroxylase
HO
OH
7α-Hydroxycholesterol
CoA-SH
Glycine
Glycochenodeoxycholic acid
Taurochenodeoxycholic acid
Taurine
CoA-SH
Chenodeoxycholyl-CoA
Cholyl-CoA
Glycine
Taurine
CoA-SH
CoA-SH
Glycocholic acid
Taurocholic acid

FIG. 19.9

Synthesis of the secondary bile acids by intestinal bacteria.

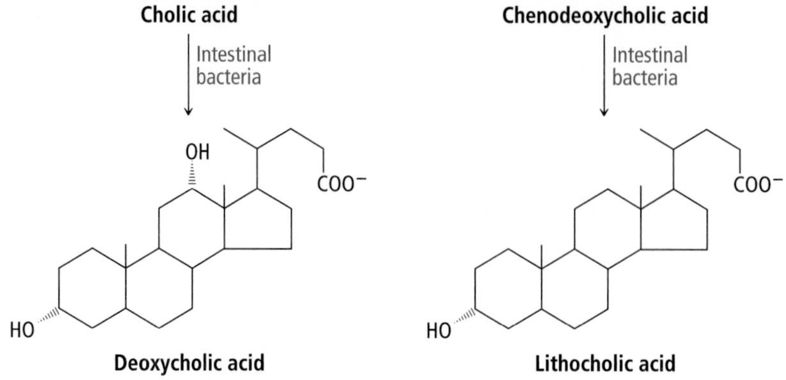

hydroxylase. The reaction is of the monooxygenase type, requiring molecular oxygen, NADPH, and cytochrome P-450. Ascorbate also seems to be involved. Ascorbate deficiency (scurvy) impairs the formation of bile acids and causes cholesterol accumulation and atherosclerosis, at least in guinea pigs.

Bile acids reduce the level of 7α-hydroxylase by inhibiting the transcription of its gene. Interestingly, bile acids also decrease the activity of HMG-CoA reductase; dietary cholesterol induces 7α-hydroxylase at the level of transcription in addition to its inhibitory action on HMG-CoA reductase. These regulatory effects ensure the maintenance of an adequate pool of free cholesterol in the liver.

Thyroid hormones induce the synthesis of 7α-hydroxylase. This effect may well be related to the observed increase of the plasma cholesterol level in patients with hypothyroidism.

Bile acids are subject to extensive enterohepatic circulation

As the primary bile acids reach the lower parts of the small intestine, they are modified by bacterial enzymes. First they are deconjugated by hydrolytic cleavage of the amide bond between the bile acid and glycine or taurine. This is followed by the reductive removal of the 7α-hydroxy group. The **secondary bile acids** formed in these reactions are **deoxycholic acid** and **lithocholic acid** (Fig. 19.9).

Approximately 98% of the bile acids are absorbed by a sodium cotransport mechanism in the ileum. *Both the primary and the secondary bile acids are returned to*

the liver through the portal circulation; they then are conjugated and secreted in the bile. Because of this *enterohepatic circulation* (Fig. 19.10), both primary and secondary bile acids are present in the bile.

The enterohepatic circulation of the bile acids is necessary for their efficient use: only 0.5 g is synthesized per day, and approximately 3 to 5 g are present in the liver, bile, and intestine at any time. The daily secretion of bile acids, however, amounts to 20 to 30 g. An average bile acid molecule is recycled five to eight times every day, and it remains in the system for approximately a week before it finally is excreted.

Bile acids in peripheral blood are measured in the clinical laboratory for the assessment of hepatobiliary function. Their levels are highest after a meal: although they are synthesized at all times, the release of bile from the gallbladder is intermittent, being stimulated by cholecystokinin after a fatty meal. After their absorption from the ileum, a very small fraction of the bile acids escapes uptake by the liver and appears in the systemic circulation. The serum bile acid levels are massively elevated in patients with biliary obstruction. Bile acids are not very toxic, but they cause a distressing itching (pruritus) in these patients.

Most gallstones consist of cholesterol

Besides water and electrolytes, the bile contains cholesterol, bile acids, phospholipid (mostly as phosphatidylcholine), and the heme-derived bile pigments. *The least soluble of these components is cholesterol.*

FIG. 19.10

Disposition of bile acids and cholesterol in the enterohepatic system.

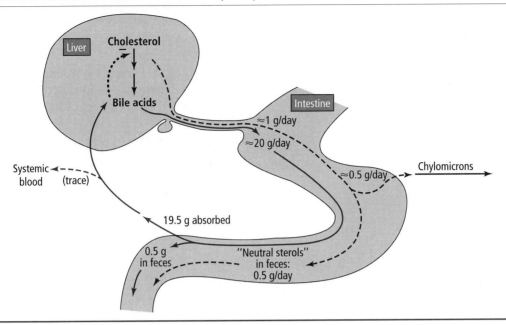

Although less abundant than some other constituents of bile (Table 19.2), *cholesterol can be kept in solution only by being incorporated in mixed bile salt/phospholipid micelles.*

The precipitation of cholesterol from these mixed micelles is the most common cause of **gallstones** (cholelithiasis). This condition, which is most common in fat, fertile females, afflicts approximately 20% of all people in Western countries sooner or later in their lives. Some gallstones contain both cholesterol and bile pigments, but others are essentially pure cholesterol. Only some 10% of all gallstones consist of substances other than cholesterol, principally bilirubin and other bile pigments. Unlike kidney stones, which in most cases are calcified and therefore visible on plain X-rays, gallstones are usually radiolucent. However, they can be visualized by cholecystography after the injection of a contrast medium. Most gallstones form in the gallbladder, where the hepatic bile becomes concentrated: inorganic ions are removed from the bile by active transport across the gallbladder epithelium, followed by passive water flux. Except for inorganic ions, all solids therefore are more concentrated in bladder bile than in hepatic bile.

The formation of cholesterol stones depends on the relative concentrations of cholesterol, bile salts,

TABLE 19.2

Approximate composition of hepatic bile and bladder bile

Component	Hepatic bile	Bladder bile
Total solids	2.5%	10%
Inorganic salt	0.85%	0.85%
Bile acids	1.2%	6%
Cholesterol	0.06%	0.4%
Lecithin	0.04%	0.3%
Bile pigments	0.2%	1.5%
pH	7.4	5.0-6.0

and phospholipid (lecithin): *either an increased concentration of cholesterol or a decreased concentration of bile salts or lecithin results in supersaturation, and the eventual precipitation of cholesterol crystals.* Unless they are rapidly flushed down the common bile duct, the cholesterol crystals grow into stones that cause irritation and obstruction of the common bile duct. Figure 19.11 is a "solubility triangle," showing the solubility of cholesterol at different concentrations of bile salts and lecithin.

Cholelithiasis most often is treated by cholecystectomy. Postoperatively, lipid absorption is only mildly abnormal because bile acids still can reach

FIG. 19.11

Solubility of cholesterol in the presence of bile acids and phosphatidylcholine ("lecithin"). If the relative composition of bile is above the blue line, the system is supersaturated with cholesterol, and cholesterol is likely to precipitate. A total lipid concentration of 10% is assumed. Point N represents a "normal" composition of bladder bile, with 5 mol% lecithin, 85 mol% bile acid, and 10 mol% cholesterol.

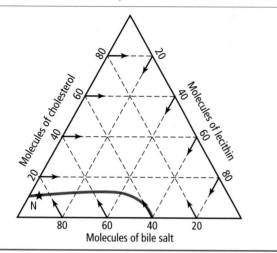

The glycosphingolipids are synthesized from ceramide and nucleotide-activated monosaccharides, and their degradation is effected by lysosomal exoglycosidases. Deficiencies of individual sphingolipid-degrading lysosomal enzymes result in lipid storage diseases.

Cholesterol is derived in part from dietary sources and in part from endogenous synthesis in liver and other tissues. Endogenous cholesterol synthesis starts with acetyl-CoA. Like most other biosynthetic pathways, cholesterol synthesis is subject to feedback inhibition. The liver releases cholesterol—mostly in the form of cholesterol esters—into the blood as a constituent of very-low-density lipoprotein (VLDL), and VLDL is a precursor of low-density lipoprotein (LDL).

Excess cholesterol can be excreted in the bile, but approximately half of the total cholesterol eventually is converted to bile acids. The bile acids, which are required in considerable quantity to facilitate intestinal lipid absorption, are subject to an extensive enterohepatic circulation.

the small intestine. Only the accurate timing of their release is no longer possible, and this limits the patient's tolerance for fatty foods. Gallstones also can be treated by the oral administration of large amounts of chenodeoxycholic acid or ursodeoxycholic acid. Through the enterohepatic circulation, these bile acids are incorporated into the bile and gradually dissolve the cholesterol stones. Unfortunately, diarrhea is such a troublesome side effect of highly dosed bile acids that cholecystectomy is still the preferred treatment.

SUMMARY

Most cells are able to synthesize phosphoglycerides, sphingolipids, and cholesterol. Phosphatidic acid, the parent compound of the phosphoglycerides, is synthesized from glycerol phosphate and CoA-activated fatty acids. Either the alcoholic substituent of the phosphoglycerides is introduced from a CDP-activated precursor, or phosphatidic acid becomes activated in the form of CDP-diacylglycerol. The phosphoglycerides are remodeled and eventually degraded by various phospholipases.

Further Reading

Barnes S: Metabolism of bile acids. In: McIntyre N, Benhamou J-P, Bircher J, Rizzetto M, Rodes J: *Oxford textbook of clinical hepatology*, vol. 1. Oxford University Press, Oxford, 1991, pp. 115–129.

Dowling RH, McIntyre N: Gallstones. In: McIntyre N, Benhamou J-P, Bircher J, Rizzetto M, Rodes J: *Oxford textbook of clinical hepatology*, vol. 2. Oxford University Press, Oxford, 1991, pp. 1107–1134.

Erlinger S: Secretion of bile. In: Schiff L, Schiff ER: *Diseases of the liver*, 7th ed., vol. 1, J. B. Lippincott, Philadelphia, 1993, pp. 85–107.

Everson GT, Kern F Jr: Bile acid and cholesterol homeostasis. In: Haubrich WS, Schaffner F, Berk JE, editors: *Gastroenterology*, 5th ed., vol. 2. W. B. Saunders, Philadelphia, 1995, pp. 984–995.

Hofmann AF: Intestinal absorption of bile acids and biliary constituents: the intestinal component of the enterohepatic circulation and the integrated system. In: Johnson LR et al, editors: *Physiology of the gastrointestinal tract*, 3rd ed., vol. 2. Raven Press, New York, 1994, pp. 1845–1865.

Kent C: Eukaryotic phospholipid biosynthesis. *Annu Rev Biochem* 64, 315–343, 1995.

Pennock CA: Lysosomal storage disorders. In: Holton JB, editors: *The inherited metabolic diseases*, 2nd ed. Churchill Livingstone, New York, 1994, pp. 205 – 242.

Scriver CR, Beaudet AL, Sly WS, Valle D, editors: *The metabolic basis of inherited disease*, 6th ed., vol. 2. McGraw-Hill, New York, 1989, pp. 1623 – 1839.

QUESTIONS

1. The ABO blood group substances are oligosaccharides in plasma membrane glycolipids of erythrocytes and other cells. The biosynthetic enzymes that are encoded by the ABO gene can be characterized as
   A. Glycosidases
   B. Glycosyltransferases
   C. Lipases
   D. Glycolipases
   E. Phospholipases

2. Gallstones can easily form when the bile contains an increased amount of
   A. Free (unesterified) fatty acids
   B. Bile salts
   C. Phospholipids
   D. Cholesterol

3. An 8-month-old child of Jewish parents is examined for failure to thrive and abnormal neurological development. The child is found to have hepatosplenomegaly and a cherry-red spot on the macula of the eye, and the chromatography of lipids from cultured leukocytes shows abnormally high levels of ganglioside G_{M2}. This child has
   A. Refsum's disease
   B. Tay-Sachs disease
   C. Gaucher's disease
   D. Metachromatic leukodystrophy

Chapter 20

Lipid Transport

Compared with glucose and the amino acids, the plasma levels of the major lipids are quite impressive, as shown in Table 20.1. They not only are higher than the normal blood glucose level of 100 mg/dL, but they also fluctuate over a wider range, depending on the nutritional state and individual constitution. This is possible because the tissues are not critically dependent on blood-derived lipids: As metabolic fuels, lipids can be replaced by glucose, ketone bodies, or amino acids in all tissues, and the membrane lipids can be synthesized locally.

Unesterified ("free") fatty acids are transported in noncovalent binding to serum albumin, but triglycerides, phospholipids, and cholesterol esters form large noncovalent aggregates with proteins that are collectively called **lipoproteins.** In this chapter we will describe not only the normal functions of lipoproteins but also their relationship to abnormal states, particularly the common ailment of atherosclerosis.

THE HIGHWAYS OF LIPID TRANSPORT

There are four highways of lipid transport in the human body:

1. *The transport of fatty acids from adipose tissue to other tissues*
2. *The transport of dietary lipids from the intestine to other tissues*
3. *The transport of endogenously synthesized lipids from the liver to other tissues*
4. *The* **reverse transport** *of cholesterol from extrahepatic tissues to the liver.* Unlike the triglycerides, phospholipids, and glycolipids, cholesterol is not de-graded locally but has to be disposed of by the hepatobiliary system.

The transport of fatty acids from adipose tissue was discussed in Chapter 18 (page 365). The following sections are concerned with the other three routes that are based on the use of lipoproteins.

Most plasma lipids are components of lipoproteins

The interactions between lipid and protein in the plasma lipoproteins are of a purely noncovalent nature. We can predict the general structure of a lipoprotein (Fig. 20.1) if we realize that *hydrophobic lipids, including triglycerides and cholesterol esters, always avoid contact with water.* They form the core of the lipoprotein. *Amphipathic lipids, including the phospholipids, prefer the interface between the aqueous solution and the hydrophobic core of the particle.* The protein components, or **apolipoproteins,** are amphipathic as well. Their most characteristic structural feature is the **amphi-**

TABLE 20.1

Typical concentrations of plasma lipids in the postabsorptive state

Lipid	Normal range (mg/dL)
Total lipid	400-800
Triglycerides	40-300
Total cholesterol	120-280
Cholesterol esters	90-200
Phospholipids	150-380
Free fatty acids	8-14

FIG. 20.1

General structure of a lipoprotein.

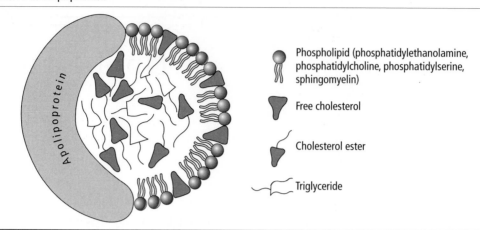

Phospholipid (phosphatidylethanolamine, phosphatidylcholine, phosphatidylserine, sphingomyelin)

Free cholesterol

Cholesterol ester

Triglyceride

pathic helix, an α helix in which one side is formed by hydrophobic, and the other by hydrophilic, amino acid side chains (see Fig. 3.3, Chapter 3). Therefore the apolipoproteins are found at the water-lipid interface. Large lipoprotein particles with a high volume/surface ratio have a high content of nonpolar lipids; small particles contain more polar lipid and protein.

The ratios of the various lipid and protein components are nonstoichiometric. Indeed, the composition of a lipoprotein particle can change rapidly in the circulation because most of the lipids and apolipoproteins are exchanged readily between different lipoprotein particles.

Besides being remodeled in the circulation, *some types of lipoproteins actually are taken up into the cells by receptor-mediated endocytosis*: the particle binds to a receptor on the cell surface, and the receptor-ligand complex then is taken up into an endocytotic vesicle. Eventually the components of the lipoprotein are digested in a secondary lysosome, and the resulting lipids and amino acids are used for the metabolic needs of the cell.

Plasma lipoproteins can be separated by either their electrophoretic mobility or their density

Electrophoresis on a thin layer plate, cellulose acetate foil, or agarose gel is the most commonly used method of protein separation in the clinical laboratory. Plasma protein electrophoresis at pH 8.6

yields five major peaks: albumin, and the α_1, α_2, β, and γ globulins, in decreasing order of mobility (see Chapter 25). In fasting serum or plasma, the two most prominent lipoprotein bands are found in the α_1 and β fractions and are designated, accordingly, as $\boldsymbol{\alpha}$- and $\boldsymbol{\beta}$-**lipoproteins.** A less prominent band, the **pre-$\boldsymbol{\beta}$-lipoproteins,** moves slightly ahead of the β-lipoproteins. After a fatty meal, but not in the fasting state, we find a fourth band, which does not move in electrophoresis. This band consists of chylomicrons (Fig. 20.2).

The behavior of lipoproteins in **density gradient centrifugation** depends on their protein/lipid ratio: nonpolar lipids have densities of approximately 0.9 g/cm³. With increasing protein content, the densities of the lipoprotein particles increase to well above 1.0 g/cm³ in the protein-rich types, from 0.9 to 0.96 in the most lipid-rich particles. According to their densities, we can distinguish the major classes of chylomicrons, very-low-density lipoprotein (VLDL), low-density lipoprotein (LDL), and high-density lipoprotein (HDL). The correspondence of these density classes with the electrophoretic separation pattern is shown in Fig. 20.2.

Lipoproteins have characteristic lipid and protein compositions

The approximate compositions of the different lipoprotein classes are shown in Table 20.2. In the fasting state, *the major triglyceride-rich lipoprotein is VLDL, and approximately 70% of the total cholesterol is in*

FIG. 20.2

Electrophoretic mobilities and density classes of plasma lipoproteins. Intermediate-density lipoprotein (IDL) is included here in LDL.

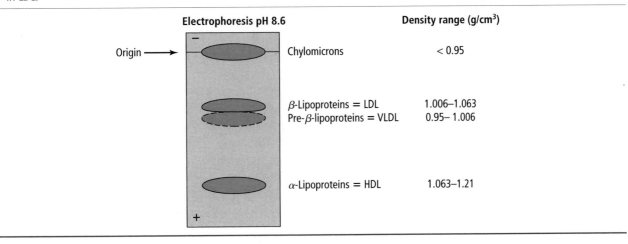

TABLE 20.2

Typical compositions of plasma lipoproteins

Lipoprotein class	Source	Diameter (nm)	Density (g/cm³)	Protein %	Trigly-cerides	Phos-pholipid	Cholesterol esters	Choles-terol
							Lipid %	
Chylomicrons	Intestine	100-1,000	0.95	1-2	86	8	3	2
Very-low-density lipoprotein (VLDL)	Liver	30-80	0.95-1.006	6-10	55	18	13	7
Intermediate-density lipoprotein (IDL)	VLDL	25-30	1.006-1.019	15-20	25	21	28	9
Low-density lipo-protein (LDL)	VLDL, IDL	20-25	1.019-1.063	22	9	20	40	8
High-density lipo-protein	Liver, intestine							
HDL₂		9-12	1.063-1.125	35-45	5	33	17	5
HDL₃		5-9	1.125-1.21	50-55	3	28	12	3

LDL (total cholesterol = free cholesterol + cholesterol esters). Therefore elevations of the plasma triglyceride level usually are caused by increased VLDL, whereas an elevated cholesterol level most often reflects an increase in the LDL fraction.

The apolipoprotein contents of the different lipoproteins are characteristic as well (Table 20.3). With the exception of the B-apolipoproteins, however, which are major structural proteins of LDL, VLDL, and chylomicrons (but not HDL), apolipoproteins can be transferred readily between different lipoprotein classes. In addition to their structural roles, the apolipoproteins participate in lipoprotein metabolism by

- *regulating enzymes of lipoprotein metabolism*, including lipoprotein lipase (LPL) and lecithin-cholesterol acyl transferase (LCAT)
- *facilitating the transfer of lipids* between different lipoprotein classes, or between lipoproteins and cells
- *mediating the cellular uptake of lipoproteins* by binding to cell surface receptors

TABLE 20.3

Characteristics of the apolipoproteins

Apolipoprotein	Mol wt	Plasma concentration (mg/dL)	Lipoproteins	Source	Function
A-I	29,000	130	HDL, chylomicrons	Liver, intestine	Major structural proteins of HDL, also in chylomicrons; apo A-I activates LCAT
A-II	17,000	40			
B-48	241,000	Variable	Chylomicrons	Intestine	Structural protein of chylomicrons
B-100	513,000	80	VLDL, LDL	Liver	Structural protein of VLDL, IDL, and LDL. Only apoprotein of LDL. Mediates tissue uptake of LDL.
C-I	6,600	6	Most lipoproteins	Liver	Readily transferred between different classes. C-II activates extrahepatic lipoprotein lipase (LPL).
C-II	8,900	3			
C-III	8,800	12			
D	19,000	10	HDL		Unknown
E	34,000	5	VLDL, IDL, chylomicrons	Liver	Mediates the uptake of chylomicron remnants and IDL by the liver

Lipids of dietary origin are transported by chylomicrons

On a typical U.S. diet, between 70 and 120 g of triglycerides have to be transported daily from the small intestine to other tissues. The chylomicrons, which carry these triglycerides, appear only after a fatty meal. They are assembled in the ER and Golgi apparatus of the mucosal cells and exocytosed into the lacteals of the intestinal villi. The chylomicrons reach the general circulation via the thoracic duct (Fig. 20.3).

Chylomicrons transport not only triglycerides but all other dietary lipids as well. Therefore their content of cholesterol, phospholipids, and fat-soluble vitamins reflects the lipid composition of the preceding meal. Chylomicrons are formed with apoB-48 and the A-apolipoproteins as their only apolipoproteins. ApoE and the C-apolipoproteins are acquired later in the bloodstream by transfer from HDL.

In adipose tissue, muscle, heart, lung, and many other extrahepatic tissues, *the chylomicron triglycerides are hydrolyzed to free fatty acids and 2-monoacylglycerol by lipoprotein lipase* (LPL, see Chapter 18). Phospholipids and apoC-II are required for LPL activity, but only

triglycerides are hydrolyzed to any great extent. The removal of 80% to 90% of the triglycerides by LPL, which is accompanied by the transfer of most of the A- and C-apolipoproteins to HDL, converts the chylomicron into a smaller particle, known as a **chylomicron remnant.**

In the liver, the remnants enter the space of Disse, where they bind first to heparan sulfate proteoglycans and then to lipoprotein receptors on the surface of hepatocytes, including the **LDL receptor** and the LDL-receptor-related protein (LRP). This binding requires apoE. After binding to one of the receptors, *the whole remnant particle is endocytosed*, and its constituent lipids and proteins are hydrolyzed by lysosomal enzymes. The whole lifetime of a chylomicron, from its secretion by the intestinal cell to the uptake of the remnant by the liver, is less than 1 h. Once in the bloodstream, the life expectancy of the chylomicron triglycerides is in the 5- to 10-minute range.

VLDL is a precursor of LDL

The liver synthesizes 25 to 50 g of triglycerides, and smaller amounts of other lipids, every day. These lipids

FIG. 20.3

Metabolism of chylomicrons. *TG,* Triglyceride; *PL,* phospholipid; *C,* free cholesterol; *CE,* cholesterol ester; *LPL,* lipoprotein lipase.

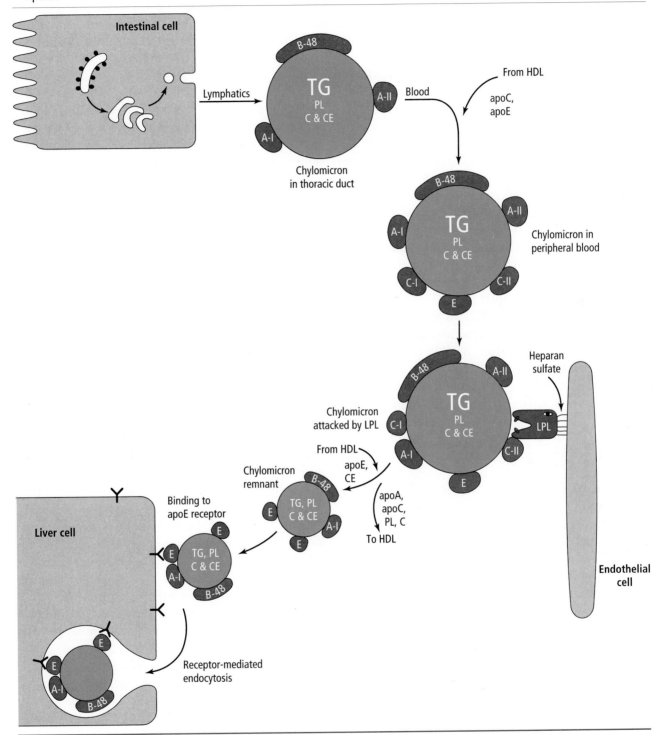

are released as constituents of VLDL. Like the chylomicrons, VLDL is synthesized in the ER and Golgi and released by exocytosis. Unlike the capillary endothelium of the intestinal mucosa, the sinusoidal endothelium of the liver is fenestrated and allows the passage of the lipoproteins into the sinusoidal blood.

Nascent VLDL contains apoB-100 and small amounts of apoE and the C-apolipoproteins. Like the chylomicrons, VLDL later acquires more apoE and C-apolipoproteins by transfer from HDL.

ApoB-100, the major apolipoprotein of VLDL, is a single polypeptide of 4536 amino acids. It is encoded by the same gene as apoB-48, a prominent apolipoprotein of chylomicrons. Indeed, apoB-48 consists of the first 2152 amino acids of apoB-100, counting from the N terminus. In the intestine, codon 2153 (CAA), which codes for glutamine, is posttranscriptionally changed into the stop codon UAA. This is an example of the *tissue-specific editing of an RNA transcript* (see Chapter 8).

Like the chylomicrons, *VLDL is metabolized initially by LPL* (Fig. 20.4). VLDL triglycerides are hydrolyzed somewhat more slowly than those in chylomicrons, with a residence time in the blood of 15 to 60 minutes, compared with 5 to 10 minutes for chylomicron triglycerides. Triglyceride hydrolysis is accompanied by the transfer of the C-apolipoproteins to HDL, but like the chylomicron remnants, VLDL remnants possess apoE, which mediates their uptake into the liver.

Approximately half of the VLDL remnants, especially the larger specimens containing multiple copies of apoE, are taken up by the liver. The smaller remnant particles appear initially as **intermediate-density lipoprotein (IDL)** and eventually are remodeled to low-density lipoprotein (LDL). This requires the hydrolysis of excess triglyceride and phospholipid by the **hepatic lipase (HL)**, as well as the transfer of excess apolipoproteins to HDL. HL, which has structural homology with LPL, is found on cell surfaces in the space of Disse, where it is anchored to heparan sulfate proteoglycans. Like LPL, it is released by heparin, but unlike LPL it is not activated by apoC-II and does not attack triglycerides in chylomicrons and VLDL. Its physiological substrates are triglycerides and phosphoglycerides in IDL and HDL. In addition to hydrolyzing lipids in these lipoproteins, it facilitates the uptake of remnant particles into hepatocytes.

LDL has a well-defined structure. Its only apolipoprotein is a solitary apoB-100 molecule, and its lipid component includes a high proportion of cholesterol and cholesterol esters (see Table 20.2).

LDL is removed by receptor-mediated endocytosis

The metabolism of LDL is rather sluggish: VLDLs and their remnants are metabolized within minutes to hours, but LDL circulates for an average of 3 days. Eventually *it is removed by receptor-mediated endocytosis*, which is initiated by binding of apoB-100 to the LDL receptor (apoB-100/apoE receptor). Approximately two-thirds of the LDL is taken up by the liver, and one third by the extrahepatic tissues. For the extrahepatic tissues, *LDL acquired through the LDL receptor is the major external source of cholesterol.*

Not all LDL is cleared by the LDL receptor. Macrophages and some endothelial cells possess alternative lipoprotein receptors, collectively known as the **scavenger receptors.** There are several of them with various affinities for native and chemically modified LDL. They mediate LDL uptake in much the same way as the LDL receptor in other cell types, but they have a four- to seven-times-higher K_m (i.e., lower affinity) for LDL. Therefore their contribution to LDL metabolism is greatest when the plasma LDL concentration is high. Interestingly, LDL that has been chemically modified by acetylating or oxidizing agents or by exposure to the cross-linking agent malondialdehyde has a higher affinity for scavenger receptors than does virgin LDL. Therefore the physiological task of these receptors may be the *removal of aberrant or aged lipoproteins* that are no longer good ligands for the other lipoprotein receptors. The scavenger receptors bind not only lipoproteins but also other particles with negative surface charges—even bacteria. Therefore these receptors may be important not only for lipoprotein metabolism but for our immune defenses as well.

More than 90% of the LDL utilization is mediated by the LDL receptor in such tissues as liver, ovary, adrenal gland, lung, and kidney. However, 44% of the LDL uptake is not mediated by the LDL receptor in the intestine, and 72% of the LDL uptake is not mediated by the LDL receptor in the spleen. These organs are rich in macrophages, which remove LDL through their scavenger receptors.

FIG. 20.4

Metabolism of VLDL and LDL. *TG,* Triglyceride; *PL,* phospholipid; *C,* free cholesterol; *CE,* cholesterol esters. *LPL,* Lipoprotein lipase; *HL,* hepatic lipase.

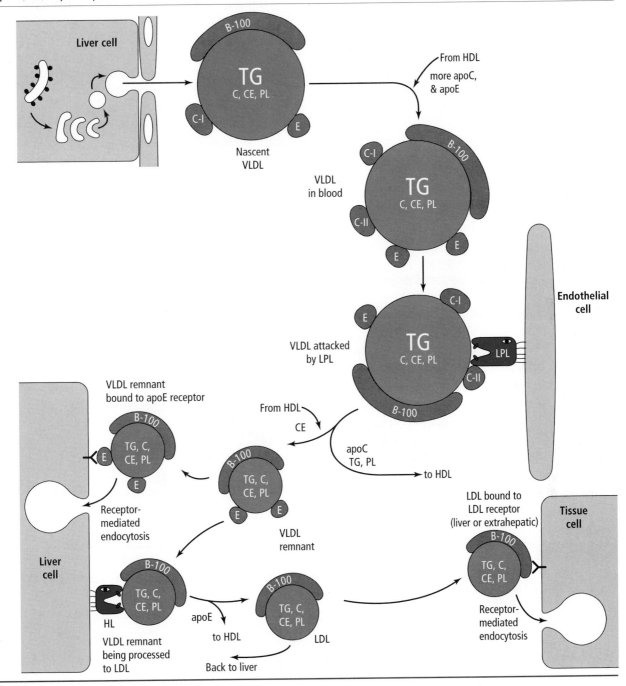

Cellular cholesterol metabolism is regulated by lipoprotein-derived cholesterol

Most cells can obtain their cholesterol either from endocytosed lipoproteins or by endogenous synthesis. Lipoprotein-derived cholesterol esters are hydrolyzed first by a nonselective acid lipase in the lysosomes that also attacks triglycerides. Together with endogenously synthesized cholesterol, the lipoprotein-derived cholesterol contributes to the free cholesterol pool of the cell. Free (unesterified) cholesterol acts on three important proteins (Fig. 20.5):

1. *It induces the enzyme ACAT*, which converts free cholesterol into highly insoluble cholesterol esters:

$$\text{Cholesterol + Acyl-CoA} \longrightarrow \text{Cholesterol ester + CoA-SH}$$

This is the form in which cholesterol is stored in the cell.

2. *It represses HMG-CoA reductase*, the rate-limiting enzyme of cholesterol biosynthesis (see Chapter 19).

3. *It reduces the synthesis, and/or accelerates the degradation, of the LDL receptor.*

These mechanisms are "designed" to ensure an adequate supply of cholesterol for the cell. Unlike the LDL receptor, the scavenger receptors of macrophages are only mildly down-regulated by excess cholesterol. Therefore macrophages accumulate cholesterol when the blood cholesterol level is high and the number of LDL receptors on other cell types is reduced.

HDL participates in reverse cholesterol transport

High-density lipoprotein (HDL) plays a key role in the reverse transport of cholesterol from the extrahepatic tissues to the liver. It occurs in several subtypes representing different stages in its metabolism. **Nascent HDL**, released from liver and intestine, is a small, phospholipid-rich particle, not spherical like the other lipoproteins but resembling a little disk of lipid bilayer with apolipoproteins at the edge (Fig. 20.6). Nascent HDL from the liver contains apoA-I,

FIG. 20.6

Hypothetical structure of nascent HDL from liver and intestine. It consists of a little piece of lipid bilayer whose edge is occupied by amphipathic helices of the apolipoproteins. The A-apolipoproteins have amphipathic α-helical portions that are separated by short, nonhelical segments.

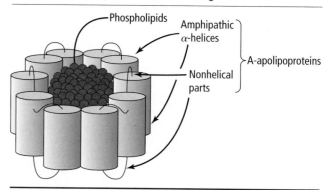

FIG. 20.5

Regulation of cholesterol metabolism by LDL-derived cholesterol in extrahepatic cells. *E*, Endosome; *L*, lysosome; *ACAT*, acyl-CoA-cholesterol acyl transferase.

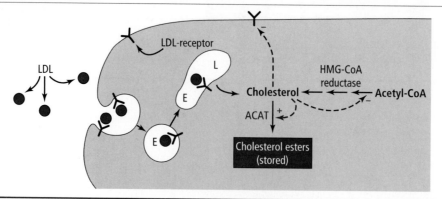

apoA-II, apoE, and the C-apolipo-proteins, but intestinal HDL is formed with only apoA-I as its principal apolipoprotein, the others being acquired later by transfer from other lipoproteins. Especially during lipolysis of the triglyceride-rich lipoproteins (VLDL and chylomicrons) by lipoprotein lipase, apolipoproteins are transferred to nascent HDL together with surface phospholipids and cholesterol. HDL does not contain the B-apolipoproteins, which are obligatory components of VLDL, LDL, and chylomicrons.

Once in the circulation, *nascent HDL attracts free, unesterified cholesterol both from other lipoproteins and from cells.* HDL particles containing only apoA-I or apoE are able to bind to cells from which they acquire free cholesterol. From these acceptor particles the cholesterol is transferred to particles containing both apoA-I and apoA-II. The further fate of cell-derived cholesterol depends on two proteins that are bound to the surface of the HDL particle:

1. **Lecithin-cholesterol acyl transferase (LCAT)** is an otherwise-soluble enzyme that binds to the surface of HDL, where it becomes activated by apoA-I. It catalyzes the reaction

$$\text{Cholesterol} + \text{Phosphatidylcholine} \longrightarrow$$
$$\text{Cholesterol ester} + \text{2-Lysophosphatidylcholine}$$

Lysophosphatidylcholine (lysolecithin) is transferred to albumin, and the hydrophobic cholesterol esters sink into the center of the HDL particle. The originally flat HDL bulges into a spherical particle called HDL_3, with a hydrophobic core of cholesterol esters.
2. **Cholesterol ester transfer protein (CETP)** effects the transfer of cholesterol esters from HDL to other lipoproteins, either alone or in exchange for triglycerides. During the lipolysis of chylomicrons and VLDL by LPL, in particular, cholesterol ester transfer from HDL to the remnant particles — mostly in exchange for triglycerides — is stimulated by the high local concentration of fatty acids. The remnant particles bring the cholesterol esters to the liver.

In the space of Disse, HDL is exposed to the hepatic lipase (HL). The hydrolysis of triglycerides and phospholipids by HL converts larger HDL particles, known as HDL_2, to the smaller HDL_3. Also, a minority of large HDL particles (HDL_c) acquire multiple copies of apoE, and this leads to their endocytotic uptake into hepatocytes. Some cholesterol and cholesterol esters also are transferred from HDL to hepatocytes, together with fatty acids and lysolecithin during lipolysis by the hepatic lipase (Fig. 20.7).

We see now that cholesterol from the extrahepatic tissues can reach the liver by three routes:

1. *By the apo-E − mediated endocytosis of remnant particles that have obtained part of their cholesterol esters from HDL*
2. *By the direct transfer of cholesterol esters from HDL during lipolysis by the hepatic lipase*
3. *By the endocytosis of large apo-E − containing HDL particles*

Of these three mechanisms, the pathway through the cholesterol ester transfer protein and remnant particles is quantitatively the most important in.humans.

LIPOPROTEINS AND ATHEROSCLEROSIS

Atherosclerosis is a set of pathological changes in the intima of large arteries that can result in serious and often fatal complications. Coronary heart disease (CHD) and acute myocardial infarction, gangrene, many cerebrovascular accidents, and some cases of senile dementia are caused by atherosclerosis. Taken together, these complications account for one third of all deaths in Western countries. In the following sections we will examine the roles of plasma lipoproteins as risk factors for atherosclerosis.

Lipoproteins are important risk factors for atherosclerosis

Atherosclerosis is defined by the presence of **atheromatous plaques,** characteristic lesions in the intima of large arteries. The typical atheromatous plaque contains a core of cholesterol esters surrounded by an area of fibrosis. The plaque impairs blood flow by narrowing the lumen of the artery, and it can lead to such complications as calcification, hemorrhage into the plaque, and thrombus formation. The early stages of plaque formation are

FIG. 20.7

Metabolism of HDL. *TG,* Triglyceride; *PL,* phospholipid; *C,* cholesterol; *CE,* cholesterol esters; *CETP,* cholesterol ester transfer protein; *LPL,* lipoprotein lipase; *HL,* hepatic lipase. All HDL apolipoproteins can be exchanged with other lipoprotein classes.

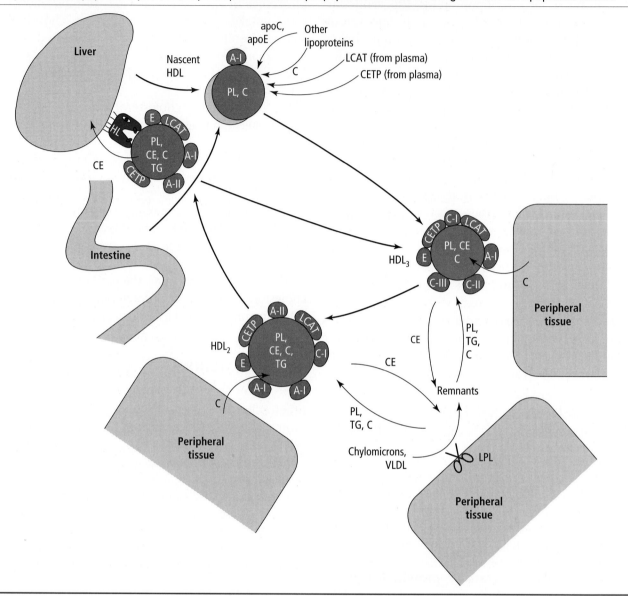

less well known, but the deposition of cholesterol esters first in tissue macrophages and later in the extracellular space is considered an early event. The **fatty streak** is an early, reversible lesion that is common even in children. Although most fatty streaks regress spontaneously, some develop into atheromatous plaques.

Many factors besides lipid deposition are important for atherogenesis. Injury to the vessel wall—for example, in response to prolonged hypertension or as a result of the microangiopathy of chronic diabetes mellitus—is thought to induce a fibroproliferative response. The recruitment of monocytes from the blood into a developing lesion, where they develop into tissue macrophages and eventually into lipid-laden **foam cells,** is thought to be important. Locally released growth factors also are thought to stimulate the deposition of a collagen-rich extracellular matrix.

The risk factors for atherosclerosis and CHD, as determined by epidemiological studies, are *age and gender* (mostly old people are affected, and males are affected earlier than females), *smoking, diabetes mellitus, hypertension, and hypercholesterolemia.* Figure 20.8 shows the relationship between the total plasma cholesterol level and the incidence of death from CHD. The total cholesterol level reflects mostly the level of LDL cholesterol, which accounts for approximately two thirds of the total plasma cholesterol. Indeed, LDL cholesterol correlates even better with CHD than does total cholesterol. High HDL cholesterol, on the other hand, is associated with a decreased risk, and *the ratio of LDL cholesterol to HDL cholesterol is an excellent predictor of disease risk.*

Lipoprotein(a) [Lp(a)] is a form of LDL in which an unusual glycoprotein, **apolipoprotein(a)**, is disulfide bonded to the apoB-100 molecule of LDL. *Elevated Lp(a) concentrations are an independent risk factor for atherosclerosis.* The plasma level of Lp(a) is determined by the rate of expression of the apolipoprotein(a) gene in the liver and may be anywhere from less than 5 to more than 100 mg/dL. Unlike ordinary LDL, Lp(a) does not seem to respond to dietary manipulations.

As shown in Fig. 20.9, most of the cholesterol esters in fatty streaks and atherosclerotic plaques are derived from LDL. The LDL particles enter the intima by transcytosis through the endothelium—the normal transport mechanism for lipoproteins across nonfenestrated endothelia—and then are endocytosed by tissue macrophages through their scavenger receptors. This uptake of LDL cholesterol has to be balanced by the transfer of excess cholesterol from the macrophages to HDL for transport to the liver, and therefore *a foam cell—and a fatty streak—develops only if the amount of cholesterol acquired from LDL exceeds the amount released to HDL.* Interestingly, premenopausal women have approximately 20% higher HDL levels than men, a circumstance that may explain the reduced incidence of CHD in women and their longer life expectancy. Some environmental effects on LDL and HDL cholesterol are summarized in Table 20.4. The mechanisms by which these manipulations affect the blood lipoprotein levels are for the most part unknown, but there is evidence that dietary and pharmacological interventions leading to increased HDL or decreased LDL actually reduce the risk of CHD.

FIG. 20.8

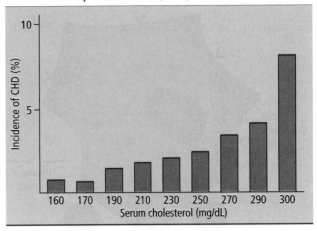

Relationship between the plasma cholesterol level and death from coronary heart disease (CHD).

In the clinical laboratory, the total cholesterol and triglyceride levels are determined directly from fresh plasma or serum. HDL cholesterol is determined after the selective precipitation of LDL and VLDL by a polyanion such as phosphotungstate. LDL cholesterol (in milligrams per deciliter) is estimated with the formula

$$\text{LDL cholesterol} = \text{Total cholesterol} - (\text{HDL cholesterol} + 0.16 \times \text{Triglycerides})$$

The reagents used for routine cholesterol determinations contain a cholesterol esterase, so the measured "cholesterol" is actually free cholesterol + cholesterol esters.

Deficiencies of individual lipoprotein classes are severe diseases

The functions of the different lipoprotein classes are highlighted by some rare genetic diseases.

Abetalipoproteinemia, a recessively inherited disease, is caused by the absence of a triglyceride transfer protein in the ER. As a result, liver and intestine are unable to assemble and secrete the triglyceride-rich, apoB-containing lipoproteins. LDL, VLDL, and chylomicrons are essentially absent, and both the

develop atherosclerosis at a very early age, and many die of CHD before age 20. The pathways in normal individuals and in FH are summarized in Fig. 20.10.

A variety of different mutations in the LDL receptor gene have been identified as causes of FH. They include complete and partial gene deletions, receptors that are not translocated from their site of synthesis in the ER to the plasma membrane, receptors that do not bind LDL, and receptors that do not trigger endocytosis even though they can bind LDL.

Reverse cholesterol transport is affected by deficiencies of LCAT and CETP

In **familial LCAT deficiency,** a rare recessively inherited condition, the cholesterol acquired by HDL cannot be esterified to cholesterol esters, and the free cholesterol/cholesterol ester ratio is increased enormously in all classes of lipoproteins. There is variable hypercholesterolemia and hypertriglyceridemia, and most of the HDL particles have the discoidal shape typical of nascent HDL. Clinical findings include severe corneal clouding, renal insufficiency with proteinuria, and prematureatherosclerosis.

CETP deficiency is a benign condition in which the cholesterol esters formed by LCAT cannot be transferred from HDL to other lipoproteins. Affected homozygotes have approximately a fourfold elevation of HDL cholesterol (100 to 250 mg/dL), but LDL cholesterol is low or normal (35 to 150 mg/dL). The HDL particles tend to be oversized, with abundant cholesterol ester and very little triglyceride. Even heterozygotes have mildly increased HDL cholesterol levels. Reverse cholesterol transport is not entirely ineffective even in homozygotes because cholesterol esters still can reach the liver by direct transfer from HDL or by the endocytosis of apoE–coated HDL particles.

CETP deficiency has been described in Japan, where approximately 1% of the population is heterozygous for an allele that causes a complete lack of cholesterol ester transfer in homozygotes. Heterozygotes have slightly elevated HDL cholesterol. Another 5% of the Japanese population is heterozygous for a CETP variant that causes moderate increases of HDL cholesterol in both homozygotes and heterozygotes. The effect of these conditions on the risk of CHD is uncertain.

The roles of various apolipoproteins, lipoprotein receptors, and enzymes of lipoprotein metabolism are summarized in Table 20.5.

Hyperlipoproteinemias are grouped into five phenotypes

Although the threshold between "normal" and "hyperlipidemic" is arbitrary, the hyperlipoproteinemias often are considered the most common biochemical abnormalities in Western populations, with a prevalence of perhaps 5% to 20%. Traditionally, the hyperlipoproteinemias are grouped into five types (Table 20.6). These five types are not diseases but rather phenotypes that occur in a variety of contexts. In rare instances—as in FH—the condition is caused by a major inherited abnormality of lipoprotein metabolism. More commonly, it is secondary to a chronic disease such as diabetes mellitus, alcoholism, or hypothyroidism. In most cases, however, the hyperlipoproteinemia is multifactorial: it results from the interaction between a lipid-elevating lifestyle and the genetic constitution.

Type I hyperlipoproteinemia, or **hyperchylomicronemia,** is a rare form (prevalence = approximately 1 in 10,000) in which the hydrolysis of chylomicron triglycerides is impaired. Some patients have an inherited deficiency of the extrahepatic LPL. Others lack apoC-II, which is required as an activator of LPL. In other cases, however, no specific cause can be identified. The hypertriglyceridemia is severe, with plasma triglyceride levels close to 1000 mg/dL. LDL, however, is decreased to 20% or less of normal, and most of the plasma cholesterol is present in VLDL rather than LDL. This shows the importance of VLDL lipolysis for the formation of LDL.

Despite the massive hypertriglyceridemia, *the type I pattern does not lead to atherosclerosis and CHD.* Patients have eruptive cutaneous xanthomas, and they complain about abdominal pain after fatty meals. If severe hypertriglyceridemia (> 2,000 mg/dL) persists for extended periods, the patient is at risk of life-threatening pancreatitis. The condition can be treated by a restriction of the dietary fat intake.

Type II hyperlipoproteinemia, or **hypercholesterolemia,** is marked by an elevation of LDL. It includes FH, but multifactorial and secondary forms are far more common, affecting 2% to 8% of the

FIG. 20.10

Metabolism of LDL in normal individuals and in patients with homozygous familial hypercholesterolemia. Υ, LDL receptor; Υ, scavenger receptor; *LPL,* lipoprotein lipase; *HL,* hepatic lipase. **A,** Normal: both liver and extrahepatic tissues obtain most Υ of their cholesterol from receptor-mediated LDL uptake. The LDL-derived cholesterol inhibits endogenous synthesis at the level of HMG-CoA reductase. **B,** Familial hypercholesterolemia (FH), homozygous. LDL is redirected from parenchymal cells in liver and extrahepatic tissue to tissue macrophages. Although most cells now depend on endogenous synthesis for their cholesterol needs, the macrophages accumulate cholesterol esters, forming foam cells. These foam cells contribute to the formation of xanthomas, fatty streaks, and atherosclerotic lesions.

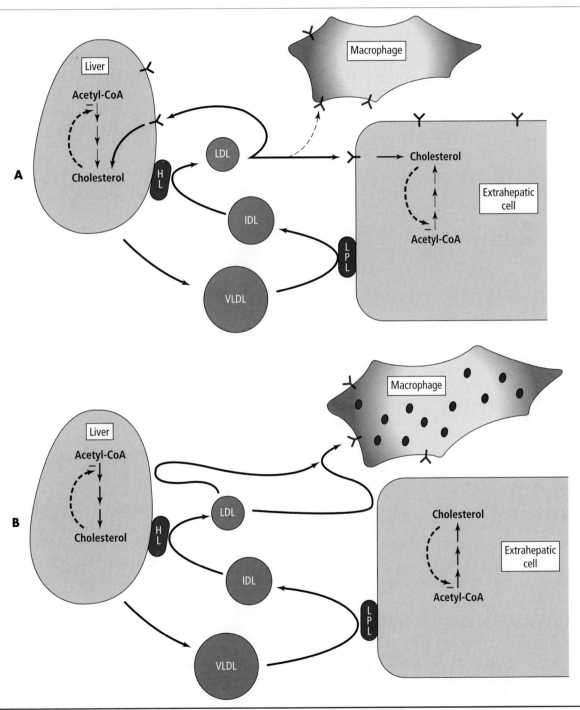

TABLE 20.5

Important determinants for hyperlipidemia and atherosclerosis

Risk factor	Normal function	Relation to plasma lipids and atherosclerosis
Lipoprotein lipase (LPL)	Hydrolysis of triglycerides in chylomicrons and VLDL	Deficiency leads to hyperchylomicronemia but no atherosclerosis
Hepatic lipase (HL)	Hydrolysis of triglycerides and phosphoglycerides in HDL and remnant particles; possibly facilitates hepatic uptake of chylomicron remnants and transfer of cholesterol esters from HDL to the liver	Activity is inversely related to the plasma HDL concentration; lower in females than in males; complete deficiency causes severe hypercholesterolemia, hypertriglyceridemia, and possibly increased atherosclerosis
ApoB-100	Major structural apolipoprotein of VLDL and LDL; ligand of the "LDL receptor"	High in patients with type II or type IV hyperlipoproteinemia; high levels are associated with high atherosclerosis risk
ApoA-I	Major apolipoprotein of HDL; mediates binding of HDL to cells, facilitates transfer of unesterified cholesterol from cell to HDL	High level of apoA-I−(but not apoA-I−*and* apoA-II−) containing HDL is associated with decreased atherosclerosis risk; higher in females than males; low in patients with CHD and their relatives; high in octagenarians
ApoE	Cellular uptake of remnant particles; stimulation of cholesterol transfer from cells to HDL	Homozygosity for apoE-2 causes dysbetalipoproteinemia; knockout mice lacking apoE have impaired flux of cholesterol from cells to HDL and develop rampant atherosclerosis
LDL receptor (apoB-100/ apoE receptor)	Cellular uptake of LDL, in both liver and extrahepatic tissues	Deficiency leads to high LDL and atherosclerosis
Lecithin-cholesterol acyl transferase (LCAT)	Formation of cholesterol esters in HDL	Homozygous deficiency leads to moderately increased atherosclerosis risk
Cholesterol ester transfer protein (CETP)	Transfer of cholesterol esters from HDL to triglyceride-rich lipoproteins; activated in the presence of LPL	Inversely related to the plasma HDL level; raised in most conditions predisposing to atherosclerosis; animal species with low CETP are at low atherosclerosis risk

total population. In some patients only LDL is elevated (type IIa); others have a combined elevation of LDL and VLDL (type IIb). Weight gain and obesity, diabetes mellitus, and a diet high in cholesterol and saturated fat are the main culprits, but genetic factors other than a deficiency of LDL receptors also are involved. *This pattern is a major risk factor for atherosclerosis and CHD.*

Type III hyperlipoproteinemia (dysbetalipoproteinemia) is caused by homozygosity for apoE2, a genetic variant of apoE that does not bind to hepatic apoE receptors. This results in the accumulation

TABLE 20.6

The five hyperlipoproteinemia phenotypes

Type	Name	Plasma lipids		Fraction elevated	Incidence	Causes
		Triglyceride	Cholesterol			
I	Hyperchylomicronemia	↑↑↑	(↑)	Chylomicrons	Rare	Inherited deficiency of LPL or apoC-II, systemic lupus erythematosus, or unknown
II	Hypercholesterolemia	(↑)	↑↑	LDL	Common	Primary: familial hypercholesterol-emia; secondary: obesity, poor dietary habits, hypothyroidism, diabetes mellitus, nephrotic syn-drome
III	Dysbetalipoproteinemia	↑	↑	Chylomicron remnants, VLDL rem-nants	Rare	Homozygosity for apoE2 (does not bind to hepatic apoE receptors), combined with poor dietary habits
IV	Hypertriglyceridemia	↑↑	↑	VLDL	Common	Diabetes mellitus, obesity, alcohol-ism, poor dietary habits
V		↑↑	↑	Chylomicrons, VLDL	Rare	Obesity, diabetes mellitus, alcohol-ism, oral contra-ceptives

of chylomicron remnants and IDL-like VLDL remnants in the blood. The presence of *cholesterol-rich, β-migrating lipoproteins with VLDL-like density* in a hyperlipidemic patient is diagnostic for type III hyperlipoproteinemia. The remnant particles are phagocytized by reticuloendothelial cells, which thereby are converted to lipid-laden foam cells. Palmar xanthomas and tuboeruptive xanthomas on knees, elbows, and buttocks are typical. Atherosclerosis shows a predilection for peripheral arteries, but CHD is increased as well. Although 1% of the population has the offending apoE genotype, only 2% to 10% of these persons

actually become hyperlipidemic. Most of them respond well to dietary management.

Elevations of VLDL (**type IV hyperlipoproteinemia**) are very common. Although triglycerides are elevated to a greater extent than is cholesterol, some hypercholesterolemia usually is present, and *the incidence of atherosclerosis is increased*. Obesity, type II diabetes mellitus, alcoholism, progesterone-rich contraceptives, and excess dietary carbohydrate (especially sugar) all can lead to elevated VLDL.

Patients with **type V hyperlipoproteinemia** have elevations of both chylomicrons and VLDL.

Although this pattern often has a familial background, it also is associated with uncontrolled diabetes mellitus, alcoholism, obesity, and kidney disease. Dietary treatment is effective.

The concept of **familial combined hyperlipoproteinemia** is derived from the observation that the two most common patterns of hyperlipoproteinemia, types II and IV, often occur in different members of the same family. This observation has been explained by the presence of a dominantly inherited gene that causes an increased synthesis of apoB-100 in the liver. Depending on a variety of genetic and environmental factors, either the type II or the type IV pattern is expressed in these patients. Approximately 1% of the population and 10% of all patients with premature CHD are thought to have this disorder.

Both diet and drugs affect plasma lipoproteins

If a hyperlipoproteinemia is caused by an underlying disease such as diabetes mellitus or alcoholism, the treatment of this disease is, of course, the principal therapeutic approach. In most other cases, dietary modification is the treatment of choice. Most hyperlipidemias respond to dietary changes, but hypertriglyceridemias often are more responsive than hypercholesterolemias. The recommendation for hypertriglyceridemic patients, who usually have the type IV pattern with increased VLDL, is *a reduction of caloric intake, alcohol, and simple carbohydrates.* In obese patients, in particular, a balanced weight-reduction diet is likely to normalize the lipoprotein pattern without the need for any further treatment.

Dietary changes are effective in many hypercholesterolemic patients as well—except those with FH, who generally require drug treatment. A diet with *reduced cholesterol and saturated fat and increased dietary fiber* is recommended, and a weight-reduction diet is indicated for obese patients.

Dietary treatment is of little practical use because most patients do not comply with a physician-imposed diet. Therefore drug treatments, which require less-dramatic lifestyle changes than a diet, often are required, especially for hypercholesterolemic patients. Two important drug classes reduce the plasma cholesterol level by interfering with critical steps in cholesterol metabolism:

1. **Lovastatin (mevinoline)** is an inhibitor of HMG-CoA reductase. Endogenous cholesterol synthesis is blocked, and the cells become dependent on the supply of cholesterol from plasma lipoproteins. Indeed, *the lack of endogenously synthesized cholesterol in the cell leads to an increased synthesis of LDL receptors* (Figs. 20.5 and 20.11). By this mechanism, *HMG-CoA reductase inhibitors reduce LDL cholesterol with little effect on HDL cholesterol.*

2. **Cholestyramine** is an insoluble, nonabsorbable anion exchanger that affects cholesterol metabolism by binding bile salts in the lumen of the small intestine. This prevents their absorption and thereby interrupts their enterohepatic circulation (see Chapter 19): instead of returning to the liver, the bile salts are excreted in the stools. Because bile acids regulate their own synthesis by feedback inhibition of 7α-hydroxylase (see Chapter 19), the diminished supply of bile acids by the enterohepatic circulation *increases the conversion of cholesterol to bile acids by the liver.* The resulting depletion of the cellular cholesterol pool leads to an *upregulation of hepatic LDL receptors* and a reduction of the LDL (but not HDL) level in the plasma (Fig. 20.11, B).

As an alternative to drug treatments, a **high-fiber diet** can be used as a moderately effective means of decreasing LDL cholesterol. At least some types of dietary fiber are thought to reduce the absorption of bile acids from the ileum, in part simply by increasing the bulk of the intestinal contents. As in

FIG. 20.11

Effects of a bile acid binding resin (cholestyramine) and an HMG-CoA reductase inhibitor (lovastatin) on cholesterol metabolism. *LPL*, Extrahepatic lipoprotein lipase; Y, LDL receptor. **A,** Normal or hyperlipidemic. **B,** Effect of cholestyramine: hepatic LDL receptors are upregulated. The liver removes an increased amount of LDL to obtain cholesterol for bile acid synthesis. **C,** Effect of lovastatin: LDL receptors are upregulated in all tissues. The cells require an increased amount of LDL cholesterol because they are unable to obtain cholesterol from endogenous synthesis.

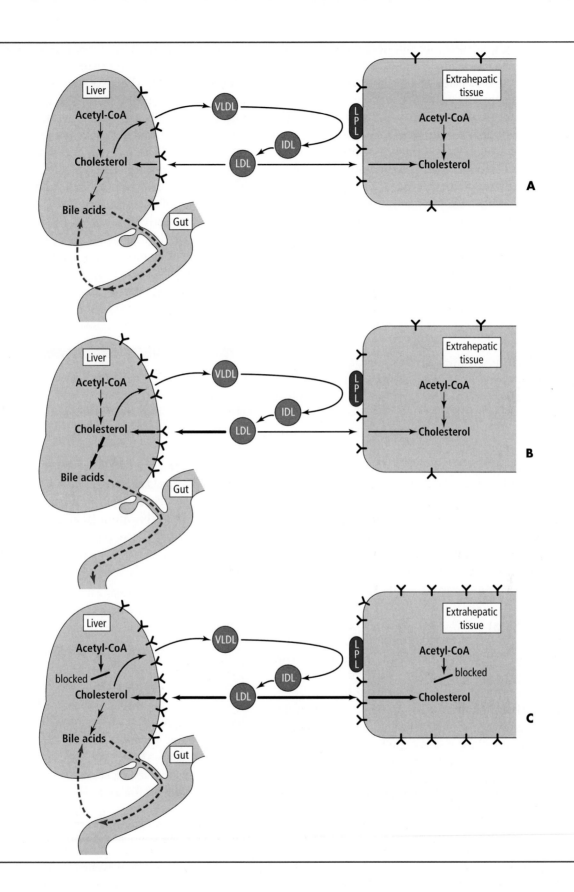

the case of cholestyramine, the increased excretion of bile acids leads to an increased conversion of cholesterol to bile acids and an upregulation of hepatic LDL receptors.

Antioxidant vitamins may be useful, too. The oxidation of LDL facilitates its uptake through macrophage scavenger receptors, so antioxidants are expected to reduce lipid accumulation in tissue macrophages, even in the face of continued high LDL levels. Antioxidant vitamins such as ascorbic acid and vitamin E are being evaluated for their possible benefit in the prevention of atherosclerosis and CHD. These agents are not only nontoxic but also less expensive than the lipid-lowering drugs.

SUMMARY

The plasma lipoproteins are noncovalent aggregates of lipid and protein that effect the interorgan transport of triglycerides, phospholipids, and cholesterol. There are three highways of lipoprotein-based lipid transport:

1. Lipids of dietary origin are transported from the intestine to other tissues as constituents of chylomicrons. Most of their triglycerides are hydrolyzed by lipoprotein lipase in adipose tissue, muscle, and other tissues, and the chylomicron remnants thus formed are endocytosed by the liver.
2. Lipids from endogenous synthesis in the liver are released as constituents of very-low-density lipoproteins (VLDLs). The VLDL triglycerides are hydrolyzed by lipoprotein lipase, and some of the resulting remnant particles are processed to low-density lipoprotein (LDL). Most of the triglyceride in normal fasting serum is present in VLDL; most of the cholesterol is in LDL. LDL is endocytosed both by the liver and by extrahepatic tissues.
3. The transport of cholesterol from extrahepatic tissues to the liver is known as reverse cholesterol transport. Cellular cholesterol is transferred to HDL, where it is esterified by the HDL-associated enzyme lecithin-cholesterol acyl transferase (LCAT). Most of the resulting cholesterol esters are transferred to other lipoproteins, which in turn are endocytosed by the liver.

Hypercholesterolemia is a risk factor for atherosclerosis. Abnormal lipid deposits in the form of a fatty streak result from the excessive uptake of LDL by macrophages in the intima of large arteries, and some fatty streaks develop into atherosclerotic lesions. Lipid accumulates only if the uptake of cholesterol from LDL exceeds its removal by HDL. Therefore an elevated level of LDL is a risk factor for the formation of abnormal lipid deposits and the development of atherosclerotic lesions. HDL, conversely, is protective.

Some hyperlipidemias are caused by major genetic defects, but most cases are the result of lipid-elevating lifestyles and polygenic inheritance, or are secondary to such diseases as diabetes mellitus, hypothyroidism, and alcoholism.

Further Reading

Bolton CH: Lipid disorders: In: Holton JB, editor: *The inherited metabolic diseases*, 2nd ed. Churchill Livingstone, New York, 1994, pp. 461-489.

Gotto AM Jr, Farmer JA: Risk factors for coronary artery disease. In: Braunwald E, editor: *Heart disease*, 4th ed., vol. 2. W. B. Saunders, Philadelphia, 1992, pp. 1125-1160.

Guyton JR, Gotto AM Jr: The pathogenesis of atherosclerosis: lipid metabolism. In: Loscalzo J, Creager MA, Dzau VJ, editors: *Vascular medicine*. Little, Brown, Boston, 1992, pp. 345-370.

Hopkins PN, Wu LL, Williams RR: Dyslipidemias. In: Noe DA, Rock RC, editors: *Laboratory medicine*. Williams & Wilkins, Baltimore, 1994, pp. 476-511.

Ross R: The pathogenesis of atherosclerosis: a perspective for the 1990s. *Nature* 362, 801-809, 1993.

Schaefer EJ: The hyperlipoproteinemias and other lipoprotein disorders. In: Loscalzo J, Creager MA, Dzau VJ, editors: *Vascular medicine*, Little, Brown, Boston, 1992, pp. 575-594.

Scriver CR, Beaudet ALB, Sly WS, Valle D, editors: *The metabolic basis of inherited disease*, 6th ed., vol. 1. McGraw-Hill, New York, 1989, pp. 1129-1302.

Tall AR: Plasma cholesterol ester transfer protein. *J Lipid Res* 34, 1255-1271, 1993.

Winder AJ: Hyperlipidaemia. In: Williams D, Marks V, editors: *Scientific foundations of biochemistry in clinical practice*, 2nd ed. Butterworth Heinemann, Oxford, 1994, pp. 601-613.

1. A pharmaceutical company wants to develop a drug for the treatment of type IV hyperlipoproteinemia. The most promising approach would be an agent that
   A. Increases the synthesis of apoB-100 in the liver
   B. Inhibits the synthesis of apoE
   C. Stimulates the hormone-sensitive adipose tissue lipase
   D. Inhibits lipoprotein lipase
   E. Inhibits triglyceride synthesis in the liver

2. The use of cholestyramine in hyperlipidemic patients is beneficial because this treatment causes an increased activity of the liver enzyme
   A. HMG-CoA reductase
   B. Lipoprotein lipase
   C. Hepatic lipase
   D. 7α-Hydroxylase
   E. Lecithin-cholesterol acyl transferase

3. Mevinoline (lovastatin) is a commonly used drug that inhibits the endogenous synthesis of cholesterol. This leads, initially, to a reduced level of free cholesterol in the cell. The reduced level of cellular cholesterol, in turn, leads to
   A. Increased activity of acyl-CoA–cholesterol acyl transferase
   B. Increased synthesis of LDL receptors in most tissues
   C. Reduced synthesis of LDL receptors in most tissues
   D. Increased transfer of cholesterol esters from the cell to HDL
   E. Increased synthesis of bile acids by the liver

4. If you are looking for ways to increase the reverse transport of cholesterol from peripheral tissues to the liver, the best bet would be a drug that
   A. Inhibits the synthesis of LDL receptors
   B. Inhibits the hepatic lipase
   C. Inhibits lipoprotein lipase
   D. Stimulates the transcription of the apoB gene
   E. Stimulates the transcription of the apoA-I gene

Chapter 21

Amino Acid
Metabolism

Amino acids are used for three major purposes:

1. *They are substrates for the generation of metabolic energy.* The catabolism of the amino acids in dietary proteins yields approximately 5.5 kcal/g, and most people in Western countries derive close to 20% of their metabolic energy from protein.
2. *They are required for protein synthesis.* Our body proteins are degraded and resynthesized continuously, so pools of free amino acids have to be maintained in all nucleated cells.
3. *They are substrates for the synthesis of many biosynthetic products* including heme, purines, pyrimidines, several coenzymes, melanin, and the biogenic amines.

Dietary proteins are a more-than-sufficient source of amino acids for most people, but 11 of the 20 amino acids also can be synthesized in the human body. Those that cannot be synthesized are known as the **essential amino acids.** They include:

Valine	Threonine
Leucine	Methionine
Isoleucine	Lysine
Phenylalanine	Histidine
Tryptophan	

The nonessential amino acids are synthesized either from common metabolic intermediates or from other amino acids. Tyrosine, for example, is made from the essential amino acid phenylalanine; cysteine requires methionine as a precursor. Therefore the nutritional requirements often are specified for "phenylalanine + tyrosine" and "methionine + cysteine."

In this chapter we discuss the fate of the amino nitrogen during amino acid catabolism, the pathways by which amino acids are degraded to simple nitrogen-free metabolic intermediates, and the biosynthesis of the nonessential amino acids.

THE FATE OF THE AMINO NITROGEN

All amino acids can be degraded to simple nitrogen-free products. The nitrogen is removed at an early stage of amino acid catabolism and eventually is converted to the excretory product **urea.** Before turning to the fates of the carbons, we have to discuss the handling of the amino nitrogen during amino acid catabolism.

Most amino acids in the body are present as constituents of proteins

Free amino acids are not abundant in tissues and body fluids. In the blood, for example, the concentrations of the 20 amino acids combined are approximately 20 to 30 mg/dL, only one quarter of the blood glucose level. Proteins, on the other hand, weigh in at approximately 10 kg in an adult human. Close to half of this is in muscle tissue.

Figure 21.1 shows the major metabolic uses of amino acids and proteins. The intake of dietary protein is variable, but approximately 100 g/day is typical for Western countries. From 250 to 300 g of body protein are synthesized per day, and the same amount of body protein is degraded. The life expectancy of an average protein molecule is there-

FIG. 21.1

Metabolic interrelationships of amino acids.

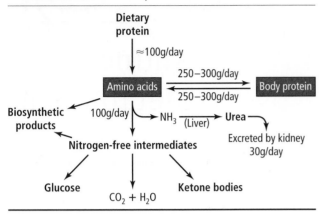

FIG. 21.2

Nitrogen balance in different normal and abnormal states. **A,** Normal adult: nitrogen equilibrium. **B,** Growth, pregnancy: positive nitrogen balance. **C,** Protein deficiency: negative nitrogen balance. **D,** Essential amino acid deficiency: negative nitrogen balance. **E,** Wasting diseases, burns, trauma: negative nitrogen balance.

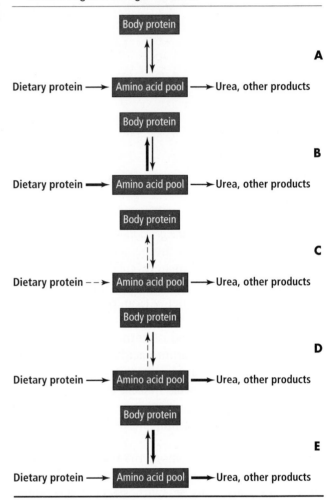

fore 35 to 40 days, but this differs widely from one protein to another: most metabolic enzymes live for only one or a few days, but most plasma proteins circulate for periods of 1 to 3 weeks. Hemoglobin survives for 120 days; collagen can last up to several years in some tissues; the lens proteins have to last for a lifetime.

When amino acids are degraded, *their nitrogen is incorporated in* **urea,** a soluble, nontoxic product that is readily excreted by the kidneys. The carbon skeletons of the amino acids are converted to simple nitrogen-free products. *The* **glucogenic amino acids** *are degraded to intermediates of TCA cycle or glycolysis, and the* **ketogenic amino acids** *are degraded to acetyl-CoA.* These products can be used for gluconeogenesis and ketogenesis, respectively. Some of the larger amino acids are both glucogenic and ketogenic.

- purely ketogenic amino acids: leucine and lysine
- both glucogenic and ketogenic: tryptophan, phenylalanine, tyrosine, isoleucine
- all other amino acids can be considered purely glucogenic

There is no specific storage of amino acids or proteins, but part of the body protein can be degraded in times of need.

The nitrogen balance is an important index of amino acid and protein metabolism

A 100-g sample of dietary protein contains approximately 16 g of nitrogen. Of this ingested nitrogen,

approximately 83% eventually leaves the body as urea, 7% as ammonium ion, and 10% as organic waste products such as uric acid and creatinine. Approximately 95% of the urea and a large majority of the other nitrogenous wastes are excreted in the urine, but 1 to 2 g of nitrogen from undigested protein also are excreted in stools.

The **nitrogen balance** is determined by comparing the nitrogen entering the body with that leaving it. A normal adult with adequate protein intake should be in *nitrogen equilibrium* (Fig. 21.2): the amounts of the incoming and outgoing nitrogen are

BOX 21.1

$$\text{Glutamate} \quad \xrightleftharpoons[\text{Glutamate dehydrogenase}]{\substack{\text{H}_2\text{O}, \\ \text{NAD(P)}^+ \qquad \text{NAD(P)H, H}^+}} \quad \alpha\text{-Ketoglutarate}$$

Glutamate

α-Ketoglutarate

equal, and the amount of body protein remains constant.

A *positive nitrogen balance* is observed when nitrogen intake exceeds nitrogen excretion; it implies that the amount of body protein increases. Growing children, pregnant women, and bodybuilders have a positive nitrogen balance. These situations are associated with an increased requirement for dietary protein.

A *negative nitrogen balance* is observed in dietary protein deficiency. Even the protein-starved body degrades 30 to 40 g of amino acids every day. This amount defines the dietary requirement: if the supply drops below this limit, a negative nitrogen balance is inevitable and body protein is lost. Essential amino acid deficiency has the same effect because protein synthesis is impaired even if only one of the essential amino acids is lacking.

A negative nitrogen balance also is seen in patients with metastatic carcinoma or severe infections, after trauma or surgery, and in burn patients. The negative nitrogen balance in these patients is caused by hormones: *the stress hormones cortisol and epinephrine favor protein degradation over protein synthesis,* and they stimulate the use of the liberated amino acids for gluconeogenesis by the liver. Also some **cytokines**—biologically active products released by white blood cells in a variety of disease states—have metabolic effects similar to those of the stress hormones.

The amino group of the amino acids is released as ammonia

During amino acid catabolism, the amino nitrogen is initially released as ammonia. The most important

ammonia-forming reaction is the oxidative deamination of glutamate by glutamate dehydrogenase as shown in Box 21.1. The enzyme is widespread in mammalian tissues, with highest activity in the liver. The reaction is freely reversible and therefore can function in both the synthesis and the degradation of glutamate. Either NAD or NADP can serve as a cosubstrate, but NAD^+ is used mainly for glutamate degradation, and NADPH for its synthesis. The glutamate dehydrogenase reaction implies that *glutamate is both a nonessential and a glucogenic amino acid.*

Most of the other amino acids do not form ammonia directly; *they transfer their α-amino group to α-ketoglutarate to form glutamate.* The enzymes catalyzing these reactions are called **transaminases** or **aminotransferases.** Examples are shown in Box 21.2. At least a dozen different transaminases, specific for different amino acid substrates, have been described in mammalian tissues. Most of them use glutamate or α-ketoglutarate as one of their substrates or products, and the reactions generally are reversible. *All amino acids except threonine, lysine, and proline can be transaminated.*

Transaminases always require **pyridoxal phosphate (PLP,** the coenzyme form of vitamin B_6) as their prosthetic group. PLP is bound to the active site of the enzyme both by electrostatic interactions and by a Schiff base bond (aldimine) with a lysine side chain of the apoprotein. The reaction follows a **ping-pong mechanism:** the prosthetic group is modified chemically during the reaction, and the first product is released before the second substrate binds (Fig. 21.3). The formation of an aldimine intermediate with the amino group of the amino acid substrate is typical for all reactions of amino acid

BOX 21.2

Alanine + α-Ketoglutarate $\xrightleftharpoons[\text{Alanine transaminase}]{B_6}$ Pyruvate + Glutamate

Alanine   α-Ketoglutarate   Pyruvate   Glutamate

Aspartate + α-Ketoglutarate $\xrightleftharpoons[\text{Aspartate transaminase}]{B_6}$ Oxaloacetate + Glutamate

Aspartate   α-Ketoglutarate   Oxaloacetate   Glutamate

BOX 21.3

$$\text{Amino acid} \xrightarrow{\quad\quad} \alpha\text{-Ketoacid}$$

H$_2$O$_2$ ← O$_2$

FAD (FMN) → FADH$_2$ (FMNH$_2$)

H$_2$O → NH$_4^+$

metabolism in which pyridoxal phosphate participates.

By successive transamination and oxidative deamination, the nitrogen of the α-amino group effectively is released as ammonia:

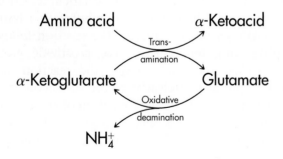

Amino acid → α-Ketoacid

Trans-amination

α-Ketoglutarate ← Glutamate

Oxidative deamination

NH$_4^+$

An alternative route is provided by L-**amino acid oxidase** and D-**amino acid oxidase,** two peroxisomal flavoproteins with broad substrate specificities as shown in Box 21.3. Both enzymes are found in liver and kidney. D-Amino acid oxidase (cofactor: FAD) is present in far higher activity than L-amino acid oxidase (cofactor: FMN). These enzymes are not important for the degradation of the common L-amino acids. Their main function is the metabolism of unusual amino acids, especially D-amino acids of bacterial origin. Thanks to D-amino acid oxidase, most L-amino acids can be replaced by their corresponding D-amino acids in the diet, for example, see Box 21.4.

FIG. 21.3

Mechanism of transamination reactions. **A,** Pyridoxal phosphate (PLP) is bound to a lysine side chain in the apoprotein by an aldimine ("Schiff base") bond. **B,** The catalytic cycle. The transaminases are a classical example of a ping-pong mechanism. Note that the transamination is actually a sequence of two reactions in which the prosthetic group of the enzyme participates as a reactant.

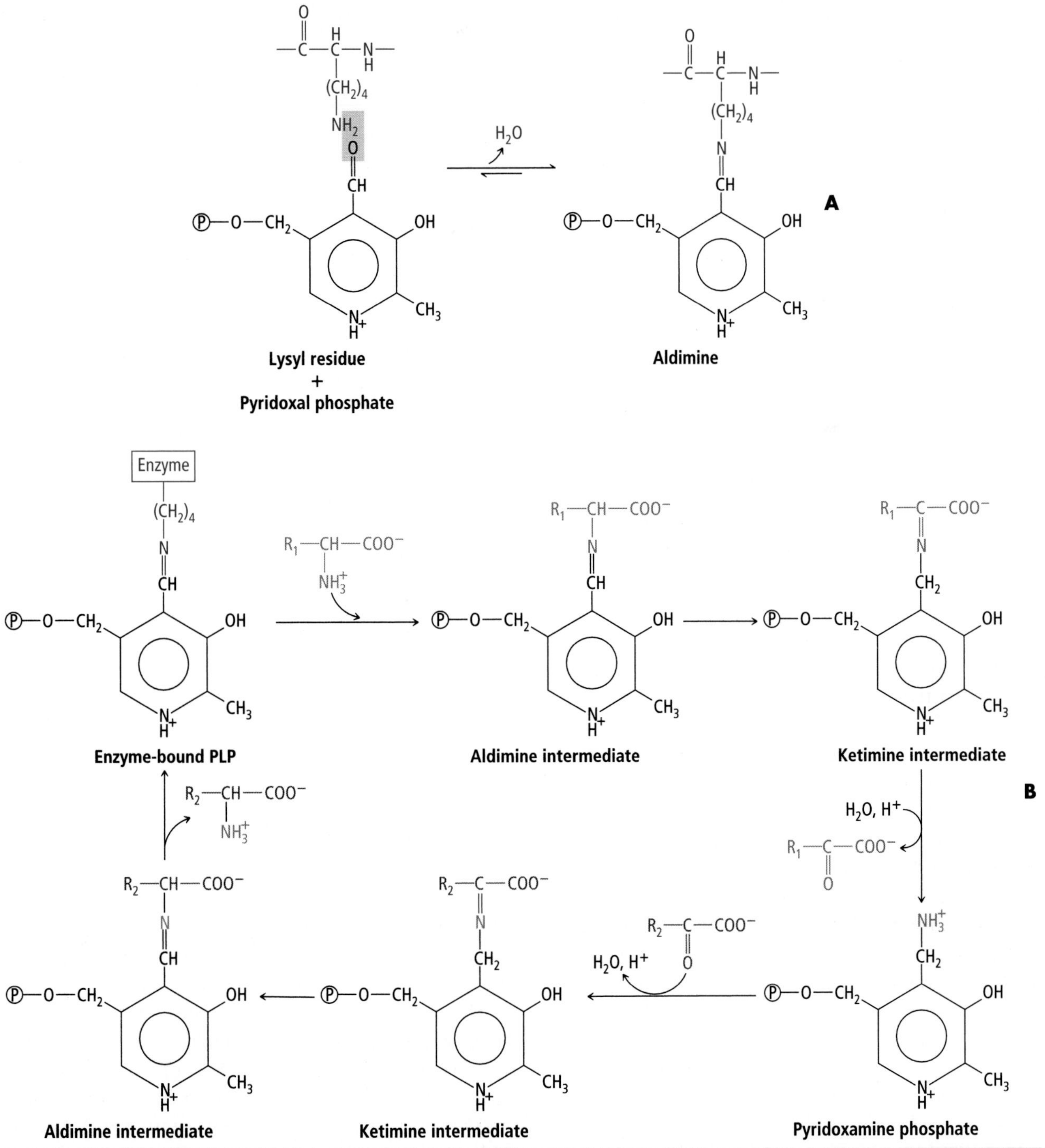

A

Lysyl residue
+
Pyridoxal phosphate

Aldimine

Enzyme-bound PLP

Aldimine intermediate

Ketimine intermediate

B

Aldimine intermediate

Ketimine intermediate

Pyridoxamine phosphate

BOX 21.4

$$\text{D-Methionine} \xrightarrow[\substack{\text{D-Amino acid}\\ \text{oxidase}}]{\substack{O_2,\\ H_2O \quad \substack{H_2O_2,\\ NH_4^+}}} \alpha\text{-Keto analog} \xrightarrow[\text{Transamination}]{\text{Glutamate} \quad \alpha\text{-Ketoglutarate}} \text{L-Methionine}$$

BOX 21.5

$$\underset{\text{Urea}}{H_2N-\overset{\overset{\textstyle O}{\|}}{C}-NH_2} \xrightarrow[2\,H_2O]{\text{Urease}} \underset{\text{Carbonic acid}}{HO-\overset{\overset{\textstyle O}{\|}}{C}-OH} + 2\,NH_3$$

BOX 21.6

$$\text{Dietary protein} \xrightarrow[\text{enzymes}]{\text{Digestive}} \text{Amino acids} \xrightarrow[\text{In tissues (liver, muscle, etc.)}]{\text{Nitrogen-free products}} NH_3 \xrightarrow[\text{Liver}]{CO_2} \text{Urea} \rightarrow \text{Urine}$$

Amino nitrogen is excreted as urea

Ammonia is a hazardous waste: it is neurotoxic even in low concentrations, and therefore it has to be disposed of without delay. Aquatic animals can release ammonia rapidly through their gills (they are **ammonotelic**), and reptiles, birds, and insects convert it to uric acid (they are **uricotelic**). We detoxify our ammonia by turning it into urea (we are **ureotelic**).

Urea is the diamide of carbonic acid. This dry statement implies that *urea can be cleaved into carbonic acid and ammonia*. This cleavage is effected by **urease**, an enzyme formed by some bacteria and plants. This reaction, shown in Box 21.5, does not occur normally in the human body, but it is important in urinary tract infections caused by the urease-producing bacterium *Proteus mirabilis*: the ammonia formed by the bacterial urease alkalinizes the urine, and this results in the precipitation of insoluble magne-

sium ammonium phosphate and the formation of large kidney stones, which can cause serious damage. The sharp smell of latrines is caused by ammonia formed by urease-producing bacteria.

Urea is formed in the liver, transported to the kidneys, and excreted in the urine as shown in Box 21.6. Urea production is directly proportional to the amount of dietary protein, reaching a respectable 33 g on a 100-g/day protein diet. Its urinary concentration is between 1% and 5%, depending on urinary volume and the amount of dietary protein.

The blood urea level is measured as **blood urea nitrogen (BUN)**. In health, the BUN is 250 to 700 μM (8 to 20 mg/dL). It is either low or normal in liver failure, when urea synthesis is impaired, and it rises sharply in patients with renal failure. This situation is called **uremia** (literally, "urine in the blood"). Although urea is not responsible for most of the clinical manifestations in uremic patients, BUN is a convenient measure of the reten-

BOX 21.7

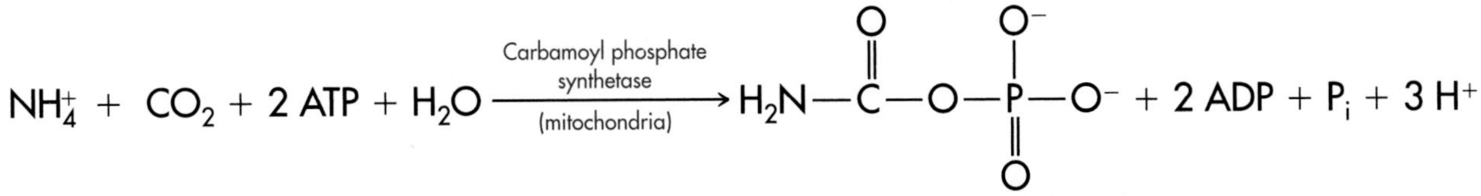

$$NH_4^+ + CO_2 + 2 \text{ ATP} + H_2O \xrightarrow[\text{(mitochondria)}]{\text{Carbamoyl phosphate} \atop \text{synthetase}} H_2N-\overset{\overset{\displaystyle O}{\|}}{C}-O-\overset{\overset{\displaystyle O^-}{|}}{\underset{\underset{\displaystyle O}{\|}}{P}}-O^- + 2 \text{ ADP} + P_i + 3 H^+$$

Carbamoyl phosphate

tion of nitrogenous wastes in patients with renal disease.

Urea is synthesized in the urea cycle

The liver synthesizes urea in the **urea cycle.** One of the substrates of the urea cycle is **carbamoyl phosphate,** which is synthesized from ammonia, carbon dioxide, and ATP as shown in Box 21.7. The use of two ATPs makes this reaction irreversible. The enzyme is present in very high concentration in liver mitochondria, and its K_m for ammonia $(250~\mu M)$ is not much higher than the physiological ammonia concentration (normal blood ammonia = 30 to 60 μM). These properties enable the enzyme *to remove ammonia quantitatively from its environment.*

In the first reaction of the urea cycle proper (Fig. 21.4), carbamoyl phosphate reacts with **ornithine** to form **citrulline.** Citrulline then forms **argininosuccinate** by reacting with aspartate. In the next reaction, the carbon skeleton of aspartate is released as fumarate while its nitrogen remains in the cycle, forming one of the nitrogens in the side chain of **arginine.** Finally, urea is formed by the hydrolytic cleavage of the guanidino group in arginine by **arginase,** and ornithine is regenerated. Only the synthesis of carbamoyl phosphate and citrulline is mitochondrial; the remaining reactions take place in the cytoplasm.

One of the two nitrogens in urea is derived from ammonia via carbamoyl phosphate, and the other is introduced by aspartate. This second nitrogen is derived either from ammonia (through the glutamate dehydrogenase reaction followed by transamination with oxaloacetate) or directly from transamination reactions as shown in Box 21.8. Four high-energy phosphate bonds are required for the synthesis of one urea molecule. Two ATPs are converted to ADPs in the carbamoyl phosphate synthetase reaction,

FIG. 21.4

The reactions of the urea cycle.

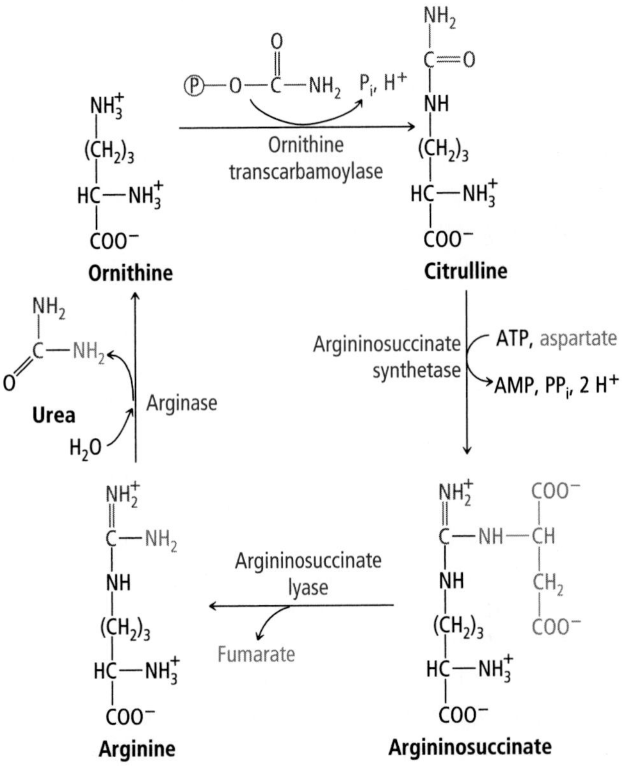

and another two phosphate bonds are consumed for the formation of argininosuccinate when one ATP is hydrolyzed to AMP and inorganic pyrophosphate. *The nitrogen is committed to urea synthesis because those two reactions by which it enters the cycle are made irreversible by ATP hydrolysis.*

Failure of the urea cycle causes hyperammonemia and CNS dysfunction

Deficiencies of urea cycle enzymes are rare, recessively inherited diseases that are characterized by

BOX 21.8

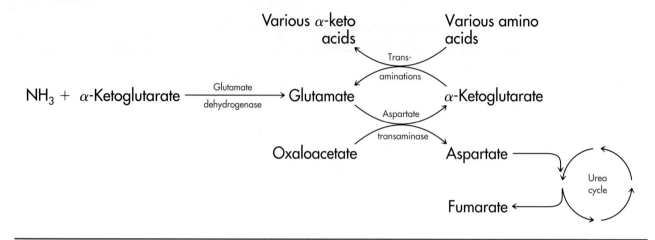

hyperammonemia and encephalopathy. Feeding difficulties, vomiting, ataxia, lethargy or irritability, poor intellectual development, and a tendency for coma and death are common to all of these disorders. The condition is aggravated by dietary protein, so many patients spontaneously develop an aversion to protein-rich foods. Besides ammonia, glutamine commonly is elevated because excess ammonia is diverted into glutamine synthesis. The immediate substrate of the deficient enzyme also is elevated in blood and urine.

A far more common cause of hyperammonemia is advanced **liver cirrhosis.** This condition is an end point of many disease processes, alcoholism being the most common cause in Western countries. It is characterized by *a progressive loss of hepatocytes, which are replaced by fibrous connective tissue.* Not only is there a loss of liver function, but the proliferating connective tissue also impairs blood flow through the liver. This results in portal hypertension and the development of a collateral circulation: venous channels in the lower esophagus and in the periumbilical, rectal, and retroperitoneal areas dilate, shunting blood from the portal vein to the systemic circulation. Portal hypertension is dangerous because it can result in fatal hemorrhage from the dilated lower esophageal veins.

The biochemical derangements in cirrhotic patients lead to **hepatic encephalopathy,** also known as **portal-systemic encephalopathy** because the shunting of blood around the cirrhotic liver is important in its pathogenesis. It is manifested by slur-

ring of speech, blurring of vision, motor incoordination (ataxia), a characteristic coarse, flapping tremor (asterixis), and mental derangements. The condition may progress to **hepatic coma** and death. Although other biochemical abnormalities have been implicated as well, *hyperammonemia is a major cause of the CNS disorder.*

For long-term management, *a low-protein diet is the mainstay of treatment.* The replacement of essential amino acids by their corresponding α-ketoacids is another effective (although expensive) dietary manipulation, aimed at reducing the total nitrogen intake without precipitating essential amino acid deficiencies. Because of the transamination reactions, most of the essential amino acids are no longer essential when their corresponding α-ketoacids are present in the diet.

Another treatment strategy is the exploitation of alternative routes of nitrogen excretion. **Benzoic acid** and **phenylacetic acid** are used clinically because they become conjugated with glycine and glutamine, respectively, as shown in Box 21.9. The conjugation products are excreted in the urine. Under normal conditions, these reactions are not important for nitrogen excretion but are part of the body's mechanisms for the disposal of unwanted organic acids from dietary sources.

Intestinal bacteria are important producers of ammonia in both health and disease: undigested dietary proteins are metabolized by bacteria in the ileum and the large intestine, and part of their nitrogen is released as ammonia. In addition, the di-

BOX 21.9

gestive secretions contain a significant amount of urea, which is cleaved to carbonic acid and ammonia by bacterial ureases. Therefore *the ammonia level is always higher in the portal blood than in the systemic circulation.* Gastrointestinal hemorrhage from peptic ulcer disease or dilated lower esophageal veins can aggravate hyperammonemia because the blood proteins entering the GI tract are a ready-made food for ammonia-producing intestinal bacteria. Sterilization of the GI tract by broad-spectrum antibiotics can be beneficial in patients with hepatic encephalopathy, although there is a danger of overgrowth by drug-resistant bacteria, with resulting enterocolitis.

Shunt surgery, in the form of a portacaval or splenorenal shunt, sometimes is performed to relieve portal hypertension and to prevent its often fatal complications. Unfortunately, these procedures can precipitate hepatic encephalopathy by further reducing hepatic blood flow. Therefore a careful evaluation of surgical candidates is absolutely essential.

THE METABOLISM OF INDIVIDUAL AMINO ACIDS

Catabolic reactions or pathways exist for all 20 amino acids, and there are biosynthetic pathways for the nonessential amino acids. In the following sections we will examine the most important reactions of individual amino acids, with special emphasis on those reactions that are affected in inborn errors of metabolism.

Alanine, aspartate, glutamate, asparagine, and glutamine are closely related to common metabolic intermediates

Some amino acids are close relatives of metabolic intermediates that we encountered in the major metabolic pathways. A typical example is alanine, which is related structurally and metabolically to pyruvate. The reversible **alanine transaminase** reaction is the only important reaction linking this amino acid to the major metabolic pathways as shown in Box 21.10. Glutamate is similarly related to α-ketoglutarate, both by transamination reactions and by oxidative deamination. Glutamine is both synthesized from and degraded to glutamate as shown in Box 21.11. Aspartate is synthesized from and degraded to oxaloacetate by reversible transamination, and asparagine is synthesized from and degraded to aspartate as shown in Box 21.12. Parenterally administered asparaginase has been used in the treatment of various malignancies. In some adult leukemias, in particular, the malignant cells are unable to synthesize asparagine and therefore have to obtain this amino acid from the blood. The injected asparagi-

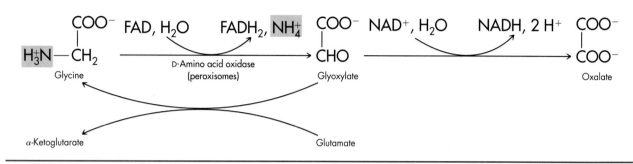

BOX 21.15

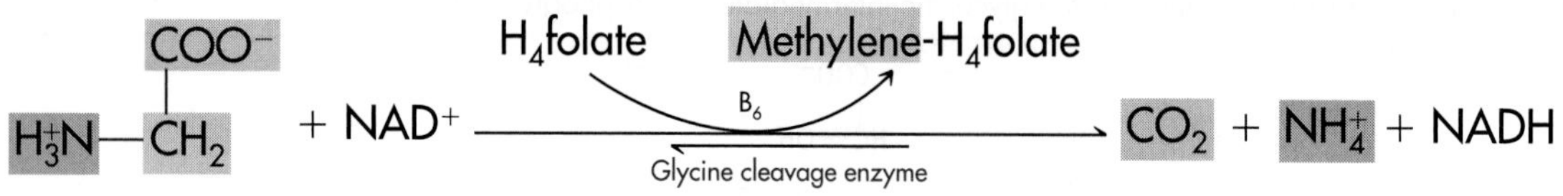

$$H_3^+N - CH_2 - COO^- + NAD^+ \xrightarrow[\text{Glycine cleavage enzyme}]{\text{H}_4\text{folate} \quad \text{Methylene-H}_4\text{folate} \atop B_6} CO_2 + NH_4^+ + NADH$$

BOX 21.16

Glycine $\xrightarrow[\text{D-Amino acid oxidase (peroxisomes)}]{\text{FAD, H}_2\text{O} \quad \text{FADH}_2, \text{NH}_4^+}$ Glyoxylate $\xrightarrow[]{\text{NAD}^+, \text{H}_2\text{O} \quad \text{NADH, 2 H}^+}$ Oxalate

α-Ketoglutarate / Glutamate

BOX 21.17

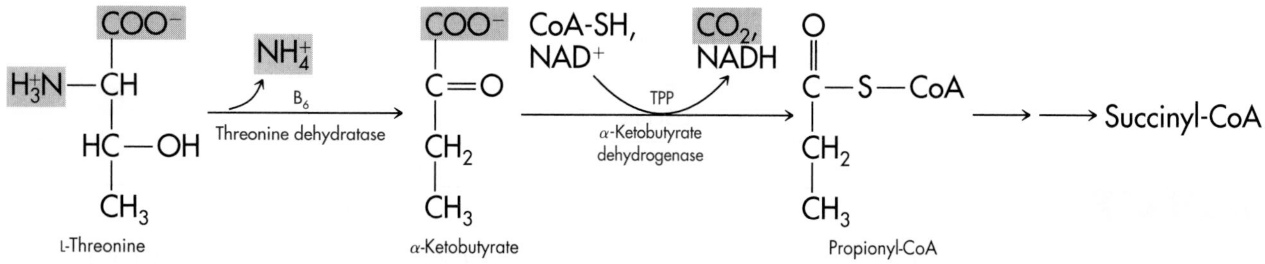

L-Threonine $\xrightarrow[\text{Threonine dehydratase}]{\text{NH}_4^+ \atop B_6}$ α-Ketobutyrate $\xrightarrow[\text{α-Ketobutyrate dehydrogenase}]{\text{CoA-SH, NAD}^+ \quad \text{CO}_2, \text{NADH} \atop \text{TPP}}$ Propionyl-CoA $\longrightarrow$ Succinyl-CoA

births) die shortly after birth with massive hyperglycinemia, and some survive with profound mental retardation.

Another reaction of glycine is the formation of **glyoxylate,** catalyzed by D-amino acid oxidase. Glyoxylate is either transaminated to glycine or oxidized to **oxalate** as shown in Box 21.16. *The precipitation of insoluble calcium oxalate is the most common cause of renal calculi.* This oxalate is derived in part from dietary sources (mostly green, leafy vegetables) and in part from endogenous synthesis.

The essential amino acid threonine can be degraded by **threonine dehydratase** in a reaction analogous to that of serine dehydratase. The resulting α-ketobutyrate is converted to propionyl-CoA by a mitochondrial multienzyme complex that re-

sembles the pyruvate dehydrogenase complex in composition, reaction mechanism, and coenzyme requirements as shown in Box 21.17. Propionyl-CoA is on the pathway of odd-chain fatty acid degradation (see Chapter 18).

Probably more important than the threonine dehydratase reaction is the oxidation to α-amino-β-ketobutyrate, which is either cleaved to acetyl-CoA and glycine or converted to pyruvate, shown in Box 21.18. Figure 21.6 summarizes the metabolic relationships of serine, glycine, and threonine.

A metabolic conversion that occurs in many bacteria but not in human tissues is the formation of **trimethylamine** from glycine shown in Box 21.19. Trimethylamine is distinguished by its scent, which resembles that of stale fish. It often is formed dur-

FIG. 21.6

Metabolism of serine, glycine, and threonine.

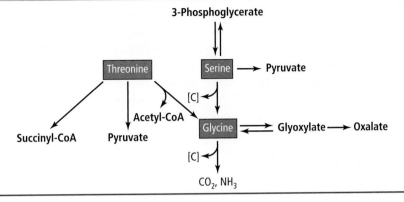

BOX 21.18

L-Threonine $\xrightarrow[\text{NAD}^+]{\text{NADH, H}^+}$ α-Amino-β-ketobutyrate

α-Amino-β-ketobutyrate $\xrightarrow{\text{CoA-SH}}$ Glycine + Acetyl-CoA

(1) Decarboxylation
(2) Transamination
(3) Oxidation
→ Pyruvate

BOX 21.19

Glycine $\xrightarrow[\text{2 SAM} \quad \text{2 SAH}]{}$ CO_2 → Trimethylamine (salt form) $\rightleftharpoons$ Trimethylamine (free base)

ing the bacterial decomposition of protein-rich substrates. The typical smell is most noticeable under alkaline conditions (for example, in the presence of soap), when the volatile free base is released from the protonated form.

Proline, arginine, ornithine, and histidine are degraded to glutamate

Proline, arginine, and ornithine are degraded to glutamate in surprisingly simple reaction sequences, as shown in Fig. 21.7. Proline can be synthesized freely from glutamate and therefore is not nutritionally essential. The capacity for arginine synthesis is limited, however, making this a "semiessential" amino acid.

Histidine is degraded to glutamate by an unrelated pathway (Fig. 21.8). Although transamination is possible, it normally is of minor importance. However, it becomes the major reaction in patients with **histidinemia**, which is caused by a recessively inherited deficiency of histidase (approximately 1 in 10,000 live births). This condition first was detected during the screening of newborns for phenylketonuria, when urinary imidazolepyruvate produced a false-positive color reaction in the ferric chloride test for urinary phenylpyruvate (see page 442). Although early reports suggested a high incidence of mental retardation and speech disorders in histidinemic children, the condition now is recognized as benign, and dietary treatment by histidine restric-

---

FIG. 21.7

Metabolism of proline, arginine, and ornithine.

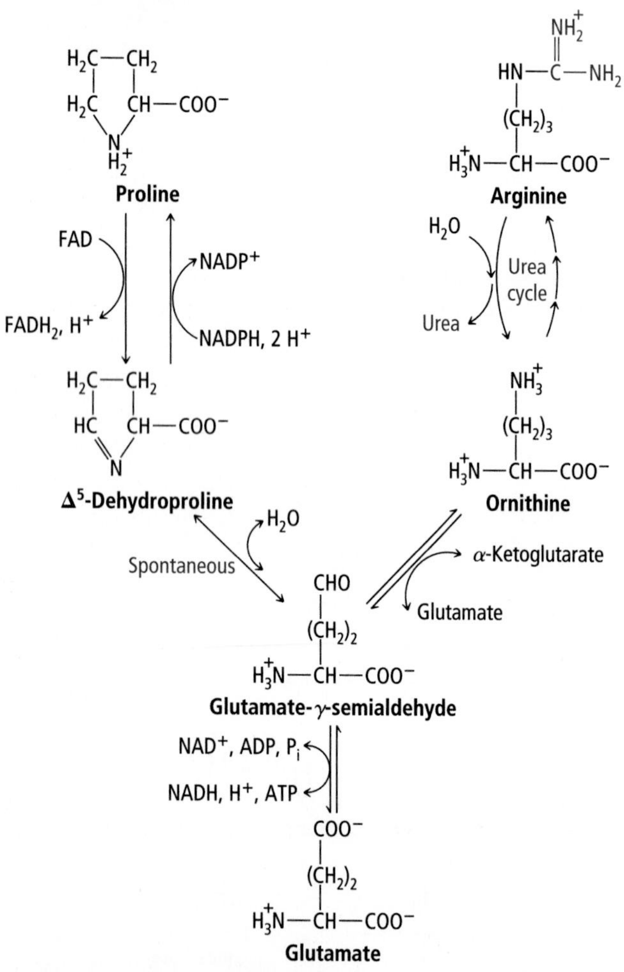

FIG. 21.8

Degradation of histidine.

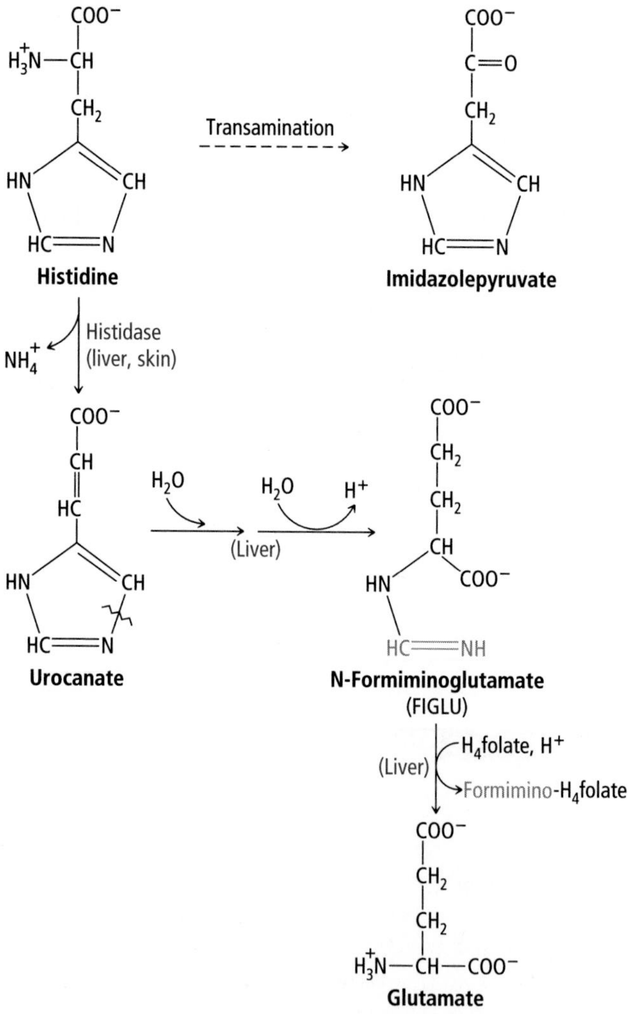

tion, which corrects the biochemical abnormality, is not required. Diagnostic procedures include the determination of serum histidine, enzyme determination in skin biopsy, and the urocanate concentration in sweat. Histidase is present only in the skin and liver, and urocanate is a normal constituent of sweat.

The last reaction in the pathway of histidine catabolism contributes a formimino group to tetrahydrofolate. The folate requirement of this reaction is exploited in a laboratory test for folate deficiency: after an oral histidine load, the excess normally is degraded without the accumulation of metabolic intermediates. In folate deficiency, however, formiminoglutamate (FIGLU) no longer is converted to glutamate and can be detected in the urine. False positives are not uncommon in this test, however, because some people lack the formimino transferase and habitually excrete FIGLU as an end product of histidine degradation. This enzyme deficiency is benign.

The catabolic pathway for histidine is irreversible, and histidine apparently cannot be synthesized in humans. Nevertheless, people can subsist on a histidine-free diet for many weeks without apparent ill effects. This is probably due to its release from **carnosine** (β-alanyl-histidine), a dipeptide that is present in large quantities in muscle tissue:

Carnosine

Carnosine is thought to function as a pH buffer in muscle tissue during contraction, when large amounts of lactic acid are formed from stored glycogen.

Methionine and cysteine are metabolically related

The essential amino acid methionine is required not only for protein synthesis but also as a precursor of S-adenosylmethionine (SAM), the most important methyl group donor in biological methylations. SAM is synthesized from methionine and ATP in an unusual reaction in which all three phosphates of ATP are released (Fig. 21.9). By donating its methyl group, SAM becomes S-adenosylhomocysteine (SAH), and SAH, in turn, is converted to homocysteine and finally back to methionine in what may be called the **SAM cycle.** The methylation reaction that converts homocysteine to methionine is important because it requires both folate (as methyltetrahydrofolate) and vitamin B_{12} (as methylcobalamin). We shall encounter this reaction later in the context of B_{12} deficiency and pernicious anemia (see Chapter 24, pages 490-491).

Cysteine is synthesized in a reaction sequence in which cystathionine first is formed from homocysteine and serine and then is cleaved to cysteine and α-ketobutyrate. Through these reactions, *cysteine is made from the carbon skeleton of serine and the sulfur of methionine.*

Cysteine is degraded by oxidation of the sulfhydryl group and transamination. Most of the sulfur is released as inorganic sulfite, which is oxidized rapidly to inorganic sulfate and is excreted in the urine. We excrete approximately 20 to 30 mmol of sulfate per day, and most of this is derived from dietary cysteine and methionine.

The most important aberration in the metabolism of the sulfur-containing amino acids is a deficiency of cystathionine synthase, which leads to **homocystinuria.** Homocysteine, homocystine, and methionine accumulate. This condition, with an estimated population incidence of 1 in 200,000, causes an increased length and decreased thickness of the long bones, osteoporosis, lens dislocation, a tendency for vascular thrombosis, and mental deficiency. The symptoms appear to be caused by the accumulation of homocysteine, not of methionine: a partial deficiency of the SAM-synthesizing enzyme, which has been observed in some individuals and which causes elevations of methionine but not of homocysteine, is a benign condition.

Homocystinuria should be treated, as early as possible, by the restriction of dietary methionine. Approximately half of the patients respond to megadoses of vitamin B_6, the cofactor of cystathionine synthase. These patients have an abnormal enzyme with a reduced affinity for pyridoxal phosphate. Supplements of vitamin B_{12} and folic acid also are often given in an attempt to boost the homocysteine $\rightarrow$ methionine reaction. Betaine (N,N,N-trimethylglycine), which is a methyl group donor in

FIG. 21.9

Metabolism of methionine and cysteine.

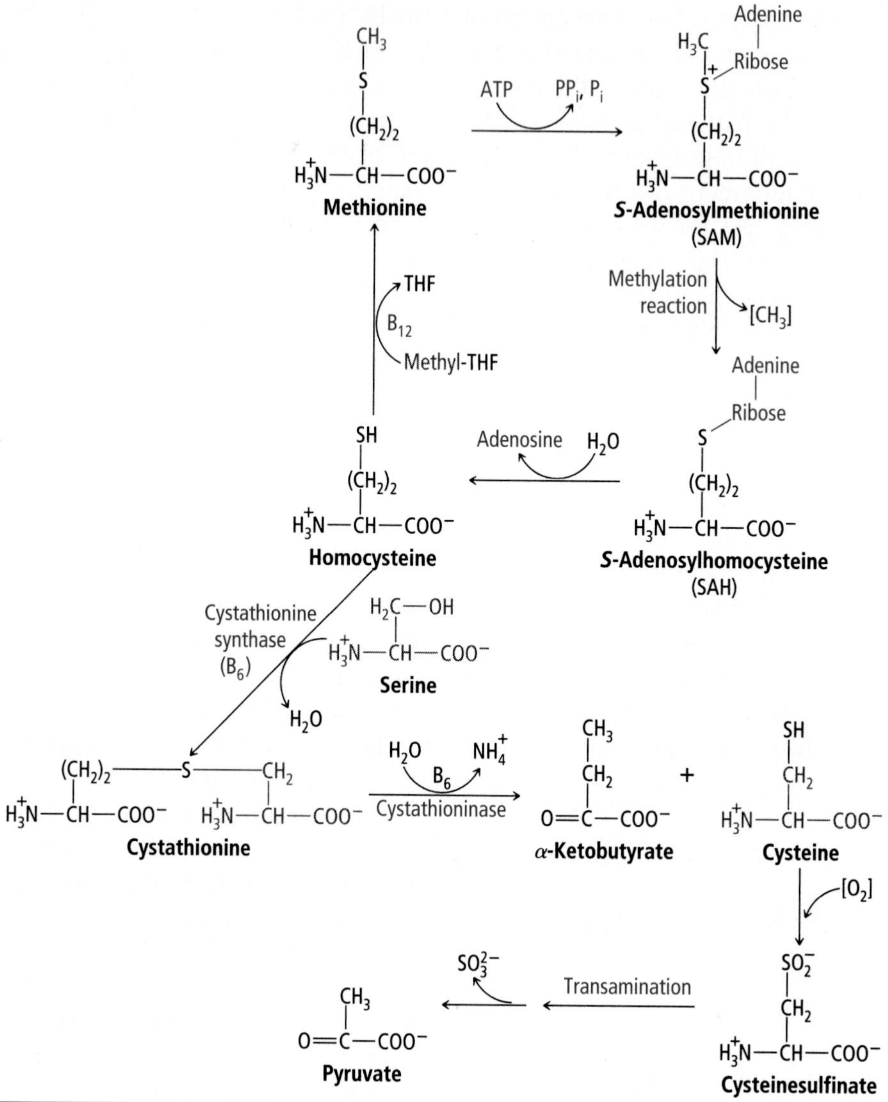

an alternative reaction for the synthesis of methionine from homocysteine, can be employed with the same reasoning.

The degradation of valine, leucine, and isoleucine is initiated by transamination and oxidative decarboxylation

The initial steps in the degradation of valine, leucine, and isoleucine are identical for all three amino acids, as shown for valine in Box 21.20.

These amino acids are transaminated in skeletal muscle and other extrahepatic tissues, and the resulting α-ketoacids are transported to the liver, where they are oxidatively decarboxylated by a mitochondrial enzyme complex. This complex resembles the pyruvate dehydrogenase complex in structure, coenzyme requirements, and reaction mechanism. In the third reaction, the bond between the α and β carbons of the CoA-thioester is oxidized to a double bond by a flavoprotein, a reaction that resembles the first step of β-oxidation (see Fig. 18.6, Chapter 18).

BOX 21.20

The remaining reactions differ for the three amino acids (Fig. 21.10). Although valine is purely glucogenic, isoleucine is both glucogenic and ketogenic, and leucine is purely ketogenic. The final reactions for valine and isoleucine are shared with the pathways of odd-chain fatty acids (see Chapter 18), threonine (threonine dehydratase), and methionine (cystathioninase).

The most important disorders of branched-chain amino acid degradation affect the first and the last reactions. The deficiency of the branched-chain α-ketoacid dehydrogenase, a rather nonselective enzyme that oxidatively decarboxylates all three branched-chain α-ketoacids, causes **maple syrup urine disease.** If the enzyme deficiency is complete, the disease leads to severe mental retardation, acidosis, sweet-smelling urine, and early death. Megadoses of thiamine are effective in only a few patients, and the treatment is based on the restriction of dietary valine, leucine, and isoleucine. The prevalence in newborns is on the order of 1 in 200,000.

The most common inherited defect in the last reactions of valine and isoleucine degradation is **methylmalonic aciduria,** in which the B_{12}-dependent methylmalonyl-CoA mutase reaction is blocked. Methylmalonic acid accumulates in the blood and is excreted in the urine. Methylmalonic aciduria can be caused by a defective enzyme protein or by an inability to convert dietary B_{12} to the coenzyme form adenosylcobalamin. It is a severe disease, with life-threatening acidosis in affected infants and children. Approximately half of the patients have a defect in cobalamin metabolism and respond to injected adenosylcobalamin. Otherwise, the restriction of dietary valine, isoleucine, threonine, and methionine is required. The inherited forms of methylmalonic aciduria occur with an overall frequency of approximately 1 in 10,000. Not surprisingly, a lack of vitamin B_{12} from dietary sources, as in patients with pernicious anemia (see page 490, Chapter 24), also is accompanied by methylmalonic aciduria.

Phenylalanine and tyrosine are both glucogenic and ketogenic

The ring systems of the aromatic amino acids cannot be synthesized in the body. Tyrosine nevertheless is considered nonessential because it is synthesized from phenylalanine in the **phenylalanine hydroxylase** reaction shown in Box 21.21. This irreversible reaction takes place only in the liver. It is a monooxygenase reaction that requires molecular oxygen and **tetrahydrobiopterin (BioH$_4$)**. BioH$_4$ becomes oxidized to dihydrobiopterin (BioH$_2$) during the reaction, and BioH$_2$ is reduced back to

FIG. 21.10

Catabolism of valine, leucine, and isoleucine.

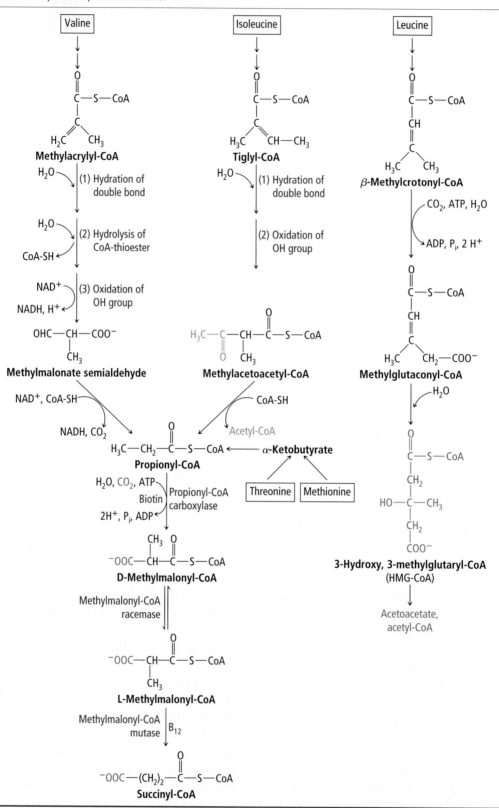

BOX 21.21

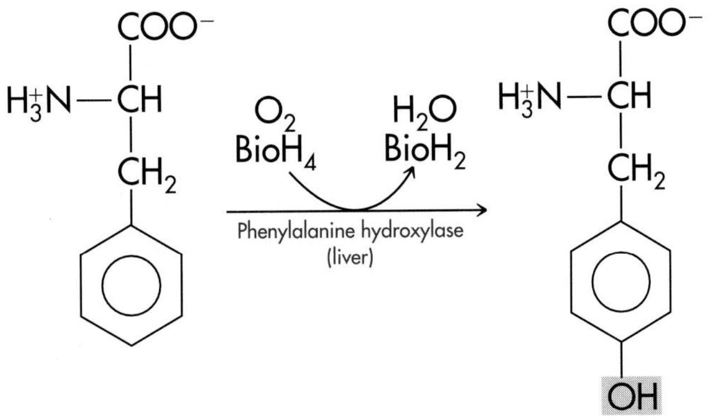

BOX 21.22

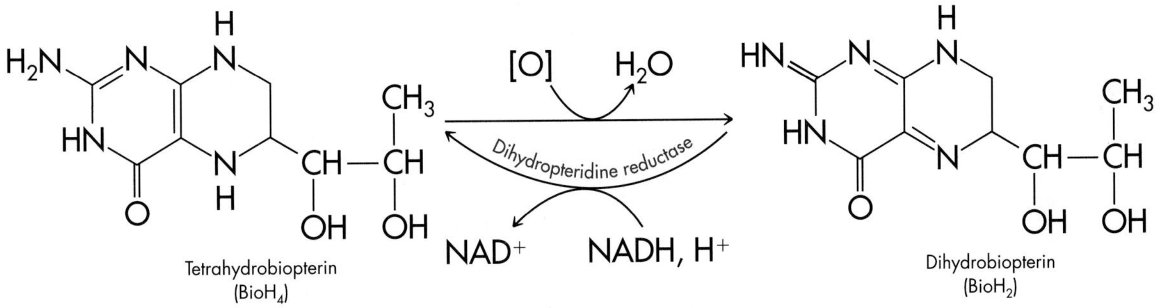

$BioH_4$ by an NADH-dependent **dihydropteridine reductase,** as shown in Box 21.22. The degradation of tyrosine, which takes place in the liver, is shown in Fig. 21.11. Several rare inborn errors of tyrosine metabolism have been described. A deficiency of homogentisate oxidase is the cause of **alkaptonuria.** The patients excrete homogentisate in their urine, an uncolored hydroquinone that is oxidized to black products on exposure to light and air. Although the ink-colored diapers of affected babies look alarming, the condition is relatively benign. Black pigments gradually accumulate in connective tissues, a condition known as **ochronosis,** and many older patients develop painful arthritis.

Two different types of **tyrosinemia** are caused by deficiencies of the cytoplasmic tyrosine transaminase (type II tyrosinemia) and of fumaryl-acetoacetate hydrolase (type I tyrosinemia). In type I tyrosinemia, which is the more common form, the accumulation of fumarylacetoacetate and related organic acids causes a cabbagelike odor, an inhibition of the early steps in tyrosine degradation, impairment of renal tubular absorption, and liver failure.

Phenylketonuria is the most important inborn error of amino acid metabolism

Phenylketonuria (PKU), in its classical form, is caused by a complete deficiency of phenylalanine hydroxylase. The immediate effect of this enzyme deficiency is the accumulation of phenylalanine in the blood. The normal blood level of this amino acid is 30 to 120 μM (0.5 to 2.0 mg/dL), but it is above 1200 μM (20 mg/dL) in phenylketonurics. Under these conditions *the direct transamination of*

FIG. 21.11

Degradation of tyrosine.

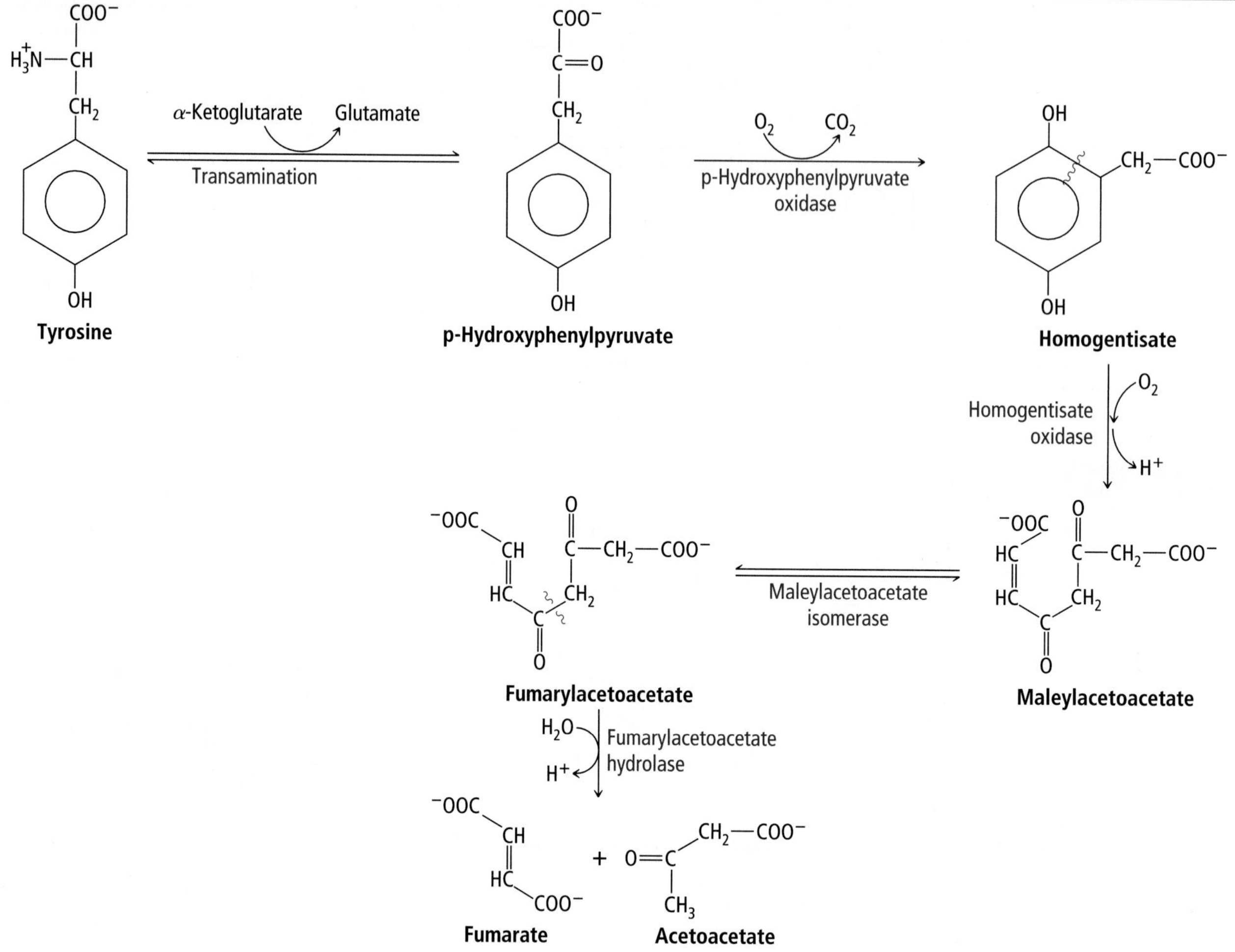

phenyl-alanine to phenylpyruvate becomes the major metabolic fate of this amino acid. Under normal conditions, direct transamination is a very minor pathway of phenylalanine metabolism. Phenylpyruvate, in turn, is converted to other products, as shown in Fig. 21.12. Phenylalanine, phenylpyruvate, phenyllactate, and phenylacetylglutamine, a conjugation product of phenylacetate, are major urinary metabolites in PKU patients.

The disease is not evident at birth because phenylalanine and its metabolites are transferred readily across the placenta, but elevated serum phenylalanine and urinary phenylpyruvate can be demonstrated within a few days after birth. *Untreated patients develop mental retardation*, with IQ values typically between 25 and 50. Neurological signs, such as spasticity and seizures, are sometimes also present. Compared with their unaffected siblings, PKU patients have a rather light complexion, because the synthesis of melanin from tyrosine is inhibited by the excessive levels of phenylalanine. The reasons for the development of mental retardation in PKU are not known.

PKU can be treated very effectively by the restriction of dietary phenylalanine. As an essential amino acid, phenylalanine cannot be omitted entirely from the diet, and frequent determinations of the blood phenylalanine level therefore are recommended. Although

FIG. 21.12

Phenylalanine metabolism in phenylketonuria (PKU).

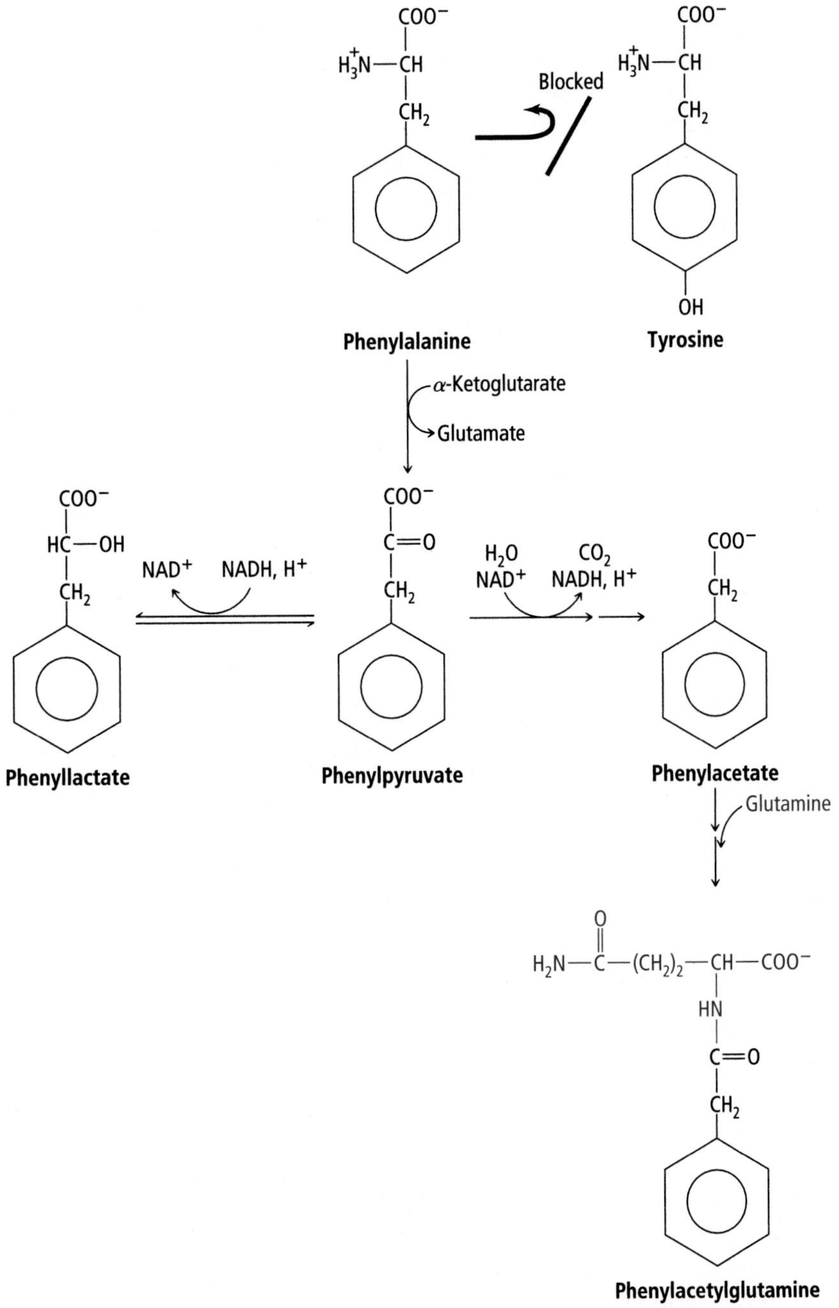

tyrosine is an essential amino acid for phenylketonurics, dietary supplements of this amino acid are not required.

Only the developing brain is vulnerable to the biochemical abnormality. Therefore the low-phenylanine diet, which is not particularly palatable, can be tapered off in older children. If dietary treatment is started within the first weeks after birth, rigorously controlled, and continued until 5 or 6 years of age, mental development is essentially normal. The artificial sweetener **aspartame** (N-aspartyl-phenyl-alanine-methylester) is a potentially dangerous source of phenylalanine for phenylketonurics.

PKU is diagnosed either by the **ferric chloride test** for urinary phenylpyruvate or, more accurately, by the determination of blood phenylalanine. The most commonly employed laboratory test is the **Guthrie bacterial inhibition assay,** in which phenylketonuric blood — but not the blood of normal individuals — supports the growth of a phenylalanine-dependent bacterial strain. *Newborn screening for PKU is mandatory in the United States.* Ideally, the test should be done not less than 2 days after birth, because false negatives are common if it is performed within the first 24 or even 48 hours. The incidence of PKU is approximately 1 in 14,000 in the white population of the United States. It is less in other racial groups (1 in 200,000 in Japan) but higher in some parts of Western Europe (1 in 5000 in Dublin).

Only a complete deficiency of phenylalanine hydroxylase causes PKU, so the disease shows recessive inheritance. Heterozygotes, who have approximately half of the normal enzyme activity, can be identified by the **phenylalanine tolerance test:** the transient increase of the blood phenylalanine level normally seen after the ingestion of a fixed amount of phenylalanine is exaggerated in the heterozygotes. Diagnosis by determination of the enzyme itself is difficult because phenylalanine hydroxylase is expressed only in the liver. Enzyme-based prenatal diagnosis, in particular, is not possible because amniotic cells, which are so valuable for the prenatal diagnosis of most other inborn errors of metabolism, do not express the enzyme. DNA-based diagnostic procedures are under study, but PKU shows extensive allelic heterogeneity: different patients have different mutations in the gene for phenylalanine hydroxylase.

Interestingly, the children of phenylketonuric mothers are mentally retarded even though most of them do not have the PKU genotype (they are heterozygotes). Phenylalanine and its metabolites are transferred from the mother to the fetus and impair fetal brain development. The management of this problem is difficult, and extremely strict dietary control throughout pregnancy probably is required. Possibly, phenylketonuric women should be advised to have no children at all.

Lysine and tryptophan have lengthy catabolic pathways

The pathway of lysine degradation is shown in abbreviated form in Fig. 21.13. Although its metabolic fates are incompletely known beyond the formation of α-ketoadipate, acetoacetyl-CoA is considered the major product, making lysine a ketogenic amino acid.

Lysine also is used for the synthesis of carnitine, the coenzyme that transports long-chain fatty acids into the mitochondrion. Carnitine is derived from protein-bound trimethyllysine, which is formed in some proteins as a posttranslational modification. After degradation of the proteins, trimethyllysine is converted to carnitine in a sequence of four reactions as shown in Box 21.23.

The degradation of **tryptophan** (Fig. 21.14) is initiated by an oxidative cleavage of the pyrrol ring, which forms N-formylkynurenine. This reaction is catalyzed by the heme protein **tryptophan pyrrolase.** After the formation of kynurenine, the pathway branches extensively: the portion of the tryptophan molecule outside the indole ring becomes alanine, and the indole ring itself is converted to a variety of other products. These include α-ketoadipate, which is on the pathway of lysine degradation, and nicotinic acid, which otherwise is considered a vitamin (see Chapter 24). Some tryptophan-derived isoquinolines, such as kynurenate and xanthurenate (Box 21.24), are not degraded further but are excreted in the urine. They are responsible in part for the yellow color of urine.

The liver is the most important organ of amino acid metabolism

Although half of our protein is present in muscle tissue, *enzymes of amino acid catabolism are most abundant in the liver.* After a meal (Fig. 21.15, A), most of the dietary glutamine and glutamate is metabolized in the intestinal mucosa. Most of the other amino acids are extracted from the portal circulation by the liver. Some are used for the synthesis of plasma proteins, but the majority are catabolized. Only the branched-chain aliphatic amino acids valine, leucine, and isoleucine are not catabolized extensively in the splanchnic system but rather are directed to

FIG. 21.13

The main catabolic pathway of lysine.

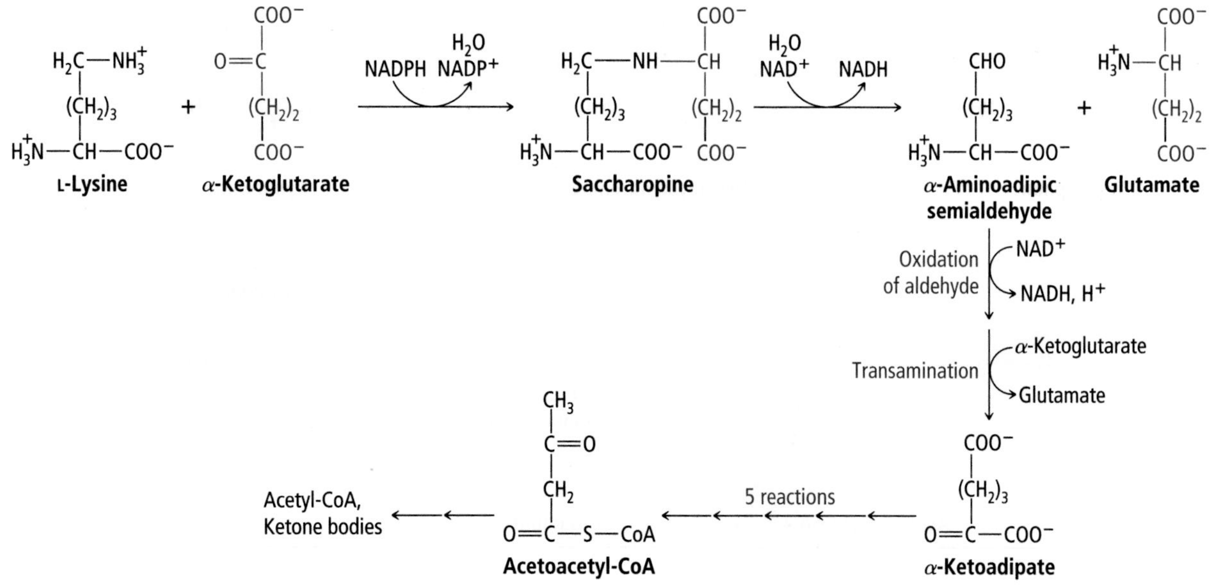

BOX 21.23

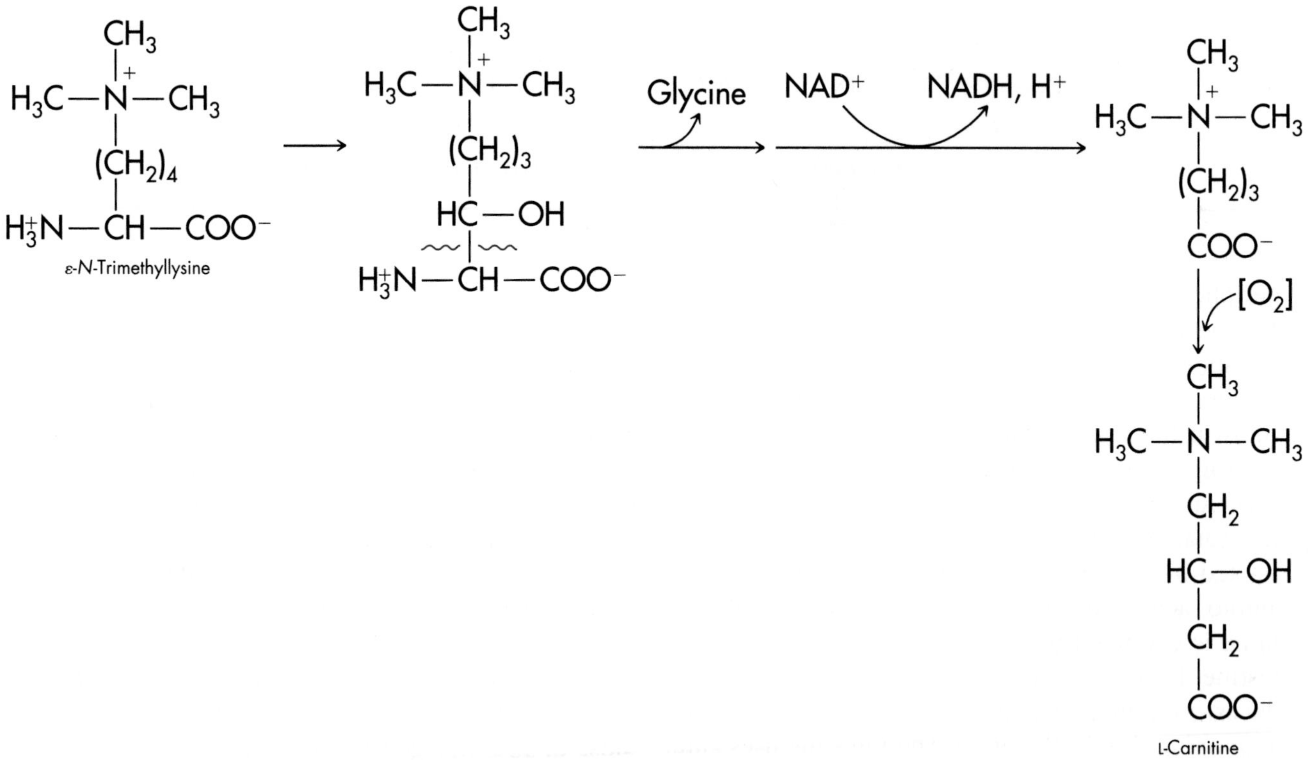

on the other hand, has bidirectional facilitated diffusion-type carriers that equilibrate the amino acids between the mucosal cell and the extracellular medium. This mechanism resembles that described before for the (re)absorption of glucose (see Fig. 11.19, Chapter 11).

Cystinuria (not to be confused with homocystinuria) is caused by a defect in the intestinal absorption and the renal reabsorption of the dibasic amino acids lysine, arginine, ornithine, and cystine. Although lysine is nutritionally essential and arginine is semiessential, signs of amino acid deficiency are not common in this condition, probably because amino acids still can be absorbed from the small intestine as di- and tripeptides (see Chapter 14). Cystine, however, is problematic: it is poorly soluble, especially under acidic conditions, and therefore *it forms kidney stones*. Cystinuria is a recessively inherited disease with an estimated population incidence of 1 in 7000, and it has to be considered in the differential diagnosis of patients with kidney stones. The diagnosis is established by the detection of abnormal quantities of dibasic amino acids in the urine. The treatment consists of measures to maintain a large urine volume and a neutral or alkaline urinary pH.

Hartnup disease is a recessively inherited defect in the transport of large neutral amino acids in renal tubules and intestinal mucosa. The clinical signs are similar to those of pellagra (niacin deficiency, see page 481, Chapter 24), with dermatitis and neurological abnormalities in the form of intermittent ataxia. These signs are caused by the *decreased availability of the amino acid tryptophan*, which normally is absorbed by the defective transporter. This results in signs of niacin deficiency, because part of the niacin requirement normally is covered by endogenous synthesis from tryptophan (see Fig. 21.14). Hartnup disease is a relatively benign disorder. Clinical signs are evident in children more often than in adults, and many individuals with the biochemical abnormality never develop any clinical signs or symptoms at all. The population incidence of Hartnup disease is approximately 1 in 24,000. It has to be considered in the differential diagnosis of children who present either with a pellagra-like skin rash or with intermittent ataxia. The treatment consists of oral niacin supplements.

Polyamines are associated with nucleic acids

The polyamines **spermidine** and **spermine** are cationic substances that are ubiquitous in both prokaryotic and eukaryotic cells. They are synthesized from ornithine and S-adenosyl methionine (Fig. 21.18).

The functions of the polyamines are not known. Because of their cationic nature, they associate with such polyanions as DNA and RNA, and they have been implicated as stimulators of both DNA and RNA synthesis. Many enzymes, including protein kinases and a topoisomerase, are either inhibited or stimulated by polyamines.

Creatine phosphate forms a store of energy-rich phosphate bonds in muscle tissue

Creatine is an amino acid–derived product that is present in muscle tissue and, to a lesser extent, in nervous tissue. **Creatine phosphate** is formed from creatine in the reversible **creatine kinase (CK)**

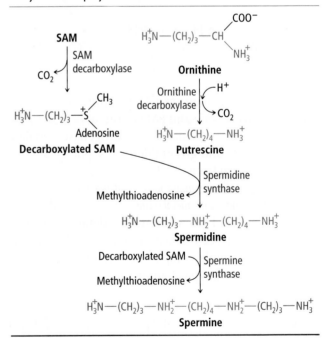

FIG. 21.18

Synthesis of polyamines.

reaction (Fig. 21.19). The phosphate bond in creatine phosphate is energy rich, with a standard free energy of hydrolysis of -10.3 kcal/mol. In the resting state, when the [ATP]/[ADP] ratio is high, most of the muscle creatine is present as creatine phosphate. During contraction, when the [ATP]/[ADP] ratio declines, *ATP is regenerated rapidly by the reversible creatine kinase reaction*. This is the most important source of ATP during the first seconds of muscle contraction. For more sustained muscular activity, however, ATP has to be regenerated by glycolysis or oxidative metabolism (see Chapter 29).

Creatine is not degraded enzymatically, but creatine phosphate cyclizes spontaneously to **creatinine,** which is released from muscle, transported to the kidneys, and excreted in the urine. It is popular for kidney function tests because its blood level is remarkably constant. Creatinine is water soluble and not protein bound, and therefore it is filtered readily through the glomerular basement membrane. It is neither secreted nor reabsorbed in the tubular system, so creatinine clearance is very convenient for the *determination of the glomerular filtration rate.*

Melanin is synthesized from tyrosine

Melanin is the dark pigment of skin, hair, the iris, and the retinal pigment epithelium. In skin and hair bulbs it is formed by melanocytes, which contain melanosomes as specialized organelles of melanin synthesis. *Melanin protects our skin* because it absorbs not only visible light but also UV radiation, which is a normal component of sunlight. UV radiation, particularly at wavelengths of 280 to 320 nm, is dangerous because it induces DNA damage and somatic mutations. This is the cause of both sunburn and skin cancer (see Chapter 9). In the eye, the melanin of the pigment epithelium underlying the sensory cells of the retina absorbs stray light, thereby enhancing visual acuity and preventing overstimulation of the photoreceptors.

Melanin is a polymeric product with a heterogeneous molecular weight and a poorly defined structure. Only the first steps in melanin synthesis are well understood: tyrosine is oxidized first to L-**dopa** (L-dihydroxyphenylalanine) and then to dopaquinone by the copper-containing enzyme **tyrosinase** shown in Box 21.25. The subsequent reactions probably are nonenzymatic.

Recessively inherited defects of melanin synthesis are the cause of **oculocutaneous albinism,** which occurs with frequencies of 1 in 50,000 to 1 in 10,000 in most parts of the world. Some albinos are lacking tyrosinase; others have a defect in the carrier that transports tyrosine across the melanosome membrane.

FIG. 21.19

Creatine and the creatine kinase reaction.

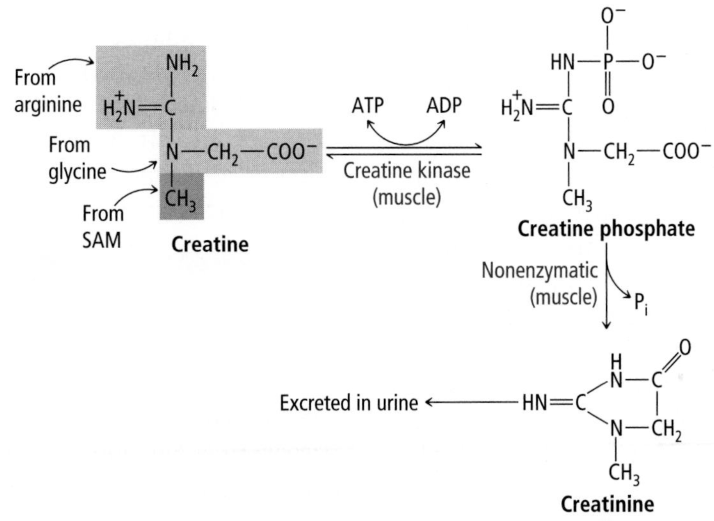

BOX 21.25

SUMMARY

Amino acids obtained from dietary sources or from endogenous protein breakdown are degraded to carbon dioxide, water, and the nitrogenous product urea. The separation of the α-amino group from the carbon skeleton is an early event in the catabolism of most amino acids. In most cases, the amino group initially is transferred to α-ketoglutarate in a transamination reaction. The glutamate formed in these reactions is deaminated oxidatively by glutamate dehydrogenase, with the formation of free ammonia. Because ammonia is toxic, it has to be converted to nontoxic urea, a water-soluble product that is excreted in the urine. Urea is synthesized only in the liver, so hyperammonemia is a typical feature of advanced liver cirrhosis. Hyperammonemia leads to hepatic encephalopathy, a condition that may proceed eventually to coma and death.

A small portion of the amino nitrogen is excreted as the ammonium ion. The excretion of the ammonium ion rather than urea is accompanied by the elimination of excess protons from the body, and the kidneys use this mechanism in acid-base regulation: they increase ammonium ion excretion when the blood pH is too low.

The carbon skeletons of the amino acids are converted to nitrogen-free metabolic intermediates.

Many deficiencies of amino acid–degrading enzymes are known, and some of them are severe diseases. The clinical manifestations of these inborn errors of amino acid metabolism are caused by the abnormal accumulation of the affected amino acid or its metabolites. Amino acids whose carbon skeletons are degraded to intermediates of TCA cycle or gluconeogenesis are called glucogenic, and those that are degraded to acetyl-CoA are called ketogenic. Most amino acids are catabolized in the liver, and the products can be channeled directly into gluconeogenesis or ketogenesis.

Several specialized products including creatine, carnitine, carnosine, melanin, and the polyamines are synthesized from amino acids. Other amino acid–derived products will be encountered in Chapters 22 (heme), 23 (purines, pyrimidines), and 26 (biogenic amines, thyroid hormones).

Further Reading

Christensen HN: Interorgan amino acid nutrition. In: Kilberg MS, Häussinger D, editors: *Mammalian amino acid transport.* Plenum Press, New York, 1992, pp. 295-304.

Conn HO: Hepatic encephalopathy. In: Schiff L, Schiff ER: *Diseases of the liver,* 7th ed., vol. 2. J. B. Lippincott, Philadelphia, 1993, pp. 1036-1060.

Herrman R, McIntyre N: Amino acid metabolism, urea production, and pH regulation. In: McIntyre N, Benhamou J-P, Bircher J, Rizzetto M, Rodes J, editors: *Oxford textbook of clinical hepatology*, vol. 1. Oxford University Press, Oxford, 1991, pp. 157-174.

Kilberg MS, Stevens BR, Novak DA: Recent advances in mammalian amino acid transport. *Annu Rev Nutr* 13, 137-165, 1993.

Morris SM Jr: Regulation of enzymes of urea and arginine synthesis. *Annu Rev Nutr* 12, 81-101, 1992.

Pollitt RJ: Amino acid disorders. In: Holton JB, editor: *The inherited metabolic diseases*, 2nd ed. Churchill Livingstone, New York, 1994, pp. 67-113.

Scriver CR, Beaudet AL, Sly WS, Valle D, editors: *The metabolic basis of inherited disease*, 6th ed. McGraw-Hill, New York, 1984, pp. 495-868, 933-944, 2479-2528, 2905-2948.

Souba WW: Glutamine: a key substrate for the splanchnic bed. *Annu Rev Nutr* 11, 285-308, 1991.

Waterlow JC: Whole-body protein turnover in humans—past, present and future. *Annu Rev Nutr* 15, 57-92, 1995.

QUESTIONS

1. A 4-month-old child is evaluated for vomiting after feeding, irritability, and delayed motor development. Blood tests show an ammonia level 10 to 20 times higher than the upper limit of normal, as well as marked elevations of ornithine and glutamine. Most likely, this child has a deficiency of the enzyme
   A. Arginase
   B. Ornithine decarboxylase
   C. Glutaminase
   D. Ornithine transcarbamoylase
   E. Ornithine transglutaminase

2. A 55-year-old alcoholic is brought to the hospital in a confused state. The ER physician notes that the patient's breath has a foul smell, but there is no sign of acute alcohol intoxication. A blood test shows an abnormally high ammonia level. The worst treatment for this patient would be to
   A. Give him a lot of good, protein-rich food
   B. Give him benzoic acid or phenylacetic acid
   C. Give him a diet low in proteins but with plenty of vitamins
   D. Give him a broad-spectrum antibiotic to eliminate intestinal bacteria

3. The mechanism for the development of mental retardation in untreated phenylketonurics is not known. All of the following substances accumulate in untreated PKU, and any of them may possibly be toxic for the brain, except
   A. Phenylalanine
   B. Tyrosine
   C. Phenylpyruvate
   D. Phenyllactate

4. Under normal conditions, the kidneys excrete a small amount of nitrogen in the form of the ammonium ion, rather than as urea. The amount of urinary ammonium ion is greatly increased in patients who suffer from
   A. Phenylketonuria
   B. Fat malabsorption
   C. Hartnup's disease
   D. Glutaminase deficiency
   E. Chronic acidosis

5. All transamination reactions require the coenzyme
   A. Tetrahydrofolate
   B. Thiamine pyrophosphate
   C. Pyridoxal phosphate
   D. Biotin
   E. S-adenosyl methionine

Chapter 22

Heme Metabolism

We have encountered heme as a tightly bound prosthetic group of such heme proteins as hemoglobin, myoglobin, catalase, and the cytochromes. It is bound to its apoproteins either noncovalently, as in hemoglobin and myoglobin, or by a covalent bond, as in cytochrome c. Chemically, heme consists of a porphyrin, known as **protoporphyrin IX,** and an iron that is chelated in the center of the porphyrin ring system. The porphyrin system consists of four pyrrole rings linked by methine (—C=) bridges shown in Box 22.1. The conjugated double bonds absorb visible light, and therefore *the heme proteins are colored.* **Porphyrinogens,** on the other hand, which are important intermediates in heme biosynthesis, are not colored because their pyrrole rings are connected by methylene (—CH$_2$—) bridges, and the double bonds are not conjugated over the whole system, which is shown in Box 22.2. Unlike the porphyrins, porphyrinogens do not chelate metal ions easily. They also lack resonance stabilization between the pyrrole rings, so *they are oxidized easily to the corresponding porphyrins.*

Although dietary sources do contain heme and a small portion of this actually is absorbed in the small intestine, *essentially all of the heme in the body is derived from endogenous synthesis.* In this chapter we encounter the pathways for the biosynthesis and degradation of heme and the diseases in which these pathways are disrupted.

Bone marrow and liver are the most important sites of heme synthesis

Most of the heme in our bodies is in hemoglobin: the 800 to 900 g of hemoglobin in the adult contains 30 to 35 g of heme. A total of 250 to 300 mg of heme has to be synthesized in the red bone marrow every day, most of this in the erythroblasts and proerythroblasts. *The bone marrow accounts for 70% to 80% of the total heme synthesis in the body.*

The second-most-important site is the liver. This organ contains high concentrations of cytochrome P-450, catalase, and cytochrome b$_5$. These heme proteins have far shorter half-lives than hemoglobin, and hepatic heme synthesis therefore is quite respectable, accounting for approximately 15% of the total.

Except for the movement of RBCs from the bone marrow to the sites of degradation in spleen and liver, there is essentially no interorgan transfer of intact heme, and *the tissues synthesize heme according to their own needs.*

Heme is synthesized from succinyl-CoA and glycine

The committed step of heme biosynthesis (Fig. 22.1) is the formation of **δ-aminolevulinate (ALA)** from succinyl-CoA and glycine. The enzyme catalyzing

BOX 22.1

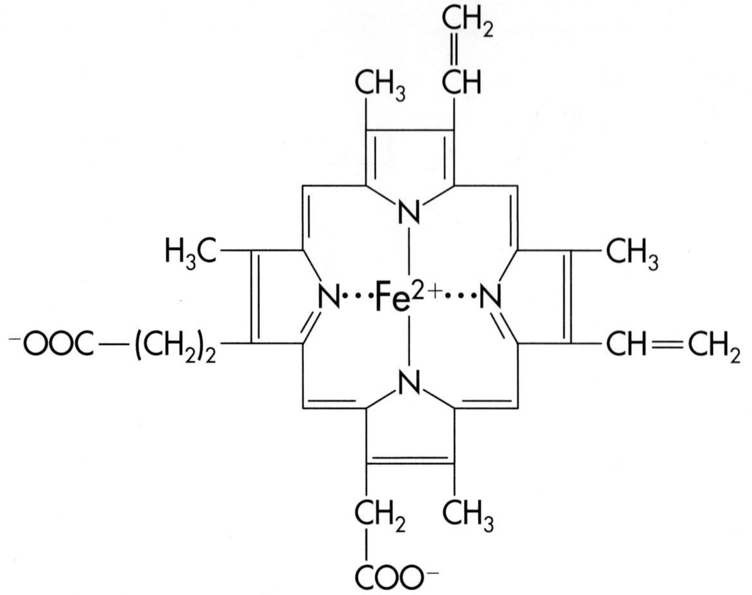

Heme
(Fe-protoporphyrin IX)

BOX 22.2

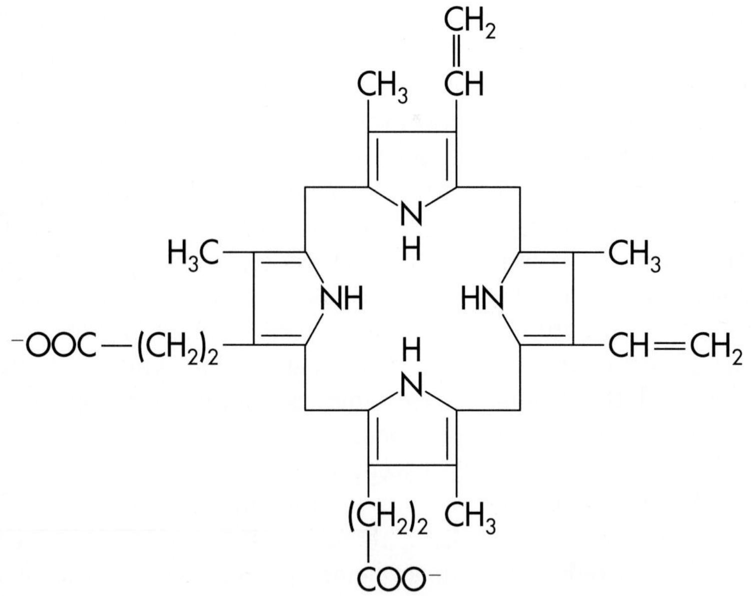

Protoporphyrinogen IX
(a porphyrinogen)

this reaction, **δ-aminolevulinate synthase (ALA synthase)**, contains a pyridoxal phosphate prosthetic group that forms a Schiff base bond with the amino group of glycine during the reaction. The second reaction, catalyzed by **ALA dehydrase**, forms the pyrrole ring of **porphobilinogen**. The enzyme contains functionally important sulfhydryl groups, so it is sensitive to inhibition by lead and other heavy metals.

In the third reaction, catalyzed by **uroporphyrinogen synthase**, one molecule of **uroporphyrinogen** is synthesized from four molecules of porphobilinogen.

FIG. 22.1

The pathway of heme biosynthesis. The numbered reactions refer to Table 22.1. *A*, Acetate (carboxymethyl) group; *P*, propionate (carboxyethyl) group; *M*, methyl group; *V*, vinyl group.

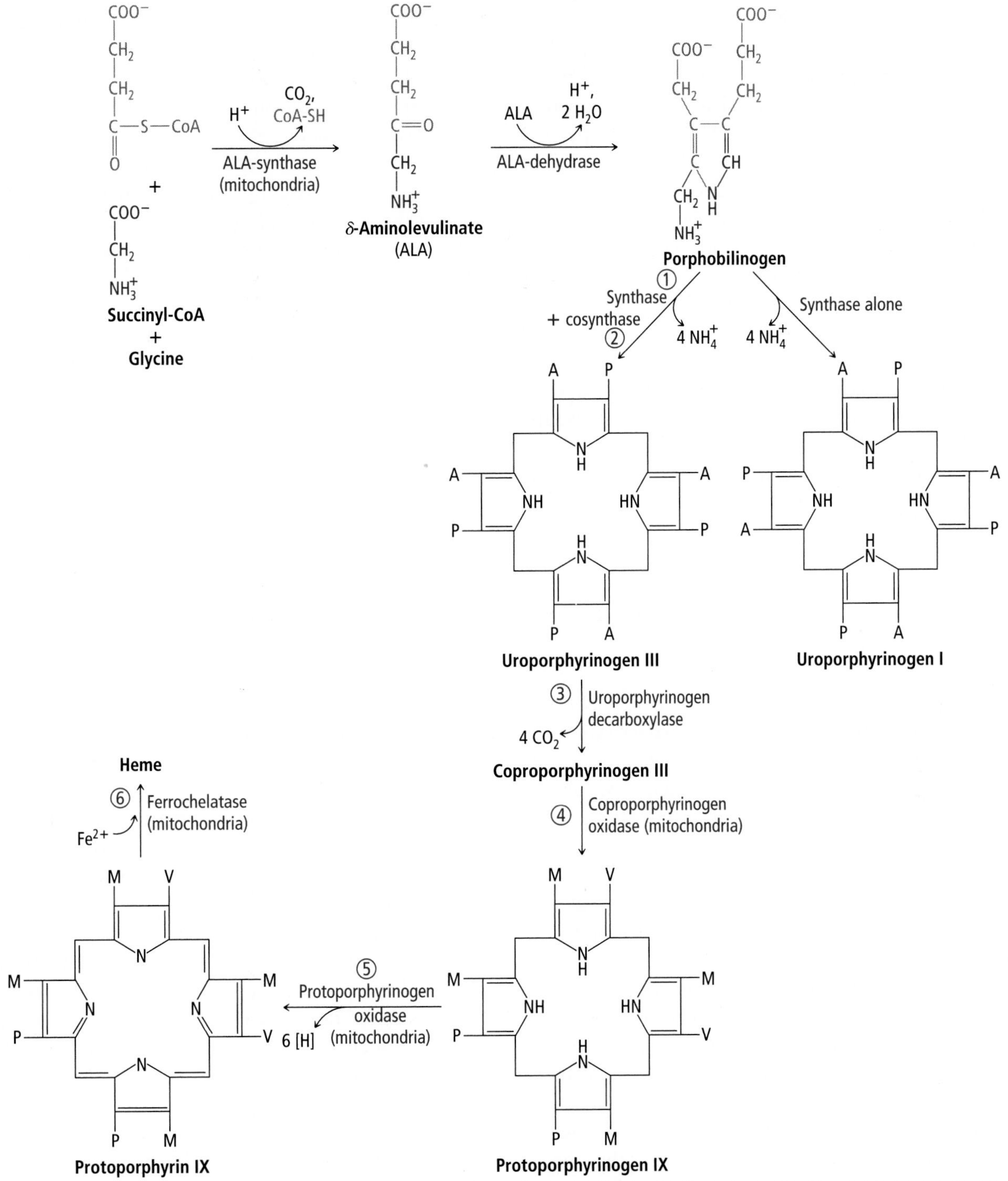

Two different products can be formed. In the absence of other proteins, the enzyme forms **uroporphyrinogen I,** a product in which the carboxymethyl (acetate) and carboxyethyl (propionate) side chains of the pyrrole rings alternate regularly. In the cell, however, a second protein, **uroporphyrinogen cosynthase,** directs the formation of the asymmetrical **uroporphyrinogen III** instead of uroporphyrinogen I by "flipping" one of the pyrrole rings. All naturally occurring porphyrins, including heme, belong to the III series. Uroporphyrinogen III finally is processed to heme by decarboxylations of the acetate and propionate groups, oxidation of the porphyrinogen to the porphyrin, and the chelation of iron in the center of the molecule.

The first reaction and the last three reactions of the pathway are mitochondrial; the remaining enzymes are cytoplasmic. *The principal regulated enzyme in the liver is ALA synthase.* This enzyme has an unusually short biological half-life of 1 to 3 hours in the liver, and *its synthesis is suppressed very effectively by heme.* Only free, non−protein-bound heme acts as a feedback inhibitor.

Porphyrias are caused by deficiencies of heme-synthesizing enzymes

The **porphyrias** are caused by a *partial deficiency of one of the heme-synthesizing enzymes other than ALA synthase.* Any one of the numbered enzymes in Fig. 22.1 may be affected. A complete deficiency would be fatal, and in many cases the inheritance is indeed autosomal dominant, with approximately 50% of the normal enzyme activity in the affected heterozygotes. According to the tissue in which the abnormality is expressed, *hepatic and erythropoietic porphyrias* can be distinguished.

Acute intermittent porphyria (AIP) is caused by a partial deficiency of uroporphyrinogen synthase, inherited as an autosomal dominant trait. The enzyme activity is reduced to 50% of normal in all tissues, but clinical manifestations are caused by impaired heme synthesis in the liver, because the activity of this enzyme relative to the other heme biosynthetic enzymes is rather low in that organ. The abnormality is asymptomatic under most conditions, and as many as 90% of individuals with the genetic trait never show clinical signs and symptoms. If problems develop, they take the form of acute attacks that last from a few days to several months but that occasionally may lead to a chronic syndrome.

The clinical manifestations of AIP are not caused directly by a deficiency of heme but by the accumulation of δ-aminolevulinate and porphobilinogen, which appear in blood, urine, and cerebrospinal fluid during the acute attack. These metabolites act on the nervous system: abdominal pain is caused by the excitation of visceral pain fibers. Constipation and cardiovascular changes (including tachycardia and increased blood pressure) are mediated by the autonomic nervous system. The involvement of peripheral nerves causes muscle weakness and, in some patients, sensory loss or paresthesias. Brain involvement is manifested by agitation, seizures, or mental derangements. Undiagnosed AIP appears to be overrepresented among patients in psychiatric institutions, where the condition often is worsened by inappropriate drug treatment.

Acute attacks of AIP can be precipitated by barbiturates, phenytoin, griseofulvin, and other drugs that induce the synthesis of **cytochrome P-450,** a family of heme proteins that contain 65% of the total heme in the liver (see Chapter 29). The increased synthesis of the apoprotein rapidly depletes the small pool of free, unbound heme, and *heme depletion leads to a derepression of ALA synthase and the accumulation of δ-aminolevulinate and porphobilinogen.*

The symptoms of AIP are not accompanied by specific physical findings, so they often are misdiagnosed as a primary neuropsychiatric disorder: the patient is treated symptomatically with sedative-hypnotics, tranquilizers, or anticonvulsants, and these drugs aggravate the condition by inducing P-450 synthesis in the liver. Some patients have died of this treatment. An adequate treatment would consist of the withdrawal of any offending drugs and the infusion of **hematin.** Hematin is a derivative of heme in which the heme iron is in the ferric form and is coordinated with a hydroxyl ion. Like heme, hematin represses the synthesis of ALA synthase. A carbohydrate-rich diet also benefits the patient by repressing (by unknown mechanisms) the synthesis of ALA synthase.

Several other porphyrias have been described. Their most important features are summarized in Table 22.1.

The most common porphyria is **porphyria cu-**

TABLE 22.1

The porphyrias

Enzyme deficiency*	Disease (and class)	Inheritance†	Signs and symptoms			Laboratory tests‡
			Visceral	Neurological	Cutaneous	
1	Acute intermittent (hepatic)	AD	++	++	−	Urinary ALA, urinary PBG
2	Congenital erythro-poietic (erythro-poietic)	AR			+++	Urinary uroporphyrin,§ urinary coproporphyrin,§ fecal coproporphyrin§
3	Porphyria cutanea tarda (hepatic)	AD¶			++	Urinary uroporphyrin, urinary uroporphyrin, coproporphyrin
4	Hereditary copro-porphyria (hepatic)	AD	+	+	(+)	Urinary ALA, urinary PBG, urinary coproporphyrin, urinary uroporphyrin
5	Variegate porphyria (hepatic)	AD	++	++	+	Urinary ALA, urinary PBG, urinary coproporphyrin, fecal protoporphyrin, fecal coproporphyrin
6	Protoporphyria (erythropoietic)	AD			+	Fecal protoporphyrin, RBC protoporphyrin

* The numbers refer to the numbered reactions in Fig. 22.1.
† AD, Autosomal dominant; AR, autosomal recessive.
‡ ALA, δ-Aminolevulinate; PBG, porphobilinogen.
§ Type I uroporphyrin and coproporphyrin are elevated.
¶ In many cases no specific inheritance can be demonstrated.

tanea tarda. Although some cases are caused by a dominantly inherited defect of uroporphyrinogen decarboxylase, this disease is expressed mostly in people with alcoholism or liver damage. Iron overload (see Chapter 24) is an important factor because the affected enzyme is sensitive to inhibition by iron salts. The clinical presentation is entirely different from that of AIP: neurological and abdominal symptoms are absent, and *the patient presents with cutaneous photosensitivity*. The condition is most common in older males during the summer months. It is treated by the avoidance of sunlight, abstinence from alcohol, and phlebotomy for the reduction of iron overload.

Cutaneous photosensitivity is typical for those porphyrias in which porphyrins or porphyrinogens accumulate. The porphyrinogens are nonenzymatically oxidized to the corresponding porphyrins, and these porphyrins become photoexcited by the action of sunlight in the skin. This leads to the formation of singlet oxygen

(a reactive form of molecular oxygen), which causes cellular damage. These porphyrias frequently result in an unusually dark or colorful urine. The color deepens when the urine is exposed to light and air because of the nonenzymatic oxidation of the porphyrinogens to porphyrins.

Porphyrias can be diagnosed biochemically by the determination of urinary metabolites. δ-Aminolevulinate and porphobilinogen are quantified by colorimetric tests, and uroporphyrin and coproporphyrin are determined fluorometrically.

Two enzymes of heme synthesis, ALA dehydrase and ferrochelatase, are sensitive to inhibition by lead. This results in increased levels of urinary δ-aminolevulinate and an increased concentration of protoporphyrin IX in erythrocytes. Some of the neurological impairments in lead poisoning may be related to this inhibition of heme biosynthesis and the resulting accumulation of metabolic intermediates.

Heme is degraded to bilirubin

Approximately 300 to 400 mg of heme are degraded in the human body per day, and close to 80% of this is derived from hemoglobin. The first reaction of heme degradation takes place in the endoplasmic reticulum of reticuloendothelial cells in the spleen and other organs. Heme is converted to the green pigment **biliverdin** in an oxygenase reaction that releases one of the CH bridges between the pyrrole rings as carbon monoxide. Heme oxygenase is the only known CO-forming enzyme in the human body. Biliverdin, still in the reticuloendothelial cell, then is converted to the yellow pigment **bilirubin** by the cytoplasmic **biliverdin reductase** (Fig. 22.2).

The stages of heme degradation can be observed in the color changes of a hematoma—for example, after a punch to the face leaves a so-called black eye. After rupture of the capillaries, RBCs are stranded in the interstitial spaces, where their hemoglobin becomes deoxygenated. Deoxy-hemoglobin is blue. Within a few days, the erythrocytes are scavenged by tissue macrophages and the heme is degraded first to biliverdin and then to bilirubin. The blue color disappears and is replaced by a greenish and finally a yellow color.

Bilirubin is conjugated and excreted by the liver

From the reticuloendothelial cells, *bilirubin is transported to the liver in tight, noncovalent binding to serum albumin.* It is taken up into the hepatocytes by a facilitated-diffusion–type carrier of high capacity and then is conjugated to the diglucuronide by two successive reactions with UDP-glucuronic acid. The water-soluble bilirubin diglucuronide is actively secreted into the bile canaliculi against a steep concentration gradient. This is an important rate-limiting step in hepatic bilirubin metabolism. The transporter is not specific for bilirubin diglucuronide, but rather secretes a variety of other anions as well, including the dye **bromosulfophthalein (BSP)**, which is used in a popular liver function test. Bile acids, however, are secreted by a different transporter.

In the intestine, bilirubin diglucuronide is deconjugated by bacterial β-glucuronidases and reduced to uncolored **urobilinogens.** Some of the urobilino-gens are oxidized to the colored **urobilins,** which are responsible for the brown color of the stools. A small amount of urobilinogen is absorbed in the terminal ileum, returned to the liver, and secreted in the bile. Only small traces (up to 4 mg/day) find their way to the kidneys to be excreted in the urine.

Elevations of serum bilirubin cause jaundice

Normal blood contains less than 17 μM (1 mg/dL) bilirubin, and most of this is unconjugated, apparently in transit from the spleen to the liver. Abnormal increases of the plasma bilirubin level are called **hyperbilirubinemia.** Either unconjugated bilirubin, conjugated bilirubin, or both are elevated. All types of hyperbilirubinemia lead to the deposition of bilirubin in the tissues, including the skin and the sclera of the eye, to which it imparts a yellow color. This condition is called **jaundice** or **icterus** and appears when the serum bilirubin level rises above 70 μM (4 mg/dL). The sclera of the eye is affected early because of its high content of elastin, for which bilirubin has a high affinity. However, there are two important differences between conjugated and unconjugated bilirubin:

1. *Only unconjugated bilirubin, which is lipid soluble, can enter the brain,* especially in infants. Bilirubin deposition in the basal ganglia can cause irreversible brain damage, a condition known as **kernicterus** (from *kern* [German], "nucleus"). Kernicterus in infants leads initially to hypotonia, and the condition may rapidly progress to atonia and death. Survivors often are left with permanent neurological impairments, including an athetoid motor disorder, mental deficiency, and various cranial nerve symptoms. At a normal albumin concentration of 4 g/dL, up to 25 mg/dL of bilirubin is transported in tight, noncovalent association with a high-affinity binding site on this plasma protein. Kernicterus develops only at bilirubin levels above this limit, when the binding capacity of albumin is exceeded.

2. *The kidneys excrete only conjugated bilirubin.* Unconjugated bilirubin cannot be excreted because it is tightly bound to albumin, but conjugated bilirubin is water soluble and not protein bound. Therefore it is excreted in the urine, to which

FIG. 22.2

Heme degradation and bilirubin metabolism. *M,* Methyl; *V,* vinyl.

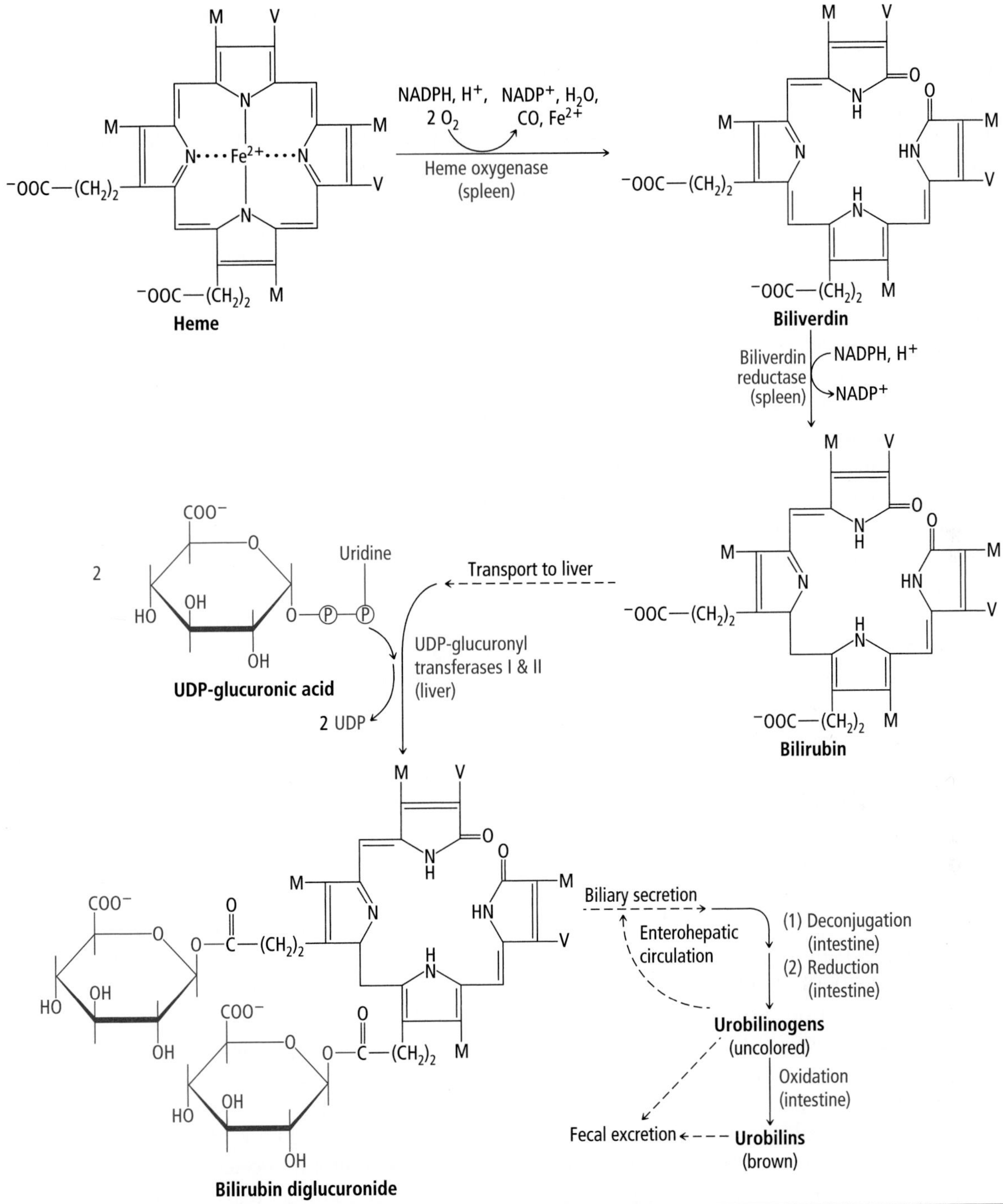

it imparts a yellow-brown color. This is called **choluric jaundice.**

In the laboratory, bilirubin traditionally is detected by the **van den Bergh method:** mixing of the plasma or serum sample with Ehrlich's diazo reagent (diazotized sulfanilic acid) results in a color reaction that is proportional to the bilirubin concentration. If an organic solvent is included in the assay solution, both conjugated and unconjugated bilirubin react rapidly. If the test is performed in water, however, only the conjugated form reacts. Conjugated bilirubin therefore is called *"direct reacting" or simply "direct" bilirubin,* whereas unconjugated bilirubin is known as *"indirect (reacting)" bilirubin.*

Urinary and fecal urobilinogen also can be determined. The levels of urinary urobilinogen depend both on the biliary supply of bilirubin diglucuronide, from which the urobilinogens are formed in the intestine, and on the functional state of the liver, which normally scavenges most of the absorbed urobilinogen from the portal circulation.

Unconjugated hyperbilirubinemia is most common in newborns

Unconjugated hyperbilirubinemia can be caused by hemolytic conditions. An increased destruction of erythrocytes leads to increased heme degradation and bilirubin formation. Fortunately the healthy adult liver has a very high capacity for bilirubin metabolism, so the hyperbilirubinemia of hemolytic diseases rarely exceeds 50 to 70 μM (3 to 4 mg/dL). The biliary excretion of conjugated bilirubin is increased in proportion to the severity of hemolysis, so the levels of fecal and urinary urobilinogen, which is derived from biliary bilirubin diglucuronide, are elevated (Fig. 22.3).

The most common type of unconjugated hyperbilirubinemia is **physiological jaundice of the newborn.** In normal infants the serum bilirubin concentration rises from a level of 17 to 35 μM (1 to 2 mg/dL) at birth to approximately 80 to 100 μM (5 to 6 mg/dL) at day 3; it gradually declines to 15 to 20 μM (1 mg/dL) over the following week. Up to 50% of all newborns become visibly jaundiced during the first 5 days after birth; 16% reach a maximal serum bilirubin concentration of 170 μM (10 mg/dL) or

above, and in 5%, the serum bilirubin rises above 250 μM (15 mg/dL).

Physiological jaundice of the newborn is caused by a relative *immaturity of the bilirubin-metabolizing system of the liver.* The uptake of unconjugated bilirubin, the activity of the conjugating enzyme system, the intracellular level of UDP-glucuronic acid, and the biliary secretion of bilirubin diglucuronide are all low in the neonate. To make matters worse, bilirubin diglucuronide is deconjugated by intestinal β-glucuronidase, but the unconjugated bilirubin thus formed is not converted to urobilinogen for lack of intestinal bacteria. Some of this unconjugated bilirubin is absorbed from the intestine and contributes to the hyperbilirubinemia.

The milder forms of physiological jaundice require no treatment. However, there is a danger of kernicterus, so *increases of serum bilirubin above 250 to 350 μM (15 to 20 mg/dL) have to be prevented.* The first line of treatment is phototherapy: the baby is exposed to ordinary, visible light. This safe, noninvasive treatment effects a photochemical isomerization of bilirubin in the skin. The geometrical isomers thus formed are more water soluble than native bilirubin and can be excreted in the bile without conjugation. The administration of phenobarbital is indicated when the bilirubin level stays dangerously high despite phototherapy. This drug induces the synthesis of the bilirubin-conjugating enzyme and some other components of the bilirubin-metabolizing system. Orally administered agar, which binds intestinal bilirubin and thereby prevents its absorption, sometimes is used.

Hemolytic conditions in the neonatal period are particularly dangerous. In **rhesus incompatibility,** severe hemolysis in the newborn is caused by a maternal IgG antibody to a fetal blood group antigen. This may require exchange transfusion immediately after birth or even in the fetus before birth.

Unusually severe or persistent jaundice in newborns always should be evaluated by the determination of hemoglobin concentration or hematocrit, both of which are decreased in hemolytic diseases, and by liver function tests or the determination of serum transaminases, which are abnormal in liver diseases.

Rare cases of unconjugated hyperbilirubinemia are caused by an inherited defect of bilirubin uptake or conjugation. In **Crigler-Najjar syndrome type I,**

FIG. 22.3

Bilirubin and urobilinogen in different types of jaundice. - - - - -, Unconjugated (indirect) bilirubin; ———, conjugated (direct) bilirubin; ----, urobilinogen. **A,** Normal pattern. **B,** Hemolysis. **C,** Biliary obstruction. **D,** Hepatitis (no cholestasis). **E,** Physiological jaundice of the newborn.

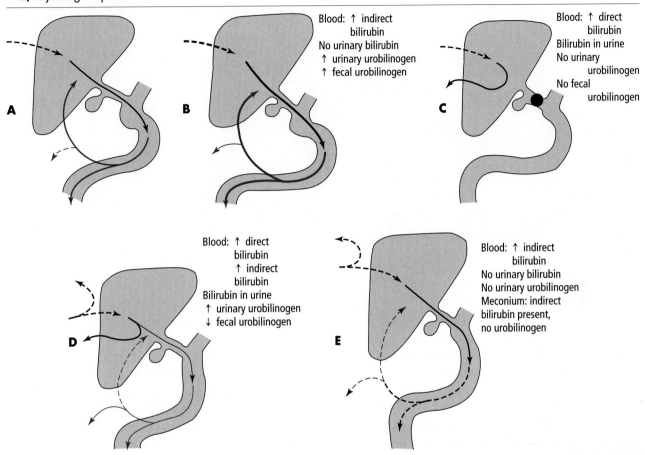

B,
Blood: ↑ indirect
     bilirubin
No urinary bilirubin
↑ urinary urobilinogen
↑ fecal urobilinogen

C,
Blood: ↑ direct
     bilirubin
Bilirubin in urine
No urinary
     urobilinogen
No fecal
     urobilinogen

D,
Blood: ↑ direct
     bilirubin
    ↑ indirect
     bilirubin
Bilirubin in urine
↑ urinary urobilinogen
↓ fecal urobilinogen

E,
Blood: ↑ indirect
     bilirubin
No urinary bilirubin
No urinary urobilinogen
Meconium: indirect
bilirubin present,
no urobilinogen

a complete deficiency of the bilirubin-conjugating enzyme, bilirubin-UDP-glucuronosyl tranferase, causes massive hyperbilirubinemia ($>350\ \mu$M) and kernicterus. Most patients with this recessively inherited disease die within weeks after birth. **Crigler-Najjar syndrome type II** is a less severe defect of bilirubin conjugation with milder hyperbilirubinemia (80 to 350 μM), and bilirubin monoglucuronide rather than the diglucuronide is the predominant form in the bile. These patients respond to phenobarbital. **Gilbert syndrome** is a diagnostic label for patients with a mild, usually asymptomatic, unconjugated hyperbilirubinemia of unknown origin.

Biliary obstruction causes conjugated hyperbilirubinemia

Conjugated hyperbilirubinemia has to be expected whenever the bilirubin-conjugating capacity of the liver is more or less intact but the biliary system is blocked: *the liver still conjugates bilirubin, but the bile no longer carries the product to the intestine.* Having nowhere else to go, bilirubin diglucuronide overflows into the blood. This is called **cholestatic jaundice.**

Urobilinogen, normally formed from bilirubin by intestinal bacteria, disappears from blood, stool, and urine. In complete biliary obstruction, the

FIG. 22.4

Levels of serum bilirubin (——, conjugated bilirubin; ——, unconjugated bilirubin) and urinary urobilinogen (----) in a patient with viral hepatitis. Urobilinogen is increased as long as the disease does not lead to cholestasis, but it disappears as soon as cholestasis develops.

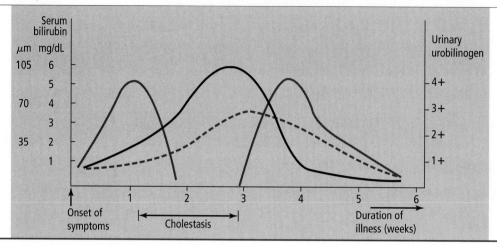

stools no longer have their normal brown color, which is caused by urobilins, but appear clay colored. The urine, on the other hand, is yellow-brown because of its content of bilirubin diglucuronide (choluric jaundice). Liver function is unimpaired in acute biliary obstruction, but longstanding cholestasis causes irreversible liver damage.

The most common cause of **extrahepatic biliary obstruction** is a dislodged gallstone. Carcinoma of the head of the pancreas is another possible cause, and cholestatic jaundice is often the first sign of this aggressive tumor. **Intrahepatic biliary obstruction** occurs in many nonspecific liver diseases in which either the bile canaliculi are blocked or the hepatocytes lose the ability for bile formation. The secretion of bile requires the energy-dependent transport of bile salts and inorganic ions across the intact hepatocyte membrane, and this may no longer be possible during severe liver diseases.

Nonspecific liver diseases such as viral hepatitis, yellow fever, and toxic liver damage result in a mixed conjugated and unconjugated hyperbilirubinemia (Fig. 22.4). The presence of cholestasis can be evaluated by the determination of urinary urobilinogen: in uncomplicated liver disease, urinary urobilinogen is elevated because the diseased liver has a reduced ability to extract absorbed urobilinogen from the portal circulation. If the disease has resulted in intrahepatic cholestasis, however, urobilinogen can no longer be formed in the intestine, and urobilinogen disappears from the urine.

Two rare genetic disorders, **Dubin-Johnson syndrome** and **Rotor's syndrome,** are associated with conjugated hyperbilirubinemia. The biliary secretion of bilirubin diglucuronide is impaired in Dubin-Johnson syndrome; the molecular defect in Rotor's syndrome is unknown.

SUMMARY

Heme is synthesized in bone marrow, liver, and other tissues that produce heme proteins. The pathway starts with the formation of δ-aminolevulinate (ALA) from succinyl-CoA and glycine. This reaction, catalyzed by ALA synthase, is feedback-inhibited by free, non−protein-bound heme. The pathway is disrupted in the porphyrias, a group of diseases in which one of the reactions leading from ALA to heme is impaired. Porphyrias and related conditions can be caused by inherited enzyme deficiencies, iron overload, or lead poisoning. The clinical manifestations are caused by the abnormal accumulation of biosynthetic intermediates and may include abdominal pain, neuropsychiatric signs, and cutaneous photosensitivity.

The degradation of hemoglobin-derived heme is initiated in reticuloendothelial cells of the spleen and other organs. Heme first is oxidized to biliverdin, and this in turn is reduced to bilirubin. Bilirubin is transported to the liver in tight binding to serum albumin. The liver conjugates bilirubin to bilirubin diglucuronide, and this product is actively secreted into the bile. Elevations of the serum bilirubin level, known as hyperbilirubinemia, result in jaundice. Unconjugated hyperbilirubinemia occurs in hemolytic conditions and in otherwise normal newborns; conjugated hyperbilirubinemia results from conditions in which bile flow is blocked (cholestasis); and a mixed hyperbilirubinemia is typical for such nonspecific liver diseases as viral hepatitis and toxic liver damage.

Further Reading

Bloomer JR, Straka JG, Rank JM: The porphyrias. In: Schiff L, Schiff ER, editors: Diseases of the liver, 7th ed., vol. 2. J. B. Lippincott, Philadelphia, 1993, pp. 1438–1464.

Crawford JM, Gollan JL: Bilirubin metabolism and the pathophysiology of jaundice. In: Schiff L, Schiff ER, editors: Diseases of the liver, 7th ed., vol. 1. J. B. Lippincott, Philadelphia, 1993, pp. 42–84.

Elder GH: The porphyrias. In: Holton JB, editor: The inherited metabolic diseases, 2nd ed. Churchill Livingstone, New York, 1994, pp. 351–378.

Fevery J, Blanckaert N: Hyperbilirubinemia. In: McIntyre N, Benhamou J-P, Bircher J, Rizzetto M, Rodes J, editors: Oxford textbook of clinical hepatology, vol. 2. Oxford University Press, Oxford, 1991, pp. 985–991.

Nordmann Y: Human hereditary porphyrias. In: McIntyre N, Benhamou J-P, Bircher J, Rizzetto M, Rodes J, editors: Oxford textbook of clinical hepatology, vol. 2. Oxford University Press, Oxford, 1991, pp. 974–985.

Sassa S, Kappas A: Disorders of heme production and catabolism. In: Handin RI, Lux SE, Stossel TP, editors: Blood. J. B. Lippincott, Philadelphia, 1995, pp. 1473–1523.

Schaffner F: Jaundice. In: Haubrich WS, Schaffner F, Berk JE, editors: Gastroenterology, 5th ed., vol. 1. W. B. Saunders, Philadelphia, 1995, pp. 129–137.

Scriver CR, Beaudet AL, Sly WS, Valle D, editors: The metabolic basis of inherited disease, 6th ed., vol. 1. McGraw-Hill, New York, 1989, pp. 1305–1408.

QUESTIONS

1. Porphyrias can be caused by a reduced activity of any of the following enzymes except
   A. Ferrochelatase
   B. Uroporphyrinogen decarboxylase
   C. Uroporphyrinogen synthase
   D. δ-Aminolevulinate synthase
   E. Protoporphyrinogen oxidase
2. A combination of elevated conjugated bilirubin, near-normal unconjugated bilirubin, and absent fecal urobilinogen in a jaundiced patient suggests
   A. Mild hepatitis
   B. Cholestasis
   C. Hemolysis
   D. Absence of UDP-glucuronyl transferase

Chapter 23

The Metabolism of Purines and Pyrimidines

We have encountered the purine and pyrimidine bases, as shown in Box 23.1, as constituents of nucleotides and nucleic acids. The **ribonucleotides**, ATP, GTP, CTP, and UTP (for nucleotide structures, see Chapter 1), are important coenzymes. They are present in millimolar concentrations in the cell. The **deoxyribonucleotides** dATP, dGTP, dCTP, and dTTP are required only for DNA replication and DNA repair.

They are present in micromolar concentrations, and their abundance varies with the cell cycle, being highest in the S phase when the DNA is replicated. Although dietary nucleic acids and nucleotides are digested to nucleosides and free bases in the intestine, the products are poorly absorbed. Also, especially in the case of the purines, the absorbed bases are not delivered to the tissues but rather are degraded within the intestinal mucosa. Therefore *we*

BOX 23.1

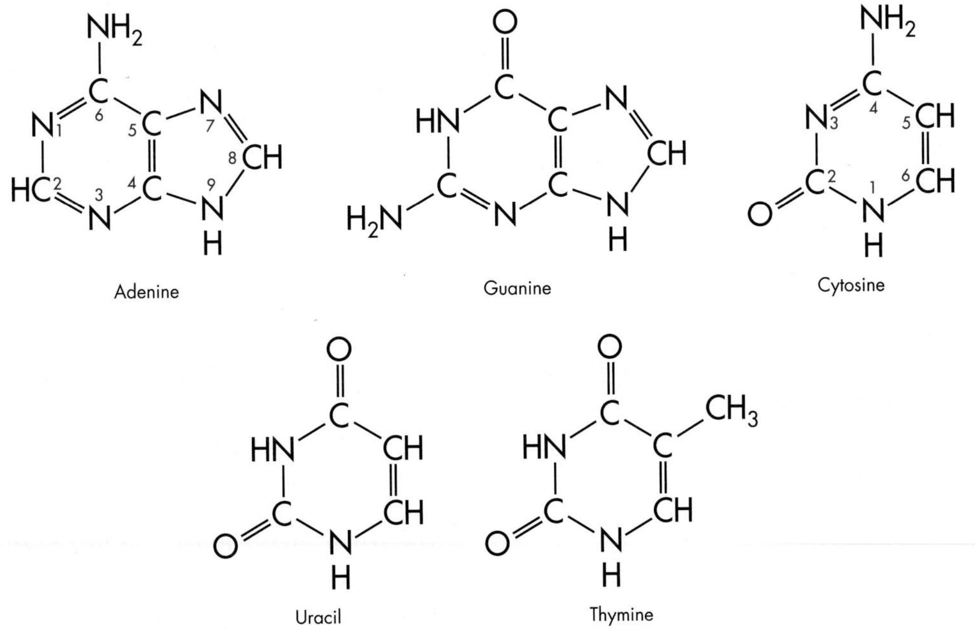

Adenine

Guanine

Cytosine

Uracil

Thymine

FIG. 23.1

The de novo pathway of purine biosynthesis.

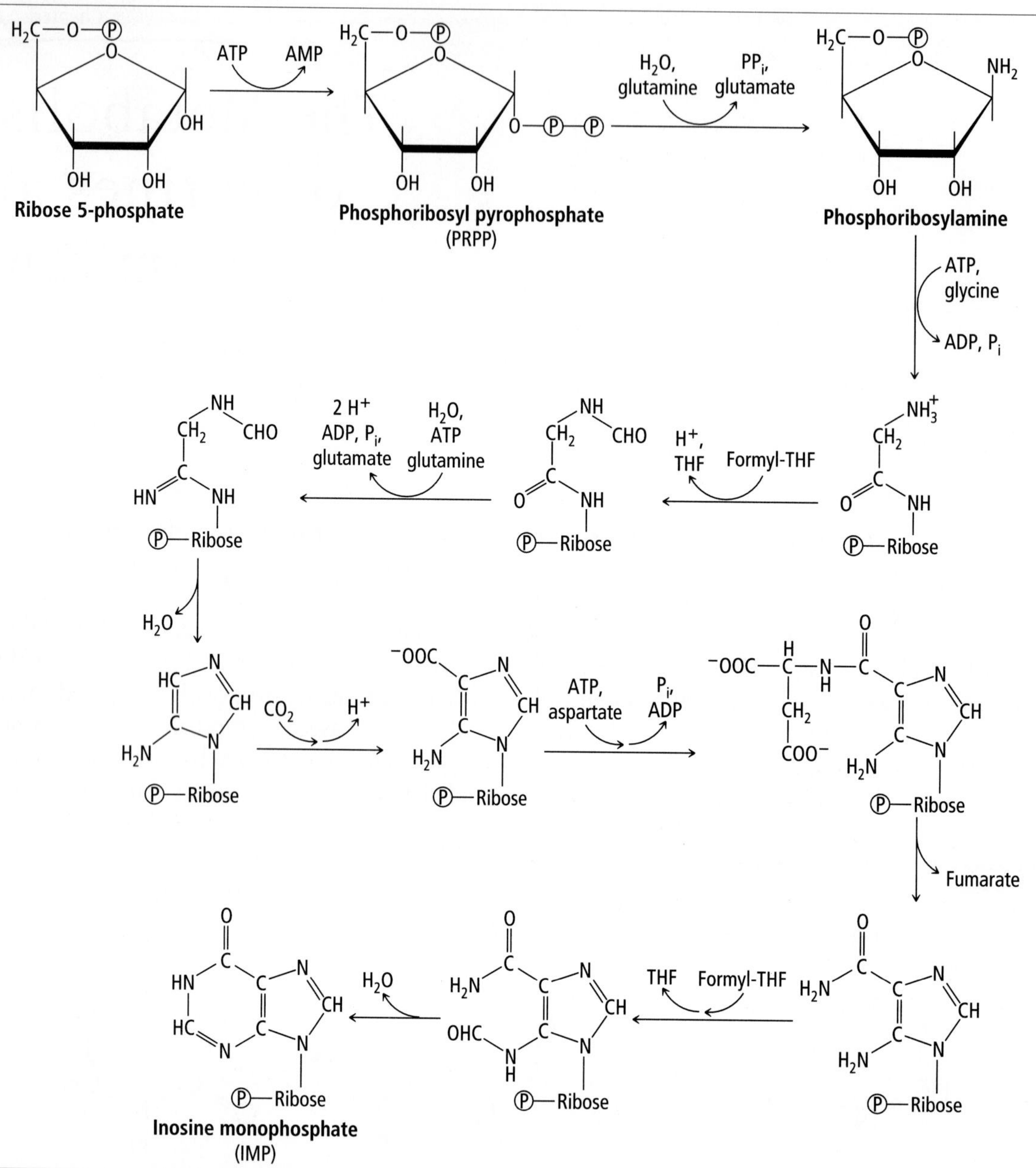

Ribose 5-phosphate → **Phosphoribosyl pyrophosphate (PRPP)** → **Phosphoribosylamine** → ... → **Inosine monophosphate (IMP)**

depend on the endogenous synthesis of purines and pyrimidines. This chapter is concerned with the pathways for the synthesis and degradation of the nucleotides.

Purine synthesis starts with ribose 5-phosphate

The de novo synthesis of purines is most active in the liver, which exports the bases and nucleosides to other tissues. The starting point for the biosyn-

thetic pathway (Fig. 23.1) is **ribose 5-phosphate**, a product of the pentose phosphate pathway (see Chapter 17). In the reactions of the pathway, all of them cytoplasmic, *the elements of the purine ring system are added step by step, using C-1 of ribose 5-phosphate as a primer.*

The first enzyme of the pathway, **PRPP synthetase**, transfers a pyrophosphate group from ATP to C-1 of ribose 5-phosphate, forming **5-phosphoribosyl-1-pyrophosphate (PRPP)**. Effectively, C-1 of

FIG. 23.2

Synthesis of AMP and GMP from IMP.

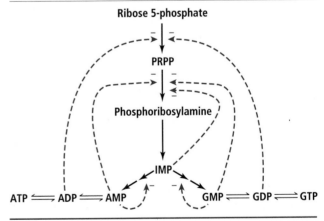

Adenylosuccinate

Inosine monophosphate (IMP)

Xanthosine monophosphate (XMP)

Adenosine monophosphate (AMP)

Guanosine monophosphate (GMP)

ribose 5-phosphate becomes activated by this reaction, and indeed *PRPP is used as an activated form of ribose for the synthesis of all purine and pyrimidine nucleotides.* In the next reaction, catalyzed by **PRPP amidotransferase,** a nitrogen from the side chain of glutamine is transferred to C-1 of PRPP, and inorganic pyrophosphate is released. *This reaction is the committed step of purine biosynthesis.* In the next reactions of the pathway, the purine ring is constructed from simple precursors. You, the student, should be aware of the sources for the carbons and nitrogens in the purine ring:

Glutamine supplies two nitrogens, and tetrahydrofolate supplies two carbons. We shall see later that

FIG. 23.3

Feedback inhibition of de novo purine biosynthesis by nucleotides.

drugs that interfere with the utilization of either glutamine or tetrahydrofolate are inhibitors of purine synthesis.

The first nucleotide formed in the pathway is **inosine monophosphate (IMP),** which contains the base **hypoxanthine.** IMP is a branch point from which both AMP and GMP are formed (Fig. 23.2).

These nucleoside monophosphates are in equilibrium with their corresponding di- and triphosphates.

The regulation of de novo purine synthesis (Fig. 23.3) illustrates the familiar principle of feedback inhibition: *the first two enzymes of the pathway, PRPP synthetase and PRPP amidotransferase, are inhibited by the purine nucleotides.* The reactions leading from IMP to AMP and GMP are feedback-inhibited by AMP and GMP, respectively—in both cases by competitive inhibition.

Purines are degraded to uric acid

The degradation of purine nucleotides (Fig. 23.4) is initiated by the hydrolytic removal of phosphate from

FIG. 23.4

Degradation of purine nucleotides to uric acid, and the salvage of purine bases. ①, 5'-Nucleotidase; ②, AMP deaminase; ③, adenosine deaminase; ④, purine nucleoside phosphorylase; ⑤, guanine deaminase; ⑥, xanthine oxidase; ⑦, adenine phosphoribosyltransferase; ⑧, hypoxanthine-guanine phosphoribosyltransferase.

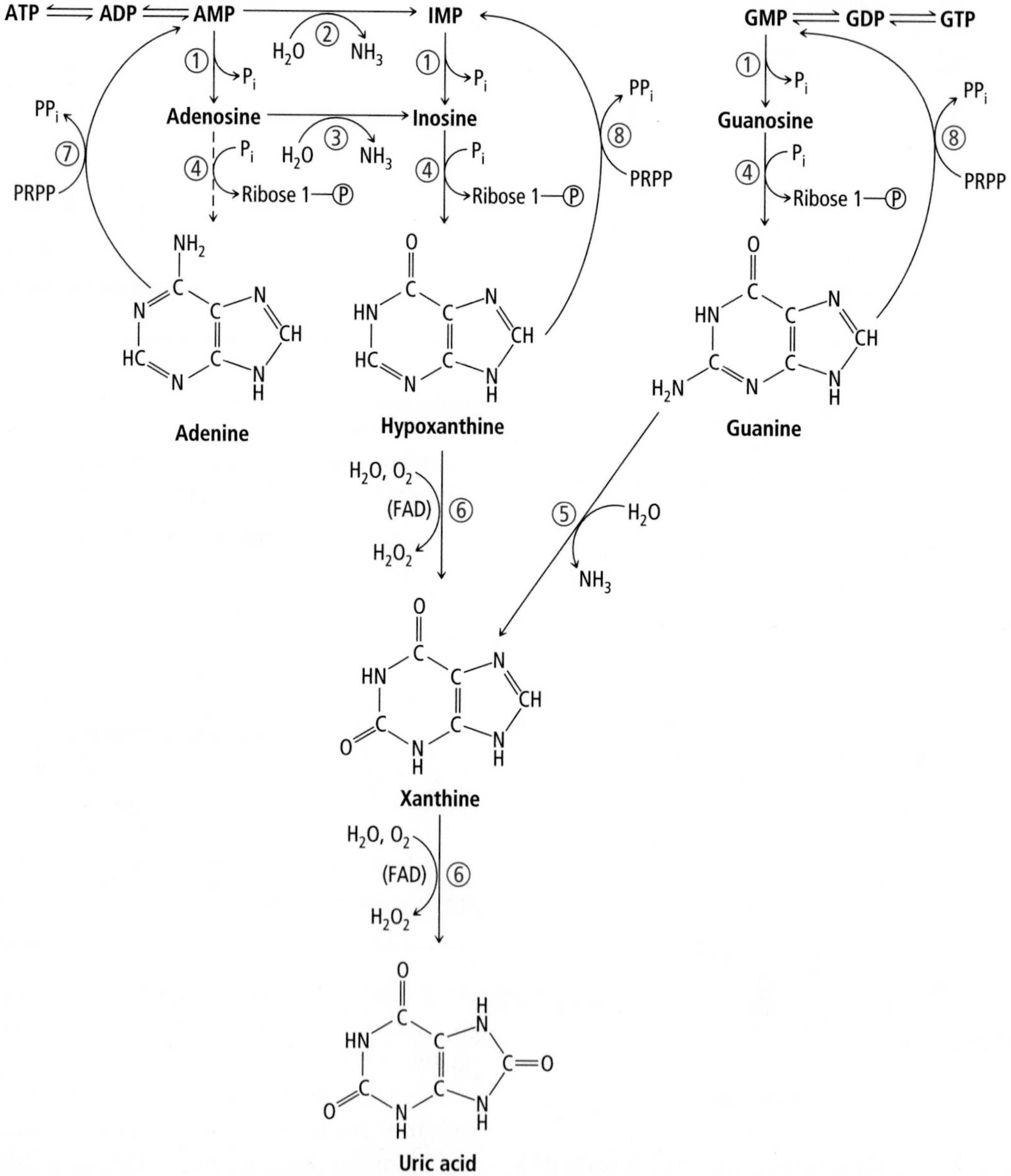

the nucleotides. The nucleosides thus formed are then cleaved into ribose 1-phosphate and the free base by the **purine nucleoside phosphorylase.** Adenosine is a poor substrate of the nucleoside phosphorylase. It therefore is first deaminated to inosine, and inosine is cleaved to hypoxanthine and ribose 1-phosphate. Alternatively, the adenine nucleotides can be degraded via IMP.

Uric acid is the final product of purine degradation in humans. Hypoxanthine, derived from the adenine nucleotides, is oxidized to xanthine, and xanthine to uric acid, by **xanthine oxidase.** This enzyme contains FAD, non-heme iron, and molybdenum. Like many other flavoproteins, it regenerates its FAD by the transfer of hydrogen from $FADH_2$ to molecular oxygen, forming hydrogen peroxide.

Free purine bases can be salvaged

The free bases can be degraded to uric acid, but they also can be used to resynthesize the nucleotides. This requires the PRPP-dependent salvage enzymes **hypoxanthine-guanine phosphoribosyltransferase (HGPRT)** and **adenine phosphoribosyltransferase (APRT):**

$$\text{Hypoxanthine + PRPP} \xrightarrow{\text{HGPRT}}$$
$$\text{Inosine monophosphate (IMP)}$$

$$\text{Guanine + PRPP} \xrightarrow{\text{HGPRT}}$$
$$\text{Guanosine monophosphate (GMP)}$$

$$\text{Adenine + PRPP} \xrightarrow{\text{APRT}}$$
$$\text{Adenosine monophosphate (AMP)}$$

The salvage reactions reduce the requirement for the energetically costly de novo biosynthesis, and they are an essential source of purine nucleotides for those tissues (most notably the brain) in which the de novo pathway is absent or poorly developed. HGPRT is quantitatively by far the more important salvage enzyme. It is competitively inhibited by IMP and GMP; APRT is inhibited by AMP.

Pyrimidines are synthesized from carbamoyl phosphate and aspartate

The pathway of pyrimidine biosynthesis is shown in Fig. 23.5. In contrast to purine synthesis, *the pyrimidine biosynthetic pathway synthesizes the ring system of the base first, before ribose 5-phosphate is introduced from PRPP.* The pathway starts with carbamoyl phosphate and aspartate, and **orotic acid** is formed as the first pyrimidine. Orotic acid is processed to the uridine nucleotides, and these are the precursors of the cytidine nucleotides. The enzymes of the pathway are cytosolic except for the dihydroorotate dehydrogenase (reaction ④ in Fig. 23.5), which is on the outer surface of the inner mitochondrial membrane.

Although carbamoyl phosphate is used both for pyrimidine synthesis and for the urea cycle (see Chapter 21), its sources are different: the carbamoyl phosphate synthetase of the urea cycle is mitochondrial and uses free ammonia as its nitrogen source, whereas the enzyme of pyrimidine synthesis is cytoplasmic and uses the nitrogen from the carboxamide of glutamine.

The pathway is feedback-inhibited by CTP, which inhibits the cytoplasmic carbamoyl phosphate synthetase (step ① in Fig. 23.5). The CTP synthetase also is inhibited by CTP.

Inherited deficiencies of the orotate phosphoribosyltransferase or the orotidylate decarboxylase or both (reactions ⑤ and ⑥ in Fig. 23.5) are the cause of **familial orotic aciduria.** This rare condition is characterized by growth retardation, megaloblastic anemia, and a crystalline sediment of orotic acid in the urine. The important clinical signs are caused not by the accumulation of orotic acid but by the lack of pyrimidines. The patients are pyrimidine auxotrophs who can be treated quite effectively by large doses of orally administered uridine.

Mild orotic aciduria also is seen in ammonia toxicity and in patients with ornithine transcarbamoylase deficiency. These conditions lead to an accumulation of carbamoyl phosphate in liver mitochondria, and some of this leaks into the cytoplasm, where it is converted to orotic acid.

The pyrimidines are degraded to water-soluble products that either are excreted as such or are oxidized to carbon dioxide and water (Fig. 23.6).

Deoxyribonucleotides have to be provided as substrates of DNA synthesis

Deoxyribonucleotides are synthesized from the corresponding ribonucleotides. Two reactions have to

FIG. 23.5

Biosynthesis of pyrimidine nucleotides. ①, Carbamoyl phosphate synthetase II; ②, aspartate transcarbamoylase; ③, dihydroorotase; ④, dihydroorotate dehydrogenase; ⑤, orotate phosphoribosyltransferase; ⑥, orotidylate decarboxylase; ⑦, CTP synthetase.

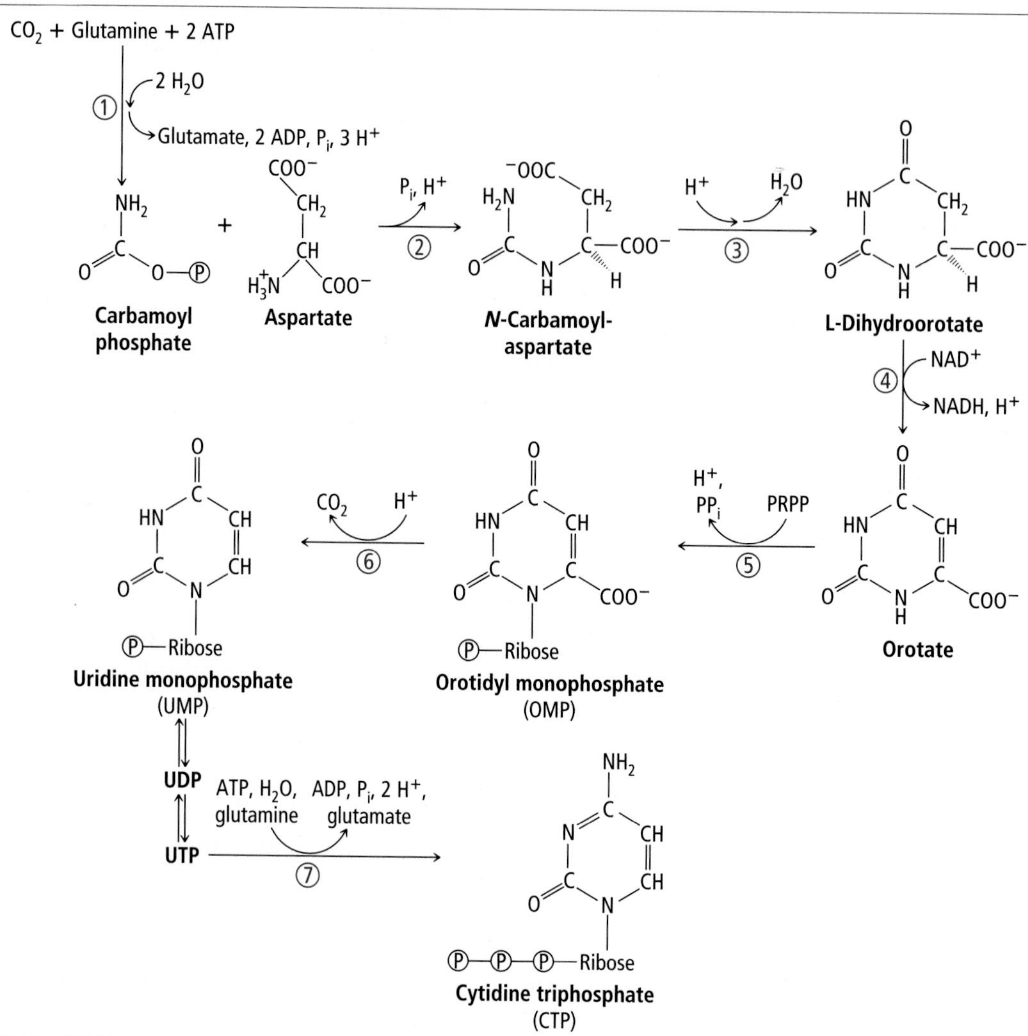

take place: *the ribose has to be reduced to 2-deoxyribose, and uracil has to be methylated to thymine.*

Ribonucleotide reductase reduces the ribose residues in all four ribonucleoside diphosphates as shown in Box 23.2. The level of ribonucleotide reductase increases immediately before the S phase of the cell cycle. The enzyme also is subject to an intricate allosteric control: dATP is a negative effector for all reactions, whereas other nucleotides modulate the substrate specificity and thereby guarantee a balanced production of the deoxyribonucleotides.

Thymine is synthesized by **thymidylate synthase** as shown in Box 23.3. This methylation reaction re-

quires methylene-tetrahydrofolate. The methylene group is reduced to a methyl group during its transfer to dUMP; tetrahydrofolate is oxidized to dihydrofolate (DHF). Dihydrofolate has to be reduced by **dihydrofolate reductase** to regenerate the active coenzyme form as shown in Box 23.4.

Many antineoplastic drugs interfere with nucleotide metabolism

The development of drugs with selective toxicity for tumor cells is difficult because neoplastic cells share most of their biochemical activities with the

FIG. 23.6

Degradation of pyrimidines.

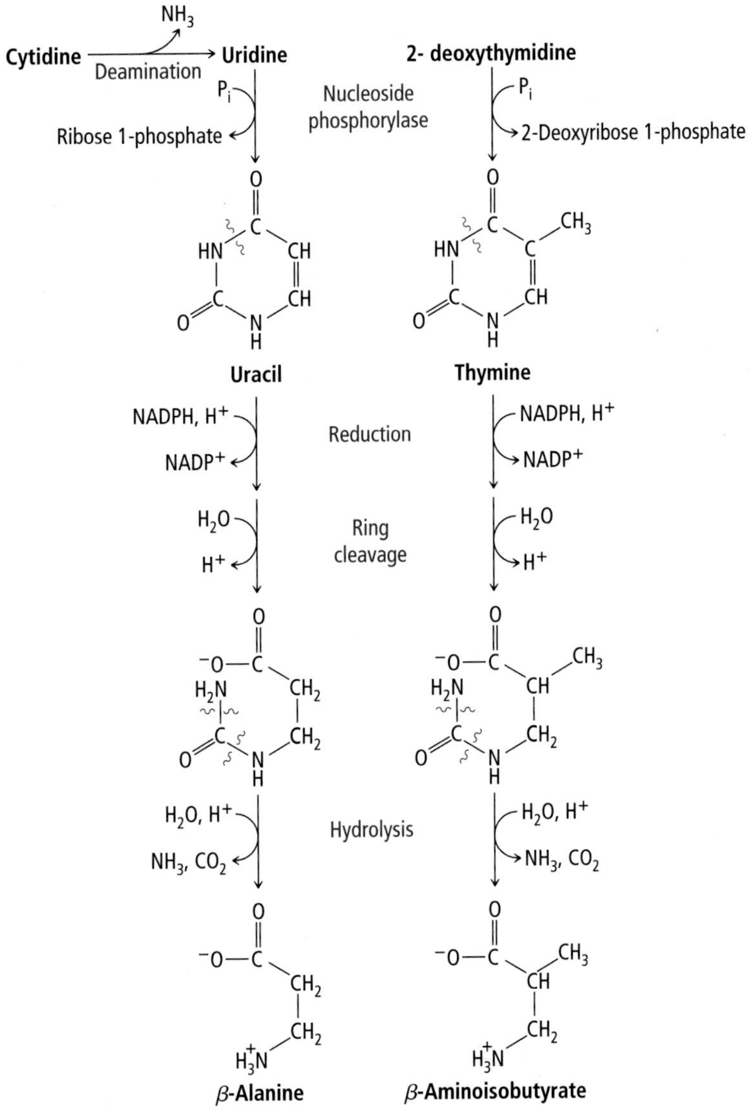

normal cells from which they are derived. Agents that are toxic for cancer cells therefore are likely to be just as toxic for normal cells. Tumor cells, however, do have a higher mitotic rate than normal cells, and therefore *they have a higher requirement for DNA synthesis.*

With this in mind, drugs have been developed as antagonists of nucleotide synthesis:

- *Glutamine antagonists*, exemplified by **azaserine** (shown in Box 23.5), inhibit those steps in purine and pyrimidine synthesis in which glutamine

donates a nitrogen: the incorporation of N-3 and N-9 into the purine ring, and the IMP → GMP and UTP → CTP reactions.

- Several *structural analogs of bases or nucleosides* are useful as antineoplastic drugs. They act either as inhibitors of individual reactions in nucleotide metabolism or through their incorporation into DNA or RNA. A typical example for this type of drug is **5-fluorouracil**, a uracil analog that has been used in the treatment of several solid tumors. This drug is converted enzymatically to fluorodeoxyuridine monophosphate in the body,

BOX 23.2

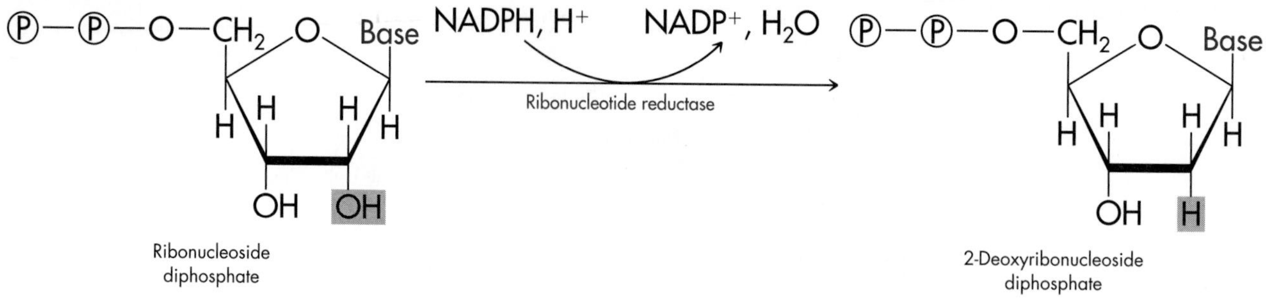

$$\text{Ribonucleoside diphosphate} \xrightarrow[\text{Ribonucleotide reductase}]{\text{NADPH, H}^+ \quad \text{NADP}^+, \text{H}_2\text{O}} \text{2-Deoxyribonucleoside diphosphate}$$

P—P—O—CH₂—O—Base

Ribonucleoside
diphosphate

2-Deoxyribonucleoside
diphosphate

BOX 23.3

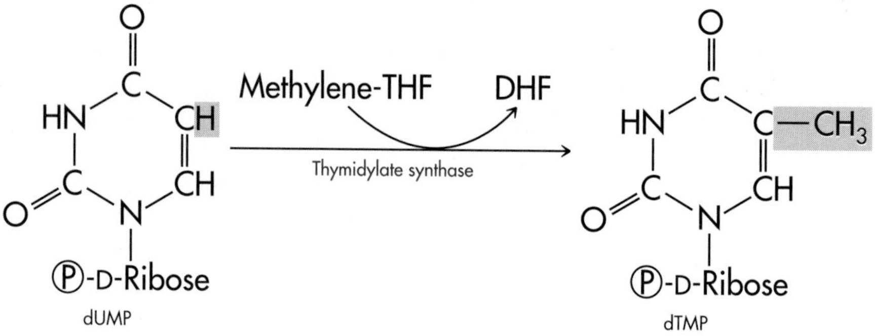

$$\text{dUMP} \xrightarrow[\text{Thymidylate synthase}]{\text{Methylene-THF} \quad \text{DHF}} \text{dTMP}$$

P-D-Ribose
dUMP

P-D-Ribose
dTMP

BOX 23.4

$$\text{Dihydrofolate} \xrightarrow[\substack{\text{Dihydrofolate} \\ \text{reductase}}]{\text{NADPH, H}^+ \quad \text{NADP}^+} \text{Tetrahydrofolate}$$

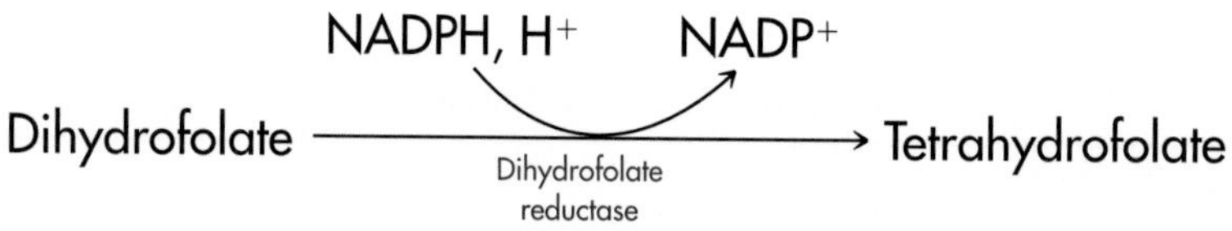

as shown in Box 23.6. This product binds tightly to thymidylate synthase as a structural analog of its natural substrate dUMP. Eventually it reacts covalently with the enzyme, resulting in irreversible inhibition. Fluorouracil also is incorporated into RNA in place of uracil. Indeed, the simultaneous administration of thymidine antagonizes the general toxicity of this drug to a greater extent than its action on tumor cells. This suggests that, for unknown reasons, fluorouracil's incorporation into RNA is more damaging for tumor cells than for normal cells, whereas the inhibition of thymidylate synthase is equally damaging for all cells.

■ *Antifolates* are best exemplified by **amethopterine (methotrexate)** as shown in Box 23.7.

BOX 23.5

Glutamine

Azaserine

BOX 23.6

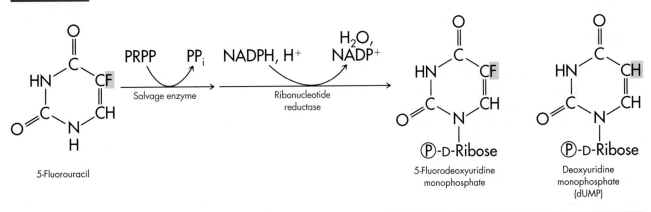

5-Fluorouracil

PRPP → PP$_i$ — Salvage enzyme

NADPH, H$^+$ → H$_2$O, NADP$^+$ — Ribonucleotide reductase

Ⓟ-D-Ribose
5-Fluorodeoxyuridine monophosphate

Ⓟ-D-Ribose
Deoxyuridine monophosphate (dUMP)

BOX 23.7

Amethopterine (methotrexate)

Folic acid

Methotrexate inhibits dihydrofolate reductase competitively. Thymidylate synthase is the only important enzyme that converts a tetrahydrofolate coenzyme to dihydrofolate. Therefore rapidly dividing cells, with their high activity of this enzyme, are rapidly depleted of tetrahydrofolate in the presence of methotrexate.

Needless to say, these anticancer drugs are highly toxic for all rapidly dividing cells in the body, including those in bone marrow, intestinal mucosa, and hair bulbs. Therefore bone marrow depression, diarrhea, and hair loss are common side effects of cancer chemotherapy.

Some immunodeficiency diseases are caused by defects in nucleotide metabolism

Inherited immunodeficiency diseases in which both B cells and T cells are defective are known as **severe combined immunodeficiency (SCID)**. Some patients with recessively inherited SCID have been found to be deficient in **adenosine deaminase.** This enzyme deaminates adenosine to inosine and deoxyadenosine to deoxyinosine (Fig. 23.7). Both adenosine and deoxyadenosine also can be phosphorylated to the corresponding nucleoside monophosphate. However, AMP can be deaminated to IMP by adenylate deaminase, but dAMP has no alternative route of degradation. Therefore it accumulates, together with its di- and triphosphate derivatives. dATP is thought to cause the immunodeficiency by its powerful inhibition of ribonu-

cleotide reductase, thus depriving the cell of the precursors for DNA synthesis. The selective impairment of lymphocytes but not of other cell types in this condition, however, remains an enigma.

The deficiency of **purine nucleoside phosphorylase** results in a different type of immunodeficiency, in which only T cells but not B cells are affected. The mechanism of the selective T-cell impairment in this condition is unknown (Table 23.1).

Uric acid has limited water solubility

The precipitation of uric acid crystals is the cause of **gouty arthritis** and of **uric acid nephropathy.** Uric acid is a weak acid with a pK of 5.7 whose water solubility depends on its ionization state as shown in Box 23.8. The protonated form usually is less soluble than the deprotonated form, but even the deprotonated form is poorly soluble in the presence of a high sodium concentration when sodium urate precipitates. The solubility in urine at pH 5.0 is approximately 0.9 mM (15 mg/dL); the solubility in pH 7.0 urine is on the order of 9 mM (150 mg/dL). Therefore, when uric acid precipitates in the urinary tract, it will be at the level of the collecting ducts where the urine becomes acidified, and the insoluble product will be free uric acid. Approximately 5% to 10% of all kidney stones consist of uric acid. In plasma and interstitial fluids, however, with a pH of 7.3 to 7.4 and a high sodium concentration, sodium urate is most likely to precipitate. Its solubility in the serum is approximately 0.4 mM (7 mg/dL). "Normal" serum urate levels in adults are between 3 and 7 mg/dL, so *even a moderate*

FIG. 23.7

The role of adenosine deaminase in the metabolism of adenine nucleotides. The ribonucleotides can be catabolized by AMP-deaminase, but the deoxyribonucleotides accumulate in adenosine deaminase deficiency.

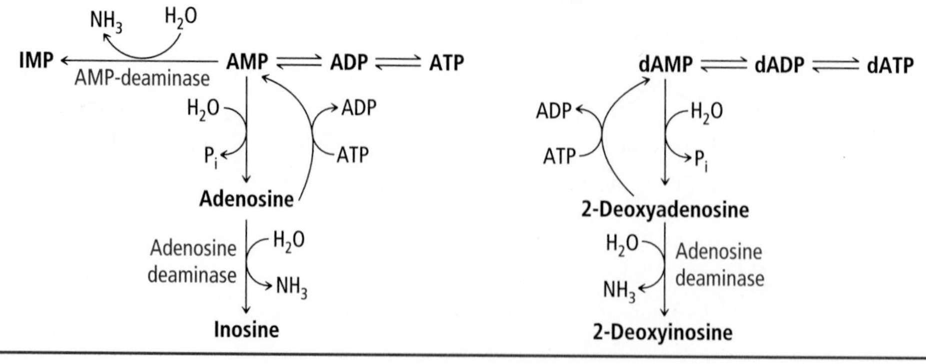

increase of the serum urate concentration will exceed the limit of solubility. The average uric acid level is higher in males than in females by approximately 1 mg/dL and rises with increasing age.

Elevated levels of uric acid cause gout

Elevations of serum uric acid above the limit of solubility are called **hyperuricemia,** and sustained hyperuricemia will lead eventually to the precipitation of sodium urate crystals. Focal deposits of sodium urate in subcutaneous tissues, known as **tophi,** are asymptomatic, but sodium urate crystals in the joints trigger the inflammatory response of **gouty arthritis.** This disease is most common in middle-aged and older males, with a prevalence of between 0.4% and 0.8% in this population group in the United States. It is very rare in premenopausal women.

Gouty arthritis is marked by acute attacks of severe joint pain and inflammation, separated by long asymptomatic intervals. The disease has a predilec-

BOX 23.8

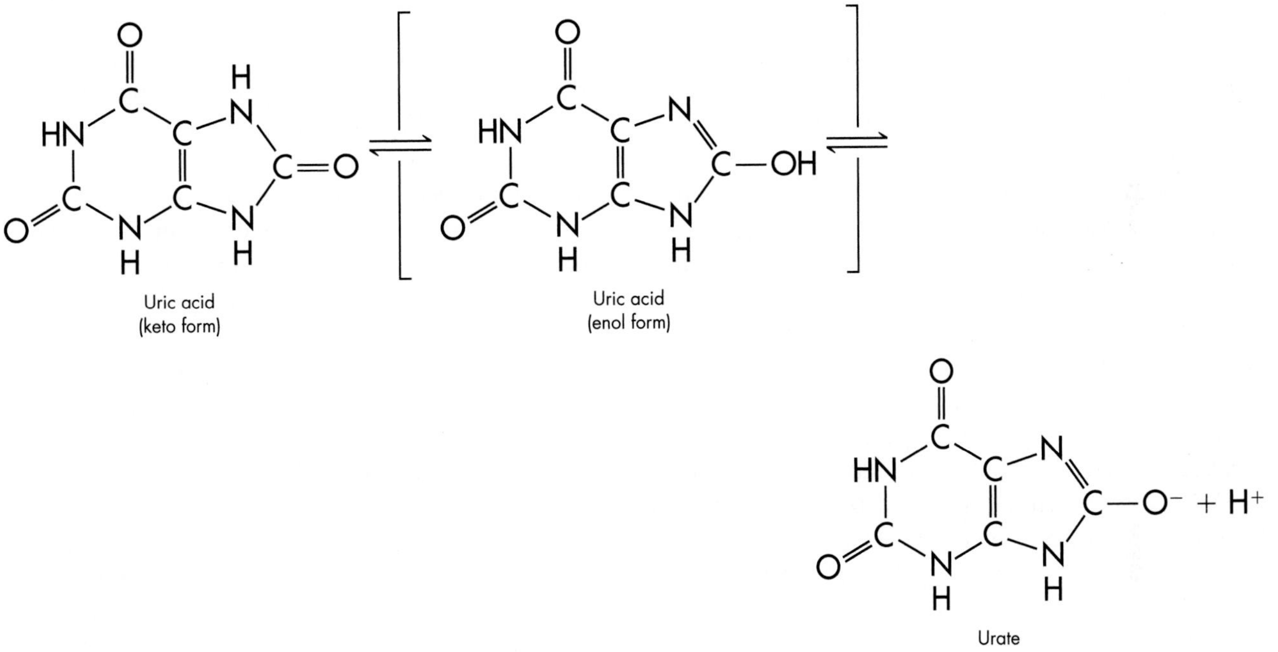

Uric acid
(keto form)

Uric acid
(enol form)

Urate

TABLE 23.1

Inherited disorders of purine and pyrimidine metabolism

Disease	Enzyme deficiency	Signs and symptoms
Adenosine deaminase deficiency	Adenosine deaminase	Severe combined immunodeficiency
Purine nucleoside phosphorylase deficiency	Purine nucleoside phosphorylase	Immunodeficiency with T-cell defect
Familial orotic aciduria	Orotate phosphoribosyltransferase	Accumulation of orotic acid in blood and urine, failure to thrive
Lesch-Nyhan syndrome	Hypoxanthine-guanine phosphoribosyltransferase	Mental retardation with self-mutilation, hyperuricemia

tion for small peripheral joints, and the metatarsophalangeal joint of the big toe is affected initially in approximately half of the patients. The solubility of sodium urate is temperature dependent: crystals form in the coldest parts of the body first.

Any sustained hyperuricemia is likely to cause gouty arthritis, but uric acid levels are somewhat variable over time. On random sampling, 2% to 18% of the healthy population has uric acid levels above the solubility limit of 7 mg/dL, and 10% to 20% of gouty patients have values below this limit at the time of their first attack.

More important than the determination of serum uric acid is **synovial fluid analysis** from an acutely inflamed joint. Gouty patients have needle-shaped, optically birefringent crystals of sodium urate in affected joints, frequently within polymorphonuclear leukocytes. These cells phagocytize sodium urate crystals, and these undigestible crystals damage their lysosomes, eventually killing the cell.

Secondary hyperuricemia is caused by an underlying disease, but most cases of **primary hyperuricemia** are of unknown etiology. Secondary hyperuricemia is typical for conditions with increased cell turnover, including psoriasis, chronic hemolytic anemias, pernicious anemia, and malignancies. Radiation treatment or chemotherapy of neoplastic diseases can cause massive hyperuricemia, with the formation of widespread urate deposits in the kidneys. This is known as **uric acid nephropathy** and may very well terminate in renal failure. In the chemotherapy of hematological malignancies it is common practice to start treatment for hyperuricemia before cytotoxic drugs are given.

Uric acid production also is increased in metabolic disorders in which the activity of the pentose phosphate pathway is increased. Thus, some gouty patients have been found to have an increased activity of the NADPH-consuming enzyme glutathione reductase (Chapter 17). Patients with type I glycogen storage disease (von Gierke's disease; see Chapter 17) also have hyperuricemia. In these conditions, an increased supply of ribose 5-phosphate through the pentose phosphate pathway leads to an increased rate of de novo purine biosynthesis. Purines cannot be stored in the body, so *any increase in the rate of their de novo synthesis has to be matched by an increased rate of degradation to uric acid.*

Primary hyperuricemia is caused either by an *over-production of uric acid* or by an *impairment of its renal excretion*, or both. The production of uric acid can be assessed by its measurement in a 24-hour urine sample: levels in excess of 600 mg/day are an indication of uric acid overproduction. Approximately 15% to 25% of patients with primary gout are overproducers. Impaired renal excretion is the likely cause of hyperuricemia in patients with normal production. The handling of uric acid by the kidney is complex. It is subject to glomerular filtration, and both active secretion and reabsorption occur in the tubular system.

Some gouty patients have abnormalities of purine-metabolizing enzymes

Specific enzymatic abnormalities have been identified in a minority of gouty patients with uric acid overproduction. Two enzymes may be affected:

1. *An increased activity of PRPP synthetase*, inherited as an X-linked trait, has been seen in several patients. The resulting overproduction of purine nucleotides has to be balanced by their increased breakdown to uric acid. High levels of IMP, GMP, and AMP, derived from increased de novo biosynthesis, inhibit the salvage enzymes and thereby favor uric acid formation. The finding of hyperuricemia in patients with an increased activity of PRPP synthetase shows that this enzyme is normally rate limiting in de novo purine synthesis. The rate of the amidotransferase reaction depends largely on the concentration of its rate-limiting substrate PRPP.

2. *A decreased activity of the salvage enzyme HGPRT*, also inherited as an X-linked trait, has been found in several patients with early onset of gout. This enzyme deficiency causes hyperuricemia because the substrates of the deficient enzyme accumulate while the levels of its products are reduced:

- *The cellular levels of the free bases are increased*, thus providing more substrate for the uric acid–producing enzymes.
- *The cellular PRPP level is increased* because of decreased consumption in the salvage reactions, and more substrate is available for the PRPP amidotransferase of the de novo pathway.

- *The cellular concentrations of the nucleotides are decreased,* and the regulated enzymes of the de novo pathway therefore are disinhibited.

The result is an increased rate of de novo synthesis, balanced by an equally increased rate of uric acid formation.

Partial deficiencies of HGPRT cause only hyperuricemia, but a complete deficiency results in **Lesch-Nyhan syndrome.** This rare, X-linked recessive disorder is characterized by choreoathetosis, spasticity, mental retardation, and a bizarre pattern of self-mutilating behavior: the patients chew off their lips and fingers or jam their hands into the spokes of their wheelchairs. The presence of uric acid crystals in the urine is an early sign of the disease, and most patients die sooner or later of uric acid nephropathy. The CNS involvement, however, is not caused by uric acid. The brain has an extremely low capacity for de novo purine biosynthesis, so a complete absence of the salvage enzyme damages the brain by depriving it of purine nucleotides.

Most animals other than the higher primates avoid the problems associated with uric acid by degrading it to water-soluble products. Why do we use uric acid as the final product of purine metabolism, and why is our uric acid level so high that we are often teetering on the brink of gout? One possible explanation can be found in the chemical reactivity of uric acid: it is an effective antioxidant that scavenges reactive oxygen derivatives such as hydroxy radicals, superoxide radicals, and singlet oxygen. Thus it may contribute to the body's defenses against oxidative damage.

Drugs are very effective in the treatment of gout

The short-term goal in the treatment of gout is the alleviation of the excruciating pain of the acute attack. Long-term treatment is aimed at reducing serum uric acid levels.

The most important drug treatments are:

- *Antiinflammatory drugs.* **Colchicine** is the classical treatment for the acute attack. It is not very effective in other forms of arthritis, and it therefore can be used for the differential diagnosis of gout. This approach, in which the response to the treatment confirms (or refutes) a preliminary diagnosis, is called a diagnosis *ex juvantibus.* Because of gastrointestinal side effects, however, colchicine has been largely replaced by nonsteroidal antiinflammatory drugs such as indomethacin and ibuprofen.
- *Uricosuric agents* increase the renal excretion of uric acid. **Probenecide** is a typical example.
- *Inhibition of xanthine oxidase* is effected by **allopurinol.** This purine analog initially is oxidized to alloxanthine by xanthine oxidase, as shown in Box 23.9, and alloxanthine inhibits the enzyme by tight, noncovalent binding. As a result, the formation of uric acid is reduced while hypoxanthine and xanthine are excreted. Gout and renal problems are improved because the mix of xanthine, hypoxanthine, and uric acid is more soluble than uric acid alone.

In patients with intact HGPRT, allopurinol also decreases the de novo synthesis of purines, because hypoxanthine and xanthine are salvaged to

BOX 23.9

Allopurinol   Alloxanthine

IMP and xanthosine monophosphate (XMP), respectively. These reactions consume PRPP and produce nucleotides that feedback-inhibit the regulated enzymes of the de novo pathway.

Are there dietary treatments for gout? Dietary purines mostly are degraded to uric acid in the intestinal mucosa. Indeed, the consumption of 4 g of yeast RNA per day raises blood urate levels to those found in gout. On the other hand, eliminating all purines from a typical Western diet would reduce the serum urate level by only 1 mg/dL. A low-protein diet often is recommended in the belief that an excess of precursor amino acids increases de novo purine synthesis. Alcohol should be avoided because of associated dehydration and because the increased lactate levels during alcohol intoxication (see Chapter 29) may impair the renal excretion of uric acid. Acute attacks of gouty arthritis often are triggered by an alcoholic binge.

pecially in acidic urine, and more widespread urate deposits in the kidney can lead to dangerous uric acid nephropathy.

Further Reading

Emmerson BT: Hyperuricemia and gout. In: Noe DA, Rock RC, editors: *Laboratory medicine.* Williams & Wilkins, Baltimore, 1994, pp. 512–524.

Kelley WN, Schumacher HR Jr: Gout. In: Kelley WN, Harris ED, Ruddy S, Sledge CB, editors: *Textbook of rheumatology,* 4th ed., vol. 2. W. B Saunders, Philadelphia, 1993, pp. 1291–1336.

Scriver CR, Beaudet AL, Sly WS, Valle D, editors: *The metabolic basis of inherited disease,* 6th ed., vol. 1. McGraw-Hill, New York, 1989, pp. 965–1126.

Simmonds HA: Purine and pyrimidine disorders. In: Holton JB, editors: *The inherited metabolic diseases,* 2nd ed. Churchill Livingstone, New York, 1994, pp. 297–349.

Stone TW, Simmonds HA: *Purines: basic and clinical aspects.* Kluwer Academic Publishers, Dordrecht, 1991.

SUMMARY

The vast majority of the purines and pyrimidines in our nucleotides and nucleic acids are derived from endogenous synthesis rather than from the diet. The heterocyclic ring systems are assembled from simple precursors, and the ribose portion is introduced from 5-phosphoribosyl-1-pyrophosphate (PRPP), the activated form of ribose 5-phosphate. The first reactions of the biosynthetic pathways are feedback-inhibited by the nucleotides. The ribonucleotides are synthesized first, and they are the precursors of the corresponding 2-deoxyribonucleotides, the substrates of DNA synthesis. Many antineoplastic drugs are inhibitors of nucleotide synthesis. These agents are useful because they are most toxic for rapidly dividing cells.

Purine nucleotides are catabolized to the free bases first, and these are either oxidized to the excretory product uric acid or converted back to the corresponding nucleotides in PRPP-dependent salvage reactions. Uric acid is problematic because of its low water solubility. Even moderate elevations of its plasma level lead to the precipitation of sodium urate crystals in the joints, causing gouty arthritis. Uric acid also can form kidney stones, es-

QUESTIONS

1. An enzyme abnormality that can predispose people to hyperuricemia and gouty arthritis is
   A. Reduced activity of PRPP synthetase
   B. Reduced activity of xanthine oxidase
   C. Reduced activity of hypoxanthine-guanine phosphoribosyltransferase
   D. Reduced activity of PRPP amidotransferase
   E. Reduced activity of dihydroorotate dehydrogenase

2. A tetrahydrofolate derivative is required for
   A. The de novo synthesis of pyrimidines
   B. The synthesis of thymine-containing nucleotides from uracil-containing nucleotides
   C. The synthesis of xanthine from purine nucleotides
   D. The cleavage of the purine ring in uric acid by an enzyme in the human liver
   E. The reduction of ribonucleotides to 2-deoxyribonucleotides

Chapter 24

Vitamins and Minerals

Vitamins are organic nutrients that are required in small quantities in the diet. Unlike the major nutrients, they are not used for the generation of metabolic energy, but rather serve specialized functions in the body. **Minerals** are inorganic nutrients. The **macrominerals,** such as sodium, calcium, and phosphate, are required in quantities of more than 100 mg/day. They are components of the body fluids and the inorganic matrix of bone. The **microminerals,** or **trace minerals,** on the other hand, are required only in small quantities and serve specialized biochemical functions. Only the vitamins and trace minerals will be discussed in this chapter.

The dietary requirements for vitamins and minerals are specified in terms of a **recommended daily allowance (RDA).** RDAs are published by the Food and Nutrition Board of the National Academy of Sciences in the United States and by similar agencies in other countries. The RDA defines not a minimal requirement but *a dietary intake that is considered optimal under ordinary conditions.* There is not always perfect agreement about "optimal" levels of intake, so RDAs are revised frequently. The requirement also depends on such variables as sex, age, body weight, diet, and physiological status. Thus, increased dietary intakes of many nutrients are recommended during pregnancy and lactation. Many diseases also require special nutritional considerations that are beyond the scope of this book. Figure 24.1 summarizes the RDAs of the most important vitamins and minerals for the 70-kg "textbook" male.

THE WATER-SOLUBLE VITAMINS

The water-soluble vitamins are the largest class of essential micronutrients. Although their biological functions are very diverse, *most water-soluble vitamins are biosynthetic precursors of coenzymes.* They are absorbed readily from the intestine and are transported to the tissues, where they are converted to the active coenzyme forms. The water-soluble vitamins can be excreted by the kidneys, so they cannot accumulate easily to toxic levels.

Riboflavin is required for the synthesis of FAD and FMN

Riboflavin (vitamin B_2) consists of a dimethylisoalloxazine ring that is covalently bound to ribitol, a sugar alcohol related to ribose. It has only one biological function: *it is a precursor of FAD and FMN,* the prosthetic groups of the flavoproteins. Both free riboflavin and the flavin coenzymes are yellow in their reduced form, with an absorption band at 450 nm (Latin *flavus,* "yellow"). The oxidized form is strongly fluorescent. Although riboflavin and its derivatives are heat stable, they are degraded rapidly to inactive products on exposure to visible light.

Dietary riboflavin is absorbed by an energy-dependent transport system in the upper small intestine and transported to the tissues, where it is converted to FMN and FAD (Fig. 24.2). The excess is excreted in the urine or metabolized by microsomal enzymes in the liver.

The adult male RDA of riboflavin is set at 1.4 to 1.7 mg/day, and most people readily obtain this amount from their diet. Good dietary sources include liver, yeast, eggs, meat, enriched bread and cereals, and milk (both human and cow's milk). Riboflavin deficiency usually occurs together with other vitamin deficiencies and is most common in alcoholics. The symptoms include glossitis (magenta tongue), angular stomatitis, sore throat, and a moist (seborrheic) dermatitis of the scrotum and nose. This may be accompanied by a normochromic normocytic anemia.

Riboflavin deficiency can occur in infants who are under phototherapy for hyperbilirubinemia (see Chapter 22). Not only bilirubin but also riboflavin is destroyed by light in the skin, so riboflavin supplements are given routinely in this situation.

The dietary status can be assessed by the fluorometric or microbiological determination of urinary riboflavin. Alternatively, the activity of erythrocyte glutathione reductase (see Chapter 17) is determined in freshly lysed RBCs before and after the addition of its coenzyme FAD: in patients with riboflavin deficiency, the apoenzyme is not saturated completely with its cofactor, and the enzymatic activity therefore is increased by added FAD.

FIG. 24.1

Recommended daily allowances of vitamins and minerals for a young, healthy, 70-kg male.

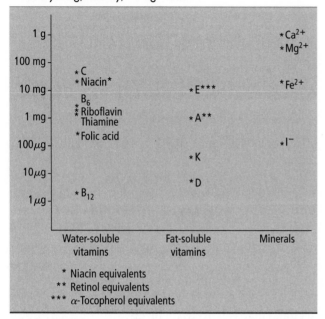

1 g
100 mg
10 mg
1 mg
100μg
10μg
1μg
*C
Niacin
B6
Riboflavin
Thiamine
*Folic acid
*B12
*E***
*A**
*K
*D
*Ca2+
*Mg2+
*Fe2+
*I−
Water-soluble vitamins
Fat-soluble vitamins
Minerals
* Niacin equivalents
** Retinol equivalents
*** α-Tocopherol equivalents

Niacin is a precursor of NAD and NADP

The term **niacin**, originally applied to nicotinic acid, now is often used as a generic term for the vitamin-active pyrimidine derivatives **nicotinic acid** and **nicotinamide:**

FIG. 24.2

Synthesis of FMN and FAD from dietary riboflavin.

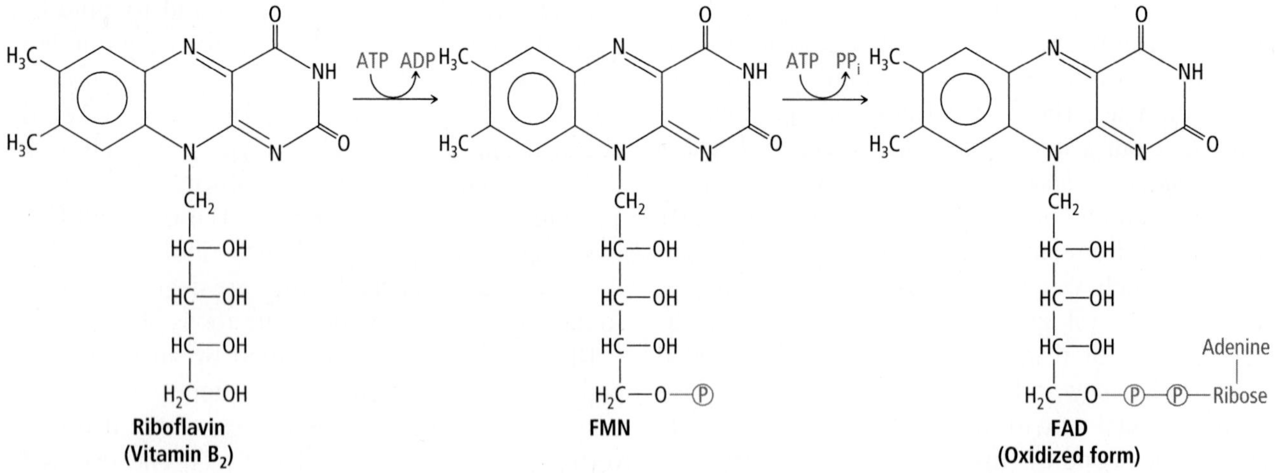

ATP ADP
ATP PPi
Adenine
Ribose
Riboflavin
(Vitamin B2)
FMN
FAD
(Oxidized form)

Nicotinic acid (niacin)   Nicotinamide (niacinamide)

Both in the human body and in dietary sources, *niacin is present as a constituent of NAD and NADP.* The dietary coenzymes are hydrolyzed in the GI tract, and free nicotinic acid and nicotinamide are absorbed in the small intestine. After their transport to the tissues, the vitamin forms are incorporated into the coenzymes (Fig. 24.3). Excess niacin is excreted by the kidneys, partly as unchanged nicotinic acid and nicotinamide and partly in the form of various metabolites.

NAD and NADP can be synthesized endogenously from tryptophan, but the pathway is inefficient: approximately 60 mg of dietary tryptophan, which is nutritionally essential itself, is required for the synthesis of 1 mg of niacin. The pathway of endogenous niacin synthesis requires riboflavin, thiamine, and pyridoxine, and it therefore may be impaired in patients with multiple vitamin deficiencies.

Niacin deficiency, known as **pellagra** (the name is Italian and means "rough skin"), is seen only on a diet low in both niacin and tryptophan. Corn-based diets, in particular, are associated with this deficiency: maize protein has a low tryptophan content, and the niacin, which actually is present in moderate amounts, is poorly absorbed because it is tightly bound to other constituents of the grain.

Early deficiency signs include weakness, lassitude, anorexia, indigestion, and a glossitis that resembles that of riboflavin deficiency. The signs of severe deficiency are dermatitis, diarrhea, and dementia. The dermatitis presents as a symmetrical erythematous rash on sun-exposed parts of the skin. Diarrhea is caused by widespread inflammation of mucosal surfaces. The mental changes, which initially are quite vague, can progress to a profound encephalopathy with confusion, memory loss, and overt organic psychosis. In severe cases, mental deterioration can become irreversible. Although pellagra was widespread in the southern United States during the early years of the twentieth century, niacin deficiency is now rare in industrialized countries.

The adult male RDA is 15 to 20 niacin equivalents (NEs), with one NE corresponding to the biological activity of 1 mg of niacin. On a typical diet, between 8 and 16 NEs are derived from dietary tryptophan, and approximately the same amount from niacin. Good sources of niacin include yeast, meat, liver, peanuts and other legume seeds, and enriched cereals.

Nicotinic acid is used in pharmacological doses (several grams daily) for the treatment of hyperlipidemias. The pharmacological effects of these doses include an immediate peripheral vasodilation and, on prolonged treatment, a decreased release of free fatty acids from adipose tissue and a decreased formation of VLDL by the liver. These effects are unrelated to the vitamin activity of nicotinic acid.

Thiamine is required for carbonyl transfers

Dietary **thiamine** is absorbed readily and is transported to the tissues, where it is phosphorylated to its coenzyme form **thiamine pyrophosphate (TPP)** in an ATP-dependent reaction. Approximately 30 mg of the vitamin is present in the body, 80% of this in the form of TPP as shown in Box 24.1. The TPP-dependent reactions are *aldehyde transfers,* in which the aldehyde is bound covalently to one of the carbons in the thiazole (sulfur-and-nitrogen) ring of the coenzyme. One reaction type, the *oxidative decarboxylation of α-ketoacids,* is catalyzed by mitochondrial multienzyme complexes. The decarboxylations of pyruvate, α-ketoglutarate, branched-chain α-keto acids and α-ketobutyrate (see Chapter 21) all follow the reaction mechanism that was described for pyruvate dehydrogenase in Chapter 16. A different reaction type is encountered in the cytoplasmic *transketolase reaction* (see Chapter 17), in which TPP transfers a glycolaldehyde from one monosaccharide to another. It is the major catabolic, energy-producing pathways that are particularly dependent on TPP.

Mild thiamine deficiency is associated with gastrointestinal complaints, weakness, and burning feet. Peripheral neuropathy, abnormalities of mental

FIG. 24.3

Synthesis of NAD and NADP.

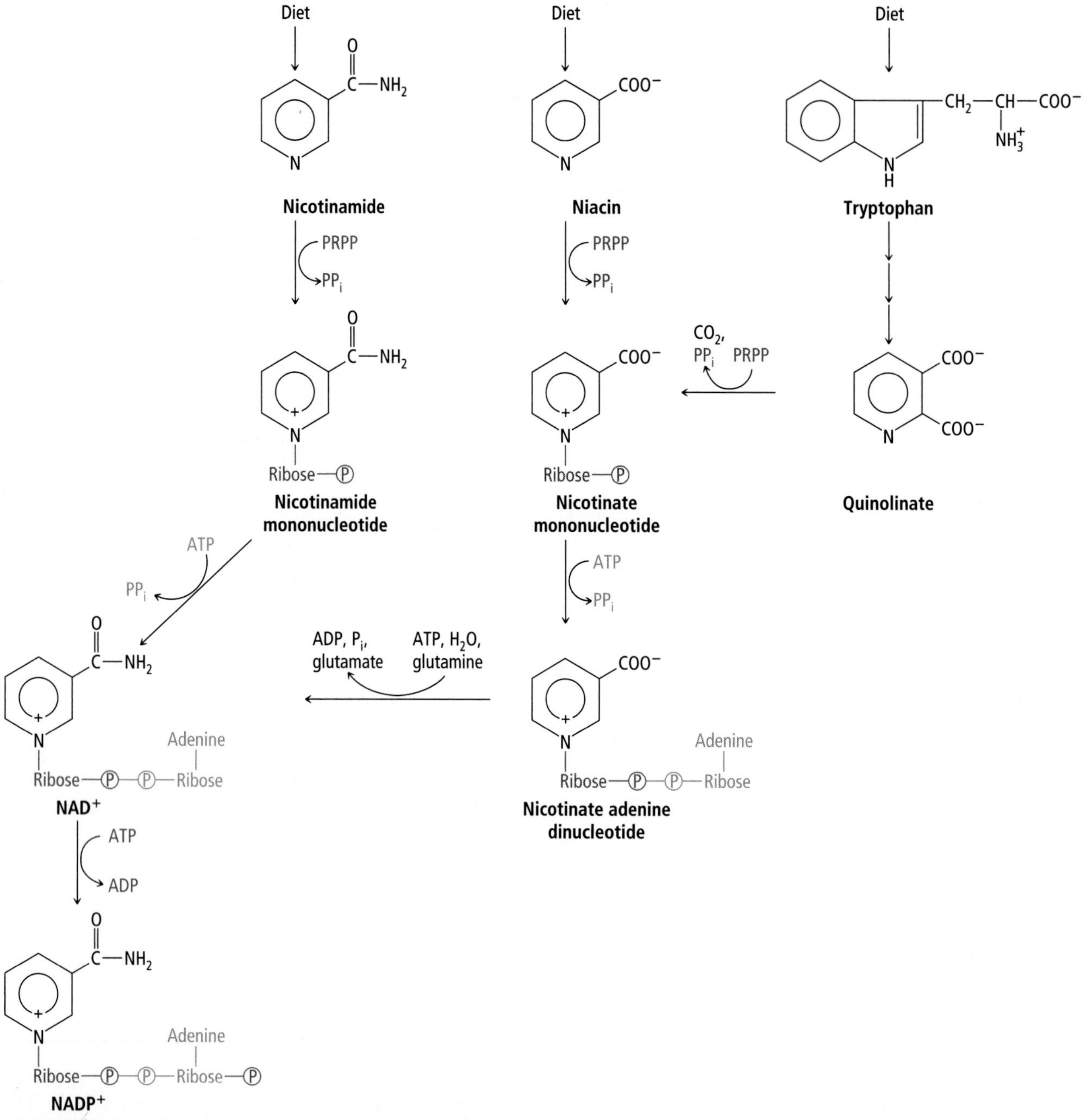

status, and ataxia develop in moderate deficiency; full-blown deficiency, known as **beriberi**, presents with *advanced neuromuscular and cardiovascular disorders*: delirium, muscle weakness and muscle wasting, oph-thalmoplegia (paralysis of the eye muscles), and memory loss are typical and are accompanied by peripheral vasodilation and an increased venous re-

turn to the heart. Thiamine deficiency also impairs myocardial contractility, and death may result from high-output cardiac failure.

Beriberi became a prominent health problem in some parts of Asia at the end of the nineteenth cen-tury, when the milling and polishing of rice were introduced in these countries. The thiamine of rice

BOX 24.1

Thiamine pyrophosphate
(TPP)

is present in the outer layers of the grain, which are removed by polishing, so beriberi became the scourge of poor people who had to subsist on a rice-based diet.

The dietary thiamine requirement depends on the caloric intake, with a recommended daily allowance of 0.5 mg/1000 kcal. Thiamine deficiency is not common in developed countries *except in alcoholics*, who have poor intestinal absorption in addition to an inadequate dietary intake.

Thiamine deficiency in alcoholics does not result in beriberi but rather in **Wernicke-Korsakoff syndrome**. In the acute stage of this disease, known as **Wernicke's encephalopathy**, the patient presents with mental derangements and delirium, ataxia (motor incoordination), and ophthalmoplegia. The chronic stage, known as **Korsakoff psychosis**, is a severely debilitating condition that is dominated by anterograde amnesia. *Korsakoff psychosis is the most common form of amnestic syndrome in the United States.* The disease is related to a recognizable pattern of brain damage: at autopsy, focal lesions are found in the periventricular areas of the thalamus and hypothalamus, the periaqueductal gray of the midbrain, and in the mamillary bodies. The reasons for this pattern of brain damage are unknown.

Wernicke's encephalopathy can be treated by thiamine injections, but *timely diagnosis and immediate treatment are essential* because the amnestic syndrome, once established, is irreversible.

The thiamine status can be evaluated by the measurement of urinary thiamine excretion, but the determination of transketolase activity in whole blood or erythrocytes, both before and after the addition of thiamine pyrophosphate, is the preferred diagnostic procedure. In addition, the plasma levels of lactate and pyruvate can be determined after an oral glucose load. These acids accumulate because of the decreased activity of pyruvate dehydrogenase.

Vitamin B_6 plays a key role in amino acid metabolism

Vitamin B_6 is the generic name for the dietary precursors of the active coenzyme form, **pyridoxal phosphate (PLP)**. They include **pyridoxine, pyridoxal,** and **pyridoxamine,** as well as their phosphorylated derivatives as shown in Box 24.2. The phosphate derivatives are hydrolyzed by intestinal alkaline phosphatase, and the dephosphorylated forms are absorbed. The synthesis of the active coenzyme form is shown in Fig. 24.4. The total body content of PLP is approximately 25 mg in adults, and pyridoxal and pyridoxal phosphate are the major circulating forms of the vitamin.

The aldehyde group of PLP forms aldimine derivatives with primary amino groups of amino acids. The aldimine is stabilized by an intramolecular hydrogen bond with the phenolic hydroxy group as shown in Box 24.3. Several dozen enzymes of amino acid metabolism in human tissues contain PLP as a tightly bound prosthetic group.

Glycogen phosphorylase also contains PLP. In this case, however, the phosphate group of PLP participates in the catalytic mechanism as a general acid to promote the attack of the substrate phosphate on the glycosidic bond in glycogen. More than half of the B_6 in the human body is present in glycogen phosphorylase.

Liver, fish, whole grains, nuts, legumes, egg yolk, and yeast are good sources of B_6. The dietary requirement is proportional to the protein content of the diet, and 1.6 to 2.0 mg/day is recommended on a 100-g/day protein intake. More serious forms of de-

BOX 24.2

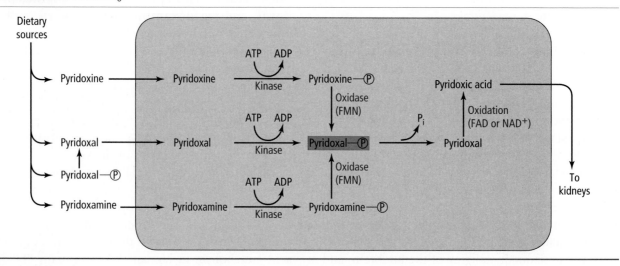

Pyridoxine

Pyridoxal

Pyridoxamine

Pyridoxal phosphate
(PLP)

FIG. 24.4

Metabolism of vitamin B$_6$.

Dietary
sources

Pyridoxine → Pyridoxine $\xrightarrow[\text{Kinase}]{\text{ATP ADP}}$ Pyridoxine—P

Pyridoxic acid

Oxidase
(FMN)

Pyridoxal → Pyridoxal $\xrightarrow[\text{Kinase}]{\text{ATP ADP}}$ Pyridoxal—P $\xrightarrow{\text{P}_i}$ Pyridoxal

Pyridoxal—P

Oxidation
(FAD or NAD$^+$)

Oxidase
(FMN)

To
kidneys

Pyridoxamine → Pyridoxamine $\xrightarrow[\text{Kinase}]{\text{ATP ADP}}$ Pyridoxamine—P

BOX 24.3

ficiency, which are rare, are characterized by *peripheral neuropathy*, and epileptic seizures may appear, especially in children. Some of the neurological derangements may be the result of the impaired activity of the PLP-dependent enzyme glutamate decarboxylase, which forms the inhibitory neurotransmitter GABA (see Chapter 26). Dermatitis, glossitis, and **sideroblastic anemia** are other abnormalities in B_6 deficiency. Sideroblastic anemia is a microcytic hypochromic anemia, similar to iron deficiency anemia (see Chapter 24) but in the presence of normal serum iron. The utilization of iron for heme synthesis is impaired, however, probably because of the PLP requirement of ALA synthase (see Chapter 22). As a result, the iron storage proteins ferritin and hemosiderin accumulate in sideroblasts (ferritin-laden macrophages) within the bone marrow.

B_6 *deficiency is most common in alcoholics*, contributing to the development of sideroblastic anemia and peripheral neuropathy. Some drugs, including **isoniazid** (a tuberculostatic) and **penicillamine** (a metal chelator, also used in rheumatoid arthritis) can precipitate B_6 deficiency. These drugs react nonenzymatically with the aldehyde group of pyridoxal or pyridoxal phosphate.

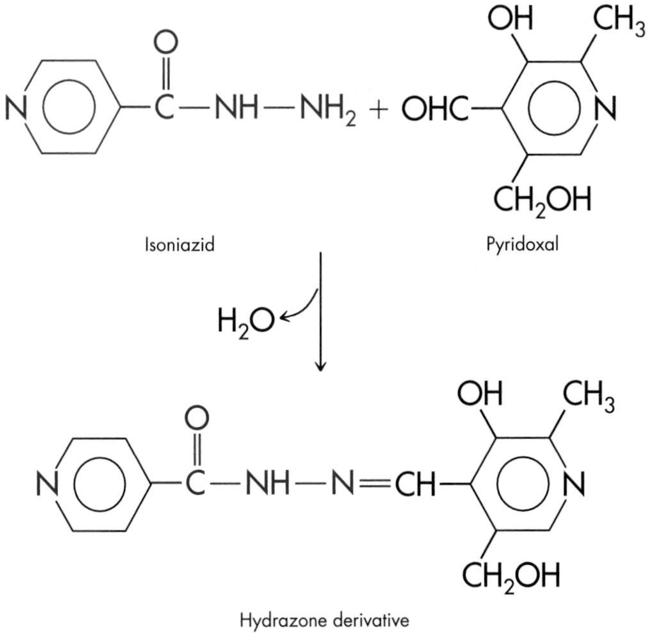

Isoniazid

Pyridoxal

H_2O

Hydrazone derivative

Unlike the other water-soluble vitamins, *vitamin B_6 is toxic when used in very high doses*. The daily consumption of more than 500 mg of pyridoxine for several

months leads to a *peripheral sensory neuropathy*, which is reversible after discontinuation of the vitamin. Doses of 100 to 150 mg/day are used for the symptomatic treatment of carpal tunnel syndrome, a painful nerve entrapment syndrome. These high-dose "therapeutic" effects are, in all likelihood, unrelated to the vitamin character of pyridoxine but could be related to its "toxic" effects.

B_6 status can be evaluated by determining the plasma level of PLP (normal range = 5 to 23 ng/mL) or the urinary excretion of the PLP metabolite 4-pyridoxic acid. Alternatively, the urinary excretion of xanthurenic acid can be determined after an oral load of 2 to 5 g of tryptophan. B_6 deficiency impairs the major catabolic pathway of this amino acid at the level of the PLP-dependent kynureninase (see Fig. 21.14, page 444, Chapter 21), and an increased fraction of tryptophan is catabolized to the yellow product xanthurenic acid, which can be measured easily in the urine.

Pantothenic acid is a building block of coenzyme A

Pantothenic acid consists of pantoic acid and β-alanine as shown in Box 24.4. Pantothenic acid occurs as *a constituent of coenzyme A* and of the phosphopantetheine group in the fatty acid synthase complex (see Chapter 18). The structure and synthesis of coenzyme A from dietary pantothenic acid are summarized in Fig. 24.5.

Pantothenic acid deficiency has never been observed under ordinary conditions, and an isolated deficiency in humans could be induced only under rigorously controlled experimental conditions. A daily intake of 4 to 7 mg appears to be adequate, and this amount is supplied readily by ordinary diets.

Biotin is a coenzyme in carboxylation reactions

Biotin is a *prosthetic group of ATP-dependent carboxylases* including pyruvate carboxylase (see Chapter 16), acetyl-CoA carboxylase (see Chapter 18), and propionyl-CoA carboxylase (see Chapter 18). These multisubunit enzymes contain biotin covalently bound to the ϵ-amino group of a lysine residue. In these reactions, biotin functions as a carrier of a bicarbonate-derived carboxy group as shown in Box 24.5.

BOX 24.4

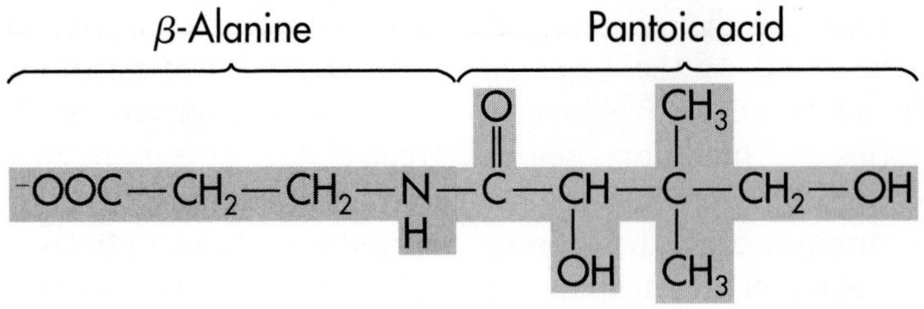

β-Alanine   Pantoic acid

Pantothenic acid

FIG. 24.5

Structure and biosynthesis of coenzyme A. **A,** Structure of the coenzyme. **B,** Biosynthetic pathway.

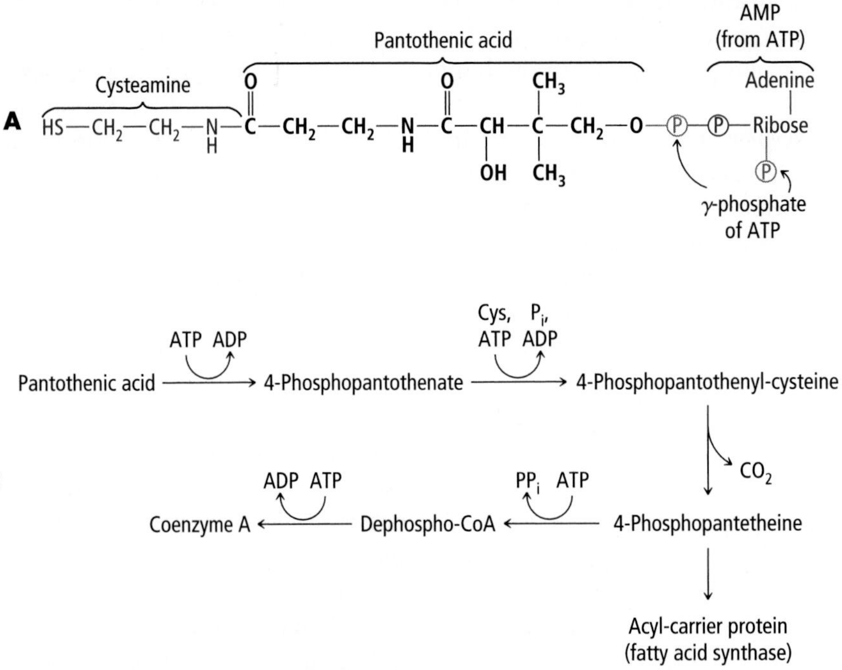

BOX 24.5

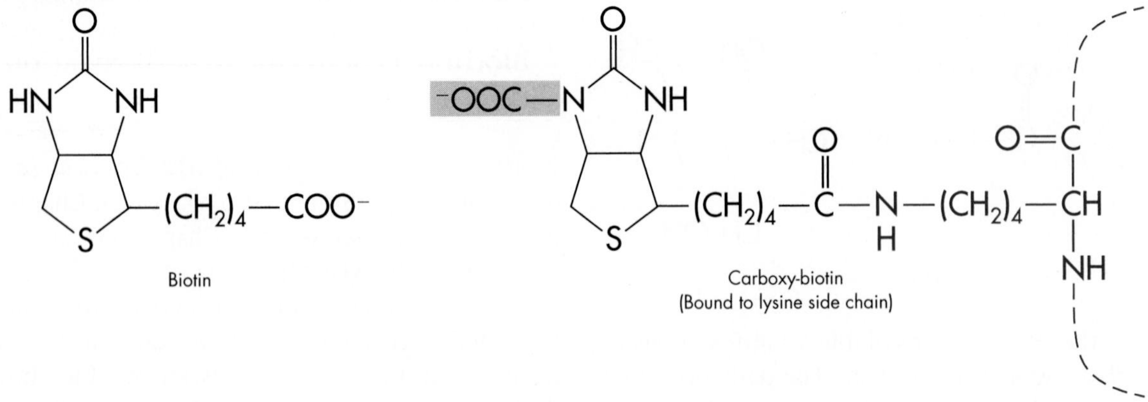

Biotin

Carboxy-biotin
(Bound to lysine side chain)

Yeast, liver, eggs, peanuts, milk, chocolate, and fish are good sources of biotin, and intestinal bacteria make a sizeable contribution. Biotin deficiency does not occur under ordinary conditions, but raw egg white contains the protein **avidin**, which binds biotin avidly in the GI tract, thereby preventing its absorption. People who eat more than 20 raw egg whites per day are likely to get biotin deficiency. The dietary requirement is on the order of 100 μg/day.

The proteolytic degradation of biotin-containing enzymes, both in the intestinal lumen and in the tissues, produces **biocytin** (Fig. 24.6), a product in which biotin is bound to the ϵ-amino group of lysine. Biotin is released from biocytin by **biotinidase,** and *a deficiency of this enzyme causes nondietary biotin deficiency.* Affected infants present with hypotonia, seizures, optic atrophy, dermatitis, and conjunctivitis. Biotinidase deficiency can be diagnosed by enzyme assay in fresh serum or, as a screening test, on a strip of blood-soaked filter paper. Because the condition can be cured readily by regular biotin supplements, *biotinidase deficiency often is included in newborn screening programs* for treatable congenital diseases, together with such disorders as

phenylketonuria, galactosemia, maple syrup urine disease, and congenital hypothyroidism.

Folic acid deficiency causes megaloblastic anemia

Folic acid consists of pteroic acid (pteridine + para-aminobenzoic acid) and one to seven γ-linked glutamate residues as shown in Box 24.6. Dietary polyglutamate forms of folic acid are hydrolyzed to pteroyl monoglutamate in the intestinal lumen, and the monoglutamate is reduced to the active coenzyme form **tetrahydrofolate (THF)** by **dihydrofolate reductase** in the intestinal mucosa. The monoglutamate conjugate of methyl-tetrahydrofolate is the most important circulating form of THF; intracellular THF is present in the form of polyglutamate conjugates, which are more potent coenzyme forms than the monoglutamate (Fig. 24.7).

THF functions as a carrier of one-carbon units that are bound to one or both of two nitrogens in the molecule, N-5 and N-10 (Fig. 24.8):

1. *A one-carbon unit is acquired by THF during a catabolic reaction.* The major one-carbon sources are serine

---

FIG. 24.6

Recycling of biotin. These reactions are required both for the utilization of dietary biotin and for the recycling of biotin during the degradation of biotin-containing carboxylase enzymes in the tissues.

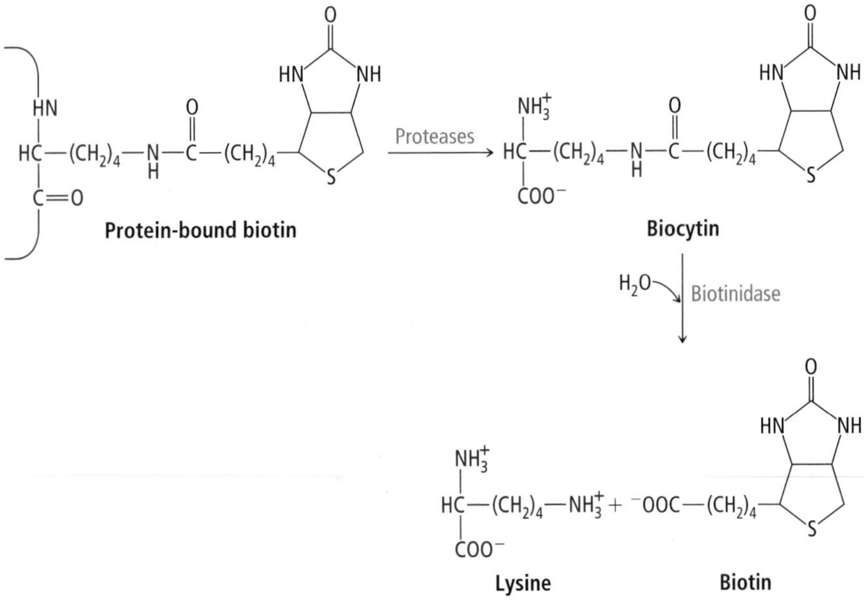

BOX 24.6

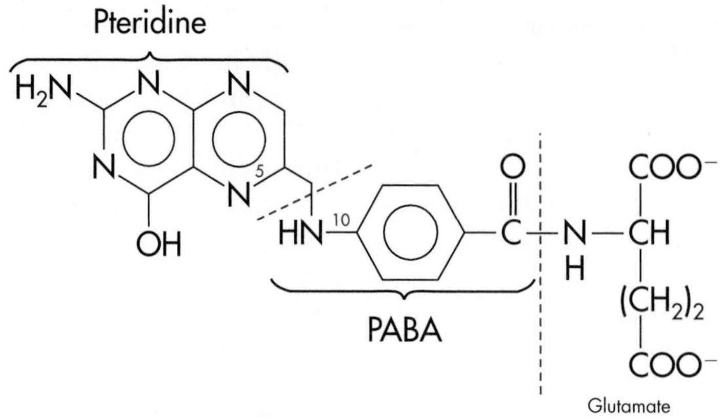

Pteridine

PABA

Glutamate

Pteroyl-monoglutamate
(the absorbed form of folic acid)

FIG. 24.7

From folate to methyltetrahydrofolate. Dihydrofolate reductase is present in all tissues, including the intestinal mucosa.

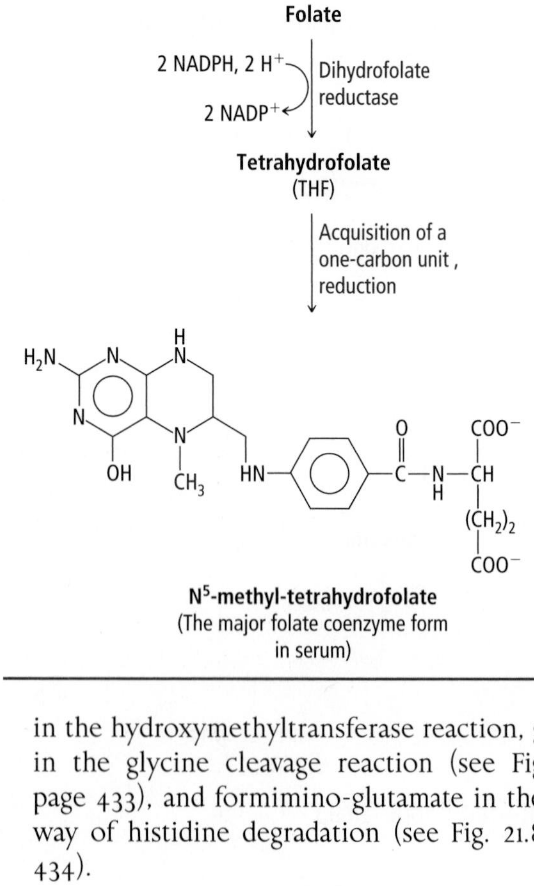

Folate

2 NADPH, 2 H$^+$ — Dihydrofolate reductase
2 NADP$^+$

Tetrahydrofolate
(THF)

Acquisition of a one-carbon unit, reduction

N^5-methyl-tetrahydrofolate
(The major folate coenzyme form
in serum)

in the hydroxymethyltransferase reaction, glycine in the glycine cleavage reaction (see Fig. 21.6, page 433), and formimino-glutamate in the pathway of histidine degradation (see Fig. 21.8, page 434).

2. Once bound to THF, *the one-carbon unit can be oxidized or reduced enzymatically.*

3. *The one-carbon unit is transferred from THF to an acceptor molecule* during a biosynthetic reaction. THF-dependent biosynthetic processes include the synthesis of purine nucleotides, the thymidylate synthase reaction (see Chapter 23), and the methylation of homocysteine to methionine (see Fig. 21.9, page 436).

The clinical expressions of folate deficiency are caused by an *impairment of DNA replication,* resulting from a shortage of purine nucleotides and thymine. The cytoplasm of the folate-deficient cell grows at a normal rate, but DNA replication and cell division are delayed. Rapidly dividing cells of the bone marrow and certain epithelia show *megaloblastic changes,* with oversized cells that have an abnormally large amount of cytoplasm. The hematological changes may progress to a condition known as **megaloblastic anemia** or **macrocytic anemia,** which is readily distinguished from iron deficiency anemia by the presence of unusually large erythrocytes (macrocytes; megaloblasts are oversized RBC precursors in the bone marrow).

Inhibitors of folate synthesis in bacteria (Fig. 24.9) are bacteriostatic: the **sulfonamides** act as structural analogs of para-aminobenzoic acid (PABA) to inhibit the synthesis of pteroic acid from pteridine and PABA in bacteria, and **trimethoprim** is an

FIG. 24.8

Tetrahydrofolate as a carrier of one-carbon units. FIGLU, Formiminoglutamate (formed during histidine degradation).

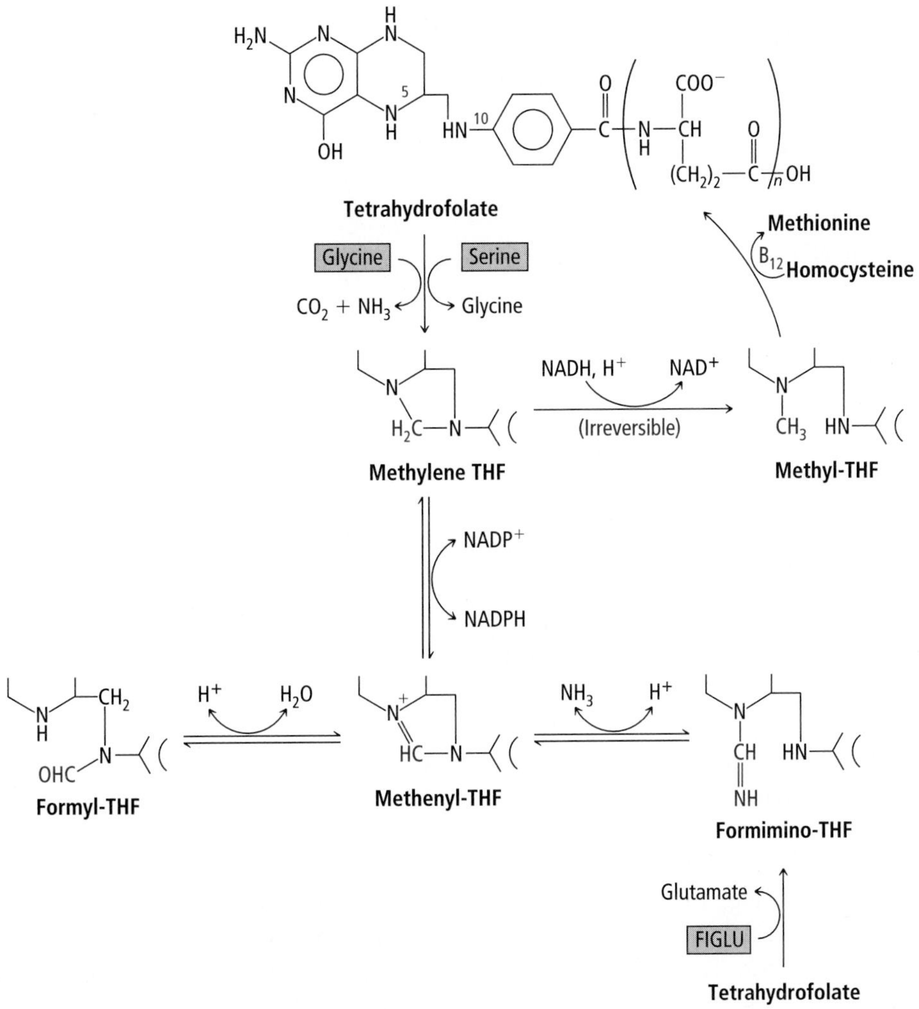

inhibitor of bacterial but not of human dihydrofolate reductase. The combination of trimethoprim with the sulfonamide sulfamethoxazole is popular for the treatment of urinary tract infections.

Good dietary sources of folic acid include yeast, liver, some fruits, and green vegetables (Latin *folium*, "leaf"). Folate is, however, heat labile, and losses during food processing may be extensive. The recommended daily intake is 200 μg, but this is increased to 300 μg during lactation and to 400 to 500 μg in the third trimester of pregnancy. Low levels of serum folate often are encountered in late pregnancy, and *megaloblastic anemia can be precipitated by pregnancy* in women on marginally folate-deficient diets. Alcoholism and malabsorption diseases are two other situations in which folate deficiency is common.

Folate supplements are recommended for the prevention of **neural tube defects** (spina bifida and anencephaly), severe congenital malformations that are present in approximately 1 of every 400 births. The current recommendation of the U.S. Public Health Service is that *all women who might possibly become pregnant should consume 400 μg of folic acid per day* to reduce the risk of a neural tube defect in their child.

FIG. 24.9

Pharmacological inhibition of tetrahydrofolate synthesis in bacteria.

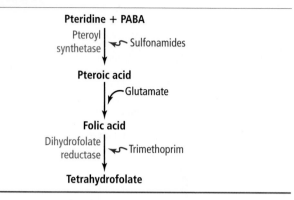

Pteridine + PABA

Pteroyl synthetase ←— Sulfonamides

Pteroic acid

←Glutamate

Folic acid

Dihydrofolate reductase ←—Trimethoprim

Tetrahydrofolate

FIG. 24.10

Structure of methylcobalamin.

The folate status can be evaluated by the determination of folate levels in serum and erythrocytes. In subacute deficiency, the serum "folate" (actually methyl-tetrahydrofolate) declines within days, followed much later by a decrease of RBC folate. *Deficiency signs appear only when the intracellular stores are depleted.*

Pernicious anemia is caused by the malabsorption of vitamin B_{12}

Vitamin B_{12}, or **cobalamin,** is chemically the most complex of all vitamins (Fig. 24.10). It contains a corrin ring system, with a cobalt ion complexed to four nitrogens in its center. The cobalt ion forms two more bonds, one with the nitrogen of a dimethylbenzimidazole group and one with a variable substituent that is either a methyl or a deoxyadenosyl group in the active coenzyme forms. This complex structure is synthesized only by some microorganisms. Plants do not contain vitamin B_{12}, and *the dietary requirement has to be covered from animal products.* A small amount is synthesized by colon bacteria, but its absorption is negligible.

*The absorption of dietary B_{12} requires **intrinsic factor,*** a 50-kDa glycoprotein secreted by the parietal cells of the stomach (Fig. 24.11). B_{12} binds tightly to intrinsic factor, and in this form it is absorbed from the ileum. The cobalamin in the blood is tightly bound to **transcobalamin** II and other plasma proteins. The cobalamin-transcobalamin II complex is taken up into the cells by receptor-mediated endocytosis. The binding to plasma proteins not only directs the

vitamin to the tissues where it is needed, it also prevents its renal excretion. B_{12} is a scarce and valuable resource, so renal losses have to be avoided by any means.

Only two reactions are known to require cobalamin in human tissues: the cytoplasmic *methylation of homocysteine to methionine* (see Chapter 21) requires methylcobalamin, and the mitochondrial *methylmalonyl-CoA mutase reaction* (see Chapter 18) depends on deoxyadenosylcobalamin.

B_{12} deficiency causes two types of abnormalities: a *megaloblastic anemia* develops that is hematologically indistinguishable from that of folate deficiency, and demyelination in peripheral nerves and the spinal cord leads to *neurological dysfunction.* A similar neurological disorder is not seen in patients with folate deficiency. The megaloblastic anemia is explained by the **methyl folate trap** hypothesis: during the metabolism of one-carbon units, a small amount of methylene-tetrahydrofolate is reduced irreversibly to methyl-tetrahydrofolate (Fig. 24.8). Being useless for the synthesis of purines or thymine, methyl-THF has to be converted back to one of the other coenzyme forms. *The only important reaction of methyl-THF is the methylation of homocysteine to methionine,* which re-

FIG. 24.11

Absorption, transport, and tissue utilization of vitamin B_{12}. *IF*, Intrinsic factor; *TC II*, transcobalamin II.

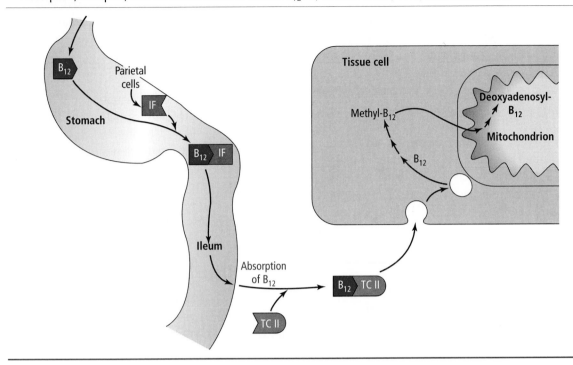

generates free THF. This reaction requires B_{12}, so methyl-THF accumulates in B_{12} deficiency—to the detriment of the other coenzyme forms that are sorely needed for nucleotide synthesis. The methyl folate trap hypothesis explains the megaloblastic anemia of B_{12} deficiency, but the mechanism of the demyelination is unknown.

The RDA for vitamin B_{12} is set at 2 μg, but as little as 0.1 to 0.2 μg/day is probably sufficient to prevent deficiency signs. Because essentially all dietary B_{12} is derived from animal products, *strict vegetarians are at risk of B_{12} deficiency* unless their food is habitually contaminated with bacteria or fecal matter. Between 1 and 10 mg of B_{12} is stored in the body, mostly in the liver. Therefore a sudden switch to a B_{12}-free diet will cause serious deficiency only after several decades.

Impaired intestinal absorption, on the other hand, results in deficiency signs within 2 to 6 years: every day, 1 to 10 μg of B_{12} is secreted into the bile, and the absorption of this biliary B_{12} depends on intrinsic factor. Therefore *most cases of B_{12} deficiency are caused by malabsorption rather than by insufficient dietary intake*. **Pernicious anemia** is caused by an atrophic gastritis in which the parietal cells of the stomach are destroyed by autoimmune mechanisms. The resulting lack of intrinsic factor prevents the absorption of both dietary and biliary cobalamin. This disease was uniformly fatal until 1926, when the oral administration of liver extracts was found to be curative: even in the absence of intrinsic factor, 0.1% to 1% of orally administered B_{12} is absorbed by nonspecific mechanisms, and the large amount of B_{12} in the liver extracts was sufficient to correct the deficiency. Pernicious anemia now is treated either by large oral B_{12} supplements or by monthly injections of more moderate doses.

The plasma levels of cobalamin can be determined by bacteriological methods or radioimmunoassay.

Vitamin C is an important water-soluble antioxidant

During recorded history, **scurvy** has been possibly the second-most-important nutritional deficiency, after protein-calorie malnutrition. The structure of the antiscorbutic agent, now known as **ascorbic acid** or **vitamin C**, was determined in 1932 after its isolation from lemon juice and other natural sources. Its structure is simple, resembling a monosaccharide, and most animals are indeed able to synthesize ascorbic acid in one of the minor pathways of carbohydrate metabolism (see Fig. 17.25, Chapter 17). Only primates, guinea pigs, and some fruit bats have lost the ability to synthesize ascorbic acid.

Ascorbic acid is a reducing agent and a scavenger of free radicals (Fig. 24.12). Thus, the oxidation of LDL is prevented by ascorbate. The formation of potentially carcinogenic nitrosamines from dietary nitrite and nitrate in the stomach also is suppressed, and a protective effect against stomach cancer and several other cancers has been suggested by epidemiological studies. More specific actions on individual en-

zymatic reactions are attributed to a protective effect on oxidizable groups in the enzyme protein. Some metal-containing enzymes, in particular, depend on ascorbate. Only some of the many ascorbate-dependent reactions can be mentioned here:

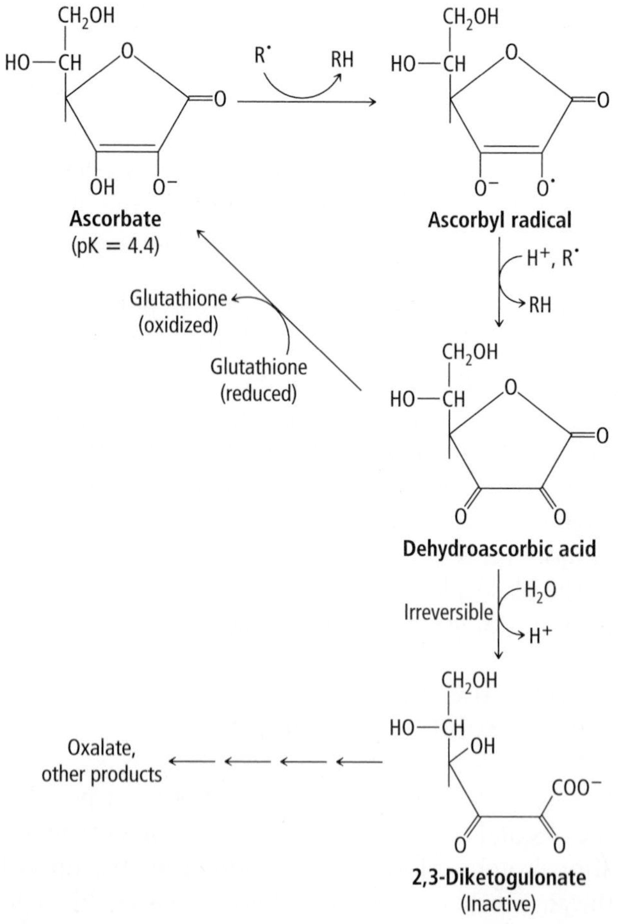

1. *The hydroxylation of prolyl and lysyl residues in procollagen* (see Chapter 13) requires ascorbate. The impairment of these reactions accounts for the prominent connective tissue abnormalities of scurvy.
2. *Carnitine synthesis* (see Chapter 21) requires two Fe^{2+}-containing, ascorbate-dependent dioxygenases. Carnitine deficiency may contribute to the fatigue and lassitude characteristic of scurvy.
3. *The synthesis of norepinephrine from dopamine* (see Chapter 26) requires ascorbic acid.
4. *The 7α-hydroxylase reaction*, which initiates the conversion of cholesterol to bile acids in liver microsomes (see Chapter 19), depends on ascorbic acid.

Dietary vitamin C is absorbed by a saturable, sodium-dependent transport mechanism that has a maximum capacity of approximately 1 g of ascorbate per day. *The plasma level is almost linearly related to the dietary intake*, up to intakes of approximately 150 mg/day. Thus, a plasma level of 11 μM (0.2 mg/dL) is expected on a 20-mg/day diet, and 45 to 55 μM (0.8 to 1.0 mg/dL) is typical on a 100-mg/day diet. The total body store is approximately 1.5 g on a 45-mg/day diet and 4 g on a 120-mg/day diet. Excess ascorbic acid is excreted in the urine together with several water-soluble metabolites, including oxalic acid.

After a sudden switch to a vitamin C–free diet, the first signs of scurvy become evident after 2 to 3 months, when the plasma level has dropped to 3 μM and the total pool is reduced to 300 to 400 mg. *Cutaneous petechiae and purpura* (small and medium-sized hemorrhages) develop, together with *follicular hyperkeratosis* (gooseflesh). Dry mouth and eyes, decaying and peeling gums, and loose teeth are seen in more advanced cases. Wound healing and scar formation are disrupted, and bleeding from old scars may occur. The patient experiences weakness and lethargy, sometimes accompanied by arthralgia (joint pain) and aching of the legs.

A daily intake of 20 mg of vitamin C is sufficient to prevent and even to cure scurvy. Fresh fruits and vegetables are the major dietary sources under ordinary conditions. Unfortunately, vitamin C is not excessively stable under neutral or alkaline conditions,

FIG. 24.12

Structure and antioxidant action of ascorbic acid (vitamin C). The standard reduction potential of ascorbate/dehydroascorbate is + 0.08 V; that of glutathione is − 0.23 V.

and it is oxidized easily to inactive products by boiling in the presence of oxygen and catalytic amounts of heavy metal ions.

Vitamin C does not only prevent scurvy. High intakes have been associated with a reduced incidence of coronary heart disease (CHD), marginally reduced plasma cholesterol levels, and even a reduced incidence of various cancers. Not all of these effects are well established, however, and the literature abounds with contradictory claims. The RDA currently is set at 60 mg.

The benefits of megadoses of vitamin C had been popularized by the late Linus Pauling, whose name is linked forever not only to the structure of the α-helix (see Chapter 2) but also to the claim that large daily doses of vitamin C can prevent the common cold. Between 1978 and 1994, this latter claim was investigated in at least 21 placebo-controlled studies with doses of at least 1 g per day. The results were rather consistent: although the number of colds seemed to be unaffected, most studies showed that the duration of the episodes and the severity of the symptoms were indeed reduced. Although the advisability of very large doses is still controversial, Pauling lived to an age of 97 years, consuming several grams of vitamin C per day for his last 40 years.

THE FAT-SOLUBLE VITAMINS

Chemically, the fat-soluble vitamins are isoprenoids that are synthesized by plants or bacteria. Unlike the water-soluble vitamins, *they require bile salt micelles for their intestinal absorption*, and therefore they often are deficient in patients with fat malabsorption. For the same reason, supplements of fat-soluble vitamins are most effective when taken with a fatty meal. The interorgan transport of the fat-soluble vitamins is effected either by plasma lipoproteins or by specific transport proteins. They cannot be excreted by the kidneys, so they tend to accumulate—sometimes to toxic levels—in lipid-rich structures of the body when their dietary intake is excessive.

Retinol, retinal, and retinoic acid are the active forms of vitamin A

The biologically active forms of vitamin A are the **retinoids** as shown in Box 24.7. Foods of animal origin contain most of their vitamin A in the form of *esters between retinol and a long-chain fatty acid*. The retinol esters are hydrolyzed by a pancreatic enzyme in the small intestine and, in the presence of bile acids, free retinol is absorbed with an efficiency of 40% to 80%. Within the mucosal cell, most of the retinol becomes esterified with a long-chain fatty acid, and the retinol esters thus formed are incorporated in chylomicrons. Most of this reaches the liver as a constituent of chylomicron remnants (see Chapter 20). Up to 100 mg of retinol esters is stored in the liver, mostly within the stellate cells (Fig. 24.13).

β-Carotene, the orange pigment of carrots and many other vegetables, is the major vitamin A precursor in plants. It is cleaved by β-carotene dioxy-

BOX 24.7

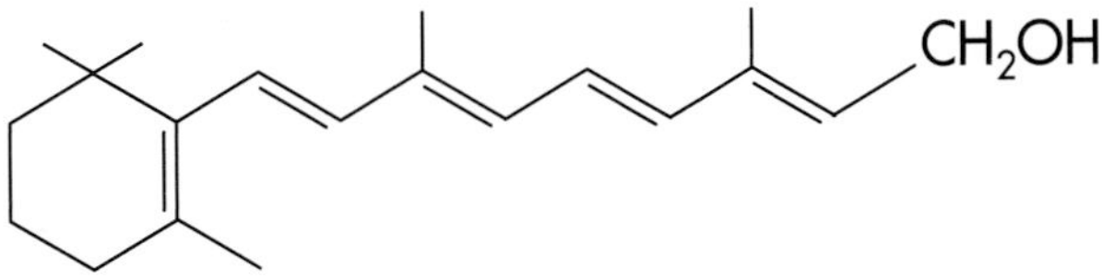

All-*trans*-retinol

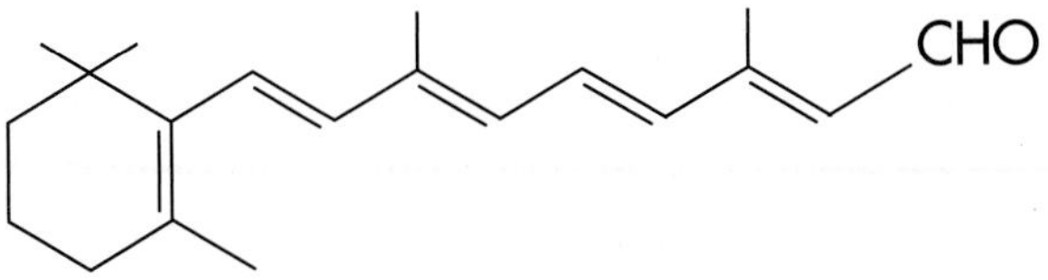

All-*trans*-retinal

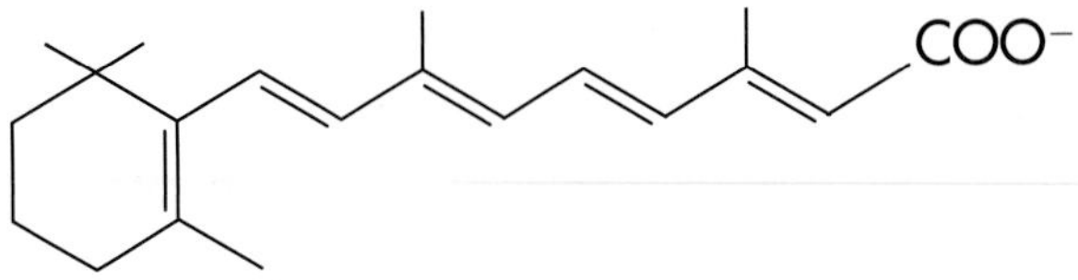

All-*trans*-retinoic acid

FIG. 24.13

Transport and metabolism of retinoids. *RBP*, Retinol binding protein; *LPL*, lipoprotein lipase. Retinol is esterified by two different enzymes that use acyl-CoA and lecithin, respectively, as a source of the fatty acid.

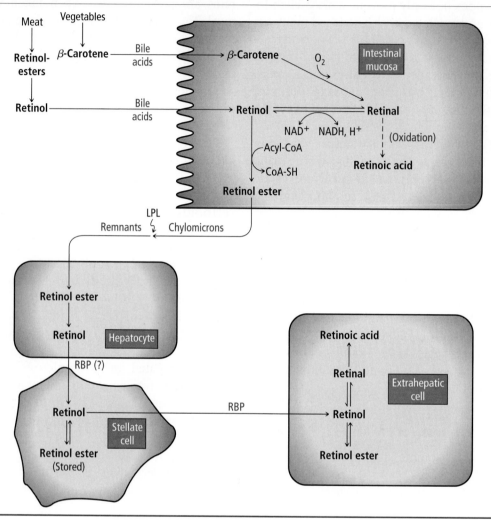

genase in the cytoplasm of the intestinal mucosal cell as shown in Box 24.8. Absorption and cleavage are not very efficient, and therefore approximately 6 mg of β-carotene is required to produce 1 mg of retinal.

Other carotenes, including α- and γ-carotene, also are cleaved by β-carotene dioxygenase, as shown in Box 24.9, but yield only one molecule of retinal. They have, therefore, only half of the provitamin A activity of β-carotene. Retinal is in equilibrium with retinol through a reversible, NADH-dependent dehydrogenase reaction, and a small amount is irreversibly oxidized to **retinoic acid** (Fig. 24.13).

Retinol is transported from the liver to the extrahepatic tissues in tight binding to **retinol binding protein (RBP)**. Epithelial cells are the main destination of RBP-bound retinol. Like the intestinal mucosa, the target tissues can oxidize retinol to retinal and retinal to retinoic acid. Retinal and retinoic acid are the most important biologically active forms.

Retinal is the *prosthetic group of the rhodopsins*, the visual pigments of rods and cones (see Chapter 27). For this reason vitamin A deficiency causes night blindness.

Retinoic acid (RA) binds to nuclear receptor proteins, and *the receptor-RA complex regulates gene expression*

BOX 24.8

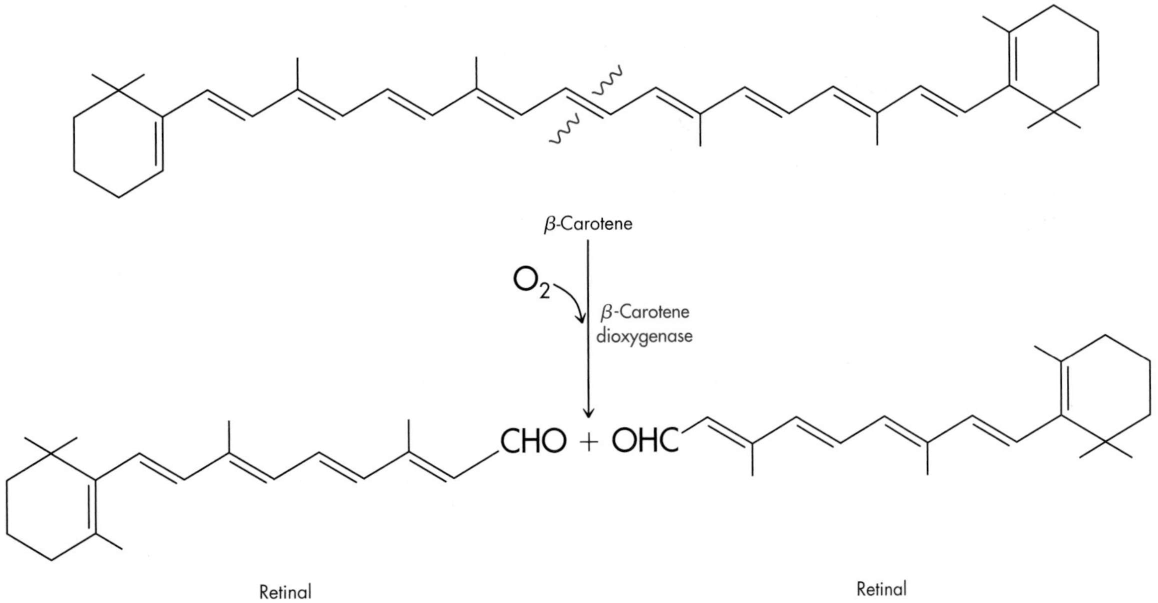

β-Carotene

β-Carotene dioxygenase

CHO + OHC

Retinal   Retinal

BOX 24.9

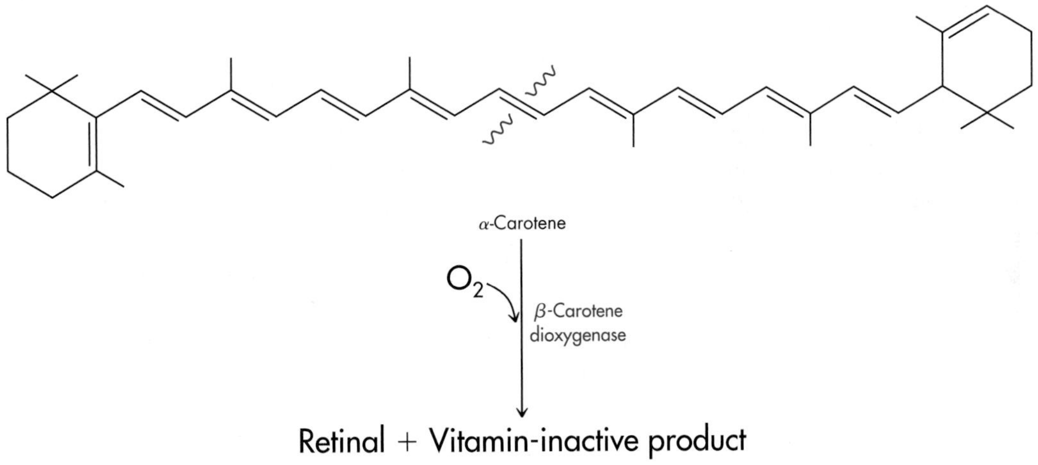

α-Carotene

β-Carotene dioxygenase

Retinal + Vitamin-inactive product

by binding to response elements on the DNA. This mechanism resembles the action of the steroid hormones on their target tissues (see Chapter 27), and indeed the RA receptors belong to the same superfamily of ligand-regulated transcription factors as the steroid hormone receptors.

RA is important for the maintenance of epithelial tissues. Vitamin A deficiency is characterized by the transformation of columnar epithelia into heavily keratinized squamous epithelia, a process known as **squamous metaplasia.** Follicular hyperkeratosis (gooseflesh) is an early sign. In more advanced cases the conjunctiva of the eye loses its mucus secreting cells and becomes keratinized, and the glycoprotein content of the tears is reduced as well. These changes disrupt the fluid film that normally bathes the cornea. This condition, known as **xerophthalmia** ("dry eyes"), often is complicated by bacterial or chlamydial infection, resulting in perforation of the cornea and blindness. Other abnormalities in vitamin A deficiency include night blindness, microcytic anemia, and an impairment of reproductive function in both males and females. Although rare in the United States, *serious vitamin A deficiency is common in many developing countries, where it is a leading cause of blindness.*

Liver, meat, dairy products, and the (in)famous cod liver oil provide vitamin A in the form of retinol esters; vegetables supply carotenes. The carotenes betray their presence by their color: yellow or orange vegetables and fruits such as carrots, pumpkins, mangoes, and papayas are excellent sources, whereas less colorful ones, such as peeled apples and pears, have little or no vitamin A activity. The carotenes also are accessory pigments of photosynthesis and therefore are present in all green leafy vegetables. The adult male RDA is set at 1000 retinol equivalents (1 mg of retinol).

A single dose of more than 200 mg of retinol or retinal, or the chronic consumption of more than 40 mg per day, causes nonspecific signs of toxicity. More importantly, *vitamin A is a potent teratogen,* causing major malformations when taken early during pregnancy. Embryonic tissues maintain gradients of retinoic acid, and through its nuclear receptors, retinoic acid is thought to participate in the regulation of gene expression during normal embryogenesis. Vitamin A preparations are used in the treatment of various skin diseases, including common acne, and all it takes for a major prenatal disaster is an acne-plagued teenage girl taking high doses of retinoids and becoming unexpectedly pregnant.

Carotenes are not toxic, but they can accumulate in the tissues. Adipose tissue often acquires a yellow tint that is caused by dietary carotenes, and an orange-yellow discoloration of the skin is seen in babies who have been overfed with carrot juice.

The vitamin A status can be evaluated by the determination of serum retinol. Values between 10 and 100 μg/dL are considered normal, with lower and higher values suggesting vitamin A deficiency and toxicity, respectively.

Both the retinoids and the carotenes are effective antioxidants at the low oxygen partial pressures in the tissues, and this property may allow them to curtail oxidative processes that otherwise are likely to result in mutagenesis and carcinogenesis. However, studies about the effects of vitamin A and carotenoids on cancer risk have produced ambiguous results.

Vitamin D is a prohormone

Although vitamin D is nutritionally essential for people who stay out of the sun, *it can be synthesized photochemically in the skin* (Fig. 24.14), and with even mild sun exposure there is no need for a dietary source. Vitamin D is synthesized from **7-dehydrocholesterol**, which is present in small amount in all tissues. This steroid is photochemically cleaved to **cholecalciferol** (vitamin D_3) by radiation in the UV range.

The cholecalciferol formed in the skin is transported in tight noncovalent binding to a vitamin D−binding plasma protein. Cholecalciferol is converted to **1,25-dihydroxycholecalciferol (calcitriol)** by successive hydroxylations in liver and kidney. *Calcitriol is the major physiologically active form of vitamin D.* 25-Hydroxylation in the liver is not rate limiting, and therefore 25-hydroxycholecalciferol (**25-OH-D$_3$**), which is also bound to the D-binding protein, is the major circulating form of the vitamin. The 1α-hydroxylase in the kidney, however, is tightly regulated: its activity is increased by parathyroid hormone (PTH), byhypocalcemia, and by hypophosphatemia. Cholecalciferol and 25-OH-D$_3$ have biological half-lives on the order of 30 days, but calcitriol lives for only 2 to 4 hours.

Calcitriol is a hormonelike substance. Its receptor is a ligand-regulated transcription factor that belongs to the same superfamily as the receptors for retinoic acid, steroid hormones, and thyroid hormones. *Calcitriol upregulates the plasma calcium concentration,* an effect that it shares with PTH. In bone, *it facilitates the resorption of calcium and phosphate* by stimulating osteoclasts, acting cooperatively with PTH in this tissue. In the intestine, *it stimulates the absorption of dietary calcium and phosphate,* without the aid of PTH. In the kidney *it stimulates calcium reabsorption,* again in cooperation with PTH.

The plasma calcium level is regulated very tightly. In acute hypocalcemia, PTH restores the plasma calcium level within minutes by stimulating osteoclasts and inducing the release of calcium and phosphate from bone. It also boosts calcitriol formation by stimulating the renal 1α-hydroxylase. While PTH acts on bone to maintain the plasma calcium level

FIG. 24.14

Synthesis of calcitriol, the active form of vitamin D, from 7-dehydrocholesterol.

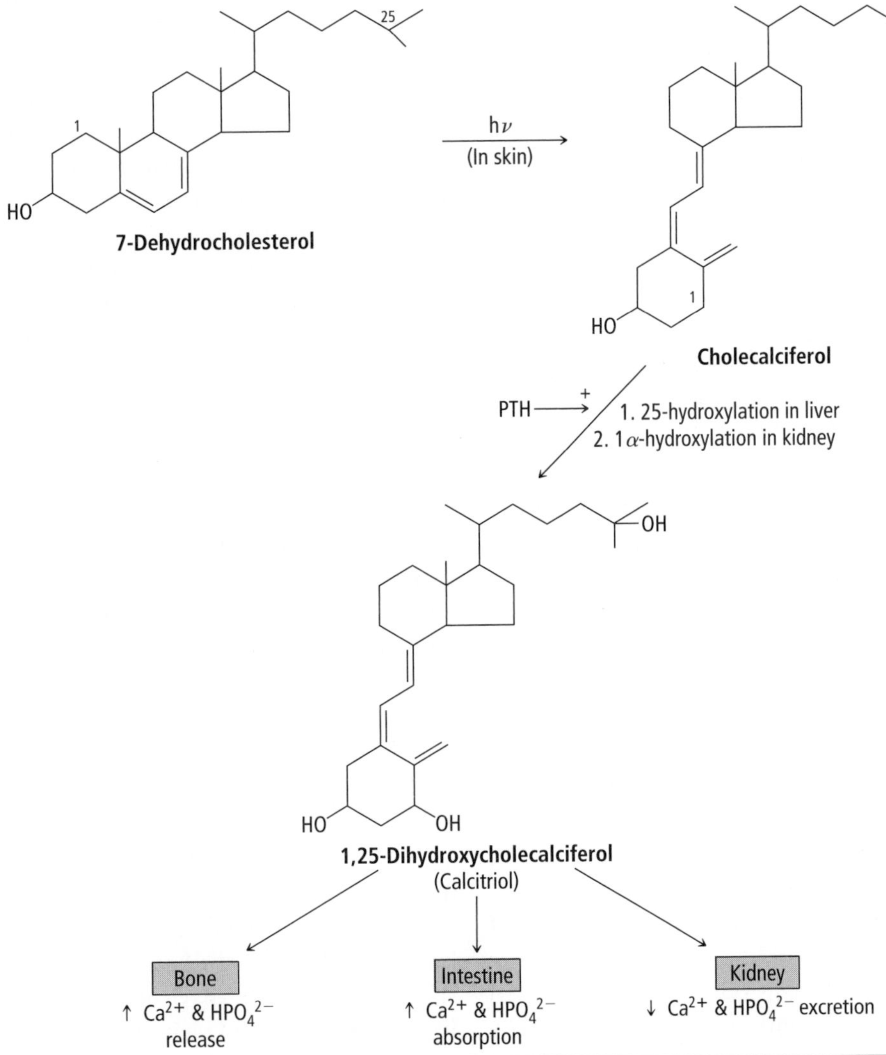

7-Dehydrocholesterol

$h\nu$
(In skin)

Cholecalciferol

PTH $\longrightarrow$ 1. 25-hydroxylation in liver
2. 1α-hydroxylation in kidney

1,25-Dihydroxycholecalciferol
(Calcitriol)

| Bone | Intestine | Kidney |

↑ Ca^{2+} & HPO_4^{2-} release | ↑ Ca^{2+} & HPO_4^{2-} absorption | ↓ Ca^{2+} & HPO_4^{2-} excretion

on a minute-to-minute basis, *calcitriol acts on intestine and kidney to increase the total amount of calcium and phosphate in the body.*

Vitamin D deficiency is called **rickets** in children and **osteomalacia** in adults. The immediate effect is a decrease of the plasma calcium concentration. This hypocalcemia is compensated by an increased release of PTH, which rapidly restores plasma calcium to near-normal levels. Even in long-term vitamin D deficiency, the plasma calcium level can be maintained by PTH—at the expense of the bones, which are tapped as a calcium reservoir and gradually are depleted of their mineral content. PTH also

reduces the level of circulating phosphate by inhibiting renal phosphate reabsorption. More than 99% of our calcium and phosphate is in the extracellular matrix of bone, and *the depletion of total body stores of calcium and phosphate in vitamin D deficiency leads to soft, poorly mineralized bones* that bend rather than break under stress.

Although rickets used to be common in cloudy countries, notably England, it is now rare. In the absence of sunlight, a daily intake of 5 to 10 μg (200 to 400 IU) of cholecalciferol is considered adequate. Vitamin D is present in only a few natural foodstuffs, including liver, egg yolk, and saltwater fish (cod liver oil!), as well as in fortified foods. The synthesis of cholecalciferol in the skin is affected by skin color: white skin produces approximately five times more vitamin D than black skin does. The protection from rickets is thought to be the main advantage of white skin in those human races that evolved in cloudy climates.

Calcitriol has been found effective in the treatment of **osteoporosis,** a common cause of pathological fractures in the elderly. Vitamin D actually may be involved in the etiology of this ailment: the calcitriol receptor occurs in two common allelic variants—B and b—in the population, and homozygosity for the B allele is associated with a high risk of the disease.

Hypervitaminosis D, caused by the overuse of vitamin D supplements, leads to rampant hypercalcemia, hypercalciuria, and metastatic calcification. The toxic state persists for a few months after discontinuation of the offending agent if the overuse of cholecalciferol is the cause, but it lasts for only a week or so if toxicity is caused by calcitriol. Chronic hypercalcemia can result in irreversible cardiovascular and renal damage.

Vitamin E is an important antioxidant

No less than eight closely related substances with vitamin E activity have been isolated from natural sources. The most abundant and most potent of these is **α-tocopherol.**

In the presence of bile salts, vitamin E is absorbed from the small intestine with an efficiency of 20% to 40%. It has no specific binding protein in the blood but is transported by plasma lipoproteins. The tissue distribution also shows little selectivity: vitamin E is enriched in all lipid-rich structures, with highest concentrations in adipose tissue.

The only recognized biological function of vitamin E is its action as an *antioxidant and scavenger of free radicals* (Fig. 24.15): in the membranes, fat depots, and lipoproteins in which it is enriched, it reacts with the free radicals that are formed during lipid peroxidation (see Chapter 18), thereby interrupting free radical chain reactions. Reducing agents such as ascorbate and glutathione prevent a rapid depletion of vitamin E by reducing the initially formed free radical and quinone intermediates back to the active form.

Unlike most other vitamins, vitamin E was discovered not by the observation of a deficiency disease in humans, but rather as a result of animal experiments. Although it has been called a "vitamin in search of a disease," human deficiency occasionally does occur. It sometimes is seen in premature infants who are born with low tissue stores and who have poor intestinal absorption for several weeks after birth. Vitamin E deficiency results in a mild hemolytic anemia, both in infants and in malabsorption syndromes of children and adults. The most serious form of vitamin E deficiency in humans occurs in patients with abetalipoproteinemia (see Chapter 20), who develop neuropathic and myopathic changes in addition to hemolysis.

Epidemiological studies suggest an inverse relationship between vitamin E intake and the risk of CHD. This protective effect tends to be more consistent than similar effects of the other antioxidant vitamins, A and C. Intervention studies have shown a reduced risk of CHD in individuals consuming vitamin E supplements on the order of 200 mg/day. Like the other antioxidant vitamins, vitamin E also is thought to be protective against some cancers, but the results of epidemiological and intervention studies are contradictory.

Intake of 10 mg of α-tocopherol per day is considered adequate, and this amount is supplied by most diets. Good sources include vegetable oils, various oil seeds, and wheat germ. Although vitamin E is a popular object of abuse by health-food enthusiasts, the dangers of overdosage are minimal: unlike vitamins A and D, vitamin E is nontoxic in doses up to 50 times the recommended intake.

Vitamin K is required for the synthesis of blood clotting factors

The name vitamin K is derived from "koagulation." Indeed, the only known physiological role of this vitamin is the posttranslational processing of some clotting factors, and the only deficiency sign is an impairment of blood clotting.

The naturally occurring forms of vitamin K are isoprenoids containing a quinoid ring structure. **Phylloquinone** is present in vegetables; **menaquinone** is produced by bacteria, including intestinal bacteria as shown in Box 24.10. **Menadione** is a synthetic analog that acts like the natural vitamin

FIG. 24.15

The action of α-tocopherol as a scavenger of free radicals. R' = free radical.

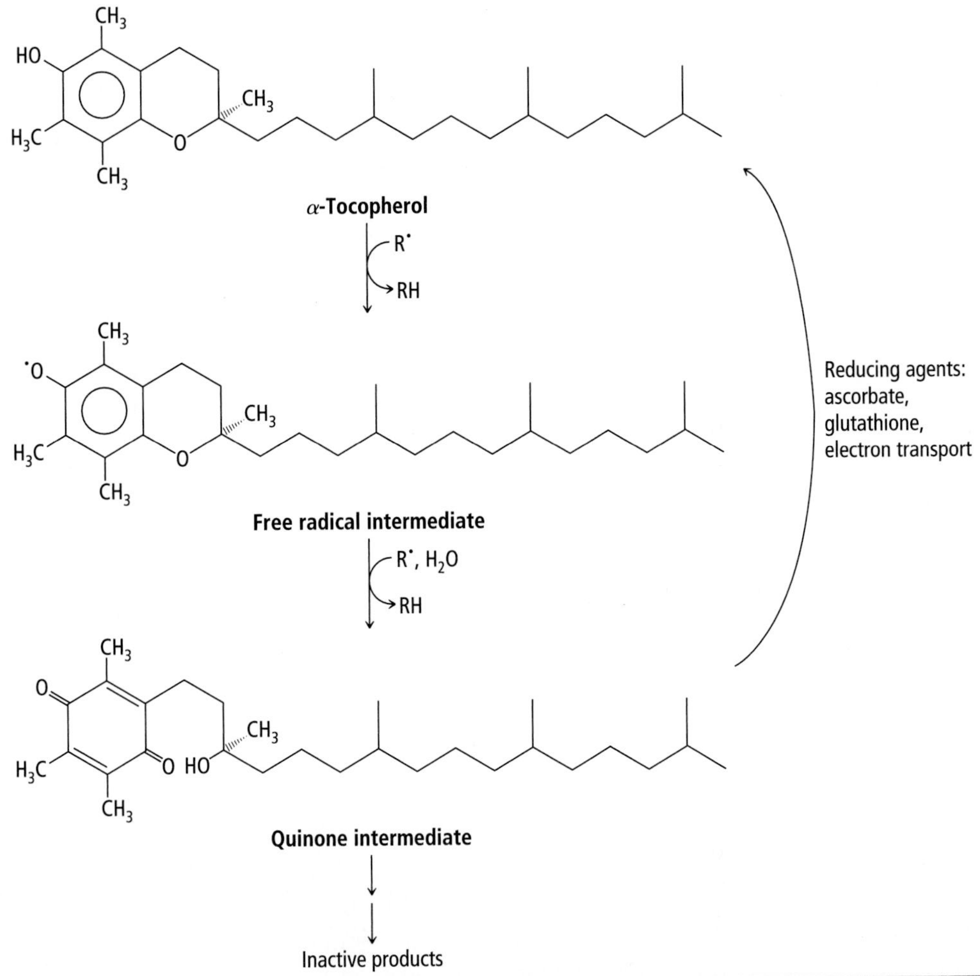

α-Tocopherol

Free radical intermediate

Quinone intermediate

Reducing agents:
ascorbate,
glutathione,
electron transport

Inactive products

forms after its enzymatic alkylation in the human body.

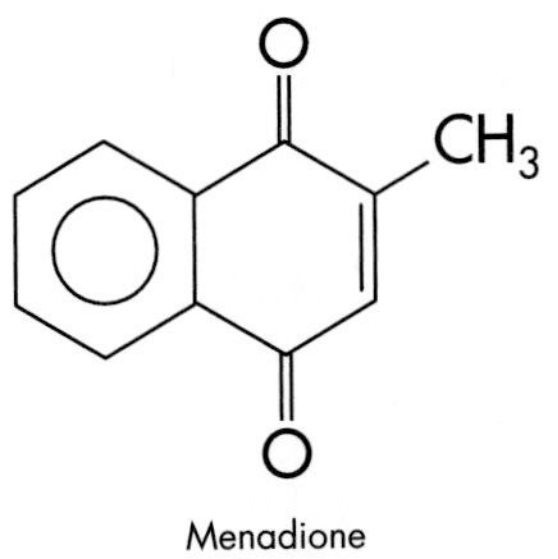

Menadione
(Vitamin K₃)

Unlike the natural forms, menadione is absorbed efficiently even in the absence of bile salts.

The vitamin K requirement is covered in part by dietary phylloquinone and in part by menaquinone, derived from bacteria in the small intestine. Colon bacteria do not make a significant contribution, because vitamin K is absorbed only in the small intestine. Like vitamin E, vitamin K has no specific binding protein in the plasma and is retailed to the tissues by chylomicrons and other plasma lipoproteins. Unlike the other fat-soluble vitamins, *vitamin K is not stored to any great extent.* Total body stores are as low as 50 to 100 μg, so *vitamin K is the first fat-soluble vitamin to be deficient in acute fat malabsorption.*

Vitamin K participates in the enzymatic carboxylation of glutamyl residues during the synthesis of prothrombin and several other blood clotting factors in the liver (Fig. 24.16). The only important deficiency sign is a clotting disorder, and the determi-

BOX 24.10

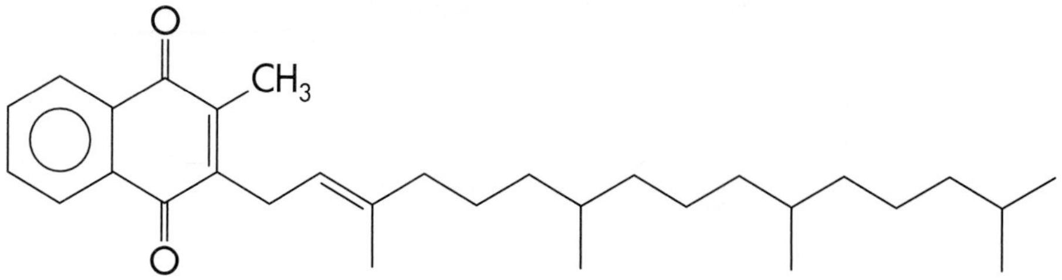

Phylloquinone
(Vitamin K₁)

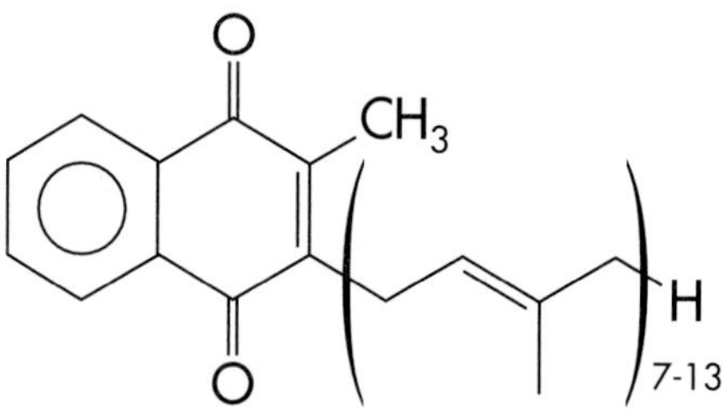

Menaquinone
(Vitamin K₂)

nation of the prothrombin time (see Chapter 25) is the most important laboratory test for the evaluation of vitamin K status.

Newborns, especially if they are premature, are prone to vitamin K deficiency: the tissue stores are low at birth, the intestinal flora is not yet established, and breast milk contains only 1 to 2 μg of vitamin K per liter. Since the newborn has a requirement of 5 μg/day (3 liters of breast milk), it is not surprising that even in normal newborns the levels of vitamin K–dependent clotting factors decline during the first 2 to 3 days after birth. In perhaps 1 of every 400 newborns, an abnormal bleeding tendency is evident at this time. This condition is known as **hemorrhagic disease of the newborn.** *It is the most common nutritional deficiency in newborns.* Most newborns in the United States now are treated with vitamin K either orally or intramuscularly, and vitamin K prophylaxis is mandatory in some states.

Vitamin K deficiency in adults usually is caused by fat malabsorption. It is, for example, common practice to administer vitamin K supplements for a few days before surgery for biliary tract obstruction because these patients have impaired vitamin K absorption, and the resulting impairment of blood clotting makes them vulnerable to surgical complications.

Because of the contribution made by intestinal bacteria, a dietary requirement is hard to define.

The RDA is set at 60 to 80 μg, but many people consume as much as 300 to 500 μg/day.

THE TRACE MINERALS

Almost a dozen trace minerals are known or suspected to be nutritionally essential. Most are metals that are essential components of individual proteins. Although required in the diet, *most trace minerals are toxic at higher doses.* Indeed, most metal ions, including iron, zinc, and copper, are complexed with specific intracellular binding proteins that not only store the mineral but also prevent toxicity by scavenging any free, unbound metal ions. In the following sections we will focus on those trace minerals that are most important in medical practice.

Iron is conserved very efficiently in the body

By virtue of its ability to change readily between the ferrous (Fe^{2+}) and the ferric (Fe^{3+}) states, *iron can function as a redox system.* Both the non-heme iron in the iron-sulfur proteins and the heme iron of the cytochromes are used this way. *Iron also is able to bind a variety of ligands,* including cyanide, carbon monoxide, molecular oxygen, and the free electron pairs

FIG. 24.16

Carboxylation of glutamate residues during the posttranslational modification of clotting factors in the endoplasmic reticulum of the liver. Unlike other carboxylations, this reaction does not require biotin and ATP; it is driven by the exergonic oxidation of the vitamin K cofactor. R = variable side chain.

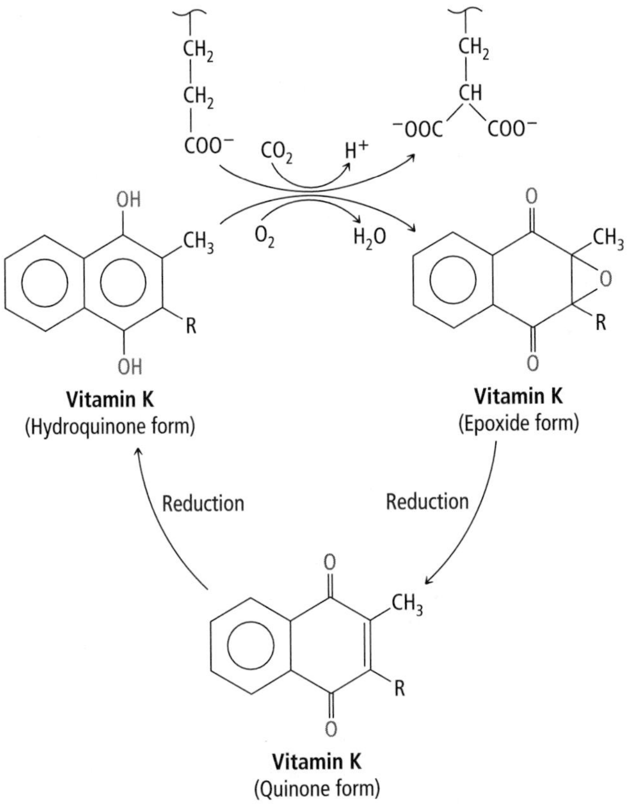

TABLE 24.1

Distribution of body iron in a "typical" 70-kg male and 55-kg female

| Protein | Amount (g) in: | |
	70-kg man	55-kg woman
Hemoglobin	2.5	1.7
Myoglobin	0.15	0.1
Enzymes, cytochromes, Fe-S-proteins	0.15	0.1
Storage iron		
Ferritin	0.5	0.3
Hemosiderin	0.5	0.1
Transferrin	0.003	0.002
Total	3.8 g	2.3 g

on nitrogen atoms in organic molecules. This property is exploited in such oxygen-binding proteins as hemoglobin, myoglobin, and cytochrome oxidase. When present in excess or in the wrong place, however, iron is quite toxic: like other heavy metals it binds to many proteins, disrupting their structure and biological properties. Even worse, it can initiate oxidative damage by forming reactive hydroxyl and peroxide radicals in the presence of molecular oxygen (see Fig. 18.16, Chapter 18). Therefore *the concentration of free, unbound iron has to be kept at a minimum.* This is achieved by iron-binding proteins that are not fully saturated under physiological conditions.

The body of an adult man contains 3 to 4 g of iron (Table 24.1). Two thirds of this is present in hemoglobin, and most of the rest is in **ferritin** and

hemosiderin, two intracellular iron storage proteins that abound in liver, spleen, bone marrow, intestinal mucosa, pancreas, the myocardium, and other tissues. The amount of stored iron is highly variable. It may reach several grams in some older males, but storage iron is nearly absent in many children and menstruating women.

Ferritin contains two slightly different polypeptide chains (MW 19 kDa and 21 kDa) that form a shell of 24 polypeptide subunits. This shell of apoferritin, with an external diameter of 13 nm and an internal cavity 6 nm across, is riddled with pores that allow the access of ionized iron and other low-molecular-weight substances. The hollow core of the molecule can accommodate up to 4500 ferric irons in the form of ferric oxide hydroxide (FeOOH) crystals, but actually it rarely contains more than 3000.

Hemosiderin, the second iron storage form, contains ferric oxide hydroxide and the same polypeptide subunits as ferritin, but it is distinguished from ferritin by its water insolubility. Ferritin is the more abundant storage form when the tissue stores are low; hemosiderin predominates when tissue stores are high. A small amount of ferritin, consisting mostly of apoferritin with little bound iron, also is present in the blood. This ferritin is released during normal cell turnover in the liver and other tissues.

*Essentially all the serum iron is tightly bound to **transferrin,*** a liver-derived β-globulin with a molecular weight of 78 kDa and a plasma concentration of approximately 300 mg/dL. The single polypeptide chain of transferrin ("apotransferrin") contains two sites that bind ferric (but not ferrous) iron with extremely high affinity. Only approximately one third of the iron-binding sites normally are occupied. This is expressed as an **iron saturation** of 33%. In the laboratory, the transferrin concentration is measured as the **total iron-binding capacity (TIBC)**.

Transferrin-bound iron is utilized by *receptor-mediated endocytosis* (Fig. 24.17). The **transferrin receptor** in the plasma membrane binds the iron-transferrin complex in preference to apotransferrin, and binding is followed by endocytosis. The endocytotic vesicle becomes acidified to a pH of approximately 5.0, forming an organelle known as a **CURL** (compartment of uncoupling of receptor and ligand). Under the low-pH conditions in the CURL, iron dissociates from apotransferrin and is transported into the cytoplasm. The vesicle itself is recycled to the cell surface, and the apotransferrin can resume its voyage through the circulatory system.

Most people consume between 10 and 50 mg of iron per day. A large part of this is derived not from the foodstuffs themselves but from the cooking utensils used for food preparation. The replacement of iron cooking ware by aluminum products, and the increasing use of Teflon-coated pots and pans, are considered important for the incidence of iron deficiency.

Only ferrous iron can be absorbed, mostly in the duodenum. The reduction of the ferric iron in food is favored by the low pH in the stomach and the presence of reducing substances, particularly ascorbic acid. Therefore iron absorption is enhanced by vitamin C−rich fruit juices, and it is reduced in patients with achlorhydria (lack of gastric acid) or after gastrectomy (surgical removal of the stomach). Iron absorption also is reduced by tannins, oxalate, phytate (inositol hexaphosphate), large quantities of inor-

---

FIG. 24.17

Utilization of transferrin-bound iron by receptor-mediated endocytosis. In this variation of the endocytotic pathway, the endosome is acidified to a pH of approximately 5.0. In this acidified organelle, known as CURL (compartment of uncoupling of receptor and ligand), iron is released from transferrin. While iron is transported into the cytoplasm, the receptor-bound apotransferrin is returned to the cell surface. $\vataxis$, Apotransferrin; •, Fe^{3+}; Y, transferrin receptor.

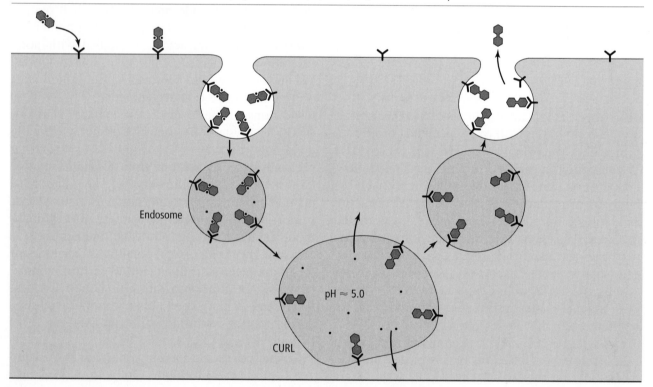

ganic phosphate, and certain antacids that form insoluble or nonabsorbable iron complexes. *Only approximately 5% of dietary non-heme iron is absorbed by normal individuals*, but this rate is more than doubled in response to iron deficiency. Indeed, *any anemic state, irrespective of its cause, enhances intestinal iron absorption.* Heme iron, which accounts for a significant portion of iron in meat and other animal products, is absorbed by separate mechanisms and with an efficiency of 20% to 25%.

The mechanism and regulation of iron absorption are poorly known. The absorbed iron initially is bound to ferritin in the intestinal mucosal cell. From intracellular ferritin either it is transferred to circulating transferrin, or it returns to the intestinal lumen when the mucosal cell is sloughed off from the epithelium at the end of its 2- to 6-day lifespan.

Iron transport in the body is dominated by the need for the redistribution of iron from the spleen and other sites of RBC destruction to the bone marrow (Fig. 24.18). Compared with the 15 mg of iron that is transported from spleen to bone marrow every day, the amount absorbed or excreted by the intestinal mucosa is quite unimpressive.

Cells throughout the body have to regulate their iron uptake according to their needs. Thus, a resting cell needs far less iron from circulating transferrin than a dividing cell, which has to double the amount of its iron proteins with each mitotic cycle.

Cells regulate their iron uptake by adjusting the number of transferrin receptors in the plasma membrane: when iron is abundant in the cell, the number of transferrin receptors is reduced; when the cell's stores are running low or an increased amount is required, the number of transferrin receptors increases. The synthesis of transferrin receptors is regulated at the mRNA level (Fig. 24.19): in the iron-deficient state, a 90-kDa regulatory protein (**IRE-BP,** iron response element binding protein) binds to an **iron response element** in the 3'-untranslated region of the transferrin receptor mRNA. This prolongs the lifespan of the mRNA by protecting it from cellular nucleases. Iron acts by poorly understood mechanisms to convert IRE-BP to an inactive form.

The synthesis of apoferritin is regulated by IRE-BP, too: in the iron-depleted state, the regulatory protein binds to an iron response element in the 5'-untranslated region of apoferritin mRNA, thereby blocking the initiation of translation. This mechanism ensures that *an increased amount of apoferritin is produced when iron is plentiful*, thus protecting the cell from the toxic effects of unbound iron.

FIG. 24.18

Daily transport of iron in the body.

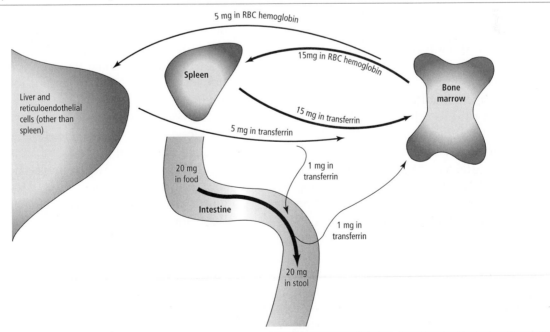

5 mg in RBC hemoglobin

15mg in RBC hemoglobin

15 mg in transferrin

5 mg in transferrin

Spleen

Bone marrow

Liver and reticuloendothelial cells (other than spleen)

20 mg in food

1 mg in transferrin

Intestine

1 mg in transferrin

20 mg in stool

FIG. 24.19

Cellular adaptations in the iron-deficient state: more transferrin *(Tf)* receptors are synthesized to acquire iron from circulating transferrin, and the synthesis of apoferritin is inhibited. *IRE,* Iron response element; *IRE-BP,* iron response element binding protein. IRE is a regulatory sequence of approximately 30 nucleotides in the mRNAs for the transferrin receptor and apoferritin. In iron deficiency, IRE-BP is converted to an active form that binds the IREs with high affinity.

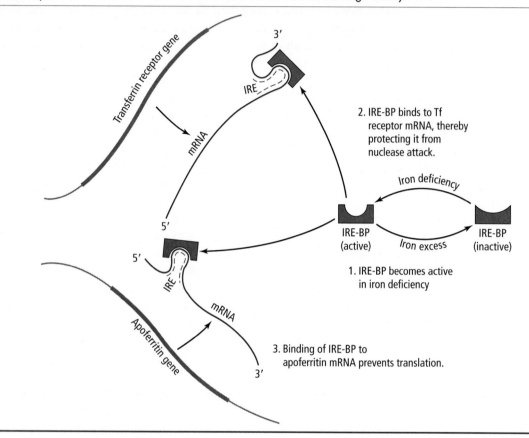

Iron deficiency is the most common nutritional deficiency worldwide

Only 1.0 mg of iron per day is absorbed in men, and 1.5 mg/day in menstruating women. On an iron-free diet (which is hard to achieve because iron is present in most foods), *storage iron is mobilized first,* before the levels of hemoglobin and other essential iron proteins are affected. Deficiency signs therefore would appear only after one or a few years, when ferritin and hemosiderin are depleted. Iron deficiency therefore is rarely caused by dietary deficiency alone. The typical situations are:

1. *Acute massive hemorrhage.* With a blood loss of 1 liter, 500 to 550 mg of iron is drained from the body. In most people, however, a blood loss of this magnitude does not result in lasting iron deficiency anemia, because storage iron is mobilized for use by the bone marrow, and the hematocrit returns to normal within a few weeks. Iron supplements are required only if the body stores are low.

2. *Chronic hemorrhage.* Most women lose 20 to 40 mL of blood during each menstrual period. This amount contains 11 to 22 mg of iron (0.35 to 0.7 mg/day), which has to be replaced from dietary sources. "Occult" blood loss (discounting vampires) most often is caused by chronic hemorrhage into the alimentary canal from esophageal varices, peptic ulcer, hemorrhoids, blood-sucking intestinal parasites, or tumors. Iron deficiency anemia in adult males always should be evaluated carefully because it may be the first sign of a malignancy.

3. *Growth.* Adults require iron only for the replace-

ment of daily losses, but growing children have to maintain a positive iron balance as the blood volume expands. The iron content of breast milk is low, and the blood hemoglobin concentration therefore normally declines from 18% to 20% at birth to 10% to 14% at 5 months. Oxygen delivery is not much affected by this decline, because fetal hemoglobin is replaced by adult hemoglobin during this time period, and adult hemoglobin is the better oxygen carrier after birth. Iron supplements sometimes are given at this time to prevent a decline below 10%, which is arbitrarily considered the lower limit of the "normal" range.

4. *Pregnancy and lactation*. Approximately 250 to 300 mg of iron is transferred to the fetus during pregnancy, and the additional iron loss in the placenta and cord and in blood loss at the time of birth may range anywhere from 80 to 400 mg. Another 100 to 180 mg is lost during lactation. The drain is minimal during the first months of pregnancy, but up to 5 mg/day is transferred to the fetus during the third trimester. Because many women have negligible iron stores, supplements routinely are given during late pregnancy.

Iron deficiency results in a *microcytic hypochromic anemia* (microcytic = small RBCs; hypochromic = low hemoglobin content per cell). The most important differential diagnoses are the thalassemias (see Chapter 9), which should be excluded before the initiation of iron therapy because iron supplements are contraindicated in thalassemia. Pallor, weakness, and lassitude are typical manifestations of iron deficiency. Not all symptoms are necessarily caused by the anemia, however. Not only the hemoglobin concentration in blood but also the levels of myoglobin, cytochromes, and other iron-containing proteins are reduced in iron deficiency.

Iron deficiency anemia is treated with iron supplements, most commonly in the form of ferrous sulfate. Some of the commonly used iron supplements contain both an iron salt and ascorbic acid, which improves the absorption of iron in the upper portions of the small intestine. The treatment is given for several months, and it should be continued for some months after hematological improvement to allow for the formation of adequate tissue stores.

Iron deficiency is most prevalent in growing children and in menstruating or pregnant women. Depending on the diagnostic criteria, nutritional habits in the population, and the use of iron-fortified foods, the prevalence of iron deficiency anemia in these groups often is reported as between 2% and 15% in industrialized countries and 10% to 50% in developing countries. *With the exception of protein-calorie malnutrition, iron deficiency is the most prevalent nutritional deficiency worldwide*, with a total of at least half a billion people affected. Biochemical indices of iron deficiency anemia are summarized in Table 24.2. The level of serum ferritin, determined by radioimmunoassay, is considered the most sensitive indicator of iron deficiency because it reflects the amount of tissue stores that decline in iron deficiency before any detectable decrease of the metabolically active iron in hemoglobin and transferrin.

Hemochromatosis is caused by abnormal iron accumulation

Apart from the normal turnover of intestinal mucosal cells, which contain iron in the form of ferritin, *there are no effective mechanisms of iron excretion*. If in an adult the amount of absorbed iron exceeds the losses for many years, iron accumulates in the tissues initially as ferritin and later as hemosiderin. This is called **hemosiderosis**. Although initially asymptomatic, *excessive iron accumulation is dangerous because it assists in the formation of destructive free radicals* (see Chapter 18). The longer lifespan of females may have to do with the fact that they have lower iron stores than males.

Hemochromatosis is an iron overload syndrome with progressive hemosiderosis and resulting organ damage. *Liver damage, diabetes mellitus* resulting from pancreatic involvement, *cardiomyopathy, hyperpigmentation* of the skin, and *arthralgia* (joint pain) are its most frequent signs. The condition often is associated with homozygosity for an incompletely recessive gene. Approximately 1 of every 400 white Americans is homozygous for this gene, and approximately 10% are heterozygous. *Hemochromatosis is the most common inherited metabolic disorder in the white population.*

The diet is important, too, and with excess dietary iron, hemochromatosis can develop in the absence of the predisposing gene. The iron fortification of staple foods, which has reduced the incidence

TABLE 24.2

Biochemical indices of iron deficiency and iron overload

Index	Normal	Changes in:	
		Iron deficiency	Iron overload
Hematocrit			
Male	43%-49%	Decreased	Normal
Female	41%-46%		
Blood hemoglobin			
Male	14%-18%	Decreased	Normal
Female	12%-16%		
Total plasma iron	50-160 μg/dL	Decreased	Increased
Total iron binding capacity	250-400 μg/dL	Increased	Increased
% Transferrin saturation	20%-55%	Decreased	Increased
Serum ferritin			
Male	5-30 μg/dL	Decreased	Increased
Female	1.2-10 μg/dL		

of iron deficiency anemia in many parts of the world, is not necessarily good for those older males who are at risk of iron overload. Alcohol also appears to increase iron absorption. Many South African Bantus, for example, developed hemochromatosis from the lifelong consumption of iron-rich alcoholic beverages. The excessive iron was derived from the steel vats in which these local brews were fermented.

Signs of hemochromatosis are most common in middle-aged and older males, who may accumulate 20 to 40 g of iron in the course of several decades. Premenopausal women are protected by menstruation and childbearing, but those homozygous for the gene defect can develop clinical signs of iron overload after menopause. The prevalence of clinically significant hemochromatosis, probably between 0.1% and 0.5% in older males, is uncertain because most cases are misdiagnosed as "alcoholic" cirrhosis, diabetes mellitus, or "idiopathic" or alcoholic cardiomyopathy. Elevated iron levels are common in liver biopsies of patients with "alcoholic cirrhosis," and it is not always clear whether iron overload is the cause or the result of the liver disease. *Hemochromatosis is treated by repeated phlebotomy.* This is indeed the only disease in which use of the traditional leech is the treatment of choice.

A secondary form of hemochromatosis is encountered in patients with hemolytic anemias who have been treated with repeated blood transfusions (see Chapter 9). These cases, of course, are not treated by phlebotomy. They require **desferrioxamine.** This iron chelator forms a soluble iron complex that is excreted in the urine.

Zinc is present in many enzymes

Next to iron, zinc is the most abundant trace mineral, with total body stores of 1.5 to 2.5 g. It is most important as a *constituent of the zinc metalloenzymes,* which include, among others, carbonic anhydrase, the extramitochondrial superoxide dismutase (which contains both copper and zinc), alcohol dehydrogenase, carboxypeptidases A and B, and DNA and RNA polymerases.

Zinc is obtained from meat, nuts, beans, wheat germ, and a variety of other foods, and the daily diet should contain 10 to 20 mg. Its absorption from the upper portions of the small intestine is incomplete, depending largely on the presence or absence of interfering substances in the food. There is no specific binding protein in the blood, and zinc is transported in association with serum albumin. In the cells it is stored in the form of the metalloprotein **metallothionein,** which also binds copper and some other heavy metals. Metallothionein is present in many tissues, and its synthesis is induced by heavy metals including zinc, cadmium, bismuth, and arsenic. It protects the cells from the toxic effects of the free, unbound metal ions. Zinc is present in pancreatic secretions, and the stools are the major route for its excretion. Compared with the fecal losses, the amounts lost in urine (0.5 mg/day), sweat (0.2 to 2 mg/day), and seminal fluid (up to 1 mg/ejaculate) are of minor importance. The adult male RDA is set at 15 mg/day.

Zinc deficiency has been described as a cause of poor growth, testicular atrophy, and delayed sexual development in children. Both children and adults show poor wound healing and dermatitis in zinc deficiency, as well as neuropsychiatric impairments and decreased taste acuity.

Acrodermatitis enteropathica is a rare, recessively inherited disease characterized by dermatitis, diarrhea, and alopecia (hair loss). It is caused by an impairment of intestinal zinc absorption. High doses of orally administered zinc are curative.

Copper participates in reactions of molecular oxygen

Copper also functions primarily as a component of metalloenzymes. The copper-containing enzymes, as a rule, *use either molecular oxygen or an oxygen derivative* as one of their substrates. Examples include cytochrome oxidase, dopamine β-hydroxylase, tyrosinase, Δ^9-desaturase, lysyl oxidase, and the cytoplasmic superoxide dismutase.

The total copper stores in the body amount to 80 to 110 mg, and the dietary requirement has been estimated as between 1 and 3 mg/day. The major route of copper excretion is the bile, which carries 1.5 to 2.0 mg/day. Sixty percent of the copper in the serum is tightly bound in **ceruloplasmin,** and the rest is loosely bound to albumin or complexed with histidine.

Copper deficiency, which occasionally has been observed in patients on total parenteral nutrition and in infants on copper-deficient formulas—but rarely in other situations—is characterized by a microcytic hypochromic anemia, leukopenia, hemorrhagic vascular changes, bone demineralization, hypercholesterolemia, and neurological problems.

Menkes' syndrome, also known as **kinky-hair syndrome,** is a rare, X-linked recessive disease caused by the deficiency of an ATP-dependent membrane transporter for copper. The transfer of copper from the intestinal mucosal cells to the blood is blocked, and its intracellular transport is abnormal as well. This fatal disease is characterized by growth retardation, mental deficiency, seizures, arterial aneurysms, bone demineralization, and brittle hair. It can be treated by the administration of the copper-histidine complex.

Wilson's disease (hepatolenticular degeneration) is a rare (incidence = 1 in 30,000), recessively inherited deficiency of a different copper transporter. The biliary excretion of copper is blocked, and copper accumulation in liver and brain leads to liver damage or neurological degeneration, or both. This disease responds to D-penicillamine, a copper chelator that permits urinary excretion by forming a soluble copper complex.

Some trace elements serve very specific functions

Most trace minerals other than iron, zinc, and copper serve extremely specialized functions. Those for which a dietary requirement is reasonably well established include:

Manganese: This metal stimulates the activity of many enzymes but can be replaced, in most cases, by magnesium. An adequate intake is 2 to 5 mg/day. Excess manganese is toxic, causing psychosis and parkinsonism ("manganese madness").

Molybdenum: Occurs in a few oxidase enzymes, including xanthine oxidase.

Selenium: In the form of selenocysteine, this element occurs in glutathione peroxidase. Both selenium deficiency and toxicity have been described. **Keshan disease,** an endemic cardiomyopathy in parts of China, is caused by the low selenium content of locally grown foodstuffs. The selenium content of the soil varies widely in different parts of the world, and this is reflected in the selenium content of the food plants grown in these soils.

Chromium: This metal is a component of "glucose tolerance factor," a poorly characterized complex that facilitates the action of insulin on its target tissues. Only a minority of diabetics show a favorable response to chromium, however.

Fluorine: Although not absolutely essential, fluorine strengthens teeth and bones by being incorporated in their inorganic crystal structure. It may have some protective effect in osteoporosis.

SUMMARY

Vitamins are essential micronutrients that serve very specific functions in metabolism. Most of the water-soluble vitamins are precursors of coenzymes: riboflavin, for example, is required for the synthesis of the flavin coenzymes, niacin for NAD and NADP, thiamine for thiamine pyrophosphate, pantothenic acid for coenzyme A, and folic acid for tetrahydrofolate.

Other vitamins, notably vitamin C (ascorbic acid), vitamin E, and vitamin A, are antioxidants that limit the extent of free radical–mediated oxidative reactions. They prevent lipid peroxidation, and they may have antimutagenic properties. High doses of these vitamins may provide protection from atherosclerosis (presumably by inhibiting the oxidation of LDL) and possibly from cancer (by preventing somatic mutations).

A third type of vitamin action is exhibited by vitamins A and D: they are converted to the active forms retinoic acid and calcitriol, respectively, and these act as physiological regulators, much like hormones. Indeed, their mechanism of action closely parallels that of the steroid and thyroid hormones.

Of the minerals, the macrominerals are bulk constituents of the body fluids, and the microminerals serve specific functions, most of them as constituents of proteins. Iron, in particular, is required as a constituent of a large number of heme proteins and iron-sulfur proteins.

Nutritional deficiencies of individual vitamins and minerals cause deficiency diseases whose symptoms can be traced, in some cases, to specific metabolic functions of the missing nutrient. Vitamin C deficiency (scurvy), for example, results in connective tissue problems because of impaired collagen synthesis, and iron deficiency results in anemia because of impaired hemoglobin synthesis. Although the incidence of severe nutritional deficiencies has declined in industrialized countries, vitamin and mineral nutrition is still a major public health concern, especially for such at-risk groups as infants, pregnant women, alcoholics, and the elderly.

Further Reading

Aggett PJ: Metal disorders. In: Holton JB, editor: *The inherited metabolic diseases*, 2nd ed. Churchill Livingstone, New York, 1994, pp. 491–522.

Blomhoff R, Green MH, Norum KR: Vitamin A: physiological and biochemical processing. *Annu Rev Nutr* 12, 37–57, 1992.

Brissot P, Deugnier Y-M: Normal iron metabolism. In: McIntyre N, Benhamou J-P, Bircher J, Rizzetto M, Rodes J, editors: *Oxford textbook of clinical hepatology*, vol. 1. Oxford University Press, Oxford, 1991, pp. 221–225.

Byers T, Perry G: Dietary carotenes, vitamin C, and vitamin E as protective antioxidants in human cancers. *Annu Rev Nutr* 12, 139–159, 1992.

Combs GF Jr: *The vitamins: fundamental aspects in nutrition and health*. Academic Press, San Diego, 1992.

Dickerson JWT: Nutritional disorders. In: Williams D, Marks V, editors: *Scientific foundations of biochemistry in clinical practice*, 2nd ed. Butterworth Heinemann, Oxford, 1994, pp. 1–24.

Gudas LJ: Retinoids and vertebrate development. *J Biol Chem* 269 (22), 15399–15402, 1994.

Gutierrez JA, Wessling-Resnick M: Molecular mechanisms of iron transport. *Crit Rev Eukaryot Gene Expr* 6 (1), 1–14 (1996).

Handin RI, Lux SE, Stossel TP, editors: *Blood*. J. B. Lippincott, Philadelphia, 1995, pp. 1383–1472.

Harford JB, Rovault TA, Huebers HA, Klausner RD: Molecular mechanisms of iron metabolism. In: Stamatoyannopoulos G, Nienhuis AW, Majerus PW, Varmus H, editors: *The molecular basis of blood diseases*. W. B. Saunders, Philadelphia, 1994, pp. 351–378.

Holick MF: Vitamin D: photobiology, metabolism, and clinical applications. In: De Groot LJ et al, editors: *Endocrinology*, 3rd ed., vol. 2. W. B. Saunders, Philadelphia, 1995, pp. 990–1014.

Johnson LR et al, editors: *Physiology of the gastrointestinal tract*, 3rd ed., vol. 2. Raven Press, New York, 1994, pp. 1935–2026, 2133–2202.

Krinsky NI: Actions of carotenoids in biological systems. *Annu Rev Nutr* 13, 561–587, 1993.

Leibold EA, Guo B: Iron-dependent regulation of ferritin and transferrin receptor expression by the iron-responsive element binding protein. *Annu Rev Nutr* 12, 345–368, 1992.

Powell LW, Summers KM, Halliday JW: Hemochromatosis. In: Haubrich WS, Schaffner F, Berk JE, editors: *Gastroenterology*,

5th ed., vol. 3. W. B. Saunders, Philadelphia, 1995, pp. 2325–2339.

Scriver CR, Beaudet AL, Sly WS, Valle D, editors: *The metabolic basis of inherited disease*, 6th ed. McGraw-Hill, New York, 1989, pp. 1411-1462, 2029-2045, 2049–2103.

Shils ME, Olson JA, Shike M, editors: *Modern nutrition in health and disease*, 8th ed., vol. 1. Lea & Febiger, Philadelphia, 1994, pp. 144–448.

Sternlieb I, Scheinberg IH: Wilson's disease. In: Schiff L, Schiff ER, editors: *Diseases of the liver*, 7th ed., vol. 1. J. B. Lippincott, Philadelphia, 1993, pp. 659–668.

Tavill AS: Hemochromatosis. In: Schiff L, Schiff ER, editors: *Diseases of the liver*, 7th ed., vol. 1. J. B. Lippincott, Philadelphia, 1993, pp. 669–691.

QUESTIONS

1. A finding that would support a diagnosis of iron deficiency anemia in a 25-year-old female patient with a hematocrit of 28% is
   A. The presence of oversized erythrocytes
   B. A low iron saturation of transferrin
   C. A reduced serum transferrin concentration
   D. An increased level of serum ferritin
   E. A reduced level of metallothionein in a liver biopsy

2. Retinoic acid in high doses sometimes is used for the treatment of skin diseases, including common acne. Retinoic acid can cause many toxic effects at high doses. The most important of these toxic effects is
   A. Bone demineralization leading to pathological fractures
   B. Connective tissue weakness with multiple small subcutaneous hemorrhages
   C. Teratogenic effects during the first trimester of pregnancy
   D. Peripheral neuropathy
   E. Amnestic syndrome

3. Vitamin D can be produced by the action of sunlight on 7-dehydrocholesterol in the skin, but it has to be converted to its biologically active form by hydroxylation reactions in
   A. Lung and brain
   B. Endothelium and intestine
   C. Skeletal muscle and adrenal cortex
   D. Adipose tissue and bone
   E. Liver and kidney

4. Some vitamins have antioxidant properties and therefore are considered useful for the prevention of atherosclerosis and, possibly, for the prevention of somatic mutations leading to cancer. Antioxidant properties have been demonstrated for all of the following vitamins except
   A. Thiamine (vitamin B_1)
   B. α-Tocopherol (vitamin E)
   C. Ascorbic acid (vitamin C)
   D. Retinol (vitamin A)

5. Thiamine deficiency can cause both acute encephalopathy and an irreversible memory impairment. These problems are most often seen in thiamine-deficient
   A. Newborns
   B. Alcoholics
   C. Diabetics
   D. Vegetarians
   E. Medical students

PART FIVE

INTEGRATION

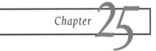

Chapter **25**

Plasma Proteins

The proteins of our blood plasma are a heterogeneous mixture of approximately a dozen major and innumerable "minor" components, with a total concentration of approximately 7 g/100 mL. These proteins serve a variety of functions:

1. *The maintenance of the colloid osmotic pressure* is a function of all plasma proteins. The colloid osmotic pressure is required to counteract the pressure filtration of fluid from the vascular space into the interstitial spaces.
2. **Binding proteins** bind and transport small molecules. They are used *to deliver nutritive and regulatory molecules to their proper destinations, and to bring waste products to reticuloendothelial cells* for endocytosis and lysosomal degradation.
3. **Protease inhibitors** are required *to curtail the ac-*

tions of proteases that are released during inflammatory processes, and to participate in the regulation of those physiological processes in which proteases participate, including the blood clotting system.
4. The **immunoglobulins,** or **antibodies,** participate in the defenses against infection by *binding foreign molecules, known as **antigens.*** Binding to the antibody is the first step in the elimination of the antigen.
5. The **clotting factors** protect us from excessive blood loss by *forming a fibrin clot at the sites of vascular injury.*

Tissue proteins that are released from dying cells during normal cell turnover also are present in small quantities. Tissue-derived enzymes are useful for the diagnosis of many diseases because their plasma levels are substantially increased after tissue damage. This chapter will give an overview of the most important plasma proteins, their physiological roles, and their diagnostic uses.

THE MAJOR PLASMA PROTEINS

With the exception of the immunoglobulins, which are derived from plasma cells, the quantitatively major plasma proteins are secreted into the blood by the liver. They are important in the clinical laboratory because their levels are affected by a variety of diseases.

Plasma is the soluble fraction of blood

Some diagnostic tests are performed on whole blood. Hemoglobin determinations, in particular, which are essential for the diagnosis of anemia, require virgin, uncentrifuged blood. For most other purposes, however, the blood is centrifuged first to separate the packed cells from the soluble fraction. Blood can be collected under conditions that inhibit blood clotting. Either heparin or a calcium chelator such as EDTA, citrate, or oxalate is used for this purpose. *If clotting is avoided, the supernatant obtained after centrifugation is called **plasma.*** It contains all plasma proteins including fibrinogen and the other clotting factors. However, if a blood clot forms before centrifugation, the supernatant no longer contains fibrinogen, and some of the other clotting factors are consumed as well. *This solution is called **serum.*** For most diagnostic tests, either plasma or serum can be used.

Plasma and serum are clear, yellow fluids that contain proteins in addition to inorganic ions and small metabolites (Table 25.1). A pink color suggests hemolysis, either in the patient or, more often, in the test tube as a result of careless handling of the sample. A milky appearance, or the formation of a fatty layer during centrifugation, shows that the patient had a fatty meal before the blood was taken (chylomicrons!), and a turbid appearance suggests a hypertriglyceridemia with elevated VLDL.

Once released into the blood, the plasma proteins circulate with half-lives on the order of some days before they finally are destroyed. **Pinocytosis** (see Chapter 8) is a nonselective mechanism of removal. A more specific mechanism is the *uptake of asialogly-*

TABLE 25.1

Reference values for some plasma constituents

Plasma constituent	Reference value
Gases and electrolytes	
pO$_2$ arterial	95-100 mm Hg
CO$_2$ arterial	21-28 mmol/L
CO$_2$ venous	24-30 mmol/L
HCO$_3^-$	21-28 mmol/L
Cl$^-$	95-103 mmol/L
Na$^+$	136-142 mmol/L
K$^+$	3.8-5.0 mmol/L
Ca^{2+} (total)	2.3-2.74 mmol/L
Mg^{2+}	0.65-1.23 mmol/L
pH	7.35-7.44
Metabolites	
Glucose (fasting)	3.9-6.1 mmol/L (70-110 mg/dL)
Ammonia	7-70 μmol/L (12-120 mg/dL)
Urea nitrogen	2.9-8.2 mmol/L (8-23 mg/dL)
Uric acid	0.16-0.51 mmol/L (2.7-8.5 mg/dL)
Creatinine	53-106 μmol/L (0.6-1.2 mg/dL)
Bilirubin (total)	2-20 μmol/L (0.1-1.2 mg/dL)
Bile acids	0.3-3 mg/dL
Lipids (total)	400-800 mg/dL
Acetoacetic acid	20-100 μmol/L (0.2-1 mg/dL)
Acetone	50-340 μmol/L (0.3-2 mg/dL)
Proteins	
Total protein	6-8 g/dL
Albumin	3.2-5.6 g/dL (52-65% of total)
α_1-Globulins	0.1-0.4 g/dL (2.5-5% of total)
α_2-Globulins	0.4-1.2 g/dL (7-13% of total)
β-Globulins	0.5-1.1 g/dL (8-14% of total)
γ-Globulins	0.5-1.6 g/dL (12-22% of total)

coproteins by the liver (Fig. 25.1): with the only important exception of albumin, the plasma proteins are glycoproteins. Most of the complex N-linked oligosaccharides of these plasma glycoproteins end with a sialic acid (N-acetylneuraminic acid) residue bound to galactose. During the lifetime of the plasma glycoprotein, these terminal sialic acid residues gradually are chewed off by endothelial neuraminidases. After the loss of the sialic acid, the exposed galactose at the end of the oligosaccharide binds to the **asialoglycoprotein receptor** on the surface of

FIG. 25.1

Removal of terminal sialic acid residues *(Sia)* from a typical *N*-linked oligosaccharide in a plasma protein exposes galactose residues that mediate the binding of the protein to the hepatic asialoglycoprotein receptor.

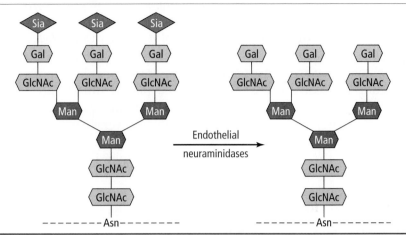

hepatocytes, followed by receptor-mediated endocytosis and lysosomal degradation.

Electrophoresis is the most important method for the separation of plasma proteins

For most diagnostic applications, the plasma proteins have to be separated into different fractions. The most important method for the separation of plasma proteins in the clinical laboratory is **electrophoresis** (Fig. 25.2). The procedure usually is performed at a mildly alkaline pH value at which all major plasma proteins carry a net negative charge: they all move to the anode, but at different speeds. The commonly used procedures employ solid or semisolid support media such as cellulose acetate foil or agarose gels, and *they separate the proteins on the basis of their charge/mass ratio rather than by molecular weight*. The separated proteins are visualized by suitable stains such as Coomassie brilliant blue, ponceau S, or amido black, and the stained fractions are quantified by densitometric scanning. Most procedures separate the proteins into five fractions: albumin, and the α_1, α_2, β, and γ globulins.

Albumin prevents edema

Of the five fractions seen in plasma protein electrophoresis, *only the albumin peak consists of a single major protein*. Albumin constitutes approximately 60%

FIG. 25.2

Electrophoretic separation of plasma proteins on cellulose acetate foil at pH 8.6, densitometric scan. The electrophoretic pattern depends somewhat on the separation conditions, including support medium, pH, and ionic strength.

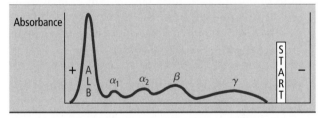

of the total plasma proteins. It is derived almost exclusively from the liver, where it accounts for approximately 25% of the total protein synthesis (12 g of albumin per day), and it circulates with a half-life of approximately 17 days.

Albumin is a tightly packed globular protein, consisting of a single polypeptide with 585 amino acids. Unlike most other plasma proteins, *it does not contain covalently bound carbohydrate*. Its compact structure is important hemodynamically: globular proteins with a compact shape do not increase the plasma viscosity to the same extent as more elongated proteins of the same molecular weight. With its molecular weight of 66,000, *albumin is large enough to avoid renal excretion. Smaller proteins are filtered through the glomerular basement membrane*, with resultant proteinuria. Indeed, most plasma proteins are either similar in size to albumin or larger (see Table 25.2).

Albumin crosses the vascular endothelium of most tissues to a limited extent. Therefore it is present in interstitial fluid and lymph, but at a lower concentration than in the plasma. Because the interstitial fluid volume is much larger than the plasma volume (12% versus 4.5% of the body volume), the total amount of albumin in the interstitial space slightly exceeds that in the vascular compartment. This albumin is returned to the blood by the lymph flow.

Albumin provides approximately 80% of the colloid osmotic pressure of the plasma, so it plays a key role in the regulation of fluid transfer across the endothelial lining: the hydrostatic pressure of the blood leads to the pressure filtration of fluid from the blood into the interstitial spaces, but the high albumin concentration in the plasma draws water back into the blood vessels (Fig. 25.3). The fluid balance across the endothelium is maintained as long as these two forces cancel each other.

If the serum albumin concentration drops to less than 2%, fluid accumulates in the interstitial spaces. This condition is called **edema.** Hypoalbuminemia and a variety of other conditions can cause edema. These include an increase in capillary permeability; venous obstruction; impaired lymph flow; and congestive heart failure with an increased venous pressure.

Albumin binds many small molecules

As a binding protein, albumin is a jack-of-all-trades: it has binding sites for fatty acids, thyroxin, cortisol, heme, bilirubin, and many other metabolites. At least half of the serum calcium also is albumin bound. Not only metabolites and inorganic ions, but also many foreign substances bind noncovalently to albumin. Most importantly, *many drugs bind to serum albumin with various affinities. Only the free, unbound fraction of a drug is pharmacologically active.* This is important in the management of patients who are chronically treated with a potentially toxic drug and whose plasma drug levels therefore are monitored at regular intervals. Being noncovalent, albumin binding is reversible:

$$\text{Albumin} \cdot \text{Drug} \rightleftharpoons \text{Albumin} + \text{Drug}$$

The dissociation constant K_d for the release of the drug from albumin is defined as

1

$$K_d = \frac{[\text{Alb}] \times [\text{Drug}]}{[\text{Alb} \cdot \text{Drug}]}$$

This can be rearranged to

2

$$\frac{[\text{Drug}]}{[\text{Alb} \cdot \text{Drug}]} = \frac{K_d}{[\text{Alb}]}$$

If the molar concentration of albumin is far higher than that of the drug, the concentration of free, unbound albumin [Alb] approximates the total serum albumin concentration. We can deduce from Equation 2 that in a patient whose albumin concentration is only half of normal, the ratio of free drug to

FIG. 25.3

Importance of the colloid osmotic pressure for fluid exchange across the capillary wall. A net flow of water into the interstitium is observed at the arterial end of the capillary. This is balanced by a net flow into the capillary at its venous end.

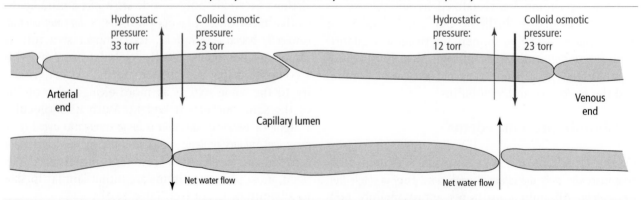

Hydrostatic pressure: 33 torr

Colloid osmotic pressure: 23 torr

Hydrostatic pressure: 12 torr

Colloid osmotic pressure: 23 torr

Arterial end

Venous end

Capillary lumen

Net water flow

Net water flow

bound drug is doubled. This becomes important when the plasma level of a chronically administered drug such as warfarin (see page 543) or a cardiotonic steroid (see Chapter 11) is measured: *if the patient has severe hypoalbuminemia, an otherwise desirable plasma level actually may be in the toxic range,* because an increased fraction of the drug is in the biologically active, unbound form. The commonly employed laboratory tests for plasma drug levels do not distinguish between the free and bound fractions. A similar situation is encountered in serum calcium determinations: in a severely hypoalbuminemic patient, a "normal" concentration of total serum calcium indicates hypercalcemia.

Many plasma proteins bind small organic molecules

Table 25.2 gives an overview of some of the more abundant or important plasma proteins. Many of these proteins are physiological binding proteins that participate in the transport of endogenous substances.

Transthyretin, also called **prealbumin** because it moves slightly ahead of albumin during electrophoresis, participates in the transport of retinol from its major storage site in the liver (see Chapter 24) to the extrahepatic tissues: a complex of retinol and retinol binding protein (RBP) is released from the liver into the blood, where it forms a ternary complex with transthyretin. The formation of this ternary complex is important because RBP (MW 21,000) is too small to escape renal excretion. The ternary complex, however, is large enough to avoid this tragic fate.

Transthyretin also binds thyroxine with a 1:1 stoichiometry. The major transport protein for thyroxine, however, is **thyroxine-binding globulin (TBG)**, which binds thyroxine with a 100-times-higher affinity than does transthyretin. An increased level of transthyretin leads to an increased level of total circulating thyroid hormone; its congenital absence leads to abnormally low levels. In both cases, however, the patient remains euthyroid. This example illustrates an important principle: *when the con-*

TABLE 25.2

Characteristics of some plasma proteins

Protein	Fraction	Concentration (mg/dL)	Mol wt	Properties
Transthyretin	Prealbumin	15-35	55,000	Retinol transport, binds T_4
Albumin	Albumin	4000-5000	66,000	Colloid osmotic pressure, binding protein
Retinol-binding protein	α_1	3-6	21,000	Retinol transport
α_1-Antiprotease	α_1	85-185	54,000	Protease inhibitor
Thyroxine-binding globulin	α_1	1-3.5	58,000	Major binding protein for T_3 and T_4
Transcortin	α_1	3-3.5	52,000	Binds glucocorticoids
α-Fetoprotein	α_1	0.002 (adults) 200-400 (fetus)		Elevated in adults with hepatoma
Ceruloplasmin	α_2	20-40	132,000	Contains copper
α_2-Macroglobulin	α_2	150-400	725,000	Protease inhibitor
Haptoglobin	α_2	100-300	85,000*	Binds hemoglobin
Transferrin	β	200-400	89,000	Binds iron
Hemopexin	β	50-120	60,000	Binds heme
Fibrinogen	β	200-400	340,000	Clot formation
C-reactive protein	γ	1.0	110,000	Acute phase reactant
Immunoglobulins	γ	700-1500	150,000-950,000	Very heterogeneous

* One genetic variant forms higher molecular weight polymers (MW > 200,000).

centration of the binding protein changes, the level of the free, unbound hormone is kept in the physiological range by homeostatic mechanisms.

Steroid hormones have their own binding proteins: most of the circulating glucocorticoids are bound to **transcortin,** and androgens and estrogens are bound to a **sex hormone binding globulin.** Because only the unbound fraction is biologically active, *variable levels of the binding proteins can complicate the interpretation of hormone levels measured in the clinical laboratory.* The separate measurement of bound and unbound hormone is technically demanding, so typically only the total circulating hormone concentration is measured.

Haptoglobin, a major component of the α_2 globulin fraction, binds hemoglobin that is released from RBCs during intravascular hemolysis. The hemoglobin-haptoglobin complex is cleared by the reticuloendothelial system (Fig. 25.4). Because haptoglobin is degraded together with hemoglobin by lysosomal enzymes in the reticuloendothelial cells, *the serum haptoglobin level is depressed in all hemolytic conditions,* sometimes to near zero. In sudden, massive hemolysis—for example, after a transfusion with incompatible blood—the binding capacity of haptoglobin may be exceeded. After dilution in the plasma, the released hemoglobin dissociates into $\alpha\beta$ dimers that are small enough (MW 33,000) to be excreted in the urine.

Haptoglobin does not bind myoglobin, which is released from damaged muscle tissue in many muscle diseases. Therefore the haptoglobin concentration, measured as the **hemoglobin-binding capacity** in the clinical laboratory, is not decreased in patients with myoglobinuria. Because the common laboratory tests for "blood" in the urine do not dis-

---

FIG. 25.4

The fate of hemoglobin *(Hb)* after intravascular hemolysis. *Hpt,* Haptoglobin; *Hpx,* hemopexin.

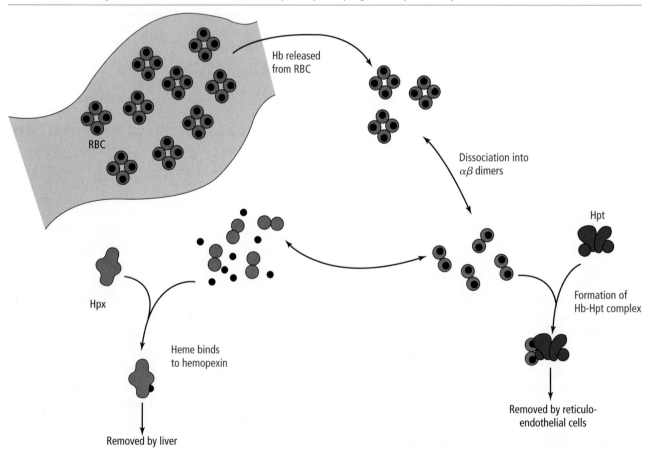

tinguish between hemoglobin and myoglobin, *the serum haptoglobin level can be determined to distinguish between hemoglobinuria and myoglobinuria.* Haptoglobin is not essential for life, and patients with a congenital absence of this protein are able to salvage hemoglobin by alternative mechanisms.

After intravascular hemolysis, heme tends to dissociate from the released hemoglobin. The ferrous iron of the heme group is oxidized rapidly to the ferric state, giving rise to **hematin.** *Both heme and hematin are bound by the β-globulin* **hemopexin,** and the complex thus formed is endocytosed in the liver. In severe hemolysis, the binding capacity of hemopexin is exceeded, the hemopexin concentration drops, and excess hematin binds loosely to albumin, forming methemalbumin. After several hours, when the hemopexin level recovers as a result of new synthesis by the liver, hematin is transferred back from albumin to hemopexin.

The presence of transferrin (see Chapter 24), haptoglobin, and hemopexin is important for the conservation of iron: *renal losses of this scarce mineral are avoided very efficiently by the binding of inorganic iron to transferrin, hemoglobin to haptoglobin, and heme to hemopexin.*

Deficiency of α_1-antiprotease causes lung emphysema

Protease inhibitors are important in the regulation of many processes, including the blood clotting system, and they limit the action of proteases released during inflammatory processes. The most abundant protease inhibitors in the plasma are α_2-macroglobulin and α_1-antiprotease.

α_2-**Macroglobulin,** one of the largest plasma proteins (MW 725,000), is a major component of the α_2-globulin fraction. It binds a great variety of proteases, and the protease-inhibitor complexes are ingested by reticuloendothelial cells, where they are digested by lysosomal enzymes.

α_1-**Antiprotease** is also known as α_1-**antitrypsin.** Actually, however, it inhibits a large number of serine proteases, including elastase and collagenase from white blood cells. In the laboratory, its activity is measured as the **trypsin inhibitory capacity (TIC).** More than 50 genetic variants of α_1-antiprotease are known, and one of these, the Z allele, codes for a protein product that cannot be

secreted from the hepatocytes where it is synthesized, resulting in a very low TIC. Heterozygotes are healthy, but *homozygosity for the Z allele has been demonstrated in young adults with lung emphysema.* In this disease, which otherwise is common only in old people with a lifelong habit of heavy smoking, the septa of the lung alveoli degenerate and the surface area available for gas exchange is reduced. Emphysema is associated with bronchitis, and the pathological changes are thought to result from the smoldering inflammatory process of chronic bronchitis.

The observation of early-onset lung emphysema in individuals with α_1-antiprotease deficiency suggests that *excessive proteolytic activity is an important mediator of tissue damage in chronic bronchitis and emphysema:* in inflammation, lysosomal proteases are released by macrophages and neutrophils either during phagocytosis or after cell death. These enzymes attack not only extracellular matrix proteins but also membrane proteins on the cell surfaces, thereby causing cell death and tissue necrosis. These proteolytic activities normally are checked by α_1-antiprotease. The lungs are exposed continuously to inhaled bacteria and other foreign particles, which are phagocytized by alveolar macrophages and other phagocytic cells.

α_1-Antiprotease, which is present not only in the blood but in bronchial secretions as well, *can be inactivated by cigarette smoke:* a methionine residue in the protein becomes oxidized to methionine sulfoxide by components of cigarette smoke. This chemical change, which impairs the protease-inhibiting activity, may be important for the development of chronic bronchitis and emphysema in smokers, even those without a genetic defect in the protease inhibitor system.

The prevalence of α_1-antiprotease deficiency in the white population of the United States is approximately 1 in 7000, and 80% of these persons eventually will develop emphysema, many of them at an early age. The strict avoidance of smoking is, of course, essential in the management of these patients.

Some patients with α_1-antiprotease deficiency develop neonatal hepatitis or infantile cirrhosis. In all likelihood this is caused not by a lack of protease inhibition but rather by the accumulation of nonsecretable α_1-antiprotease in vesicles within the hepatocytes.

Levels of plasma proteins are affected by many diseases

Plasma protein electrophoresis is a valuable aid in the diagnosis of many diseases. Figure 25.5 summarizes some typical patterns. The deficiency or excess of a major plasma protein affects the height of the corresponding peak. Thus an elevation of transferrin in iron deficiency anemia increases the height of the β-globulin peak, whereas α_1-antiprotease deficiency depresses the α_1-globulin fraction.

The levels of some plasma proteins, known as the **acute phase reactants,** *increase within 1 or 2 days after acute inflammation, trauma, or surgery.* These proteins include fibrinogen, α_1-antiprotease, haptoglobin, C-reactive protein, and ceruloplasmin. The size of the α_2 peak often is increased in these conditions because of its haptoglobin content (Fig. 25.5, *B*). The most sensitive acute phase reactant, however, is C-reactive protein. Its plasma level increases up to 100-fold in bacterial infections and to a lesser degree in some other diseases or after trauma or surgery. Transthyretin, on the other hand, is a negative acute phase reactant: its concentration may drop to less than 20% of normal during acute inflammation.

Slight to moderate decreases of serum albumin are seen in many diseases. The levels of γ-globulins, on the other hand, are increased in many chronic diseases including infections, malignancies, and liver cirrhosis, apparently by a nonspecific stimulation of immunoglobulin synthesis (Fig. 25.5, *C* and *D*). This condition is called **polyclonal gammopathy.** A **monoclonal gammopathy,** on the other

---

FIG. 25.5

Plasma protein electrophoresis in various disease states. **A,** Normal; **B,** immediate response pattern; **C,** delayed response pattern; **D,** liver cirrhosis; **E,** protein-losing conditions (nephrotic syndrome, protein-losing enteropathy); **F,** monoclonal gammopathy ("paraprotein").

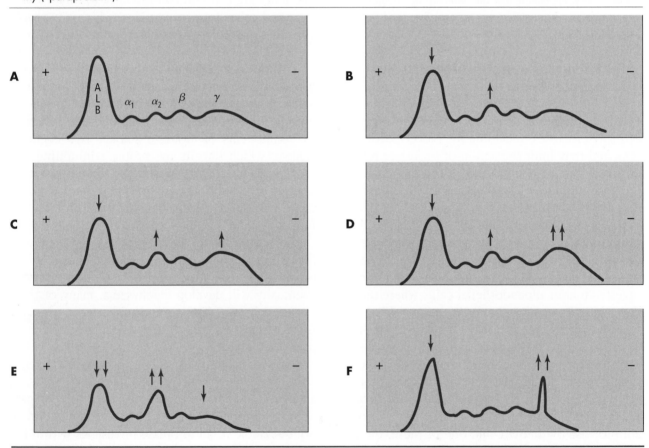

hand, is a disease in which a single immunoglobulin is overproduced by a single plasma cell clone (Fig. 25.5, F).

Nephrotic syndrome is a protein-losing condition in which *plasma proteins are lost in the urine*. This protein loss is affected by molecular size: small proteins are preferentially lost; large ones are retained. This causes decreases in the albumin peak and most of the globulin peaks, but the α_2 fraction is increased (Fig. 25.5, E). The α_2-macroglobulin in this fraction is so large (MW 725,000) that it is retained while the smaller plasma proteins are lost. Similar patterns of decreased albumin and increased α_2-globulin are seen in protein-losing enteropathy when plasma proteins are lost through a large inflamed area in the intestine, and in extensive burns when plasma proteins seep through the denuded body surface.

Disease-produced changes in the concentrations of minor plasma proteins do not change the electrophoretic pattern and have to be determined by radioimmunoassay (RIA; see Chapter 26, page 565) or other sensitive methods. α-**Fetoprotein** (α-FP), for example, which is synthesized in the fetal liver, occurs only in trace amounts in normal adult blood. *Its levels are increased in most patients with hepatocellular carcinoma*. A different use of α-FP, is the *prenatal diagnosis of open neural tube defects*. In these severe malformations, α-FP leaks from the fetal blood into amniotic fluid, where it can be detected after amniocentesis.

Blood components are used for transfusions

Blood transfusions are a time-honored treatment modality, but they require blood group matching and involve a substantial risk of disease transmission, most notably AIDS and hepatitis. Moreover, not every patient requires the same blood component. An anemic patient requires RBCs, a patient with nephrotic syndrome will benefit from albumin, and a patient with a clotting disorder needs clotting factors.

Table 25.3 lists some of the most important plasma products and their uses. Not only plasma products, but also RBCs, platelets, and granulocytes are, of course, available to the modern physician.

| CLINICAL ENZYMOLOGY |

Some enzymes are secreted normally into the plasma, where they play roles in lipoprotein metabolism, the blood clotting system, and other processes. Most metabolic enzymes, on the other hand, are intracellular, and only trace amounts of them are released into the blood during normal cell turnover.

TABLE 25.3

Plasma components available for therapeutic use

Product	Uses	Comments
Fresh frozen plasma	Multiple clotting factor deficiencies: liver cirrhosis, disseminated intravascular coagulation	Danger of disease transmission
Cryoprecipitate	Clotting disorders: hypofibrinogenemia, hemophilia, von Willebrand disease	Produced by freezing and thawing of plasma. Enriched in fibrinogen, factor VIII and fibronectin
Factor VIII concentrate	Hemophilia A	Some danger of hepatitis transmission
Albumin 5%	Hypovolemic shock	No danger of hepatitis or AIDS transmission; no blood group antibodies present
Albumin 25%	Cerebral edema	
Immune serum globulin	Immunodeficiency states affecting B cells; passive immunization against hepatitis, tetanus, etc.	For IV or IM injection

Tissue damage causes the release of cellular enzymes into the blood

Cell death is the most common cause of elevated plasma levels of cellular enzymes, but metabolic stress without necrosis can leave its mark as well, apparently by a transient increase of the membrane permeability. Neoplastic diseases also lead to elevated enzyme levels: the tumor cells represent an increased tissue source of the enzyme, tumor-invaded tissues are destroyed, and areas of tumor necrosis can develop when the tumor outgrows its blood supply.

Once released into the blood, the tissue enzymes have half-lives on the order of 1 day to 1 week (Table 25.4).

Ideally, a "useful" enzyme should be specific for a particular tissue or even for a disease. Few enzymes, however, meet this requirement. The enzymes of the major metabolic pathways, in particular, are represented in most tissues. Fortunately, *many of these enzymes occur as different **isoenzymes** in different tissues.* Isoenzymes catalyze the same reaction but are formed from structurally different polypeptides. They can be separated from each other by electrophoresis or other analytical methods, they have different kinetic properties, and they may have different sensitivities to inhibitors.

Enzymes are convenient for the clinical chemist because they can be quantified by measurements of their catalytic activities: under fixed pH and temperature conditions, an enzyme is incubated with saturating concentrations of its substrates, and either the decrease in substrate concentration or the formation of the product is measured. The V_{max}, which is determined this way (see Chapter 4), is proportional to the amount of the enzyme. Enzyme activities can be expressed in **international units (IU):** *one IU corresponds to the amount of enzyme that catalyzes the conversion of one micromole (μmol) of substrate to product per minute.*

Serum enzymes are useful for the diagnosis of many diseases

Levels of only a limited number of enzymes are determined on a routine basis in most clinical laboratories (see Table 25.5). The most important are:

1. *Plasma cholinesterase.* This enzyme differs from the acetylcholinesterase of cholinergic synapses (see Chapter 26, page 571) by its broader substrate specificity. Unlike the other diagnostically important enzymes, it normally is secreted by the liver and therefore is always present in the plasma. Its physiological role is uncertain, but it participates in the metabolism of some drugs, including succinylcholine and cocaine.

   Cholinesterase levels are decreased in parenchymatous liver diseases, including viral hepatitis and liver cirrhosis. More important is its use in the diagnosis of **organophosphate poisoning.** The organophosphates, which include many of the commonly used insecticides, are toxic for both insects and humans because they inhibit the acetylcholinesterase at cholinergic synapses irreversibly. Not only the tissue enzyme but also the plasma cholinesterase is inhibited by these agents.

   Another specific use of this enzyme is in patients treated with **succinylcholine,** a peripherally acting muscle relaxant that is used as an adjunct in general anesthesia. This drug is inactivated by plasma cholinesterase but not by the tissue enzyme. Some otherwise normal people are deficient in plasma cholinesterase, and they may develop fatal apnea after a standard dose of the drug. Therefore a determination of plasma cholinesterase may be prudent before exposing the patient to succinylcholine.

2. *Alanine transaminase (ALT) and aspartate transaminase (AST).* Like most other enzymes of amino acid metabolism, the transaminases are most abundant in the liver. They are not secreted into the blood, so any elevation of their plasma levels is the result of leakage from damaged cells.

TABLE 25.4

Plasma half-lives of some enzymes

Enzyme	$T\frac{1}{2}$ (days)
Plasma cholinesterase*	12-14
Lactate dehydrogenase	6.8
Alanine transaminase	6.3
Aspartate transaminase	2.0
Creatine kinase	1.4

* This enzyme normally is secreted into the blood by the liver.

Measurement of the transaminases is used for the diagnosis of liver diseases. In viral hepatitis, in particular, the plasma levels of both enzymes may be 20 to 50 times above the upper limit of the normal range. The enzyme elevations are proportional to the extent of the ongoing tissue damage, and they can be detected before hyperbilirubinemia and jaundice develop. The transaminases are elevated only mildly in patients with liver cirrhosis.

Substantial elevations of alanine transaminase are quite specific for liver damage, but aspartate transaminase also is moderately elevated in some extrahepatic diseases, including muscular dystrophy and acute myocardial infarction.

3. *Alkaline phosphatase and acid phosphatase.* The phosphatases are enzymes with broad substrate specificities that cleave a variety of organic phosphate esters. **Acid phosphatase (ACP)** and **alkaline phosphatase (ALP)** are distinguished by their pH optima, which are near pH 5 and 9, respectively. They therefore can be assayed separately, even using the same substrates.

ALP is most abundant in bone, placenta, intestine, and the hepatobiliary system. These organs contain different isoenzymes with different electrophoretic mobilities. The bone and liver enzymes are the most abundant in normal serum. The bone enzyme is derived from osteoblasts, and *its serum level is increased in those bone diseases in which osteoblastic activity is increased*: rickets, osteomalacia, hyperparathyroidism, osteitis deformans, neoplastic diseases with bone metastases, and healing fractures. The liver enzyme, which normally is secreted in bile, is *increased in patients with biliary obstruction*. Ascertaining the clinically important distinction between the bone and liver enzymes is possible by electrophoresis or by differential heat inactivation. During heating at 56°C for 15 minutes, the bone enzyme is destroyed to a greater extent than is the liver enzyme.

ACP originally was described in 1925 as a constituent of normal urine. It soon became evident that its concentration was far higher in male than in female urine and that its major source was the

TABLE 25.5

Changes in serum enzyme levels in different diseases

| Enzyme | Change in enzyme level in: | | | | | Neoplastic disease metastasis to | | |
	Viral hepatitis	Biliary obstruction	Muscular dystrophy	Acute myocardial infarction	Acute pancreatitis	Liver	Bone	Other
Plasma cholinesterase	↓↓	− or ↓	−	−	−	↓↓	−	Organophosphate poisoning
Alanine transaminase	↑↑↑	↑	− or ↑	− or ↑	−	↑	−	
Aspartate transaminase	↑↑↑	↑	↑	↑↑	−	↑↑	−	
Alkaline phosphatase	↑	↑↑↑	−	−	−	↑↑	↑↑↑	Bone diseases, fractures
Acid phosphatase	−	−	−	−	−	−	− or ↑	Prostatic carcinoma
Lactate dehydrogenase	↑	↑	↑↑	↑↑	−	↑↑↑	− or ↑	Megaloblastic anemia, shock
Creatine kinase	−	−	↑↑↑	↑↑	−	−	−	
Lipase	−	−	−	−	↑↑↑	−	−	Perforation of the small intestine
Amylase	−	−	−	−	↑↑↑	−	−	
γ-Glutamyltransferase	↑	↑↑↑	−	−	−	↑↑	−	

−, No change; ↑, increased; ↓, decreased.

prostate gland. RBCs, platelets, liver, and bone also contain various forms of ACP.

The only established clinical use of ACP measurement is *the diagnosis and follow-up of metastatic prostatic carcinoma*. The enzyme is not elevated in the early stages of the disease, however, so measuring it cannot replace rectal digital exam as a method for early diagnosis. The main use of ACP determination is in the follow-up of patients with established prostatic cancer, when the success or failure of treatments is reflected in the serum levels of this enzyme.

ACP is present in seminal fluid, and its detection in vaginal specimens has been used forensically to substantiate allegations of rape. The enzyme is also remarkably stable and can be detected in stains even after several weeks.

4. *Lactate dehydrogenase (LDH)*. As an enzyme of anaerobic glycolysis, LDH is present in all tissues; therefore its plasma level is elevated in a wide variety of diseases. Fortunately, different tissues contain different isoenzymes. The isoenzymes are formed from two different subunits, designated H (heart) and M (muscle). These two subunits have essentially the same molecular weight (34,000), but they differ in their charge patterns. LDH itself is a tetrameric protein, and *a total of five isoenzymes can be formed with various combinations of H and M subunits (Table 25.6)*. The isoenzymes can be separated by electrophoresis. Isoenzyme 1, consisting of four H subunits, is fastest; isoenzyme 5, consisting of four M subunits, is the slowest at pH 8.6.

The isoenzyme patterns of the tissues depend on the relative amounts of H and M subunits pro-

duced by the cells. Thus, myocardium and bone marrow produce mostly H subunits; liver and skeletal muscle produce mostly M subunits, and most other tissues (lung, brain, kidney, pancreas) produce both.

For differential diagnosis, either the separate determination of the isoenzymes or the simultaneous determination of other enzymes can be used in many cases. In the differential diagnosis of myocardial infarction and pulmonary infarction, for example, elevations of isoenzymes 1 and 2, measured 1 or 2 days after an episode of chest pain, suggest myocardial infarction, and elevations of isoenzymes 3, 4, and 5 have to be expected after pulmonary infarction. Also, combined increases of LDH, AST, and creatine kinase (CK) suggest myocardial infarction, and elevated LDH with more-or-less-normal AST and CK is typical for pulmonary infarction.

5. *Creatine kinase (CK)*. The main disadvantage of LDH is its wide tissue distribution, but creatine kinase (CK), also known as **creatine phosphokinase (CPK)**, is a reasonably specific muscle enzyme. The creatine kinase reaction

$$\text{Creatine} + \text{ATP} \rightleftharpoons \text{Creatine phosphate} + \text{ADP}$$

is important as an immediate source of ATP in contracting muscle (see Chapter 29). Besides muscle tissue, only the brain contains appreciable amounts of CK.

Like LDH, CK has tissue-specific isoenzymes. Active CK is a dimer, and two slightly different monomers occur in the tissues: skeletal muscle

TABLE 25.6

Occurrence of LDH isoenzymes in different tissues

Isoenzyme no.*	Composition	Presence in:				
		Myocardium	Erythrocytes	Skeletal muscle	Liver	Kidney
1	H_4	++++	+++	−	−	+
2	H_3M	++++	+++	−	−	+
3	H_2M_2	+	+	+	+	++
4	HM_3	−	−	++	++	++
5	M_4	−	−	++++	++++	++

* Enzyme 1 has the highest, and enzyme 5 the lowest, anodic mobility on electrophoresis at slightly alkaline pH values.

contains M subunits, the brain contains B subunits, and the myocardium contains mostly M but also some B subunits. Three different isoenzymes can be formed. They are numbered according to their electrophoretic mobility (Table 25.7), CK-1 (BB) having the greatest anodic mobility at pH 8.6.

The brain enzyme rarely is elevated in the blood, even after cerebrovascular accidents, although it is increased in the cerebrospinal fluid of patients with various CNS diseases. *The main use of CK measurement is in the diagnosis of muscle diseases.* Injuries, intramuscular injections, vigorous physical exercise, dermatomyositis, polymyositis, and the muscular dystrophies all increase the serum CK level, as well as increasing LDH, AST, and myoglobin. CK levels are normal in patients with neurogenic muscle diseases, including peripheral denervation and the upper and lower motor neuron syndromes.

Elevations of CK-2 are most revealing in the diagnosis of acute myocardial infarction. *Besides LDH and AST, CK is the most useful enzyme to measure for the diagnosis of acute myocardial infarction.* As shown in Fig. 25.6, the time courses for these enzymes are different: CK typically rises to a maximum within 24 hours, followed shortly by AST. LDH reaches its peak only after 48 to 72 hours. CK and AST levels return to normal within 2 to 3 days, but LDH remains elevated for 1 or 2 weeks. LDH typically shows the **flipped LDH** response: although LDH-2 (derived from erythrocytes) is the most abundant isoenzyme in normal serum, LDH-1 is higher than LDH-2 during the first few days after myocardial infarction.

What are the advantages of enzyme determinations over other diagnostic methods for acute myocardial infarction? The electrocardiogram (ECG), in particular, is more revealing than enzyme determinations for the diagnosis of myocardial damage: the biochemist can only estimate the extent of the damage by determining the levels of myocardial enzymes in the blood, but the electrocardiologist actually can locate the site of the infarction. On the other hand, the ECG does not distinguish between old defects and a recent infarction; enzyme elevations are specific for recent tissue damage.

6. *Lipase and amylase.* Lipase and amylase are digestive enzymes from the pancreas, and their serum levels are elevated in patients with acute pancreatitis. The main reason for measuring their levels is for *the differential diagnosis of patients who present with severe abdominal pain of sudden onset.* In these abdominal emergencies, acute pancreatitis has to be differentiated from a variety of other disorders that include, for example, the complications of peptic ulcer disease and cholelithiasis.

Amylase and lipase are elevated in some extra-

TABLE 25.7

Isoenzymes of creatine kinase (CK)

Isoenzyme	Subunit structure	Electrophoretic mobility	Present in:
CK-1	BB	Fast	Brain
CK-2	BM	Medium	Myocardium
CK-3	MM	Slow	Skeletal muscle, myocardium

FIG. 25.6

Enzyme elevations after acute myocardial infarction. *CK,* Creatine kinase; *AST,* aspartate transaminase; *LDH,* lactate dehydrogenase.

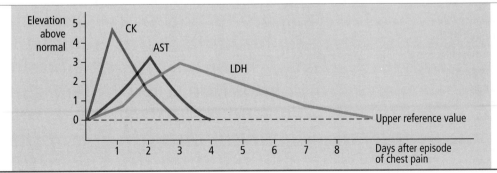

pancreatic diseases as well, including intestinal infarction or perforation, and in peritonitis. Amylase may even be elevated in patients with mumps or other forms of parotitis.

THE IMMUNOGLOBULINS

Approximately 20% of the plasma proteins move in the γ-globulin region during electrophoresis. Most of these γ globulins, and some of the β and $α_2$ globulins as well, are **immunoglobulins** (Table 25.8). These proteins, derived from plasma cells, act as **antibodies** by combining noncovalently with foreign macromolecules, known as **antigens**.

Immunoglobulins are able to bind specific antigens

All immunoglobulins are able to bind tightly to an antigen to form an **antigen-antibody complex.** An antigen is, by definition, a molecule that induces the formation of a matching antibody. To be an effective antigen, a molecule has to fulfill two requirements:

- *It has to be large*, with a molecular weight of at least 10,000, and
- *It has to be a foreign molecule.* We normally do not form antibodies to our own macromolecules—except in autoimmune diseases, when serious damage can be done by **autoantibodies** attacking normal components of our bodies.

The antigen-antibody complex is formed only by noncovalent interactions. The tightness of binding is described by the **affinity constant K_{aff}**, which is defined as the equilibrium constant for the formation of the antigen-antibody complex:

$$Ag + Ab \rightleftharpoons Ag \cdot Ab$$

$$K_{aff} = \frac{[Ag \cdot Ab]}{[Ag] \times [Ab]}$$

Typical values for the affinity constant are 10^7 to 10^{11}

TABLE 25.8

Properties of the different immunoglobulin classes

Immunoglobulin class	IgG	IgM	IgA	IgD	IgE
H chain class	γ	μ	α	δ	ε
H chain subclasses	$γ_1$, $γ_2$, $γ_3$, $γ_4$	—	$α_1$, $α_2$	—	—
Polymeric forms	—	Pentamer	Mono-, di- or trimer (serum), dimer (secreted)	—	—
Molecular weight	150,000	950,000	180,000 (monomer) 400,000 (secreted)	180,000	190,000
Carbohydrate content (%)	2-3	12	7-11	9-14	12
Serum concentration (mg/dL)	1200	120	300	3	0.005
Serum half-life (days)	21	7	6	3	2
Complement fixation (classic)	++*	+++	—	—	—
Binding to monocytes/ macrophages	++†	+	—	—	++
Binding to neutrophils	+‡	—	++	—	—
Binding to mast cells	—	—	—	—	+++
Secretion across epithelia	—	—	+++	—	—
Placental transfer	+++	—	—	—	—

Binding to monocytes/macrophages and neutrophils is important for the stimulation of phagocytosis, and binding to mast cells is important for the stimulation of histamine release during allergic responses.
* Except IgG_4.
† Except IgG_2.
‡ IgG_1 and IgG_3 only.

liters/mol. This means that at a concentration of the free antigen of 10^{-7} to 10^{-11} mol/liter, the concentration of the antigen-antibody complex equals that of the free antibody (compare with hormone-receptor binding, Chapter 27, pages 577-578).

The formation of the antigen-antibody complex is the first step in the elimination of the antigen. The complex may be endocytosed by reticuloendothelial cells, where both the antigen and the antibody fall prey to lysosomal enzymes. If the antigen-antibody complex is formed on the surface of a solid particle—for example, a virus or a bacterium—the antibody-coated particle can be phagocytized by macrophages or neutrophils: the bound antibody acts as a tag that marks the particle for phagocytosis. This stimulation of phagocytosis is called **opsonization.** Antibody-labeled cells also can be destroyed by the **complement system**, which consists of soluble plasma proteins: the first component of the complement system binds to the antigen-antibody complex on the cell surface, and this is followed by a proteolytic cascade. Eventually a cytolytic complex is formed that creates a gap junction ("drills a hole") in the membrane.

The most astounding property of the immunoglobulins is their diversity: each individual has *at least a million structurally different antibodies, each with its own unique antigen-binding specificity.* This diversity en-

---

FIG. 25.7

Structure of human IgG_1. Each domain (V_L and C_L in the light chains; V_H, C_H1, C_H2, and C_H3 in the heavy chains) is actually a globular portion of the molecule, stabilized by an intrachain disulfide bond.

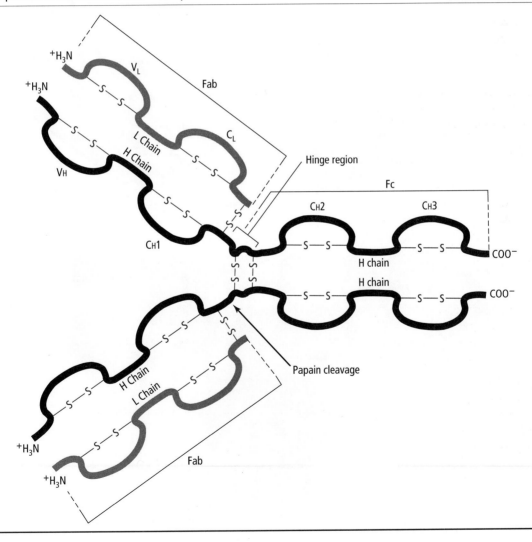

ables the body to recognize and eliminate almost any imaginable foreign macromolecule.

Antibodies consist of two light chains and two heavy chains

Despite the great diversity of their antigen-binding specificities, all immunoglobulin molecules have the same general structure. Figure 25.7 shows the structure of IgG_1, the most abundant subclass of immunoglobulin: there are two identical heavy (H) chains with molecular weights of approximately 53,000 each, and two identical light (L) chains with molecular weights of 23,000 each. These four polypeptides are held together both by noncovalent forces and by disulfide bonds. The molecule has the shape of the letter Y: each of the two arms of the Y is formed by the amino-terminal half of an H chain

---

FIG. 25.8

The three-dimensional structure of immunoglobulins. **A,** Ribbon model of an immunoglobulin light chain. Each domain contains two "blankets" formed from antiparallel β-pleated sheets (⟹ and ⟹). The interfaces of the two blankets are formed by hydrophobic amino acid side chains, and the structure is reinforced by a single disulfide bond. The variable domain contains two additional β-pleated sheet sequences not present in the constant domain (⟹). The antigen binds to three loops (━━) that are formed by the hypervariable regions. **B,** The three-dimensional structure of an IgG molecule. In this immunoglobulin class, N-linked oligosaccharides participate in the interactions between the heavy chains.

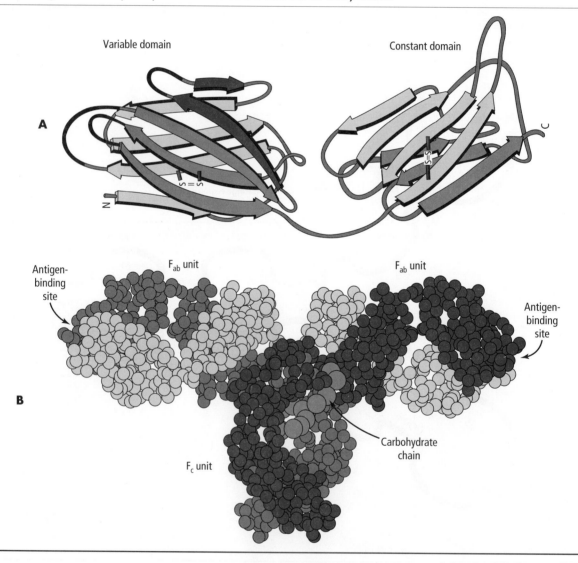

and a complete L chain. The stem consists of the carboxy-terminal halves of the two H chains. *The L chain consists of two domains* with related amino acid sequences, and *the H chain consists of four domains.* Each domain is a globular segment of approximately 110 amino acid residues, stabilized by an internal disulfide bond. All domains have a similar higher-order structure, with a characteristic arrangement of the polypeptide into two blanketlike sheets of antiparallel β-pleated sheet (Fig. 25.8). These two "blankets" are held together by a disulfide bond.

The H chain contains not only the four globular domains but also a less-compact **hinge region** between the second and third domains. The hinge region contains the disulfide bonds between the two H chains.

The amino-terminal domain of both the L chain and the H chain is special: it is a **variable domain.** When we compare the H chains of many different IgG$_1$ molecules, we find that the second, third, and fourth domains are always the same. These are the **constant domains.** The second domain of the light chain also is constant, although two different structures are found in different molecules that define the κ (kappa) and λ (lambda) types of light chain. Each immunoglobulin molecule has either two κ chains or two λ chains, but never one of each. The variable domains, however, differ widely in the different molecules: if a very skilled biochemist could isolate hundreds of different individual IgG$_1$ molecules and determine their amino acid sequences individually, he would almost never find two molecules with exactly the same amino acid sequences in the variable domains. *The great diversity of immunoglobulin structure resides, therefore, in the variable domains of the two polypeptides.* Most of the variability is concentrated in the **hypervariable regions.** There are three hypervariable regions in the variable domain of the light chain, and either three or four in the variable domain of the heavy chain.

The domain structure of the molecule is reflected in its gene structure: each domain is encoded by a separate exon, and the hinge region has its own little exon as well (see Fig. 25.14, page 531). Therefore we can assume that the genes for the immunoglobulin chains evolved from a primordial gene by exon duplication.

The important properties of the immunoglobulins include *antigen binding* and the *effector functions.* Effector functions are properties such as complement activation, opsonization, and the induction of histamine release from mast cells. The allocation of these functional properties to different regions of the molecule has been possible by partial proteolytic cleavage. Papain, a thiol protease from the latex of the papaya plant, cleaves a single peptide bond in the hinge region of IgG$_1$. This cleavage forms two types of fragments: two identical F_{ab} **fragments** (F_{ab} = antigen-binding fragment), containing a complete L chain and the amino-terminal half of an H chain; and one F_c **fragment** (F_c = crystallizable fragment), consisting of the carboxy-terminal halves of the two H chains, still linked by disulfide bonds. *Although the effector functions depend on the F_c fragment, only the F_{ab} fragment can bind antigen.*

There are two antigen-binding regions in the immunoglobulin molecule, each consisting of the variable domain of a light chain and the variable domain of a heavy chain. The three-dimensional structures of some antigen-antibody complexes have been resolved by X-ray diffraction, and the hypervariable regions have been identified as the principal sites of contact with the antigen.

FIG. 25.9

Formation of antigen-antibody complexes. **A,** Antibody excess: small complexes, no precipitation. **B,** Equivalence zone: large complexes, precipitation. **C,** Antigen excess: small complexes, no precipitation.

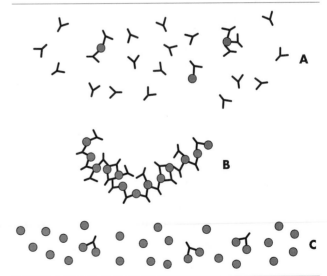

The presence of two antigen-binding sites facilitates the formation of large aggregates consisting of a latticework of interconnected antigen and antibody molecules. These aggregates are insoluble, so *the reaction between a soluble antigen and an antibody results in precipitation.* The size and solubility of the complexes depend on the relative concentrations of antigen and antibody: small, soluble complexes predominate in antigen excess and in antibody excess, but large insoluble complexes are formed in the **equivalence zone,** with equimolar concentrations of antigen and antibody (Fig. 25.9).

If the antigen is on a cell surface, the two antigen-binding sites of the antibody can combine with antigen on different cells, effectively gluing the cells together. *This results in agglutination,* an outcome that is observed, for example, when blood cells are mixed with an antiserum to a blood group antigen.

Different immunoglobulin classes have different properties

There are five major classes of heavy chains that define the class of the immunoglobulin: IgG has γ chains, IgM has μ chains, IgA has α chains, IgD has δ chains, and IgE has ε chains. The class of the heavy chain is defined by the amino acid sequence of its constant domains. IgG has four subclasses containing four slightly different γ chains with approximately 95% sequence homology, and IgA has two subclasses. Figure 25.10 summarizes the structural features of the immunoglobulin classes and subclasses.

Some immunoglobulins occur in oligomeric forms in which two or more units are disulfide bonded to each other. These oligomeric immunoglobulins contain a small polypeptide known as the **J chain.** Figure 25.11 shows the structure of IgM,

FIG. 25.10

Structural features of the different immunoglobulin classes and subclasses. IgM and IgE have four rather than three constant domains. Note the variability in the locations of the interchain disulfide bonds. —, Disulfide bonds.

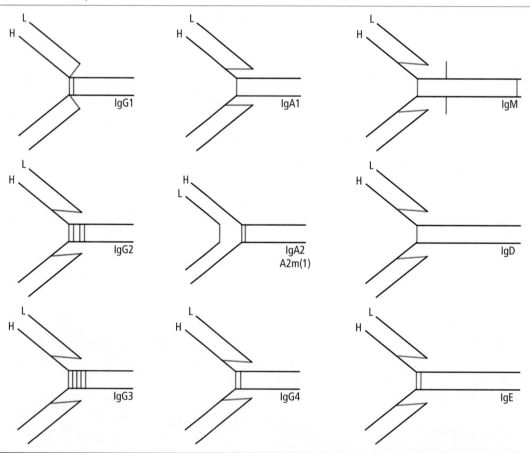

which occurs in a pentameric form in the serum: a single J chain forms disulfide bonds with two of the monomers, and the heavy chains of different monomers are disulfide bonded to each other as well.

IgA is the most abundant immunoglobulin in external secretions, including tears, saliva, bronchial mucus, intestinal and genitourinary secretions, and milk. It is secreted as a dimer, with a J chain and a noncovalently bound **secretory component.** The secretory component is a glycoprotein that is derived from the extracellular part of a membrane glycoprotein on the surface of epithelial cells (Fig. 25.12). Secretory IgA is synthesized in submucosal lymphatic tissues such as the tonsils in the throat and Peyer's patches in the intestine.

IgA is able to enter external secretions, but *only IgG can cross the placental barrier.* Maternal IgG therefore is able to protect the fetus from intrauterine infections. Indeed, almost all immunoglobulin in the fetus is maternally derived IgG.

IgE is the most troublesome immunoglobulin because *it mediates allergic reactions.* It binds avidly to the surface of basophils and mast cells, where it acts as an antigen receptor. The binding of the antigen to surface IgE induces the release of stored histamine from the cell. Most of the allergic symptoms are mediated by the released histamine, and most an-

---

FIG. 25.11

Structure of IgM, which is present as a pentamer of molecular weight 900,000 in the serum. IgM on the surface of B cells, however, is present in a monomeric form. —, Disulfide bonds.

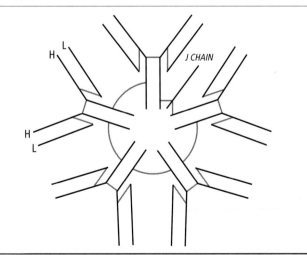

---

tiallergic drugs act by blocking the effects of histamine on its target cells.

Immunoglobulins are present on the surface of B lymphocytes

The B lymphocytes do not secrete their antibody but rather *incorporate it in their plasma membrane*, with the antigen-binding sites exposed to the extracellular environment (Fig. 25.13). The membrane-bound and secreted forms of the immunoglobulin differ in the amino acid sequences at the carboxy end of the heavy chain: the membrane-bound form contains a transmembrane helix that is lacking in the secreted antibody. This structural difference results from the optional use of a small exon 3' of the last constant domain exon (Fig. 25.14). Most importantly, *of the millions of B cells in the human body, each produces its own personal antibody with its own distinctive antigen-binding specificity.* The surface immunoglobulin enables the B cell to recognize specifically "its" antigen.

During its development, *the B cell is able to change the class of its antibody without changing the antigen-binding specificity.* The first immunoglobulin to appear on the surface of the developing B cell is an IgM antibody. IgM often is followed by IgD, and eventually IgG, IgA, or IgE may appear. This phenomenon, known as **class switching,** takes place either before or (more commonly) after exposure to the antigen. It is stimulated by **lymphokines,** soluble proteins that are released by activated helper T cells during infections and some other disease processes.

B cells become activated by the binding of antigen to the surface immunoglobulin and by exposure to helper T cells. The activated B cell divides and produces a large number of progeny cells that actively secrete their antibody. These antibody-secreting cells are called **plasma cells.** The secreted antibody of the plasma cell has exactly the same antigen-binding specificity as the original surface immunoglobulin of the ancestral B cell.

Antigen-dependent plasma cell differentiation is the basis of **clonal selection:** *a foreign molecule entering the body binds only to those few B lymphocytes that carry a matching antibody on their surface. Only these B lymphocytes develop into mature, antibody-secreting plasma cells.*

The T cells, which constitute approximately 70% of the lymphocytes in humans, do not produce antibodies. They possess, however, a membrane-

FIG. 25.12

Synthesis of secretory IgA. The dimeric form of IgA, which is derived from plasma cells in submucosal lymphatic tissue, is transported across the epithelial cell by transcytosis after binding to a cell surface receptor. On the lumenal surface, the extracellular domain of the receptor is cleaved from the membrane-spanning domain and remains bound to the secreted IgA as the "secretory component."

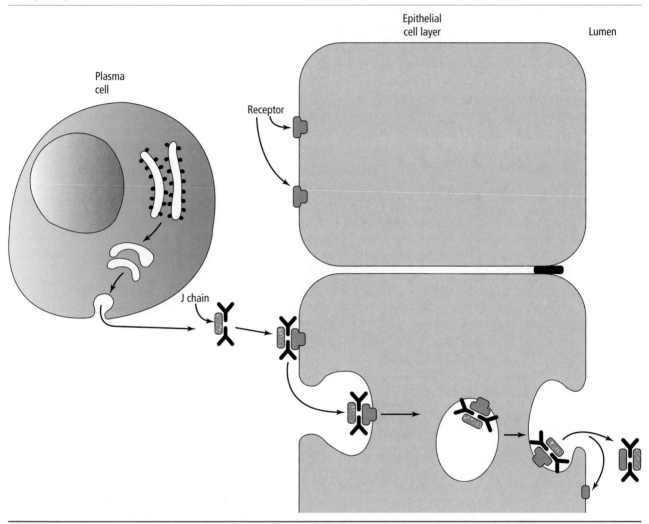

bound **T-cell receptor.** The T-cell receptor has antigen-binding domains and is functionally equivalent to the surface antibodies of B cells. *Only B lymphocytes and T lymphocytes possess antigen receptors on their surface that enable them to respond specifically to a matching antigen.*

The immunoglobulin genes are rearranged during B-cell differentiation

How can the genes for some million different antibodies find space in the human genome? This task is not as formidable as it seems, because the antigen-binding site is formed by two different polypeptides. Theoretically, a thousand different H chains and a thousand different L chains, encoded by a total of 2000 genes, would be sufficient to make a million different antibodies. Also, only the variable domains, which measure approximately 110 amino acids each, but not the constant domains come in many different variants.

The immunoglobulin chains are encoded by three separate gene clusters for κ light chains (on chromosome 2), λ light chains (on chromosome 22), and heavy chains (on chromosome 14). In the germline,

FIG. 25.13

Differentiation of a B lymphocyte. Class switching can occur either before or after antigen exposure.

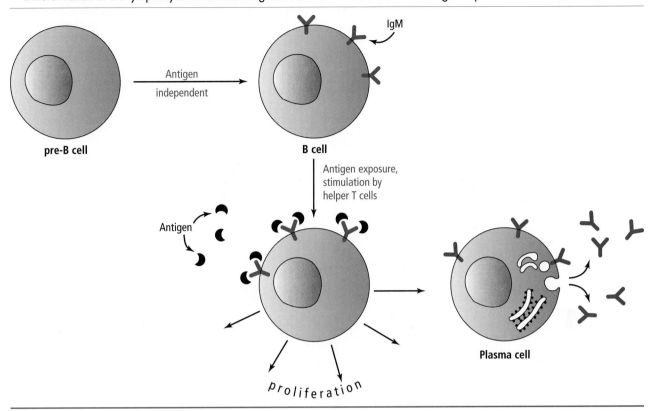

FIG. 25.14

The intron-exon structure of a γ-chain gene is shown schematically. The signal sequence, the four domains, and the hinge region are encoded by separate exons. The exon for the membrane attachment region *(M)* is included in the membrane-bound IgG but not in secreted IgG. Exon L (for leader) encodes the signal sequence.

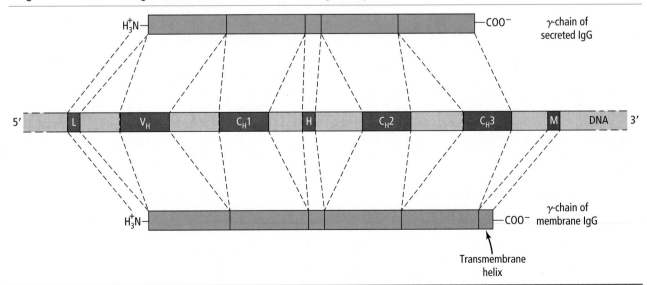

FIG. 25.15

Rearrangement and expression of the κ light-chain genes. The gene rearrangement takes place early in the development of B lymphocytes, before any antigen exposure. During the gene rearrangement, the intervening DNA (in this case the DNA between gene V_x and J3) is deleted.

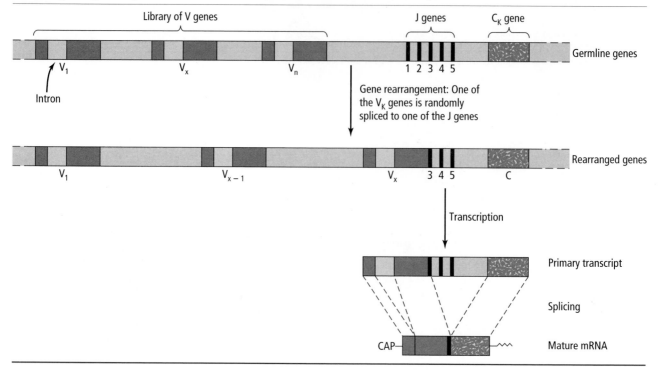

these gene clusters contain separate genes for the variable and constant domains. During the development of the B lymphocyte, *these separate genes have to be combined into a single transcription unit that codes for a complete L or H chain.*

Figure 25.15 shows the situation for the κ light chain: a single gene codes for the constant domain, which starts with amino acid 109. Most of the variable domain, reaching from amino acids 1 to 95, is encoded by a **V gene** (V for variable), and residues 96 to 108 are encoded by a small **J gene** (J for joining). The germline contains a whole library of 5 J genes and approximately 50 V genes. Each V gene starts with a small exon coding for the signal sequence, followed by an intron and a large exon coding for amino acids 1 to 95.

During B-cell development, *one of the V genes is selected at random from the library of V genes and spliced to one of the J genes* to form a complete variable-domain gene. This variable-domain gene is transcribed together with the constant-domain gene. The sequence between the J gene and the constant-do-main gene is treated as an intron and is spliced out of the primary transcript, together with the intron in the V gene.

The H-chain genes are assembled the same way, but the heavy-chain gene cluster contains a set of approximately 30 **D genes** (D for diversity) in addition to the V, J, and C_H genes (Fig. 25.16). Class switching is effected by the successive joining of the complete variable-domain gene (V + D + J) to the different constant-domain genes (Fig. 25.17). The successively produced antibodies have the same variable domains, but the constant domains of the heavy chain are different.

The use of separate genomic libraries for the assembly of the variable-domain genes is the major mechanism for the generation of antibody diversity. Additional mechanisms include a high rate of somatic mutations in the variable-domain genes, imprecise joining of segments, and even the enzymatic addition of random nucleotides by a template-independent DNA polymerase during splicing of the D genes with the J

FIG. 25.16

Rearrangements of heavy chain genes in developing B lymphocytes. The process is similar to the rearrangement of κ light chains shown in Fig. 25.15, but an additional small gene, the D (diversity) gene, contributes in addition to the V (variable), J (joining), and C (constant domain) genes. The introns in the V_H and C_μ genes are not shown.

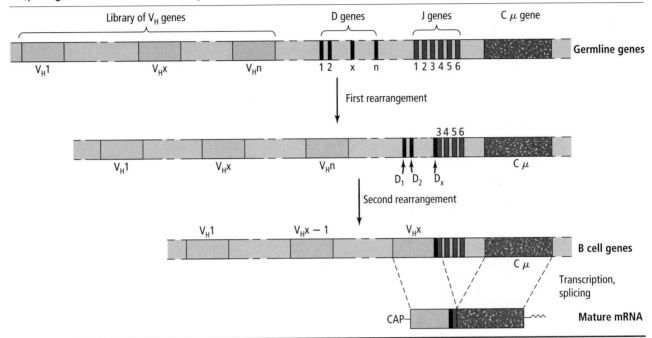

Patients with plasma cell dyscrasias overproduce a single immunoglobulin

Broad elevations in the γ-globulin fraction (Fig. 25.5, page 518) are seen in many diseases, ranging from chronic infections and autoimmune diseases to liver cirrhosis. This is thought to reflect a nonspecific stimulation of B cells by T cell−derived lymphokines and other mediators. On the other hand, decreased levels of immunoglobulins (**hypogammaglobulinemia**), or their complete absence (**agammaglobulinemia**), are encountered in several inherited immunodeficiency diseases in which B cells are affected.

Monoclonal gammopathies, also known as **plasma cell dyscrasias**, are neoplastic conditions in which *a single plasma cell clone proliferates abnormally.* Being derived from a single ancestral B cell, the proliferating plasma cells all produce the same antibody. This condition can be recognized on plasma protein electro-

phoresis by the presence of a sharp peak (a "paraprotein") in the γ-globulin fraction or, less commonly, in the β- or α_2-globulin fraction (Fig. 25.5, *F*).

In **multiple myeloma**, which is a malignant disease, the paraprotein is *a monoclonal IgG, IgA, or, sometimes, IgD antibody.* In some patients the malignant cells produce only light chains of either the κ or the λ type, which not only are found in the serum but also are excreted in the urine. These overproduced light chains are known as **Bence Jones protein.** The malignant plasma cells grow in the bone marrow, where they cause bone pain, pathological fractures, and radiological abnormalities.

Waldenström's macroglobulinemia is a malignant plasma cell dyscrasia in which *an IgM antibody is overproduced.* Because of its high molecular weight, this IgM antibody causes a dangerous increase of the blood viscosity.

Benign monoclonal gammopathy is an asymptomatic condition in which a paraprotein can be detected on plasma protein electrophoresis but signs of malignant disease are absent. *It is very common in the geriatric age group.* The evaluation of monoclonal

FIG. 25.17

Class switching, in this case from IgM (μ chain) to IgG_1 (γ_1 chain). Class switching takes place after the rearrangements shown in Figs. 25.15 and 25.16. It can be triggered by cytokines that are released from activated T lymphocytes, and it can occur either before or after antigen exposure. The intervening genes (in this case μ, δ, and γ_3) are released as a cyclic product known as a "switch circle." Each gene is preceded by a switch region (Ⅰ). Recombination takes place between the switch regions of two C_H genes.

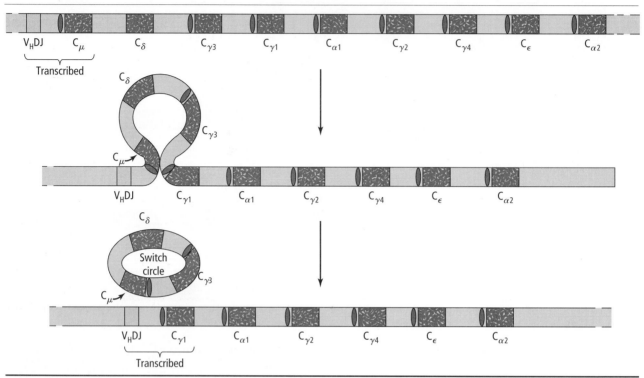

gammopathies is one of the most common indications for plasma protein electrophoresis in the clinical laboratory.

THE BLOOD CLOTTING SYSTEM

The mechanisms of **hemostasis,** which prevent excessive blood loss after vascular injury, culminate in the formation of an insoluble clot that plugs the leak in the vascular wall. Blood clotting is essential for life, but it is not without danger: a **thrombus** is formed when blood clotting takes place inappropriately within a major blood vessel, causing vascular occlusion and tissue infarction. Thrombus formation is the immediate cause for many cases of acute myocardial infarction and cerebrovascular accidents. Therefore the blood clotting system has to be tightly controlled to maintain the delicate balance between uncontrolled hemorrhage and thrombus formation.

Blood clotting requires an interplay among endothelial cells, subendothelium, platelets, and clotting factors

Before discussing the mechanisms of blood coagulation, we have to introduce the principal actors:

1. The intact **endothelial cells** inhibit blood clotting. They provide a surface structure that is not conducive to platelet adhesion, they display membrane proteins that inhibit the clotting system, and they form prostacyclin (see Chapter 26, pages 568-569), an inhibitor of platelet adhesion and aggregation.
2. The **subendothelial tissues** contain membrane proteins and extracellular matrix proteins that normally are not in contact with the blood. When exposed to the blood after injury, *platelets and clotting factors adhere to components of the subendothelial tissue, where they become activated.*

3. *Platelets* bind to components of the subendothelial tissue. They subsequently bind clotting factors, which become activated on their surface.

4. The **clotting factors** are soluble plasma proteins. Most of them are serine proteases that circulate as inactive precursors. *The blood clotting system is a proteolytic cascade in which the clotting factors become activated by selective proteolytic cleavage,* leading eventually to the formation of *insoluble fibrin from soluble fibrinogen.* The clotting factors are designated by Roman numerals. The subscript letter *a* denotes the proteolytically activated form of the clotting factor.

The adhesion of platelets to subendothelial tissue is an early event in hemostasis

Platelets bind avidly to the exposed subendothelial tissue after vascular injury. This phenomenon, known as **platelet adhesion,** is mediated by **von Willebrand factor (vWF),** a protein that is present both in the plasma and in the matrix of the subendothelial tissue. vWF binds both to a receptor on the platelet membrane and to collagen fibers in the subendothelial tissue. **Platelet activation** invariably occurs in the adherent platelets. This process is stimulated by a variety of agents that increase the calcium concentration in platelets, including thrombin and thromboxane (Fig. 25.18).

During activation, a receptor for fibrinogen becomes exposed on the platelet membrane: *fibrinogen molecules glue the platelets together,* and platelet adhesion is followed by **platelet aggregation.** Activated (but not resting) platelets release a wealth of chemicals: ADP, ATP, 5-hydroxytryptamine, and calcium are released from the dense core granules, and the α granules release a variety of proteins including fibrinogen, von Willebrand factor, factor V, factor XIII, platelet-derived growth factor (PDGF), and platelet factor 4. Thromboxane (see Chapter 26, pages 568-569) also is released. While the released clotting factors contribute to the formation of the fibrin clot, PDGF helps in the healing process and platelet factor 4 prevents the formation of an active thrombin inhibitor from heparin and antithrombin III (this will be described later in the chapter).

The effect of the released mediators is an example of *positive feedback,* which ensures a rapid and efficient formation of the platelet plug. Even the membrane lipids become rearranged during platelet activation. Phosphatidyl serine, in particular, which normally is concentrated in the inner leaflet of the plasma membrane, flip-flops to the outer leaflet, where it plays a role in the binding of prothrombin and other clotting factors.

The importance of the platelet plug is shown by the observation that *patients with unusually low platelet counts* ($<40,000/\mu L$) *develop spontaneous hemorrhages.* Normal platelet counts range between 100,000 and 400,000/μL.

Insoluble fibrin is formed from soluble fibrinogen

The platelet plug alone is sufficient to seal very small lesions, but larger injuries require the formation of a stable fibrin clot. **Fibrin,** being insoluble, is not a constituent of normal blood, but its precursor **fibrinogen** is present at concentrations averaging 300 mg/dL. With a molecular weight of 340,000, it is larger than most plasma proteins, and it is more extended, with dimensions of 9×45 nm. Fibrinogen contains three different polypeptide chains, designated Aα, Bβ, and γ. The molecule consists of two identical halves, each containing one copy of each chain, and these halves are disulfide bonded to each other. The complete molecule has three globular domains that are connected by coiled-coils of three α helices each (Fig. 25.19).

The protease **thrombin** *converts fibrinogen to fibrin* by cleaving two peptide bonds near the amino termini of the Aα and Bβ chains. These cleavages release two small peptides, fibrinopeptides A (20 amino acids) and B (18 amino acids). The remaining protein, which still has 97% of the molecular weight of fibrinogen, is called a **fibrin monomer.** Once formed, the fibrin monomers aggregate into fibrous structures. Why is fibrinogen soluble and fibrin insoluble? The reason is that the fibrinopeptides carry many negative charges on aspartate and glutamate side chains. In fibrinogen, these negative charges keep the molecules apart and prevent the formation of fibrous aggregates.

Although insoluble, the fibrin monomers form only a soft gel rather than a solid clot. For structural strength, *fibrin requires covalent crosslinking* between

FIG. 25.18

Formation of the platelet plug. **A,** Platelets adhere to exposed subendothelium. The binding is mediated by von Willebrand factor, but direct binding to tissue fibronectin or other tissue components may be important as well. **B,** Platelets become activated after binding to the subendothelial tissue and exposure to thrombin (**T**), resulting in shape change and degranulation. Functional fibrinogen receptors are assembled on the cell surface. **C,** Continued thrombin exposure, together with some of the released mediators (ADP, thromboxane), activates more and more platelets. The platelets are glued together by fibrinogen, and the platelet plug forms. The action of thrombin on fibrinogen forms insoluble fibrin, and the platelets become enmeshed in the fibrin clot.

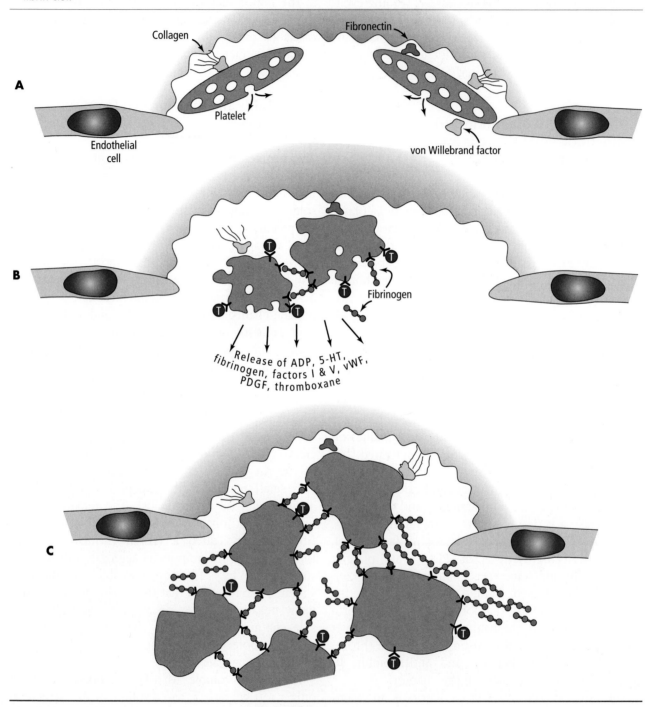

FIG. 25.19

Structure of fibrinogen. **A,** Schematic representation of fibrinogen. The coiled-coil regions, each 150 to 160 nm in length, are formed by three α-helical portions of the Aα, Bβ, and γ chains. **B,** Aggregation of fibrin monomers. **C,** Transglutaminase (factor XIIIa) strengthens the clot by forming covalent crosslinks.

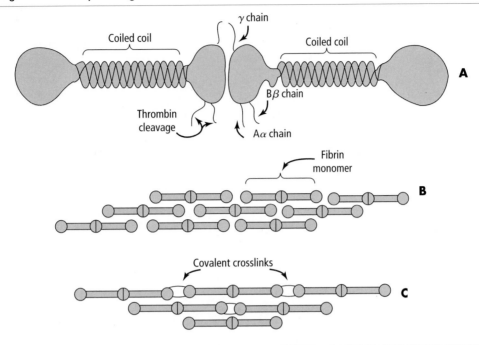

glutamine and lysine side chains. This reaction is catalyzed by **transglutaminase,** also known as **clotting factor XIII$_a$** as shown in Box 25.1.

Thrombin is derived from prothrombin

The key event in clot formation is the proteolytic removal of the fibrinopeptides by the serine protease thrombin. Because its substrate fibrinogen is a circulating plasma protein and fibrin formation has to be restricted to the site of injury, active thrombin normally should not be present in the blood. Ideally, *it should be formed only locally at the site of the injury.* Indeed, active thrombin is formed from the inactive precursor **prothrombin,** which is a circulating plasma protein. Prothrombin, a single polypeptide with 582 amino acids, is almost twice the size of active thrombin (Fig. 25.20). The cleavage of two peptide bonds by **factor X$_a$** produces active thrombin and a catalytically inactive amino-terminal fragment of 274 amino acids.

This amino-terminal fragment contains an unusual structural feature: it contains 10 γ-**carboxyglutamate** residues that are derived from glutamate residues by vitamin K–dependent carboxylation reactions in the ER of the hepatocytes, where prothrombin is synthesized. Unlike glutamate, γ-carboxyglutamate is a strong calcium chelator.

γ-Carboxyglutamate and calcium are required for the targeting of prothrombin to the site of the injury: through its bound calcium ions, *prothrombin becomes anchored to phosphatidyl serine on the surface of activated platelets.* On this phospholipid surface, prothrombin comes in contact with factor X$_a$, a serine protease that is likewise bound to the platelet membrane in close association with **factor V$_a$** (Fig. 25.21). *Factor X$_a$ activates prothrombin on the surface of the activated platelet.* Active thrombin no longer adheres to the platelet lipids, but it binds to fibrin and becomes enmeshed in the fibrin network, where it retains its enzymatic activity. Factors VII, IX, and X also contain γ-carboxyglutamate. *All γ-carboxyglutamate–*

BOX 25.1

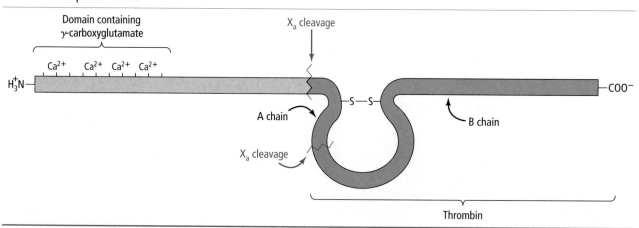

FIG. 25.20

Structure of prothrombin.

containing clotting factors bind to phospholipids on the surface of activated platelets.

Factor X can be activated by the extrinsic and intrinsic pathways

The last reactions of the clotting cascade, from factor X_a to fibrin, are known as the **final common pathway.** Not surprisingly, factor X_a has to be generated from its inactive zymogen, factor X, by a proteolytic cleavage reaction. This activation can be achieved through either the **extrinsic pathway** or the **intrinsic pathway** (Fig. 25.22).

The only protease of the extrinsic pathway is **factor VII$_a$**, which can be formed from its zymogen by thrombin or factor X_a. Proteolytic activation is not

FIG. 25.21

Activation of prothrombin by factor X_a on the surface of the platelet membrane. The membrane phospholipids facilitate the reaction by bringing prothrombin and factor X_a together on the surface of the lipid bilayer and factor V_a enhances the catalytic activity of X_a.

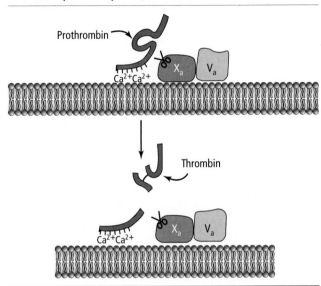

sufficient, however: VII_a is active only in the presence of **tissue factor,** a membrane glycoprotein in subendothelial tissue. *Tissue factor and factor VII come in contact only after vascular injury.* In the presence of calcium, factor VII quickly binds to tissue factor, either before or after its activation to VIIa. Not only factor X but also factor IX of the intrinsic pathway is activated by tissue factor–bound VII_a.

The intrinsic pathway derives its name from the fact that it can be induced in the test tube in the absence of an "extrinsic" tissue component, requiring only factors already present in the blood. Both in the test tube and in vivo, however, *the intrinsic pathway becomes activated only on contact with a negatively charged surface.* In the body, this surface is provided by constituents of the extracellular matrix after vascular injury.

The initiating reactions of the intrinsic pathway are known as **contact-phase activation.** They require the proteases **kallikrein** and factor XII_a, as well as the activator protein **high-molecular-weight kininogen (HMW-K).** While kallikrein acts on factor XII to produce factor XII_a, factor XII_a acts on prekallikrein to produce kallikrein. Factor XII_a, finally, activates factor XI (Fig. 25.22). These re-

actions take place only when the components are bound to a negatively charged surface. Factor XI also can be activated by thrombin and factor XI_a. Factor XI_a, finally, activates factor IX, and factor IX_a activates factor X. This latter reaction requires **factor VIII$_a$,** a potent activator protein that increases the reaction rate 200,000-fold.

We realize now that the blood clotting system is designed for a highly localized response: *the initiating reactions depend on components of the exposed subendothelial tissue, and the final steps require a lipid surface provided by activated platelets.*

Negative controls are required to prevent thrombus formation

The blood clotting system shows several examples of *positive feedback* (Fig. 25.22): kallikrein and XII_a activate each other, XI_a acts on its own zymogen to produce more XI_a, and, most importantly, thrombin activates several zymogens (VII, XI) and activator proteins (V, VIII) in the earlier steps of the system. These positive feedback loops permit a quick response to injury, but without inhibitory controls the process would progress until all our blood vessels were filled with a solid fibrin clot.

Some control, of course, is exerted by the fact that the initiating reactions (formation of XI_a and the action of VII_a) require exposed subendothelial tissue components and therefore cannot occur in intact blood vessels. Also, activated clotting factors that escape from the area of the clot are diluted rapidly in the blood, where they are easy prey for circulating protease inhibitors. Most clotting factors can be inactivated by nonselective protease inhibitors such as α_1-antiprotease and α_2-macroglobulin, but **antithrombin III** is most important under normal conditions. This protease inhibitor (Fig. 25.23), which has structural homology with α_1-antiprotease, is present in a concentration of approximately 15 mg/dL in the plasma. It is stimulated by the glycosaminoglycan **heparin,** which binds to the inhibitor by means of electrostatic interactions. A specific positioning of sulfate groups on the polysaccharide chains of heparin is necessary for antithrombin III activation. This required structure is present in approximately 30% of all heparin molecules and also in a small proportion of the heparan sulfate molecules on the endothelial cell surface. *It*

FIG. 25.22

The blood clotting system. *HMW-K,* High-molecular-weight kininogen; [ ], surface of activated platelets; *TF,* tissue factor; --→, proteolytic activation.

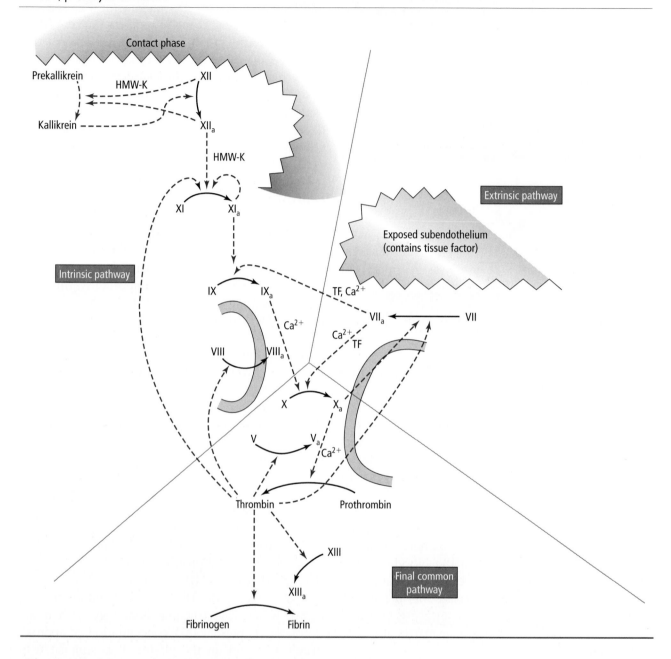

therefore is likely that the action of antithrombin III is facilitated by contact with intact endothelial cells in vivo. Most proteases of the intrinsic and final common pathway are inhibited by heparin/antithrombin III (Table 25.9).

A different anticoagulant mechanism is employed by **thrombomodulin** (Fig. 25.24), a protein of the intact endothelial cell surface that binds circulating thrombin. Once bound to thrombomodulin, thrombin no longer is able to act on fibrin, factor VIII, factor V, or factor XIII. Instead it activates **protein C,** a plasma protein that circulates as an inactive zymogen. Once activated to an active protease by thrombomodulin-bound thrombin, it acts as a powerful anticoagulant by degrading factors V$_a$ and VIII$_a$. Because of its requirement for thrombomodulin, a

FIG. 25.23

Proposed mechanism for the inhibition of thrombin by antithrombin III.

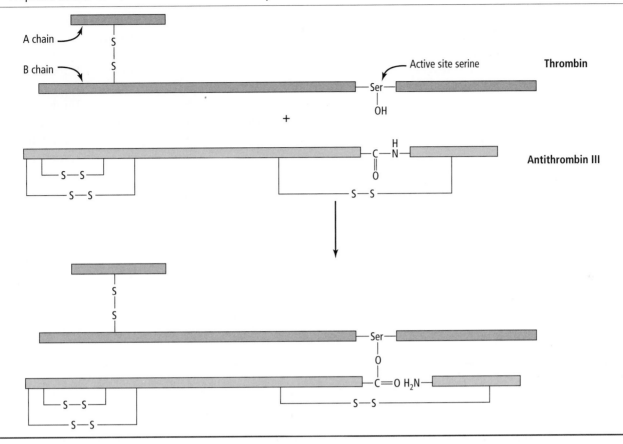

component of the intact endothelial cell surface, *this mechanism prevents the encroachment of clot formation on areas with an intact endothelial lining.*

The importance of anticoagulant mechanisms is demonstrated by the observation that some patients with thrombotic disorders have inherited deficiencies of anticoagulant proteins. Dominantly inherited deficiencies of antithrombin III and protein C have been observed repeatedly, and these patients develop thrombotic disease even though they still possess approximately 50% of the normal amount of the affected protein.

Plasmin degrades the fibrin clot

A blood clot is an ephemeral structure that has to be removed during wound healing. The principal enzyme of fibrin degradation is the protease **plasmin,** which is formed from its inactive precursor **plasminogen** by a proteolytic cleavage. Plasminogen,

which circulates in the plasma in a concentration of 10 to 20 mg/dL, binds with high affinity to the fibrin clot. In this form it can be activated by **tissue-type plasminogen activator (tPA),** a serine protease that, like plasminogen, binds avidly to fibrin. tPA does not require a proteolytic activation step, but its activity is minimal in the absence of fibrin. Therefore *active plasmin is formed only in the fibrin clot where it is needed* (Fig. 25.25).

Plasminogen can be activated not only by tPA but also by **urokinase,** a kidney-derived protein that is present in normal urine. An active urokinase-related protease also is present in the plasma, where its concentration approaches that of tPA (0.5 to 1 μg/dL). Unlike tPA, however, urokinase does not bind to the fibrin clot.

Streptokinase is a bacterial protein (from streptococci) that activates plasminogen without proteolytic cleavage: by binding to the zymogen, it induces a conformational change that exposes its

TABLE 25.9

Properties of the blood clotting factors

Factor	Functions in	Protease precursor	Mol wt	Plasma concentration (mg/dL)	Vitamin K dependent	Heparin inhibited	Activated by
Fibrinogen (I)	Common pathway	No	330,000	150-400	No	No	Thrombin
Prothrombin (II)	Common pathway	Yes	72,000	8-9	Yes	Yes	X_a
V	Common pathway	No	330,000		No	No	Thrombin
X	Common pathway	Yes	59,000	0.6	Yes	Yes	IX_a, VII_a
XIII	Common pathway	No*	320,000		No	No	Thrombin
VII	Extrinsic pathway	Yes	50,000	0.05	Yes	No	Thrombin, X_a
VIII	Intrinsic pathway	No	330,000	0.02	No	No	Thrombin,
IX	Intrinsic pathway	Yes	57,000	0.4	Yes	Yes	XI_a, VII_a
XI	Intrinsic pathway	Yes	160,000	0.5	No	Yes	Thrombin XI_a, XII_a
XII	Intrinsic pathway	Yes	76,000	3	No	Yes	Kallikrein
Prekallikrein	Intrinsic pathway	Yes	82,000	4	No	No	XII_a
High-molecular-weight kininogen	Intrinsic pathway	No	108,000	7-10	No	No	—

* Yields a fibrin-crosslinking enzyme.

FIG. 25.24

The roles of intact endothelium and exposed subendothelial tissue are evident when the effects of tissue factor and thrombo-modulin are compared. Tissue factor triggers the clotting system through the extrinsic pathway (compare Fig. 25.22); thrombomodulin blocks the process. Thrombin, which is otherwise a "procoagulant," becomes effectively an "anticoagulant" after binding to thrombomodulin. *TF*, Tissue factor; *TM*, thrombomodulin; *Thr*, thrombin; --►, proteolytic activation; ⤳, proteolytic inactivation.

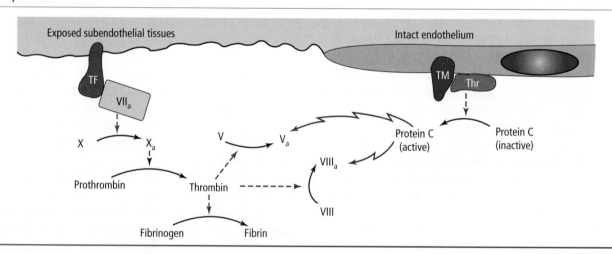

active site. Streptokinase and urokinase are established treatments for patients with thrombotic diseases. Acute myocardial infarction, for example, usually is caused by a thrombus formed on an atherosclerotic lesion within a coronary artery. In these patients thrombolytic therapy can limit the size of the infarction if it is administered within an hour after vascular occlusion, before the damage has become irreversible. Genetically engineered tPA is available as well. Although tPA should be superior to

FIG. 25.25

The fibrinolytic system. Plasminogen *(PLG)* is a circulating zymogen that binds to the fibrin clot. Tissue-type plasminogen activator *(tPA)* also binds to the clot, where it activates plasminogen by proteolytic cleavage, exposing its active site (✂). Urokinase activates circulating plasminogen by proteolysis while the bacterial protein streptokinase *(Str)* activates plasminogen without proteolytic cleavage, by inducing a conformational change in the zymogen.

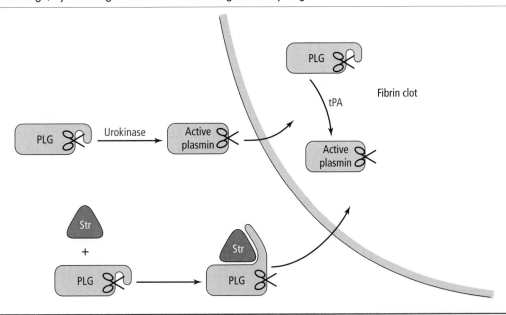

streptokinase because of its binding to the fibrin clot, the clinical evidence about the relative merits of the two treatments is equivocal.

Heparin and the vitamin K antagonists are the most important anticoagulants

In the test tube but not in vivo, *blood clotting can be inhibited readily by the removal of calcium ions.* Citrate, oxalate, and EDTA all can be used to bind calcium. Calcium is required for the function of all γ-carboxyglutamate–containing clotting factors (prothrombin, VII, IX, X). In addition, the catalytic activity of thrombin requires calcium, although thrombin no longer contains γ-carboxyglutamate.

Heparin, acting through antithrombin III (see Fig. 25.23), is an effective anticoagulant both in vivo and in vitro. Although it is not active when taken orally—because of a lack of intestinal absorption—it is used clinically as a *short-acting, injectable anticoagulant.*

Coumarin-like anticoagulants such as **warfarin** and **dicumarol** act by an entirely different mechanism: as competitive inhibitors of vitamin K, *they prevent the formation of γ-carboxyglutamate* during the posttranslational processing of prothrombin and of factors VII, IX, and X in the ER of liver cells. These drugs are not able to prevent clotting in the test tube. Their action is very sluggish: the vitamin K–dependent clotting factors have plasma half-lives of 1 to 5 days, so several days of treatment are required before the old, normal clotting factors are replaced by the abnormal, uncarboxylated factors that are produced in the presence of the drug.

The coumarin-type drugs are used not only for the management of patients with thrombotic disease but also as rat poisons. Their slow action is an advantage for this use because their lack of immediate toxicity causes the animal to eat the poison repeatedly until death ensues from internal hemorrhage. Poisons with immediate toxicity invariably cause a conditioned taste aversion in rats after a first exposure to a nonlethal dose.

Although most coumarin-type rat poisons have a low acute toxicity, their accidental ingestion should be treated with menadione, an injectable form of vitamin K. If abnormal clotting develops, the transfusion of fresh frozen plasma may be required.

The function of the blood clotting system can be assessed by various clotting tests:

1. *Bleeding time.* Bleeding time is measured after a standardized, small skinprick lesion in the fingertip or earlobe. *It is prolonged in platelet disorders.*
2. *Activated partial thromboplastin time.* Citrated plasma is treated with kaolin, a phospholipid preparation, and excess calcium. The kaolin activates the contact factors of the intrinsic pathway, and the phospholipid substitutes for platelet membranes. *This procedure tests the functioning of the intrinsic and final common pathways.* It can be used to monitor the heparin effect.
3. *Prothrombin time.* A tissue factor containing extract from brain or lung is added to citrated plasma together with excess calcium. *The prothrombin time is prolonged in deficiencies of the extrinsic and final common pathways.* It is used routinely to monitor patients on treatment with coumarin-type anticoagulants.

Clotting factor deficiencies cause bleeding disorders

The most common inherited deficiency of a blood clotting factor is **hemophilia A,** an X-linked disease that affects close to 1 in every 12,000 males. It is a serious bleeding disorder, caused by a *complete or near-complete deficiency of factor VIII,* one of the components of the intrinsic pathway (Fig. 25.22). Unlike patients with platelet disorders, hemophiliacs rarely are plagued by spontaneous hemorrhages. They show, however, prolonged bleeding from small wounds. Repeated bleeding into joints, which may lead to arthritis in later life, also is common. Bleeding episodes can be treated with cryoprecipitate, factor VIII concentrate, or genetically engineered factor VIII. Hemophiliacs are unpopular with health insurers because of the considerable cost of these treatments.

Factor IX deficiency (**hemophilia B**) causes the same clinical manifestations as hemophilia A. This is not surprising because factors VIII and IX both are required for the same reaction (Fig. 25.22). Factor XI deficiency causes a milder bleeding disorder, and deficiencies of factor XII, prekallikrein, or high-molecular-weight kininogen do not cause abnormal bleeding, although the activated partial thromboplastin time is prolonged.

Deficiencies in the final common pathway tend to be more serious than those in the intrinsic pathway. The absence of fibrinogen (**afibrinogenemia**) causes a severe clotting disorder that often is fatal in childhood, and the same is true for deficiencies of prothrombin, factor V, and factor X. Clotting factor deficiencies generally are inherited as recessive disorders.

The formation of the platelet plug also is impaired in some inherited diseases. In von Willebrand disease, inherited as an autosomal dominant trait, platelet adhesion is impaired because of a decreased concentration of von Willebrand factor. The level of factor VIII, which is bound noncovalently to von Willebrand factor in the circulation, is decreased. Defects of the receptors for either von Willebrand factor or fibrinogen on the platelet membrane are known as well. These impair platelet adhesion and platelet aggregation, respectively.

SUMMARY

The protein concentration in normal plasma and serum is between 6% and 8%. Most of these proteins, with the important exception of the immunoglobulins, are produced by the liver. Albumin is the most abundant of these, accounting for approximately 60% of the total plasma proteins. Albumin provides most of the colloid osmotic pressure of the plasma. It is also a binding protein for several physiological substances such as calcium, fatty acids, and bilirubin, and for many drugs. Many of the other plasma proteins also are physiologically important binding proteins for small molecules. The substances that are transported in binding to specific proteins include retinol, vitamin D, cobalamin, iron, and the steroid and thyroid hormones. Heme and hemoglobin, released from RBCs after intravascular hemolysis, also bind to specific plasma proteins. Protein binding facilitates the transport of water-insoluble compounds, prevents the renal excretion of water-soluble compounds, and directs nutritive substances to the sites where they are needed. Plasma protein determinations are important for the diagnosis of many diseases.

The plasma also contains trace amounts of proteins that are not secreted into the blood but rather are released from dying cells during normal cell turnover. Of these cellular proteins, several enzymes are diagnostically important because their plasma levels are elevated in tissue-destructive diseases.

The immunoglobulins, or antibodies, are a group of plasma proteins that are derived from plasma cells. They play an important role in our defenses against infections because they combine noncovalently with foreign macromolecules, called antigens, to form antigen-antibody complexes. The antigen-antibody complexes subsequently are destroyed, either intracellularly after endocytosis or phagocytosis, or through the action of soluble plasma proteins. The antigen-binding specificities of the immunoglobulins are determined by variable domains in their constituent polypeptides. There are more than one million antibodies with different antigen-binding specificities in the human body. Each B cell or plasma cell produces only one antibody. The genes that encode the polypeptides of this antibody have to be assembled by somatic gene rearrangements during the development of the B cell. These rearrangements do not require antigen exposure, but the binding of antigen to the surface-bound immunoglobulin of the B cell is a prerequisite for clonal expansion and the for-mation of fully differentiated, antibody-secreting plasma cells.

The blood clotting system employs a cascade of proteolytic activation reactions in which active proteases are generated from their inactive precursors by highly selective proteolytic cleavage reactions. These reactions culminate in the formation of the protease thrombin, which converts soluble fibrinogen into insoluble fibrin. The blood clotting cascade is initiated by the contact of circulating clotting factors with exposed subendothelial tissue components, and the final reactions take place on the surface of activated platelets that adhere to the exposed subendothelial tissue at the site of the injury.

Further Reading

Broze GJ Jr: Tissue factor pathway inhibitor and the revised theory of coagulation. *Annu Rev Med* 46, 103–112, 1995.

Carroll WL, Korsmeyer SJ: Immunoglobulins. In: Frank MM, Austen KF, Claman HN, Unanue ER, editors: *Samter's immunologic diseases*, 5th ed., vol. 1. Little, Brown, Boston, 1995, pp. 33–51.

Eriksson S, Carlson J: α_1-Antitrypsin deficiency and related disorders. In: McIntyre N, Benhamou J-P, Bircher J, Rizzetto M, Rodes J, editors: *Oxford textbook of clinical hepatology*, vol. 2. Oxford University Press, New York, 1991, pp. 958–966.

Handin RI, Lux SE, Stossel TP: *Blood*. J. B. Lippincott, Philadelphia, 1995, pp. 949–1355.

Henry JB et al: *Clinical diagnosis and management by laboratory methods*. W. B. Saunders, Philadelphia, 1991, pp. 215-228, 250-284, 734–757.

Kaplan MM: Laboratory tests: In: Schiff L, Schiff ER, editors: *Diseases of the liver*, 7th ed., vol. 1. J. B. Lippincott, Philadelphia, 1993, pp. 108–144.

Kirsch R, Bass N, Arias I: Biochemical evaluation of liver disease. In: Kirsch R, Robson S, Trey C, editors: *Diagnosis and management of liver disease*. Chapman & Hall Medical, London, 1995, pp. 9–21.

Lee-Lewandrowski E, Lewandrowski K: The plasma proteins. In: McClatchey KD, editor: *Clinical laboratory medicine*. Williams & Wilkins, Baltimore, 1994, pp. 239–258.

Loscalzo J, Creager MA, Dzau VJ, editors: *Vascular medicine*. Little, Brown, Boston, 1992, pp. 205–242, 307–333.

Mackiewicz A et al, editors: *Acute phase proteins*. CRC Press, Boca Raton FL, 1993.

Potter KN, Capra JD: Immunoglobulin genes and proteins. In: Rich RR et al, editors: *Clinical immunology*, vol. 1. Mosby, St. Louis, 1996, pp. 50–68.

Schwarzenberg SJ, Sharp HL: α_1-Antitrypsin deficiency. In: Schiff L, Schiff ER, editors: *Diseases of the liver*, 7th ed. vol. 1. J. B. Lippincott, Philadelphia, 1993, pp. 692–706.

Scriver CR, Beaudet AL, Sly WS, Valle D, editors: *The metabolic basis of inherited disease*, 6th ed., vol. 2. McGraw-Hill, New York, 1988, pp. 2107–2218, 2409–2438.

Stamatoyannopoulos G, Nienhuis AW, Majerus PW, Varmus H, editors: *The molecular basis of blood diseases*. W. B. Saunders, Philadelphia, 1994, pp. 381–424, 565–785.

Sun T: *Interpretation of protein and isoenzyme patterns in body fluids*. Igaku-Shoin, New York, 1991.

Whicher JT: Abnormalities of the plasma proteins. In: Williams D, Marks V, editors: *Scientific foundations of biochemistry in clinical practice*, 2nd ed. Butterworth Heinemann Ltd., Boston, 1994, pp. 464–494.

Wu AHB: Diagnostic enzymology. In: McClatchey KD, editor: *Clinical laboratory medicine*. Williams & Wilkins, Baltimore, 1994, pp. 259–286.

1. A complete IgG molecule contains
   A. Two antigen-binding regions
   B. A hinge region between the variable domain and the first constant domain of the heavy chain
   C. One kappa light chain and one lambda light chain
   D. A J-chain
   E. Disulfide bonds between the two light chains

2. You are not sure whether an anemic patient suffers from iron deficiency or chronic hemolysis. To evaluate the possibility of chronic hemolysis, you should determine the plasma level of
   A. Ferritin
   B. α_2-Macroglobulin
   C. Ceruloplasmin
   D. Haptoglobin
   E. C-reactive protein

3. Classical hemophilia is caused by an inherited deficiency of clotting factor VIII. This deficiency blocks
   A. The intrinsic pathway of blood clotting
   B. The extrinsic pathway of blood clotting
   C. The final common pathway of blood clotting
   D. The fibrinolytic system
   E. Contact-phase activation

4. Patients with nephrotic syndrome are deficient in most plasma proteins, but one plasma protein fraction actually is increased. This fraction is
   A. Albumin
   B. α_1-Globulin
   C. α_2-Globulin
   D. β-Globulin
   E. γ-Globulin

5. You suspect that an elderly patient with prostatic hypertrophy has prostatic cancer. Therefore you should determine the serum level of
   A. Acid phosphatase
   B. Creatine kinase
   C. Alkaline phosphatase
   D. Alanine transaminase
   E. Lactate dehydrogenase

Chapter 26

Extracellular Messengers

The transmission of chemical signals from cell to cell can take three different forms:

In **endocrine** signaling, the messenger is a hormone that is synthesized in a specialized tissue called an endocrine gland. It is transported by the blood and induces a physiological response in a distant target tissue (Fig. 26.1). This type of signaling is exquisitely suited for the orchestration of physiological responses throughout the body.

In **paracrine** signaling, the messenger is not transported by the blood but diffuses to neighboring cells in the same tissue, where it induces a physiological response.

In **autocrine** signaling, the released messenger acts on the synthesizing cell itself.

The same messenger can be used for more than one type of signaling. Norepinephrine, for example, is a classical hormone when released from the adrenal medulla together with epinephrine, and it is a specialized paracrine agent when released as a neurotransmitter from postganglionic sympathetic nerve terminals. Testosterone is a hormone when it acts on hair follicles in the face, but a paracrine messenger when it acts, in much higher concentration, on the epithelium of the seminiferous tubules in the testis.

This chapter is concerned with the metabolism of extracellular messengers. The actions of these agents on their target cells will be discussed in Chapter 27.

THE STEROID HORMONES

The steroids are employed as classical hormones. The adrenal steroids participate in the regulation of energy metabolism (glucocorticoids) and mineral balance (mineralocorticoids); the gonadal steroids are concerned primarily with sexual development and reproduction.

Steroid hormones are made from cholesterol

All steroid hormones are synthesized from cholesterol. The endocrine cells obtain cholesterol in part from endogenous synthesis—on a weight basis, some of the steroid hormone–producing glands have the highest rates of cholesterol synthesis in the body—and in part from LDL. Cholesterol esters also are stored abundantly in the cells. Hormonal stimulation by such tropic hormones as ACTH (adrenal cortex), LH (corpus luteum, Leydig cells), and FSH (ovarian follicle) activates not only the hormone-synthesizing enzymes but also a cholesteryl esterase that provides a quick supply of cholesterol to meet the increased demand. The synthesis of LDL receptors also is induced by the tropic hormones.

The major chemical and biological classes of steroid hormones, each with a typical representative, are summarized in Table 26.1. We can recognize a few structural features that are relevant for the biosynthetic pathways:

FIG. 26.1

The three types of cell-to-cell signaling. **A,** Endocrine signaling. **B,** Paracrine signaling. **C,** Autocrine signaling.

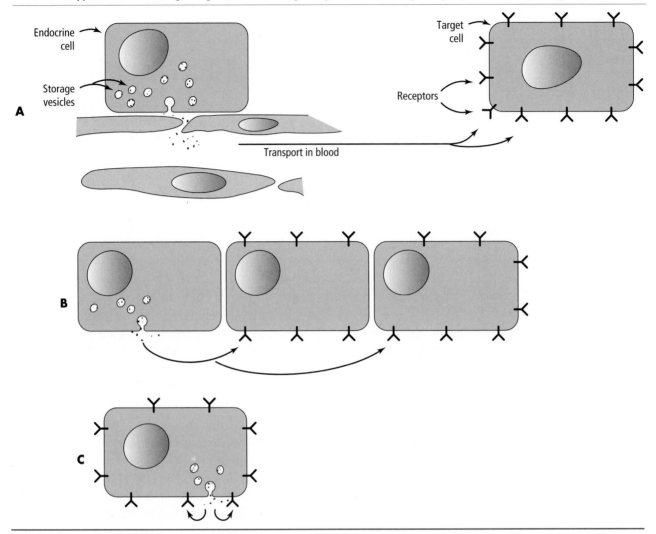

1. The steroid nucleus of cholesterol remains intact, but *the side chain at carbon 17 is either shortened to two carbons (progestins, corticosteroids) or lost entirely (androgens, estrogens).* Therefore we have to expect **side chain cleavage reactions** during steroid hormone biosynthesis.

2. Hydroxy or keto groups are present in positions 3 (all), 11 (corticosteroids), 17 (glucocorticoids, androgens, estrogens), and 21 (corticosteroids). The C-3 hydroxy group is inherited from cholesterol, but *the other oxygen functions have to be introduced by* **hydroxylation reactions.**

3. **Mineralocorticoids** can be recognized by the *aldehyde group at C-18.*

4. **Estrogens** are distinguished by *the aromatic nature of ring A.*

Progestins are the biosynthetic precursors of all other steroid hormones

The *precursor relationships* of the steroid hormones can be summarized as shown in Box 26.1. The synthesis of the progestins (Fig. 26.2) is initiated by the mitochondrial **side chain cleavage enzyme,** also known as **desmolase.** This enzyme system hydroxylates carbons 20 and 22 before the carbon-carbon bond is cleaved. The product of the side chain

TABLE 26.1

Structures of some representative steroids

Steroid class	Source	Synthesis stimulated by	Example
Cholesterol	Ubiquitous	—	Cholesterol
Progestins	Corpus luteum,* placenta	LH	Progesterone
Glucocorticoids	Adrenal cortex	ACTH	Cortisol
Mineralocorticoids	Adrenal cortex (zona glomerulosa)	Angiotensin II, ACTH	Aldosterone
Androgens	Leydig cells (major) Adrenal cortex (minor)	LH ACTH	Testosterone
Estrogens	Ovarian follicle (granulosa cells)†	FSH	Estradiol

* Progestins also are released in small quantities by the adrenal cortex and other steroid-producing glands, where they are intermediates in the synthesis of the other hormones.
† Also formed in small quantities in the corpus luteum, and by the aromatization of androgens in nonendocrine tissues.

BOX 26.1

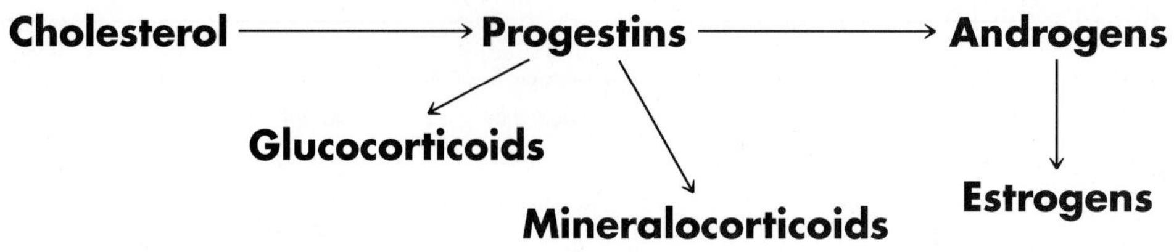

Cholesterol ⟶ Progestins ⟶ Androgens

Glucocorticoids

Mineralocorticoids

Estrogens

FIG. 26.2

Synthesis of progesterone.

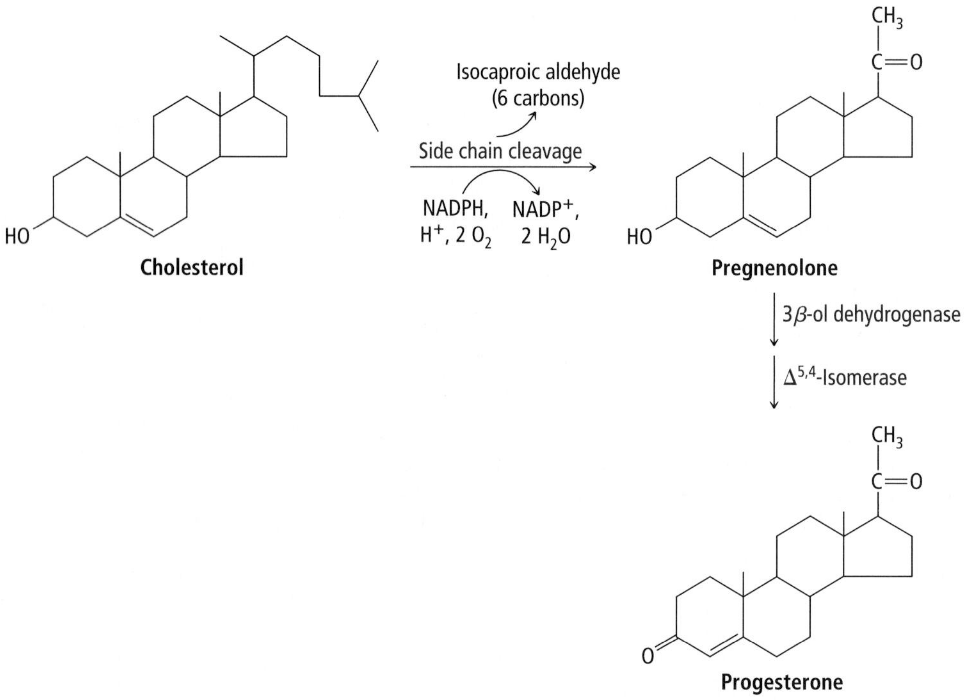

Cholesterol

Isocaproic aldehyde
(6 carbons)

Side chain cleavage

NADPH,   NADP+,
H+, 2 O2   2 H2O

Pregnenolone

3β-ol dehydrogenase

$\Delta^{5,4}$-Isomerase

Progesterone

cleavage reaction, **pregnenolone**, is converted to **progesterone** by microsomal and cytoplasmic enzymes.

Progesterone is the major end product in the corpus luteum and the placenta, but in the other endocrine glands *pregnenolone and progesterone are precursors of the other steroid hormones.* The synthesis of the major adrenal steroids is shown in Fig. 26.3.

Androgens are synthesized in the testis and, to a lesser extent, in the adrenal cortex and the theca cells at the periphery of the ovarian follicle (Figs. 26.3 and 26.4). **Testosterone** is the major androgen from the interstitial cells of the testis (Leydig's cells), where it is synthesized from pregnenolone

and progesterone by an array of microsomal enzymes. Its production in normal men is approximately 5 mg/day. The adrenal cortex contributes the far-less-potent **androstenedione** as its major androgen, at a rate of approximately 3 mg/day. In the target tissues and, to a lesser extent, in the testis itself, testosterone is converted to **dihydrotestosterone (DHT)** by the enzyme 5α-reductase. The plasma level of DHT is only some 10% of the testosterone concentration, but *DHT is a considerably more potent androgen than testosterone.* Therefore testosterone acts, in part at least, as a precursor, or *prohormone*, of the active hormone DHT.

A small amount of estrogen also is formed in

FIG. 26.3

Synthesis of adrenal steroids.

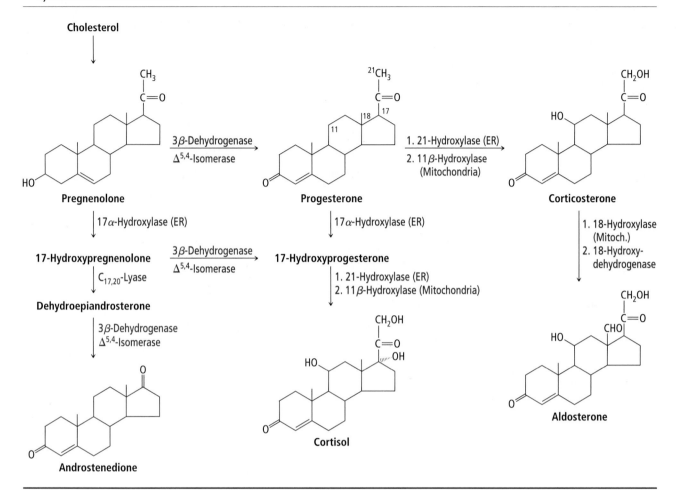

BOX 26.2

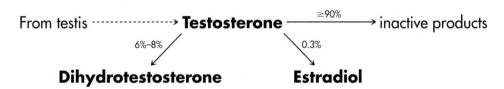

males: 65 μg of estrone and 45 μg of estradiol are produced per day by the aromatization of androstenedione and testosterone, respectively. This reaction is catalyzed by the microsomal enzyme system **aromatase.** Except for a very small quantity of estradiol that is released by the testis, the estrogens in the male are produced in adipose tissue, liver, skin, the brain, and other nonendocrine tissues. We realize now that *testosterone is a precursor of two other hormones, DHT and estradiol* as shown in Box 26.2.

Females of reproductive age produce most of their estrogen in the granulosa cells of the ovarian follicles, and the placenta is the main source during pregnancy. The main estrogen in postmenopausal women is estrone, derived from the adrenal androgen androstenedione.

FIG. 26.4

The major pathways for the synthesis of gonadal steroids. ⟶ , All steroid-producing cells; ⟶ , ovary, theca cells; ⟶ , ovary, granulosa cells; ⟶ , testis. ①, 17α-Hydroxylase/C$_{17,20}$-lyase; ②, 17β-hydroxy-steroid dehydrogenase; ③, 3β-dehydrogenase and △^{5,4}-isomerase; ④, aromatase; ⑤, 16α-hydroxylase; ⑥, 5α-reductase.

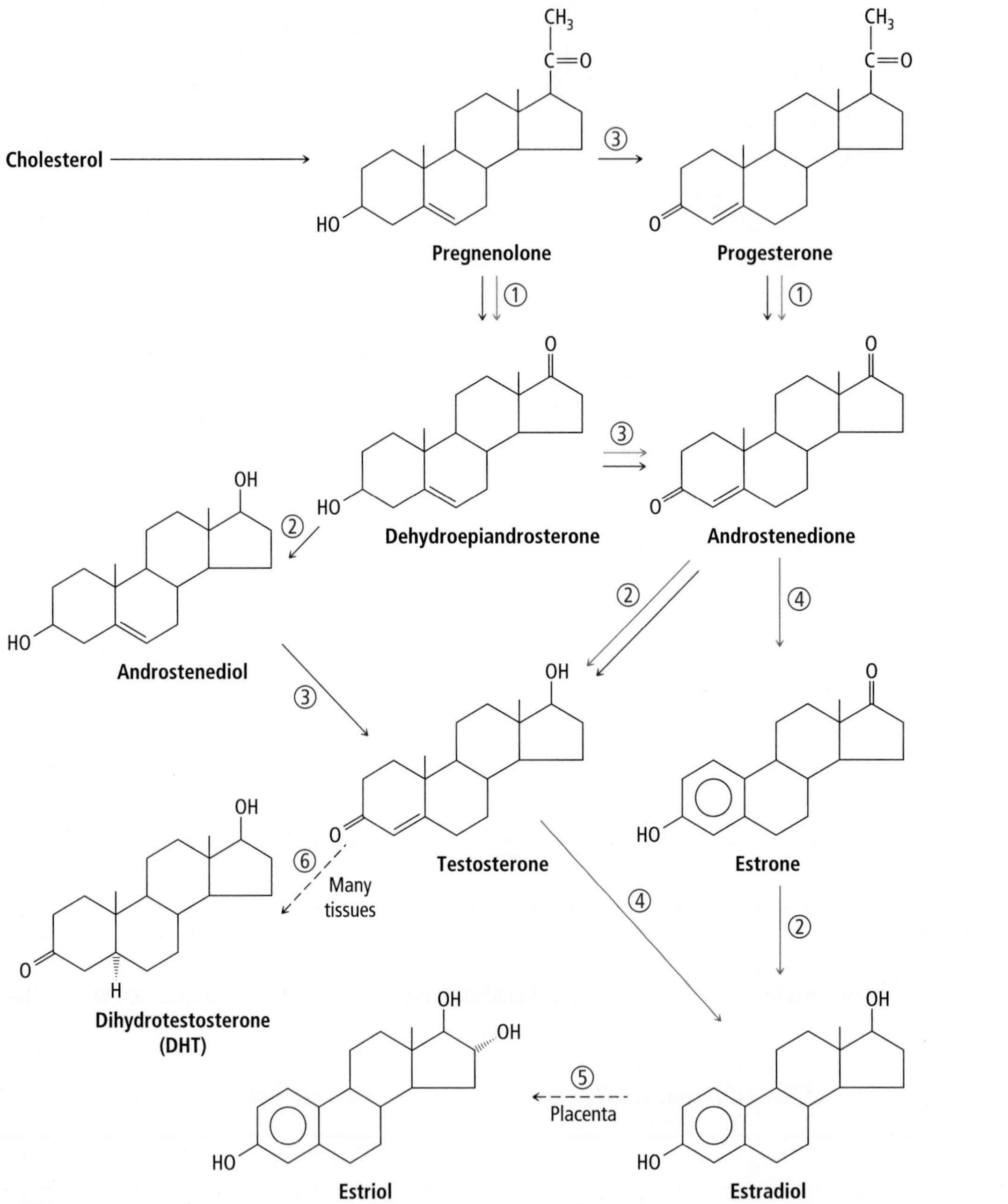

The hydroxylations in steroid hormone synthesis are *monooxygenase reactions* with the overall balance

$$\text{Steroid-H} + O_2 + \text{NADPH} + H^+ \longrightarrow$$
$$\text{Steroid-OH} + \text{NADP}^+ + H_2O$$

These reactions require **cytochrome P-450** *as an intermediate electron carrier.* This protein, which occurs in many different molecular forms in different hydroxylating enzyme systems, is an integral protein of the inner mitochondrial membrane and the ER

BOX 26.3

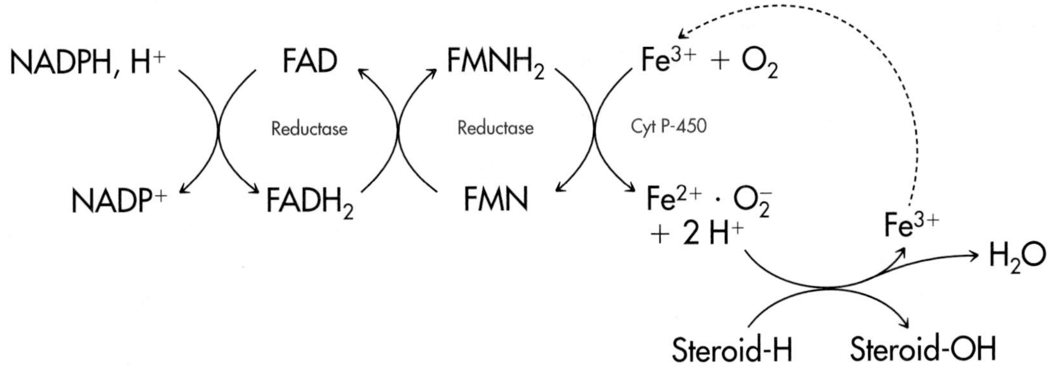

$$NADPH, H^+ \rightarrow FAD \rightarrow FMNH_2 \rightarrow Fe^{3+} + O_2$$
$$NADP^+ \rightarrow FADH_2 \rightarrow FMN \rightarrow Fe^{2+} \cdot O_2^- + 2\,H^+$$

Reductase   Reductase   Cyt P-450

$$Fe^{3+} \rightarrow H_2O$$

Steroid-H   Steroid-OH

BOX 26.4

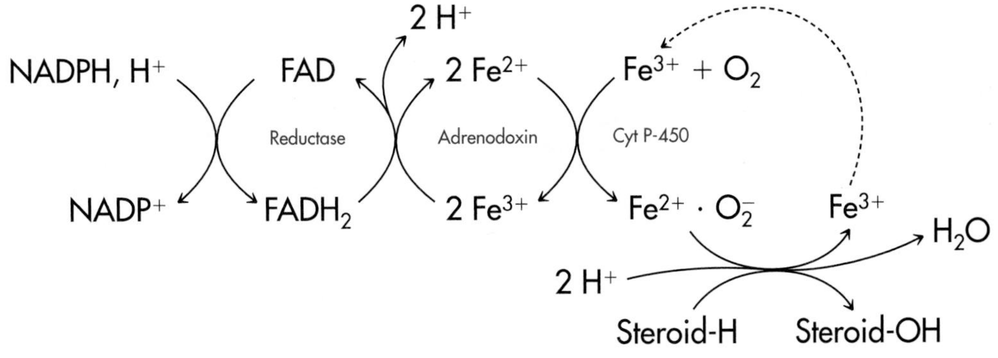

$$2\,H^+$$
$$NADPH, H^+ \rightarrow FAD \rightarrow 2\,Fe^{2+} \rightarrow Fe^{3+} + O_2$$
$$NADP^+ \rightarrow FADH_2 \rightarrow 2\,Fe^{3+} \rightarrow Fe^{2+} \cdot O_2^-$$

Reductase   Adrenodoxin   Cyt P-450

$$Fe^{3+} \rightarrow H_2O$$
$$2\,H^+$$

Steroid-H   Steroid-OH

membrane. The microsomal forms are reduced by **cytochrome P-450 reductase,** a flavoprotein containing both FAD and FMN. Through this flavoprotein, the electrons are channeled from NADPH to the heme iron of P-450 and to molecular oxygen, which binds to the ferrous form of this heme iron. The heme-bound oxygen, activated by the electron transfer, reacts with the substrate molecule as shown in Box 26.3. The mitochondrial forms of cytochrome P-450 receive their electrons through an FAD-containing flavoprotein and the iron-sulfur protein **adrenodoxin,** which are both peripheral membrane proteins as shown in Box 26.4.

Defects of steroid hormone synthesis can cause abnormalities of sexual development

Inherited deficiencies have been described for almost all of the steroid hormone−synthesizing enzymes.

The most important of these affect the synthesis of the androgens, which are required for virilization both during fetal development and at puberty.

The deficiency of **5α-reductase,** the enzyme that converts testosterone to DHT, results in a peculiar abnormality of sexual development: the external appearance of genetically male infants is predominantly female at birth, but the gonads are developed as testes and the internal wolffian duct structures, including epididymis, vas deferens, and seminal vesicles, are male. Virilization does take place at puberty, though, so 5α-reductase deficiency sometimes is referred to as the "penis-at-12 syndrome." This rare disorder, inherited as an autosomal recessive trait, shows that testosterone itself is sufficient for the embryonic development of the wolffian duct structures, but *DHT is required for the prenatal development of the external male genitalia.*

Congenital adrenal hyperplasia, or **adrenogenital syndrome,** (incidence = 1 in 10,000) is caused

FIG. 26.5

Adrenal steroid synthesis in adrenogenital syndrome.
A, Normal. **B,** Untreated adrenogenital syndrome.
C, Adrenogenital syndrome treated with cortisol (+ mineralocorticoid).

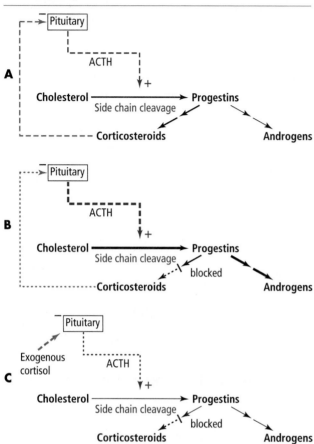

by the deficiency of either 21-hydroxylase or 11β-hydroxylase. These two enzymes are required for the synthesis of corticosteroids but not of androgens (Fig. 26.3). The resulting lack of glucocorticoids leads to a disinhibition of ACTH-release from the anterior pituitary gland, and the excess ACTH causes adrenal hyperplasia and stimulates the side chain cleavage reaction. With the pathway of corticosteroid synthesis blocked, *the initially formed progestins are diverted into androgen synthesis* (Fig. 26.5). This disorder causes precocious puberty in males; affected females are born with ambiguous external genitalia.

A partial deficiency of either 11β- or 21-hydroxylase causes only virilization, but complete deficiencies lead to dangerous hyponatremia and hyper-

kalemia as well. Both the virilization and the electrolyte imbalances can be cured by the regular administration of corticosteroids.

THE THYROID HORMONES

The thyroid hormones are produced only by the thyroid gland. They participate both in the long-term regulation of the metabolic rate and in the regulation of growth and development.

Thyroid hormones are synthesized from protein-bound tyrosine

The thyroid hormones are the only biomolecules in humans and higher animals that contain organically bound iodine as shown in Box 26.5. Iodine, in the form of the iodide ion (I^-), is derived from dietary sources that supply approximately 100 μg/day. The plasma concentration of iodide is not more than 0.2 μg/dL, but the thyroid gland concentrates the ion actively against a steep electrochemical gradient. Iodide uptake is a rate-limiting step for the synthesis of the thyroid hormones. From the follicular cell, iodide can enter the lumen of the thyroid follicle by facilitated diffusion (Fig. 26.6, page 556).

The second ingredient for thyroid hormone synthesis, besides iodine, is **thyroglobulin,** a large glycoprotein (MW 2 × 330,000) that is secreted into the lumen of the thyroid follicle by the follicular cells. Up to 40 tyrosine side chains in this protein become iodinated, but no more than 8 to 10 of these are processed to the active hormones.

The iodination of the tyrosine side chains requires **thyroperoxidase,** a heme-containing enzyme on the apical (lumenal) surface of the plasma membrane (Fig. 26.6). Besides iodide, this enzyme requires hydrogen peroxide, which is generated by an NADPH-dependent oxidase. The iodine reacts with tyrosine side chains in ortho-position to the phenolic hydroxy group, and the protein-bound hormones subsequently are formed by the coupling of two iodinated tyrosine side chains (Fig. 26.7, page 557).

The thyroid follicle stores a considerable amount of the hormones, covalently bound in the amino acid sequence of thyroglobulin. *Their release requires the pinocytotic uptake of thyroglobulin into the follicular cell,* followed by the proteolytic degradation of the whole molecule by lysosomal proteases. While the

BOX 26.5

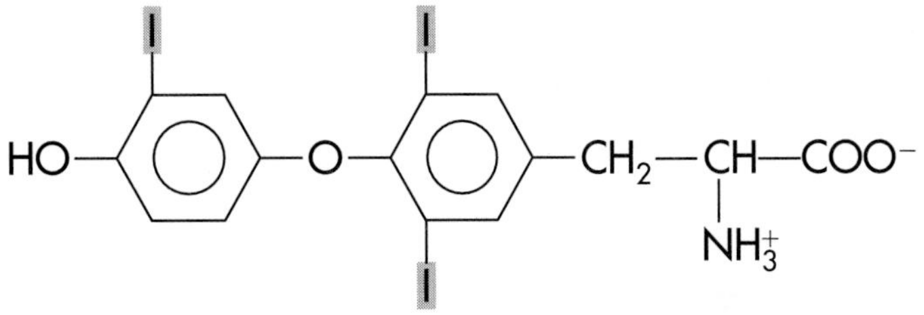

Triiodothyronine
(T₃)

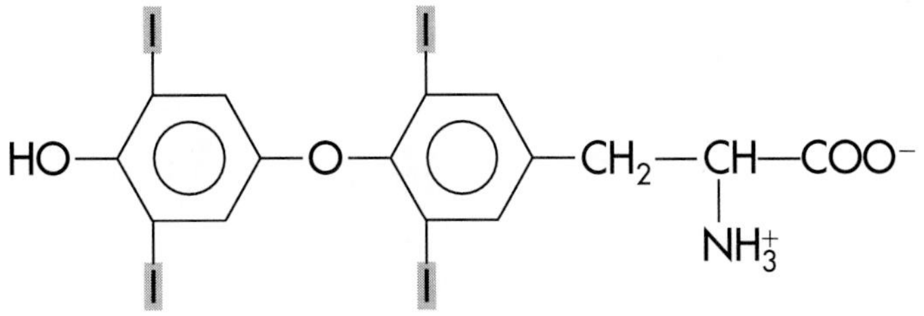

Thyroxine
(T₄)

hormones are released from the gland, the mono- and diiodotyrosines that also are present in thyroglobulin are deiodinated in the cell, and the iodine is recycled.

All steps in thyroid hormone synthesis are stimulated by **thyroid-stimulating hormone (TSH)** from the anterior pituitary gland, including iodide uptake, thyroglobulin synthesis, iodination, coupling, and the pinocytosis of thyroglobulin.

More than 99% of T_3 and more than 99.9% of T_4 are bound to plasma proteins in the blood (see Chapter 25). This extensive protein binding protects the hormones from enzymatic attack and renal excretion, so their biological half-lives are remarkably long: 6.5 days for T_4 and 1.5 days for T_3. Although the total plasma level of T_4 is approximately 50 times higher than that of T_3 (80 versus 1.5 ng/mL), the relative concentrations of free, unbound hormone are more balanced because T_3 is less extensively bound to plasma proteins than is T_4.

Approximately 90% of the hormone released from the thyroid gland is T_4 and 10% is T_3, but part of the T_4 is deiodinated to T_3 in the target tissues. Alternatively, T_4 is deiodinated to the biologically inactive reverse T_3 as shown in Box 26.6 (page 558).

Indeed, two thirds of the circulating T_3 are derived not directly from the thyroid gland but rather by the deiodination of T_4 in peripheral tissues. Of the two hormones, T_3 is approximately four times more potent than T_4 in most bioassays. Therefore *T_4 is, in part at least, a prohormone for the more potent T_3 in much the same way that testosterone is a prohormone for the more potent DHT.*

Both hypo- and hyperthyroidism are common in clinical practice

The insufficient formation of thyroid hormone is known as **hypothyroidism.** If it occurs in adults, it leads to **myxedema,** with widespread subcutaneous edema, decreased basal metabolic rate, bradycardia, and sluggishness of mental activity. Hypothyroidism in infants can be catastrophic, with severe and irreversible mental deficiency, stunted growth, and multiple physical deformities. This condition is called **cretinism.** Congenital hypothyroidism, which occurs in approximately 1 in 4000 newborns, can be caused by inherited defects of thyroid hormone synthesis, but most cases are of unknown etiology. Because the dire consequences of congenital hypothyroidism can be prevented readily by the oral administration of thyroxine, *newborn screening for congenital hypothyroidism is performed routinely in many parts of the world.* Indeed, some 9 million newborns are

FIG. 26.6

Cellular compartmentation of thyroid hormone synthesis. *TG,* Thyroglobulin; *MIT,* monoiodotyrosine; *DIT,* diiodotyrosine; *TP,* thyroperoxidase.

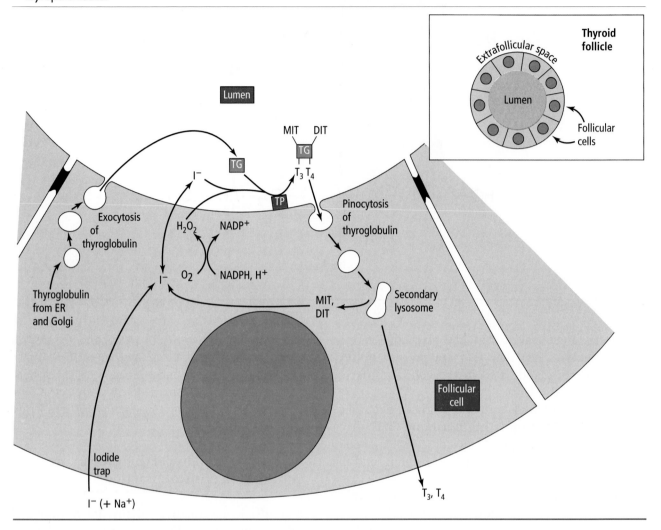

screened every year throughout the industrialized world.

Iodine deficiency is an important cause of hypothyroidism in many mountainous areas of the world, where the soil and the plants grown on it are often deficient in this mineral. It was, for example, endemic in the Alps until the early part of the twentieth century. Iodine deficiency essentially has disappeared from industrialized countries because of the routine use of iodized salt, but it is still prevalent in some mountainous areas of the developing world. There is, for example, still an extensive "goiter belt" in the Himalaya mountains.

If hypothyroidism is the result of iodine defi-ciency or a defect within the thyroid gland, it is likely to result in hypertrophy and hyperplasia of the follicular cells and the accumulation of excess thyroglobulin in the follicular lumen. This phenomenon, known as **simple goiter** or **diffuse goiter,** results from an overstimulation of the thyroid gland by TSH. *TSH release from the anterior pituitary gland is disinhibited whenever the levels of circulating thyroid hormones are abnormally low.*

Graves' disease, which affects approximately 0.4% of the population, is the most common cause of **hyperthyroidism.** Enlargement of the thyroid gland and excessive hormone production in this disease are caused by an IgG autoantibody known as

FIG. 26.7

Synthesis of thyroid hormones from iodinated tyrosine residues in thyroglobulin. These reactions take place on the lumenal surface of the follicular cells in the thyroid gland.

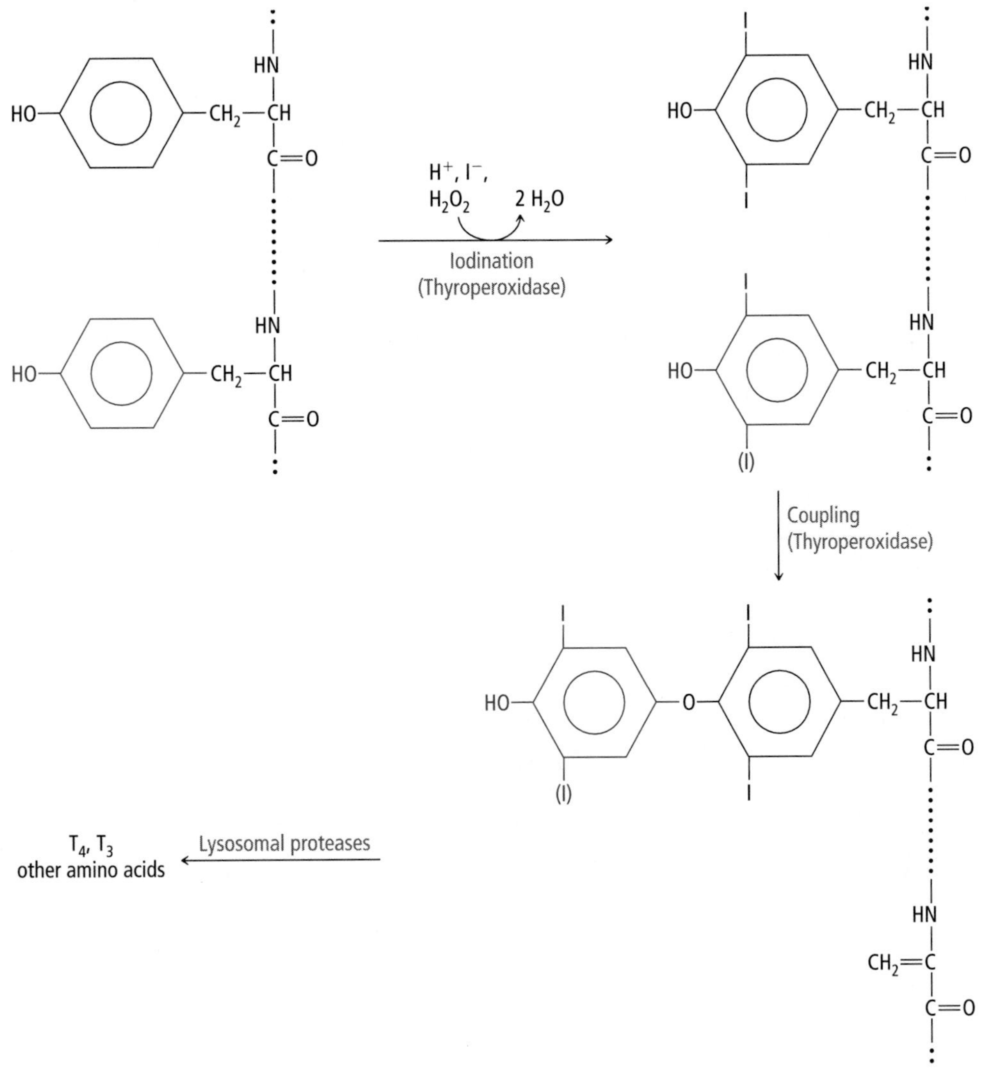

LATS (long-acting thyroid stimulator), which binds and stimulates the TSH receptor in the thyroid gland.

THE BIOGENIC AMINES

The biogenic amines **5-hydroxytryptamine (5-HT, serotonin), histamine,** and the **catecholamines** are synthesized by the *pyridoxal phosphate–dependent decarboxylation of aromatic amino acids.* Unlike the steroid and thyroid hormones, they are water-soluble products that are stored in membranous vesicles within the synthesizing cell before they are released by exocytosis.

The catecholamines are synthesized from tyrosine

The synthesis of the catecholamines dopamine, norepinephrine (noradrenaline), and epinephrine (adrenaline) is shown in Fig. 26.8. The initial reactions, up to dopamine, take place in the cytoplasm, whereas the formation of norepinephrine and epinephrine is catalyzed by enzymes within the storage

BOX 26.6

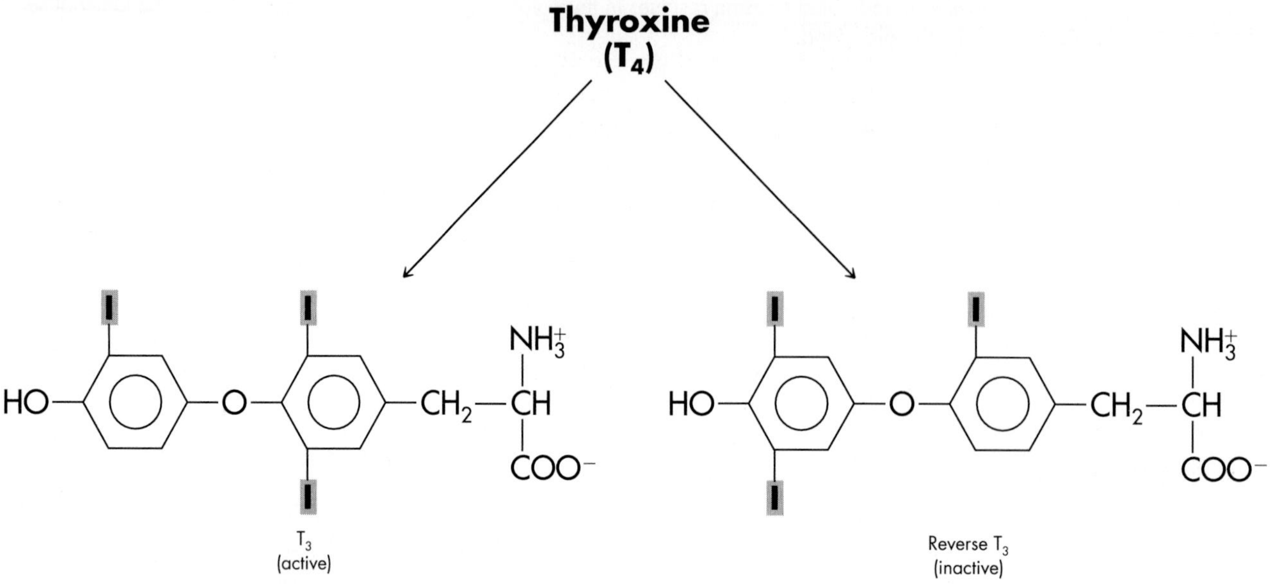

Thyroxine
(T₄)

T₃
(active)

Reverse T₃
(inactive)

FIG. 26.8

The pathway of catecholamine biosynthesis.

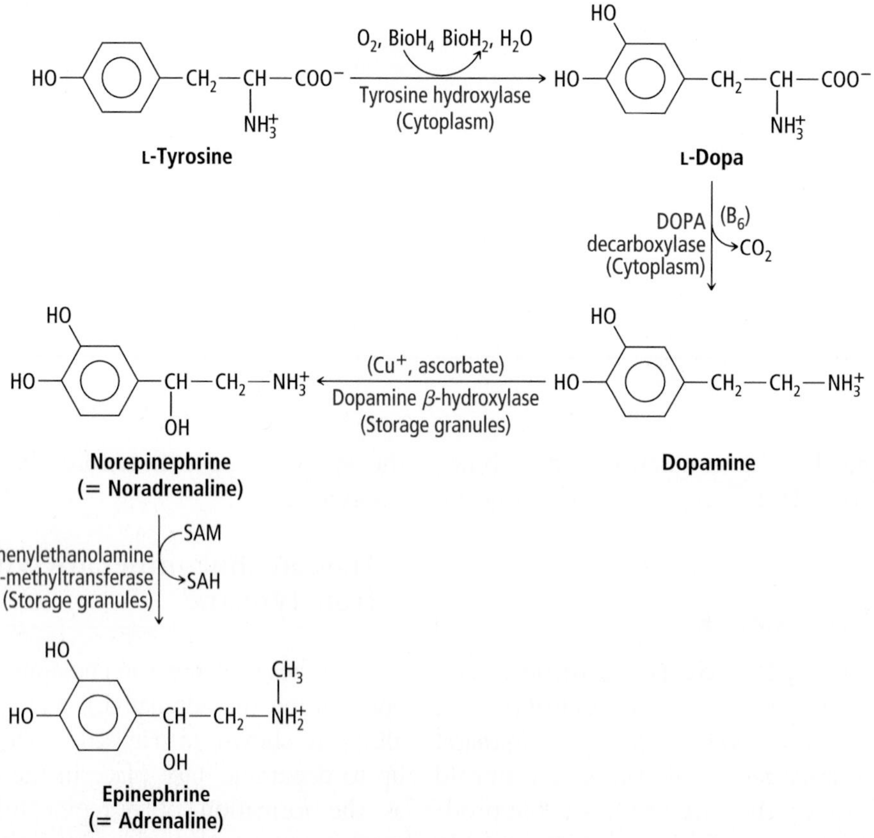

vesicles—chromaffin granules in the adrenal medulla and synaptic vesicles in neurons. The committed step in this pathway is the **tyrosine hydroxylase** reaction, which is feedback-inhibited by the amines. The end product depends on the enzymatic outfit of the cell. The dopaminergic neurons of the nigrostriatal system, for example, have only tyrosine hydroxylase and DOPA decarboxylase, but the adrenal medulla has the enzymes for the complete pathway.

There are two degrading enzymes for the catecholamines, **monoamine oxidase (MAO)** and **catechol O-methyltransferase (COMT)**. MAO, a flavoprotein enzyme of the outer mitochondrial membrane, inactivates its substrates by *oxidative deamination*: the amino group is released as ammonia, and the nitrogen-bound carbon is oxidized to an aldehyde group. The protein-bound FAD, which is reduced to $FADH_2$ during the reaction, is regenerated by molecular oxygen with the formation of hydrogen peroxide (H_2O_2). MAO removes not only the primary amino groups of dopamine and norepinephrine but also the secondary amino group of epinephrine (Fig. 26.9).

COMT *methylates one of the phenolic hydroxy groups* in its substrates, thereby greatly reducing their biologi-

---

FIG. 26.9

Enzymatic inactivation of catecholamines. Besides enzymatic inactivation, which is mostly intracellular, the rapid uptake of catecholamines into the cell is critically important for the termination of their biological actions. *MAO,* Monoamine oxidase; *COMT,* catechol O-methyltransferase.

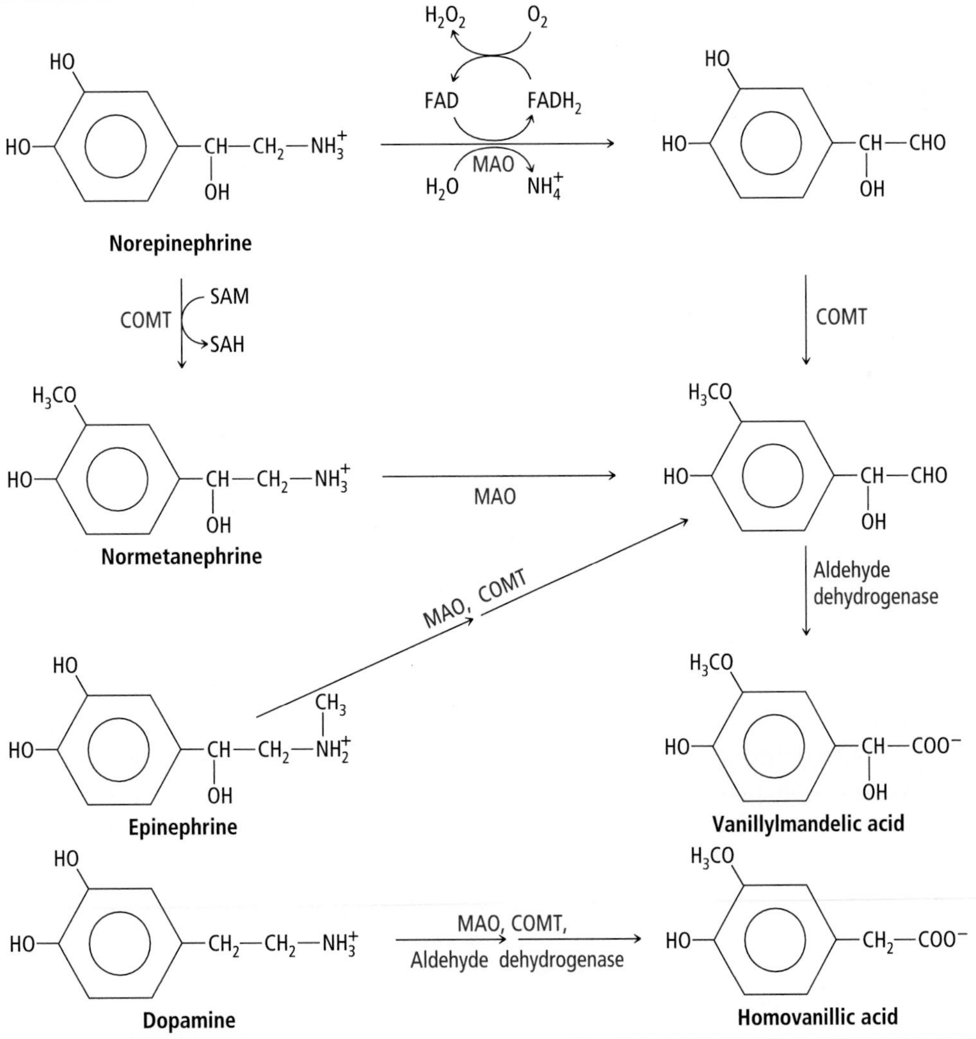

FIG. 26.10

Synthesis and degradation of 5-hydroxytryptamine (5-HT, or serotonin).

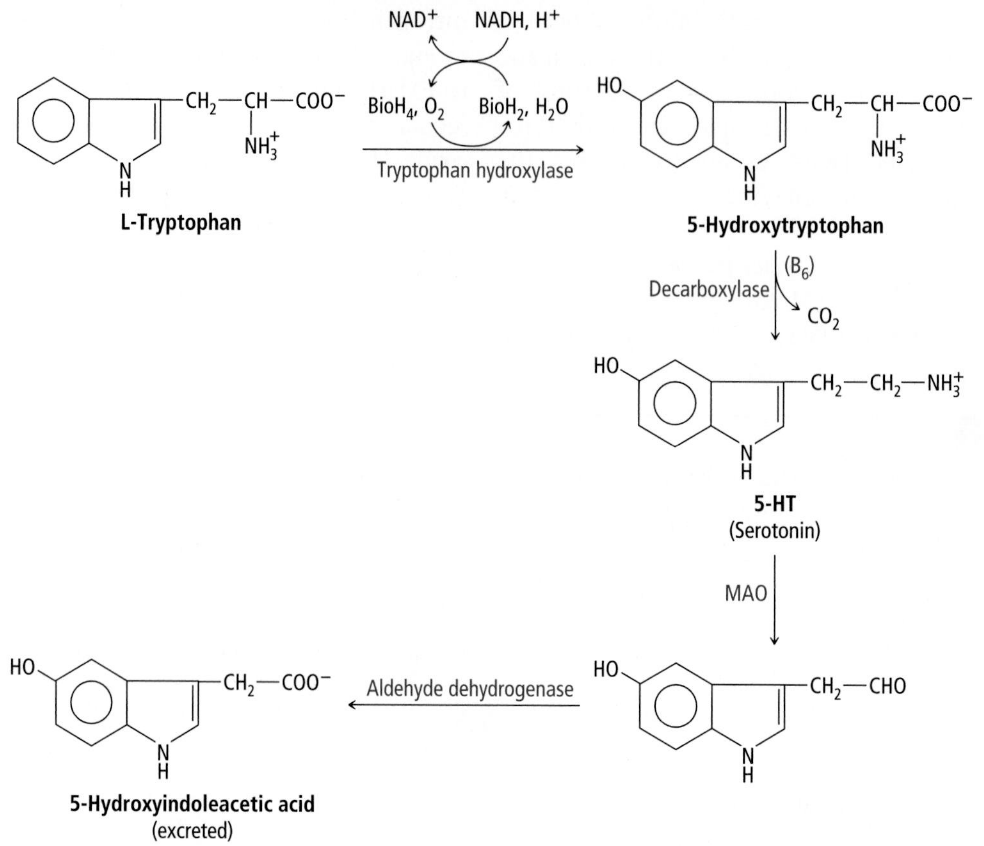

cal activities. Both MAO and COMT have broad substrate specificities, and the two reactions can occur in either sequence. Dopamine is metabolized to **homovanillic acid,** and norepinephrine and epinephrine are metabolized to **vanillylmandelic acid.** These products are excreted in the urine.

5-HT is the major indolamine

5-HT, also known as serotonin, is synthesized from tryptophan in the enterochromaffin cells of the lungs and digestive tract, in platelets, and in neurons of the central nervous system. Its biosynthetic pathway (Fig. 26.10) resembles that of the catecholamines.

Only MAO—not COMT—inactivates serotonin. Humans have two isoenzymes of MAO: MAO-A acts on serotonin and MAO-B acts on dopamine. Norepinephrine is inactivated by both.

Histamine is produced by mast cells and basophils

As a major mediator of allergic responses (type I hypersensitivity reactions), *histamine is released by circulating basophils and by their sedentary cousins, the mast cells,* typically in response to antigenic stimulation of surface-bound IgE (see Chapter 25). Histamine dilates small blood vessels, increases capillary permeability, contracts bronchial and intestinal smooth muscle, stimulates gastric acid secretion and nasal fluid discharge, and regulates the cells of the immune system. Its synthesis and degradation are summarized in Fig. 26.11.

PEPTIDES AND PROTEINS

The majority of the extracellular messengers that we know about are oligopeptides, proteins, or gly-

FIG. 26.11

Synthesis and degradation of histamine.

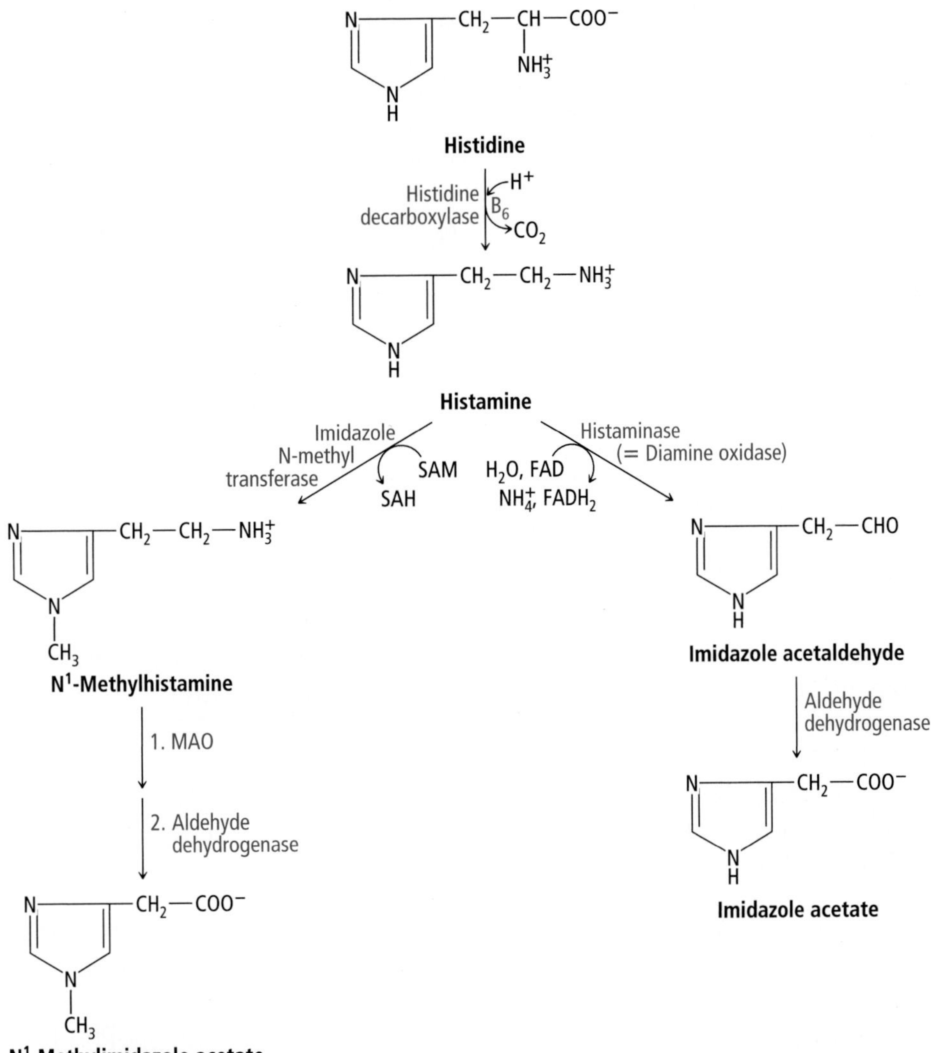

coproteins. These include not only "classical" hormones but also a variety of neurotransmitters, locally acting growth factors, and **cytokines** that are released by activated lymphocytes or monocytes/macrophages during inflammatory reactions.

Peptide hormones are synthesized from prohormones

Protein and glycoprotein hormones qualify as secreted proteins, and *they are synthesized and processed like any other secreted protein*: after their synthesis by ribosomes on the rough ER, they are channeled through the smooth ER and Golgi, packaged into secretory vesicles, and finally released by exocytosis. They can be posttranslationally modified during their passage through these organelles.

Small peptide hormones are derived from larger polypeptides, known as prohormones, that are cleaved into hormonally active fragments by specific endopeptidases in ER, Golgi, or secretory vesicles. The prohormone itself is not hormonally active.

Like other secreted proteins, *prohormones are synthesized with a signal sequence at their amino end, which directs them to the ER* (see Chapter 8), and the first step in

FIG. 26.12

Processing of prohormones at pairs of basic amino acid residues, in this case Lys-Arg. These reactions take place in the Golgi and secretory vesicles of the endocrine cell. They require enzymes with trypsinlike and carboxypeptidase B–like cleavage specificities.

$$H_3^+N\text{-}AA_1\text{-}..........\text{-}AA_n\text{-}Lys\text{-}Arg\text{-}AA_{n+3}\text{-}..........\text{-}AA_\omega\text{-}COO^-$$

↓ "Trypsin-like" enzyme

$$H_3^+N\text{-}AA_1\text{-}..........\text{-}AA_n\text{-}Lys\text{-}COO^- + Arg + H_3^+N\text{-}AA_{n+3}\text{-}..........\text{-}AA_\omega\text{-}COO^-$$

↓ "Carboxypeptidase B-like" enzyme

$$H_3^+N\text{-}AA_1\text{-}..........\text{-}AA_n\text{-}COO^- + Lys$$

prohormone processing is the removal of the signal sequence. Further proteolytic processing takes place at *pairs of basic amino acid residues that serve as preformed cleavage sites,* as shown in Fig. 26.12.

Insulin is released together with the C peptide

Mature insulin, the product of the pancreatic β cells, consists of two polypeptides: the A chain, with 21 amino acids, and the B chain, with 30 amino acids. There are three disulfide bonds: two between the A and B chains and one within the A chain (Fig. 26.13).

The polypeptide synthesized by the ribosomes, known as **preproinsulin,** is a single polypeptide with 103 amino acids. The first 24 amino acids at the amino terminus are the signal sequence. They are removed by signal peptidase in the ER during or immediately after translation. The remaining structure, known as **proinsulin,** is cleaved at paired basic amino acid residues by enzymes in the secretory granules. These cleavages release a hormonally inactive fragment, the **C peptide** (C for connecting). *Insulin and the C peptide, being formed in the same secretory vesicle, are released together into the blood.* The plasma level of the C peptide can be determined in the clinical laboratory to assess β cell function in diabetic patients under insulin treatment: although the circulating insulin of these patients comes in part from their own pancreas and in part from insulin injections, the C peptide level is directly pro-

portional to the insulin release from the patient's β cells.

The insulins of various vertebrate species are structurally similar to human insulin. Thus, the insulins from pig and cattle, which are used for the treatment of diabetic patients, differ from human insulin by only one and three amino acid substitutions, respectively. The sequence of the hormonally inactive C peptide is far less conserved. *This portion of the prohormone is required for the proper folding of proinsulin and the formation of the correct disulfide bonds:* in the test tube, the correct disulfide bonds can be regenerated easily when reduced proinsulin is treated with oxidizing agents. When, on the other hand, a mixture of reduced A and B chains is exposed to the proper reagents, disulfide bonds are formed at random and biologically inactive polymers are the main products. During insulin biosynthesis in the pancreatic β cells, disulfide bonds obviously are formed before the C peptide is removed from proinsulin.

Some prohormones form more than one active product

Some prohormones are processed to more than one hormone molecule. An example for this type of prohormone is **proenkephalin,** the precursor of the **enkephalins:**

Tyr-Gly-Gly-Phe-Met
Met-enkephalin

Tyr-Gly-Gly-Phe-Leu
Leu-enkephalin

Met-enkephalin and leu-enkephalin belong to a group of biologically active peptides known as opioid peptides or **endorphins** because they act on the same receptors as the opiates. They are neurotransmitters in brain, spinal cord, and peripheral nerve plexuses, and also are formed in the chromaffin granules of the adrenal medulla, from which they are released together with epinephrine and norepinephrine.

Proenkephalin contains six copies of the met-enkephalin sequence and one copy of the leu-enkephalin sequence, each flanked on both sides by pairs of basic amino acid residues (Fig. 26.14). Despite the multiple copies, the processing of proenkephalin is not exceedingly

FIG. 26.13

Synthesis of insulin from preproinsulin. Mature insulin consists of two disulfide-bonded polypeptides, the A chain and the B chain. During prohormone processing, the signal sequence (●●) and the C peptide (○○) are removed proteolytically. The proteolytic cleavages are performed by the signal peptidase in the rough ER (⇥→) and by enzymes with trypsinlike (⟶) carboxypeptidase B–like (--→) specificities in the storage granules. Note that pairs of basic amino acid residues serve as and preformed cleavage sites for the excision of the C peptide.

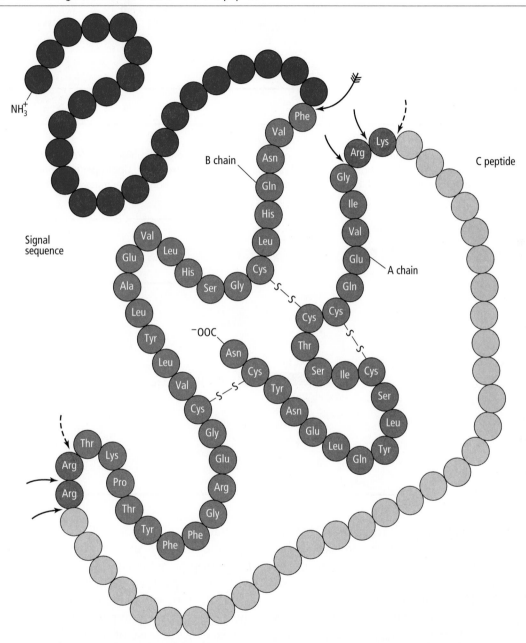

efficient: only 35 of the 267 amino acids in the precursor form useful products.

Proopiomelanocortin *is a precursor of ACTH, β-endorphin, and various forms of melanocyte-stimulating hormone (MSH) in the pituitary gland.* Peptides with a stim-ulatory action on the hormone-sensitive adipose tissue lipase, known as **lipotropins,** also are formed from this prohormone.

The processing of proopiomelanocortin is tissue specific (Fig. 26.15). ACTH and β-endorphin are the main

FIG. 26.14

Structure of human (pre-)proenkephalin.

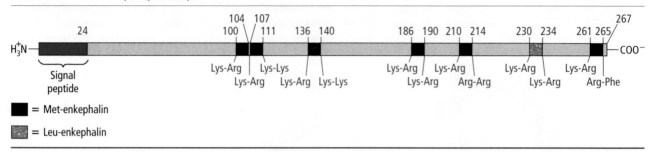

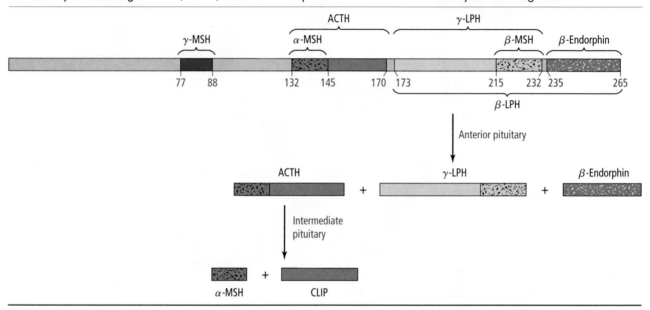

FIG. 26.15

Structure and processing of proopiomelanocortin in the pituitary gland. As in proenkephalin (Fig. 26.14), the active fragments are framed, in most cases, by pairs of basic amino acid residues (not shown here). *LPH*, Lipotropic hormone; MSH, melanocyte-stimulating hormone; ACTH, adrenocorticotropic hormone. CLIP is a hormonally inactive fragment.

products in the anterior pituitary gland. They are stored in the same vesicles and are coreleased in response to stimulation by corticotropin-releasing factor and other stimuli. Although β-endorphin is a powerful activator of opiate receptors, its physiological roles as a hormone are not well understood. In the pars intermedia of the pituitary gland, ACTH is processed further to α-MSH and a biologically inactive peptide called CLIP. As in proinsulin and proenkephalin, the hormonally active sequences of proopiomelanocortin are framed by pairs of basic amino acid residues.

In humans, where the intermediate lobe of the pituitary gland is not well developed, MSH activity is contained mostly in the larger fragments β-lipotropin, γ-lipotropin, and ACTH. In patients with Cushing's disease (an adenoma of the pituitary corticotrophs) or Addison's disease (destruction of the adrenal glands), hyperpigmentation is caused by the excessive release of these peptides.

Angiotensin is formed from circulating angiotensinogen

In the examples that we have encountered so far, the active hormone was formed from a precursor

FIG. 26.16

Synthesis of angiotensin II from circulating angiotensinogen.

H_3^+N—Asp-Arg-Val-Tyr-Ile-His-Pro-Phe-His-Leu—Angiotensinogen

↓ Renin
(from kidney)

H_3^+N—Asp-Arg-Val-Tyr-Ile-His-Pro-Phe-His-Leu—COO^-

**Angiotensin I
(inactive)**

↓ Converting enzyme
(In lung capillaries)

H_3^+N—Asp-Arg-Val-Tyr-Ile-His-Pro-Phe—COO^-

**Angiotensin II
(active)**

↓ Angiotensinases
(Vascular endothelium)

Inactive fragments,
free amino acids

protein within the endocrine cell. In the case of **angiotensin,** however, *the hormonally active peptide is formed by proteolytic cleavage outside the synthesizing cell.* The prohormone of angiotensin is **angiotensinogen,** a plasma protein from the liver. The rate-limiting step in angiotensin formation is the proteolytic cleavage of a dekapeptide, called **angiotensin I,** from the amino terminus of angiotensinogen. This step is catalyzed by **renin,** a protease from the juxtaglomerular cells of the kidney that is released in response to norepinephrine, hypovolemia, hyponatremia, and renal ischemia. Angiotensin I is biologically inactive. It has to be processed to biologically active angiotensin II by **angiotensin converting enzyme,** an endothelial enzyme in lung capillaries (Fig. 26.16).

Angiotensin II has powerful hypertensive effects: it contracts vascular smooth muscle both directly and indirectly by enhancing the release of norepinephrine from sympathetic nerve endings. It also stimulates aldosterone secretion from the zona glomerulosa cells. Renin release and angiotensin formation are increased in a variety of renal diseases. The resulting hypertension can be treated with **captopril,** an inhibitor of angiotensin converting enzyme.

Angiotensin II is very short lived: it is easy prey for endothelial peptidases, and its biological half-life is less than 1 min. *Short lifespans are typical for most biologically active peptides.* Very small peptides, in particular, often are viciously attacked by peptidases on the surface of capillary endothelial cells. The lifespans of oxytocin and vasopressin (nine amino acids), for example, are in the 1- to 10-minute range, and those of injected enkephalins (five amino acids) are measured in seconds. Even circulating insulin is degraded within 1 to 5 minute.

Radioimmunoassay is the most versatile method for the determination of hormone levels

The determination of circulating hormone levels is important for the diagnosis of endocrine disorders. Hormone determinations are difficult because the plasma levels of most hormones are extremely low and because it is rarely possible to separate the hormone from other plasma components that may interfere with the assay. Some typical plasma levels are included in Table 26.2.

The most generally applicable procedure for hormone determinations is **radioimmunoassay (RIA).** The principle of this method is illustrated in Fig. 26.17 (page 567). It requires a specific antibody to the hormone and a radiolabeled version of the hormone that contains tritium, radioactive iodine, or some other suitable radioisotope. When the patient's serum is ad-ded to the complex of the antibody with the radiolabeled hormone, *the (unlabeled) hormone in the patient's serum competes with the radiolabeled hormone for binding to the antibody.* After incubation for some minutes, the free unbound hormone has to be separated from the hormone-antibody complex. The higher the hormone concentration in the patient's serum, the more radioactive hormone is displaced from binding to the antibody and appears as free, unbound radioactivity.

This general procedure can be used for a variety of hormones, in particular the peptide and protein hormones. Other proteins also can be determined by RIA. During acute myocardial infarction, for example, the damaged myocardium releases not only enzymes such as lactate dehydrogenase, creatine kinase, and aspartate transaminase (see Chapter 25), but also various other proteins including myoglobin and troponin. The determination of these proteins by RIA is a valuable aid in the diagnosis of myocar-

TABLE 26.2

Typical plasma levels of some hormones

Hormone	Normal levels	Increased in	Decreased in	Assay method*
Cortisol	50-250 ng/mL	Cushing's disease, adrenal adenoma, or iatrogenic	Addison's disease, hypopituitarism	Fluorometric, RIA, HPLC
Aldosterone	40-310 pg/mL	Cushing's disease, adrenal adenoma	Addison's disease	RIA
ACTH	50 pg/mL	Cushing's disease	Hypopituitarism	RIA
Testosterone	3-12 ng/mL (male) 0.3-0.9 ng/mL (female)		Hypogonadism	RIA
Insulin	180-1000 pg/mL	Obesity, insulinoma	Type I diabetes mellitus	RIA
Growth hormone	1 ng/mL	Acromegaly	Hypopituitarism	RIA
Vasopressin	1-5 pg/mL	Inappropriate ADH secretion	Diabetes insipidus	RIA
Epinephrine	≤140 pg/mL	Pheochromocytoma		HPLC
Norepinephrine	70-1500 pg/mL			

* HPLC = high-pressure liquid chromatography.

BOX 26.7

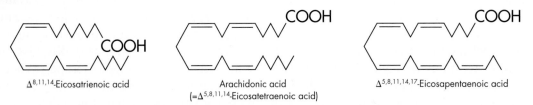

$\Delta^{8,11,14}$-Eicosatrienoic acid   Arachidonic acid ($=\Delta^{5,8,11,14}$-Eicosatetraenoic acid) $\Delta^{5,8,11,14,17}$-Eicosapentaenoic acid

dial damage. More importantly, some neoplastic cells release proteins into the blood that can be used as tumor markers. Most liver cancers, for example, release α-fetoprotein. **Carcinoembryonic antigen** is a glycoprotein of embryonic epithelia that is released by many epithelial cancers in the adult, and **prostate-specific antigen** is a prostatic protein that is widely used as a marker for prostatic cancer. All of these proteins can be assayed readily by RIA.

THE EICOSANOIDS

The eicosanoids are biologically active lipids that are derived from polyunsaturated, 20-carbon fatty acids. They are not derived from specialized endocrine tissues, but all cells except RBCs and lym-

phocytes are able to produce one or several eicosanoids. Most are short lived, with biological half-lives in the range of 10 seconds to 5 minutes, and they are not transported by the blood but rather act as paracrine and autocrine messengers within their tissue of origin.

Two major pathways lead from arachidonic acid to biologically active products

The precursors of the eicosanoids are 20-carbon fatty acids with three, four, or five double bonds as shown in Box 26.7. Any of these three fatty acids can be used as a substrate, but *arachidonic acid is by far the most important precursor simply because it is far more abundant than the others.* In the cell, these fatty acids

FIG. 26.17

The general procedure for the radioimmunoassay of a hormone. 1. After mixing a specific antibody (Y) with the labeled hormone (H*), a radioactive antigen-antibody complex is formed. 2. The patient's serum is added. The unlabeled hormone in the patient's serum (H) competes with the labeled hormone for binding to the antibody: Antibody·H* + H $\rightleftharpoons$ Antibody·H + H* 3. Free hormone and antibody-hormone complex are separated from each other. The radioactivity of the free, unbound hormone is determined in a scintillation counter. A large amount of hormone in the patient's serum leads to a high specific radioactivity of the free hormone.

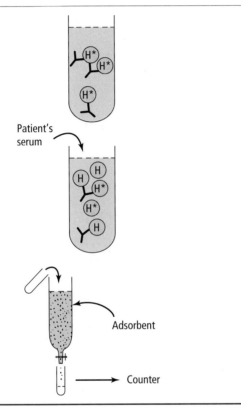

Patient's serum

Adsorbent

Counter

are encountered in position 2 of membrane phosphoglycerides, from which they are released by the action of **phospholipase A$_2$**. Alternatively, they can be released by the successive action of **phospholipase C** and a diglyceride lipase (Fig. 26.18).

Arachidonic acid can be salvaged by an acyl-CoA synthetase for reesterification, or it can be processed to eicosanoids by two alternative pathways. *The* **cyclooxygenase pathway** *produces the prostanoids, which include the prostaglandins prostacyclinand thromboxane; the* **lipoxygenase pathway** *produces, among other products, the leukotrienes* (Fig. 26.19).

Prostaglandins are synthesized in almost all tissues

The **prostaglandins** are 20-carbon compounds containing a cyclopentane ring. Prostaglandin I, also known as **prostacyclin**, contains a five-membered oxygen-containing ring as well; the **thromboxanes** have a six-membered oxygen-containing ring instead of the cyclopentane ring (Fig. 26.20). The different types of prostaglandins are designated by a capital letter according to the nature of the substituent on the cyclopentane ring. They are characterized further by a subscript indicating the number of double bonds outside the cyclopentane ring. For example see Box 26.8. The different types of prostaglandin, as designated by the capital letter, have different and sometimes antagonistic biological effects. The number of double bonds, on the other hand, affects the potency of the product but not the kind of effect on a particular target tissue.

The key enzyme of prostaglandin synthesis is the microsomal **prostaglandin synthase complex**,

BOX 26.8

PGE$_1$

PGE$_2$

PGE$_3$

FIG. 26.18

The release of free arachidonic acid from membrane phosphoglycerides.

Phospho-lipase A₂

Phospholipase C

Diglyceride lipase

FIG. 26.19

The major fates of arachidonic acid. Cyclooxygenase and 5-lipoxygenase are the key enzymes for the synthesis of the biologically active eicosanoids.

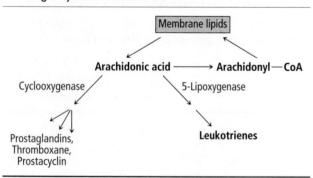

Membrane lipids

Arachidonic acid ⟶ Arachidonyl—CoA

Cyclooxygenase

5-Lipoxygenase

Prostaglandins, Thromboxane, Prostacyclin

Leukotrienes

which consists of **cyclooxygenase** and **peroxidase** components. The H-prostaglandin formed in this reaction is converted to the other prostanoids by cell-specific enzymes (Fig. 26.20). *Each cell type produces only one or a few major prostanoids.* Thus the platelets

produce thromboxane, and the vascular endothelium produces PGE and PGI.

The prostanoids participate in many physiological processes

Almost every cell in the human body responds to one or several types of prostaglandins. Only a few of the more interesting actions can be mentioned here:

1. *Aggregating platelets release thromboxane A_2 (TXA$_2$),* which causes vasoconstriction and promotes further platelet aggregation. This action is short lasting, however: within 30 to 60 seconds, TXA$_2$ is hydrolyzed to an inactive product. The actions of TXA$_2$ on platelets and vascular smooth muscle are antagonized by PGI$_2$ (prostacyclin), which is released by intact endothelial cells. Like TXA$_2$, PGI$_2$ is short lived: it is hydrolyzed within approximately 3 minutes. *PGI$_2$ from intact endothelium*

FIG. 26.20

Synthesis of prostaglandins and thromboxanes by the cyclooxygenase pathway. *GSH,* Reduced glutathione; *GSSG,* oxidized glutathione; *PG,* prostaglandin; *TX,* thromboxane.

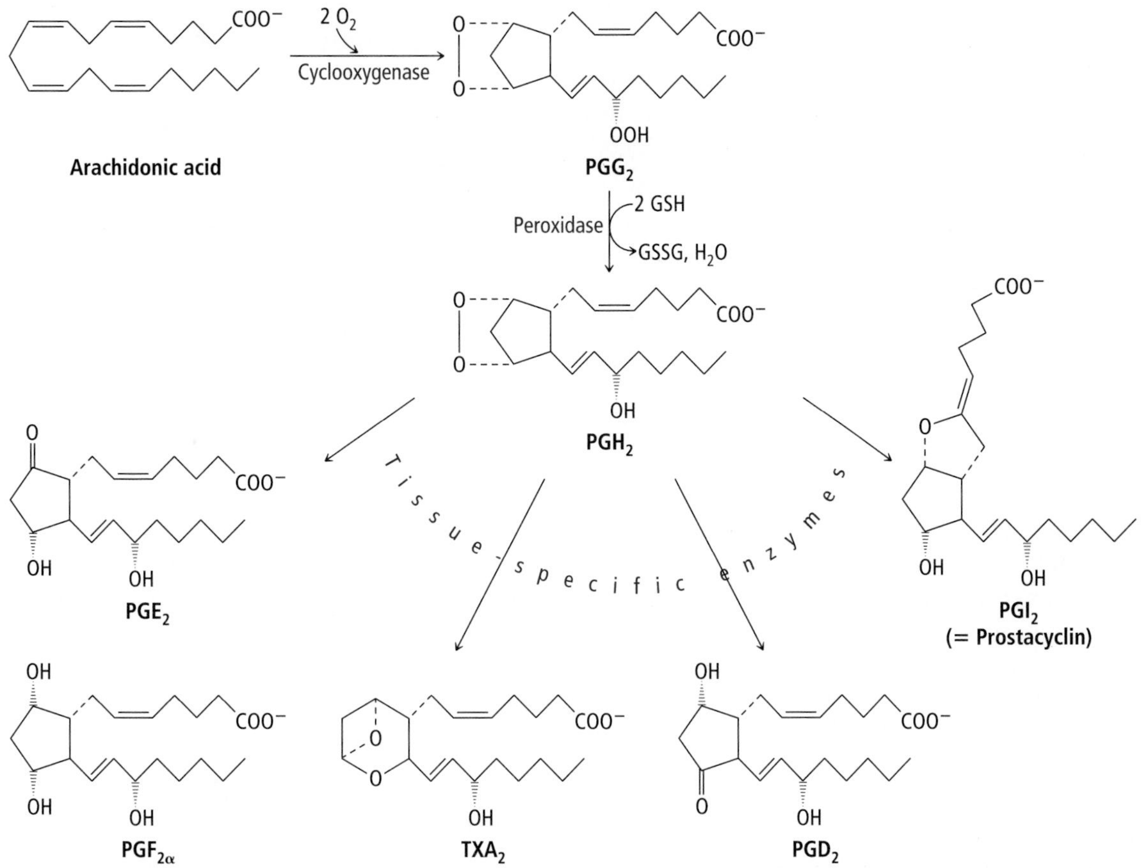

prevents platelet aggregation and thrombus formation. When the endothelial covering is lost, however, thrombus formation is promoted by the unopposed action of TXA_2.

2. PGE and PGI, which normally are formed by the vascular endothelium, are potent vasodilators. Although they cannot be used as antihypertensives because of their rapid inactivation and numerous extravascular effects, *PGE$_1$ can be used in infants with pulmonary stenosis to maintain the patency of the ductus arteriosus until surgical correction can be performed.*

3. PGE$_2$ and PGF$_{2\alpha}$, which are synthesized in the endometrium, induce uterine contraction. Their excessive production during menstruation has been identified as a cause of dysmenorrhea. Prostaglandin levels in amniotic fluid are low during pregnancy, but they increase massively at parturition. Together with oxytocin, *they participate in the normal induction of labor.* Unlike oxytocin, the prostaglandins contract the uterus not only at term of pregnancy but at all times, so *they are suitable for the induction of abortion.* Both PGE$_2$ and PGF$_{2\alpha}$ are used for this purpose via intravenous, intravaginal, or intraamniotic administration.

4. *PGE$_2$ and TXA$_2$ are formed by macrophages and other cells as local mediators of inflammation.* Together with histamine, bradykinin, the leukotrienes, and a variety of white blood cell–derived cytokines, they mediate the cardinal signs of inflammation.

5. *Fever is mediated by the cytokine **interleukin-1 (IL-1)**,* which is released from stimulated monocytes and macrophages. IL-1 binds to vascular receptors in the preoptic area of the hypothalamus, where

it induces the formation of PGE$_2$. PGE$_2$ causes fever by a direct action on the thermoregulatory center.

The actions of prostaglandins are mediated through second messenger systems (see Chapter 27). Thus, the relaxation of vascular smooth muscle by prostaglandins E and I is mediated by increases of the intracellular cAMP level, and thromboxane-induced vasoconstriction is mediated by increased intracellular calcium and decreased cAMP.

The leukotrienes are produced by the lipoxygenase pathway

The **lipoxygenases** are dioxygenases that produce hydroperoxy derivatives known as **hydroperoxyeikosatetraenoic acids** (**HPETEs**) from arachidonic acid. According to the position of the hydroperoxy group, we distinguish a 5-, a 12-, and a 15-lipoxygenase. The HPETEs are reduced rapidly to the more stable **hydroxyeikosatetraenoic acids** (**HETEs**). 5-HPETE, the product of the 5-lipoxygenase, is converted to the **leukotrienes,** in white blood cells and other cell types (Fig. 26.21). The HETEs, which are strong chemoattractants, are concerned mostly with the regulation of white blood cell activity. The leukotrienes, on the other hand, are powerful constrictors of bronchial and intestinal smooth muscle. Both types of products are involved in hypersensitivity reactions and inflammation. Unlike the other eicosanoids, *the leukotrienes are relatively stable and persist for a few hours in the tissue.* LTC$_4$, LTD$_4$, and LTE$_4$, which originally were characterized as the **slow-reacting substance of anaphylaxis,** are responsible for the protracted bronchoconstriction in asthmatic patients.

Antiinflammatory drugs inhibit the synthesis of eicosanoids

Two important antiinflammatory drug classes are in current use: the **glucocorticoids,** which include the natural steroids cortisol and cortisone as well as a host of synthetic analogs, and the **nonsteroidal antiinflammatory drugs** (**NSAIDs**), which are represented by aspirin, indomethacin, and ibuprofen. Both of these drug classes act on the synthesis of eicosanoids: *the steroids inhibit the action of phospholipase A$_2$,* which normally is rate limiting in

eicosanoid synthesis, and *the NSAIDs are inhibitors of cyclooxygenase:*

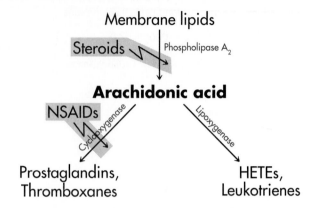

The steroids reduce the synthesis of all eicosanoids, but the NSAIDs inhibit only the synthesis of the prostanoids. The synthesis of HETEs and leukotrienes is not affected and may even be increased because more arachidonic acid is available for the lipoxygenase pathway. Aspirin, for example, is useful in the treatment of arthritis, a disease in which prostaglandins are important mediators of inflammation. However, aspirin is contraindicated in asthma, a disease in which bronchoconstriction is induced by leukotrienes rather than prostaglandins.

| NEUROTRANSMITTERS |

Neurotransmitters are extracellular messengers that transmit a targeted message from a neuron to a responding cell. They are released at specialized cell-cell contacts called synapses. A "classical" neurotransmitter:

- Is synthesized in the presynaptic cell
- Is stored in membrane-bound vesicles
- Is released from the presynaptic cell in response to membrane depolarization
- Mediates the postsynaptic effects of presynaptic nerve stimulation
- Is inactivated rapidly in the area of the synapse

Acetylcholine is the neurotransmitter of the neuromuscular junction

The **neuromuscular junction,** or **motor endplate,** is the synapse between the terminal of an α-motorneuron and a skeletal muscle fiber (Fig. 26.22). Its neurotransmitter **acetylcholine** is formed

FIG. 26.21

The products of 5-lipoxygenase: hydroperoxyeicosatetraenoic acid (HPETE), hydroxyeicosatetraenoic acid (HETE), and the leukotrienes (LTs).

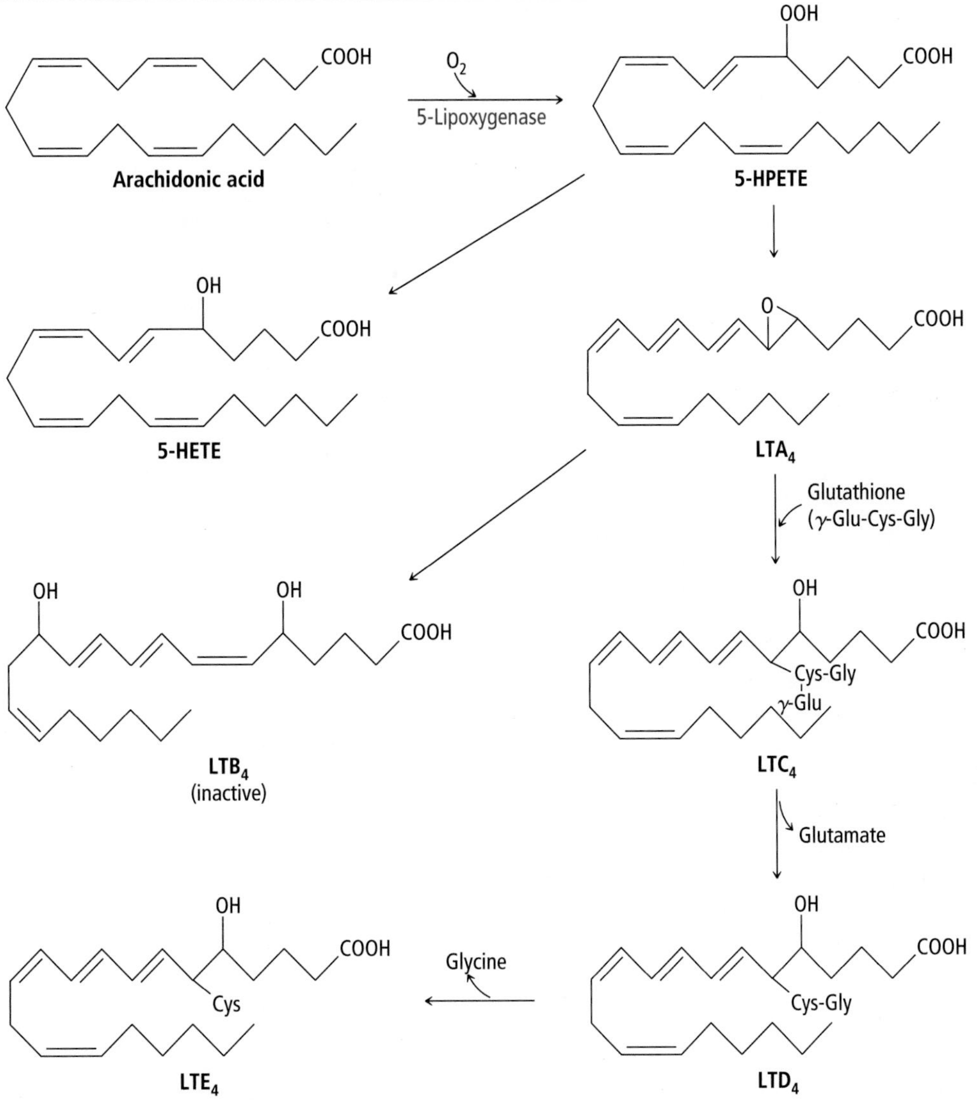

by the cytoplasmic enzyme **choline-acetyltransferase** in the nerve terminal as shown in Box 26.9. Acetylcholine is packaged in synaptic vesicles (diameter 40 nm), from which it is released into the synaptic cleft by exocytosis. Exocytosis is triggered by membrane depolarization: the nerve terminal contains a voltage-gated calcium channel that opens in response to depolarization. Calcium enters the cell and induces the fusion of synaptic vesicles with the plasma membrane. Not only acetylcholine release but *the release of all neurotransmitters is calcium dependent.*

Within approximately 1 millisecond, acetylcholine diffuses across the synaptic cleft, a distance of 50 nm. After acting on its receptor in the postsynaptic membrane (see Chapter 21), *acetylcholine is degraded by* **acetylcholinesterase.** This enzyme hydrolyzes its substrate by a mechanism that closely resembles that of the serine proteases (see Chapter 4) as shown in Box 26.10. This reaction takes place in the synaptic cleft. The breakdown products, choline and acetate, are taken up rapidly into the nerve terminal, where they are used for the resynthesis of acetylcholine.

FIG. 26.22

The neuromuscular junction: an example of a cholinergic synapse. ●, Acetylcholine; ■, acetylcholine receptor; ✂, acetyl-cholinesterase.

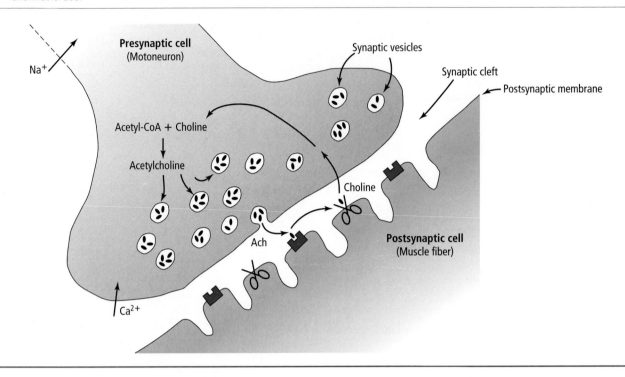

BOX 26.9

Several biogenic amines, amino acids, and peptides are used as neurotransmitters

The catecholamines, 5-HT, and perhaps histamine are used as neurotransmitters. Like acetylcholine, these biogenic amines are stored in synaptic vesicles and are released by a depolarization-induced, calcium-dependent mechanism. Their synaptic inactivation, however, is different: unlike acetylcholine, the biogenic amines are not degraded in the synaptic cleft. *Their synaptic action is terminated by sodium-*

BOX 26.10

Enzyme—Ser—OH + H₃C—N⁺(CH₃)(CH₃)—CH₂—CH₂—O—C(=O)—CH₃ ⟶

Acetylcholine

Enzyme—Ser—O—C(=O)—CH₃ + H₃C—N⁺(CH₃)(CH₃)—CH₂—CH₂—OH

Choline

↓ H₂O

↘ H⁺

Enzyme—Ser—OH + ⁻OOC—CH₃

FIG. 26.23

A noradrenergic synapse: the transmitter is taken up into the presynaptic nerve terminal by sodium-dependent, high-affinity uptake. Once in the nerve terminal, it is either recycled into the synaptic vesicles or degraded by monoamine oxidase (MAO). Y, Postsynaptic receptor; ■, norepinephrine; ✄, MAO.

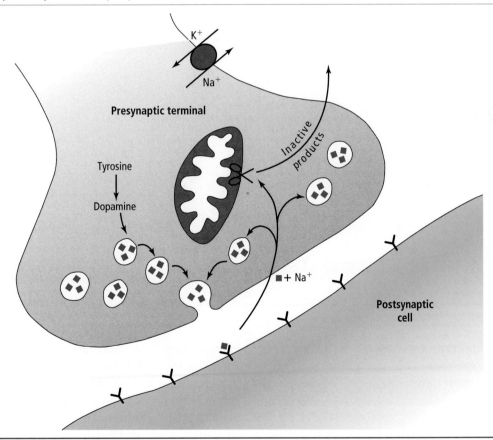

FIG. 26.24

Metabolism of γ-aminobutyric acid (GABA). **A,** Reactions. **B,** Compartmentation. ①, Glutamate decarboxylase; ②, vesicular storage; ③, release by exocytosis; ④, sodium-dependent, high-affinity uptake; ⑤, GABA transaminase. ▼, GABA; Y, postsynaptic receptors.

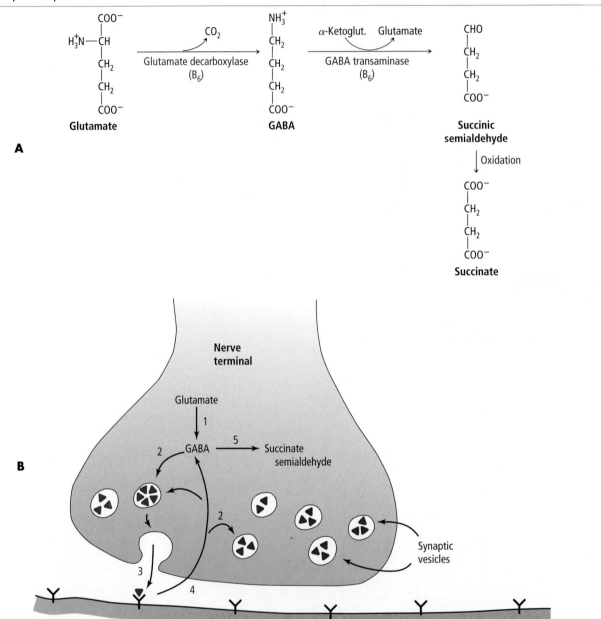

dependent, high-affinity uptake back into the nerve terminal. Once back in its home cell, the amine transmitter can be repackaged into a synaptic vesicle for release. Alternatively, it is degraded by MAO, the major inactivating enzyme in nervous tissue (Fig. 26.23).

Only 1% to 2% of the neurons in the brain use a catecholamine or 5-HT as their neurotransmitter. Amino acids are far more popular. Indeed, glutamate and aspartate are the major excitatory neurotransmitters throughout the central nervous system, and glycine is an important inhibitory neurotransmitter in spinal cord and brainstem. These amino acids

TABLE 26.3

Neurotransmitters as targets of drugs and toxins

Agent	Mechanism of action	Effects
1. Drugs		
L-Dopa	Catecholamine precursor	Antiparkinsonian
MAO inhibitors	Inhibits the degradation of catecholamines and 5-HT	Antidepressant
Reserpine	Inhibits vesicular storage of catecholamines and 5-HT	Antihypertensive, sedative, depressant
Tricyclics	Inhibits synaptic uptake of norepinephrine and/or 5-HT	Antidepressant
Cocaine	Inhibits synaptic uptake of dopamine, norepinephrine, and 5-HT	Psychostimulant
Amphetamine	Releases nonvesicular (cytoplasmic) dopamine, norepinephrine, and 5-HT	Psychostimulant
Opiates	Agonist action on opiate (endorphin) receptors	Narcotic analgesic
Neuroleptics	Antagonist action on D2 dopamine receptors	Antipsychotic
Benzodiazepines	Sensitization of GABA-A receptors	Sedative, anxiolytic, anticonvulsant
2. Bacterial toxins		
Tetanus toxin	Inhibition of glycine release in spinal cord	Lockjaw, convulsions
Botulinum toxin	Inhibition of acetylcholine release at motor endplate	Flaccid paralysis
3. Chemical toxins		
Organophosphates	Irreversible inhibition of acetylcholinesterase	Autonomic nervous effects, CNS effects
Curare	Blocks acetylcholine receptors in neuromuscular junction	Flaccid paralysis

are packaged into synaptic vesicles and released by the usual mechanisms, and *their actions are terminated by sodium-dependent, high-affinity uptake* without the need for synthesizing and inactivating enzymes.

γ-Aminobutyric acid (GABA) is an amino acid neurotransmitter that is produced by the decarboxylation of glutamate. It is removed from its receptors by high-affinity uptake into nerve terminals and surrounding glial cells, followed by transamination to biologically inactive succinic semialdehyde (Fig. 26.24).

Small peptides, including the enkephalins, substance P (an undecapeptide in primary afferents and the basal forebrain), cholecystokinin octapeptide, vasoactive intestinal polypeptide (VIP), somatostatin, and several dozen more, also are well-established neurotransmitters. Their high-molecular-weight precursors are synthesized at the rough ER in the perikaryon, packaged into vesicles, and transported to the nerve endings by fast axoplasmic transport. En route, the active transmitter is formed by proteolytic cleavage reactions. Their synaptic inactivation is effected by peptidases on the surface of neurons and glial cells.

Neurotransmitter systems are eminently important in neuropharmacology and neurotoxicology. Some important examples of neurotransmitter-directed drugs and toxins are listed in Table 26.3.

SUMMARY

Several classes of agents are employed by the body to transmit signals from one cell to another. The **steroids,** which function as classical hormones, are synthesized from cholesterol by side chain cleavage, hydroxylations, and other reactions. The **thyroid hormones** are derived from protein-bound tyrosine, and their synthesis requires iodine. The **biogenic amines** are water-soluble products that are produced by the decarboxylation of aromatic amino acids. The most important biogenic amines are the catecholamines, which serve as neurotransmitters in the central and peripheral nervous systems and as hormones in the adrenal medulla. **Protein hormones** are products of the secretory pathway that are processed through ER, Golgi apparatus, and secretory vesicles. Smaller peptide hormones are derived from large precursors called prohormones. Prohormone processing is effected by endopeptidases in the organelles of the secretory pathway. The **eicosanoids** are 20-carbon lipids that are derived from arachidonic acid and related polyunsaturated fatty acids. Most of them are short lived and act only locally in their tissue of origin. They are important mediators of inflammation, and agents that inhibit their synthesis are important antiinflammatory drugs. **Neurotransmitters** are small, water-soluble messengers that are released by neurons. Acetylcholine, the biogenic amines, some amino acids, and a variety of peptides are used as neurotransmitters. Most neuropharmacological drugs interfere with the actions of individual neurotransmitters.

Further Reading

de Groot LJ et al, editors: *Endocrinology*, 3rd ed. W. B. Saunders, Philadelphia, 1995, vol. 2, pp. 1630–1641.

de Groot LJ et al, editors: *Endocrinology*, 3rd ed. W. B. Saunders, Philadelphia, 1995, vol. 3, pp. 2019–2030.

Ford-Hutchinson AW, Gresser M, Young RN: 5-Lipoxygenase. *Annu Rev Biochem* 63, 383–417, 1994.

Scriver R, Beaudet AL, Sly WS, Valle D, editors: *The metabolic basis of inherited disease*, 6th ed., vol. 2. McGraw-Hill, New York, 1989, pp. 1843–2028.

Sundberg DK: Chemical messenger systems. In: Conn PM, editor: *Neuroscience in medicine*, J. B. Lippincott, Philadelphia, 1995, pp. 403–430.

QUESTIONS

1. Phaeochromocytoma is a tumor of catecholamine-secreting cells that causes dangerous hypertension in patients. To prevent these hypertensive episodes, you may try an inhibitor of
   A. Monoamine oxidase (MAO)
   B. Tyrosinase
   C. Catechol O-methyltransferase (COMT)
   D. The sodium-dependent norepinephrine carrier in sympathetic nerve terminals
   E. Tyrosine hydroxylase

2. The pancreatic β-cells secrete not only insulin, but also an equimolar amount of
   A. Glucagon
   B. C peptide
   C. Cyclic AMP
   D. Proopiomelanocortin
   E. Enkephalin

3. The adrenal cortex contains a sizeable collection of enzymes for steroid hormone synthesis. Two of these enzymes are required for the synthesis of glucocorticoids but not of androgens, so their deficiency leads to an overproduction of adrenal androgens. These two enzymes are
   A. 7α-Hydroxylase and 17-hydroxylase
   B. Desmolase and HMG-CoA reductase
   C. 11β-Hydroxylase and 21-hydroxylase
   D. 17-Hydroxylase and adrenodoxin
   E. 18-Hydroxylase and aromatase

4. A pharmacological inhibitor of lipoxygenase would be useful for the treatment of asthma, because it prevents the formation of
   A. Prostaglandins
   B. Gamma-aminobutyric acid (GABA)
   C. Thromboxanes
   D. Prostacyclin
   E. Leukotrienes

Chapter 27

Intracellular Messengers

In the previous chapter we encountered agents that transmit messages from cell to cell. These messengers can control almost any aspect of cellular function, but some of the most prominent targets are:

1. *Ion channels in the plasma membrane.* Neurotransmitters, in particular, affect the membrane potential by opening or, less commonly, closing individual ion channels.
2. *Metabolic enzymes.* We have encountered several examples in which hormones or other extracellular messengers regulate metabolic enzymes. These effects usually are mediated by phosphorylation of the regulated enzyme.
3. *Cytoskeletal proteins.* Although the cytoskeleton is affected by external agents in all cells, the most conspicuous example is the regulation of muscle contraction.
4. *Nuclear transcription factors.* Many agents affect the expression of individual sets of genes, thereby regulating the amounts of the protein products.

In this chapter we will examine the signaling pathways through which external agents affect these cellular targets.

| RECEPTORS |

For the physiologist, a "receptor" is a sensory cell. For the biochemist, on the other hand, *a receptor is a cellular protein that binds an extracellular messenger and thereby initiates the physiological response.* The receptors for water-soluble messengers are integral proteins of the plasma membrane. The hormone binds to an extracellular domain of the receptor, and the receptor transmits its message across the membrane. Lipid-soluble hormones, in contrast, can diffuse through the plasma membrane and act on intracellular receptors, either in the nucleus or in the cytoplasm. Most of these intracellular receptors, after binding their ligands, affect gene transcription directly by binding to regulatory DNA sequences (Fig. 27.1).

Receptor-hormone interactions are noncovalent, reversible, and saturable

Like the binding of a substrate to its enzyme, or of an antigen to its antibody, *hormone-receptor binding is always effected by noncovalent interactions.* Because of its noncovalent nature, this binding is reversible:

$$R + H \rightleftharpoons R \cdot H$$

where R = unoccupied receptor; H = unbound hormone; R · H = receptor-hormone complex.

The dissociation constant K_D of the receptor-hormone complex is defined as:

$$K_D = \frac{[R] \times [H]}{[R \cdot H]} = \frac{k_1}{k_{-1}}$$

You may note that K_D has the dimension of moles per liter, and when we rearrange this equation we see that *the K_D corresponds to the hormone concentration [H] at which half of the receptor molecules are converted to receptor-hormone complex ([R] = [R · H])*:

$$\frac{K_D}{[H]} = \frac{R}{[R \cdot H]}$$

The dissociation constant for hormone-receptor bind-

ing resembles the Michaelis constant of enzyme kinetics (see Chapter 4). It describes the affinity between the hormone and its receptor. Dissociation constants between 10^{-9} and 10^{-11} mol/liter are typical for hormone-receptor interactions.

Hormone binding shows *saturation kinetics* (Fig. 27.2): at a hormone concentration far above the K_D, more or less all receptors are occupied. The physio-

---

FIG. 27.1

Cellular locations of receptors for hormones and other extracellular messengers. ▭, Thyroid hormone receptor; ◡, glucocorticoid receptor; Y and Y, cell surface receptors.

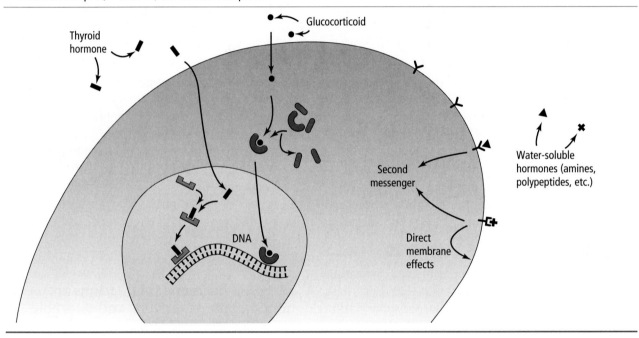

FIG. 27.2

Receptor binding at various hormone concentrations. The maximal binding B_{max} corresponds to the total number of receptors.

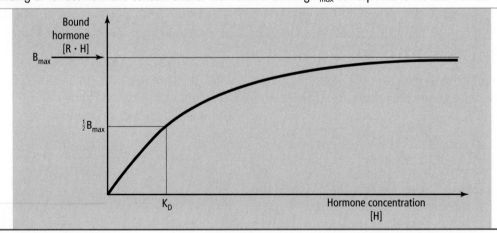

logical response is maximal, and a further increase of the hormone concentration will not result in an increased response. This situation is equivalent to the zero-order reaction in enzyme kinetics. *The maximal binding (B_{max}) corresponds to the number of receptor molecules in the cell.*

The biological response depends on the number of receptor-hormone complexes. If receptors are scarce, the maximal biological response requires that all receptors be engaged by their hormonal ligands. If the receptors are plentiful, however, a response is maximal even when only a small percentage of the cellular receptors are occupied. In the latter case, we speak of **spare receptors**: the cell has many more receptors than it actually needs for a maximal response. *Spare receptors allow the cell to respond maximally even to hormone concentrations well below the K_D.* The importance of spare receptors is evident when we imagine that a cell loses half of its receptors: in the absence of spare receptors, the maximal response is reduced by 50%. However, if the cell has many spare receptors to begin with, the maximal response still is obtained, but it requires twice the original hormone concentration.

Many neurotransmitter receptors are ion channels

Some receptors induce their cellular response by a direct mechanism, without the need for lengthy signaling cascades. Neurotransmitters, in particular, which are water soluble and therefore not able to enter the cell, induce a postsynaptic membrane potential—either stimulatory or inhibitory—by manipulating ion channels in the plasma membrane. Although they can achieve this by a variety of mechanisms, *the fastest and most direct mechanism is the binding of the neurotransmitter to a ligand-gated ion channel in the plasma membrane.*

The **nicotinic acetylcholine receptor** in the neuromuscular junction, for example, is a channel for the monovalent cations sodium and potassium (Fig. 27.3). It consists of five membrane-spanning subunits with the subunit structure α_2, β, γ, δ. Each of the subunits has four transmembrane helices, and one helix of each subunit lines the central pore of the channel. This channel is closed in the absence of acetylcholine. The extracellular domains of the α subunits contain the acetylcholine-binding sites, and the binding of this ligand opens the channel. As a result,

---

FIG. 27.3

Structure of the nicotinic acetylcholine receptor in the neuromuscular junction. This receptor is a ligand-gated channel for small cations (Na$^+$, K$^+$). Acetylcholine binds with positive cooperativity to the two α subunits. Each of the five polypeptides traverses the membrane four times, and one of the transmembrane helices in each subunit contributes to the "gate" in the channel. (© Cell Press.)

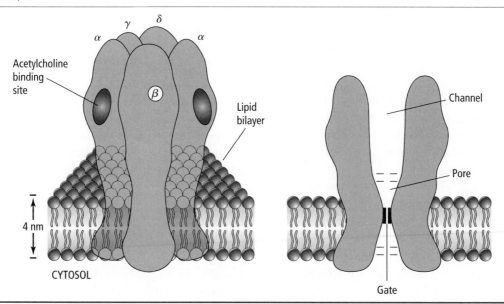

sodium enters the cell down its electrochemical gradient and the membrane becomes depolarized.

There is a whole family of ligand-gated ion channels. They all consist of five subunits but differ both in their ligand-binding specificities and in their ionic selectivities. Whereas *many excitatory neurotransmitters open sodium or calcium channels, some inhibitory neurotransmitters open chloride channels.* The GABA-A receptor in the brain, for example, is a ligand-gated chloride channel. Incidentally, this channel not only binds GABA but has binding sites for barbiturates and benzodiazepines as well. Although these agents are drugs rather than physiological messengers, endogenous ligands have been described for the benzodiazepine-binding site, and these ligands may play physiological roles in the regulation of the channel.

The ligand-gated ion channels illustrate that *receptors are allosteric proteins that change their conformation in response to ligand binding.* Cooperativity between two or more bound ligands is possible if the receptor possesses more than one ligand-binding site.

The ligand-gated ion channels—and many other receptors—come in many different variants. The subunits of the nicotinic acetylcholine receptors in the nervous system, for example, are slightly different from those of the receptor in the neuromuscular junction. Indeed, different populations of neurons possess different combinations of subunits that are either encoded by separate genes or obtained by the differential processing of gene transcripts. *This diversity is important for drug development because the different receptor subtypes respond differently to drugs.* Low doses of **nicotine,** for example, stimulate nicotinic receptors in the nervous system but not in the neuromuscular junction. The arrow poison **curare,** on the other hand, blocks the receptor in the neuromuscular junction but not in the nervous system. An agent that, like nicotine, activates a receptor is called an **agonist,** and an agent that, like curare, blocks a receptor is called an **antagonist.** *Like enzymes, receptors are subject to competitive, noncompetitive, or irreversible inhibition by drugs and toxins.*

The steroid and thyroid hormone receptors are transcription factors

Unlike neurotransmitters and protein hormones, the steroid and thyroid hormones are able to diffuse across the cellular membranes. They encounter their receptors either in the cytoplasm or in the nucleus. The unstimulated glucocorticoid receptor, for example, resides in the cytoplasm, complexed to cytoplasmic proteins that mask its DNA-binding domain. After hormone binding, the receptor releases its cytoplasmic binding proteins, and the DNA-binding site is exposed. Together with the bound hormone, *the activated receptor moves to the nucleus, where it binds to specific DNA sequences* known as **hormone response elements (HREs).** They are located next to the hormone-regulated genes, usually within a few hundred base pairs upstream of the start site for transcription. They are not part of the core promoter because their distance from the transcriptional initiation site is variable in different genes, and they may be on either the coding or the noncoding strand.

Binding of the activated receptor increases or, in some cases, decreases the rate of transcription. This effect is specific: in a glucocorticoid-responsive cell, less than 1% of all genes possess the response element and are affected by the receptor-hormone complex. On the other hand, every gene possessing the response element seems to be regulated by the hormone. With recombinant DNA methods, an HRE can be attached to any gene, even to genes of bacterial origin. After transfection into cultured human cells, the expression of this "reporter gene" is affected by the hormone—provided, of course, that the cultured cells possess the hormone receptor. At this point, we can recognize two levels of targeting: *only those cells that possess the receptor can respond to the hormone, and within the cell only those genes that possess the hormone response element are regulated.*

The glucocorticoid receptor is a zinc-finger protein (see Chapter 8) that belongs to the same superfamily of regulatory DNA-binding proteins as the other steroid hormone receptors and the receptors for thyroid hormones, calcitriol, and retinoic acid. Like most other transcriptional regulators, it binds to its target DNA in a dimeric form. The dimeric nature of the activated receptor is reflected in the base sequence of its response elements, which contain a conserved palindrome.

The details of subcellular location and receptor activation differ in different cases. Thus the receptors for thyroid hormones and, probably, the estrogen receptor are intranuclear rather than cytoplasmic. In all cases, however, *the receptor is a ligand-regulated transcription factor.*

The inherited deficiency of a receptor makes the cells unable to respond to the corresponding hormone. This is most impressively seen in patients with **testicular feminization**. Genetically male individuals with this disorder grow up with an entirely female external appearance, although they possess testes rather than ovaries, and the müllerian duct structures (uterus and fallopian tubes) are absent. This syndrome is caused by an inherited defect of the androgen receptor: although androgens are released by the testes both during fetal development and in later life, the target tissues are unable to respond to the circulating hormones, and a female phenotype develops by default.

SIGNALING CASCADES: G PROTEINS, SECOND MESSENGERS, AND PROTEIN KINASES

Being unable to enter their target cells, water-soluble hormones have to deliver their messages at the cell surface. Their receptors are integral membrane glycoproteins with three functional domains: the *extracellular domain* binds the hormone; one or several *transmembrane α helices* penetrate the lipid bilayer; and the *intracellular domain* is coupled with an effector mechanism. These receptors have to transmit their signal through cascades of protein-protein interactions, and they employ small, diffusible molecules known as **second messengers** for long-distance signaling across the cytoplasmic space.

The seven-transmembrane receptors are coupled to G proteins

Whereas the "fast" actions of neurotransmitters are mediated by ligand-gated ion channels, *most hormone receptors belong to a family of membrane glycoproteins with seven membrane-spanning α helices* (Fig. 27.4). These crisscrossing membrane proteins do not form a channel, nor do they possess enzymatic activities. Their intracellular domain, however, is associated with a guanine nucleotide-binding protein, or **G protein.** The G protein consists of three subunits designated α (MW 45,000), β (MW 35,000), and γ (MW 7,000). The α subunit has a guanine nucleotide-binding site that can accommodate either GDP or GTP. The β and γ subunits are tightly

FIG. 27.4

The β-adrenergic receptor is an integral membrane protein with seven membrane-spanning α helices. Note that the binding site for β-adrenergic agonists is on the extracellular side, whereas the binding site for the G_s protein is on the cytoplasmic side of the plasma membrane. All G protein–coupled receptors resemble the β-adrenergic receptor in their amino acid sequence and membrane topography.

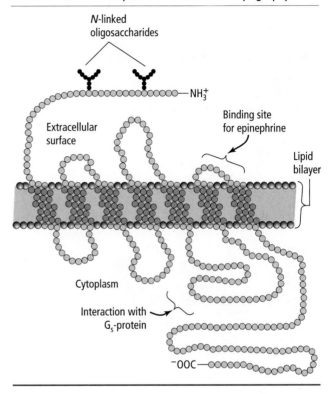

bound to each other and function as a single unit; the α subunit is associated only loosely with βγ.

The function of the G protein is shown in Fig. 27.5. In the resting state, the complete G protein is associated with the unstimulated receptor, with GDP bound to the guanine nucleotide-binding site. Binding of the hormone to the receptor induces a conformational change both in the receptor and in the attached G protein. This conformational change greatly reduces the affinity of the α subunit for GDP. GDP therefore dissociates away and is replaced quickly by GTP. Once GTP is bound, the α subunit loses its affinity both for the receptor and for the βγ complex: the G protein dissociates from the receptor, and it breaks up into the α-GTP subunit and the βγ complex. Both α-GTP and βγ are peripheral membrane proteins that diffuse along the inner sur-

FIG. 27.5

Coupling of a hormone receptor *(R)* to effector proteins *(E₁, E₂)* in the plasma membrane through a G protein. The most important effectors of hormone-regulated G proteins are second messenger–synthesizing enzymes such as adenylate cyclase and phospholipase C, but some calcium and potassium channels also are regulated by this mechanism. By an allosteric mechanism, the activation of the receptor causes GDP-GTP exchange and the dissociation of the heterotrimeric G protein into $\beta\gamma$ and α-GTP subunits. These subunits act allosterically on the effectors. The stimulation of the effector is terminated when the α subunit hydrolyzes its bound GTP.

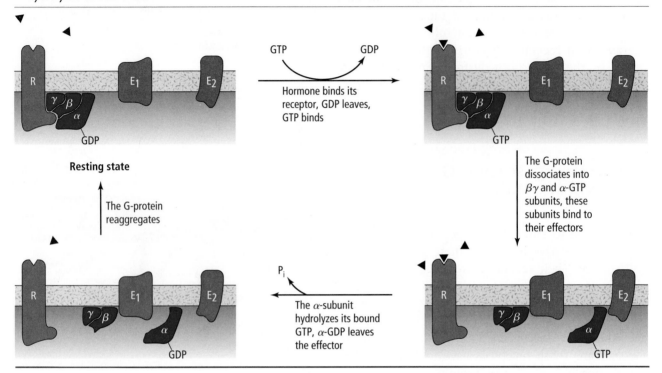

face of the plasma membrane. Both products can bind to target proteins in the plasma membrane, known as **effectors,** whose properties they affect by allosteric mechanisms. *The components of the G protein are membrane-bound messengers that transmit a signal from the receptor to the effector.*

How is this signal terminated? *The α subunit possesses a GTPase activity that hydrolyzes the bound GTP to GDP and inorganic phosphate.* This GTPase activity is stimulated by the binding of the α subunit–GTP complex to the effector. GDP remains bound to the α subunit, but the α-GDP complex no longer acts on the effector. Instead, it diffuses back to the $\beta\gamma$ complex, and the complete, heterotrimeric G protein again associates with the receptor. Note that *all G proteins exist in two forms, an active GTP-bound form that acts on the effector and an inactive GDP-bound form that does not.*

Humans have approximately 20 different G protein α subunits, 5 different β subunits, and 10 γ subunits, which are expressed in various combinations in different cell types. According to the structure and function of their α subunit, we distinguish four families of G proteins:

1. **G$_s$ proteins** (s for stimulatory) stimulate adenylate cyclase, the enzyme that synthesizes the second messenger cyclic AMP (cAMP).
2. **G$_i$ proteins** (i for inhibitory) inhibit adenylate cyclase.
3. **G$_q$ proteins** stimulate a phosphatidylinositol-specific phospholipase C, which forms the second messengers inositol 1,4,5-trisphosphate (IP$_3$) and 1,2-diacylglycerol (DAG).
4. **G$_{12}$ proteins** regulate ion channels.

BOX 27.1

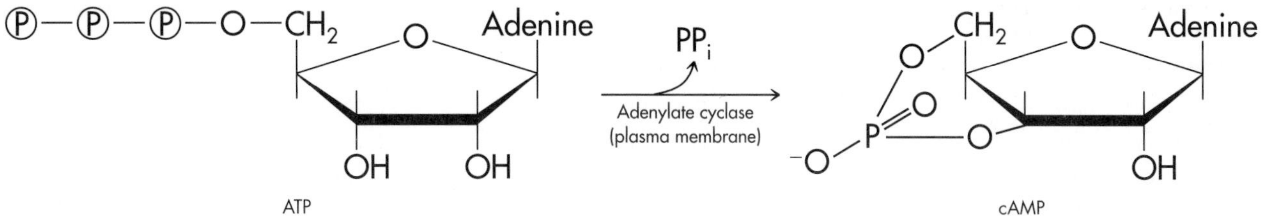

BOX 27.2

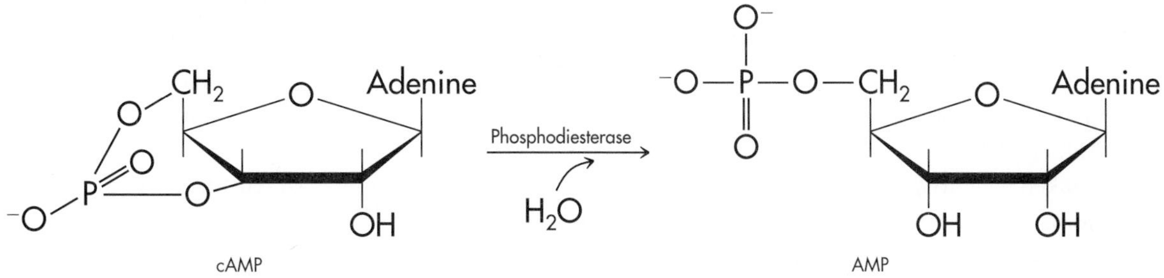

Besides the G_{12} proteins, some members of the G_s and G_i families regulate calcium or potassium channels in various cell types.

Cyclic AMP is the second messenger of many hormones

The hormone-activated G proteins carry messages along the plasma membrane, but they do not cross the cytoplasmic space. *To send a signal into the interior of the cell, the G protein has to induce the synthesis of a small, diffusible molecule known as a* **second messenger.** One of the most commonly used second messengers is cyclic AMP (cAMP). cAMP is synthesized from ATP by adenylate cyclase, an enzyme of the plasma membrane that is always under hormonal control as shown in Box 27.1. The inorganic pyrophosphate (PP_1) is rapidly hydrolyzed by pyrophosphatases, making the reaction irreversible. Approximately eight different adenylate cyclases, differing in their regulatory properties, have been described in mammalian tissues. All of them are integral membrane proteins with 12 transmembrane helices. *The adenylate cyclases are stimulated by the α_s subunit of the G_s proteins.*

cAMP is degraded by a group of enzymes known collectively as **phosphodiesterases** as shown in Box 27.2. Phosphodiesterases can be inhibited pharmacologically by **methylxanthines** such as caffeine, theophylline, and aminophylline, which thereby potentiate the cAMP-mediated effects. After a cup of coffee, for example, the level of plasma free fatty acids is increased because lipolysis in adipose tissue is stimulated by cAMP.

After its hormone-induced formation on the inner surface of the plasma membrane, cAMP diffuses throughout the cytoplasmic space. *It affects cellular function by stimulating the cAMP-dependent* **protein kinase A.** In the absence of cAMP, two catalytic subunits of this enzyme are bound tightly to two regulatory subunits. This form of the enzyme is inactive. The two regulatory subunits (R), which do not possess any enzymatic activity, can bind up to four cAMP molecules. cAMP binding, in turn, causes a conformational change that leads to the release of the two catalytic subunits (C):

TABLE 27.1

Substrates of protein kinase A

Protein	Tissue	Effect of phosphorylation
Glycogen synthase	Liver, muscle	Inhibition
Phosphorylase kinase	Liver, muscle	Stimulation
Acetyl-CoA carboxylase	Liver	Inhibition
Hormone-sensitive lipase	Adipose tissue	Stimulation
Inhibitor-1	Liver	Stimulation
6-Phosphofructo-2-kinase*	Liver	Inhibition
	Muscle	Stimulation
Fructose 2,6-bisphosphatase*	Liver	Stimulation
	Muscle	Inhibition
Pyruvate kinase	Liver	Inhibition
Phenylalanine hydroxylase	Liver	Stimulation
Microtubular subunits	Kidney	Formation of "water channels"
Transcription factors of the CREB family	All tissues	Stimulation
Many G_s-linked receptors	All tissues	Desensitization

* These two enzyme activities are present on the same polypeptide (see Chapter 17).

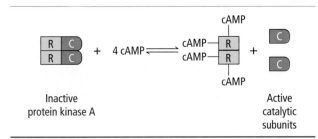

Inactive protein kinase A

Active catalytic subunits

The active catalytic subunits phosphorylate their protein substrates on serine or threonine side chains. The enzyme is quite selective, and only a very small proportion of the cellular proteins serve as substrates. Table 27.1 lists some of the proteins that are phosphorylated by protein kinase A.

The cAMP cascade amplifies the hormonal stimulus (Fig. 27.6). The interaction of a single epinephrine molecule with a β-adrenergic receptor, for example, leads to the activation of up to 20 G_s proteins; each α_s-GTP, in turn, acts on adenylate cyclase long enough to cause the synthesis of hundreds of cAMP molecules; and although four cAMP molecules are required to activate two catalytic subunits of protein kinase A, each active subunit can phosphorylate hundreds or thousands of substrate proteins before it reassociates with the regulatory subunits.

The G_s protein can couple to more than one kind of hormone receptor, so *more than one hormone can stimulate adenylate cyclase in any given cell.* The G_s-protein and adenylate cyclase are present in all cells, but *the responsiveness of the cell to an individual hormone depends on the presence of the hormone receptor.*

Some hormones inhibit adenylate cyclase through an inhibitory G protein

Some hormones do not stimulate but rather inhibit adenylate cyclase (Table 27.2). This negative coupling is mediated by the α_i subunit of the inhibitory G protein G_i. Most cells possess both G_s-linked and G_i-linked hormone receptors, and *the actual activity of adenylate cyclase depends on the balance between the stimulatory and inhibitory hormones* (Fig. 27.7).

Some bacterial toxins modify G proteins

Cholera is an intestinal infection that leads to a severe and often fatal diarrhea. The offending bacterium, *Vibrio cholerae*, does not invade the tissue but rather causes the diarrhea by producing a potent en-

FIG. 27.6

The cyclic AMP *(cAMP)* cascade. Receptor and adenylate cyclase are coupled by the stimulatory G protein G_s, which consists of the α_s, β, and γ subunits. All known cAMP effects in humans are mediated by protein kinase A. This protein kinase phosphorylates a variety of protein substrates in the cytoplasm and the nucleus.

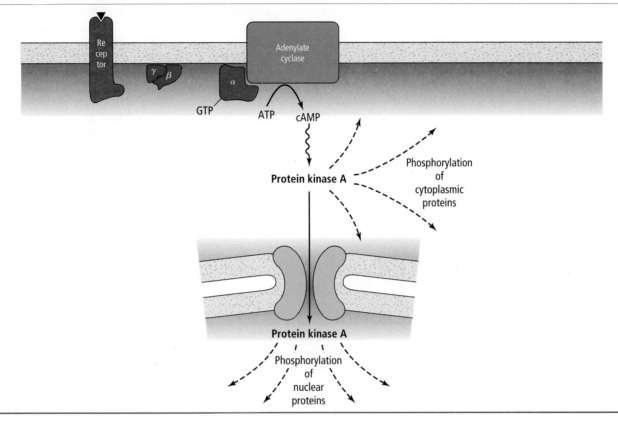

BOX 27.3

terotoxin. This enterotoxin is a secreted protein with an A_1 subunit, an A_2 subunit, and five B subunits. The B subunits bind to ganglioside GM_1 on the surface of intestinal mucosal cells, and the A_1 subunit enters the cell, where it acts as an enzyme, catalyzing the covalent modification of an arginine side chain in the α subunit of the G_s protein as shown in Box 27.3. The ADP-ribosylated α subunit still can bind GTP and stimulate adenylate cyclase. Its GTPase activity, however, is blocked: *the protein has lost its "off" switch and is locked in the active, GTP-bound form.* With continued stimulation of adenylate cyclase, *the cell soon is flooded with cAMP.* Fortunately, cholera toxin is not carried to distant organs; its effects remain confined to the intestine. In the intestinal mucosa, however, the excessive levels of cAMP cause a profuse secretion of water and electrolytes. Not only cholera toxin but also one of the enterotoxins of enterotoxigenic *E. coli*—the cause of the dreaded traveler's diarrhea (known locally un-

TABLE 27.2

Roles of cAMP in different tissues

Tissue/cell type	Agents increasing cAMP	Agents decreasing cAMP	Effects of elevated cAMP
Liver	Glucagon, epinephrine	Insulin*	Glycogen degradation, gluconeogenesis
Skeletal muscle	Epinephrine		Glycogen degradation, glycolysis
Adipose tissue	Epinephrine	Insulin*	Lipolysis
Renal tubular epithelium	Antidiuretic hormone		Water reabsorption
Intestinal mucosa	Vasoactive intestinal polypeptide, adenosine, epinephrine	Endorphins	Water and electrolyte secretion
Vascular smooth muscle	Epinephrine (β receptor)	Epinephrine (α_2 receptor)	Relaxation, growth inhibition
Bronchial smooth muscle	Epinephrine (β receptor)		Relaxation
Platelets	Prostacyclin, prostaglandin E		Maintenance of inactive state
Adrenal cortex	ACTH		Hormone secretion

* Insulin does not act through a G protein; it decreases cAMP levels by alternative routes.

FIG. 27.7

Regulation of adenylate cyclase by the α subunits of the stimulatory and inhibitory G proteins. Some isoforms of adenylate cyclase are affected by $\beta\gamma$-complexes of the G proteins as well. R, Receptor; Cyc, adenylate cyclase.

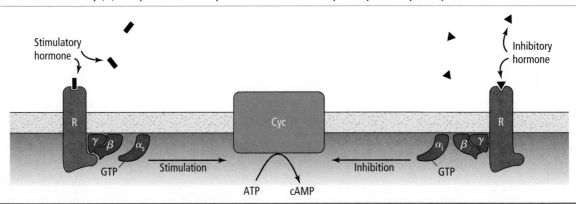

der such names as Tehranitis, Kabulitis, or Montezuma's revenge)—acts by the covalent modification of the G_s protein.

Under ordinary conditions, the cAMP levels in the intestinal mucosa are controlled by peptide hormones and neurotransmitters from the local nerve plexuses. Thus vasoactive intestinal polypeptide (VIP) stimulates, and the endorphins inhibit, cAMP formation. **Pancreatic cholera** is not an infection but rather a neoplastic disease in which severe diar-

rhea is induced by a VIP-secreting pancreatic tumor. Morphine, on the other hand, which inhibits adenylate cyclase by stimulating endorphin receptors, is an excellent antidiarrheal agent.

The inhibitory G protein is also the target of an important bacterial toxin: **pertussis toxin** ADP-ribosylates a cysteine side chain in the α_i subunit of G_i. This covalent modification makes G_i unable to inhibit adenylate cyclase. The effect is the same as with cholera toxin: the cell is flooded with cAMP.

Bordetella pertussis, which produces pertussis toxin, is the cause of whooping cough.

Responses to hormones can be blocked at several levels

Many hormones can act on more than one receptor type, and these receptors may be coupled to different G proteins. Epinephrine, for example, can either stimulate cAMP synthesis by an action on β-adrenergic receptors, or inhibit cAMP synthesis by an action on α_2-adrenergic receptors. In addition, each type of G protein can couple with more than one hormone receptor. *The blockade of a hormone receptor prevents the cAMP response to the normal ligand of the receptor, but other hormones still can act on the cell.* β-Adrenergic receptor blockers, for example, make adipose cells unable to respond to epinephrine. If, however, the cell possesses receptors for other adenylate cyclase–activating hormones such as ACTH, glucagon, and β-lipotropin, then these hormones still can induce cAMP synthesis and lipolysis.

A defective or inhibited G_s or G_i protein, on the other hand, will make the cell unable to respond to any hormone that stimulates or inhibits adenylate cyclase. An example of this situation is seen in **pseudohypoparathyroidism.** Patients with this inherited disorder have hypocalcemia like those with true hypoparathyroidism, but their parathyroid hormone (PTH) levels are either normal or elevated. Some of these patients have an abnormal G_s protein that couples poorly between hormone receptor and adenylate cyclase. Hypocalcemia is present because PTH is one of those hormones that act by stimulating adenylate cyclase (Table 27.2). Not surprisingly, patients with this disorder have associated abnormalities such as short stature and poor intellectual development, because the actions of many hormones other than PTH are impaired as well. Some patients with pseudohypoparathyroidism have a normal G_s protein. They may have abnormalities in adenylate cyclase or protein kinase A.

Cytoplasmic calcium is an important intracellular signal

The distribution of calcium ions in different compartments is remarkable: although the extracellular calcium concentration is on the order of 2 mM, its cytoplasmic concentration is close to 0.2 μM. Why do cells maintain this 10,000-fold concentration difference? The most elementary reason is that phosphate is the principal inorganic anion in the intracellular space. Phosphate, however, forms insoluble salts with calcium, as it does in bones (see Chapter 12), and at an intracellular calcium concentration similar to that in blood and extracellular fluid, the cell soon would be filled with noxious calcium phosphate crystals.

Despite the low cytoplasmic concentrations, *the ER and the mitochondria store a considerable amount of calcium.* The calcium gradients have to be maintained by active transport. The ER and the sarcoplasmic reticulum of muscle cells accumulate calcium by means of a Ca^{2+} ATPase (see Chapter 11); mitochondrial calcium transport is fueled by ATP, the membrane potential, or the proton gradient across the inner membrane; and the plasma membrane contains either a Na^+/Ca^{2+} antiporter or a Ca^{2+} ATPase or both.

Many external agents mediate their cellular effects by inducing a transient increase of the cytoplasmic calcium concentration. They can achieve this by several mechanisms:

1. *The extracellular messenger binds directly to a ligand-gated calcium channel in the plasma membrane.* The NMDA (N-methyl-D-aspartate) type of glutamate receptor in the brain is a ligand-gated calcium channel.
2. *A receptor-coupled G protein opens a calcium channel in the plasma membrane.* Myocardial cells, for example, possess a voltage-gated calcium channel that is positively regulated by the α_s subunit of the G_s protein in response to norepinephrine.
3. *An extracellular stimulus depolarizes the plasma membrane, thereby opening voltage-gated calcium channels.* This mechanism is commonplace in all excitable cells. In nerve terminals, for example, depolarization induces transmitter release by opening voltage-gated calcium channels in the plasma membrane of the nerve terminal. The plasma membrane of smooth muscle cells also is riddled with voltage-gated calcium channels. The voltage-gated calcium channels in vascular smooth muscle cells and in the conducting system of the heart are the targets of verapamil and other **calcium channel blockers.** These drugs are used for the treatment of hypertension, vasospastic

FIG. 27.8

Formation of the second messengers 1,2-diacylglycerol and IP$_3$ from phosphatidylinositol 4,5-bisphosphate. ———, Allosteric stimulation.

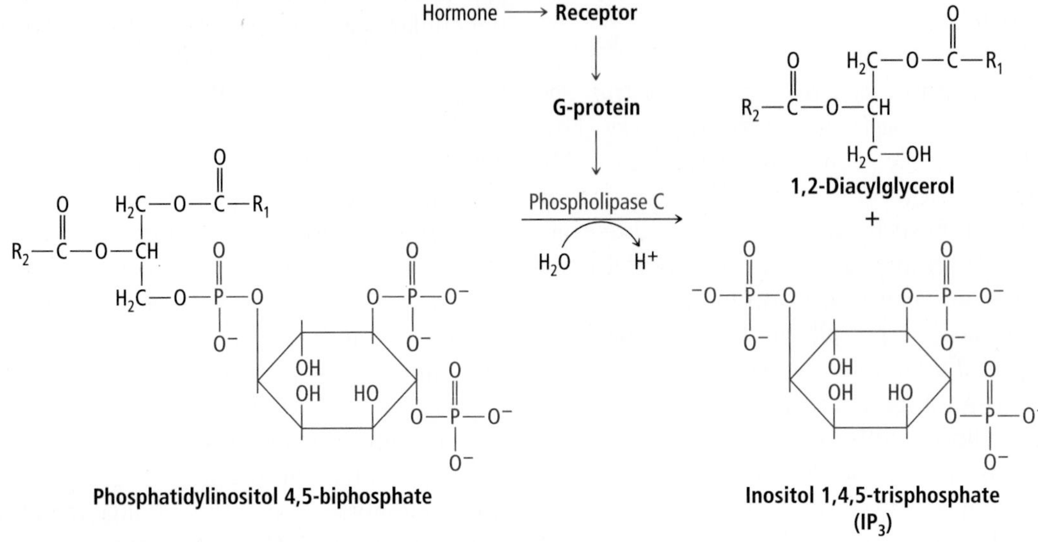

Phosphatidylinositol 4,5-biphosphate

Inositol 1,4,5-trisphosphate (IP$_3$)

disorders, angina pectoris, and cardiac arrhythmias.

4. *An extracellular agent induces the release of calcium from the ER.* This mechanism will be discussed in the following section.

Phospholipase C generates two second messengers

Most calcium-elevating hormones induce the release of calcium from intracellular stores, either from the ER or from ER-derived vesicles. A key event in this signal transduction pathway is the stimulation of a membrane-bound **phospholipase C (PLC)** that is specific for inositol-containing phosphoglycerides (Fig. 27.8). *Like adenylate cyclase, PLC is stimulated by hormone-activated G proteins:* the α-GTP subunits of various G proteins in the G$_q$ family are powerful activators of PLC. These proteins are different from the G$_s$ and G$_i$ proteins that regulate adenylate cyclase. In addition, $\beta\gamma$ complexes derived from G$_i$ proteins are known to stimulate this enzyme.

The hormone-stimulated phospholipase C acts on phosphatidylinositol and its phosphorylated derivatives, which are all present in the inner leaflet of the plasma membrane. Phosphatidylinositol 4,5-bisphosphate is the most important substrate because its cleavage forms the second messenger **inositol**

1,4,5-trisphosphate (IP$_3$; Fig. 27.8). *IP$_3$ induces the release of stored calcium from the ER by binding to a calcium channel in the ER membrane.*

IP$_3$ itself is converted to inositol by successive dephosphorylations, either directly or after an initial phosphorylation to inositol 1,3,4,5-tetrakisphosphate (IP$_4$). IP$_4$ may participate in the system itself, possibly by stimulating further calcium influx through the plasma membrane.

1,2-Diacylglycerol, the second product of phospholipase C, also is a second messenger: in the presence of calcium and phosphatidylserine, it stimulates the membrane-bound enzyme **protein kinase C** (Fig. 27.9). Like protein kinase A, protein kinase C phosphorylates serine and threonine side chains of proteins. Although some proteins, including glycogen synthase (see Chapter 17), can be phosphorylated by both enzymes, the substrate specificities of the two kinases are quite different. In many cells, the phosphorylation of proteins by protein kinase C promotes cell growth (see Chapter 28). **Phorbol esters,** which are naturally present in croton oil, act as tumor promoters by activating protein kinase C.

Calcium induces its effects by binding to specific regulatory proteins. In striated muscle, for example, we encountered troponin C as a calcium sensor on the thin filaments (see Chapter 12). A second calcium-binding protein, **calmodulin** (MW 17,000), which is

FIG. 27.9

G protein–coupled receptors *(R₁, R₂ . . .)* and their second messenger systems. Note that more than one hormone receptor (🔲) can couple to an effector in the plasma membrane (⬛). The effector produces the second messenger, and the second messenger stimulates intracellular targets (▦). Note also that some receptors can couple to more than one G protein (G_i and G_q in the case of R_3) and thereby act on different effectors. *AC,* Adenylate cyclase; *PLC,* phosphatidylinositol-specific phospholipase C; *cAMP,* cyclic AMP; *PIP₂,* phosphatidylinositol 4,5-bisphosphate; *IP₃,* inositol 1,4,5-trisphosphate; *DAG,* 1,2-diacylglycerol; *IP₃-R,* IP₃ receptor (an IP₃-regulated calcium channel in the ER); *PKC,* protein kinase C.

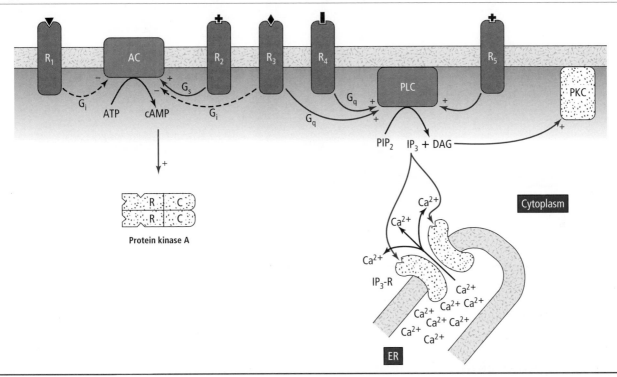

related structurally to troponin C, is present not only in striated muscle but in all nucleated cells. In a Ca^{2+} concentration range of 10^{-7} to 10^{-6} M, *calmodulin forms a calcium complex that functions as an activator of many enzymes.* Examples of Ca^{2+}-calmodulin–activated enzymes include phosphorylase kinase (see Chapter 17), the Mg^{2+}/Ca^{2+} ATPase in the sarcoplasmic reticulum (see Chapter 11), and the myosin light-chain kinase in smooth muscle cells. The Ca^{2+}-calmodulin–regulated enzymes include a family of protein kinases that phosphorylate serine and threonine side chains and have substrate specificities different from those of protein kinases A and C.

Both cAMP and calcium affect gene transcription

After their release from the regulatory subunits in the presence of cAMP, the active catalytic subunits of protein kinase A are able to translocate to the nu-

cleus, where they phosphorylate several transcription factors, including the **CREB protein** (**c**yclic AMP **r**esponse **e**lement **b**inding). These transcription factors form homo- and heterodimers that bind to the **cAMP response element**, a palindromic sequence (TGACGTCA) in the promoters and enhancers of the cAMP-regulated genes. Although even dephosphorylated CREB is bound to the response element, *it stimulates transcription only after the phosphorylation of a single serine residue (Ser-133) by protein kinase A.*

Calcium also can act on the cAMP-regulated genes (Fig. 27.10): a calcium-calmodulin–activated protein kinase, CaMK II, phosphorylates a different serine residue (Ser-142) in CREB, and this phosphorylation prevents transcriptional activation. Both CaMK II and another calcium-calmodulin–dependent protein kinase, CaMK IV, also can phosphorylate Ser-133 and thereby activate transcription. As a result, *calcium can act either synergistically or antagonistically with cAMP in the regulation of gene expression,* depending on

FIG. 27.10

Actions of the protein kinase A catalytic subunit *(PKA)* and of calcium-calmodulin–activated protein kinases (CaMK II, CaMK IV) on the CREB protein, which mediates cAMP effects on transcription. The phosphorylation of Ser-133 is thought to induce transcription through a CREB-binding protein *(CBP)* that binds both to phosphorylated CREB and to transcription factor IIB in the transcriptional initiation complex. The phosphorylation of Ser-142 is thought to prevent this interaction. ⟶, Allosteric stimulation; ⟿, activating phosphorylation; ⟿, inhibitory phosphorylation.

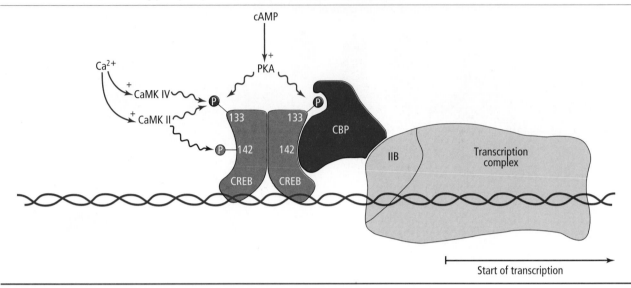

the presence of individual calcium-calmodulin–regulated protein kinases in the cell.

Muscle contraction and exocytosis are triggered by calcium

Muscle contraction is always calcium dependent. Striated muscle contraction requires the binding of calcium to troponin C on the thin filaments (see Chapter 12), but smooth muscle cells do not have troponin. Their contraction is calcium dependent, too, but *the calcium-sensing protein in smooth muscle is calmodulin, not troponin C* (Fig. 27.11). The Ca^{2+}-calmodulin complex activates **myosin light-chain kinase,** and this enzyme causes contraction by phosphorylating a pair of light chains on the globular head of myosin. cAMP decreases the calcium concentration by unknown mechanisms, probably by inducing the phosphorylation of several proteins involved in calcium homeostasis. A direct action of the α_s-GTP subunit on voltage-gated calcium channels also has been described in some types of smooth muscle. For these reasons, *smooth muscle is contracted by agents that increase cytoplasmic calcium or decrease cAMP, and it is relaxed by cAMP-increasing agents* (Table 27.2 and 27.3).

Bronchial smooth muscle, for example, is contracted by the calcium-elevating agents histamine, acting through H$_1$ receptors, and acetylcholine, acting through muscarinic receptors. β-Adrenergic agonists, on the other hand, relax bronchial smooth muscle by increasing cAMP. Therefore epinephrine and other β agonists can be used for the treatment of asthma and other obstructive pulmonary diseases. Phosphodiesterase inhibitors such as theophylline and aminophylline also are useful in asthma because they elevate intracellular cAMP.

Like muscle contraction, *the release of water-soluble products by exocytosis is always triggered by calcium.* Examples include the release of neurotransmitters from nerve terminals, zymogens from the pancreas, insulin from pancreatic β cells, and histamine from mast cells (Table 27.3).

Cyclic GMP is a second messenger in the retinal rod cell

Besides cAMP, **cyclic GMP (cGMP)** is an important second messenger in many cells. The synthesis and degradation of cGMP are analogous to the corresponding steps in cAMP metabolism:

FIG. 27.11

Regulation of smooth muscle contraction by calcium. Calcium enters the cytoplasm either from the extracellular space through voltage-gated calcium channels or through the IP_3-operated channel in the ER. Voltage-gated calcium channels are regulated indirectly by neurotransmitters that act on ligand-gated ion channels. However, they also are regulated by hormone-operated G proteins, and they can be phosphorylated by protein kinases that are themselves under the control of second messengers. R_1, R_2, G protein–linked hormone receptors; *PLC*, phospholipase C; *MLC-kinase*, myosin light-chain kinase.

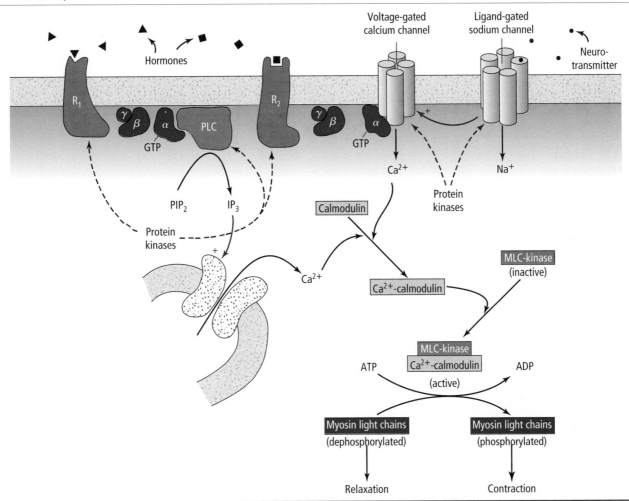

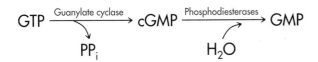

Several guanylate cyclases and phosphodiesterases have been identified in different tissues, and some of these are under the control of hormones or other external stimuli.

In retinal rod cells, cGMP functions as a link in the processing of the visual stimulus. In the absence of light, the membrane of the rod cell is half depolarized, and the cell releases its transmitter continuously. This state is maintained by the presence of cGMP, which is synthesized by a constitutively active guanylate cyclase. cGMP binds to a sodium channel in the plasma membrane, maintaining this channel in the open state. *In response to light, the cGMP level declines, the sodium channel closes, the membrane hyperpolarizes, and transmitter release is curtailed.*

The light-sensing molecule in the retinal rod cell is **rhodopsin.** This protein is located in the optic discs, a membrane system in the outer segment of the rod cell (Fig. 27.12). Rhodopsin is an integral membrane protein with seven transmembrane helices, and it is indeed a distant relative of the β-adrenergic receptor and the other seven-transmembrane

TABLE 27.3

Effects of elevated cytoplasmic calcium levels in different tissues

Tissue/cell type	Agents inducing release from ER	Effects
Pancreatic acinar cells	Cholecystokinin, acetylcholine	Zymogen secretion
Intestinal mucosa	Acetylcholine	Water and electrolyte secretion
Platelets	Thromboxane, collagen, thrombin, platelet-activating factor, ADP	Shape change, degranulation
Endothelial cells	Histamine, bradykinin, ATP, acetylcholine, thrombin	Nitric oxide synthesis
Vascular smooth muscle cells	Epinephrine (α_1 receptor), angiotensin II, vasopressin	Contraction
Bronchial smooth muscle cells	Histamine	Contraction
Thyroid gland	TSH	Hormone synthesis and release
Corpus luteum	LHRH	Hormone synthesis
Liver	Epinephrine (α_1 receptor)	Glycogen degradation

receptors. The vitamin A derivative **11-*cis* retinal** is the light-absorbing part of rhodopsin. It is bound in the center of the molecule, interacting with the membrane-spanning α helices. The aldehyde group of 11-*cis* retinal is linked to a lysine residue in the apoprotein by a protonated Schiff base bond.

*Visible light isomerizes 11-cis retinal to all-*trans*-retinal* (Fig. 27.13). This photoisomerization switches rhodopsin to an activated, "photoexcited" conformation known as **metarhodopsin II (R*)**. The Schiff-base bond between all-*trans* retinal and the apoprotein in R* then hydrolyzes, and all-*trans* retinal dissociates from the apoprotein.

Before the bond between all-*trans* retinal and opsin in R* is hydrolyzed, however, the photoexcited rhodopsin does something useful: *it activates the G protein **transducin**,* a member of the G_i family of heterotrimeric G proteins. The α subunit–GTP complex dissociates from the $\beta\gamma$ subunits and activates a cGMP-specific phosphodiesterase. Thereby *the light stimulus decreases the cellular cGMP concentration.* The decreased cGMP level, in turn, leads to closure of the sodium channels, hyperpolarization, and decreased transmitter release.

The light-induced stimulus is highly amplified: a single photoexcited rhodopsin molecule activates approximately 500 transducin molecules; each transducin-activated phosphodiesterase molecule hydrolyzes approximately 1000 cGMP molecules per second; and cGMP inhibition of a single sodium channel prevents the influx of thousands of sodium ions. Therefore a single photon can prevent the influx of more than a million sodium ions and can hyperpolarize the cell by approximately 1 mV.

The somewhat exotic environment of the retinal rod cell shows some interesting variations on the theme of signal transduction. We have encountered:

- *A receptor* (rhodopsin) that responds not to a hormone but to photons
- *A G protein* (transducin) that activates not adenylate cyclase or phospholipase C but a cGMP-specific phosphodiesterase
- *A second messenger* (cGMP) whose cellular level is adjusted by regulation not of its synthesis but of its degradation
- *An ion channel* that is regulated neither by the membrane potential nor by a neurotransmitter, G protein, or protein kinase, but rather by the direct binding of a second messenger.

RECEPTORS WITH ENZYMATIC ACTIVITIES

Although all extracellular messengers affect the activities of cellular enzymes indirectly, some can do so directly, by binding to receptors that are themselves enzymes. These receptors are simply allosteric enzymes for which the extracellular messenger is an allosteric effector.

FIG. 27.12

Signal transduction in the retinal rod cell. **A,** Structure of the retinal rod cell. **B,** The visual cascade. *R,* Rhodopsin; *R*,* photoexcited rhodopsin; *hν,* visible light; *PDE,* cGMP phosphodiesterase.

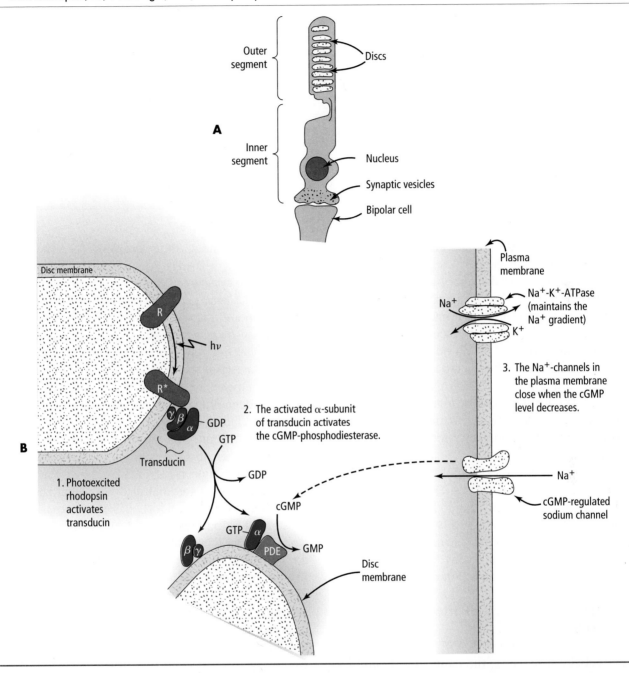

The receptor for atrial natriuretic factor is a membrane-bound guanylate cyclase

Phosphodiesterase activity controls the cGMP level in retinal rod cells (as we described earlier). **Guanylate cyclase** is the more important regulated enzyme in most other cells.

In some tissues, cGMP is regulated by **atrial natriuretic factor (ANF)**, a peptide hormone (28 amino acids) that is released from the atrium of the heart in response to increased blood volume, increased blood pressure, and increased salt intake. It acts on the kidney to increase glomerular filtration rate, urine volume, and sodium excretion. It also decreases renin re-

FIG. 27.13

Photoisomerization of 11-*cis* retinal to all-*trans* retinal. Retinal is the prosthetic group of rhodopsin in the rod cells and of the related "color vision" pigments in the cone cells.

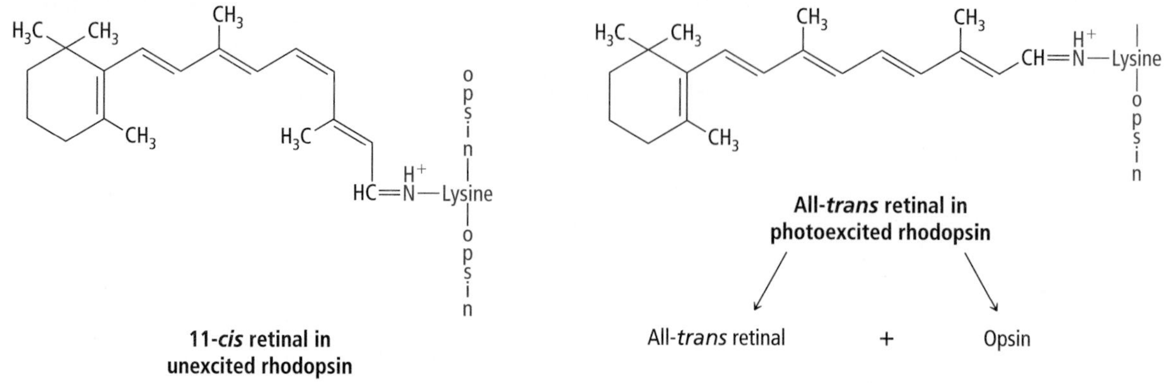

**11-*cis* retinal in
unexcited rhodopsin**

**All-*trans* retinal in
photoexcited rhodopsin**

All-*trans* retinal   +   Opsin

lease from the juxtaglomerular cells and aldosterone release from the zonaglomerulosa of the adrenal cortex, and it relaxes vascular smooth muscle.

The ANF receptor is a membrane protein with an extracellular ligand-binding domain, a single transmembrane helix, and an intracellular domain that acts as a guanylate cyclase, all on the same polypeptide. *The intracellular guanylate cyclase domain requires the binding of ANF to the extracellular domain for its catalytic activity.* Once formed, *cGMP activates a protein kinase that is conveniently named* **protein kinase G.** It mediates most of the cGMP effects by phosphorylating a variety of cellular proteins.

The cyclic nucleotides are not entirely specific for their respective protein kinases. Thus, cAMP can cause vasodilation by activating protein kinase G in vascular smooth muscle cells. High levels of cGMP in the intestinal mucosa, on the other hand—induced, for example, by bacterial enterotoxins—can cause fluid secretion and diarrhea by an action on protein kinase A.

Nitric oxide and cGMP mediate vasodilation

ANF acts by stimulating the membrane-bound form of guanylate cyclase, which is actually the intracellular domain of the ANF receptor. Although some vascular beds are relaxed by ANF, the principal guanylate cyclase of vascular smooth muscle is a soluble, cytoplasmic enzyme. This cytoplasmic guanylate cyclase is not activated by ANF but by **nitric oxide (NO)**, which is synthesized in endothelial cells from one of the nitrogens in the side

chain of arginine as shown in Box 27.4. The endothelial NO synthase is stimulated by calcium-calmodulin, so *synthesis of NO is stimulated by agents that elevate the cytoplasmic calcium concentration in endothelial cells.*

As a membrane-permeant paracrine messenger, *NO diffuses from the endothelial cells to the underlying smooth muscle cells, where it activates the cytoplasmic guanylate cyclase* (Fig. 27.14). NO is chemically unstable and decomposes within a few seconds, without the need for degrading enzymes. The **nitro-vasodilator drugs,** including nitroglycerine and nitroprusside, relax vascular smooth muscle because they form NO during their metabolism. These drugs, shown in Box 27.5, are time-honored treatments for angina pectoris and other vascular disorders. Pharmacological inhibitors of the endothelial NO synthase cause substantial blood pressure increases. This shows that *formation of NO is important for blood pressure regulation under ordinary conditions.* Physiological agents such as histamine, acetylcholine, bradykinin, thrombin, and ATP relax vascular smooth muscle by increasing the intracellular calcium concentration and stimulating NO synthesis in endothelial cells.

In the corpora cavernosa of the penis (Fig. 27.15), we encounter a vascular bed that is expected to respond to parasympathetic nerve stimulation by profound vasodilation. **Vasoactive intestinal polypeptide (VIP),** released from the nerve terminals to-gether with acetylcholine, acts directly on the smooth muscle cells to stimulate adenylate cyclase through the stimulatory G protein. **Acetylcholine,** on the other hand, acts indirectly: it increases the cytoplasmic calcium concentration in endothelial

FIG. 27.14

Formation of cyclic GMP *(cGMP)* in vascular smooth muscle cells. The atrial natriuretic factor *(ANF)* receptor is present not only in vascular smooth muscle but in the kidney and some other tissues as well. Nitric oxide *(NO)* acts as "endothelium-derived relaxing factor." ——▶, Allosteric stimulation; *R,* ANF receptor.

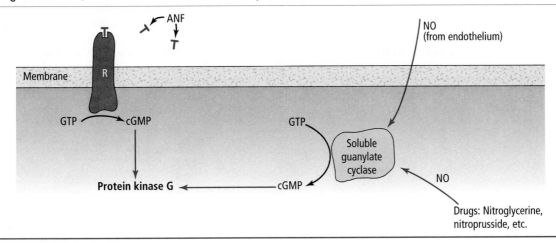

BOX 27.4

Arginine + NADPH → Hydroxyarginine + Citrulline + NO

BOX 27.5

Nitroglycerine   Nitroprusside

FIG. 27.15

Signaling pathways that mediate vasodilation and erection in the corpora cavernosa of the penis. Acetylcholine *(Ach)*, vasoactive intestinal polypeptide *(VIP)*, and possibly other neurotransmitters are released from parasympathetic nerve terminals during sexual arousal. While VIP acts directly on smooth muscle cells to induce cAMP synthesis, acetylcholine signals through muscarinic receptors on endothelial cells to increase cytoplasmic calcium. The calcium-calmodulin−stimulated NO synthase produces NO, which diffuses to the underlying smooth muscle cells, where it stimulates guanylate cyclase. The nerve terminals in this tissue also contain NO synthase, which may be stimulated by calcium entering through voltage-gated calcium channels. It is not known whether cAMP induces its effects through protein kinase A *(PKA)* or protein kinase G *(PKG)* in this tissue. *Arg*, Arginine; *Cit*, citrulline; *AC*, adenylate cyclase; *PLC*, phospholipase C.

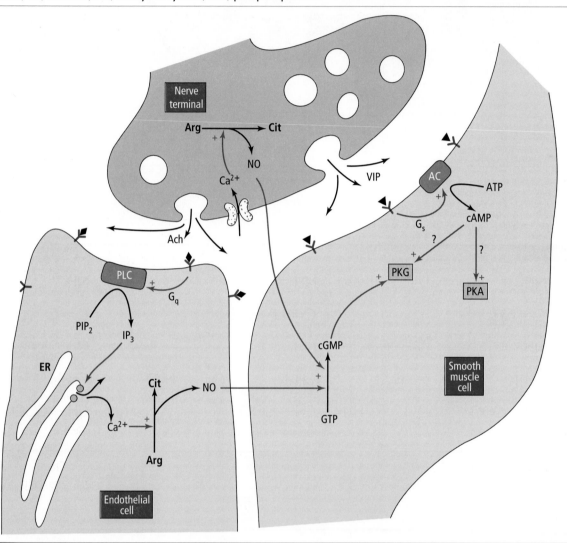

cells, thereby activating the endothelial NO synthase. In this tissue, NO synthase is also present in parasympathetic nerve terminals, where its activity is stimulated by the influx of calcium through voltage-gated calcium channels. This example shows how three different cell types, using separate signal transduction pathways, can cooperate productively in the pursuit of a noble cause.

Receptors for insulin and growth factors contain a protein tyrosine kinase domain

The insulin receptor, as well as the receptors for a variety of growth factors, are membrane glycoproteins with an unusual enzymatic activity: after binding of the ligand to the extracellular domain, *the in-*

FIG. 27.16

Receptor for epidermal growth factor *(EGF)*. Ligand binding induces dimerization or oligomerization of the receptor, followed by autophosphorylation on tyrosine side chains. Most growth factors act by this general mechanism. Their actions are terminated by tyrosine-specific protein phosphatases that dephosphorylate the receptor and its substrates.

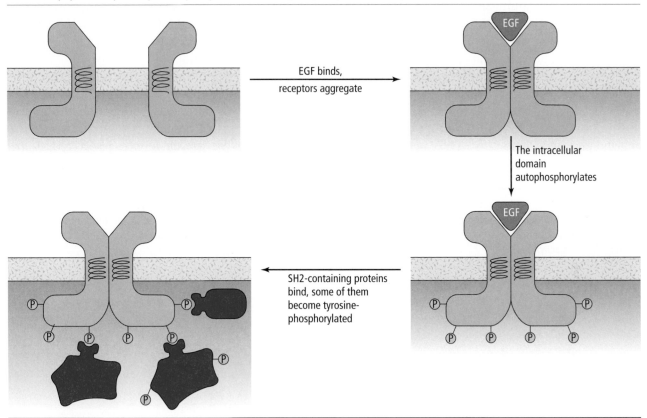

EGF binds, receptors aggregate

The intracellular domain autophosphorylates

SH2-containing proteins bind, some of them become tyrosine-phosphorylated

tracellular domain phosphorylates proteins on tyrosine side chains (Figs. 27.16 and 27.17). The protein kinases that we have encountered so far, on the other hand, including the hormone-stimulated protein kinases A, C, and G, all phosphorylate serine and threonine residues in their substrates. In resting cells, less than 0.1% of the protein-bound phosphate is on tyrosine side chains. The substrate specificity of these receptors is unusual as well: after ligand binding, *the receptors aggregate in the membrane and phosphorylate each other.* This activity is called **autophosphorylation.**

Most tyrosine protein kinase receptors can autophosphorylate on several tyrosine side chains, sometimes more than a dozen in a single receptor molecule. The effect of autophosphorylation is twofold: *it stimulates the receptor kinase activity toward external substrates,* and *it creates docking sites for various cytoplasmic and membrane-associated proteins.* Most of these proteins bind to tyrosine-phosphorylated sites

through a specialized domain, the **SH2 domain** (SH for *src* homology). Because each protein tyrosine kinase receptor has a unique combination of autophosphorylation sites, *each receptor can interact with a unique set of SH2-containing binding proteins.* Binding to the autophosphorylated receptor can have several consequences:

1. *Soluble cytoplasmic proteins are recruited to the plasma membrane,* where they serve specialized functions, either as enzymes or as links in signaling pathways.
2. *Receptor binding can affect the biological properties of the bound molecules allosterically.* The activities of enzymes, for example, may change once they are bound to the autophosphorylated receptor.
3. *The bound proteins may become tyrosine phosphorylated by the receptor,* and this phosphorylation is likely to affect their biological properties.

Insulin receptor signaling (Fig. 27.17) shows a variation on this theme: although autophosphorylation stimulates the tyrosine protein kinase activity of the receptor, it does not create effective docking sites for SH2-containing proteins. Instead, the receptor binds a 131-kDa phosphoprotein called **IRS-1** (insulin receptor substrate 1), which becomes extensively phosphorylated on approximately 20 tyrosine residues. *These phosphotyrosine residues are the docking sites for the SH2-containing proteins.* The signaling pathways for the metabolic effects of insulin are still poorly known beyond the point of IRS-1 binding and phosphorylation.

Many receptors become desensitized after overstimulation

Many cells lose their responsiveness when they are exposed to high concentrations of an extracellular messenger. This process of **desensitization** can occur rapidly within seconds to minutes, or gradually in the course of several hours or days.

The β-adrenergic receptor, for example, becomes unable to activate the G$_s$ protein within minutes of agonist exposure, although it still can bind the hormone. The receptor desensitizes because *the intracellular domain of the receptor becomes phosphorylated after*

FIG. 27.17

The insulin receptor. Unlike the growth factor receptors, which are monomers in the unstimulated state, the insulin receptor is a disulfide-bonded tetramer. Also, the insulin receptor does not bind SH2-containing signaling proteins itself but rather recruits IRS-1 for this purpose.

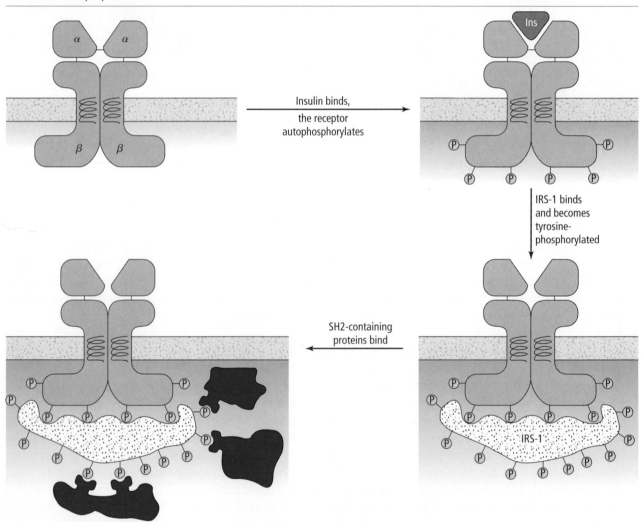

FIG. 27.18

Desensitization of β-adrenergic receptors by phosphorylation. *BARK*, β-Adrenergic receptor kinase. Only the ligand-stimulated receptor is phosphorylated by BARK. Note that the receptor can be desensitized not only by β-adrenergic agonists but also by other cAMP-elevating agonists that act through protein kinase A. The phosphorylated receptor still can bind its ligand, but it is uncoupled from the G_s protein. ——→, Allosteric activation; ⌇→, inhibitory phosphorylation.

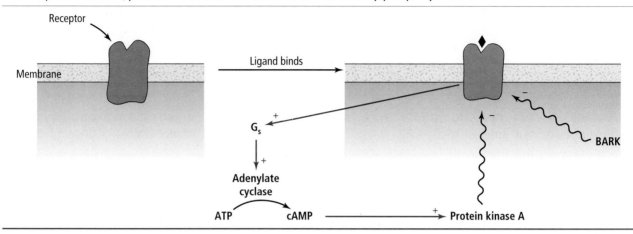

FIG. 27.19

Down-regulation by receptor-mediated endocytosis. ⊺, Receptor; ▼, hormone.

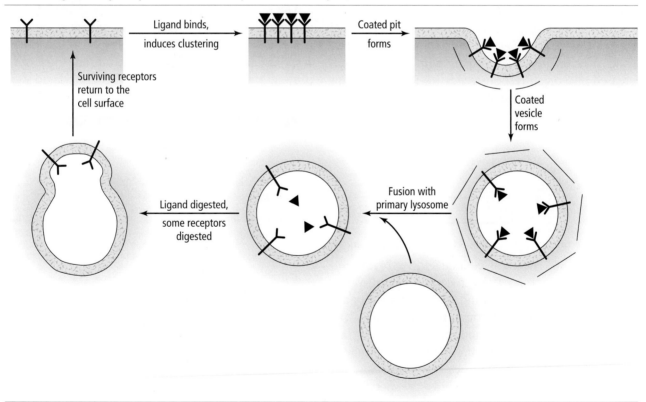

agonist exposure (Fig. 27.18). This phosphorylation can be effected by a specific **β-adrenergic receptor kinase (BARK)**, which phosphorylates the stimulated but not the unstimulated receptor. Protein kinase A also phosphorylates the activated receptor, thereby forming a negative feedback loop. Indeed, many G_s-linked receptors are phosphorylated by protein kinase A. *This type of desensitization can be reversed by the action of protein phosphatases*, which gradually remove the phosphate groups from the desensitized receptor.

Another type of desensitization results from **receptor-mediated endocytosis** (Fig. 27.19). In this process, ligand-stimulated receptors aggregate on the cell surface and are internalized in an endocytotic vesicle. Eventually, this vesicle fuses with a lysosome, where the bound ligand is degraded. Although some of the receptors are returned to the cell surface, receptor recycling is not very efficient for many hormone receptors, and some of the endocytosed receptors fall victim to the lysosomal enzymes themselves. In the case of the epidermal growth factor (EGF) receptor, for example, only approximately half of the internalized receptors return safely to the cell surface. *The loss of receptors by internalization and subsequent degradation can be remedied only by the synthesis of new receptors.* This long-term type of desensitization is called **down-regulation.** The decreased end-organ responsiveness to insulin in many patients with type II diabetes mellitus, for example (see Chapter 29), is thought to result at least in part from an inability to replace insulin receptors that have been lost by receptor-mediated endocytosis.

SUMMARY

Hormones, neurotransmitters, and other extracellular messengers initiate their cellular effects by binding to specific receptors. These receptors are allosteric proteins that bind their ligand with high affinity and selectivity. The receptors for steroid hormones, thyroid hormones, calcitriol, and retinoic acid are transcription factors that encounter their hormonal ligand either in the cytoplasm or in the nucleus. The receptor-hormone complex binds to specific response elements in the regulatory sites of genes and affects the rate of transcription.

Water-soluble agents have to bind to receptors on the cell surface. For many neurotransmitters, the receptor is a ligand-gated ion channel. Most hormones, on the other hand, act on plasma membrane receptors that are coupled to a heterotrimeric G protein. Hormone binding to the receptor activates the G protein, and the components of the activated G protein act on effector proteins in the plasma membrane.

Most hormones induce the formation of a second messenger. Second messengers are small, diffusible molecules such as cyclic AMP, cyclic GMP, inositol 1,4,5-trisphosphate, and 1,2-diacylglycerol, which are suitable for long-distance signaling throughout the cell. cAMP is synthesized by adenylate cyclase, an enzyme in the plasma membrane that can be both stimulated and inhibited by receptor-controlled G proteins. Adenylate cyclase affects intracellular targets by stimulating protein kinase A. IP_3 is synthesized by a hormone-activated phospholipase C. This second messenger induces the release of calcium from the ER. cGMP is synthesized either by a membrane-bound guanylate cyclase that functions as a receptor for atrial natriuretic factor, or by a cytoplasmic enzyme that is stimulated by nitric oxide.

The receptors for insulin and many growth factors are membrane proteins with an intrinsic tyrosine protein kinase activity. They autophosphorylate in response to ligand binding and transmit signals via protein binding to the tyrosine-phosphorylated sites.

Further Reading

Andersson K-E, Wagner G: Physiology of penile erection. *Physiol Rev 75* (1), 191−236, 1995.

Bootman MD, Berridge MJ: The elemental principles of calcium signaling. *Cell 83*, 675−678, 1995.

Bredt DS, Snyder SH: Nitric oxide: a physiological messenger molecule. *Annu Rev Biochem 63*, 175−195, 1994.

Casey PJ: Protein lipidation in cell signaling. *Science 268*, 221−225, 1995.

Clapham DE: Calcium signaling. *Cell 80*, 259−268, 1995.

Conti M, Nemoz G, Sette C, Vicini E: Recent progress in understanding the hormonal regulation of phosphodiesterases. *Endocrine Rev 16* (3), 370−389, 1995.

D'Arcangelo G, Curran T: Smart transcription factors. *Nature 376*, 292−293, 1995.

de Groot LJ et al, editors: *Endocrinology*, 3rd ed., vol. 1. W. B. Saunders, Philadelphia, 1995, pp. 3–147, 1656–1667.

Furuichi T, Mikoshiba K: Inositol 1,4,5-trisphosphate receptor-mediated calcium signaling in the brain. *J Neurochem* 64 (3), 953–960, 1995.

Garbers DL, Lowe DG: Guanylyl cyclase receptors. *J Biol Chem* 269 (49), 30741–30744, 1994.

Ghosh A, Greenberg ME: Calcium signaling in neurons: molecular mechanisms and cellular consequences. *Science* 268, 239–247, 1995.

Graves LM, Lawrence JC Jr: Insulin, growth factors and cAMP: antagonism in the signal transduction pathways. *Trends Endocrinol Metabol* 7, 43–50, 1996.

Hein L, Kobilka BK: Adrenergic receptor signal transduction and regulation. *Neuropharmacology* 34 (4), 357–366, 1995.

Howe LR, Weiss A: Multiple kinases mediate T-cell receptor signaling. *Trends Biochem Sci* 20, 59–64, 1995.

Lauffenburger DA, Linderman JJ: *Receptors: models for binding, trafficking and signaling.* Oxford University Press, New York, 1993.

Lincoln TM: *Cyclic GMP: biochemistry, physiology and pathophysiology.* R. G. Landes, Austin TX, 1994.

Lismaa TP, Biden TJ, Shine J: *G protein-coupled receptors.* R. G. Landes, Austin TX, 1995.

Marks F, editor: *Protein phosphorylation.* Weinheim, New York, 1996.

Mochly-Rosen D: Localization of protein kinases by anchoring proteins: a theme in signal transduction. *Science* 268, 247–251, 1995.

Myers MG Jr, Sun XJ, White MF: The IRS-1 signaling system. *Trends Biochem Sci* 19, 289–293, 1994.

Neer EJ: Heterotrimeric G proteins: organizers of transmembrane signals. *Cell* 80, 249–257, 1995.

Spiegel AM, Jones TLE, Simonds WF, Weinstein LS: *G proteins.* R. G. Landes, Austin TX, 1994.

Sundberg DK: Postsynaptic receptors. In: Conn PM, editor: *Neuroscience in medicine.* J. B. Lippincott, Philadelphia, 1995, pp. 115–133.

Wera S, Hemmings BA: Serine/threonine protein phosphatases. *Biochem J* 311, 17–29, 1995.

Yarfitz S, Hurley JB: Transduction mechanisms of vertebrate and invertebrate photoreceptors. *J Biol Chem* 269 (20), 14329–14332, 1994.

Yau K-W: Cyclic nucleotide-gated channels: an expanding new family of ion channels. *Proc Natl Acad Sci USA* 91, 3481–3483, 1994.

Zenner G, zur Hausen JD, Burn P, Mustelin T: Towards unraveling the complexity of T cell signal transduction. *Bioessays* 17 (11), 967–975, 1995.

QUESTIONS

1. Vascular smooth muscle contracts when the cytoplasmic calcium level increases. Nevertheless, many natural agents that stimulate the phosphatidylinositol/calcium system (including acetylcholine, histamine, and bradykinin) are potent vasodilators. Why?
   A. In the vascular smooth muscle cell, calcium rapidly equilibrates across the plasma membrane.
   B. The calcium-calmodulin complex blocks voltage-gated calcium channels in vascular smooth muscle.
   C. An increased cytoplasmic calcium concentration in endothelial cells causes the transfer of calcium from smooth muscle to endothelial cells through gap junctions.
   D. The calcium-calmodulin complex stimulates nitric oxide synthase in endothelial cells.
   E. The calcium-calmodulin complex inhibits adenylate cyclase in vascular smooth muscle cells.

2. The activation of the phosphatidylinositol/calcium system leads to growth stimulation in many cells, both normal cells and cancer cells. To inhibit this second messenger system, you could try to develop a drug that
   A. Inhibits the dephosphorylation of inositol 1,4,5-trisphosphate
   B. Stimulates protein kinase C
   C. Reacts chemically with the α subunits of the G_q proteins, thereby making them unable to bind to phospholipase C
   D. Inhibits the GTPase activity of the G_q proteins
   E. Inhibits the active transport of calcium in the plasma membrane

3. The expression of many genes is increased in the presence of a high cytoplasmic cAMP concentration. How does cAMP affect gene expression?
   A. It induces the phosphorylation of transcription factors.

B. It binds directly to cAMP response elements in promoters and enhancers.

C. It mediates this effect by increasing the calcium concentration in the cytoplasm and the nucleus.

D. It binds to nuclear transcription factors whose DNA binding and transcriptional activation are affected by the bound cAMP.

4. Most growth factor receptors are able to phosphorylate tyrosine side chains of proteins. Although the substrates of the activated receptors differ, one protein always becomes tyrosine phosphorylated. This protein is

A. Adenylate cyclase

B. Inositol trisphosphate

C. Protein kinase C

D. Protein kinase A

E. The receptor itself

Chapter 28

Cellular Growth Control and Cancer

The genetic information of somatic cells, which ultimately is derived from the fertilized ovum, or **zygote,** has to be passed down through a chain of mitotic events. The progression through repeated cycles of cell division requires a meticulously timed sequence of regulatory events. Superimposed on this intrinsic system of cell cycle progression, the cell has to adjust its growth to its environment: it has to respond to external signals. These signals regulate two aspects of cell growth: *they increase or decrease the rate of cell proliferation,* and *they induce and maintain the differentiated state of the diverse cell types.* The regulation of cell growth and differentiation is of particular interest for the medical sciences because *derangements of cellular growth control are the cause of cancer,* and cancer accounts for approximately 20% of all deaths in industrialized countries. Indeed, the molecular mechanisms of neoplastic diseases are unraveling at a breathtaking pace, and even now the process of carcinogenesis can be described, in part, in molecular terms. In this chapter we will encounter the elements of cell cycle control, the responses of the cell to growth-regulating stimuli, and the principles of carcinogenesis.

CELL CYCLE CONTROL

The cells in embryonic tissues, as well as in many adult tissues, proceed through repeated rounds of cell division. The replicative cycle of these cells, known as the **cell cycle,** requires a carefully timed sequence of events that include cyclic alterations in gene expression and protein phosphorylation.

The cell cycle is regulated at two important checkpoints

Routine cytological examination reveals two principal stages of the cell cycle: **interphase** and **mitosis** (Fig. 28.1). Interphase is the period between cell divisions when the cell possesses an intact nuclear membrane, with chromatin dispersed throughout the nucleus. Mitosis is the stage of cell division. It takes approximately 1 hour and consists of a well-defined sequence of events: the chromatin condenses into chromosomes, the nuclear membrane disintegrates into numerous small vesicles, the mitotic spindle forms, and the replicated chromosomes are pulled to opposite poles of the cell. Finally the cytoplasm divides to form two daughter cells.

Based on biochemical rather than cytological events, interphase is subdivided into G_1, **S,** and G_2 phases. During G_1 (G for gap), which follows mitosis, the cellular genome is in the **diploid** state: each chromosome, and each gene, is present in two copies. This is followed by S phase (S for synthesis), during which the DNA is replicated, and finally by G_2.

The cell makes two important all-or-none decisions during the cell cycle: the first decision, made late in G_1, is the *entry into S phase.* DNA replication

FIG. 28.1

The cell cycle. G_1 + S + G_2 = interphase. The DNA is replicated during the S (synthesis) phase; the chromosomes segregate during mitosis (M). Nondividing cells are in G_0.

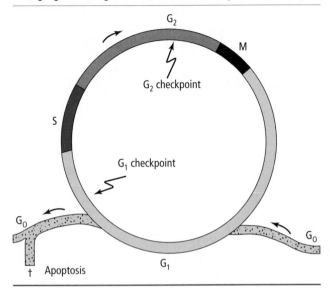

should be embarked on only when the cell is ready to progress through the complete cell cycle, and it should be initiated only after any DNA damage that may have been sustained during the preceding stages has been thoroughly repaired. The second all-or-none decision is the *entry into mitosis.* Mitosis should be initiated only after the completion of DNA replication and only if the replicated chromosomes are structurally intact; once initiated, mitosis has to proceed through all stages. These two all-or-none decisions define the **G_1 checkpoint** and the **G_2 checkpoint,** respectively.

Only dividing cells proceed through the cell cycle. Nondividing cells are said to be in **G_0.** Some nondividing cells, such as neurons and skeletal muscle fibers, are unable to re-enter the cell cycle. Others, such as fibroblasts, hepatocytes, and lymphocytes, are usually in G_0 but can be activated by external agents. Fibroblasts, for example, can be stimulated into the cell cycle by platelet-derived growth factor or by other growth factors during wound healing, and lymphocytes in peripheral blood divide after exposure to antigen and to cytokines released from helper T cells.

Cells also can commit suicide by programmed cell death, or **apoptosis.** Apoptosis is a normal event during embryonic development, but it also occurs in response to severe cellular damage, viral infections, and somatic mutations. *Apoptosis is a protective mechanism that eliminates many virus-infected and genetically altered cells.* It is especially important for the elimination of somatically mutated cells that have the potential of evolving into cancer cells. Although apoptosis is induced by many damaging agents that also can induce "ordinary" cell death, or **necrosis,** apoptosis and necrosis can be distinguished cytologically. Unlike necrosis, apoptosis depends on the selective induction of specific proteases and nucleases that degrade the cellular proteins and nucleic acids.

The cell cycle can be studied in cultured cells

Cells in the living organism are not amenable to observation, biochemical analysis, and experimental manipulations, so most studies on cell cycle control in humans and other mammals have to rely on cultured cells. Cells suitable for culture include, for example, white blood cells, fibroblasts, and various types of epithelial cells. Typical features of these cultured cells include:

1. *The cells grow only in the presence of **mitogens.*** Most physiological mitogens are **growth factors**—soluble extracellular proteins that are required in minute quantities for cell growth and cell division. The mitogen requirement can be fulfilled by the addition of serum, of purified growth factors, or of nonphysiological mitogens that mimic the actions of physiological growth factors.
2. *Cells divide only if they are anchored to a solid support.* Because of this **anchorage dependence,** cells dispersed in solution rarely if ever divide. Only white blood cells, which are suspended naturally, can be cultured readily without support.
3. *Cells are growth inhibited by contact with other cells of the same kind.* This **contact inhibition** causes cultured cells to stop dividing once a continuous monolayer has been formed.
4. *Cells have a finite lifespan.* Cultured fibroblasts, for example, divide between 30 and 80 times until they finally stop growing and die. Interestingly, fibroblasts taken from a baby have, on average, a higher life expectancy in culture than those taken from an aged individual. This suggests that the senescence of cultured cells and the aging

FIG. 28.2

Cyclins and cyclin-dependent kinases *(Cdk, Cdc)* during the cell cycle. Most cyclins are short lived, and their levels fluctuate with the stages of the cell cycle. The cyclin-dependent kinases and cyclin D, on the other hand, are present throughout the cell cycle. G_1, S, G_2, and M are the stages of the cell cycle (see Fig. 28.1).

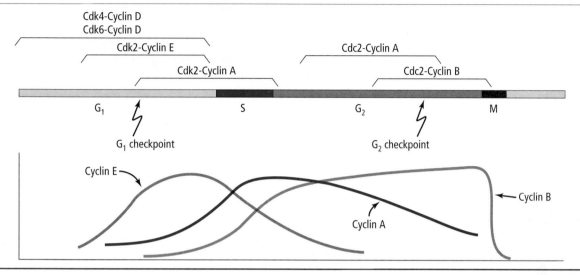

process of the individual are not merely superficially analogous.

These limitations on the growth of cultured cells apply only to normal cells, not to cancer cells. Cells from malignant tumors can grow in the absence of growth factors; their growth is anchorage independent; they are not subject to contact inhibition; and they are immortal.

Cell cultures are useful for diagnosis as well as in research. Cultured white blood cells, fibroblasts, and, for prenatal diagnosis, amniotic cells are used for the cytological diagnosis of chromosome aberrations, for DNA-based diagnostic procedures, and for enzyme assays.

Cyclin-dependent protein kinases play key roles in cell cycle control

Cell cycle progression requires both *adjustments in the steady-state levels of various proteins* and the *regulation of preexisting proteins by phosphorylation/dephosphorylation.* The synthesis of dihydrofolate reductase (see Chapter 23), thymidylate kinase, the DNA polymerase δ subunit PCNA (proliferating cell nuclear antigen), and DNA polymerase α (see Chapter 8), for example, is induced in late G_1 and during S phase when these enzymes are required for DNA synthesis. Phospho-

rylations of chromosomal scaffold proteins, histone H1, and the nuclear lamins, on the other hand, have to take place when the cell enters mitosis.

The main puppetmasters in these processes are a family of nuclear protein kinases whose activities depend on regulatory subunits called **cyclins.** Most of the cyclins, and some of the **cyclin-dependent kinases (CDKs),** have half-lives of 1 hour or less, and their expression is affected by the cell cycle (Fig. 28.2).

The first cyclin to form active protein kinase complexes is **cyclin D,** which associates with the catalytic subunits **Cdk4** and **Cdk6** (Cdk = cyclin-dependent kinase) during mid- to late G_1. Unlike the other cyclins, whose levels vary predictably with the cell cycle, cyclin D may be present at any time. *The expression of cyclin D is controlled not by the cell cycle, but by mitogens.* A little later, in late G_1 and at the G_1 to S transition, **cyclin E** is expressed and forms a catalytically active complex with **Cdk2.** Cyclin A, which also forms a complex with Cdk2, is expressed shortly after cyclin E. **Cyclin B,** finally, is expressed first during S phase, accumulates throughout G_2, and is degraded suddenly during mitosis. It forms an active complex with the catalytic subunit **Cdc2** (cell division cycle gene product), and this protein kinase is required for the entry into mitosis.

The retinoblastoma protein controls the G₁ checkpoint

The cyclin-dependent protein kinases are positive regulators of cell cycle progression, but inhibitory controls are required as well. Indeed, the cyclin-dependent protein kinases require not only the association with a cyclin for their activity, but also the phosphorylation of a single threonine residue (Thr-160 in Cdk2 and Thr-161 in Cdc2). Phosphorylations at other sites inhibit their activity, and they also are controlled by **CDK inhibitors,** which form catalytically inactive complexes with the kinase subunits.

The most important inhibitor of cell cycle progression, however, is the **retinoblastoma protein (pRb),** a nuclear phosphoprotein that controls the G₁ checkpoint. Although its steady-state levels fluctuate somewhat during the cell cycle, *pRb is controlled primarily by changes in its phosphorylation state* (Fig. 28.3): during G₀ and early G₁, pRb is present in a hypophosphorylated form, and *this form is an inhibitor of cell cycle progression, preventing entry into S phase.* During late G₁, pRb becomes phosphorylated and thereby inactivated by complexes of cyclin D with Cdk4 and Cdk6, and of cyclin E with Cdk2, and the cell can proceed into S phase. pRb remains in the inactive

hyperphosphorylated form for the rest of the cell cycle until the cell emerges from mitosis.

How does pRb prevent cell cycle progression? Although it does not bind to DNA itself, pRb has a binding pocket for the transcription factor **E2F.** Together with its dimerization partner **DP,** *E2F is a transcriptional activator for many genes that are required for cell cycle progression.* Throughout G₀ and early G₁, E2F/DP is tightly complexed with hypophosphorylated pRB, and this complex acts as a transcriptional repressor rather than as an activator. At the checkpoint, however, both pRb and E2F become phosphorylated by cyclin-Cdk complexes, and E2F/DP, now freed from pRb, becomes a transcriptional activator. Several cell cycle–dependent genes are induced by this transcription factor, including those for thymidine kinase, dihydrofolate reductase, DNA polymerase α, the protooncogenes *c-myc* and *N-myc, cdc2* (the gene for the Cdc2 protein kinase), the genes for cyclins E and A, and even the E2F gene itself. *Through its interaction with E2F/DP, pRb acts as the guardian of the G₁ checkpoint.*

Now we can trace the events by which quiescent cells enter the cell cycle: mitogenic stimulation induces the synthesis of cyclin D. The cyclin D/Cdk complexes then start phosphorylating pRb, and this

---

FIG. 28.3

Function of the retinoblastoma protein *(pRb)* in the control of the G₁ checkpoint. The phosphorylation of pRb by cyclin-dependent protein kinases *(Cdk)* releases the transcription factor E2F/DP from inhibitory control, thus enabling the transcription of genes for cell cycle progression. Growth-inhibiting stimuli prevent pRb phosphorylation indirectly by increasing the activity of cyclin/Cdk inhibitors. TGF-β, transforming growth factor-beta; P, phosphate groups.

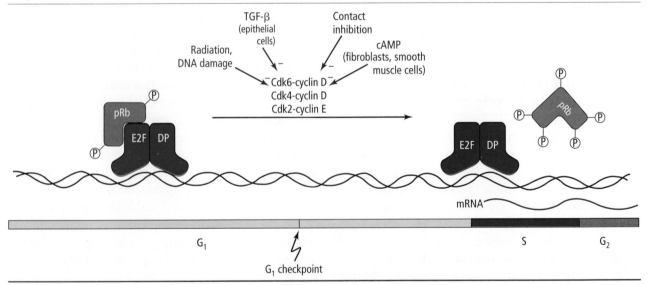

in turn activates the E2F-regulated genes, including those for cyclin E, cyclin A, and E2F itself. The Cdk complexes of cyclin E and cyclin A cause further pRb phosphorylation, thereby further activating the E2F-regulated genes. These events amount to a *positive feedback* that carries the cell through the G₁ checkpoint. Only the initial events, which are mediated by cyclin D, require mitogenic stimulation. The remaining steps are autonomous.

DNA damage causes either growth arrest or programmed cell death

Most growth-inhibiting external stimuli, including cell-cell contact and growth-inhibiting hormones, do not act directly on pRb but rather *induce the synthesis or promote the activity of various CDK inhibitors that prevent the action of cyclin-CDK complexes on pRb* (Fig. 28.3). Not only physiological stimuli, but also radiation and other DNA-damaging agents cause growth arrest. In some cell types and in some situations, this growth arrest is followed by apoptosis.

The key integrator of the DNA-damage response is the nuclear phosphoprotein **p53**, named after its molecular weight of 53,000. p53 is a short-lived protein ($T_{\frac{1}{2}}$ less than 1 hour in unstressed cells) that

is present in low concentrations at all times. By poorly understood posttranslational mechanisms, DNA damage causes a sharp increase in the nuclear p53 level. *p53 is a transcription factor that drives the expression of genes for growth arrest, DNA repair, and apoptosis.* The mechanisms of p53-induced apoptosis are poorly understood, but the p53-dependent cell cycle arrest is known to depend on the CDK inhibitor **p21,** a nuclear phosphoprotein (MW 21,000) that inhibits various cyclin-CDK complexes, including those that phosphorylate pRb (Fig. 28.4). *p53 has antimutagenic properties* because it delays DNA replication until DNA damage has been repaired. By inducing apoptosis, *it prevents the survival of genetically defective cells.* Because of these properties, p53 has been called the "guardian of the genome." p53 is not required for normal development, however: knockout mice that are lacking both copies of the *p53* gene develop normally, although they get cancers later in life (see Table 28.3, page 630).

MITOGENIC SIGNALING

Most cells of the developing embryo are dividing actively, and their proliferation is tightly linked to cell differentiation: immature stem cells divide more

---

FIG. 28.4

Role of the p53 protein in the response to DNA damage. p53 is a transcription factor whose steady-state level increases sharply after exposure to radiation or other DNA-damaging agents. It induces genes for DNA repair, and it causes cell cycle arrest by inducing the synthesis of the cyclin-CDK inhibitor p21 (Waf-1).

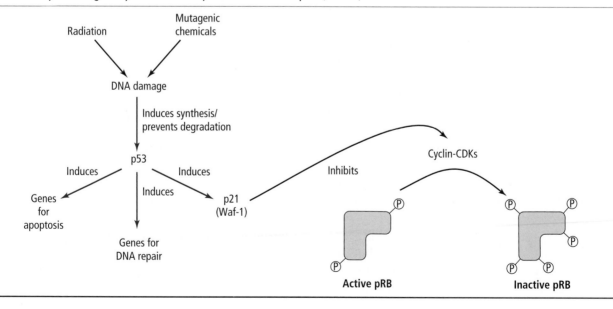

or less continuously, but *once the stem cell develops into a terminally differentiated cell type, it withdraws from the cell cycle.* For some cells, including neurons and skeletal muscle fibers, the withdrawal into G_o is final. Others, however — for example, hepatocytes and fibroblasts — behave like Sleeping Beauty: they can be restored to reproductive life by external agents. The prince's kiss that causes these cells to abandon G_o and re-enter the cell cycle is delivered by agents called mitogens. Mitogenic stimuli can be provided by anchorage to extracellular matrix constituents — as in the anchorage dependence of cultured cells — but the best-understood mitogens are soluble extracellular agents commonly referred to as growth factors. In the following sections, we shall examine how these growth factors affect the growth and differentiation of their target cells.

Cell proliferation is regulated by a large number of growth factors

Constructing and maintaining the architecture of a multicellular organism is a daunting task, requiring complex external signals for the regulation of cell growth and differentiation. Contacts with the surfaces of neighboring cells and with constituents of the extracellular matrix allow the cell to respond to its immediate environment. The responses to these stimuli may consist of growth stimulation, growth inhibition, shape changes, crawling toward or away from the external stimulus, differentiation into another cell type, or apoptosis.

Most of the responses to physical contact with the extracellular matrix depend on cell surface receptors of the **integrin** type. Matrix-bound integrin receptors are clustered in specialized structures called **focal adhesions.** Through peripheral membrane proteins, the integrins of the focal adhesions interact with actin microfilaments, thereby linking the extracellular matrix to the cytoskeleton. In addition to their mechanical function, however, the focal adhesions contain protein kinases and G-proteins (see Chapter 27) that transmit stimuli not only for the organization of the cytoskeleton but also for cell cycle progression.

Cell-matrix interactions usually are mitogenic, leading to anchorage-dependent growth, but cell-cell contacts usually are antimitogenic. Cell-cell contact appears to lead to an increased expression of various CDK inhibitors, but the signaling cascades that mediate contact inhibition are not well known.

Soluble growth factors allow the cell to respond to signals from more distant sources. There are many growth factors. Some of them affect a wide variety of cell types; others have narrow specificities. Most act as mitogens, but others cause their target cells to migrate, to differentiate, or to grow to large size without dividing. Growth factors even can induce opposite effects in different cell types — causing some cells to proliferate, for example, and others to stop growing or to undergo terminal differentiation. Some examples of growth factors are:

1. *Platelet-derived growth factor (PDGF).* This polypeptide growth factor is present in the α granules of platelets, from which it is released during platelet activation. Acting on a large number of cell types, including fibroblasts and smooth muscle cells, *it participates in wound healing.* The discovery of PDGF followed the observation that added serum stimulates the growth of cultured cells to a greater extent than does plasma. This serum effect was found to be caused by PDGF, which is released from activated platelets during blood clotting.

2. *Epidermal growth factor (EGF).* This growth factor also acts on a broad spectrum of cell types, being most active on epithelial cells. It is synthesized by a variety of cells and acts primarily in its tissues of origin.

3. *Fibroblast growth factor (FGF).* Like EGF, FGF acts mostly in the tissues in which it is synthesized. It stimulates fibroblasts as well as many other cells. The inherited deficiency of an FGF receptor, which makes chondroblasts in epiphyseal cartilage unable to respond normally to FGF, leads to **achondroplasia,** a dominantly inherited form of short-limbed dwarfism with abnormal development of epiphyseal cartilage and impaired growth of the long bones.

4. *Insulinlike growth factor-1 (IGF-1).* IGF-1 is released from the liver in response to growth hormone. Pygmies are said to have just as much growth hormone as taller people, but they release less IGF-1. This shows that at least part of the normal growth-promoting effect of growth hormone is mediated by IGF-1.

5. *Erythropoietin.* This growth factor is released from the kidney in response to hypoxia. It stimulates specifically the development of RBC precursors in the bone marrow.

6. *Nerve growth factor (NGF).* NGF acts only on specific populations of neurons. Its most conspicuous effect is the stimulation of growth and differentiation of postganglionic sympathetic neurons. Being released by sympathetically innervated tissues during embryonic development, it stimulates the growth and differentiation—but not cell division—of immature sympathetic neurons, causes the outgrowth of dendrites and axons, and acts as a chemoattractant for the growing axons, directing them to their proper destinations.

Mitogens act by promoting gene expression

G_0 is not simply an extended G_1. Proliferating cells express many genes for cell cycle progression, including those for most of the CDKs and for cyclin D, at more or less all times during the cell cycle. *Cells in G_0, on the other hand, do not express the genes for these positive regulators of cell cycle progression.* These genes have to be induced by mitogens before the cell can enter the cell cycle.

When a quiescent cell is stimulated by a mitogen (Fig. 28.5), some previously repressed genes become active within as little as 15 minutes. The activation of these **early-response genes** is mediated by the

---

FIG. 28.5

Cellular response to mitogens.

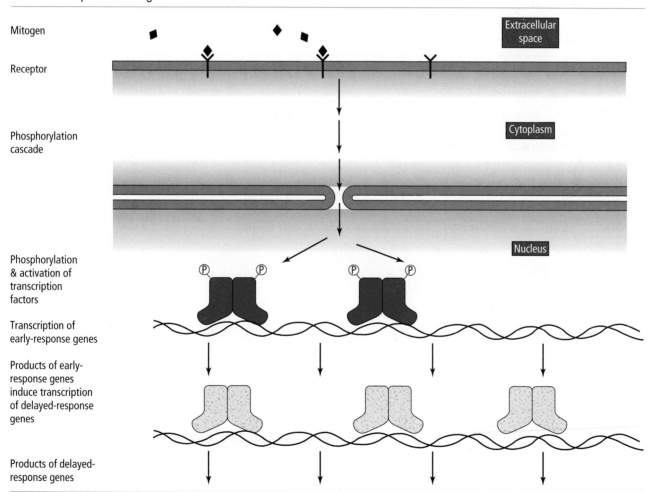

Mitogen

Receptor

Extracellular space

Phosphorylation cascade

Cytoplasm

Nucleus

Phosphorylation & activation of transcription factors

Transcription of early-response genes

Products of early-response genes induce transcription of delayed-response genes

Products of delayed-response genes

posttranslational regulation of existing transcription factors and does not require ongoing protein synthesis. Indeed, *the mitogens trigger signaling cascades that lead to the phosphorylation of transcription factors and the derepression of the early-response genes.* Because of a variety of negative feedback mechanisms, the mitogen-induced levels of early-response gene expression usually are not maintained but drop either to near zero or to a less-than-maximal steady-state level within a few hours after the initial exposure to the mitogen, even if the mitogen is still present in undiminished quantity.

The **delayed-response genes** are induced within approximately 1 hour of mitogen exposure, and their induction depends on ongoing protein synthesis. The products of some of the early-response genes are themselves transcription factors, and *these gene products induce the transcription of the delayed-response genes.* The products of the delayed-response genes, in turn, include the cyclins, CDKs, and other essential components of the cell cycle machinery.

Most growth factor receptors are tyrosine protein kinases

Most growth factor receptors possess an intracellular domain that acts as a tyrosine-specific protein kinase (see Fig. 27.16, Chapter 27). The binding of the growth factor to the extracellular domain of its receptor causes receptor aggregation and autophosphorylation of the intracellular tyrosine kinase domain. *The autophosphorylated receptor initiates signaling pathways by binding specific proteins that contain a phosphotyrosine-binding SH2 domain.*

Some of the receptor-bound proteins become tyrosine phosphorylated by the activated receptor. The γ-isoenzyme of the phosphoinositide-specific phospholipase C (**PLC-γ**), for example, which generates the second messengers IP$_3$ and diacylglycerol, becomes tyrosine phosphorylated and thereby activated by receptor tyrosine kinases. The β-isoenzyme (**PLC-β**), on the other hand, is activated not by receptor tyrosine kinases but rather by receptor-operated G

FIG. 28.6

The phospholipase C *(PLC)*-dependent second messenger system. The phosphoinositide-specific phospholipase C occurs in several isoforms. PLC-β is stimulated by receptor-controlled G proteins of the G$_q$ family; PLC-γ is stimulated by tyrosine phosphorylation. PLC activation has mitogenic effects in many cells. These mitogenic effects are mediated, in part, by various isoenzymes of protein kinase C *(PKC)*. The PKC isoenzymes are activated by 1,2-diacylglycerol *(DAG)* or by DAG + calcium. *PIP$_2$,* Phosphatidylinositol 4,5-bisphosphate; *IP$_3$,* inositol 1,4,5-trisphosphate. Compare with Fig. 27.9.

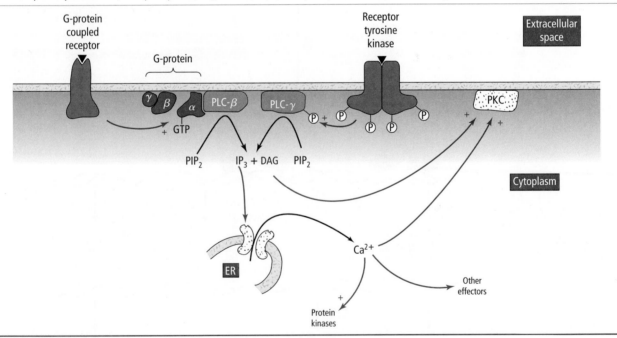

proteins (see Fig. 27.9). We realize now that *the IP₃/diacylglycerol/calcium second messenger system can be activated both by receptor tyrosine kinases and by G protein–coupled receptors* (Fig. 28.6). This signaling chain makes a major contribution to the mitogenic effects of receptor tyrosine kinase stimulation. The activation of protein kinase C (see Chapter 27), in particular, participates in mitogenic signaling in many cells.

Several other cytoplasmic and membrane-associated proteins besides PLC-γ become tyrosine phosphorylated by activated receptor tyrosine kinases. **Phosphoinositide 3-kinase,** for example, is a membrane-associated enzyme that phosphorylates phosphatidylinositol (PtlIns), PtlIns-4-phosphate, and PtlIns-4,5-bisphosphate. The resulting phosphorylated products are second messengers that activate some protein kinase C isoenzymes as well as other protein kinases. This system stimulates mitosis and prevents apoptosis in many cell types.

The MAP kinase pathway uses the Ras protein and a phosphorylation cascade

One of the major mitogenic signaling pathways, the **MAP kinase cascade,** is shown in Figs. 28.7 and 28.8. It is initiated by the SH2-containing adapter protein **Grb2,** which binds to autophosphorylated growth factor receptors without becoming phosphorylated itself. Grb2, in turn, binds the **Sos** protein (<u>s</u>on <u>of</u> <u>s</u>evenless, named after a mutant in the fruit fly *Drosophila*), effectively recruiting this otherwise-soluble cytoplasmic protein to the plasma membrane. Sos, finally, binds to the **Ras protein,** a G protein that is anchored to the inner leaflet of the plasma membrane by a covalently attached isoprenoid group.

Like the heterotrimeric G proteins that mediate the effects of most hormones (see Chapter 27), *the Ras protein cycles between an inactive GDP-bound form and an active GTP-bound form.* However, the Ras protein (MW 21,000) is far smaller than the heterotrimeric G proteins, and it consists of a single polypeptide. The Sos protein acts on the Ras protein to catalyze the removal of GDP and its replacement by GTP. Effectively, *the autophosphorylated receptor, Grb, Sos, and Ras form a bucket brigade of protein-protein interactions that convert the Ras protein to its active, GTP-bound form.*

Rather than diffusing through the cytoplasm, *the Ras protein continues the signal chain by assisting in the activation of cytoplasmic serine/threonine kinases.* The most important of these is **Raf-1.** This protein kinase becomes translocated to the plasma membrane as it binds to Ras-GTP. Once at the plasma membrane in association with Ras, Raf-1 becomes activated by phosphorylation. Some isoenzymes of protein kinase C are able to activate Ras-bound Raf, and thereby the phospholipase C system (Fig. 28.6) feeds into the MAP kinase pathway.

Raf phosphorylates and thereby activates the protein kinase **MEK** (<u>M</u>APK/<u>E</u>RK <u>k</u>inase). MEK is a dual-

---

FIG. 28.7

Activation of the Ras protein by growth factors *(GF)*. The sequence of events is: dimerization or oligomerization of the stimulated growth factor receptor ⟶ receptor autophosphorylation ⟶ binding of an SH2-containing adapter protein *(Grb2)* ⟶ recruitment of a nucleotide exchange factor *(Sos)* to the plasma membrane ⟶ activation of Ras. The hydrolysis of the bound GTP by Ras is stimulated by GTPase-activating proteins (Ras-GAP, neurofibromin).

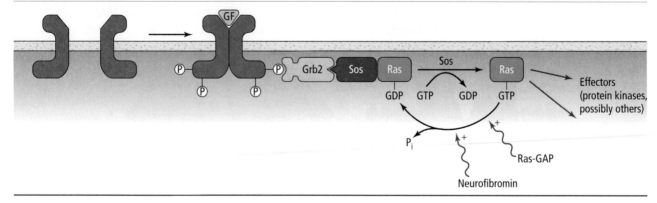

FIG. 28.8

MAP kinase pathways. In the "classical" pathway, the activated Ras protein (Ras-GTP) binds Raf-1 and aids in its activation. Raf-1 phosphorylates and activates MEK (MAP kinase/ERK kinase); MEK phosphorylates and activates the ERKs (extracellular signal regulated kinases); and the ERKs phosphorylate numerous cytoplasmic and nuclear proteins. The second pathway uses MEKK (MEK kinase), SEK, and the ERK-related kinases JNK (Jun-N-terminal kinase) and SAPK (stress-activated protein kinase). A third signaling chain ends with the protein kinase p38 (38-kDa protein). Some isoenzymes of protein kinase C (PKC) are known to phosphorylate and activate Raf-1.

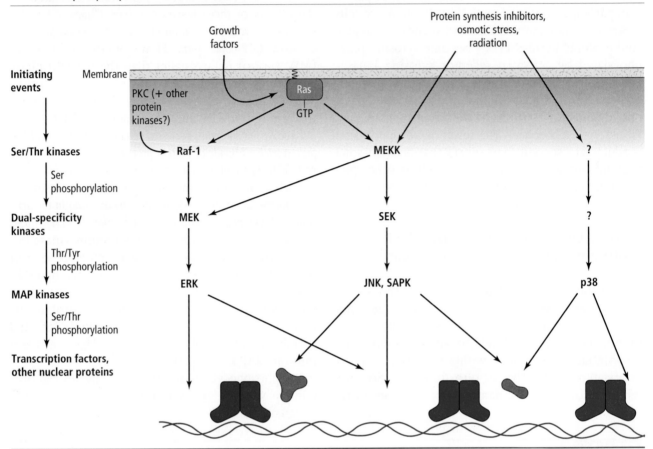

specificity kinase that phosphorylates a third set of kinases known as **ERK** (<u>e</u>xtracellular signal <u>r</u>egulated <u>k</u>inases) on threonine and tyrosine residues in the sequence Thr-Glu-Tyr. Together with some other serine/threonine kinases, the ERKs belong to the family of <u>m</u>itogen-<u>a</u>ctivated <u>p</u>rotein kinases (**MAP kinases**).

Once activated by this dual phosphorylation, the ERKs phosphorylate a wide variety of cytoplasmic and membrane-associated proteins on serine and threonine side chains. Most importantly, *they translocate to the nucleus, where they induce the transcription of the early-response genes.* Some of these effects are achieved by the direct phosphorylation of transcrip-

tion factors, but others are indirect, mediated by nuclear protein kinases that are themselves phosphorylated and activated by the MAP kinases. The products of some of the early-response genes, including **Jun, Fos,** and the members of the **Myc** family, are transcription factors themselves that stimulate the transcription of the delayed-response genes.

How is the mitogenic cascade switched off? *The most important terminators are protein phosphatases that reverse the mitogen-induced phosphorylations at all levels,* from the autophosphorylated receptors all the way to the phosphorylated transcription factors. Tyrosine phosphorylations, in particular, are very short lived because of an abundance of tyrosine-specific protein phosphatases in the cell. Some protein phosphatases are constitutively active, but others are controlled by extracellular signals. Some tyrosine-specific protein phosphatases are integral membrane proteins. They are thought to function as receptors, although their extracellular ligands still are unknown.

The Ras protein, like other G proteins, switches itself off by hydrolyzing its bound GTP. This GTPase activity is stimulated by various regulatory proteins, including **Ras-GAP** (GAP = <u>G</u>TPase-<u>a</u>ctivating protein) and **neurofibromin,** the product of the *NF-1* tumor suppressor gene.

The major mitogenic pathway actually is quite complex. There are, for example, three different isoforms of Ras and three different isoforms of Raf. MEK can be activated not only by Raf but also by a set of **MEK kinases (MEKKs)** and possibly by other kinases as well. There are as many as four different MEKKs in some cells. The **ERKs** also come in two isoforms, which differ in their regulatory properties and substrate specificities.

The Ras-Raf-MEK-ERK pathway is the most important mitogenic signaling pathway in many cells, but two parallel pathways have been described as well (Fig. 28.8). These pathways are activated either by mitogens or by stressful conditions such as high osmolarity, heat shock, or inhibitors of protein synthesis.

Even the classical MAP kinase cascade plays different roles in different cells. Most commonly, it recruits the cell into the cell cycle. In immature neurons, however, the activation of this cascade by nerve growth factor results in terminal differentiation rather than proliferation. The reasons for these cell-type–specific effects are not known.

The T-cell receptor recruits cytosolic tyrosine protein kinases

In Chapter 25, we saw that B lymphocytes proliferate and differentiate into plasma cells after the binding of antigen to their surface immunoglobulins. Indeed, *the antigen acts like a growth factor on B lymphocytes, and the surface immunoglobulin behaves like a growth factor receptor.* The T lymphocytes do not have a surface immunoglobulin, but are equipped with a **T-cell receptor** instead. *Like the surface immunoglobulin of the B cells, the T-cell receptor is able to recognize a specific*

antigen. The two antigen-binding polypeptides of the T-cell receptor are called α and β (Fig. 28.9). Like the variable domains of the immunoglobulins, the peripheral domains of the α and β chains come in many different variants. Like the B cells, each individual T cell expresses only one of these variants. Once exposed to the antigen – as well as to cytokines from helper T cells—the T cell becomes activated and proliferates.

Although both the surface immunoglobulin of the B cells and the T-cell receptor behave like growth factor receptors, they possess no intrinsic tyrosine protein kinase activity. The signaling pathways are best understood for the T-cell receptor. Besides the antigen-recognizing α and β chains, this receptor contains a dimer of two ζ (zeta) chains, as well as the **CDC3** complex, consisting of a γ chain, a δ chain, and two ϵ chains (Fig. 28.9).

Antigen binding induces a conformational change that exposes the cytoplasmic tails of the γ, δ, ϵ, and ζ chains to the action of a *tyrosine-specific protein kinase of the Src family.* The Src family protein kinases (named after avian sarcoma, a virally induced cancer in chickens) are not constituents of cell surface receptors, but are attached to the inner surface of the plasma membrane by a covalently bound myristoyl group. Besides Src itself, there are eight different Src-related protein kinases in different cells, and two of them, known as Lck and Fyn, are the major kinases phosphorylating the T-cell receptor.

Once it has been tyrosine phosphorylated by the Src family kinases, the T-cell receptor binds a second type of tyrosine protein kinase, known as **ZAP-70** (ZAP = <u>z</u>eta-<u>a</u>ssociated protein). ZAP-70 has two SH2 domains, and these domains anchor the kinase to the tyrosine-phosphorylated T-cell receptor. *The receptor-associated ZAP-70 phosphorylates target proteins and thereby mediates most of the effects of receptor stimulation.* It phosphorylates, for example, phospholipase C-γ (PLC-γ). *The resulting elevations of cytoplasmic diacylglycerol (DAG), inositol trisphosphate (IP$_3$), and calcium mediate mitogenesis in lymphocytes.*

An inherited deficiency of ZAP-70 has been identified as a cause of severe combined immunodeficiency in some patients. Although signaling through the surface immunoglobulin of B cells does not require ZAP-70 but rather relies on other protein kinases, B cells are crippled as well because their activation requires helper T cells in addition to antigen.

FIG. 28.9

Signaling through the T-cell receptor. The intracellular tails of the γ, δ, ϵ, and ζ chains possess antigen-recognition activation motifs (ARAMs, ‑\/\/\/\‑) that become tyrosine phosphorylated by tyrosine protein kinases of the Src family. The extracellular portions of the α, β, γ, and δ chains contain immunoglobulinlike domains, but only the α and β chains have variable domains for antigen recognition. T cells can respond specifically to an antigen on the surface of a presenting cell. Like many other signal transducing proteins, ZAP-70 has SH2 domains ( ) that bind to tyrosine-phosphorylated sites.

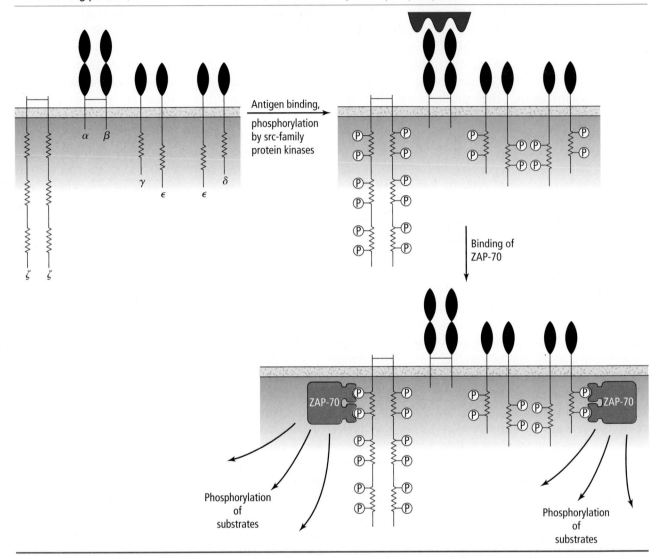

Antigen receptors are not the only receptors that affect cell growth by recruiting soluble cytoplasmic tyrosine protein kinases. The receptors for **growth hormone, prolactin, erythropoietin, leptin,** and some **cytokines,** including the interleukins and interferons, also are lacking enzymatic activities. After ligand binding, these receptors associate with a type of tyrosine protein kinase called **janus kinase,** and these janus kinases phosphorylate target proteins.

The molecular basis of neoplastic disease

The normal controls on cell proliferation ensure that each cell behaves unselfishly throughout its limited lifespan: during embryonic development, the cells divide and finally differentiate in highly coordinated and disciplined ways to form the tissues and organs of the body. Some of them die dutifully, by apoptosis, once their task is fulfilled. The cells of the adult body divide only to replace those cells that are lost from their tissue.

Derangements of cellular growth control can result in excessive proliferation and in the accumulation of an abnormal cell mass called a **tumor.** This type of disease is called **neoplasia** (Greek for "new growth"). If the growth of the tumor is self limited, it is said to be **benign.** If, however, the cells proliferate indefinitely, the tumor is said to be **malignant,** and the resulting disease is called a **cancer.** In the following sections we will examine the molecular lesions that lead to abnormal cell proliferation and cancer.

Essentially all cancers are monoclonal in origin

Malignant tumors are derived from normal somatic cells by a process called **malignant transformation,** and they are classified according to the normal cell type from which they are derived. Indeed, to a varying extent the malignant cells maintain morphological and biochemical features typical for their cells of origin. Some tumors of epithelial origin, for example, known as **carcinomas,** still produce keratins; connective tissue tumors, known as **sarcomas,** still may produce constituents of the extracellular matrix; and some endocrine tumors still secrete hormones. However, there are typical differences between malignant neoplastic cells and the normal cells from which they are derived:

1. *Cancer cells have an abnormally high mitotic rate.* The abundance of mitotic cells in histological specimens is used diagnostically to estimate the malignant potential of tumors.
2. *Cancer cells show signs of de-differentiation and assume features of immature stem cells.* The cells in epithelial cancers (carcinomas), for example, lose the normal squamous, cuboidal, or columnar shape of their normal progenitors and assume an undifferentiated, embryonic appearance.
3. *Cancer cells show disordered growth patterns.* Rather than growing as an integral part of their tissue, malignant cells show no respect for anatomical boundaries but grow as a chaotic mass of cells, spreading and sprawling in all directions. The de-differentiation and disordered growth of cancerous cells are called **anaplasia.** The degree of anaplasia can be determined histologically. It predicts

the malignant behavior of the cells—and the survival chances of the patient.

4. *Cancer cells can colonize distant tissues.* Cells can break loose from a primary tumor to be carried away by either the lymph or the blood. These cells can establish themselves in far-off tissues to form secondary growths called **metastases.** Metastatic spread requires poor adherence to neighboring cells in the tumor, as well as the ability to adhere to components of distant tissues, to cross basement membranes, and to grow in an environment different from the cell's tissue of origin.
5. *Many cancer cells show gross genomic abnormalities.* Aberrations in chromosome number (**aneuploidy**) are common in malignant tumors; there may be major deletions or translocations, gene amplifications, or even extrachromosomal genetic elements. Quite obviously, the malignant cells suffer from genomic instability and are afflicted by frequent mutations.
6. *Cancer cells can grow in the absence of normal mitogenic stimuli.* This property is readily evident in cell cultures where neoplastic cells, unlike their normal counterparts, can grow under conditions of growth factor deprivation and in the absence of a solid support.
7. *Cancer cells are immortal.* Both in cell culture and in the body, cancer cells escape the normal process of senescence. Many neoplastic cells also have lost the ability for apoptosis in response to growth factor deprivation, DNA damage, or other environmental insults—they do not commit suicide in hopeless situations.
8. *The malignant phenotype is heritable.* Cancer cells can be propagated through many mitotic divisions and under a variety of environmental conditions without losing their neoplastic features. This shows that cancer is caused by heritable changes in the cellular genome.

Are the cells of a malignant tumor derived from a single aberrant somatic cell, or from a whole cell population? Some malignant tumors possess readily identifiable genetic markers. Most patients with chronic myelogenous leukemia, for example, have a characteristic translocation between chromosomes 9 and 22 that is known as the **Philadelphia chromosome.** This strictly heritable aberration is present in all tumor cells, but not in the normal somatic cells of the patient. This suggests that all malignant cells in the patient are descended from a single cell carrying this translocation. Observations of this kind indicate that *all cells of the tumor are derived by successive mitotic divisions from a single aberrant somatic cell: malignant tumors are monoclonal in origin.*

Malignant transformation can be caused by the activation of growth-promoting genes or the inactivation of growth-inhibiting genes

Some elements of cellular growth control promote cell proliferation; others are inhibitory. Growth factors, their receptors, and the components of the MAP kinase pathway, for example, promote growth and cell division, whereas cyclin-CDK inhibitors, the retinoblastoma protein pRb, and the p53 protein are inhibitory. *The common cancers are caused by somatic mutations in genes that code for growth-promoting or growth-inhibiting protein products.* Therefore we can envisage two kinds of molecular accidents by which a cell can be transformed to malignancy (Fig. 28.10):

1. *A gene that codes for a growth-promoting protein becomes abnormally activated by a somatic mutation.* Such activation can be achieved in several ways: a point

---

FIG. 28.10

The difference between an oncogene and a tumor suppressor gene. **A,** The products of cellular protooncogenes (████) are growth-stimulating proteins. A single activating mutation ("gain-of-function" mutation) is sufficient to produce abnormal cell growth. **B,** The products of tumor suppressor genes (▨▨▨) are growth-inhibiting proteins. Two inactivating mutations ("loss-of-function" mutations) are required to produce abnormal cell growth.

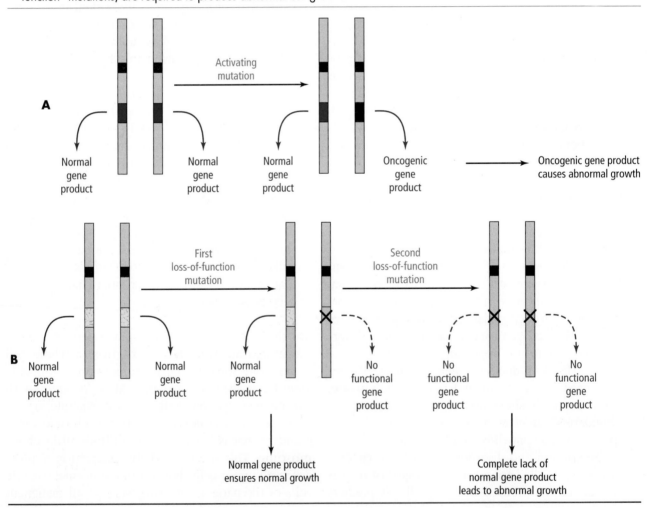

mutation, for example, can create a "superactive" product, or a mutation in a regulatory site of the gene can cause the excessive or uncontrolled synthesis of a structurally normal gene product. Less-conventional mutations also are common. Thus a gene can become amplified, or it can become translocated to a site where it is overexpressed under the influence of the enhancers or promoters of other genes (Fig. 28.11). The mutationally activated form of a growth-promoting gene is called an **oncogene,** and the corresponding normal gene is called a **protooncogene.**

2. *A gene that codes for a growth-inhibiting product becomes*

inactivated by a somatic mutation. This type of mutation also is common in neoplastic diseases. The inactivating mutation can be a missense mutation, splice site mutation, nonsense mutation, frameshift mutation, or a large deletion that removes the whole gene together with the surrounding chromosomal region. The normal gene that becomes inactivated is called a **tumor suppressor gene.**

The formation of an active oncogene can transform the cell even if only one copy of a growth-promoting gene in the diploid somatic cell becomes acti-

---

FIG. 28.11

Oncogenic activation of a cellular protooncogene.

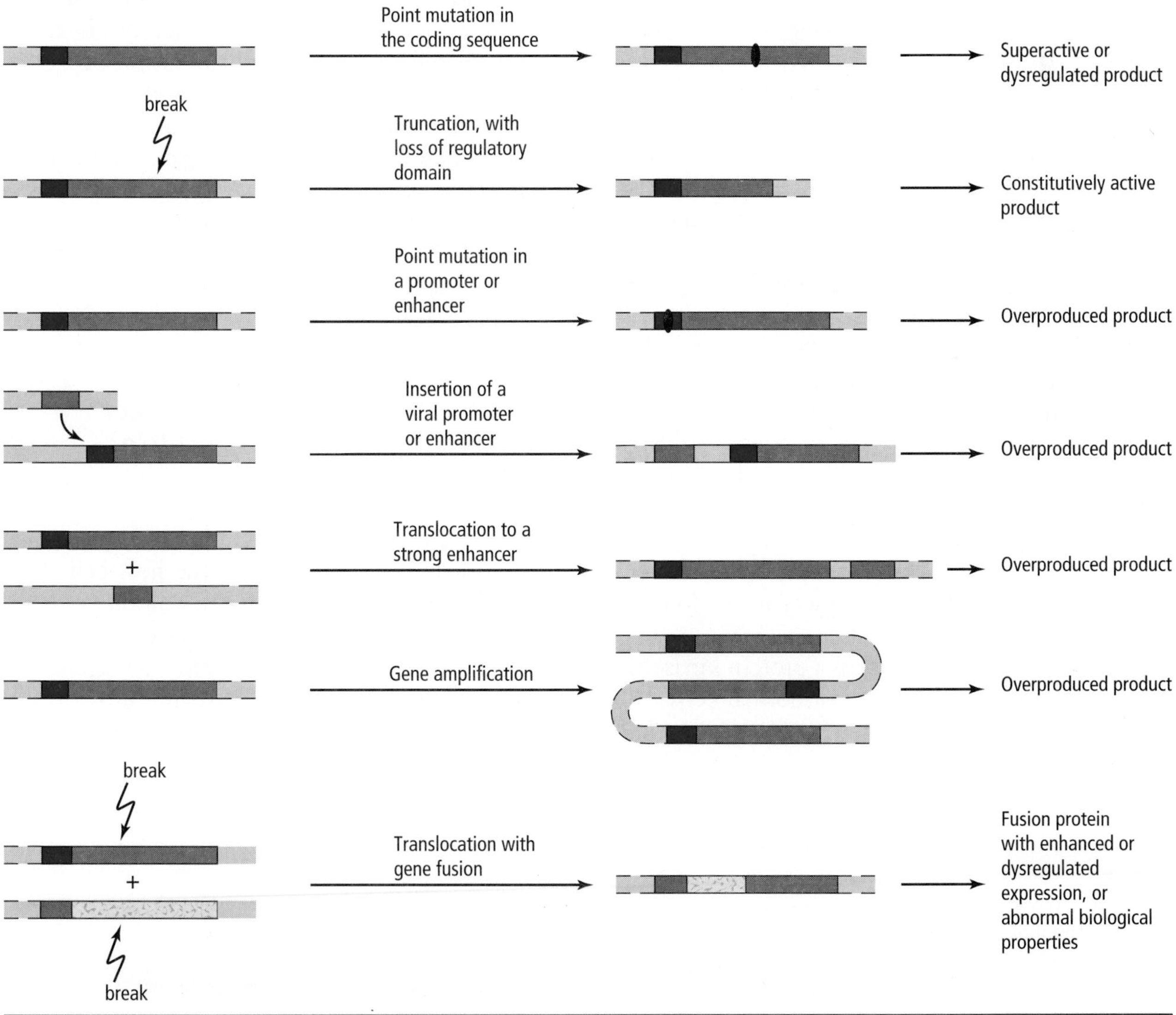

Point mutation in the coding sequence	Superactive or dysregulated product
Truncation, with loss of regulatory domain	Constitutively active product
Point mutation in a promoter or enhancer	Overproduced product
Insertion of a viral promoter or enhancer	Overproduced product
Translocation to a strong enhancer	Overproduced product
Gene amplification	Overproduced product
Translocation with gene fusion	Fusion protein with enhanced or dysregulated expression, or abnormal biological properties

vated. The inactivation of a tumor suppressor gene, on the other hand, is effective only if both copies of the gene are inactivated: a single active gene still can produce enough of the tumor-suppressing protein product to guarantee normal growth.

The common cancers contain not just a single somatic mutation but a combination of several mutations that include both activated oncogenes and inactivated tumor suppressor genes. Only the combined effects of these mutations drive the cells into malignancy.

Some retroviruses cause malignant transformation by introducing an oncogene

The vast majority of cancers result from somatic mutations, but *some viruses can cause cancer by introducing a **viral oncogene.*** Although virally induced cancers are rare, viral oncogenes were among the first to be identified. As early as 1910, Peyton Rous established the transmissible nature of a rare connective tissue tumor in chickens. Much later the transmissible agent, now known as the **Rous sarcoma virus (RSV)**, was identified as a retrovirus. Like other retroviruses (see Chapter 7), RSV has a small RNA genome with three major genes that are essential for viral reproduction: *gag*, *pol*, and *env*. Besides these three genes, RSV has a fourth gene whose product is not required for viral replication. *This gene, known as the src gene (src for sarcoma), or v-src gene (v for viral), is a viral oncogene* (Fig. 28.12). During retroviral infection, a cDNA copy of the *src* gene is inserted into the host-cell DNA together with the rest of the viral genome and is expressed at a high rate under the direction of the viral promoter and enhancer in the long terminal repeats.

The v-*src* oncogene codes for a protein kinase that is closely related to a protein in normal cells. How can a retrovirus carry a gene that is closely related to a normal cellular gene? Apparently, the virus acquired the gene accidentally during a previous infectious cycle. *This hijacked gene, slightly mutated and grossly overexpressed, turns the virus-infected cell into a tumor cell.* The product of both the normal cellular *src* protooncogene and the v-*src* oncogene is a nonreceptor tyrosine protein kinase that is loosely bound to cellular membranes with the aid of a covalently bound myristic acid residue. The normal cellular Src kinase becomes activated after binding to activated growth factor receptors or to proteins in focal adhesions. It stimulates mitosis by phosphorylating many of the same substrates that are phosphorylated also by activated growth factor receptors. We encountered Src-related protein kinases earlier, in the signal transduction pathways of the antigen receptors (Fig. 28.9, page 614).

Some other retroviral oncogenes besides v-*src* have been identified (Table 28.1), and all of them are closely related to normal cellular protooncogenes. *All retroviral oncogenes transform cells only after being incorporated in the cellular genome.* Rous sarcoma virus is fully infective, but the other oncogenic retroviruses are defective because they have lost some of the essential retroviral genes during acquisition of their oncogene. These viruses can reproduce only if their host cell is also infected by a second, intact retrovirus that supplies the missing gene products.

Retroviruses also can cause cancer by inserting themselves next to a cellular protooncogene

Retroviruses integrate a cDNA copy of their genome at more-or-less-random sites in the host-cell DNA. Even if the retrovirus does not carry an oncogene, it can cause cancer if it inserts itself next to a cellular protooncogene. Although the protooncogene remains structurally intact, the retroviral provirus can boost the transcription of the neighboring pro-

FIG. 28.12

The genome of Rous sarcoma virus. *LTR*, Long terminal repeat. Whereas *gag*, *pol*, and *env* are required for virus replication, *src* causes malignant transformation. The total length of the provirus is approximately 11,000 base pairs.

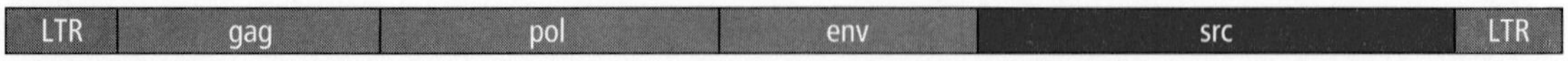

| LTR | gag | pol | env | src | LTR |

TABLE 28.1

Examples of retroviral oncogenes

Oncogene	Protein product	Tumor (species)
sis	Truncated version of platelet-derived growth factor (PDGF)	Simian sarcoma (monkey)
erb-B	Epidermal growth factor (EGF) receptor	Erythroblastosis (chicken)
src	Nonreceptor tyrosine kinase	Sarcoma (chicken)
abl	Nonreceptor tyrosine kinase	Leukemia (mouse), sarcoma (cat)
H-ras K-ras	Ras protein (a G protein)	Sarcoma, erythroleukemia (rat)
raf	Raf protein (a serine/threonine protein kinase)	Sarcoma (chicken, mouse)
myc	Transcription factor of the helix-loop-helix family	Sarcoma, myelocytoma (chicken)
erb-A	Thyroid hormone receptor	Erythroblastosis (chicken)
fos jun	DNA-binding proteins, components of the heterodimeric transcription factor AP-1 (activator protein 1)	Sarcoma (mouse, chicken), erythroblastosis (chicken)

FIG. 28.13

Activation of a cellular protooncogene by an integrated retrovirus. The two long terminal repeats *(LTRs)* of the provirus are identical. Note that the protooncogene is not damaged during retroviral integration, but its rate of transcription is increased. **A,** Promoter insertion. The promoter in the downstream LTR is used for the transcription of the protooncogene. **B,** Enhancer insertion. The viral enhancer stimulates transcription from the normal promoter even if inserted downstream of the protooncogene, or if inserted with opposite polarity.

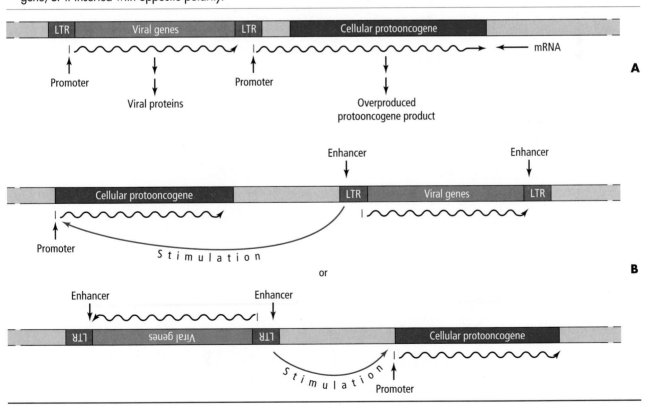

tooncogene in some cases. This can be effected by two mechanisms (Fig. 28.13):

1. In **promoter insertion,** the retroviral DNA is lodged immediately upstream of the protoonco-gene, and the promoter in the downstream long terminal repeat is used to initiate the transcription of the protooncogene—at an abnormally high rate and without the negative controls that normally regulate the rate of transcription.

2. In **enhancer insertion,** the enhancer in the long terminal repeats of the retrovirus stimulates the transcription of the neighboring protooncogene. This can occur even if the retroviral genome is inserted some distance away from the protoonco-gene—up to 10,000 base pairs in some cases.

Like the normal cellular enhancers (see Chapter 8), the retroviral enhancers can act over considerable distances.

Many oncogene products are links in mitogenic signaling pathways

Cellular oncogenes are derived from normal protooncogenes by somatic mutations that either change the structure of the gene product or lead to its overexpression. The questions that we have to examine now are: Which proteins are encoded by the protooncogenes? What roles do these protooncogenes and their products play in normal growth control? How can the protooncogene be activated to produce uncontrolled cancerous growth? Because

FIG. 28.14

Autocrine stimulation of a neoplastic cell. Some tumor cells express both a growth factor and the corresponding receptor, thereby stimulating their own growth.

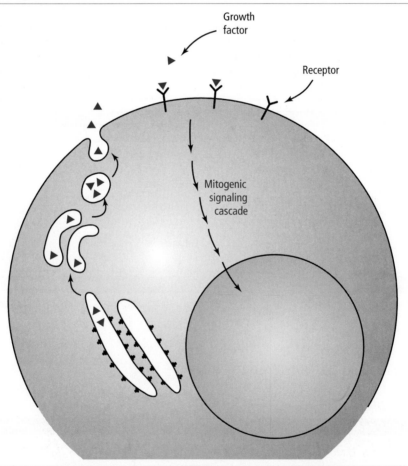

abnormal cell proliferation is the hallmark of cancerous growth, we can expect that oncogene products are involved in the transmission of mitogenic stimuli. Indeed, *most oncogene products are links in mitogenic signaling cascades.* They include:

1. *Growth factors:* Only one viral oncogene, the *sis* oncogene (<u>si</u>mian <u>s</u>arcoma), codes for a growth factor. *Many spontaneous human tumors, however, secrete growth factors that stimulate the tumor cells through an autocrine loop* (Fig. 28.14). Many sarcomas and glial tumors, for example, express both PDGF and the PDGF receptor. Many malignant melanomas—but not normal melanocytes—produce FGF, which stimulates the proliferation of both normal and transformed melanocytes.

2. *Receptor tyrosine kinases.* Overexpressed or structurally altered growth factor receptors are relatively common in malignant tumors. The *erb*-B oncogene of the avian erythroblastosis virus, for example, codes for a truncated version of the EGF receptor that has lost the extracellular ligand-binding domain (Fig. 28.15).

   The gene product has an intact tyrosine protein kinase domain, but this domain no longer is controlled by the ligand; it phosphorylates substrates at all times, even in the absence of EGF. The *neu* oncogene, on the other hand, which has been identified in some spontaneous, nonviral neuroblastomas in rodents, differs from its normal counterpart only by a single amino acid substitution at one end of the transmembrane helix. This point mutation disrupts the coupling between the extracellular ligand-binding domain and the intracellular protein kinase domain: the protein kinase is active at all times, irrespective of ligand binding. The normal ligand for the Neu receptor still is not known with certainty. These two examples illustrate an important principle: *oncogenically mutated growth factor receptors are switched on at all times, even in the absence of their ligands.* Besides structurally abnormal receptors, overexpressed receptors are common in various cancers. Many squamous cell carcinomas and glioblastomas, for example, have an overexpressed or amplified gene for the EGF receptor.

3. *Nonreceptor tyrosine protein kinases.* The cellular equivalent of the v-*src* oncogene (Fig. 28.12), known as c-*src*, is a tyrosine-specific protein kinase that transmits mitogenic stimuli from both activated

---

FIG. 28.15

Abnormal growth factor receptors as oncogene products. The intracellular protein tyrosine kinase domains of the abnormal receptors are constitutively active, even in the absence of the ligand.

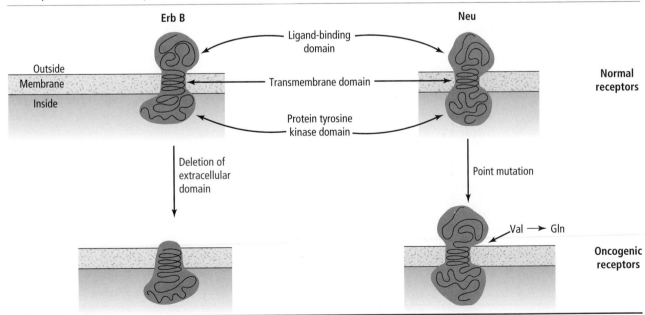

growth factor receptors and activated integrin receptors in focal adhesions. Therefore *it mediates mitogenic responses to both growth factors and contact with the extracellular matrix*. It complements the MAP kinase pathway by acting on a different set of early-response genes (Fig. 28.16). c-*src* is mutated in many spontaneous, nonviral cancers.

The Src protein kinase itself is inhibited by tyrosine phosphorylation, and under ordinary conditions more than 90% of Src is in the inactive, tyrosine-phosphorylated form. Normally, Src activity is increased transiently by interactions of Src with activated growth factor receptors or constituents of focal adhesions. These interactions lead to the removal of the inhibitory phosphate by protein phosphatases.

Some of the structurally altered oncogenic forms of Src are mutated at the tyrosine phosphorylation site and therefore are permanently activated. The simple overexpression of a structurally normal cellular *src* gene also is not uncommon in spontaneous cancers. Because the Src protein kinase relays mitogenic stimuli both from growth factor receptors and from focal adhesions, *src* mutations can contribute to both the mitogen

independence and the anchorage independence of malignant cell growth.

A different situation is encountered with the *abl* gene. The nonreceptor tyrosine kinase encoded by this gene normally is located in the nucleus, where it acts as a suppressor rather than a stimulator of cell proliferation. The oncogenically mutated forms, however, reside in the cytoplasm, where they have access to a different set of substrates. The phosphorylation of these substrates causes excessive cell proliferation. In patients with chronic myelogenous leukemia, the *abl* protooncogene is fused with an unrelated gene as a result of a chromosomal translocation (the "Philadelphia chromosome"), and the resulting fusion protein contributes to malignant transformation.

4. *Cytoplasmic serine/threonine kinases*. Activating mutations of the *raf* protooncogene are encountered in some tumors. The Raf protein kinase encoded by this gene (see Fig. 28.8, page 612) is regulated by phosphorylations at multiple sites, some of them activating and some inhibitory. Oncogenic forms of Raf frequently have point mutations that destroy negative phosphorylation sites, or they

FIG. 28.16

Two hypothetical signaling cascades that are triggered by the activation of growth factor receptors and the binding of integrin receptors to extracellular matrix proteins in focal adhesions. Both the Ras protein (a small, GTP-binding protein) and the Src protein (a tyrosine-specific protein kinase) are activated abnormally in many cancers. ⟶+, Induction; ⟶, repression.

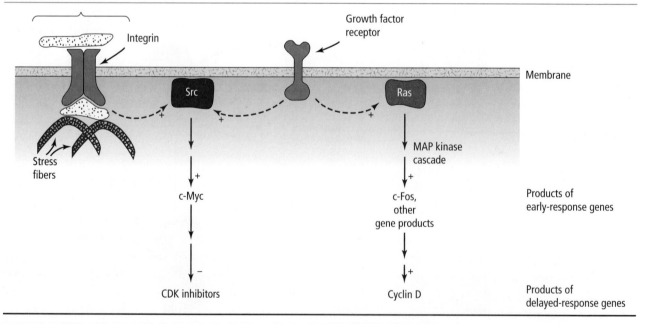

have lost part or all of their regulatory domain. *These mutations leave the kinase in a permanently activated state.*

5. *G proteins.* Oncogenic forms of the *ras* gene are among the most common genetic alterations in malignant cells. They occur, for example, in 30% to 50% of all lung and colon cancers and in 90% of all pancreatic cancers. Most oncogenic forms of the *ras* gene have point mutations that either disrupt the GTPase activity of the encoded Ras protein or make it insensitive to the action of GTPase-activating proteins. *These oncogenic Ras proteins have lost their "off" switch and remain in the active state at all times.*

Heterotrimeric G proteins also are involved in some neoplastic conditions. cAMP has growth-inhibitory effects in some cells, including fibroblasts and smooth muscle cells, but it stimulates the growth of many endocrine cells. Indeed, mutations in the α subunit of either the G_s or the G_i protein are not uncommon in benign adenomas of the pituitary somatotrophs, the thyroid gland, and the adrenal cortex. These mutations eliminate the GTPase activity of the α_s subunit or prevent the action of the α_i subunit on adenylate cyclase. As a result, *the affected cells are flooded with cAMP, proliferate, and secrete excessive amounts of hormone.*

6. *Nuclear transcription factors.* Many oncogene products are nuclear proteins. The *myc* genes are especially important. There are three cellular counterparts to the viral oncogene v-*myc* (Table 28.1), which have been dubbed c-*myc*, N-*myc*, and L-*myc*. They are early-response genes that are induced in response to growth factors and cell-matrix contact (see Fig. 28.16). *The myc genes are amplified in many malignant tumors,* with a corresponding overexpression of the gene product. c-*myc* is amplified in a great variety of tumors, including many breast, colon, and stomach cancers, small-cell lung cancers, and glioblastomas; N-*myc* is amplified in some neuroblastomas, retinoblastomas, and small-cell lung carcinomas; and L-*myc* is amplified in some small-cell lung carcinomas.

The *myc* amplifications frequently occur late during tumor progression and are associated with an aggressively malignant phenotype. The isolated overexpression of a *myc* gene in an otherwise normal cell can lead to abnormal proliferation, but many cells undergo apoptosis in response to this

abnormality. This illustrates the importance of apoptosis in the prevention of cancer: cells with a dangerous somatic mutation are eliminated before they can accumulate additional mutations that lead to a frankly malignant phenotype.

A different mode of c-*myc* activation is observed in patients with **Burkitt's lymphoma.** In this B-cell malignancy, the c-*myc* gene on chromosome 8 is translocated into the locus for immunoglobulin kappa chains (on chromosome 2), lambda chains (chromosome 22), or heavy chains (chromosome 14). *The translocation places the myc gene into a transcriptionally active spot of the genome, where it is overexpressed under the influence of local enhancers.*

The inactivation of tumor suppressor genes is more common than the formation of active oncogenes in spontaneous cancers

Oncogenes can be identified in many but not all spontaneous cancers. This may mean simply that there are oncogenes that we do not know about (close to 100 have been described already), but it also suggests that the inactivation of tumor suppressor genes is a crucial event in many cancers. The importance of tumor suppressor genes first was recognized in experiments performed in the late 1960s by molecular biologist Henry Harris and his colleagues at Oxford University. These investigators fused cultured cancer cells, which were able to form tumors in animals, with normal somatic cells. In most cases, the resulting hybrid cells were unable to form tumors in animals.

These experiments suggested that *the malignant phenotype of the tumor cells was caused not by a dominantly acting oncogene but by the homozygous loss of a tumor suppressor gene.* Once the tumor suppressor gene was reintroduced by the normal cell, the cells no longer could form tumors (Fig. 28.17).

If this model is correct, then a hybrid cell should become tumorigenic again if it loses the tumor suppressor gene of the normal parental cell. Indeed, when somatic cell hybrids are propagated in culture for many generations, they tend to lose individual chromosomes: they become aneuploid. Some of these aneuploid cells have been found to regain their tumorigenic properties, and this has been associated with the loss of individual chromosomes. These ex-

FIG. 28.17

The importance of tumor suppressor genes, as demonstrated by somatic cell hybridization. Only the chromosome with the tumor suppressor gene *(TS)* is shown. The tumorigenicity of the cells can be assessed by injecting them into immunodeficient mice. The original cancer cell is able to cause tumors, but the hybrid cell is not. The hybrid cell becomes tumorigenic only if the chromosomes with the intact tumor suppressor gene are lost during prolonged culturing. The product of the tumor suppressor gene has growth-inhibiting properties, so progeny cells that have lost the normal chromosomes with the intact tumor suppressor gene by mitotic nondisjunction gradually outgrow the normal hybrid cells in culture.

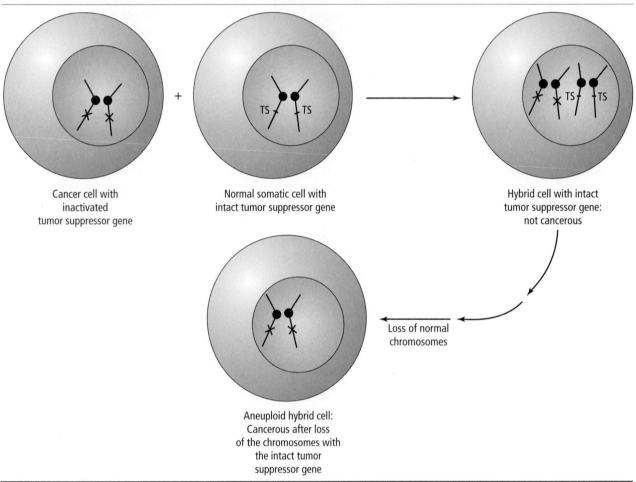

Cancer cell with
inactivated
tumor suppressor gene

Normal somatic cell with
intact tumor suppressor gene

Hybrid cell with intact
tumor suppressor gene:
not cancerous

Loss of normal
chromosomes

Aneuploid hybrid cell:
Cancerous after loss
of the chromosomes with
the intact tumor
suppressor gene

periments showed that *the presence of certain chromosomes from normal somatic cells suppresses the malignant phenotype in the cell hybrids.* These tumor-suppressing chromosomes carry tumor suppressor genes.

Retinoblastoma is caused by the inactivation of a tumor suppressor gene

Retinoblastoma is a rare, malignant tumor of immature retinal cells (retinoblasts) that occurs in children during the first 5 years of life, with a population incidence of approximately 1 in 20,000. Sixty percent of the patients have a sporadic form of the disease. These patients, who always have only a single primary tumor, have no affected family members, and the tumor apparently is not heritable. Approximately 40% of all patients, however, have a form of the disease that is heritable as an autosomal dominant trait. *These patients are heterozygous for the predisposing gene defect.* Children with the inherited predisposition have a 90% chance of getting the disease. Most of them develop more than one retinal tumor, and their tumors are often bilateral (in both eyes).

FIG. 28.18

Homozygous inactivation of the *Rb* gene on chromosome 13 in the spontaneous and the inherited forms of retinoblastoma. **A,** Spontaneous tumor: two inactivating mutations are required for malignant transformation. **B,** Inherited tumor: the first mutation is already present in the germline. A single somatic mutation in a retinoblast is sufficient for malignant transformation.

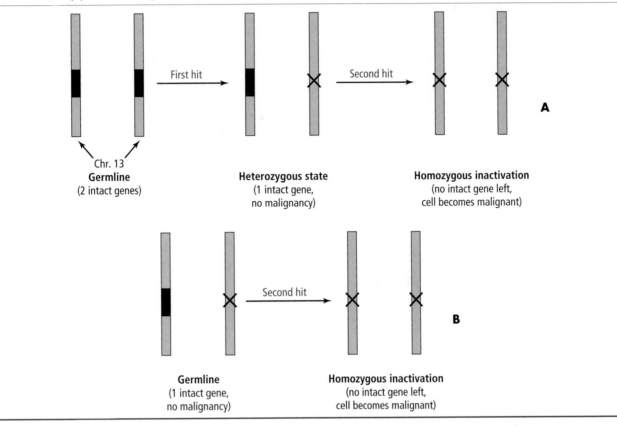

In both the sporadic and the inherited forms of the disease, *the tumor cells are unable to synthesize functional retinoblastoma protein (pRb).* pRb is the "guardian of the G_1 checkpoint" (Fig. 28.3). It prevents cell cycle progression, so its inactivation can be expected to increase the mitotic rate. The homozygous (but not the heterozygous) inactivation of *Rb* in an immature retinal cell causes malignant transformation. Cells with only a single copy of the intact gene are normal. Therefore *two mutational hits in the Rb gene are required for malignant transformation* (Fig. 28.18).

In patients with the sporadic form of the disease, both mutations take place in the retinoblast. These mutations are rare events, and sporadic retinoblastoma is indeed rare. Patients with the inherited form of the disease, however, are born with a defect in one copy of their *Rb* gene. *All of their somatic cells have only one intact copy of the gene,* so a single mutation in one of the million or so retinoblasts is suffi-cient to create a malignant cell. This event may oc-cur by chance in more than one retinoblast; there-fore the tumors in the inherited disease often are multifocal.

In most cases the second hit in patients with in-herited retinoblastoma is not an independent small mutation but rather a large deletion, loss of the nor-mal chromosome, or the replacement of the normal gene by the defective one by homologous recombi-nation during mitosis (Fig. 28.19). These events lead to a characteristic **loss of heterozygosity,** both for the *Rb* gene and for genetic markers (for example, restriction fragment length polymorphisms, RFLPs) close to it.

Note that although the disease is inherited as an autosomal dominant trait at the level of the individ-ual, the mutation is recessive at the cellular level: *Rb inactivation causes malignant transformation only if the cell loses both copies of the gene.*

FIG. 28.19

Loss of the intact *Rb* gene in patients with inherited retinoblastoma. All of the mechanisms shown here, except the first, lead to a loss of heterozygosity both for the gene itself and for closely linked genetic markers. The loss of heterozygosity for genetic markers (for example, restriction fragment length polymorphisms) of known chromosomal location in tumor cells is an important aid in the mapping of tumor suppressor genes. **A,** Independent small mutation; **B,** large deletion; **C,** loss of the intact chromosome by mitotic nondisjunction; **D,** somatic recombination by mitotic crossing-over.

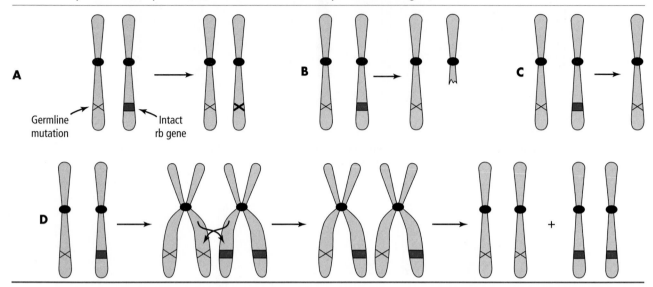

The retinoblastoma protein is expressed in all nucleated cells, so we may wonder whether patients with an inherited *Rb* mutation are at risk for cancers other than retinoblastoma. Indeed, some patients surviving the disease in childhood develop osteosarcoma (bone cancer) in later life. We also may wonder whether somatic mutations of the *Rb* gene are involved in spontaneous cancers other than retinoblastoma. Indeed, the homozygous inactivation of this gene is observed in some common cancers. These mutations occur, for example, in most small-cell lung carcinomas and in approximately one third of all breast and bladder cancers. This suggests that *in cells other than retinoblasts, the loss of Rb gene function can contribute to malignant transformation but is not sufficient by itself to cause cancer.*

Components of the cell cycle machinery are abnormal in most cancers

The mechanisms of cell cycle control are exceedingly complex, and they differ in different cell types. There are, for example, three different isoforms of cyclin D (D1, D2, and D3); besides pRb,

there are two other "pocket proteins," p107 and p130, that bind to transcription factors of the E2F type; and there are five isoforms of E2F and two of its dimerization partner DP. The different E2Fs have similar but not identical affinities for the E2F response elements of different genes, and each of them is regulated by one or two of the three pocket proteins. The cyclin-dependent kinases are inhibited by many CDK inhibitors. Whereas p21 is induced by p53 (see Fig. 28.4, page 607), other growth-inhibitory stimuli can be mediated by the related inhibitor p27, and there is a whole family of CDK inhibitors that includes INK4a, INK4b, INK4c, and INK4d. These four inhibitors are specific for the cyclin complexes of Cdk4 and Cdk6 (INK4 = <u>in</u>hibitor of <u>k</u>inase <u>4</u>).

Cyclin-Cdks, CDK inhibitors, pocket proteins, and E2F/DP cooperate in the regulation of the G₁ checkpoint (Fig. 28.20). The inactivation of pRb in many cancers suggests that other control elements of the G₁ checkpoint may be important in carcinogenesis as well (Table 28.2). Of the pocket proteins, however, only pRb is abnormal in many cancers; p107 and p130 generally are normal.

At the G₁ checkpoint, pRb normally is inactivated

FIG. 28.20

Abnormalities of the G₁ checkpoint in human cancers. For explanations, see text.

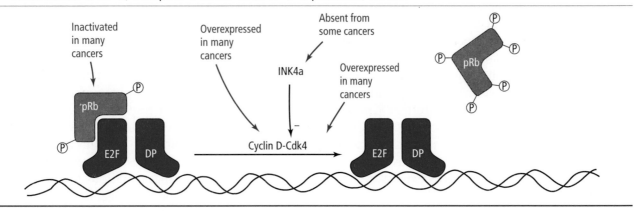

TABLE 28.2

Cell cycle regulators in cancer

Protein	Normal function	Abnormalities in cancer cells
Cyclin D1	Major G₁ cyclin; responds to mitogens	Overexpressed in many cancers
Cyclin D2 Cyclin D3	G₁ cyclins	None known
Cyclin E	Entry into S phase	None known
Cyclin A	Entry into S phase and progression toward mitosis	Rarely overexpressed in cancers
Cdk4	Major catalytic partner of the D cyclins	Amplification in sarcomas and gliomas; activating mutations in some melanomas
INK4a	Inhibitor of Cdk4, induced by growth-inhibiting stimuli	Deleted or mutated in many cancers
INK4b INK4c INK4d	Similar to INK4a	None known
pRb	"Pocket protein"; controls E2F	Mutated or deleted in many cancers
p107, p130	Similar to pRb	None known
E2F	Transcription factors; regulated by pocket proteins	None known

by cyclin-dependent phosphorylation. Indeed, *cyclin D1 is overexpressed in many cancers.* Amplifications of the cyclin D1 gene have been found in 43% of squamous cell carcinomas of the head and neck, 34% of esophageal cancers, and 10% of small-cell lung cancers and liver cancers. More than 50% of breast cancers overexpress cyclin D1, although the gene in most cases is not amplified. Also, *Cdk4, the most important catalytic partner of the D cyclins, is overexpressed or structurally abnormal in some cancers.*

Of the CDK inhibitors, the p53-induced p21 protein is rarely affected in cancers, but *mutations that in-*

activate INK4a are very common. For example, 55% of gliomas and mesotheliomas, 50% of biliary tract cancers, 40% of nasopharyngeal carcinomas, and 30% of esophageal cancers and acute lymphocytic leukemias, as well as many sarcomas and bladder and ovarian cancers, have lost functional INK4a. In addition, some patients with familial melanoma have been found to have inactivating germline mutations in the INK4a gene. Evidently, *the INK4a gene is a true tumor suppressor gene*, just as the genes for pRb and p53 are. Interestingly, tumors that overexpress cyclin D1 or are deficient in INK4a usually retain pRb, whereas those with pRb loss express cyclin D1 and INK4a normally.

The cyclin-Cdks, CDK inhibitors, and pocket proteins induce most of their effects by controlling the E2F transcription factors. Therefore we might expect overexpression of E2F in tumor cells. Actually, however, mutations of this kind have not been observed in human cancers. Experimentally, cultured cells that were transfected with overexpressed E2F genes did indeed increase their mitotic rate, but this was followed by apoptosis. Quite possibly, activating E2F mutations are not seen in cancers because such mutations lead to apoptosis. This shows that the cyclin-Cdks and pRb affect cell cycle progression and survival not only by regulating E2F, but by other mechanisms as well.

Mutations in the *p53* tumor suppressor gene are the most common genetic changes in spontaneous cancers

When the cellular DNA is damaged, the nuclear phosphoprotein p53 induces the transcription of genes that are required for growth arrest, DNA repair, and apoptosis (Fig. 28.4, page 607). Despite this seemingly specialized function, *mutations in the p53 gene (p53) have been identified in 50% to 60% of all spontaneous human cancers*. For example, these mutations are found in 70% of all colorectal cancers, 50% of lung cancers, and 40% of breast cancers. This is the most common genetic change in spontaneous tumors. Although the *p53* mutations are inactivating, they are different from the typical retinoblastoma (*Rb*) mutations: most *Rb* mutations are nonsense mutations, frameshift mutations, or large deletions, whereas 70% to 80% of the *p53* mutations are missense mutations. The mutant forms of the p53 pro-

tein are conformationally changed, fail to activate gene transcription, and in most cases are longer lived than authentic p53, which has a half-life of less than 1 hour in unstressed cells. Indeed, elevated levels of p53 are suggestive of an inactivating mutation.

Why are mutations that disrupt the p53 protein carcinogenic? The normal p53 protein has two major functions: it suppresses S-phase entry, and it induces apoptosis, both in response to DNA damage. The action at the G_1 checkpoint is known to be mediated by the CDK inhibitor p21. If this action is important for the tumor-suppressing action of normal p53, we would expect that mutations that inactivate the p21 protein would be tumorigenic as well. Actually, however, such mutations have been found in only a few prostatic cancers and seem otherwise rare in malignant tumors. It appears, therefore, that the apoptosis-suppressing effect of p53 is more important for the prevention of cancer than is the inhibition of S-phase entry: without functional p53, aberrant cells can survive and evolve into fully malignant cells.

p53 mutations have implications for cancer treatment, too: p53 is required for apoptosis in response to DNA damage. Therefore, *tumor cells without p53 are more likely to survive after radiation or DNA-damaging chemicals than are normal cells*. Indeed, the loss of functional p53 often is associated with treatment resistance.

The lack of functional p53 in many common cancers is the result of somatic mutation. Some individuals, however, are born with a mutation in one of their *p53* genes. These inherited defects give rise to the **Li-Fraumeni syndrome,** a rare (approximately 1 in 30,000), dominantly inherited cancer susceptibility syndrome with a high incidence of sarcomas, breast cancer, leukemias, brain tumors, and adrenocortical carcinomas. Half of the patients develop invasive cancers by age 30, and 90% do so by age 70. Although the normal somatic cells of these patients are heterozygous for the mutant *p53*, *their tumor cells have lost the second, intact copy of the gene*. Therefore the two-hit model shown in Fig. 28.18 for retinoblastoma applies to the Li-Fraumeni syndrome as well.

Most of the *p53* mutations—both in the common tumors and in the germline of patients with Li-Fraumeni syndrome—lead to single–amino acid substitutions in the DNA-binding domain. *These mutant p53 proteins are not necessarily inactive.* In some cases they can form transcriptionally inactive complexes with normal p53, thereby inactivating the normal p53 protein in a heterozygous cell. Normal p53 binds DNA as a tetramer, and the incorporation of mutant p53 in these tetramers disrupts their biological activity. Some mutant p53 proteins even stimulate cell proliferation by unknown mechanisms, making these mutations behave like true oncogenes.

Not only p53 itself but also proteins that interact with p53 sometimes are involved in cancer. **Mdm2,** for example, the protein product of the *mdm2* gene, binds to a site on p53 that overlaps with the transcriptional activation domain, thereby inhibiting p53's effect on gene transcription (Fig. 28.21). *mdm2* is a protooncogene that is amplified in perhaps 30% of all soft-tissue sarcomas, as well as in some glial tumors. Although these tumor cells possess normal p53, they show the same phenotypic features as cells with inactivated p53.

Although the loss of functional p53 contributes to malignant transformation, observations in p53 knockout mice show that p53 is not required for

FIG. 28.21

Interaction between p53 (■■■■) and Mdm2 (■■■■), the product of the *mdm2* (proto-) oncogene. The transcriptional activation by p53 can be disrupted by *p53* mutations that prevent sequence-specific DNA binding, the formation of transcriptionally active p53 oligomers, or the interaction with the transcriptional machinery. It also can be disrupted by the overexpression of the Mdm2 protein, which binds to p53 and thereby prevents its interaction with the transcriptional initiation complex. **A,** Normal p53 stimulates gene transcription, and this action is antagonized by Mdm2. **B,** Mutant *p53* fails to bind to its response elements in the promoters of regulated genes and to stimulate transcription. **C,** When the *mdm2* gene is amplified and its product is overexpressed, most of the p53 is tied up in complexes with Mdm2 and is not available for transcriptional activation.

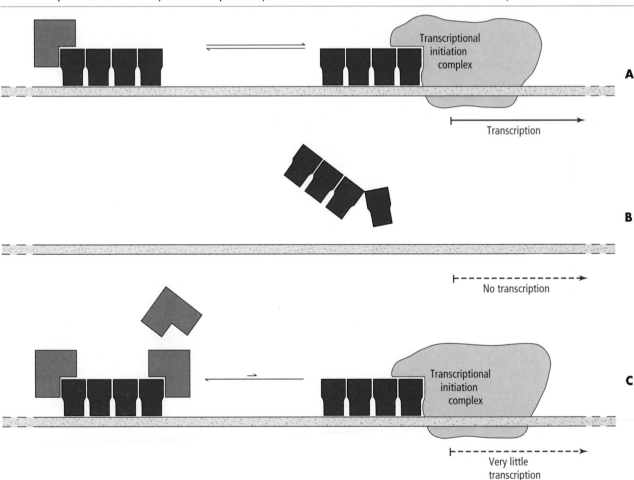

TABLE 28.3

Abnormalities in knockout mice that are homozygously deficient in cell cycle regulators

Protein	Viability of mice	Tumors
Regulators of the G_1 checkpoint		
Cyclin D1	Viable, but small size and behavioral abnormalities	None
pRb	Death at gestational day 14	—
p27*	Viable, but increased body size and female sterility	Pituitary tumors
INK4a*	Viable	Tumors by 6 months of age
E2F-1†	Viable, but T cell hyperplasia	None
Components of the DNA damage response		
p53	Viable, few abnormalities	Tumors by 3 months of age
p21*	Normal	None
Mdm2	Embryos dying at implantation‡	—
Mitogenic signal transducers		
N-Ras	Viable, no gross abnormalities	None
c-Src	Viable, but osteoclast malfunction (osteopetrosis)	None
c-Myc	Early death	—

* CDK inhibitors.
† An isoform of E2F that is regulated by pRb but not by p107 and p130.
‡ Mice lacking both Mdm2 and p53 are viable.

normal development. Its dysregulated expression in *mdm2* knockouts, however, is fatal (Table 28.3). Although p53 is important as a molecular policeman, it apparently is not required for normal embryonic development. Knockout mice lacking other important cell cycle regulators often are surprisingly normal. This suggests that many elements of cellular growth control are redundant.

Some DNA viruses possess oncogenes whose products neutralize the products of cellular tumor suppressor genes

Retrovirally induced cancers are extremely rare in humans. Some of the common cancers, however, are associated with DNA viruses. Some DNA viruses can promote cancer simply by causing chronic tissue damage, which leads to a stimulation of cell division in the surviving cells. This increases the pool of mitotic cells that potentially can acquire oncogenic mutations.

Unlike the retroviruses, *DNA viruses do not habitually integrate their DNA into the host-cell genome*. The integration of viral DNA into a host-cell chromosome, however, does occur as a rare accident during viral infection. *These viruses can induce cancer when their DNA becomes integrated into the host-cell DNA*. Like retroviral insertion (see Fig. 28.13), this occasionally can activate a cellular protooncogene by promoter insertion or enhancer insertion. **Hepatitis B virus,** for example, can insert at random sites in the genome. *Chronic infections by hepatitis B virus are an important risk factor for hepatocellular carcinoma*, although the virus does not carry an oncogene.

The **human papillomavirus** (wart virus), however, which infects the cells of squamous epithelia in the skin and mucous membranes, has its own oncogenes. This virus is a genetic pauper, with a small, circular, double-stranded DNA genome of approximately 8000 base pairs that codes for approximately half a dozen proteins. For its own reproduction, the virus has to rely heavily on DNA polymerases, helicases, and other proteins of the host cell. These host-cell proteins, however, are produced only in dividing cells, so it is in the virus' best interest to induce cell division in its host. The virus achieves this goal through the products of its two oncogenes, **E6** and **E7.** *These viral oncogene prod-*

FIG. 28.22

The molecular mechanism by which human papillomavirus stimulates the growth of infected cells. The viral E6 and E7 proteins bind to the p53 protein and the retinoblastoma protein (pRB), respectively, tying them up in inactive complexes. The resulting changes in gene transcription lead to increased cell proliferation and an increased rate of somatic mutations. In ordinary warts, the viral DNA exists as a plasmidlike episome, but in most cervical cancers the viral *E6* and/or *E7* genes are integrated in the host-cell DNA. Although the product of the *E6* gene acts like the product of the cellular *mdm2* gene (see Fig. 28.21), the two proteins are not structurally related.

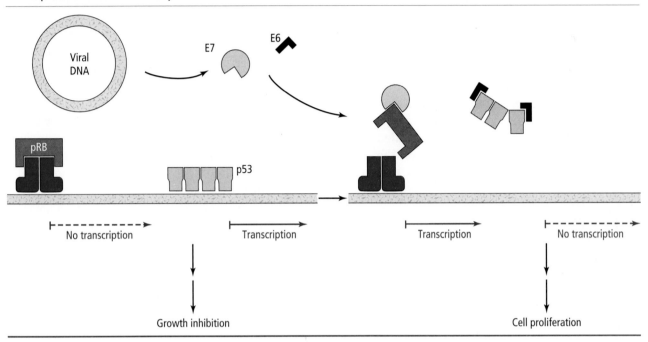

ucts inactivate the products of the major cellular tumor suppressor genes: E6 binds tightly to p53, and E7 ties up the retinoblastoma protein pRB (Fig. 28.22). After binding to the viral proteins, the tumor suppressor proteins are destroyed by normal cellular proteases. The infected cell now can proceed through the cell cycle, producing deoxyribonucleotides and enzymes of DNA replication that can be abused by the virus for the replication of its own DNA. Unlike the retroviral oncogenes, the oncogenes of the papillomavirus and other DNA viruses are not related to normal cellular protooncogenes.

Ordinarily, infection by the papillomavirus results in a common wart, with abnormally proliferating epithelial cells that contain viral DNA as plasmidlike entities. Although these cells grow abnormally, their growth is benign, and eventually they will either die or lose their virus. Rarely, however, portions of the viral DNA, including the *E6* and/or *E7* genes, become integrated into a host-cell chromosome. *These cells cannot lose the viral DNA, and some of them accumulate additional mutations that lead to a malignancy.* The papillo-

mavirus plays a sinister role in the origin of most cervical cancers. In as many as 93% of all cervical cancers worldwide, the cells contain fragments of the papillomavirus DNA integrated in their own genome. *They express the viral E6 and/or E7 proteins*, and these viral oncoproteins contribute to malignant growth by effectively depriving the cells of their p53 and pRB proteins. The papillomavirus can be transmitted by sexual intercourse, so cervical cancer can be considered a "sexually transmitted cancer." More than 50% of other anogenital cancers, as well as many nonmelanoma skin cancers and some cancers of the oral cavity, also contain the viral oncogenes.

Defective mismatch repair leads to cancer

Any condition that increases the frequency of somatic mutations is likely to increase the cancer risk. Indeed, we already have encountered inherited defects of nucleotide excision repair as a cause of skin cancer in patients with xeroderma pigmentosum (Chapter 9).

A different type of repair defect is the cause of **hereditary nonpolyposis colon cancer (HNPCC).** This dominantly inherited cancer susceptibility syndrome has a prevalence of 1 in 400 and is responsible for approximately 6% of all cases of colorectal cancer. Individuals with this syndrome also have a mildly increased risk for cancers of other tissues, including the small bowel, stomach, endometrium, urinary tract, biliary system, and ovary.

Patients with HNPCC are defective in a DNA repair system that removes base mismatches and small insertions/deletions after DNA replication. This repair system is the eukaryotic equivalent of the well-studied methyl-directed mismatch repair system of *E. coli* (Chapter 9). It requires a mismatch-recognizing protein called hMSH2 (human mutS homolog-2, named after the corresponding protein in *E. coli*) and at least three other proteins. Any of them can be mutated in patients with HNPCC.

The normal somatic cells of HNPCC patients contain a defective copy of one of the mismatch repair genes (most often the *hMSH2* gene) besides an intact copy, and their mismatch repair is near normal. Once a somatic cell loses its second, intact copy of the repair gene, however, *it becomes genetically unstable, accumulating mutations at least 100 times faster than normal cells do.* Most of these cells are doomed to die sooner or later of the rapidly accumulating genetic defects, but *some cells acquire mutations that lead to malignancy.* The potent mutator phenotype of the resulting tumor cells can be recognized by DNA fingerprinting (see Chapter 10): the microsatellite sequences of the tumor cells often differ from those of normal somatic cells of the patient, indicating that mutations occurred in the repair-deficient tumor cells.

The number of known tumor suppressor genes is increasing rapidly

Approximately two dozen tumor suppressor genes have been cloned, and the chromosomal locations have been described for many more (Table 28.4). Some of the more important features of the known tumor suppressor genes are:

1. *The encoded proteins are very heterogeneous.* Some tumor suppressor genes encode nuclear proteins that are concerned with the regulation of gene expression or the cell cycle machinery (pRb, p53, WT-1, INK4). Others encode plasma membrane proteins that may be involved in the contact inhibition or anchorage dependence of cell growth (DCC, VHL). Some are cytoskeleton-associated proteins (NF2, APC). In many cases we do not know how the tumor suppressor affects cell growth.

2. *For most tumor suppressor genes, germline mutations are known that lead to a dominantly inherited cancer susceptibility syndrome.* In the inherited diseases, the patient's somatic cells are heterozygous for the mutated and the normal ("wild-type") allele. *The tumor cells, however, usually have lost the wild-type allele.* Overall, only a minority of tumors, including 4% to 10% of all breast and colon cancers, occur in the context of an inherited cancer susceptibility syndrome.

3. *Most inherited defects of tumor suppressor genes are associated with a narrow range of tumors.* Defects of the APC gene and of postreplication mismatch repair, for example, greatly increase the risk of colorectal cancers but not of other malignancies; carriers of *BRCA1* or *BRCA2* mutations get only cancers of the breast and ovary. In some cases, the normal expression of the gene is most conspicuous in those cells that are affected by the tumors. The *WT-1* gene, for example, is associated with familial Wilms' tumor (nephroblastoma), a rare childhood tumor (incidence approximately 1 in 20,000) that arises from immature kidney cells. This gene normally is expressed in the urinary tract, but not in most other organ systems. Most other tumor suppressor genes, on the other hand, are expressed in many tissues, but only some of these are affected by the inherited disease.

4. *Most tumor suppressor genes can be inactivated either by somatic mutation or by an inherited defect.* Some, however, like the DCC (deleted in colon cancer) gene, are lost or mutated often in spontaneous tumors but rarely if ever in the germline. Although the genes that are inactivated in the heritable cancer susceptibility syndromes usually are also mutated in some spontaneous tumors, these are not necessarily the same as in the inherited syndrome. *Rb* mutations, for example, occur in many spontaneous lung and bladder cancers, although these tumors are not typical for patients with inherited retinoblastoma.

TABLE 28.4

Examples of tumor suppressor genes

Gene	Location*	Encoded protein	Inherited disease†	Inactivation or lack of expression in spontaneous tumors
Rb	13q	Nuclear phosphoprotein	Retinoblastoma	Retinoblastoma, lung, and bladder cancers
p53	17p	Nuclear phosphoprotein	Li-Fraumeni syndrome	50% of all cancers
hMsh2	2p	Mismatch repair protein	Hereditary nonpolyposis colon cancer (HNPCC)	Some colon cancers, rarely in other cancers
WT-1	11p	Nuclear protein	Wilms' tumor	Rare
NF1	17q	Neurofibromin, a Ras-GTPase activating protein	Neurofibromatosis-1	Some tumors of neural crest origin
NF2	22q	Cytoskeleton-associated peripheral membrane protein	Neurofibromatosis-2	Rare
APC	5q	Cytoskeleton-associated protein	Adenomatous polyposis coli (APC)	Most colon cancers
DCC	18q	Membrane protein	?	Most colon cancers, many other solid tumors
INK4a	9p	An inhibitor of Cdk4	Some familial melanomas	Some esophageal and pancreatic cancers
BRCA1	17q	DNA-binding protein (?)	Familial breast and ovarian cancer	Some sporadic breast cancer
BRCA2	13q	?	Familial breast and ovarian cancer	20-40% of spontaneous breast cancers
nm23	17q	Transcription factor (?)	?	Many metastatic cancers
VHL	3p	Cell surface protein (?)	von Hippel-Lindau disease	Some renal cell carcinomas

* p, Short arm; q, long arm of the chromosome.
† These diseases are inherited as autosomal dominant traits.

Carcinogenesis is a multistep process

Neoplastic diseases show a great deal of diversity, and even tumors that are derived from the same cell type vary greatly in their growth habits and clinical behaviors. Moreover, a neoplastic disease in an individual patient may change its character over time. A benign mole, for example, occasionally may turn into a malignant melanoma; a slowly progressive chronic leukemia may transform suddenly into a rapidly fatal acute stage ("blast crisis") that kills the patient within weeks; and a longstanding, indolent astrocytoma or oligodendroglioma may give rise to a highly aggressive, rapidly fatal glioblastoma.

Events of this type are called **tumor progression.**

Tumor progression occurs when a new mutation arises in an already abnormal, neoplastic cell population. *Neoplastic cells behave like any other population of living creatures: those variants that reproduce at a higher rate gradually replace those that reproduce at a lower rate.* In a population of cancerous cells, especially if these cells are afflicted by genetic instability and a high mutation rate, mutations that increase mitotic rate or invasiveness are bound to occur over time, and the more-malignant cells outgrow their less-malignant companions.

The molecular basis of tumor progression has been worked out for only a few tumors. Colorectal cancers, for example, are common, and they can be studied readily by colonoscopy and tissue biopsy.

BOX 28.1

Normal epithelium $\xrightarrow{APC\ inactivation}$ Small polyp $\xrightarrow{K\text{-}ras\ activation}$ Large polyp

p53 inactivation
and/or
DCC inactivation

Metastasis $\xleftarrow{nm23\ inactivation}$ Carcinoma

Most of these tumors develop from benign polyps. Some of these polyps gradually grow larger and become more anaplastic (disordered) in their histological appearance until a frankly invasive and finally metastatic cancer is established. A typical sequence of mutational events for this cancer looks as shown in Box 28.1. Of these mutations, only the homozygous inactivation of the APC (adenomatous polyposis coli) gene appears to be essential for the formation of a polyp and the further development of invasive cancer. Normal people have occasional intestinal polyps, but in patients with inherited adenomatous polyposis coli, the whole colonic mucosa becomes studded with thousands of polyps. Activating mutations of the K-ras protooncogene are not common in small polyps, but are seen in 40% of large polyps and carcinomas. Loss of the DCC gene or the p53 gene, or both, appears to mark the transition from a benign polyp to a true carcinoma. Many metastatic cancers, finally, show a loss or reduced expression of the nm23 tumor suppressor gene.

Some molecular markers are useful for the prognosis of cancer. The deletion of the long arm of chromosome 18 in the tumor cells, for example, is associated with decreased survival in patients with colorectal cancer. This chromosome arm harbors the DCC tumor suppressor gene. A reduced or absent expression of the nm23 gene is always associated with a high metastatic potential, not only in colorectal cancers but in many other malignancies as well. Molecular markers not only can be used for fortune telling, *they also give valuable information for the selection of treatment strategies.* If molecular markers indicate a poor prognosis, for example, aggressive treatment may be indicated; if the markers point to a high metastatic potential, systemic treatments such as chemotherapy may be indicated at an early stage in addition to local treatments such as surgery or radiation.

SUMMARY

Cell division requires an ordered sequence of events that is known as the cell cycle. The DNA is replicated during the S phase of the cell cycle, and the replicated chromosomes are distributed to the daughter cells during mitosis. There are two gaps, G_1 and G_2, from mitosis to S phase and from S phase to mitosis, respectively. The events during the cell cycle are controlled by the cyclin-dependent protein kinases (CDKs) and by their regulatory subunits, the cyclins. During G_1, the initiation of DNA replication is suppressed by the retinoblastoma protein pRB, but in dividing cells this inhibition is overcome by the CDK-induced phosphorylation and inactivation of pRB. Most of the CDKs and cyclins are not expressed in nondividing cells, which are said to be in G_0. Many cells also can undergo programmed cell death, or apoptosis, under adverse conditions.

Both cell proliferation and terminal differentiation are affected by external stimuli, including cell-cell contact, cell-matrix interactions, and exposure to soluble growth factors. Most growth factor receptors are ligand-activated, tyrosine-specific protein kinases in the plasma membrane. The most important growth-regulating signaling cascade triggered by these receptors is the MAP kinase pathway. It involves the membrane-bound Ras protein and a protein kinase cascade. This pathway affects cell growth by inducing the phosphorylation of nuclear transcription factors, thereby regulating the expression of genes for cell cycle progression and terminal differentiation.

Derangements of cellular growth control lead to neoplastic diseases, including cancer. Almost all cancers are monoclonal in origin, and they usually are caused by the cumulative effects of several mutations in a somatic cell. In one type of mutation, a growth-promoting gene becomes overexpressed or structurally altered to form a superactive product. This type of mutation produces an oncogene, and it affects cell growth even if only one copy of the growth-promoting gene becomes mutationally activated. In another type of mutation, a growth-inhibiting gene known as a tumor suppressor gene becomes inactivated by a somatic mutation. This type of mutation is effective only if both copies of the tumor suppressor gene become inactivated. Inherited defects of tumor suppressor genes occur, and they lead to familial cancer susceptibility syndromes. Some viruses can cause cancer. Most of these viruses introduce a viral oncogene that becomes covalently integrated into the cellular DNA.

Further Reading

Assoian RK: Anchorage-dependent cell cycle progression. *J Cell Biol* 136 (1), 1−4, 1997.

Bates S, Vousden KH: p53 in signaling checkpoint arrest or apoptosis. *Curr Opin Genet Dev* 6, 12−19, 1996.

Beijersbergen RL, Bernards R: Cell cycle regulation by the retinoblastoma family of growth inhibitory proteins. *Biochim Biophys Acta* 1287, 103−120, 1996.

Bellacosa A, Genuardi M, Anti M, Viel A, Ponz de Leon M: Hereditary nonpolyposis colon cancer: review of clinical, molecular genetics and counseling aspects. *Am J Med Genet* 62, 353−364, 1996.

Benz CC, Brandt BH, Zänker KS: Gene diagnostics provide new insights into breast cancer prognosis and therapy. *Gene* 159, 3−7, 1995.

Brown MT, Cooper JA: Regulation, substrates and function of src. *Biochim Biophys Acta* 1287, 121−149, 1996.

Carpenter CL, Cantley LC: Phosphoinositide 3-kinase and the regulation of cell growth. *Biochim Biophys Acta* 1288, M11−M16, 1996.

Claesson-Welsh L: Platelet-derived growth factor receptor signals. *J Biol Chem* 269 (51), 32023−32026, 1994.

Clark EA, Brugge JB: Integrins and signal transduction pathways: the road taken. *Science* 268, 233−239, 1995.

Dedhar S: Integrin mediated signal transduction in oncogenesis: an overview. *Cancer Metastasis Rev* 14, 165−172, 1995.

Desbarats L, Schneider A, Muller D, Burgin A, Eilers M: Myc: a single gene controls both proliferation and apoptosis in mammalian cells. *Experientia* 52, 1123−1128, 1996.

Dunlop MG: Mutator genes and mosaicism in colorectal cancer. *Curr Opin Genet Dev* 6, 75−80, 1996.

Eisenman RN, Cooper JA: Beating a path to myc. *Nature* 378, 438−439, 1995.

Fearon ER: DCC: is there a connection between tumorigenesis and cell guidance molecules? *Biochim Biophys Acta* 1288, M17−M23, 1996.

Gottlieb TM, Oren M: p53 in growth control and neoplasia. *Biochim Biophys Acta* 1287, 77−102, 1996.

Harper JW, Elledge SJ: Cdk inhibitors in development and cancer. *Curr Opin Genet Dev* 6, 56−64, 1996.

Jiricny J: Colon cancer and DNA repair: have mismatches met their match? *Trends Genet* 10 (5), 164−168, 1994.

Kamb A: Cell-cycle regulators and cancer. *Trends Genet* 11 (4), 136−140, 1995.

Karp JE, Broder S: Molecular foundations of cancer: new targets for intervention. *Nature Med* 1 (4), 309−320, 1995.

Malik RK, Parsons JT: Integrin-mediated signaling in normal and malignant cells: a role of protein tyrosine kinases. *Biochim Biophys Acta* 1287, 73−76, 1996.

Malkin D: p53 and the Li-Fraumeni syndrome. *Biochim Biophys Acta* 1198, 197−213, 1994.

Momand J, Zambetti GP: Mdm-2: "big brother" of p53. *J Cell Biochem* 64, 343−352, 1997.

Müller R: Transcriptional regulation during the mammalian cell cycle. *Trends Genet* 11 (5), 173−178, 1995.

Rabbitts TH: Chromosomal translocations in human cancer. *Nature* 372, 143−149, 1994.

Reddy JC, Licht JD: The WT1 Wilms' tumor suppressor gene: how much do we really know? *Biochim Biophys Acta* 1287, 1−28, 1996.

Sherr CJ: D-type cyclins. *Trends Biochem Sci* 20, 187−190, 1995.

Sherr CJ: Cancer cell cycles. *Science* 274, 1672−1677, 1996.

Yonish-Rouach E: The p53 tumour suppressor gene: a mediator of a G1 growth arrest and of apoptosis. *Experientia* 52, 1001−1005, 1996.

zur Hausen H: Papillomavirus infections—a major cause of human cancers. *Biochim Biophys Acta* 1288, F55−F78, 1996.

QUESTIONS

1. An activating mutation in the *ras* gene most likely will
   A. Prevent the autophosphorylation of growth factor receptors
   B. Inhibit the release of calcium from the ER
   C. Increase the activity of the MAP kinases
   D. Activate the Src protein kinase
   E. Reduce the nuclear concentration of cyclin D

2. Which type of structural/functional change would be most likely in an oncogenically activated variant of the Ras protein?
    A. Inability to interact with the Raf-1 protein kinase
    B. Reduced GTPase activity
    C. A point mutation in a transmembrane helix
    D. Enhanced GTPase activity
    E. An increased ability to tyrosine-phosphorylate proteins

3. Most of the cyclins are induced and repressed periodically during the cell cycle. One cyclin, however, is controlled primarily by mitogens rather than by the cell cycle machinery. This mitogen-sensing cyclin is
    A. Cyclin A
    B. Cyclin B
    C. Cyclin C
    D. Cyclin D
    E. Cyclin E

4. The retinoblastoma protein (pRb) is a major control element of the cell cycle. pRb normally becomes
    A. Transcriptionally induced at the G_1 checkpoint
    B. Dephosphorylated at the G_1 checkpoint
    C. Phosphorylated at the G_1 checkpoint
    D. Phosphorylated at the G_2 checkpoint
    E. Transcriptionally induced at the G_2 checkpoint

5. The homozygous loss of a cell cycle regulator or signaling molecule may contribute to malignant transformation. This is most likely for the homozygous loss of
    A. The Cdk4 protein kinase
    B. Cyclin E
    C. A peripheral membrane protein that is required for the normal interaction between integrin receptors and the Src protein
    D. A MAP kinase
    E. The CDK inhibitor INK4

6. Some strains of the human papillomavirus contribute to malignant transformation by producing oncogene products that
    A. Induce the transcription of early-response genes
    B. Bind and inactivate the retinoblastoma and p53 proteins

    C. Activate growth factor receptors in the absence of the normal ligand
    D. Activate cyclin-dependent kinases by direct binding to the catalytic subunit
    E. Act as protein kinases that phosphorylate many of the same proteins as the MAP kinases

7. The entry into mitosis is accompanied by the phosphorylation of histone H1, chromosomal scaffold proteins, and nuclear lamins. The protein kinase that is responsible for these phosphorylations is known to be regulated by all of the following except
    A. Binding of a regulatory cyclin
    B. Activating phosphorylations
    C. Inhibitory phosphorylations
    D. Protein phosphatases
    E. The reversible binding of a GTP molecule to a regulatory site

8. Mutations in the *p53* gene are the most common aberrations in spontaneous human cancers. The normal p53 protein participates in normal cell cycle regulation by
    A. Inducing cell cycle arrest and apoptosis in response to DNA damage
    B. Inducing the phosphorylation of the retinoblastoma protein in response to mitogens
    C. Directly inhibiting CDK inhibitors in response to cell-cell contact ("contact inhibition") and other growth-inhibiting stimuli
    D. Increasing the activity of cyclin-dependent protein kinases by inducing their phosphorylation
    E. Binding and thereby inactivating the products of many early-response genes

9. The first event in signal transduction by the PDGF (platelet-derived growth factor) receptor is:
    A. Opening of a calcium channel in the plasma membrane
    B. Opening of a calcium channel in the ER membrane
    C. The phosphorylation of the Ras protein on serine side chains
    D. The autophosphorylation of the receptor on tyrosine side chains
    E. The activation of a heterotrimeric G protein

Chapter 29

Integration of Metabolism

Metabolic activity has to satisfy both the needs of the individual cell and those of the organism as a whole. The main concern of the individual cell is the supply of metabolic energy in the form of ATP. More altruistic mechanisms, however, have to operate in the interest of the body as a whole. Glycogenolysis in hepatocytes and lipolysis in adipocytes, for example, are required not for the well-being of these cells but for the nourishment of distant tissues.

Metabolic activity has to adapt to a fluctuating nutrient supply and to changing physiological needs. We have to adjust the activities of our metabolic pathways to conditions of overeating and starvation; sometimes we have to engage in vigorous muscular activity; and we have to deal with noxious environmental chemicals that have to be metabolized and excreted. Most of these challenges require close cooperation among the different tissues and organs whose activities have to be coordinated by hormonal and neural mechanisms. In this chapter we are concerned with the metabolic adaptations to environmental challenges and varying physiological needs. We will encounter the hormonal mechanisms of metabolic regulation and some clinical conditions in which these regulatory mechanisms are deranged.

EXTRACELLULAR MESSENGERS AS METABOLIC REGULATORS

Metabolic pathways can be regulated directly by the supply of nutrients. Such nutrients as glucose and fatty acids are not only substrates of the pathways, they also are able to regulate metabolic activity at the level of enzyme synthesis or enzyme activity. A far more elaborate system of metabolic regulators, however, is available in the form of hormones, neurotransmitters, and other extracellular messengers. *These messengers are released in specific physiological situations* to coordinate metabolic activities in different parts of the body.

Insulin is a satiety hormone

After a hearty meal, the body is flooded with monosaccharides, amino acids, and triglycerides. Not all of this bounty can be used immediately for the energy needs of the tissues, and *the excess nutrients have to be stored away as glycogen and triglycerides.*

Most adaptations to the well-fed state are mediated by **insulin**. *The synthesis and release of this hormone are powerfully stimulated by glucose*, and this effect is potentiated by amino acids. Therefore *the plasma level of insulin is highest after a carbohydrate-rich mixed meal.*

The metabolic effects of insulin are summarized in Table 29.1. The attentive reader will notice immediately that *insulin stimulates the utilization of dietary nutrients* including glucose, amino acids, and triglycerides. Some of these nutrients are used for the synthesis of glycogen and triglycerides, the principal energy reserves of the body.

Insulin regulates the blood glucose level by its actions on liver, muscle, and adipose tissue. *In skeletal muscle and adipose tissue, the uptake of glucose into the cell*

TABLE 29.1

Metabolic effects of insulin

Tissue	Affected pathway	Affected enzyme
Liver	↑ Glucose phosphorylation	Glucokinase
	↑ Glycolysis	Phosphofructokinase-1,† pyruvate kinase*
	↓ Gluconeogenesis	PEP-carboxykinase, fructose 1,6-bisphosphatase,† glucose 6-phosphatase
	↑ Glycogen synthesis	Glycogen synthase*
	↓ Glycogenolysis	Glycogen phosphorylase*
	↑ Fatty acid synthesis	Acetyl-CoA carboxylase,* ATP-citrate lyase, malic enzyme
	↑ Pentose phosphate pathway	Glucose 6-phosphate dehydrogenase
Adipose tissue	↑ Glucose uptake	Glucose carrier
	↑ Glycolysis	Phosphofructokinase-1
	↑ Pentose phosphate pathway	Glucose 6-phosphate dehydrogenase
	↑ Pyruvate oxidation	Pyruvate dehydrogenase*
	↑ Triglyceride utilization (from lipoproteins)	Lipoprotein lipase
	↑ Triglyceride synthesis	Glycerol 3-phosphate acyl transferase
	↓ Lipolysis	Hormone-sensitive lipase*
Skeletal muscle	↑ Glucose uptake	Glucose carrier
	↑ Glycolysis	Phosphofructokinase-1
	↑ Glycogen synthesis	Glycogen synthase*
	↓ Glycogenolysis	Glycogen phosphorylase*
	↑ Protein synthesis	Translational initiation complex

* Insulin acts by promoting the dephosphorylation of the enzyme.
† Insulin acts indirectly by promoting the dephosphorylation of phosphofructokinase-2/fructose 2,6-bisphosphatase, thereby increasing the level of fructose 2,6-bisphosphate.
Most of the other insulin effects included here are actions on the rate of synthesis or degradation of the affected enzyme.

is the rate-limiting step of glucose metabolism. In unstimulated adipose tissue, only a small fraction of the glucose carriers are present in the plasma membrane, and these carriers are not fully active (Fig. 29.1). Most of the glucose transporters are in the membranes of small intracellular vesicles, where they are kept in reserve until needed. The binding of insulin to its receptor induces the fusion of these vesicles with the plasma membrane in a process analogous to exocytosis. At the same time, the carriers already present on the cell surface become fully active. The overall result is a *ten- to twentyfold increase in the V_{max} of glucose uptake within a few minutes after insulin exposure.*

The liver has an insulin-independent glucose transporter that is not rate limiting, but *the glucose-metabolizing enzymes are stimulated by insulin.* The levels of the regulated glycolytic enzymes gradually increase within several hours after insulin exposure as a result of increased de novo synthesis, while the levels of the gluconeogenic enzymes decline. In addition, the glucose-consuming activities of glycolysis and glycogen synthesis are stimulated on a minute-by-minute basis while the opposing activities of gluconeogenesis and glycogen degradation are inhibited. These short-term effects are mediated by the dephosphorylation of metabolic and regulatory enzymes.

Glucose metabolism in brain and erythrocytes is not insulin dependent, so these tissues keep consuming glucose even during fasting, when the insulin level is low. Unlike muscle, adipose tissue, and the liver, brain cells and RBCs cannot easily switch to alternative fuels; they depend on glucose at all times.

Insulin is important for lipid metabolism, too. *It*

FIG. 29.1

Effect of insulin on the glucose carriers in adipocytes. A similar mechanism is thought to operate in skeletal muscle. **A,** In the resting state, most glucose carriers are present in the membrane of intracellular vesicles. **B,** After insulin binding and receptor autophosphorylation, the carrier-containing vesicles fuse with the plasma membrane. This leads to an increased V_{max} of glucose transport across the plasma membrane.

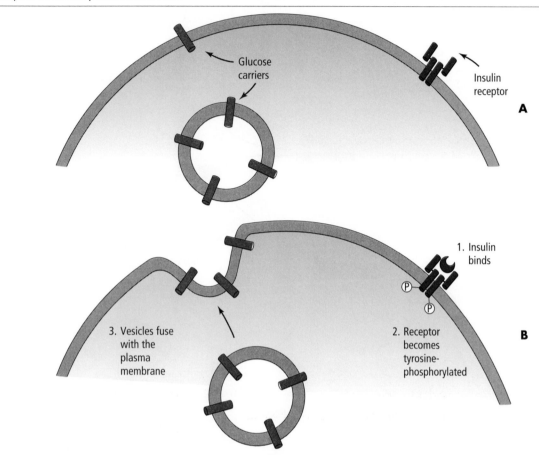

helps to direct dietary triglycerides to adipose tissue by inducing lipoprotein lipase in this tissue and by facilitating triglyceride synthesis (see Chapter 18). At the same time, *it prevents the hydrolysis of stored triglycerides* by potently inhibiting the hormone-sensitive adipose tissue lipase.

The mechanisms of the insulin effects on carbohydrate and lipid metabolism are poorly understood. Although insulin signaling is initiated by receptor autophosphorylation (see Chapter 27), and insulin-stimulated protein kinases are known (see, for example, Fig. 18.14), most of the metabolic insulin effects are mediated by the dephosphorylation of metabolic enzymes. Insulin also lowers the cAMP concentration in many tissues, including liver and adipose tissue, by incompletely known mechanisms.

The utilization of amino acids also is stimulated by insulin. In many tissues, *insulin stimulates protein synthesis by a direct action on the translational machinery.* This effect is mediated by the MAP kinase pathway (see Chapter 28), which is activated not only by growth factors but also by insulin (Fig. 29.2).

Glucagon maintains the blood glucose level

The secretion of glucagon from the pancreatic α cells is increased two- to threefold by hypoglycemia and is reduced to half of the basal release by hyperglycemia. Acting through its second messenger cAMP, *glucagon upregulates the blood glucose level whenever dietary carbohydrate is in short supply.* Its actions on the pathways

FIG. 29.2

Stimulation of ribosomal protein synthesis in adipose cells by insulin. Like the growth factors (see Figs. 28.7 and 28.8), insulin stimulates the activity of the MAP kinases. The MAP kinases phosphorylate the 12-kDa protein PHAS-1. The unphosphorylated form of PHAS-1 is bound to the initiation factor eIF-4E. Once phosphorylated by the MAP kinases, PHAS-1 no longer binds the initiation factor, which is now free to attach itself to the cap at the 5' end of the mRNA. The binding of eIF-4E to the cap is required for the initiation of translation.

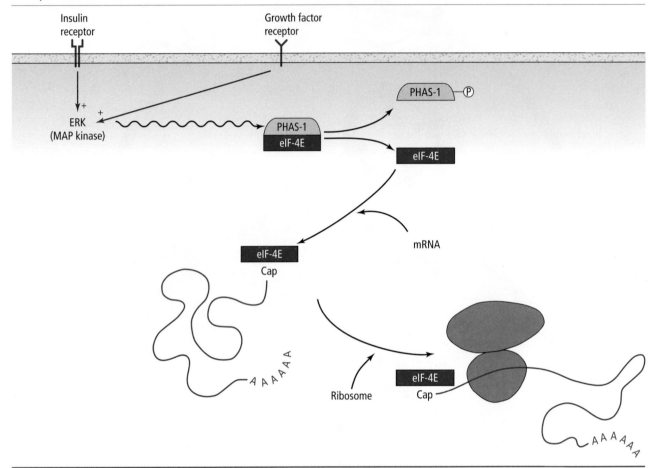

of glucose metabolism are opposite to those of insulin (Table 29.2), but unlike insulin, *glucagon acts almost exclusively on the liver*, with negligible effects on adipose tissue, muscle, and other extrahepatic tissues.

Catecholamines mediate the flight-or-fight response

Norepinephrine is the principal neurotransmitter of postganglionic sympathetic neurons, and both epinephrine and norepinephrine are released from the adrenal medulla in response to nerve stimulation.

The catecholamines are released in response to physical and psychological stress. Physical exertion is always accompanied by catecholamine release, as is cold exposure. A purely psychological stress, such as taking a biochemistry exam, also results in catecholamine release.

The catecholamines can elevate the cellular cAMP level by an action on β-adrenergic receptors, and they can elevate cytoplasmic calcium by an action on α_1-adrenergic receptors. Whereas β receptors are the principal adrenergic receptors in skeletal muscle and adipose tissue, the α_1 receptors prevail in the liver.

TABLE 29.2

Metabolic effects of glucagon on the liver*

		Enzyme affected by		
Effect on pathway	Affected enzyme	Enzyme induction/repression	Enzyme phosphorylation	Other
↓ Glycolysis	Glucokinase	+		
	Phosphofructokinase			+†
	Pyruvate kinase	+		
↑ Gluconeogenesis	PEP-carboxykinase	+		
	Fructose 1,6-bisphosphatase	+		+†
	Glucose 6-phosphatase	+		
↓ Glycogen synthesis	Glycogen synthase		+	
↑ Glycogenolysis	Glycogen phosphorylase		+	
↓ Fatty acid synthesis	Acetyl-CoA carboxylase	+	+	
↑ Fatty acid oxidation	Carnitine-palmitoyl transferase-1	+		

* Both the enzyme phosphorylations and the effects on gene expression are mediated by cAMP.
† Mediated by the cAMP-dependent phosphorylation of phosphofructokinase-2/fructose 2,6-bisphosphatase and a decreased cellular concentration of fructose 2,6-bisphosphate.

TABLE 29.3

Metabolic effects of norepinephrine and epinephrine

Tissue	Affected pathway	Affected enzyme	Second messenger
Adipose tissue	↑ ↑ ↑ Lipolysis	Hormone-sensitive lipase*	cAMP
	↓ Triglyceride utilization (from lipoproteins)	Lipoprotein lipase	?
Liver	↓ Glycolysis	Phosphofructokinase-1†	cAMP
	↑ Gluconeogenesis	Fructose 1,6-bisphosphatase†	
	↓ ↓ Glycogen synthesis	Glycogen synthase*	Ca²⁺, cAMP
	↑ ↑ ↑ Glycogenolysis	Glycogen phosphorylase*	
	↓ Fatty acid synthesis	Acetyl-CoA carboxylase*	cAMP
Skeletal muscle	↑ ↑ ↑ Glycolysis	Phosphofructokinase-1†	cAMP
	↓ ↓ Glycogen synthesis	Glycogen synthase*	
	↑ ↑ ↑ Glycogenolysis	Glycogen phosphorylase*	
	↑ Triglyceride utilization (from lipoproteins)	Lipoprotein lipase	?

↑ and ↓, Weak or inconsistent effect; ↑ ↑ and ↓ ↓, moderately strong effect; ↑ ↑ ↑ and ↓ ↓ ↓, strong effect.
* Effects mediated by enzyme phosphorylation.
† Mediated indirectly by phosphorylation of phosphofructokinase-2/fructose 2,6-bisphosphatase.

The metabolic actions of the catecholamines are summarized in Table 29.3. These actions, which appear within seconds, are part of the **flight-or-fight response**: *the catecholamines mobilize the body's fat and glycogen reserves for use by the contracting muscles.* In mus-cle tissue itself, *an abundant ATP supply is secured by a powerful stimulation of glycogen degradation and glycolysis.* As in the liver (see Chapter 17), glycolysis in skele-tal muscle is stimulated by fructose 2,6-bisphos-phate, which acts as a potent allosteric activator of phosphofructokinase-1. The phosphofructokinase-2/fructose 2,6-bisphosphatase of skeletal muscle, however, is different from the liver enzyme: its kinase activity is not inhibited but rather stimulated by cAMP-induced phosphorylation. Therefore the catecholamines, acting through β receptors and cAMP, stimulate rather than inhibit glycolysis in muscle tissue.

The catecholamines are functional antagonists of insulin. They increase, for example, the blood glucose level and the concentration of plasma free fatty acids. They are not very important for blood glucose regulation under ordinary conditions, but they become important in metabolic emergencies because *their release is potently stimulated by hypoglycemia.* Indeed, hypoglycemic episodes in a variety of metabolic diseases always are accompanied by signs of excessive sympathetic activity such as pallor, sweating, and tachycardia.

Glucocorticoids are released in chronic stress

Cortisol and other glucocorticoids are released in response to neural stimuli that reach the adrenal cortex through corticotropin-releasing factor and ACTH. *Their release is increased in chronic stress,* and many of their metabolic actions can be understood best as adaptations to life in a dangerous world.

Many of these metabolic actions, summarized in Table 29.4, are synergistic with those of epinephrine. However, there is one important difference: the epinephrine effects are mediated by the second messengers cAMP and calcium, which affect metabolic enzymes within seconds. Glucocorticoids, on the other hand, induce the synthesis of new enzyme proteins, so their effects have a slower onset and are longer lasting.

Cortisol assists in the mobilization of adipose tissue triglycerides by inducing the synthesis of the hormone-sensitive lipase. This does not cause excessive lipolysis under ordinary conditions, but the action of epinephrine is potentiated. In addition, *gluconeogenesis is stimulated at all levels:* increased protein breakdown in skeletal muscle and other extrahepatic tissues supplies amino acid precursors; in the liver, transaminases and other enzymes of amino acid metabolism are induced together with PEP-carboxykinase. Part of the glucose 6-phosphate formed by gluconeogenesis is diverted into glycogen synthesis, and *liver glycogen stores are increased.*

We now can see how cortisol and epinephrine cooperate in a stressful situation: during an extended hunting expedition by a Stone Age caveman, cortisol induces the hormone-sensitive lipase in his adipose tissue, and it builds up the glycogen stores in his liver. As soon as our hunter is attacked by a cave bear, epinephrine comes into play: the hormone-sensitive lipase now releases fatty acids from his adipose tissue, and his liver glycogen is converted to glucose. Thanks to the supply of these fuels to his muscles, our caveman manages to dodge the cave bear's attack, kill the animal with his club, and have a fine dinner that night.

The stress hormones are important in contemporary settings as well. In patients suffering from infections, autoimmune diseases, malignancies, injuries, and indeed any illness, we have to expect increased levels of glucocorticoids and catecholamines. *Any seriously ill patient is likely to have a negative nitrogen balance* because of the cortisol-induced protein and amino acid catabolism, and muscle

---

TABLE 29.4

Important metabolic actions of cortisol and other glucocorticoids*

Tissue	Affected pathway	Affected enzyme
Adipose tissue	↑ Lipolysis	Hormone-sensitive lipase
Muscle tissue	↑ Protein degradation	?
Liver	↑ Gluconeogenesis	Enzymes of amino acid catabolism, PEP-carboxykinase
	↑ Glycogen synthesis	Glycogen synthase

* The glucocorticoid effects are mediated by altered rates of enzyme synthesis.

wasting is inevitable in protracted diseases. Well-meaning dieticians try, of course, to counteract this effect with a protein-rich diet. Because the stress hormones oppose the effects of insulin on carbohydrate metabolism, *insulin resistance and poor glucose tolerance have to be expected.* The management of insulin-dependent diabetics during otherwise harmless infections or other illnesses is difficult because their insulin requirement increases substantially.

Some cytokines, which are released by white blood cells during infections and some other diseases, also have metabolic effects. **Interleukin-1**, for example, stimulates proteolysis in skeletal muscle, and **tumor necrosis factor** is thought to promote lipolysis in adipose tissue. These mediators may be important for the weight loss that is common in patients with malignancies or chronic infections.

FEEDING AND FASTING

Unlike ruminants and some other animals, most people do not eat continuously, but rather in well-spaced meals. For a few hours after a meal, the dietary nutrients are more than sufficient to provide for the energy needs of the body, but stored energy reserves have to be mobilized during fasting. In the following sections we will encounter the metabolic adaptations that enable us to survive in the face of a fluctuating nutrient supply.

Energy and glucose have to be supplied during fasting

Adipose tissue triglycerides contain most of the stored energy—almost 100 times more than the combined glycogen stores (Table 29.5). Therefore glycogen cannot be used as an energy source during prolonged fasting. Indeed, *triglycerides are a "savings account"* for use during long-term fasting, but *glycogen is a "checking account"* from which withdrawals are made on an hour-by-hour basis. Triglycerides are more suitable than glycogen for storage because of their higher caloric density.

Why, then, do we need glycogen at all? The muscles take advantage of the fact that *glycogen, unlike fat, can provide ATP under anaerobic conditions.* The liver, on the other hand, uses glycogen as *a ready-made source of free glucose.* All cells in the human body can utilize glucose, but not every cell can oxidize fatty acids. The brain, in particular, cannot utilize fatty acids from adipose tissue, so it depends on liver-supplied glucose during fasting. Under ordinary conditions, the brain covers almost all of its energy needs from glucose—some 120 g every day. Therefore *an adequate blood glucose level has to be maintained for this fastidious eater at all times.*

Unlike glycogen and triglycerides, proteins are not a specialized energy storage form. Although it serves important functions of its own, much of the protein in muscle and other tissues can be degraded during fasting. *Protein breakdown is required to supply amino acid substrates for gluconeogenesis.* Even-chain fatty acids, which account for 95% of the energy value of triglycerides, cannot be used for gluconeogenesis. Therefore *the progressive loss of protein from muscle and other tissues is inevitable during prolonged periods of fasting.*

The levels of nutrients and hormones are affected by feeding and fasting

Figure 29.3 shows some of the changes in blood chemistry during the transition from the well-fed state to starvation. The most important hormonal factor is *the balance between insulin and its antagonists,*

TABLE 29.5

Energy reserves of the "textbook" 70-kg male

Stored nutrient	Tissue	Amt stored (kg)	Energy value (kcal)
Triglyceride	Adipose tissue	10-15	90,000-140,000
Glycogen	Muscle	0.3	1200
	Liver	0.08*	320*
Protein	Muscle	6-8	30,000-40,000

* After a meal. Liver glycogen is approximately 20% to 30% of this value after an overnight fast of 12 hours.

FIG. 29.3

Plasma levels of hormones and nutrients at different times after the last meal.

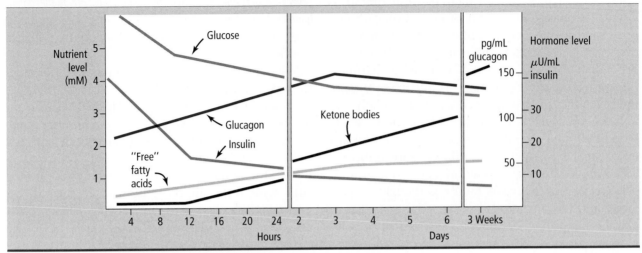

particularly glucagon. During fasting, the plasma level of insulin decreases while those of first epinephrine, then glucagon, and finally cortisol increase.

The blood glucose level decreases only to a limited extent even during prolonged fasting, but free fatty acids increase four- to eightfold, and ketone bodies (β-hydroxybutyrate and acetoacetate) increase up to 100-fold. *Blood glucose, unlike fatty acids and ketone bodies, has to be tightly regulated because the brain and RBCs require it as an essential fuel.*

The metabolism of adipose tissue changes dramatically in different nutritional states

Both triglyceride synthesis and triglyceride hydrolysis (lipolysis) in adipose tissue are affected by the nutritional state (Fig. 29.4). Triglyceride synthesis depends on the supply of glycerol phosphate, which has to be synthesized from glucose via dihydroxyacetone phosphate (see Fig. 18.3). *The insulin-dependent uptake of glucose into the cell is the most important rate-limiting step in this pathway.*

Chylomicrons are the principal source of fatty acids for triglyceride synthesis after a mixed meal. The utilization of chylomicron triglycerides depends on **lipoprotein lipase.** This enzyme is insulin inducible in adipose tissue but not in skeletal or cardiac muscle, so *lipoprotein triglycerides are routed preferentially to adipose tissue in the well-fed state but not during fasting.*

Lipolysis is controlled by the catecholamines, which stimulate the hormone-sensitive lipase, and by insulin, which opposes this effect. Adipose tissue is more sensitive than most other tissues to insulin, and *lipolysis is inhibited even at moderately high insulin levels during the early stages of fasting.*

The liver converts dietary carbohydrates to glycogen and fat

Whereas adipose tissue is the most important destination of dietary triglycerides, *the liver metabolizes 20% to 30% of the dietary glucose* after a carbohydrate-rich meal (Fig. 29.5). Because of the high K_m of glucokinase (see Fig. 17.8, Chapter 17), *hepatic glucose utilization is controlled by substrate availability.* Insulin facilitates glucose phosphorylation by inducing the synthesis of glucokinase, an effect that is maximal after 2 or 3 days on a high-carbohydrate diet.

A good deal of the glucose 6-phosphate is used for glycogen synthesis after a carbohydrate-rich meal, and most of the rest is metabolized by glycolysis. The liver has only a moderately high capacity for glycolysis, and after a mixed meal amino acids are a more important source of metabolic energy than is glucose. *In the liver, glycolysis is the first step in the conversion of carbohydrate to fat.* Triglycerides, phospholipids, and cholesterol esters are released by the liver as constituents of VLDL. The carbohydrate-to-fat conversion is coordinated by insulin, which

FIG. 29.4

Metabolism of adipose tissue after a mixed meal and during fasting. **A,** After a meal. Insulin-stimulated or insulin-inhibited steps are marked by + or −, respectively. LPL, lipoprotein lipase; IDL, intermediate-density lipoprotein (VLDL remnant). **B,** During fasting.

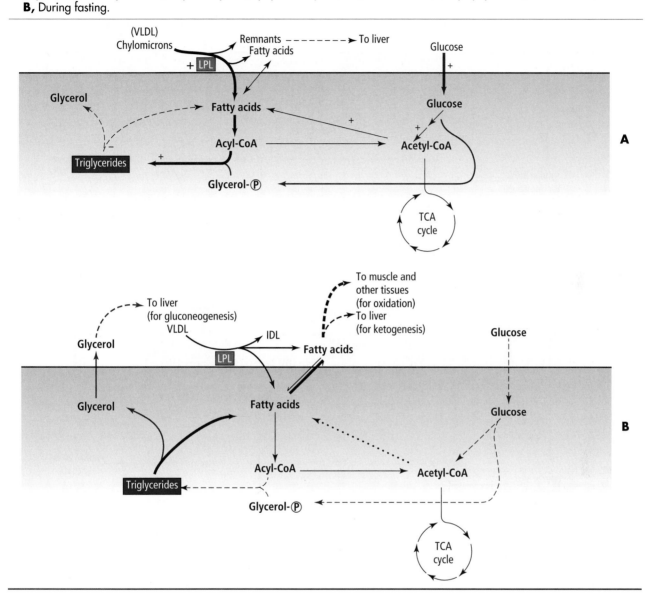

stimulates both glycolysis and fatty acid synthesis after a carbohydrate-rich meal.

The liver has no lipoprotein lipase, so *it is not a major consumer of dietary triglycerides*. It still obtains some dietary triglyceride, together with other dietary lipids, by the uptake of chylomicron remnants (see Fig. 20.3). The levels of plasma free fatty acids are low after a mixed meal, because lipolysis in adipose tissue is inhibited and most of the fatty acids released by lipoprotein lipase are esterified to triglycerides in adipose tissue or oxidized directly in other extrahepatic tissues.

The liver supplies glucose and ketone bodies during fasting

In the fasting state, *the liver has to keep the glucose-dependent tissues alive by releasing glucose into the blood*. The brain is the most avid consumer of glucose both after a meal and during fasting. It is the most aristo-

FIG. 29.5

The yo-yo dieter's liver. **A,** After a meal. Pathways that are stimulated or inhibited by insulin are marked by + or −, respectively. **B,** Twelve hours after the last meal.

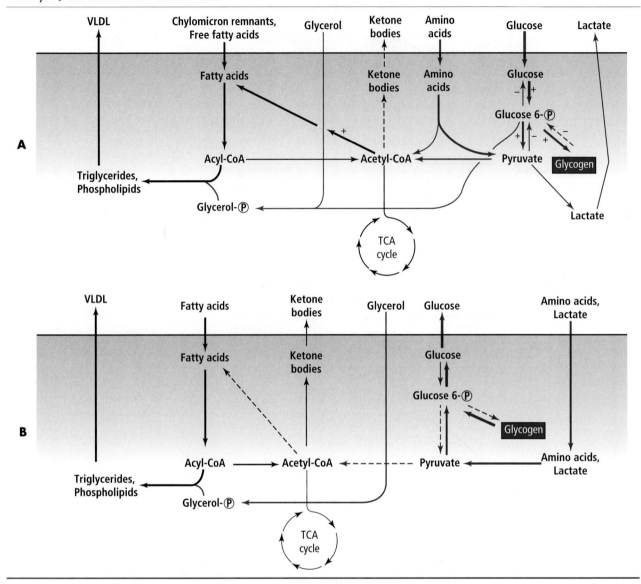

cratic organ in the body, and like any aristocrat it requires a large share of the communally owned resources: although it accounts for only 2% of the body weight in an adult, it consumes almost 30% of the total energy in the resting body. This large energy demand is covered almost exclusively from glucose under ordinary conditions, and from glucose and ketone bodies during prolonged fasting. The brain oxidizes approximately 120 g of glucose per day in the well-fed state and 50 g during long-term fasting.

Within 3 to 5 hours after a meal, the liver becomes a net producer of glucose. The glucose initially is formed by glycogen breakdown, but *liver glycogen is depleted within a day*, so gluconeogenesis is the only source of glucose during extended fasting. Lactate, glycerol, and amino acids are the substrates, and the rate of gluconeogenesis is determined in part by their availability. Glycerol and amino acids are supplied during fasting from lipolysis in adipose tissue and from protein degradation in skeletal muscle. Gluconeogenesis itself is stimulated hormon-

FIG. 29.5 CONT'D

C, Four days after the last meal. **D,** The first good meal after 4 days of fasting.

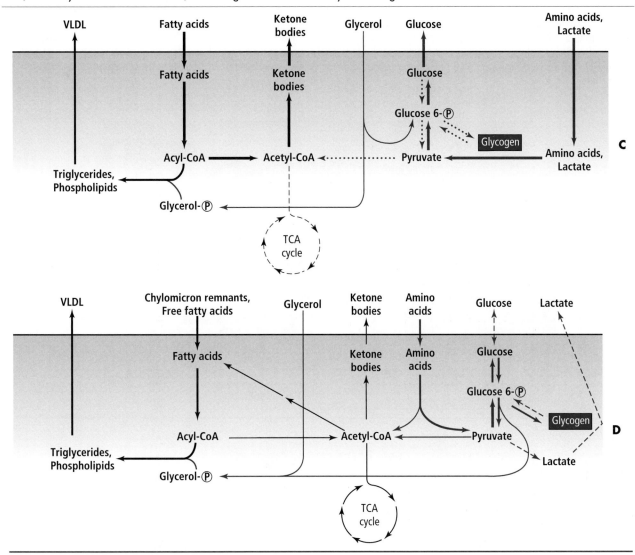

ally. It produces 100 to 180 g of glucose per day during fasting, and most of this is consumed by the brain. More than half of the glucose is synthesized from amino acids.

Ketone bodies (see Chapter 18) are another important product of the fasting liver. In theory, both carbohydrates and fatty acids can be converted into ketone bodies via acetyl-CoA. Actually, however, the maximal rate of glycolysis in the liver is no more than 2 μmol per g of tissue weight per minute, or 30 g/hr for a 3-pound liver. Because a large portion of the acetyl-CoA is used for lipogenesis and some is oxidized in the TCA cycle after a meal, very little is left for ketogenesis. The

capacity of the liver for fatty acid oxidation, on the other hand, is very high, and over a wide range of plasma levels approximately 30% of the incoming fatty acids are extracted and metabolized: *hepatic fatty acid utilization is controlled by substrate availability*. It is increased during fasting, when adipose tissue supplies large amounts of free fatty acids.

The liver has several options for the metabolism of these fatty acids (Fig. 29.6):

1. *The fatty acids are esterified in the cytoplasm or ER. The resulting triglycerides, phospholipids, and cholesterol esters are exported as constituents of VLDL.*

FIG. 29.6

Alternative fates of fatty acids in the liver. The regulated steps are: ① carnitine acyl transferase-1. This enzyme is induced in the fasting state. It also is acutely inhibited by malonyl-CoA (the product of the acetyl-CoA carboxylase reaction) when fatty acid biosynthesis is stimulated after a carbohydrate-rich meal. ② Acetyl-CoA carboxylase. This enzyme is induced in the well-fed state. It is inhibited in the fasting state by high acyl-CoA, low citrate (direct allosteric effects), and a high glucagon/insulin ratio (leading to phosphorylation and inactivation). ③ The TCA cycle is inhibited when alternative sources supply ATP and NADH. Therefore a high rate of β-oxidation reduces its activity. ④ The ketogenic enzymes are induced during fasting.

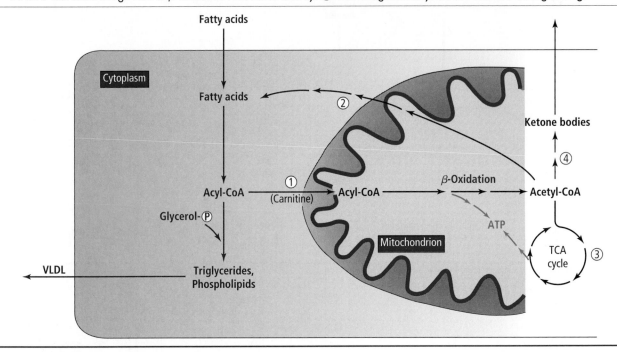

2. *The fatty acids are taken up into the mitochondrion and are β-oxidized to acetyl-CoA.* This acetyl-CoA can be (a) oxidized in the TCA cycle, (b) turned into fatty acids, or (c) turned into ketone bodies.

The first alternative is between esterification in the cytoplasm and uptake into the mitochondrion. Hepatic triglyceride synthesis is not regulated tightly. Therefore *the liver synthesizes triglycerides and releases VLDL both after a meal and in the fasting state.* Only the source of the fatty acids is different: after a meal, some of the fatty acids are synthesized from carbohydrates, whereas the fasting liver esterifies fatty acids from adipose tissue.

Fatty acid uptake into the mitochondrion, however, is stimulated in the fasting liver: carnitine-palmitoyl transferase 1, which is required for the transport of long-chain fatty acids into the mitochondrion (see Fig. 18.5), is induced by cAMP (glucagon!). Malonyl-CoA, the product of the acetyl-CoA carboxylase reaction, is a negative allosteric effector of this enzyme. In the fasting liver, acetyl-CoA carboxylase is inhibited by high levels of acyl-CoA, low levels of citrate, and a high glucagon/insulin ratio. Therefore both fatty acid synthesis and the cellular malonyl-CoA concentration are minimal, and carnitine-palmitoyl transferase 1 activity is maximal, in the fasting liver. As a result, *a larger fraction of the cytoplasmic acyl-CoA is transported into the mitochondrion rather than being esterified in the cytoplasm.*

β-Oxidation is the only major fate of fatty acids in the mitochondrion. The resulting acetyl-CoA, however, has to be partitioned between the TCA cycle and ketogenesis. The activity of the TCA cycle is regulated by the cell's need for ATP: the regulated enzymes in the cycle, including citrate synthase, isocitrate dehydrogenase, and α-ketoglutarate dehydrogenase, are inhibited by ATP and/or by a high $NADH/NAD^+$ ratio.

FIG. 29.7

Total body glucose consumption after a meal and during fasting.

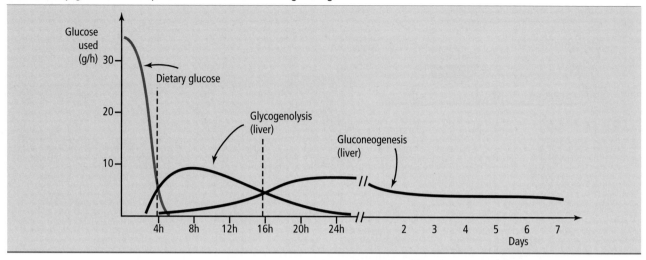

β-Oxidation produces NADH and, indirectly, ATP. Therefore *the β-oxidation of a large amount of fatty acids reduces the activity of the TCA cycle*, and an increased fraction of the mitochondrial acetyl-CoA is available for ketogenesis. Enzyme induction also is important: the activity of HMG-CoA lyase, the enzyme that forms acetoacetate from HMG-CoA, is increased greatly during fasting.

Ketogenesis amounts to an incomplete oxidation of fatty acids. Whereas the complete oxidation of one molecule of palmitoyl-CoA produces 131 ATP molecules, its conversion to acetoacetate produces 35 ATPs, and conversion to β-hydroxybutyrate produces 23 ATPs. *Ketogenesis from fatty acids is an important energy source for the fasting liver.* The conversion of 50 g of fatty acids to acetoacetate during a foodless day supplies enough energy to synthesize 190 g of glucose from lactic acid!

Why does the liver convert fatty acids to ketone bodies when carbohydrates are in short supply? The reason is that *ketone bodies are more easily metabolized than fatty acids by many tissues.* The brain, in particular, which depends almost entirely on glucose under ordinary conditions, is unable to oxidize fatty acids, but it can cover up to 70% of its energy needs from ketone bodies during prolonged fasting when ketone body levels are very high. *This reduces the need for gluconeogenesis and spares body protein* that otherwise would haveto be degraded to supply amino acids for gluconeogenesis.

Most people can survive for 3 months without food

Fatty acids supply most of the energy needs of the fasting body, and proteins are degraded to produce glucose for the brain and other glucose-dependent tissues. *The total glucose consumption decreases during prolonged fasting because most tissues switch from glucose to fatty acids and ketone bodies as their main energy sources* (Fig. 29.7). Indeed, only those tissues that depend on glucose for their energy needs, such as the brain and RBCs, still consume glucose during prolonged fasting. Glucose utilization by these tissues does not require insulin, so *glucose is rerouted from liver, muscle, and adipose tissue to brain and erythrocytes during the transition from the fed to the fasting state* (Fig. 29.8). The switch from glucose oxidation to fat oxidation is reflected in the **respiratory quotient** (see first page of Chapter 16), which declines from values of approximately 0.9 after a mixed meal to slightly above 0.7 in the fasting state. The protein reserves are not used indiscriminately: albumin and other plasma proteins are mobilized during the first days, and skeletal muscle becomes the major source during the later stages. The protein in vital organs, most notably the brain, is spared.

The **basal metabolic rate** (**BMR**) is the energy consumption in the absence of physical activity. It is on the order of 20 kcal per kg of body weight per day. It is higher in children than in adults, a little

FIG. 29.8

Interorgan transfer of nutrients after a mixed meal and during fasting. **A,** After a mixed meal; **B,** postabsorptive state, 12 hours after the last meal; **C,** one week after the last meal.

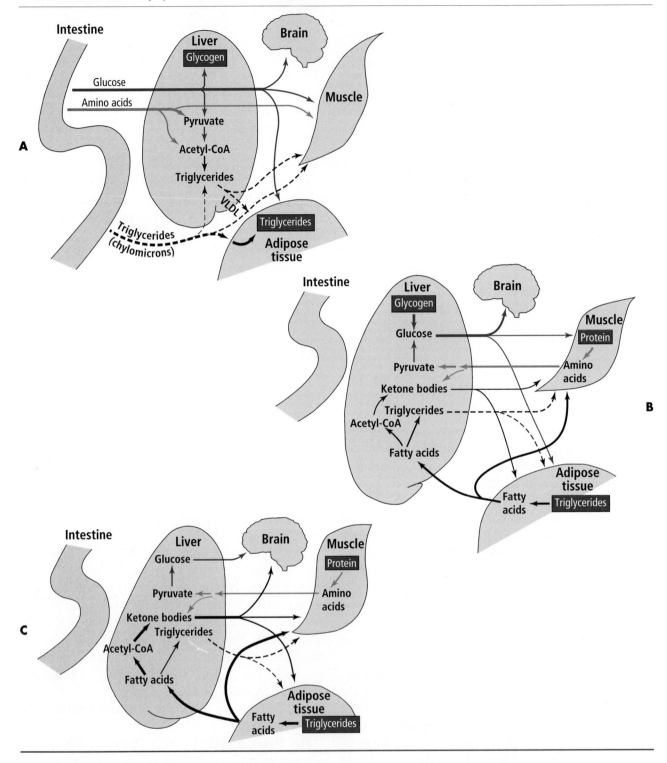

higher in young adults than in the elderly, and a lit-tle higher in males than in females. After a meal, the metabolic rate increases to a moderate extent, depending on the size and composition of the meal. This additional energy expenditure is called **postprandial thermogenesis.** During starvation, the BMR declines to values in the vicinity of 15 kcal/kg. This decline may be related to a decreased conversion of T_4 to T_3 (see Chapter 26), and to a reduced futile cycling in the major metabolic pathways.

How long can we survive without food? Experiences with people who have died in the course of hunger strikes show that death often occurs after 2 or 3 months, but there is also anecdotal evidence that obese patients can survive a "tap water and vitamin pill" diet for more than 6 months. *Survival time depends on the fat stores.* You can calculate the approximate survival time of the "textbook" 70-kg male (see Table 29.5)—and can estimate your own survival time—by comparing the caloric value of the fat reserves with the BMR.

The refeeding of severely starved patients is not entirely unproblematic: the levels of glycolytic enzymes in the liver are very low, and the patients show profound carbohydrate intolerance. Therefore *refeeding should be started slowly,* especially in advanced cases.

Obesity is the most important nutrition-related disorder in developed countries

Obesity is the most visible medical problem in Western countries. Any dietary nutrients that are not oxidized immediately are channeled into adipose tissue, and *changes in the fat depots reflect the difference between energy intake and energy expenditure.*

Eating habits are not the only determinant of obesity. On a weight basis, the BMRs of different individuals may vary by as much as 25% to 30%, and some, though not all, obese people have a low BMR. The reasons for these variations are unknown. They may include factors as diverse as body composition (relative weights of adipose tissue, muscle tissue, and internal organs), differences in the rates of futile cycling in metabolic pathways, and variations in the activities of sodium-potassium ATPase or other major energy-consuming enzymes. A feeble insulin response also may contribute to obesity: most obese patients are poorly responsive to normal levels of insulin, a condition known as **insulin resistance.** Insulin resistance in borderline diabetics is associated with reduced postprandial thermogenesis.

Postprandial thermogenesis also is reduced in some but not all obese individuals. Postprandial thermogenesis is highest after a protein meal, lowest after a fat meal, and intermediate after a carbohydrate meal. A balanced meal (protein + fat + carbohydrate) causes less thermogenesis than would be expected from the additive effects of the individual components. Postprandial thermogenesis most likely is caused by increased futile cycling in major metabolic pathways. Increased futile cycling after meals, for example, has been demonstrated for glycolysis/gluconeogenesis in the liver.

The physiological mechanisms regulating the amount of triglycerides in adipose tissue are becoming known only now: when the amount of stored fat becomes excessive, *adipocytes release the polypeptide hormone leptin* (Greek *leptos* (λεπτος), slim). This hormone increases the BMR and acts on the ventromedial hypothalamus to reduce appetite. Unlike other parts of the brain, the ventromedial hypothalamus does not possess a blood-brain barrier and therefore is able to respond to circulating peptide hormones. The ways in which leptin is involved in both the common and the morbid varieties of obesity are currently under study, and efforts are under way to use leptin as a specific antiobesity treatment.

In the meantime, however, the healthiest way to lose weight is a low-calorie diet with a balanced content of all major nutrients. Of course, hardly any obese patient ever manages to comply with this cruel and unreasonable type of diet, so more sophisticated manipulations have been proposed. A high-carbohydrate diet has been recommended because of the low caloric density of carbohydrates and their high postprandial thermogenesis when compared with fat. A fat-only diet also has been recommended. In the absence of dietary carbohydrate, the hormonal balance resembles that in the fasting state, and this leads to rampant lipolysis in adipose tissue and ketogenesis in the liver (Fig. 29.9). This diet is indeed excellent for weight reduction, especially for strong people: the caloric needs of the body are amply supplied by chylomicron triglycerides, free fatty acids, and ketone bodies, but

FIG. 29.9

Disposition of nutrients after different types of meals. **A,** Carbohydrate meal (insulin high, glucagon low); **B,** protein meal (insulin moderately high, glucagon high); **C,** fat meal (insulin low, glucagon high).

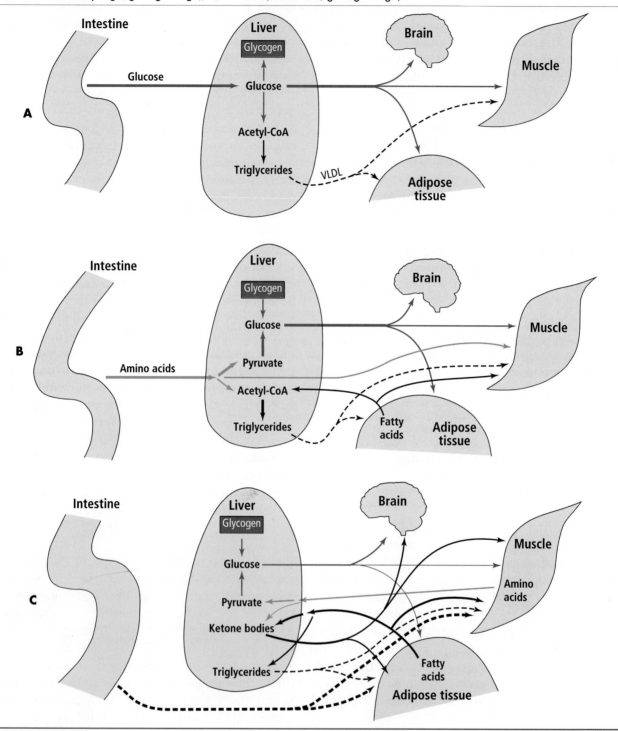

muscle protein has to be degraded for gluconeogenesis, with a resulting decrease in muscle mass and body weight.

Last but not least, many obese people have an increased number of adipocytes: *their obesity is caused not by hypertrophy but by hyperplasia of adipose tissue.* When these patients are starved to a "normal" weight, their metabolic patterns (including their BMR) become similar to those of non-obese people during periods of long starvation.

Diabetes mellitus

There are many endocrine disorders in which one of the hormones that regulate fuel utilization either is deficient or is produced in excess, but **diabetes mellitus** is by far the most common of them: close to 5% of all young people will develop diabetes as they grow older. Far from being a harmless trait, diabetes is a serious chronic disease whose long-term sequelae are among the more common causes of death and disability in Western countries.

Diabetes can be caused by insulin deficiency or insulin resistance

Diabetes mellitus is not a single disease but rather a group of metabolic disorders that are caused by a relative or absolute deficiency of insulin action. **Hyperglycemia** (abnormally elevated blood glucose) is the biochemical hallmark of diabetes mellitus, but the metabolic derangements affect the pathways of all major nutrients.

There are two primary forms of diabetes: type I and type II (Table 29.6). **Type I diabetes** has an early onset, usually in childhood or adolescence. *It is caused by the destruction of pancreatic β cells* (but not of the glucagon-producing α cells), probably by an autoimmune process. Insulin no longer is produced, and the patients require lifelong insulin injections for survival. Injections are required because insulin is not orally active. Being a protein, it is destroyed by proteases in the stomach and intestine.

Type II diabetes is a disease of middle-aged and older individuals. It is more common and less severe than type I, and it has more complex origins. The pancreatic β cells show no signs of destruction, and the plasma levels of insulin frequently are within the normal range. Type II diabetics have either *a reduction of basal or glucose-induced insulin release, or a reduced responsiveness of the target tissues to circulating insulin (insulin resistance), or both.*

Most type I diabetics are thin, especially if their disease is poorly controlled, but *most type II diabetics are obese.* Many of these obese diabetics have a decreased number of insulin receptors. The traditional explanation is simple enough: *overeating causes insulin release, and excess insulin causes insulin resistance.* Indeed, overexposure to insulin results in the receptor-mediated endocytosis of insulin receptors in the target tissues (see Chapter 27), and the overeater has to strike a new balance between a high plasma insulin level and a low density of insulin receptors in the target tissues. Those who cannot increase their insulin output sufficiently to balance the loss of insulin receptors become diabetic. This concept is

TABLE 29.6

Typical features of the two major types of diabetes mellitus

Parameter	Type I	Type II
Age of onset	< 20 years	> 20 years
Lifetime incidence	0.2-0.4%	2-6%
Heritability	≈ 50%	≈ 80%
Pancreatic β-cells	Destroyed	Normal
Circulating insulin	Absent	Normal, high, or low
Tissue response to insulin	Normal	Reduced (most patients)
Fasting hyperglycemia	Severe	Variable
Metabolic complications	Ketoacidosis	Nonketotic hyperosmolar coma
Treatment	Insulin injections	Diet, oral antidiabetics, or insulin

supported by the observation that *nondiabetic obese individuals have approximately twofold-higher insulin levels than thin people, and their tissue responsiveness is proportionately reduced*. Also, in most obese diabetics a balanced weight-reduction diet restores tissue responsiveness and corrects the metabolic derangements. Of course, not all obese diabetics stand the rigors of a low-calorie/low-carbohydrate diet, so either insulin or oral antidiabetic drugs often are required.

In diabetes, the metabolic pathways are regulated as in starvation

The release of insulin is reduced sharply during extended fasting (Fig. 29.3), and the metabolic adaptations in the starving body are, in large part, the result of the low insulin level. Therefore the insufficient insulin action in the diabetic leads to metabolic changes that otherwise are typical for the starved state (Fig. 29.10).

The hyperglycemia of diabetes mellitus is caused by both *overproduction and underutilization of glucose*: glucose is synthesized rather than consumed by the liver, and the glucose uptake into muscle and adipose tissue is reduced drastically. *There is also rampant lipolysis in adipose tissue*, leading to high levels of plasma free fatty acids. Excess fatty acids, in turn, are converted to ketone bodies by the liver. These metabolic derangements are indeed identical to the normal adaptations in severe starvation, when adipose tissue and liver have to keep all of the other tissues alive by supplying them with glucose, fatty acids, and ketone bodies. Not only does the diabetic have abnormally high plasma levels of glucose, fatty acids, and ketone bodies, but VLDL triglycerides tend to be elevated, too, because the ample supply

---

FIG. 29.10

Disposition of the major nutrients in diabetes mellitus (postabsorptive state).

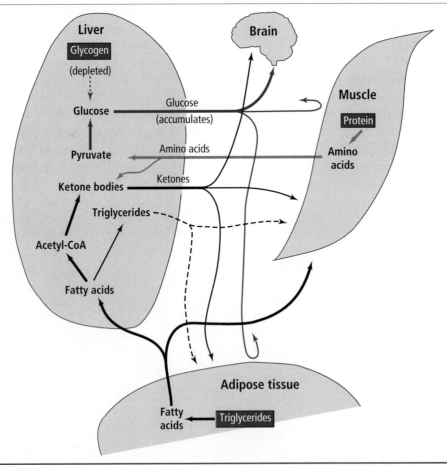

---

of fatty acids promotes triglyceride synthesis in the liver and because the activity of lipoprotein lipase in adipose tissue is reduced. For unknown reasons, hypercholesterolemia is not uncommon either.

A near-complete absence of insulin in type I diabetics leads to **diabetic ketoacidosis,** with severe ketonemia, acidosis, and blood glucose values as high as 1000 mg/dL. Large amounts of glucose are lost in the urine, and osmotic diuresis causes dehydration and electrolyte imbalances. Ketone bodies also are excreted profusely in the urine, together with such counterions as sodium and potassium. The resulting depletion of inorganic cations, which are required to buffer organic acids, leads to severe acidosis. *Diabetic ketoacidosis is an emergency condition that can be rapidly fatal.* It requires immediate fluid replacement, correction of the acidosis, and of course insulin injections to correct the underlying metabolic disorder.

Type II diabetics are not afflicted by ketoacidosis, but elderly patients may develop **nonketotic hyperosmolar coma.** This is caused by severe glucosuria with osmotic diuresis. If the patient forgets to drink, the resulting dehydration may become sufficiently severe to affect the CNS.

These two forms of diabetic coma have to be distinguished from **hypoglycemic shock.** Hypoglycemia sufficient to induce CNS dysfunction with loss of consciousness or seizures can be induced by insulin overdose or, less commonly, by the liberal use of oral antidiabetics. *The injection of glucose is a useful emergency measure in the unconscious patient* before the results of laboratory tests are available and before the cause of the problem is known. This treatment quickly resuscitates the patient with hypoglycemia while doing little harm to the patient with diabetic coma. Rarely, hypoglycemia is caused by an **insulinoma,** an insulin-secreting tumor of pancreatic β cells. The diagnosis of insulinoma is established by the measurement of elevated levels of either insulin or the C peptide (see Fig. 26.13).

Several laboratory tests are used for diagnosis and management of diabetes mellitus

Urinalysis is the most convenient screening test for diabetes mellitus. *Whenever the blood glucose level exceeds 9 to 10 mM (160 to 180 mg/dL), glucose will appear in the urine.* Ketone bodies also are excreted in the urine. There is no true renal threshold for ketone bodies, but at normal blood concentrations only trace amounts are excreted. In uncontrolled diabetes, however, substantial quantities of ketone bodies are excreted together with glucose. Urinalysis generally is performed as a semiquantitative procedure.

The quantitative determination of the fasting blood glucose level is the most important laboratory test for both the initial diagnosis and the follow-up of diabetes. A fasting blood glucose concentration of more than 7.8 mM (140 mg/dL) on two different occasions often is used as a diagnostic cutoff. The **glucose tolerance test** consists of repeated measurements of the blood glucose level immediately before and at specific time intervals after the ingestion of a glucose solution (Fig. 29.11). We have to realize, however, that both the fasting blood glucose concentration and, to a far greater extent, the glucose tolerance test show wide variations among normal individuals. Therefore the diagnostic cutoff between "normal" and "diabetic" is no less arbitrary than that between "pass" and "fail" on a biochemistry exam.

Another laboratory test determines the nonenzymatic glycosylation of hemoglobin: the free amino termini of the hemoglobin α and β chains react nonenzymatically with glucose. Although the initial reaction is reversible, a stable product, called **hemoglobin A$_{1C}$,** is formed in an intramolecular rearrangement (Fig. 29.12). *The concentration of glycosylated hemoglobin is proportional to the blood glucose level.* It is 3% to 5% in normal individuals and above 6% in diabetics. Because the lifespan of hemoglobin is approximately 4 months, this test provides information about the average severity of hyperglycemia during the weeks and months leading up to the test. An analogous glycosylation product is formed with serum albumin. The lifespan of albumin is approximately 20 days, so the determination of glycosylated albumin is used to estimate whether the blood glucose level has been controlled adequately during the preceding 2 or 3 weeks.

Longstanding diabetes leads to many pathological changes

Although acute metabolic complications can be prevented by adequate treatment, diabetics still have a markedly reduced life expectancy: in the course of

FIG. 29.11

The glucose tolerance test. Blood glucose is measured at different time intervals after the oral ingestion of a flavored glucose solution (75 g of glucose). In normal individuals, but not in diabetics, the blood glucose returns to the fasting level within 2 hours.

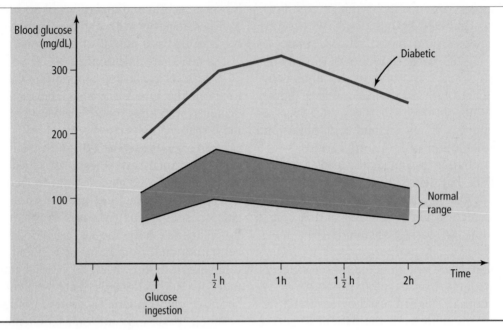

FIG. 29.12

Nonenzymatic glycosylation of the terminal amino groups in proteins. A stable fructose derivative is formed in these reactions. Hemoglobin A_{1c} and glycosylated albumin are formed this way.

many years they develop microangiopathy, nephropathy, retinopathy, cataracts, and peripheral neuropathy. Two biochemical mechanisms have been proposed for these delayed complications:

1. *The nonenzymatic glycosylation of terminal amino groups* (Fig. 29.12) interferes with the normal function or turnover of proteins. This mechanism has been suggested for the thickening of basement membranes that is observed in the renal glomeruli of diabetics.

2. In the presence of hyperglycemia, *increased amounts of sorbitol and fructose are formed by the polyol pathway* as shown in Box 29.1. The K_m of aldose reductase for

BOX 29.1

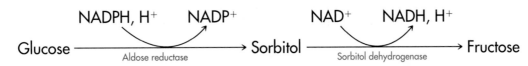

The accumulation of sorbitol and fructose is thought to interfere with the metabolism of inositol. The cellular levels of inositol have been found to be decreased in diabetics, whereas sorbitol and fructose are elevated. Aldose reductase is abundant in Schwann cells of peripheral nerves, the papillae of the kidney, and the lens epithelium, sites that are affected in diabetes.

In diabetics, the intracellular glucose concentration is not elevated in muscle and adipose tissue whose glucose uptake is insulin dependent. The tissues affected in longstanding diabetes, however, including nerve sheaths, blood vessels, kidney, and retina, have insulin-independent glucose transporters. *In these tissues the intracellular glucose concentration parallels the blood glucose concentration.*

PHYSICAL EXERCISE

Hard work requires energy. Indeed, during strenuous activity our muscles can boost their ATP production approximately twenty fold—and during short-term, all-out exercise even up to 100-fold—above the resting level. This requires a maximal stimulation of the ATP-producing pathways in the muscles themselves, and it requires the generous supply of metabolic fuels from other tissues. In the next sections we will examine the metabolic adaptations that enable us to perform vigorous physical exercise.

Contracting muscle has three main energy sources

Contracting muscle obtains its energy from three sources:

TABLE 29.7

Concentrations of some phosphate compounds in the quadriceps femoralis muscle at rest

Compound	Mmol/kg, muscle tissue
ATP	5.85
ADP	0.74
AMP	0.02
Creatine phosphate	24*
Creatine	5*

*Determined *in situ,* by nuclear magnetic resonance. In biopsy samples the ratio of phosphocreatine to creatine is approximately 3:2.

1. *The phosphagen system.* Phosphagens are energy-rich phosphate compounds that feed the contractile apparatus either directly or indirectly. ATP, as the immediate fuel for the myosin ATPase, is present at a concentration of 5 to 6 mmol/kg in resting muscle. During vigorous contraction, all ATP would be hydrolyzed to ADP and phosphate within 2 to 4 seconds. Creatine phosphate is present at a concentration of more than 20 mmol/kg in muscle tissue (Table 29.7). During exercise, when the myosin ATPase lowers the concentration of ATP and increases that of ADP, *phosphate is transferred from creatine phosphate to ADP,* thereby replenishing the ATP pool:

$$\text{Creatine phosphate} + \text{ADP} \xrightleftharpoons{\text{Creatine kinase}} \text{Creatine} + \text{ATP}$$
$$\Delta G^{0\prime} = -3.0 \text{ kcal/mol}$$

The equilibrium of this reaction favors ATP formation, so creatine phosphate is utilized while the ATP concentration is only slightly reduced from its resting level. The phosphagen system does not require oxygen or external nutrients, but *it can supply ATP only for the first 6 to 20 seconds of*

FIG. 29.13

Regulation of glycogenolysis and glycolysis in skeletal muscle. The important control points are glycogen phosphorylase, phosphofructokinase, and the glucose carrier in the plasma membrane.

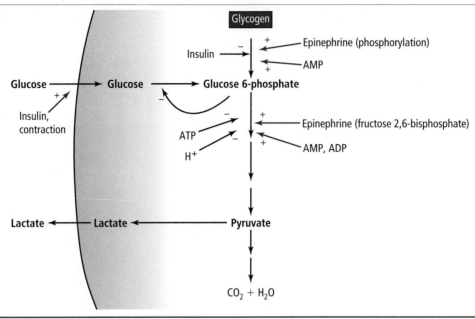

vigorous exercise. It is the main energy source for weight lifting and during a 100-meter sprint.

2. *Anaerobic glycolysis.* Muscle uses both blood glucose and its own stored glycogen for anaerobic glycolysis, but stored glycogen is quantitatively the more important substrate:

$$(Glc)_n + 3\ ADP + 3\ P_i$$

$$\downarrow$$

$$(Glc)_{n-1} + 2\ Lactate + 3\ ATP + 2\ H_2O$$

This system does not require oxygen, but *it is limited by the accumulation of lactic acid,* which acidifies the tissue and inhibits glycolysis at the level of phosphofructokinase (Fig. 29.13). Anaerobic glycolysis is the most important energy source after approximately 20 seconds to 2 minutes of vigorous exercise.

3. *Oxidative metabolism.* Oxidative metabolism is approximately 10 times more energy efficient than anaerobic glycolysis from glycogen, but *it is limited by the oxygen supply.* Muscle can oxidize stored glycogen, glucose, fatty acids, ketone bodies, and amino acids. Resting muscle relies mostly on fatty acid oxidation during the postabsorptive state, al-

though glucose is an important fuel after a carbohydrate-containing meal. Fatty acids are still the major fuel during mild to moderate physical activity, but vigorously contracting muscle depends in large part on carbohydrate oxidation (Fig. 29.14).

The catecholamines orchestrate metabolic activity during exercise

Vigorous tonic contraction, as in weight lifting, impairs the blood supply of the muscle. This type of exercise, known as **anaerobic exercise,** does not require the supply of external fuels but rather relies on creatine phosphate and the anaerobic metabolism of stored glycogen.

In **aerobic exercise,** on the other hand, such as long-distance running and swimming, blood flow to the active muscles is increased because of the effects of local mediators and of β-adrenergic stimulation of vascular smooth muscle. Therefore oxidative metabolism can function as the major energy source. Both stored glycogen and external nutrients are oxidized (Figs. 29.14 and 29.16).

The nutrient supply to exercising muscle is under neural and hormonal control. The plasma insulin concentration decreases during strenuous exercise.

FIG. 29.14

The sportsman's muscle.

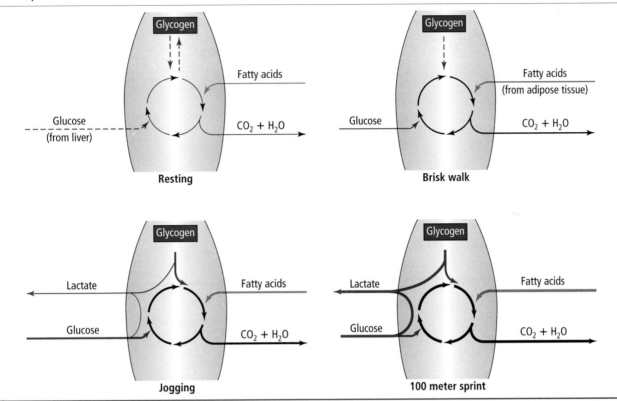

Glucagon initially is unchanged but tends to rise with prolonged vigorous activity. Most important, however, are norepinephrine and epinephrine. The plasma levels of these two catecholamines are elevated approximately ten- to twentyfold during strenuous physical activity.

In the skeletal muscle fiber itself, the main effect of the catecholamines is *a powerful stimulation of glycogen degradation and glycolysis* (Fig. 29.13). These effects are mediated by a stimulation of β-adrenergic receptors and an increased intracellular cAMP level.

In addition to their effects on muscle tissue itself, *the catecholamines mobilize stored triglycerides from adipose tissue and glycogen from the liver* (see Table 29.3, page 641). In adipose tissue they stimulate lipolysis by the cAMP-mediated phosphorylation of the hormone-sensitive lipase. Their main effect on the liver is a powerful stimulation of glycogen degradation. Also, gluconeogenesis is stimulated while glycolysis is inhibited. The liver releases substantial amounts of glucose during exercise, and most of this is derived from glycogen. Gluconeogenesis becomes important only during prolonged, all-out exercise (Fig. 29.15). Most of the substrate for gluconeogenesis actually is supplied by the muscles themselves: lactate is transported from active muscle to the liver for the resynthesis of glucose in the **Cori cycle,** and alanine makes the same journey in the **alanine cycle** (Fig. 29.16).

The plasma levels of glucose, unesterified fatty acids, and ketone bodies are elevated only mildly during physical exercise. Although these fuels are produced in quantity by adipose tissue and liver, they are consumed rapidly by the working muscles. The use of fatty acids by active muscle is proportional to the plasma free fatty acid level. The uptake of circulating glucose, which is insulin dependent in resting muscle, is stimulated directly by active contraction, even in the face of low insulin levels. Ketone bodies (from the liver) and amino acids (from protein breakdown in muscle itself) are oxidized as well, but they play minor roles, except perhaps in very extended vigorous exercise, when the glycogen stores are depleted.

FIG. 29.15

The marathoner's plight. **A,** Resting. **B,** After 10 minutes: muscle glycogen and glucose from liver glycogen are the most important fuels. **C,** After 2 hours: glycogen reserves in muscle and liver are seriously reduced. Fatty acids become more important. **D,** At the finishing line: both liver and muscle glycogen are depleted. Hypoglycemia develops. Complete exhaustion.

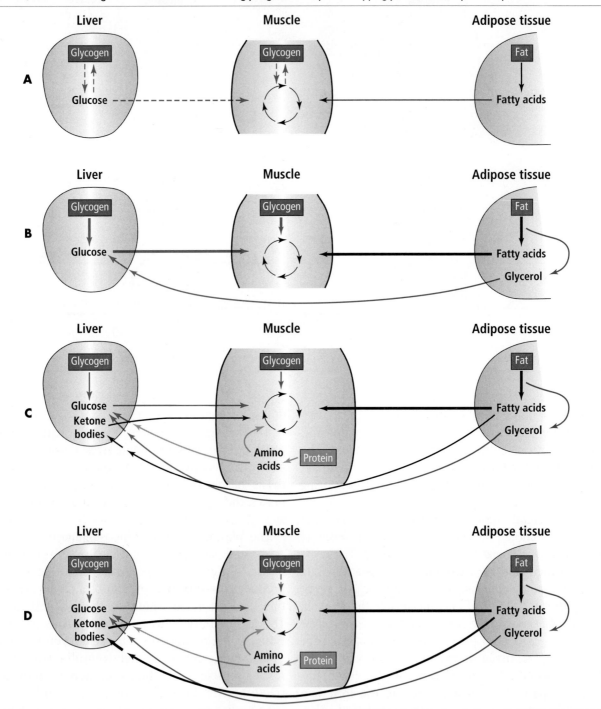

FIG. 29.16

The Cori cycle and the alanine cycle. **A,** The Cori cycle; **B,** the alanine cycle.

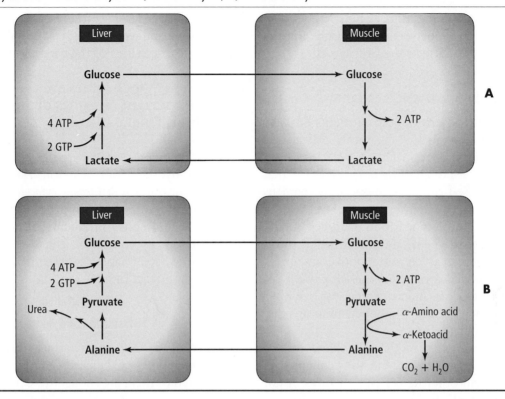

Physical endurance depends on oxidative capacity and muscle glycogen stores

Although anaerobic glycolysis from stored muscle glycogen continues unabated during extended physical exercise, prolonged activity, as in a marathon race (Fig. 29.15), depends on oxidative metabolism. The capacity for oxidative metabolism depends on the oxygen supply to the tissue, the abundance of mitochondria, the activities of oxidative enzymes, and the availability of substrates. To some extent, the muscle fibers are metabolic specialists: **fast-twitch fibers** ("white" fibers) have large glycogen stores, an abundance of glycolytic enzymes, and few mitochondria. They rely mostly on the anaerobic metabolism of their stored glycogen. **Slow-twitch fibers** ("red" fibers), on the other hand, are well equipped with mitochondria and are geared for oxidative metabolism. Fast-twitch fibers are specialized for rapid, vigorous, short-lasting contractions; slow-twitch fibers maintain their activity for prolonged periods. Our muscles consist of a mix of fast-twitch and slow-twitch fibers in variable proportions.

Regular strenuous exercise leads to important adaptive changes: endurance athletes have an increased capillary density in the trained muscles, and their muscle mitochondria are increased in size and number. The activities of enzymes for fatty acid and ketone body oxidation are increased, although the glycolytic enzymes are unchanged.

The amount of muscle glycogen is important, too. During strenuous exercise it is metabolized both aerobically and anaerobically, and its depletion leads to severe exhaustion. This occurs when, 2 or 3 hours into a marathon, the runner encounters the dreaded "wall" (Fig. 29.15). *The amount of muscle glycogen is affected by the carbohydrate content of the diet.* For this reason, methods of **carbohydrate loading** have been devised that aim at the buildup of large glycogen stores before an important athletic contest. Typically the athlete is placed on a 70% to 80% carbohydrate diet for 3 to 8 days before the event. These regimens are quite effective for endurance athletes, but they are useless in athletic performances of less than 1 or 2 hours' duration, when glycogen depletion is not a problem.

Liver glycogen does not last forever. It is depleted at approximately the same time as muscle glycogen, and the resulting hypoglycemia not only impairs muscular activity but affects the CNS as well.

THE METABOLISM OF XENOBIOTICS

The body is exposed not only to nutrients but also to a variety of nonnutritive chemicals collectively called **xenobiotics.** They include a wide variety of plant metabolites — not all of them innocuous — that have to be disposed of. More importantly, humans in their inscrutable wisdom expose themselves to a variety of drugs, intoxicants, food additives, industrial and agricultural chemicals, and pyrolysis products in such sources as cigarette smoke and fried, roasted, and smoked foods. *Water-soluble products can be excreted in urine or bile.* Indeed, some water-soluble drugs such as penicillin and amphetamine are disposed of by this simple route.

Lipophilic xenobiotics, on the other hand, cannot be excreted easily, and they tend to accumulate in adipose tissue and other lipid-rich structures. A fair amount of Δ^1-tetrahydrocannabinol (THC), for example, the active constituent of marijuana, still is present in the body several days after inhalation.

Lipophilic xenobiotics are metabolized to water-soluble products

The most important organs of xenobiotic metabolism are the liver, which is strategically located to deal with chemicals entering the body through the alimentary tract, and the lungs, which have to take care of airborne pollutants. In these organs, *lipophilic xenobiotics are metabolized to water-soluble products that can be excreted in urine or bile.* Xenobiotics are metabolized in two phases: in **phase 1 reactions,** the substance is oxidized. In most but not all cases, this oxidation takes the form of a hydroxylation reaction. The phase 1 reactions affect the biological properties of the substrate: in many cases they detoxify a toxic substance or terminate the effect of a drug. Sometimes, however, an otherwise innocuous substance is converted to a toxin (Fig. 29.17), or an inactive pro-drug is processed to a pharmacologically active metabolite. In **phase 2 reactions,** the foreign sub-

stance or its metabolite is conjugated with a hydrophilic molecule such as glucuronic acid, sulfate, glycine, glutamine, or glutathione (Fig. 29.18). The products of these conjugation reactions are not only water soluble and excretable, but they also have lost the biological activities of the parent compound.

The P-450 cytochromes are the most important enzymes of xenobiotic metabolism

The most common reaction type in phase 1 metabolism is the hydroxylation reaction. *These reactions are monooxygenase reactions that require cytochrome P-450 as an electron carrier.* We encountered this cytochrome in the steroid hormone – producing glands, where it participates in hydroxylation and side chain cleavage reactions (see Chapter 26). The balance of these hydroxylation reactions is:

$$\text{Substrate-H} + O_2 + \text{NADPH} + H^+ \longrightarrow$$
$$\text{Substrate-OH} + H_2O + \text{NADP}^+$$

Cytochrome P-450 is not a single protein but a whole superfamily of heme-containing proteins. A few hundred of them are thought to exist in humans, and the structures of many of them have been deduced from their cDNAs. They are membrane-bound proteins, either in the ER ("microsomes") or in the inner mitochondrial membrane. Approximately a dozen of them participate in normal lipid metabolism, including the synthesis of steroid hormones and the ω-oxidation of fatty acids. These species of cytochrome P-450 have tight substrate specificities.

The drug-metabolizing varieties of cytochrome P-450 are found in the smooth ER, where they help to activate molecular oxygen by the transfer of an electron from NADPH (Fig. 29.19). This electron transfer is effected by **NADPH – cyt P-450 reductase,** a membrane flavoprotein containing both FAD and FMN. The xenobiotic-metabolizing cytochrome P-450 species have broad and overlapping substrate specificities that enable them to oxidize almost any conceivable foreign molecule. As a rule, *they are inducible either by their own substrates or by other xenobiotics.* The antiepileptic drug phenobarbital, for example, induces several cytochrome P-450 species in the smooth ER of the liver, including those responsible for its own metabolism. Therefore tolerance to phenobarbital develops within approximately a week,

FIG. 29.17

Metabolic activation of carcinogens. Both benzpyrene and aflatoxin are activated to highly reactive epoxides by cytochrome P-450–containing enzyme systems. **A,** Metabolic activation of benzpyrene, a polycyclic hydrocarbon in cigarette smoke. Although benzpyrene itself is innocuous, the epoxide reacts spontaneously with DNA bases, causing point mutations. Individuals with a geneti-cally determined high activity of the activating P-450 have an increased risk of lung cancer—if they smoke. **B,** Activation of aflatoxin B$_1$, a toxin of the mold *Aspergillus flavus*. The resulting epoxide reacts spontaneously with guanine residues in DNA, causing point mutations. Besides hepatitis B virus, aflatoxins are a major risk factor for liver cancer. The offending mold thrives under hot and humid conditions, so liver cancer is common in many tropical countries.

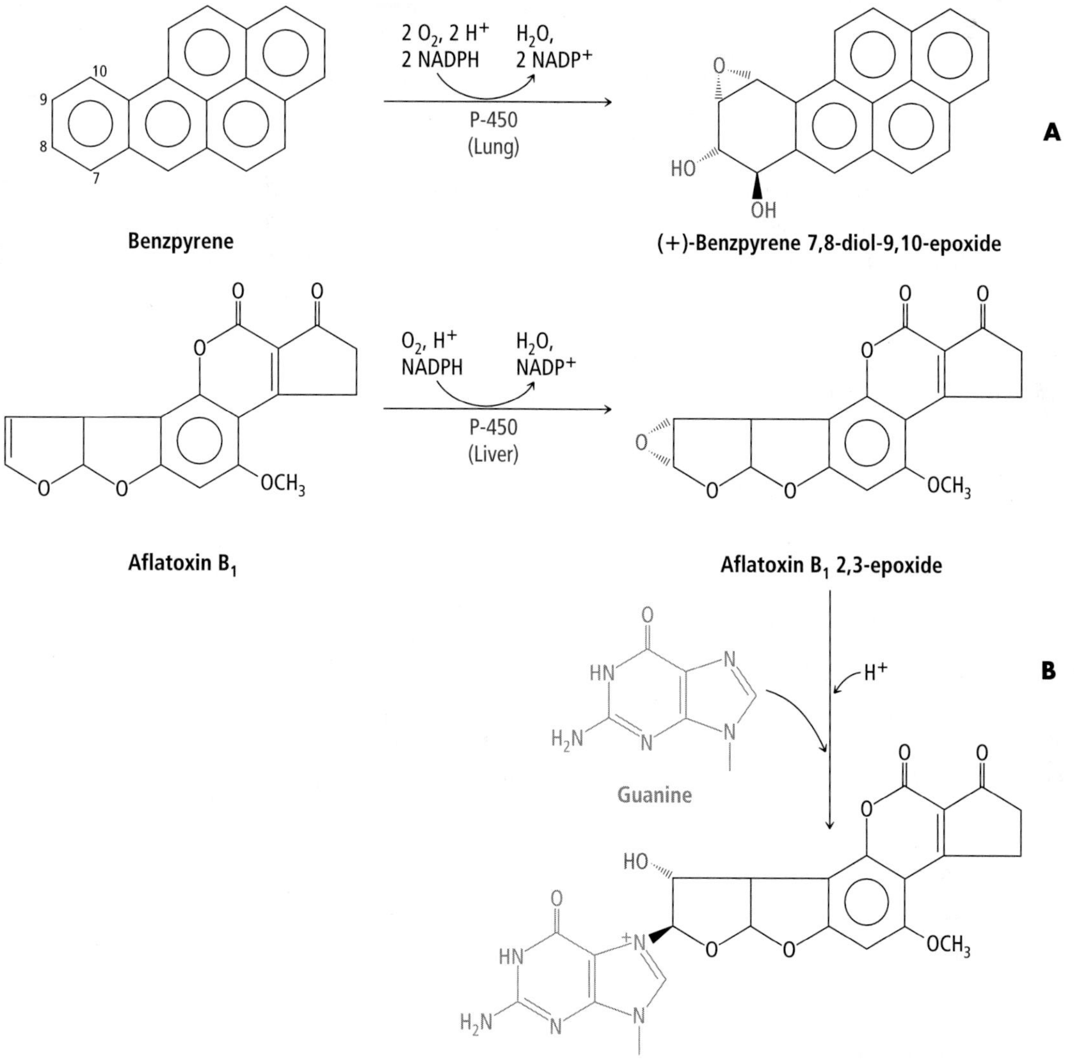

and this necessitates a three- to fourfold dosage increase to maintain the original therapeutic effect. Phenobarbital also induces P-450 species that metabolize other drugs. Thus, the metabolism of the anticoagulant dicumarol is accelerated if the patient also is treated with phenobarbital. This necessitates an increase in the dosage of the anticoagulant—and a decrease when the patient is taken off phenobarbital.

Ethanol is metabolized to acetyl-CoA in the liver

Ethanol is not only an intoxicant but a nutrient as well: the oxidation of 1 g of ethanol provides no less than 7 kcal of energy, so a person consuming 100 to 120 g of alcohol per day can cover half of his or her basal metabolic energy needs from this source alone.

FIG. 29.18

Conjugation reactions used in phase 2 of xenobiotic metabolism. Most of these reactions take place in the liver, and the water-soluble products are excreted either in the bile or in the urine.

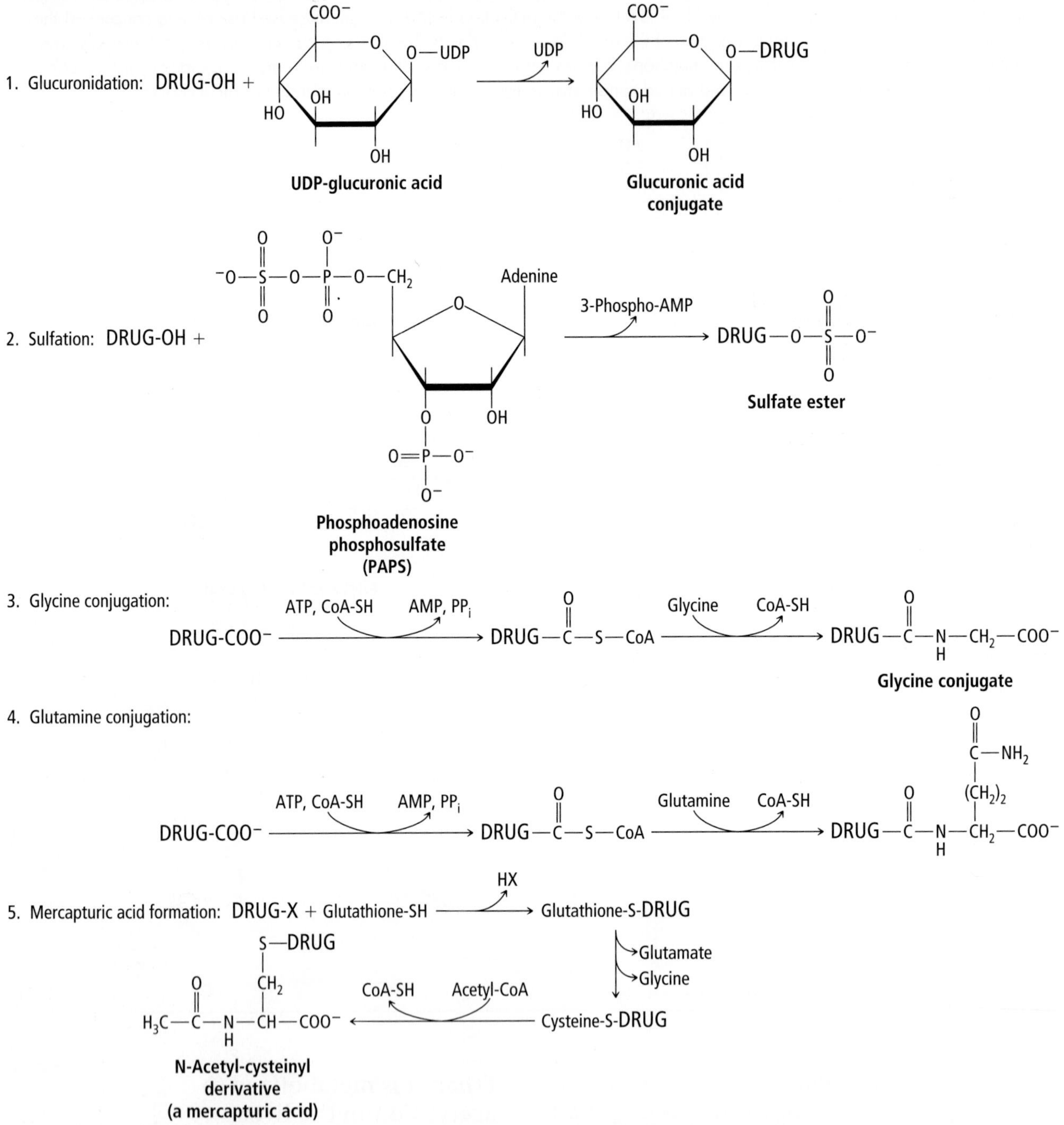

1. Glucuronidation: DRUG-OH +
COO⁻
O—UDP
OH
HO
OH
UDP-glucuronic acid
UDP
O—DRUG
Glucuronic acid conjugate
2. Sulfation: DRUG-OH +
Adenine
Phosphoadenosine phosphosulfate (PAPS)
3-Phospho-AMP
Sulfate ester
3. Glycine conjugation:
DRUG-COO⁻
ATP, CoA-SH
AMP, PPi
DRUG—C—S—CoA
Glycine
CoA-SH
Glycine conjugate
4. Glutamine conjugation:
Glutamine
5. Mercapturic acid formation: DRUG-X + Glutathione-SH
HX
Glutathione-S-DRUG
Glutamate
Glycine
Cysteine-S-DRUG
CoA-SH
Acetyl-CoA
N-Acetyl-cysteinyl derivative (a mercapturic acid)

Distilled alcoholic beverages are "empty calories," and alcoholics therefore are prone to multiple vitamin and mineral deficiencies.

Being a water-miscible organic solvent, ethanol rapidly distributes through the aqueous compartments of the body, with tissue concentrations similar to the blood alcohol level. It is metabolized by the following reactions as shown in Box 29.2. The first two reactions take place in the liver, but most of the acetate is released into the blood and oxi-

FIG. 29.19

The mechanism of cytochrome P-450–dependent hydroxylation reactions in the smooth ER. Oxygen activation by cyt P-450 involves the sequential transfer of two electrons (e^-) from the NADPH–P-450 reductase. As in hemoglobin and cytochrome oxidase, molecular oxygen binds to the ferrous (Fe^{2+}) form of the heme iron. The P-450–bound oxygen is highly reactive and can be used not only for hydroxylation reactions but also for other reactions, for example, the formation of epoxides (see Fig. 29.17).

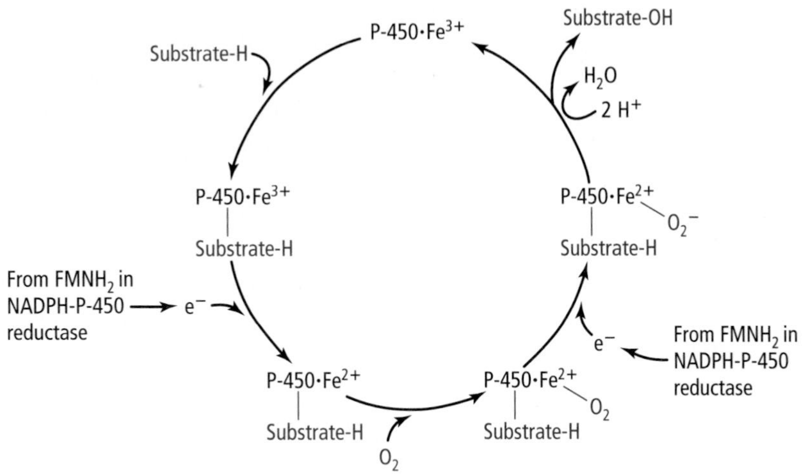

BOX 29.2

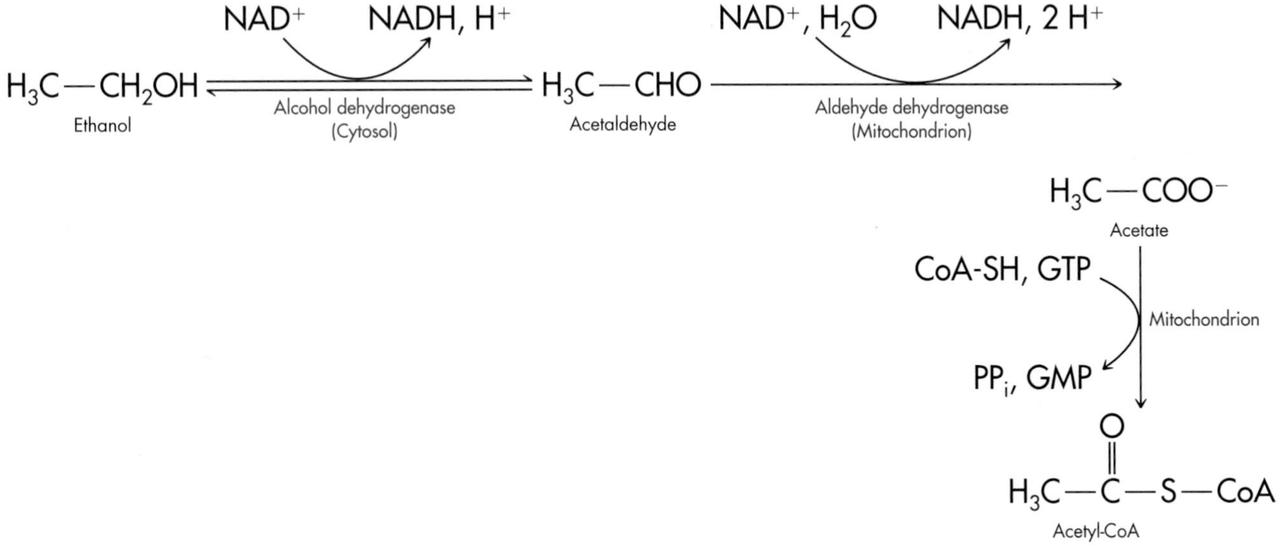

dized by extrahepatic tissues. *Alcohol metabolism is limited by the activity of alcohol dehydrogenase (ADH) and the availability of NAD$^+$*. The K_m of ADH for ethanol is on the order of 1 mM (46 mg/liter). Therefore the enzyme essentially is saturated after only one or two drinks, and *alcohol metabolism follows zero-order kinetics* (see Chapter 4). Most people metabolize approxi-

mately 10 g of alcohol per hour, and the blood alcohol level decreases by approximately 0.15 g/liter every hour. These calculations are important when a blood sample from a drunk driver has been obtained some hours after an accident.

Genetic variants of alcohol-metabolizing enzymes are common, and they contribute to individual differences in alcohol tolerance. Three genetic variants of ADH have been described with different pH optima and V_{max} values. The most interesting polymorphism, however, affects the mitochondrial aldehyde dehydrogenase, which oxidizes acetaldehyde to acetate. This enzyme normally is not rate limiting, and because of its low K_m of 10 μM for acetaldehyde, this intermediate does not accumulate to any great extent: a drunk person's blood alcohol level is between 20 and 50 mM, and the acetic acid level is between 1 and 2 mM, but acetaldehyde remains below 20 μM. Many East Asians, however, have an atypical aldehyde dehydrogenase with a single amino acid substitution (Glu → Lys) in position 487 of the polypeptide. This genetic variant behaves as a "dominant negative" mutation: even heterozygotes, who still produce the normal enzyme in addition to the defective one, have near-zero enzyme activity, possibly because the mutant enzyme forms inactive oligomers with the normal one. In these individuals, acetaldehyde is oxidized by a cytosolic aldehyde dehydrogenase whose K_m for acetaldehyde is close to 1 mM. Therefore toxic acetaldehyde accumulates to high levels after only one or two drinks. The result is the **oriental flush** response, with vasodilation, facial flushing, and tachycardia. These effects are perceived as unpleasant, and alcoholism is indeed rare in individuals with this enzyme deficiency. Some 30% to 40% of Chinese, Japanese, Mongolians, Koreans, Vietnamese, and Indonesians, and also many South American Indians, have the atypical aldehyde dehydrogenase.

The mitochondrial aldehyde dehydrogenase can be inhibited pharmacologically by **disulfiram (Antabuse)**. This drug is used in the treatment of alcoholics, but its use requires strict medical supervision: fatal reactions have occurred when the drug was mixed into an unsuspecting alcoholic's drink.

Alcohol also is metabolized by the cytochrome P-450 system in the ER:

$$H_3C\text{—}CH_2OH + O_2 + NADPH + H^+ \longrightarrow$$

Ethanol

$$H_3C\text{—}CHO + NADP^+ + 2\,H_2O$$

Acetaldehyde

This route accounts only for a small proportion of total alcohol metabolism under most conditions.

Liver metabolism is seriously affected by alcohol

Unlike carbohydrate and fatty acid oxidation, alcohol metabolism in the liver is not subject to negative controls, so *the oxidation of alcohol takes preference over the oxidation of other nutrients.* The lack of feedback inhibition suggests that the reactions of alcohol metabolism have evolved not as an energy-generating pathway but rather as a detoxification system for the small amount of alcohol that normally is formed by bacterial fermentation in the colon.

Alcohol metabolism produces acetyl-CoA, NADH, and ATP. As shown in Fig. 29.20, these products inhibit glucose metabolism at the level of phosphofructokinase and pyruvate dehydrogenase. Fatty acid oxidation is impaired by the depletion of NAD^+ and, possibly, by an elevated malonyl-CoA level, which inhibits the uptake of fatty acids into the mitochondrion. The TCA cycle is inhibited by high levels of ATP and NADH, and by the depletion of NAD^+. The TCA cycle is dispensable for the drunk liver because the respiratory chain oxidation of the two NADHs generated in the oxidation of ethanol to acetic acid is more than sufficient to provide for the energy needs of the cell.

Triglyceride synthesis, VLDL release, and plasma triglyceride level are increased, probably because fatty acid oxidation is impaired and excess fatty acids are esterified instead. Fatty acid synthesis also may be increased, especially when a high insulin/glucagon ratio stimulates the activity of acetyl-CoA carboxylase.

Despite the high levels of ATP and NADH, gluconeogenesis from pyruvate and oxaloacetate is inhibited by alcohol because the high NADH/NAD$^+$ ratio increases the lactate/pyruvate and malate/oxaloacetate ratios through the reversible lactate dehydrogenase and malate dehydrogenase reactions:

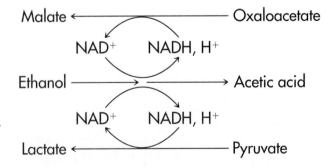

FIG. 29.20

Effects of alcohol on liver metabolism. Important control points: ① phosphofructokinase: inhibited by high energy charge; ② pyruvate dehydrogenase: inhibited by high energy charge, high NADH/NAD⁺ ratio, and high acetyl-CoA; ③ lactate dehydrogenase: high NADH/NAD⁺ ratio favors lactate formation; ④ β-oxidation: slowed down because of low NAD⁺; ⑤ malate dehydrogenase: high NADH/NAD⁺ ratio favors malate formation, oxaloacetate is depleted; ⑥ isocitrate dehydrogenase: inhibited by high energy charge and high NADH/NAD⁺ ratio; ⑦ acetyl-CoA carboxylase: may be stimulated by high citrate (accumulates because isocitrate dehydrogenase is inhibited).

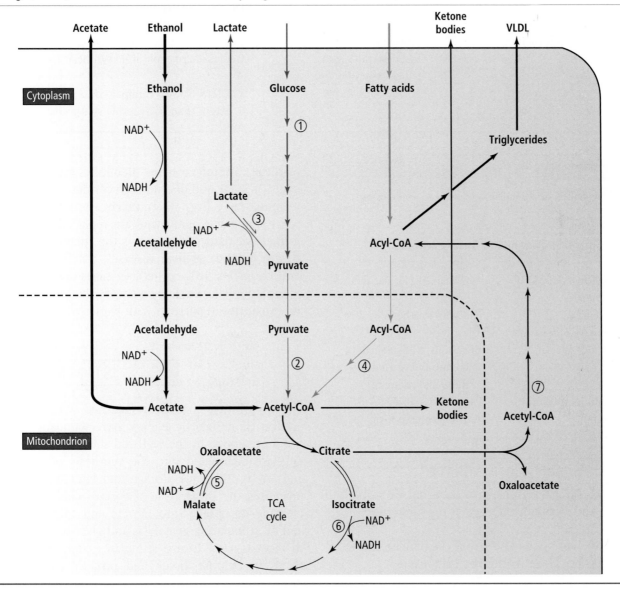

Pyruvate and oxaloacetate are depleted while the blood level of lactate is increased. *Alcohol can precipitate hypoglycemia whenever the liver glycogen stores are depleted,* for example, in a starved drinker or after a period of vigorous, exhausting physical activity.

Alcohol induces the cytochrome P-450 system, thereby increasing not only its own metabolism but also that of barbiturates and some other drugs. Therefore the sober alcoholic is not very responsive to these drugs, and problems can arise, for example, in the induction of anesthesia for surgical procedures. In the intoxicated patient, on the other hand, the metabolism of alcohol competes with that of the drug, and the responsiveness to the drug is re-

TABLE 29.8

Conditions leading to fat accumulation in the liver

Condition	Examples	Mechanism
Increased triglyceride synthesis	Starvation Diabetes mellitus	Increased supply of fatty acids from adipose tissue
	Alcoholism	Decreased fatty acid oxidation; possibly increased intrahepatic fatty acid synthesis
Decreased formation of VLDL	Protein deficiency	Decreased synthesis of VLDL apolipoprotein
	Essential fatty acid deficiency	Decreased phospholipid synthesis
	Toxic liver damage	VLDL formation is impaired to a greater extent than triglyceride synthesis

TABLE 29.9

Biochemical abnormalities in advanced liver cirrhosis

Abnormality	Impaired function
Fasting hypoglycemia	Glycogenolysis, gluconeogenesis
Prolonged clotting time	Synthesis of clotting factors
Edema	Albumin synthesis*
Hyperammonemia	Urea cycle
"Fetid" breath	Metabolism of sulfhydryl compounds formed by intestinal bacteria
Alcohol intolerance	Alcohol metabolism
Jaundice	Bilirubin metabolism

*Impaired lymph flow is another cause of abdominal edema (ascites).

stored. Fatal reactions have occurred when barbiturates and alcohol were used at the same time.

Alcoholism is the most common cause of fatty liver and liver cirrhosis

The liver synthesizes triglycerides at all times. These triglycerides are not stored but rather are released as constituents of VLDL. *A fatty liver develops in all conditions in which either triglyceride synthesis in the liver is increased or the formation of VLDL is decreased* (Table 29.8). Fatty liver is a reversible lesion, and it does not cause liver dysfunction by itself. Alcoholism, which is the most common cause of fatty liver, does not decrease VLDL formation, but it increases fat

synthesis. Therefore many alcoholics have elevated levels of VLDL and plasma triglycerides.

Unlike fatty liver, **liver cirrhosis** is irreversible: hepatocytes degenerate and are replaced by fibrous connective tissue. Cirrhosis is the final outcome of a large number of liver diseases, but in industrialized countries 60% to 70% of cases are associated with alcoholism. Table 29.9 summarizes some of the abnormalities in patients with liver cirrhosis.

SUMMARY

Those pathways that are concerned with the generation of metabolic energy have to adapt to the nutrient supply. In the well-fed state, dietary nutrients are channeled into the synthesis of glycogen and triglycerides for storage and later use. Insulin promotes the utilization of dietary glucose by increasing its uptake into muscle and adipose tissue and by stimulating glycolysis and glycogen synthesis in most tissues. It also stimulates triglyceride synthesis in adipose tissue and protein synthesis in most tissues.

Fatty acids from adipose tissue are the main energy source of the body during fasting. These fatty acids are oxidized either directly or after their initial conversion to ketone bodies by the liver. Only a few tissues, including brain and erythrocytes, require glucose during fasting. The liver maintains an adequate blood glucose level in the fasting state, initially by glycogen degradation and later by gluconeogenesis from amino acids, lactate, and glycerol.

The major metabolic pathways are deranged in many endocrine disorders. In diabetes mellitus, a relative or absolute deficiency of insulin action results in decreased glucose utilization, increased glucose production by the liver, and increased lipolysis in adipose tissue and ketogenesis in the liver.

Physical and psychological stress leads to the release of stress hormones, including the catecholamines and the glucocorticoids. The catecholamines play a central role in the acute metabolic response to physical exercise. They mobilize the body's energy stores by promoting glycogenolysis and glycolysis in muscle, lipolysis in adipose tissue, and glycogenolysis in the liver.

Nonphysiological chemicals, including drugs, toxins, food additives, and environmental pollutants, have to be eliminated from the body. Most water-soluble chemicals can be excreted by the kidneys. Most lipid-soluble chemicals, on the other hand, initially are oxidized by cytochrome P-450-containing enzyme systems and then are conjugated to water-soluble products for renal or biliary excretion. Ethanol is oxidized to acetic acid and acetyl-CoA and therefore is a substrate for the generation of metabolic energy.

Further Reading

Alpers DH, Sabesin SM, White HM: Fatty liver: biochemical and clinical aspects. In: Schiff L, Schiff ER, editors: *Diseases of the liver*, 7th ed., vol. 2. J. B. Lippincott, Philadelphia, 1993, pp. 825–855.

Barinaga M: "Obese" protein slims mice. *Science* 269, 475–476, 1995.

de Groot LJ et al, editors: *Endocrinology*, 3rd ed., vol. 2. W. B. Saunders, Philadelphia, 1995, pp. 1296–1623.

Efrat S, Tal M, Lodish HF: The pancreatic β-cell glucose sensor. *Trends Biochem Sci* 19 (12), 535–538, 1994.

Efrat S et al: Ribozyme-mediated attenuation of pancreatic β-cell glucokinase expression in transgenic mice results in impaired glucose-induced insulin secretion. *Proc Natl Acad Sci USA* 91, 2051–2055, 1994.

Felber J-P, Golay A: Regulation of nutrient metabolism and energy expenditure. *Metabolism* 44 (2. Suppl. 2), 4–9, 1995.

Flier JS: The adipocyte: storage depot or node on the energy information superhighway? *Cell* 80, 15–18, 1995.

Foster DW: Diabetes mellitus. In: Scriver CR, Beaudet AL, Sly WS, Valle D, editors: *The metabolic basis of inherited disease*, 6th ed., vol. 1. McGraw-Hill, New York, 1989, pp. 375–397.

Hoffer LJ: Starvation. In: Shils ME, Olson JA, Shike M, editors: *Modern nutrition in health and disease*, 8th ed., vol. 2. Lea & Febiger, Philadelphia, 1994, pp. 927–949.

Kinney JM, Tucker HN: *Energy metabolism: tissue determinants and cellular corollaries*. Raven Press, New York, 1991.

Kinney JM, Tucker HN, editors: *Energy metabolism*. Raven Press, New York, 1992.

Nattrass M: Diabetes mellitus. In: Williams D, Marks V, editors: *Scientific foundations of biochemistry in clinical practice*, 2nd ed. pp. 103–120. Butterworth Heinemann Ltd., Newton, 1994.

Ortiz de Montellano PA, editor: *Cytochrome p450: structure, mechanism and biochemistry*, 2nd ed. Plenum Press, New York, 1995.

Pagliassotti MJ, Cherrington AD: Regulation of net hepatic glucose uptake in vivo. *Annu Rev Physiol* 54, 847–860, 1992.

Rifkin H, Porte D, editors: *Diabetes mellitus*. Elsevier, Amsterdam, 1990.

Salaspuro M: Epidemiological aspects of alcohol and alcoholic liver disease, ethanol metabolism, and pathogenesis of alcoholic liver injury. In: McIntyre N, Benhamou J-P, Bircher J, Rizzetto M, Rodes J, editors: *Oxford textbook of clinical hepatology*, vol. 2. Oxford University Press, New York, 1991, pp. 791–810.

Schenkman JB: Cytochrome P450-dependent monooxygenase: an overview. In: Arinc E, Schenkman JB, Hodgson E, editors: *Molecular aspects of monooxygenases and bioactivation of toxic compounds*. Plenum Press, New York, 1991.

Srere P: Complexities of metabolic regulation. *Trends Biochem Sci* 19, 519–520, 1994.

QUESTIONS

1. How can you best describe the function of cytochrome P-450 in the metabolism of xenobiotics?
   A. It transfers an electron to adrenodoxin.
   B. It binds a water molecule, thereby activating it for a nucleophilic attack on the substrate.
   C. It accepts two electrons and a proton from NADPH for transfer to the substrate.
   D. It activates an oxygen molecule.
   E. It acts as an ATPase.

2. Although the brain produces most of its energy by the aerobic metabolism of glucose, during long-term fasting it can cover more than half of its energy needs from
    A. Anaerobic glycolysis
    B. Oxidation of its stored glycogen
    C. Oxidation of free fatty acids
    D. Oxidation of amino acids
    E. Oxidation of ketone bodies
3. When an insulin-dependent diabetic patient undergoes surgery (any surgery), you should monitor his blood glucose level very carefully because
    A. Stress hormones antagonize insulin, and the patient therefore may require extra insulin.
    B. Stress reduces insulin release from the pancreas, a condition known as insulin shock.
    C. Insulin not only is a metabolic hormone but also plays a crucial role in blood clotting.
    D. Any physical or psychological stress is likely to cause hypoglycemia.
4. Approximately how much glucose does a healthy adult liver produce in a 24-hour period, 2 to 3 days after the last meal?
    A. 10 grams
    B. 25 grams
    C. 60 grams
    D. 150 grams
    E. 450 grams
5. The catecholamines epinephrine and norepinephrine adjust metabolic activity throughout the body to satisfy the energy demands of the working muscles. All of the following catecholamine effects are important during physical activity except
    A. Stimulation of glycogenolysis in the liver
    B. Stimulation of glycogenolysis in skeletal muscle
    C. Inhibition of glycolysis in skeletal muscle
    D. Inhibition of glycolysis in the liver
    E. Stimulation of lipolysis in adipose tissue
6. When you get up in the morning, 12 hours after dinner, what is the main source of your blood glucose?
    A. Dietary glucose
    B. Liver glycogen
    C. Muscle glycogen
    D. Gluconeogenesis

The Mafia Boss

Once upon a time there was a Mafia boss in Chicago who had killed a great many people. He used to dispose of his victims' bodies by throwing them into a lake or river. There was one problem, however: even if he tied heavy stones to a victim, the body would be found floating 2 or 3 days later. He finally consulted a physician about this problem.

QUESTIONS

1. What is the typical density of the human body? Which tissues are lighter and which are heavier than water? Describe how the content of protein, lipid, and inorganic materials is related to the density of the tissue.
2. Are there gas-filled spaces in the body? What happens to these spaces after death?
3. What advice can you give the Mafia boss?

Viral Gastroenteritis

Benita is a 6-week-old black girl in a rural district of Alabama who was born after a normal pregnancy and weighed 3.2 kg at birth. Her parents and two older brothers were reported to be in good health. She had been breast-fed for 4 weeks, and her weight gain had been normal. The composition of human milk is as follows:

Total solids:	12%-15%
Fat:	3.5%-4%
Lactose:	7.0%

Total protein:	1.35%
Lactalbumin:	0.7%
Casein:	0.5%
Minerals:	0.2%
kcal/100 mL:	66

Her stools during this period were described as "loose" but were not considered by her mother to be abnormal. At 4 weeks of age, breast-feeding was discontinued and a commercial baby formula was substituted. Within approximately 10 days, the child developed watery diarrhea and vomiting, which was diagnosed as viral gastroenteritis. At the age of 6 weeks she was admitted to a local hospital. Physical examination at the time of admission revealed only a moderate degree of dehydration (dry mucous membranes, slight depression of the anterior fontanel, and sunken appearance of the eyes). Skin turgor seemed normal, and body weight was 3.4 kg. Urinalysis yielded a 1+ reaction for reducing substance and no reaction for glucose. The infant was hydrated with IV fluids over a period of 24 hours, and then with fluids orally for another 24 hours. During this time the diarrhea subsided and her weight increased to 3.7 kg. She then was fed the commercial formula (67 kcal/100 mL). Within 24 hours her stools became watery and were passed at the time of each feeding.

On the fourth day of hospitalization, formula X was substituted for the commercial formula. The number of stools decreased to two or three daily. They contained no reducing substance and became semiformed in character. The infant gained 40 g/day during the next 4 days. However, because of the cost and inconvenience of formula X, a single feeding of the commercial formula was given once again as a trial. The infant did not pass a stool, but a

TABLE C-1

Formula compositions

Components	Commercial formula	Formula X
Cow milk protein	+	
Casein hydrolysate		+
Corn oil	+	+
Coconut oil	+	−
Lactose	+	−
Sucrose	−	+
Arrowroot starch	−	+
Protein	1.7%	2.2%
Fat	3.4%	2.6%
Carbohydrate	6.6%	8.5%
Minerals	0.4%	0.6%

second feeding with the commercial formula 4 hours later was followed by several explosive, watery stools. The stool pH was 5.0, and it gave a positive reaction for reducing substance.

The child was switched back to formula X, and the diarrhea subsided within 24 hours. After another 2 days in the hospital, the child was discharged and the mother was given a 1-week supply of formula X. After 1 week at home, the formula X gradually was replaced by the commercial formula in the course of a few days. There was no recurrence of diarrhea, even after several months on the commercial formula. The compositions of the commercial formula and formula X are given in Table C-1.

QUESTIONS

1. Which tissues are affected in viral gastroenteritis? What kind of functional derangements can you possibly expect?
2. Why did the child show signs of dehydration when admitted to the hospital?
3. Urinalysis showed the presence of small amounts of a reducing substance. What kind of reducing substance was this? Is the presence of reducing substances in the urine normal? Do you know of other diseases in which reducing substances appear in the urine?
4. Which methods are best employed to determine the presence and concentration of glucose in urine, blood, or stool, without interference by other substances?
5. Why was a reducing substance present in the stool after the baby was fed the commercial formula but not after formula X?
6. Why was the pH of the stool in the acidic range (pH 5)? Which acids could possibly be present?
7. The bacterial fermentation of undigested carbohydrates in the intestine is accompanied by the formation of gas. Which gases are formed?
8. Do you know of an inherited enzyme deficiency that would cause diarrhea in response to the commercial formula? Is this likely in the present case?
9. Some patients, both children and adults, have gastrointestinal problems because they are hypersensitive to a dietary component. Which component of the commercial formula could possibly act as an effective antigen that can stimulate B or T lymphocytes?

Suggested Reading

Haubrich WS, Schaffner F, Berk JE: *Gastroenterology*, 5th ed., vol. 2. W. B. Saunders, Philadelphia, 1995, p. 1093.

Death In Installments

A 19-year-old man was admitted to the hospital because of a progressive CNS disorder. He had developed disturbances of motor coordination since age 14, had dropped out of college at age 17, and had been evaluated at various hospitals between ages 17 and 19, without clear diagnosis. Repeated lumbar punctures, EEGs, pneumoencephalogram, liver function tests, and ceruloplasmin level had been normal.

On admission he showed some insight into his illness, but was indifferent about his deficits. He was disoriented in relation to time but could provide information about the previous 10 years. Spasticity and ataxia were present. Verbal IQ was 83; performance IQ was 67. Pneumoencephalography disclosed ventricular dilatation. A specific diagnosis could not be established at this time.

Over the next years, the patient's condition worsened and he required total care because of inability to walk and incontinence. At age 34, a computed tomography (CT) scan showed ventricular dilatation, and there was marked peripheral neuropathy, mainly of demyelinative nature. Blood cells, electrolytes, and CO_2 were normal; a serological test for syphilis was negative. Lumbar puncture yielded clear, colorless acellular CSF under normal pressure, glucose 57 mg/100 mL, protein 150 mg/100 mL. The B_{12} level was normal. Diagnostic procedures included the determination of enzyme activities in cultured leukocytes. Some results were as follows:

Arylsulfatase A (mmol per mg of protein per hour):

Patient: 31
Normal: 77 ± 18

Sulfatidase (mmol per mg of protein per 2 hours):

Patient: 0.2
Normal: 12.9 ± 3.2

Urine sulfatide excretion (mmol per mg of creatinine)

Patient: 0.39
Normal: 0.07-0.14

QUESTIONS

1. Several diagnostic tests had been performed on the patient before a definitive diagnosis could be established. Give a rationale for each of these tests.
2. What is sulfatide, and where does it occur?
3. Arylsulfatase A and sulfatidase are the same enzyme, assayed either with a synthetic substrate (arylsulfatase A) or with the natural substrate (sulfatidase). What do the discrepancies between the two enzyme activities (each compared with normal levels) suggest?
4. Ultrastructural studies were not performed on the patient's leukocytes. If such studies had been performed, what would be the likely observation?
5. Traditionally, leukocytes are cultured in a serum-containing medium. Fresh plasma is less suitable for stimulating leukocyte growth. Do you know of a mitogen that is released from platelets when the platelets become activated during blood clotting?

6. The patient's enzyme activities were determined only in cultured leukocytes. Do you expect the enzyme deficiency to be present in other cells (cultured skin fibroblasts, for example) as well?
7. Many genetic diseases, including the patient's disease, show subtypes that vary in their severity and age of onset (infantile, juvenile, adult forms). Why?
8. What would abnormally high protein levels or low glucose levels in CSF suggest? Are the patient's values in the normal range?

Suggested Readings

Kolodny EH: Metachromatic leukodystrophy and multiple sulfatase deficiency: sulfatide lipidosis. In: Scriver CR and others, editors: *The metabolic basis of inherited disease*, Vol. 2. McGraw-Hill, New York, 1989, pp. 1721-1750.

Pennock CA: Lysosomal storage disorders. In: Holton JB, editor: *The inherited metabolic diseases*, 2nd ed. Churchill Livingstone, 1994, pp. 205-242.

A Mysterious Death*

In the summer of 1989, Patricia Stallings brought her 3-month-old son Ryan to the emergency room of Cardinal Glennon Children's Hospital in St. Louis. The child had labored breathing, uncontrollable vomiting, and gastric distress. According to the attending physician, a toxicologist, the child's symptoms indicated that he had been poisoned with ethylene glycol (an antifreeze). This suspicion was confirmed by a commercial laboratory. After he recovered, the child was placed in a foster home, and the parents were allowed to see him in supervised visits. However, when the infant became ill and subsequently died after a visit in which Stallings had been left alone briefly with him, she was charged with first-degree murder and held without bail. Both the commercial lab and the hospital lab found large amounts of ethylene glycol in the boy's blood and traces of it in a bottle of milk Stallings had fed her son during the visit.

While in custody, Patricia Stallings learned that she was pregnant. In February 1990 she gave birth to another son, David Stallings, Jr. This son was placed

---

* © American Association for the Advancement of Science.

immediately in a foster home, but within weeks he started having symptoms similar to Ryan's. Eventually David was diagnosed with methylmalonic acidemia. Despite this new evidence, Patricia Stallings was convicted of assault with a deadly weapon and sentenced to life in prison.

After hearing about the case from a television broadcast, William Sly, chairman of the Department of Biochemistry and Molecular Biology, and James Shoemaker, head of a metabolic screening lab, both at St. Louis University, became interested. Together with Piero Rinaldo, a metabolic-disease expert at Yale University School of Medicine, they analyzed Ryan's blood. Rather than ethylene glycol, they found large amounts of methylmalonic acid. They also found massive amounts of ketone bodies in the boy's blood and urine, another typical finding in methylmalonic aciduria. The bottle could not be tested because it had mysteriously disappeared. When the previous findings supporting ethylene glycol poisoning were checked, it turned out that one laboratory had claimed the presence of ethylene glycol even though Ryan's blood did not match their own profile for a sample containing ethylene glycol. The other laboratory had detected an abnormal substance in Ryan's blood and had assumed that it was ethylene glycol. Samples from the bottle had produced nothing unusual, yet the laboratory had claimed evidence of ethylene glycol in that, too.

After these findings, all charges against Patricia Stallings were dismissed on September 20, 1991.

QUESTIONS

1. What causes methylmalonic aciduria, and what signs and symptoms would you expect?
2. Can you propose a mechanism for the excessive formation of ketone bodies in this disease?
3. What treatments can you suggest for methylmalonic aciduria?
4. Some metabolic diseases can be treated with megadoses of a vitamin or coenzyme. Which vitamin or coenzyme would you try in a patient with methylmalonic aciduria?
5. Why are the signs of ethylene glycol poisoning similar to those of methylmalonic aciduria?
6. Is vomiting a sign that is specific for individual diseases? What is the function of the vomiting reflex?

Suggested Readings

Gossel TA, Bricker JD: *Principles of clinical toxicology,* 3rd ed. Raven Press, New York, 1994, pp. 85-87.

Rosenberg LE, Fenton WA: Disorders of propionate and methylmalonate metabolism. In: Scriver CR, Beaudet AL, Sly WS, Valle D, editors: *The molecular basis of inherited disease,* vol. 1. McGraw-Hill, New York, 1989, pp. 821-822, 832-840.

To Treat Or Not To Treat?

Becky Brummond was transferred to a specialized metabolic clinic at the age of 14 months. She had first presented with coma at the age of 3 days, and she had developed severe seizures at 4 weeks. Nonketotic hyperglycinemia was diagnosed at 2 months, with a plasma glycine level of 897 μM (normal: 81 to 436 μM) and normal urine organic acids. She was treated with lorazepam and phenobarbital and with sodium benzoate at 500 mg/kg/day.

At 14 months, she had severe axial hypotonia, spasticity, and frequent myoclonic seizures. She occasionally babbled and had a short attention span. Her plasma glycine level was 917 μM. The sodium benzoate dosage was increased to 640 mg/kg/day, and the plasma glycine decreased to 352 μM. Within the next 3 months she became more awake, her seizures ceased, and she made developmental progress. She learned to roll from front to back and from back to front, and to reach and take objects in her hands. When the benzoate dosage was decreased inadvertently to 64 mg/kg/day at 1 year 8 months of age, she had frequent severe seizures despite increasing doses of anticonvulsants that made her progressively drowsy. Plasma glycine level was 657 μM and CSF glycine 117 μM (normal: 3 to 10 μM). The error soon was noted, and her normal sodium benzoate dosage was reinstated. At the age of 2 years 6 months her seizures recurred when her glycine level became elevated. With an increase in the benzoate dosage to 750 mg/kg/day, good control of her plasma glycine level and seizures was achieved.

At the age of 2 years 8 months, she still had pronounced axial hypotonia with distal spasticity. She had achieved some degree of head control, she could push herself up on her hands, and she could push herself around on the floor. One year later, at the age of 3 years 10 months, no substantial developmental progress was seen: her adaptive skills were at the 8- to 16-week level, gross motor skills were at the 8- to 12-week level, fine motor skills were at the 4-week level, language skills were at the 8- to 16-week level, and personal social skills were at the 4- to 12-week level. Visual inattentiveness was striking. Magnetic resonance imaging showed a static delayed myelinization. When the plasma carnitine level was noted to be in the low-normal range at age 3, L-carnitine therapy (50 mg/kg/day) was started. After the initiation of this treatment, an increased activity level was noted.

QUESTIONS

1. Describe the metabolism of glycine and the molecular defect in nonketotic hyperglycinemia.
2. Does glycine serve any specialized functions in the brain?
3. How does benzoic acid lower the plasma glycine level? Which other diseases can be treated with benzoic acid?
4. Benzoic acid treatment induces carnitine deficiency in some patients. How? And which metabolic processes are impaired in carnitine deficiency?
5. Can you think of any ethical problems in the treatment of children who suffer from severe brain damage?

Suggested Readings

Nyhan WL: Nonketotic hyperglycinemia. In: van Hove JLK et al, editors: Benzoate therapy and carnitine deficiency in non-ketotic hyperglycinemia. *Am J Med Genet* 59, 444-453, 1995.

Scriver CR, Beaudet AL, Sly WS, Valle D, editors: *The metabolic basis of inherited disease*, vol. 1. McGraw-Hill, New York, 1989. pp. 743-752.

Yellow Eyes

Andrew Brown, a 64-year-old civil servant at the Internal Revenue Service, was in excellent health when he was told at work that the sclerae of his eyes were yellow. He ignored this for 2 weeks and then noted that his stools were pale and his urine was dark. He had slight anorexia and had lost 10 pounds.

Although he did not suffer from abdominal pain and had no fever, he consulted his physician, who noted the jaundice and found a nontender swelling in the right upper abdomen, which appeared to be a dilated gallbladder.

Mr. Brown was sent to the local hospital, where some tests were performed on his blood. The results were as follows (normal ranges are in parentheses):

Hematocrit:	48% (40-54)
Platelets:	250,000/μL (150,000-450,000)
White cells:	17,000/μL (4,500-11,000)
Prothrombin time:	26 sec (10-13)
Total bilirubin:	14.2 mg/dL (0.1-1.2)
Direct bilirubin:	12.0 mg/dL (0.1-0.4)
Alanine transaminase (ALT):	12 U/L (4-36)
α-Amylase:	200 U/L (30-220)
Alkaline phosphatase (ALP):	650 U/L (20-130)
Lactate dehydrogenase (LDH):	410 U/L (208-378)

The urine had a brown color and tested positive for bilirubin. Tests for urobilinogen in urine and stool were negative, and the stool was noted to be clay colored.

An ultrasound confirmed the presence of a dilated common bile duct, but there was no evidence of gallstones.

Exploratory laparotomy was performed 5 days later. Besides the dilatation of the gallbladder and the common bile duct, the head of the pancreas was found to be swollen, and a small amount of ascitic fluid was noted. Biopsy samples were obtained from the head of the pancreas and from five regional lymph nodes. Routine cytology established a diagnosis of pancreatic adenocarcinoma, and four of the five lymph nodes turned out to be invaded. The patient was offered combination chemotherapy with fluorouracil, methotrexate, and vincristine, but he declined when the likely outcome was explained to him. He died 4 months later, with morphine as his only medication.

QUESTIONS

1. How is bilirubin normally metabolized?
2. What are the possible causes of jaundice in adults? Is the absence of fever significant for the initial diagnosis?
3. Why were the stools "clay colored," and why was the urine brown?
4. What is urobilinogen, and why can it be used to distinguish different types of jaundice?
5. Give rationales for the laboratory tests employed.
6. Do you think that an injection of vitamin K would correct the prolonged prothrombin time?
7. Why was no attempt made to treat Mr. Brown's cancer surgically?
8. How do fluorouracil, methotrexate, and vincristine work, and would you expect any side effects?

Suggested Readings

Gertsch P, Blumgart LH: Malignant biliary tract obstruction. In: McIntyre N, Benhamou J-P, Bircher J, Rizzetto M, Rodes J, editors: *Oxford textbook of clinical hepatology*, vol. 2. Oxford University Press, Oxford, 1991, pp. 1059-1063.

Schaffner F: Jaundice. In: Haubrich WS, Schaffner F, Berk JE, editors: *Gastroenterology*, 5th ed., vol. 1. W. B. Saunders, Philadelphia, 1995, pp. 129-137.

An Abdominal Emergency

Elma Crawford is a 62-year-old retired housewife, 40 pounds overweight, who was rushed to the emergency room by her husband one Saturday morning after suddenly developing severe pain in the epigastric region. The pain had started suddenly and had become very severe over a period of only 15 minutes, followed shortly by repeated vomiting. On reaching the hospital she was pale and in obvious distress. Her blood pressure was 100/60 in a reclining position and 70/40 in the upright position. The heart rate was 110/minute, and the respiratory rate was 35/minute. Physical examination was unremarkable except for extreme tenderness in the epigastric region.

Two ampules of blood were drawn for blood tests. Because Ms. Crawford was in extreme pain, she was given 75 mg of meperidine IM, and a history was obtained from her husband. She had been in good health until that morning, but 5 years ago she had had episodes of abdominal pain, and ultrasound had shown a number of stones in her gallbladder. She had been treated with chenodiol (chenodeoxycholic acid) for 1 year, after which time the gallstones had disappeared and the treatment was discontinued.

The following results of the blood tests were available 3 hours later (normal ranges are in parentheses):

Hematocrit:	41% (38-47)
Na^+:	146 mM (136-142)
K^+:	4.6 mM (3.8-5.0)
Ca^{2+}:	2.4 mM (2.30-2.74)
Cl^-:	104 mM (95-103)
Glucose:	130 mg/dL (70-110 fasting)
Total bilirubin:	<1 mg/dL (0.1-1.2)
Blood urea nitrogen:	22 mg/dL (8-23)
Creatinine:	1.0 mg/dL (0.6-1.2)
Lactate dehydrogenase:	410 U/L (208-378)
Alanine transaminase:	16 U/L (4-36)
Creatine kinase:	55 U/L (30-135)
Alkaline phosphatase:	120 U/L (20-130)
α-Amylase:	760 U/L (30-220)

She was transferred immediately to the intensive care unit, where she was treated with IV fluids, parenteral nutrition, nasogastric suction, and cimetidine. A blood sample obtained the following morning showed the following laboratory values (again, normal values are in parentheses):

Glucose:	180 mg/dL (70-110 fasting)
Na^+:	135 mM (136-142)
K^+:	4.0 mM (3.8-5.0)
Ca^{2+}:	1.8 mM (2.30-2.74)
Mg^{2+}:	0.4 mM (0.65-1.05)
Cl^-:	92 mM (95-103)
α-Amylase:	850 U/L (30-220)

She was mildly febrile at this time (38.9°C).

At this point 10 mL of 10% calcium-gluconate and 2 mL of 50% magnesium sulfate were added to her IV replacement fluid, and intensive care treatment was continued for another 3 days. After this time her condition had improved sufficiently to permit her transfer to a regular hospital ward, and she was discharged after another 2 weeks. A cholecystectomy was scheduled for 3 weeks later. Her gallbladder was removed together with four yellow-brown stones that she took home in a glass jar to show to her family and friends.

QUESTIONS

1. What possible causes do you know for severe abdominal pain of sudden onset? Which diagnostic procedures can be used for the differential diagnosis?
2. Describe the normal composition of bile and the origin of its constituents.
3. What are the typical constituents of gallstones?
4. Can you think of biochemical and physiological conditions leading to an increased risk of gallstone formation?
5. Most gallstones form not in the bile ducts but in the gallbladder. Why?
6. Is the risk of gallstones affected by the diet, and are there any commonly used drug treatments that either increase or decrease the risk of gallstones?
7. Why can oral chenodeoxycholic acid (chenodiol) be used for the treatment of gallstones? Compare the merits of chenodiol treatment and cholecystectomy.
8. Chenodiol increases the level of LDL cholesterol but not of HDL cholesterol in some patients. Can you propose a biochemical mechanism for this?
9. How can gallstones cause pancreatitis?
10. Which pancreatic enzymes are synthesized as zymogens?
11. Can you propose rational treatments for acute pancreatitis?
12. Many patients with severe pancreatitis develop hypocalcemia and hypomagnesemia. Why?
13. One day after the onset of pain the patient had mild hyperglycemia. Why?

Suggested Readings

Banks PA: Acute pancreatitis. In: Haubrich WS, Schaffner F, Berk JE, editors: *Gastroenterology*, 5th ed., vol. 4. W. B. Saunders, Philadelphia, 1995, pp. 2888-2917.

Dowling RH, McIntyre N: Gallstones. In: McIntyre N, Benhamou J-P, Bircher J, Rizzetto M, Rodes J, editors: *Oxford textbook of clinical hepatology*, vol. 2. Oxford University Press, Oxford, 1991, pp. 1107-1134.

Ellis H: Clinical diagnosis of the acute abdomen. In: Williams D, Marks V, editors: *Scientific foundations of biochemistry in clinical practice*, 2nd ed. Butterworth Heinemann, Oxford, 1994, pp. 399-408.

Malet PF, Rosenberg DJ: Cholelithiasis: gallstone pathogenesis, natural history, biliary pain and nonsurgical therapy. In: Haubrich WS, Schaffner F, Berk JE, editors: *Gastroenterology*, 5th ed., vol. 3. W. B. Saunders, Philadelphia, 1995, pp. 2674-2729.

Marks JW, Schoenfield LJ: Formation and treatment of gallstones. In: Schiff L, Schiff ER, editors: *Diseases of the liver*, 7th ed., vol. 1. J. B. Lippincott, Philadelphia, 1993, pp. 427-447.

Shortness of Breath

Oscar Schnorr, a high-school teacher, was 53 years old when he consulted his physician for the first time with complaints of shortness of breath. He also mentioned several occasions when he felt tightness or pain in the middle of the chest that radiated to the inner side of the left arm. These episodes were always precipitated by physical activity, in several instances by climbing the stairs to his fifth-floor apartment.

Mr. Schnorr was approximately 25 pounds overweight, and he had been a pack-a-day smoker for 35 years. Physical examination was unremarkable. His blood pressure was 155/100, and his heart sounds were normal. His breath sounds were near-normal, with only mild evidence of chronic bronchitis. Laboratory tests for fasting blood glucose and lipids showed the following results:

Glucose:	105 mg/dL (normal: 70-110 mg/dL)
Total cholesterol:	240 mg/dL (normal: 140-250 mg/dL)
Triglycerides:	310 mg/dL (normal: 10-190 mg/dL)

The physician directed Mr. Schnorr initially to adopt a diet with a reduced amount of animal fat and cholesterol, to normalize his blood lipid levels. A blood test taken 4 weeks later, however, showed no improvement of his hyperlipidemia. After a telephone conversation with the dietician at the local Veterans Administration (V.A.) hospital, the physician placed Mr. Schnorr on a low-carbohydrate/

high-fiber diet. Much to everyone's surprise, Mr. Schnorr found this diet quite acceptable. He lost 10 pounds during the following year, and repeated laboratory tests showed cholesterol and triglyceride levels within the normal range.

Now, however, the patient still complains about shortness of breath and chest pain. Acting on the strong advice of the doctor, he quits smoking, and he is treated with nitroglycerin for chest pain. At age 56 he is referred to the cardiology unit of the V.A. hospital for a diagnostic workup. The EKG shows evidence of mild myocardial damage in the wall of the left ventricle, consistent with an old infarction in the area of the descending branch of the left coronary artery. A coronary arteriogram shows a severe stenotic lesion near the origin of the main left coronary artery.

Coronary bypass surgery is performed. Several weeks later the patient reports that he no longer suffers chest pain after exertion, and that he feels 20 years younger. In several counseling sessions with the dietician, he is advised to adhere to a low-saturated-fat/low-cholesterol/high-polyunsaturated-fat/low-carbohydrate/high-fiber diet.

Six weeks after surgery, he is enrolled in a double-blind, placebo-controlled clinical trial of the effects of antioxidant vitamins on late complications and survival of coronary bypass patients. He is now taking one daily capsule with 200 mg of vitamin E + 1 g of vitamin C (or placebo), and he has to go to the V.A. hospital once every 2 months to have his blood lipids and plasma ascorbic acid levels checked and to receive his supply of vitamin (or placebo?) capsules. He is still doing well 5 years after surgery.

QUESTIONS

1. What are the possible causes for "shortness of breath"? Which features in Mr. Schnorr's initial clinical presentation suggest that he has a cardiac problem?
2. How would you classify the pattern of hyperlipidemia in this patient? Which type of lipoprotein is elevated?
3. Why did the patient's hyperlipidemia improve on a low-carbohydrate diet but not on a low-fat diet?
4. Is smoking a risk factor for coronary heart dis-

ease? By what mechanisms can smoking affect the underlying disease process and its clinical expression?
5. How does nitroglycerin work (in medicine, not terrorism)?
6. What is "stenosis," and what is the likely nature of the "stenotic lesion" in the patient's coronary artery?
7. Describe the role of lipoproteins in the formation of atherosclerotic lesions.
8. There was evidence for an old infarct in one of the terminal branches of the patient's left coronary artery. Could the lesion at the root of the left coronary artery be responsible for this infarct, and if so, how?
9. How long can myocardial tissue survive under ischemic conditions?
10. Describe the biochemical consequences of ischemia.
11. ATP is required for all major energy-dependent processes in the cell. What are these energy-dependent processes in the myocardium? Failure of which of these energy-dependent processes is most likely to kill the cells during an ischemic attack?
12. Cell death during ischemia could be caused, in theory, either directly by the lack of oxygen or indirectly by the accumulation of metabolic end products. Can you design an animal experiment that distinguishes between these two possibilities?
13. Would anticoagulant therapy make sense for our patient?
14. What is a coronary bypass?
15. How are placebo-controlled, double-blind clinical trials designed?
16. Does anything in the patient's history suggest that he is particularly suitable for participation in a clinical trial?
17. During the clinical trial, the laboratory checks not only the patient's blood lipids but also his plasma ascorbate level. Why?
18. Antioxidant vitamins have been proposed as prophylactic agents for coronary heart disease. What is their proposed mechanism of action?
19. Compare the effects of lipid-lowering drugs (lovastatin, colestipol, niacin) on blood lipids with the effects of dietary manipulations. In which situations would you rely on diet, and in which situations do you use drugs?

Suggested Readings

Davies MJ: The pathology of coronary atherosclerosis. In: Schlant RC, Alexander RW, editors: *Hurst's the heart*, 8th ed., vol. 1. McGraw-Hill, New York, 1994, pp. 1009-1020.

Marks V: Chest pain. In: Williams D, Marks V, editors: *Scientific foundations of biochemistry in clinical practice*, 2nd ed. Butterworth Heinemann, Oxford, 1994, pp. 614-620.

Winder AJ: Hyperlipidaemia. In: Williams D, Marks V, editors: *Scientific foundations of biochemistry in clinical practice*, 2nd ed. Butterworth Heinemann, Oxford, 1994, pp. 601-613.

Itching

Margaret Mallon was a 55-year-old librarian at the public library when she saw her doctor with a complaint of diffuse itching at night, which had troubled her for the past 3 months. Physical examination was unremarkable except for slight liver enlargement. There was no urticaria. The patient was prescribed chlorpheniramine maleate, 6mg 4 to 5 times daily. When the patient returned 3 weeks later, commenting that the medication made her drowsy but was otherwise useless, a series of laboratory tests was performed on her blood, with the following results (normal ranges are in parentheses):

Hematocrit:	41% (38-47)
RBCs:	$4.5 \times 10^6/\mu L$ (4.2-5.4)
White cells:	$22 \times 10^3/\mu L$ (4.5-11)
Platelets:	250,000/μL (150,000-450,000)
Total protein:	6.9 g/dL (6.0-7.8)
Albumin	2.7 g/dL (3.2-4.5)
Globulin	4.2 g/dL (2.3-3.5)
Prothrombin time:	12 sec (10-13)
Glucose:	80 mg/dL (70-110)
Cholesterol:	330 mg/dL (150-250)
Triglyceride:	75 mg/dL (10-190)
Bilirubin (total):	3.5 mg/dL (<1)
Lactate dehydrogenase:	280 U/L (90-310)
Alanine transaminase:	55 U/L (4-36)
Creatine kinase:	45 U/L (30-135)
Alkaline phosphatase:	680 U/L (20-130)
γ-Glutamyl transferase:	220 U/L (5-40)
BUN:	15 mg/dL (8-23)

After these test results were in, Ms. Mallon was referred to the gastroenterology department of the local hospital for a cholangiography, a transcutaneous needle biopsy of the liver, and some additional laboratory tests. The cholangiography showed a normal morphology of the extrahepatic biliary system. The biopsy showed degeneration of intrahepatic bile ducts. There was inflammation with an infiltrate of mononuclear cells, and the ductular epithelial cells were in disarray. The bile canaliculi between the hepatocytes were dilated, and the hepatocytes adjacent to the portal tract had a swollen and foamy appearance. Excess copper was shown with a rhodamine stain. Blood tests showed a serum copper level of 85 μmol/dL (normal: 13-24) and a fasting bile acid level of 12.5 mg/dL (normal: 0.3-3.0). Immunoelectrophoresis showed mildly elevated IgG and strongly elevated IgM, and antimitochondrial antibodies could be detected.

Treatment with cholestyramine, 10 g/day, was initiated, and this improved the itching. She also was treated intermittently with cortisol and with penicillamine. She remained in reasonably good health during the next 3 years, although she retired from her job at the public library because the work was too strenuous and she felt that she needed more rest.

Four years after the initial diagnosis she was brought to the emergency room by her husband. She was in a mildly confused state, had a coarse tremor, and was unable to walk without support. In the ER, she was unable to complete a number-connection test in the allotted time of 60 seconds. The EEG showed a bilateral synchronous decrease in wave frequency and increase in wave amplitude with disappearance of the normal α-rhythm. A series of blood tests was performed, with the following results (normal ranges are in parentheses):

Hematocrit:	37% (38-47)
Total protein:	6.5 g/dL (6.0-7.8)
Albumin:	1.9 g/dL (3.2-4.5)
Globulin:	4.6 g/dL (2.3-3.5)
Prothrombin time:	25 sec (10-13)
Glucose:	100 mg/dL (70-110)
Cholesterol:	210 mg/dL (150-250)
Triglyceride:	40 mg/dL (10-190)
Bilirubin:	8.6 mg/dL (<1.0)
Alanine transaminase:	115 U/L (4-36)
Alkaline phosphatase:	450 U/L (20-130)
Ammonia:	450 μg/dL (40-80)
BUN:	16 mg/dL (8-23)

She initially was treated with mannitol enemas, followed on the next day by neomycin. Sodium phenylacetate and sodium benzoate, 10 g/day each, was given, and she was kept on a diet with 40 to 50 g of protein per day. With this treatment she regained her previous state of health within a few days, and she was discharged on a regimen of cholestyramine, vitamin K, and phenylacetate, and on a diet that provided 40 to 50 g of high-quality protein per day.

Six months later she was rushed to the hospital after throwing up copious amounts of blood. She died in the hospital a few hours later.

QUESTIONS

1. Which illness did the doctor suspect on Ms. Mallon's first visit, before the laboratory and biopsy tests established the diagnosis of a hepatobiliary disease?
2. Which of the initial laboratory test results suggested a biliary problem?
3. Why was a cholangiography performed?
4. Could the elevated IgM and the antimitochondrial antibodies be related to the cause of Ms. Mallon's disease?
5. Why were serum bile acids, cholesterol, and copper elevated?
6. What was the rationale for the use of mannitol and neomycin?
7. Is it possible that vitamin K treatment was ineffective in this patient?
8. Why was the patient treated with a low-protein diet?
9. How do sodium phenylacetate and sodium benzoate work?
10. What caused Ms. Mallon's sudden death?

Suggested Readings

Bodenheimer HC Jr: Primary biliary cirrhosis. In: Haubrich WS, Schaffner F, Berk JE, editors: *Gastroenterology*, 5th ed. vol. 3. W. B. Saunders, Philadelphia, 1995, pp. 2276-2293.

Conn HO: Hepatic encephalopathy. In: Schiff L, Schiff ER, editors: *Diseases of the liver*, 7th ed., vol. 2. J. B. Lippincott, Philadelphia, 1993, pp. 1036-1060.

Ferenzi P: Hepatic encephalopathy. In: McIntyre N, Benhamou J-P, Bircher J, Rizzetto R, Rodes J, editors: *Oxford textbook of clinical hepatology*, vol. 1. Oxford University Press, Oxford, 1991, pp. 471-483.

Kaplan MM: Primary biliary cirrhosis. In: Schiff L, Schiff ER, editors: *Diseases of the liver*, 7th ed., vol. 1. J. B. Lippincott, Philadelphia, 1993, pp. 377-410.

McIntyre N, Benhamou J-P, Bircher J, Rizzetto M, Rodes J, editors: *Oxford textbook of clinical hepatology*, vol. 2. Oxford University Press, Oxford, 1991, pp. 243-249.

McIntyre N, Rosalhi SB: Tests of the functions of the liver. In: Williams D, Marks V, editors: *Scientific foundations of biochemistry in clinical practice*, 2nd ed. Butterworth Heinemann, Oxford, 1994, pp. 383-398.

Abdominal Pain

Betty Belmaker was a 29-year-old woman who had been a secret but heavy drinker for a few years, ever since she had married a physician who neglected her in favor of his patients and his secretary. One day she developed acute pain in the lumbar region and abdomen. On the following day, she entered a hospital and initially was treated with ampicillin for suspected urinary tract infection. Shortly after admission she had two grand mal seizures. Her serum sodium was 119 mmol/liter at that time (normal: 136-142), and the EEG was mildly abnormal.

The patient was treated with hypertonic saline and phenytoin. This resulted in initial improvement, and the patient was discharged on the ninth hospital day. However, the pain persisted and muscle weakness developed.

The patient was readmitted 4 days later. Temperature, pulse rate, and blood pressure were normal, and no rash or lymphadenopathy was found. Lungs, heart, breasts, abdomen, and extremities were normal; pelvic and rectal examinations were negative. There was, however, considerable muscle tenderness and weakness. On the neurological examination the patient was alert but irritable and mildly confused. There were no signs of aphasia or apraxia.

Urine: Amber, with specific gravity of 1.022 and pH of 5.0. Few white cells and bacteria.
Stool: No occult blood.

One day after admission, several laboratory tests were performed on the patient's blood, with the following results (normal ranges are in parentheses):

Hematocrit:	38.9% (38-47)
White cells:	6300/μL (4,500-11,000)
58% Neutrophils	(56%)

40% Lymphocytes	(34%)
2% Monocytes	(4%)

Platelets:	291,000 (150,000-450,000)
Protein:	6.4 g/dL (6-7.8)
Albumin	3.7 g/dL (3.2-4.5)
Globulin	2.7 g/dL (2.3-3.5)
Urea nitrogen:	23 mg/dL (8-23)
Glucose:	123 mg/dL (70-110 fasting)
Uric acid:	3.0 mg/dL (2.7-7.3)
Bilirubin:	0.3 mg/dL (0.1-1.2)
Sodium:	138 mM (136-142)
Potassium:	4.1 mM (3.8-5.0)
Calcium:	2.3 mM (2.30-2.74)
Phosphate:	1.2 mM (0.74-1.52)
Chloride:	92 mM (95-103)
CO_2:	28 mM (22-26)
Aspartate transaminase (AST):	31 U/L (8-33)
Lactate dehydrogenase (LDH):	235 U/L (208-378)
Creatine kinase (CK):	13 U/L (30-135)
α-Amylase:	10 U/L (30-220)
Alkaline phosphatase (ALP):	54 U/L (20-130)
Heart rate:	126/min (70-95)
Chest X-ray:	normal

Lumbar puncture produced clear, colorless CSF with two red cells, one lymphocyte, and one mononuclear cell/μL; no bacteria:

Glucose	80 mg/dL (40-80)
Protein	21 mg/dL (12-60)

Plasma electrophoresis: mild increase in the γ-globulin fraction.

Immunoelectrophoresis: mild increase of IgG, mild decrease of IgA.

The patient remained afebrile. A urine sample obtained 3 days after readmission showed an orange discoloration. The sediment had few white cells and bacteria.

After a tentative diagnosis was made, phenytoin was withdrawn and the patient was treated with IV glucose and hemin (hematin). This resulted in gradual improvement over the following days.

QUESTIONS

1. Give rationales for the blood tests that were performed on this patient. Based on the normal results of most of these tests, which diseases can be excluded?
2. Do you know of diseases that cause an abnormal color of the urine?
3. Why was a lumbar puncture performed?
4. What was the tentative diagnosis—which was confirmed by the effectiveness of the treatment? Can you think of a laboratory test that would establish a definitive diagnosis?
5. What is hemin, and why was it effective?
6. Could it be that the phenytoin treatment worsened the patient's condition?

Suggested Readings

Bloomer JR, Straka JG, Rank JM: The porphyrias. In: Schiff L, Schiff ER, editors: *Diseases of the liver*, 7th ed., vol. 2. J. B. Lippincott, Philadelphia, 1993, pp. 1438-1464.

Elder GH: Haem synthesis and the porphyrias. In: Williams D, Marks V, editors: *Scientific foundations of biochemistry in clinical practice*, 2nd ed. Butterworth Heinemann, Oxford, 1994, pp. 409-419.

Kappas A, Sassa S, Galbraith RA, Nordmann Y: The porphyrias. In: Scriver CR, Beaudet AL, Sly WS, Valle D, editors: *The metabolic basis of inherited disease*, vol. 1. McGraw-Hill, New York, 1989, pp. 1320-1329.

Nordmann Y: Human hereditary porphyrias. In: McIntyre N, Benhamou J-P, Bircher J, Rizzetto M, Rodes J, editors: *Oxford textbook of clinical hepatology*, vol. 2. Oxford University Press, Oxford, 1991, pp. 974-985.

Rheumatism

Charles Fillmore is a 62-year-old racetrack bookie who saw his doctor with complaints of stiffness and pain in his hands and wrists, which troubled him during his work. An X-ray showed joint space narrowing of the metacarpophalangeal joints and chondrocalcinosis in the area of the wrist joint. A tentative diagnosis of rheumatoid arthritis was made, and aspirin was prescribed. Eight weeks later, he was in his doctor's office again with complaints of serious stomach pain that could be relieved only by eating. The X-ray showed evidence of a gastric ulcer. Aspirin was discontinued, and with Tagamet treatment (cimetidine, a histamine H_2 receptor blocker) the ulcer healed within 2 months. Subsequently Mr. Fillmore occasionally used phenacetin or Tylenol (acetaminophen) for his "rheumatism," but with little success. After another year he noticed that he felt increasingly weak and lethargic, and he had a complete lack of libido. He went for a complete medical checkup. At this time he was noted to have a brown discoloration of the skin. Echocardiography showed moderately severe ventricular enlargement, and his blood pressure was 140/95. Physical examination was normal except for a mild swelling and tenderness of the metacarpophalangeal joints, restricted mobility of the wrist joint, and some tenderness of the medial aspect of the left knee joint. A series of blood tests was performed, with the following results (normal ranges are in parentheses):

Hematocrit:	44% (40-54)
RBCs:	$5.1 \times 10^6/\mu L$ (4.6-6.2)
WBCs:	8,000/μL (4,500-11,000)
Platelets:	380,000/μL (150,000-450,000)
Hemoglobin:	14.8% (13.5-18.0)
Total protein:	7.3% (6.0-7.8)
Albumin:	2.9% (3.2-4.5)
Globulin:	4.4% (2.3-3.5)
Prothrombin time:	11 sec (10-13)
Glucose:	240 mg/dL (70-110)
Urea nitrogen:	20 mg/dL (8-23)
Bilirubin:	1.5 mg/dL (0.1-1.2)
Total iron-binding capacity (TIBC):	330 μg/dL (250-400)
Transferrin saturation:	92% (20-55)
Serum ferritin:	680 ng/mL (15-200)
Creatine kinase:	75 U/L (55-170)
Alanine transaminase:	65 U/L (4-36)
Alkaline phosphatase:	160 U/L (20-130)

He was referred to the gastroenterology unit for a liver biopsy. Histological examination showed fibrous degeneration of moderate severity. A Prussian blue stain showed extensive iron accumulation in hepatocytes, with less intense staining of Kupffer's cells. The iron concentration was determined, by atomic absorption spectroscopy, to be 320 μmol/g dry weight (normal: 5-40).

QUESTIONS

1. What disease does Mr. Fillmore have, and what is the most likely cause?
2. Which blood tests were most important for the diagnosis?
3. What treatment would you use?
4. In which tissues is iron normally stored, and why does this require specialized iron storage proteins?

5. The patient presented initially with symptoms of arthritis. What types of arthritis do you know?
6. The patient developed a gastric ulcer after using aspirin for several weeks. Can you think of a reason why aspirin is especially bad for the stomach and not for the intestine or other parts of the GI tract?

Structure of aspirin

7. The patient had a dark discoloration of the skin. Do you know of other diseases in which the color of the skin is abnormal?
8. A loss of libido in males often is caused by insufficient testosterone secretion. Malfunction of which other endocrine gland (besides the testis) can cause this, and which laboratory tests can you use to distinguish among the different possibilities?
9. Which blood tests suggest that Mr. Fillmore's prognosis is relatively favorable, provided he receives adequate treatment?

Suggested Readings

Bothwell TH, Charlton RW, Motulsky AG: Hemochromatosis. In: Scriver CR, Beaudet AL, Sly WS, Valle D, editors: *The metabolic basis of inherited disease*, 6th ed. McGraw-Hill, New York, 1989, pp. 1433-1462.

Brissot P, Deugnier Y-M: Normal iron metabolism. In: McIntyre N, Benhamou J-P, Bircher J, Rizzetto M, Rodes J, editors: *Oxford textbook of clinical hepatology*, vol. 1. Oxford University Press, Oxford, 1991, pp. 221-225.

Tavill AS: Hemochromatosis. In: Schiff L, Schiff ER, editors: *Diseases of the liver*, 7th ed., vol. 1. J. B. Lippincott, Philadelphia, 1993, pp. 669-691.

Worwood M: Disorders of iron metabolism. In: Williams D, Marks V, editors: *Scientific foundations of biochemistry in clinical practice*, 2nd ed. Butterworth Heinemann, Oxford, 1994, pp. 446-452.

TABLE C-2

Blood test results

Substance	Concentration	
	mmol/L	*mg/dL*
Alcohol	55	250
Glucose	3.0 (3.9-6.1)	54 (70-110)
Lactate	3.2 (0.6-2.2)	29 (5-20)

A Bank Manager In Trouble

John Penny, a bank manager in a small town in the Midwest, was 46 years old when he was admitted to the hospital after collapsing at a business meeting. Results of some blood tests performed immediately after admission are shown in Table C-2 (normal ranges are in parentheses).

At 4 o'clock the following morning he woke up with excruciating pain in the left big toe. On questioning, Mr. Penny reported that he had had spasmodic pain in his left big toe on a few occasions during the past few months and admitted that he had been a heavy drinker for some time. Nodules could be seen and felt in his earlobes, and the joint of his big toe was swollen and exquisitely tender. The serum urate level was determined on the same day. It was 0.6 mM, or 10.1 mg/dL (normal: 0.24 to 0.51 mM, or 4.0 to 8.5 mg/dL).

Mr. Penny was given indomethacin and allopurinol. His urate level was in the normal range when he was discharged 3 days later.

QUESTIONS

1. How is alcohol metabolized, and how is alcohol metabolism regulated?
2. How can alcohol affect the blood levels of glucose and lactate?
3. Which diseases can result in joint pain? Are there typical differences in the clinical presentation of gout versus other forms of arthritis?
4. Is an elevated serum urate level diagnostic for gout? Which laboratory test would establish a definitive diagnosis?
5. Why does gout affect small peripheral joints first?
6. Outline the rationales of pharmacological treatments for the acute attack of gouty arthritis and for the long-term maintenance of the patient.
7. What recommendations can you make to Mr. Penny concerning his diet and lifestyle?

Suggested Readings

Kelley, WN, Schumacher HR Jr: Gout. In: Kelley WN, Harris ED, Ruddy S, Sledge CB, editors: *Textbook of rheumatology*, 4th ed., vol. 2. W. B. Saunders, Philadelphia, 1993, pp. 1291-1336.

Lieber CS: Metabolism of alcohol and associated hepatic effects. In: Haubrich WS, Schaffner F, Berk JE, editors: *Gastroenterology*, 5th ed., vol. 3. W. B. Saunders, Philadelphia, 1995, pp. 2190-2214.

McCarty DJ, Koopman WJ: *Arthritis and allied conditions*, 12th ed., vol. 2. Lea & Febiger, Philadelphia, 1993, pp. 1773-1829.

Rosalki SB: The clinical biochemistry of alcohol. In: Williams D, Marks V, editors: *Scientific foundations of biochemistry in clinical practice*, 2nd ed. Butterworth Heinemann, Oxford, 1994, pp. 121-143.

Kidney Problems

Cathy Stout is a 33-year-old typist who has been diabetic since the age of 14. She controls her disease with daily insulin injections, and she has to see her physician once a month. Regular laboratory tests have shown fasting blood glucose levels anywhere between 150 and 600 mg/dL, and her insulin medication has been adjusted repeatedly for optimal blood glucose control. During this month's doctor's visit she complains about lassitude, nausea, and appetite loss, and she also mentions a distressing itching that typically appears in the late evening and interferes with sleep. She has tried unsuccessfully to self-medicate for this problem with phenacetin and sleeping pills. Her blood pressure at this time is 175/120. She is sent to the laboratory for some tests.

RESULTS OF URINALYSIS:

DIPSTICK TESTS:

Glucose: 2+
Ketones: trace
Protein: 4+
Blood: 2+

RESULTS OF URINALYSIS:

SEDIMENT:

Erythrocytes: 260/μL (normal: 3-20)
White blood cells: 210/μL (normal: 5-30)
Some casts

The 24-hour urine contains 3.7 g of protein.

A series of blood tests is performed, with the following results (normal ranges are in parentheses):

Hematocrit:	29% (38-47)
Red cells:	3.1×10^6/μL (4.2-5.4×10^6)
White cells:	12.6×10^3/μL (4.5-11.0×10^3)
Platelets:	240,000/μL (150,000-450,000)
Total protein:	6.3 g/dL (6.0-7.8)
Albumin:	2.5 g/dL (3.2-4.5)
Globulin:	3.8 g/dL (2.3-3.5)
Sodium:	148 mEq/L (136-142)
Potassium:	6.2 mEq/L (3.8-5.0)
Calcium:	4.0 mEq/L (4.6-5.5)
Magnesium:	3.9 mEq/L (1.3-2.1)
Phosphorus:	8.5 mg/dL (2.3-4.7)
Total CO_2:	18 mmol/L (24-30)
pH:	7.35 (7.35-7.45)
Glucose:	220 mg/dL (70-110)
Total bilirubin:	<1.0 mg/dL (<1.0)
BUN:	185 mg/dL (8-23)
Uric acid:	8.3 mg/dL (2.7-7.3)
Creatinine:	4.5 mg/dL (0.6-1.2)
Alanine transaminase:	8 U/L (4-36)
Alkaline phosphatase:	325 U/L (20-130)
Creatine kinase:	48 U/L (30-135)
Ferritin:	175 μg/L (15-150)

The creatinine clearance is 12 mL/min (normal: 87-107).

Ophthalmoscopy shows vascular changes with numerous microaneurysms.

At this point extra attention is given to the control of her blood glucose, with weekly determinations of the blood glucose level and occasional determination of hemoglobin A_{1C}. She also is placed on a diet with restricted protein, potassium, and sodium, and she is given sodium bicarbonate, 1.2 g/day, and calcium carbonate, 500 mg with each meal. Her hypertension is treated with captopril. After initial improvement, her condition worsens again and she is placed on hemodialysis 8 months later. She now is receiving hemodialysis three times a week while waiting for a kidney transplant.

QUESTIONS

1. Which type of diabetes does Cathy Stout have? What histologic abnormalities do you expect in her pancreas?
2. Why does the patient depend on insulin injections? Do you know of alternative methods for treating diabetes?
3. The patient complains about itching. Do you know of other diseases that cause itching?
4. Should the patient ask her doctor before she self-medicates for such problems as itching and indigestion?
5. Explain the electrolyte abnormalities in this patient.
6. Why is the level of alkaline phosphatase high?
7. The PTH level was not determined. How would you determine PTH, and what results can you expect in this patient?
8. Why is the total CO_2 low?
9. How does the kidney participate in acid-base regulation?
10. What is the BUN, and in which diseases is it elevated?
11. Why is the hematocrit low?
12. The blood pressure is elevated in many kidney diseases. Why?
13. Is there any reason to examine the eyes in patients with diabetic nephropathy?
14. Give rationales for the initial treatment.
15. What is hemodialysis?

Suggested Readings

Friedman EA: Diabetic renal disease. In: Rifkin H, Porte D Jr, editors: *Diabetes mellitus*, 4th ed. Elsevier, Amsterdam, 1990, pp. 684-709.

Payne RB: Tests of kidney function. In: Williams D, Marks V, editors: *Scientific foundations of biochemistry in clinical practice*, 2nd ed. Butterworth Heinemann, Oxford, 1994, pp. 325-337.

Shapiro JI, Schrier RW: Etiology, pathogenesis, and management of renal failure. In: Walsh PC, Retik AB, Stamey TA, Vaughan ED Jr, editors: *Campbell's urology*, 6th ed., vol. 2. W. B. Saunders, Philadelphia, 1992, pp. 2045-2064.

Tisher CC, Hostetter TH: Diabetic nephropathy. In: Tisher CC, Brenner BM: *Renal pathology*, 2nd ed., vol. 2. J. B. Lippincott, Philadelphia, 1994, pp. 1387-1412.

A Sickly Child

PART I
History

David was a 5-month-old boy who was brought by his mother to the emergency room at Children's Hospital at 8:00 a.m. after 12 hours of fever with increasing wheezing and coughing. On admission he was found to be in acute respiratory distress, with a temperature of 40.5°C (105°F). He was also somewhat underweight for his age.

David's mother reported that he had experienced several episodes of fever, congestion, and noisy breathing over the last month, which had improved with ampicillin until the day of admission. David was the product of a normal term pregnancy, labor, and delivery. His mother described him as a sickly child. She was concerned about his feeding behavior, as he would vomit frequently, particularly during the first hour after feeding. She also commented that during these times his skin became clammy and tasted salty.

Urinalysis: Glucose negative
Ketones present in moderate amounts

Gases in face mask oxygen:

$$pO_2 = 189 \text{ torr } (150 \text{ in room air})$$
$$pCO_2 = 14 \text{ torr } (36\text{-}40)$$

Blood tests:

White count:	17,150/mm^3 (6,000-12,000)
Hematocrit:	29% (33-40)
Total CO$_2$:	5 mEq/L (25-28)
pH:	7.08 (7.35-7.45)
Blood sugar:	<25 mg/dL (80-110)
ALT (alanine transaminase):	86 U/L (5-30)
LDH (lactate dehydrogenase):	587 U/L (208-378)
Total protein:	9.4 g/dL (6.4-8.1)
Total cholesterol:	270 mg/dL (110-200)
Triglycerides:	480 mg/dL (10-150)
Bilirubin:	0.5 mg/dL total, 0.1 direct (0-1.0, direct)
Uric acid:	8.5 mg/dL (3.5-7.2)
Lactate:	15 mM (0.6-1.5)

QUESTIONS

1. Is vomiting after feeding a common problem in infants? Name some possible causes.
2. Based on the history, what is the most likely acute problem that brought David to the emergency room?

PART II
Physical Examination and Laboratory Tests

On physical examination David was found to be a pale, somewhat thin, extremely weak, lethargic child who was slightly cyanotic. His respiratory rate was 80 (normal: 40), and his heart rate was 220 (normal: 90 to 100). He was clammy and was in extreme respiratory distress. His liver was palpable 10 cm below the right costal margin, and the spleen was felt 3 cm below the left costal margin. Both organs were firm and nontender. A liver scan showed profound liver enlargement without any focal lesions.

Some laboratory data were obtained (normal ranges are in parentheses):

QUESTIONS

1. David's respiratory rate was too high. Based on the history (presence of fever, "slightly cyanotic," previous response to ampicillin), what seems to be the most obvious mechanism for this? Is this mechanism confirmed by the laboratory results?
2. The patient had tachycardia, and he was "clammy." What physiological mechanism is likely to mediate these effects? Could the same mechanism explain the slight cyanosis?
3. Why was a liver scan performed?
4. Why was the patient treated with oxygen? Do you think this treatment was continued once the lab results were in?
5. Which were the most immediately life-threatening abnormalities revealed by the laboratory tests? Is there anything you can do to help this patient immediately?
6. Why were LDH, ALT, and bilirubin determined, and what do the results tell you?
7. A hematocrit of 33% to 40% is indicated as normal for a 5-month-old, whereas 40% to 50% is considered normal for adults. How does the hematocrit normally change during the first 6 months after birth?

PART III
Hospital Course

David was treated with IV antibiotics, and he became afebrile within 24 hours. The rest of his hospital course was devoted to a diagnostic workup of his hypoglycemia. He underwent an oral glucose tolerance test. With glucose at 2.5 g/kg given as a single dose via a nasogastric tube, his blood glucose rose to within normal limits (90 mg/dL), but within 4 hours it fell to 14 mg/dL. He showed no response to glucagon administered IM, with blood glucose levels remaining <14 mg/dL.

When David was given a constant glucose infusion at 0.5 g/kg/hr via a nasogastric tube, a normal blood glucose level of 90 to 100 mg/dL was maintained.

While in the hospital, David was maintained on feedings of 150 cc of 10% glucose (IV) every 4 hours in addition to his other food. Before one of the 8:00 a.m. feedings, he was noted to have twitching and jerking movements, which resolved rapidly when he was fed additional glucose.

QUESTIONS

1. How is the blood glucose level normally maintained during fasting?
2. How does glucagon affect blood glucose, and what does the complete unresponsiveness to glucagon suggest?
3. Can "twitching and jerking movements" be caused by hypoglycemia?

PART IV
Diagnosis

A GI consultation was sought, and a liver biopsy was carried out. A histological examination showed the presence of abnormal amounts of fat and glycogen within the hepatocytes. Biochemical tests included the determination of glucose 6-phosphatase activity in liver microsomes. Enzyme activity was absent both from fresh microsomes and from microsomes that had been subjected to repeated freezing and thawing.

QUESTIONS

1. Give examples of enzyme deficiencies that result in glycogen accumulation.

2. Does the liver normally produce triglycerides? What is the normal fate of liver-derived triglycerides, and under what conditions can fat accumulate in the liver?
3. What are microsomes, and how are they prepared?
4. The enzyme activity was determined both in fresh microsomes and in microsomes that had been frozen and thawed repeatedly. Can you give a rationale for this approach?
5. What diagnostic label can you attach to this patient?
6. David had increased amounts of glycogen and fat in his liver. Do you expect elevations of metabolic intermediates as well?
7. Knowing the molecular defect in the patient, how can you explain his abnormal blood chemistry, including the hypoglycemia, lactic acidemia, hyperuricemia, hyperlipidemia, and the presence of ketone bodies? Do hormones play a role in these abnormalities?

PART V
Follow-Up

David was discharged from the hospital after 2 weeks. At home, he was maintained on a regimen of lactose-free milk preparation with added glucose, approximately 2 g/kg every 4 hours. This formula was given around the clock, with a baby soft diet as tolerated. He did well on this therapy, although periodically he had hypoglycemic spells anywhere from 3 to 4 hours post-feeding.

When David was 3 years old his glucose formula gradually was tapered off, and he received cornstarch several times daily. He did well on this schedule, although nightly feeding remained a major inconvenience: it was necessary to wake him up once every night for his cornstarch porridge. Periodic blood tests showed near-normal blood lipid levels, although lactate and uric acid remained elevated. Starting at age 5, he was treated with allopurinol.

QUESTIONS

1. Why was David given lactose-free milk? Compare the metabolism of glucose and galactose. Would sucrose be better than lactose?
2. Why was he given cornstarch?
3. How does allopurinol work?

PART 6
Prenatal Diagnosis

David's parents had been told by his physician that his condition was inherited and that there was a considerable risk of the disease in future children. For this reason they refrained from having more children until, quite by accident, his mother got pregnant again when David was 4 years old, again from her husband. Fortunately the gene for glucose 6-phosphatase had been sequenced the year before, and a laboratory was located that could perform molecular studies on David's DNA. Frozen blood samples from David and his parents were sent to the laboratory. The DNA was extracted, and the coding regions and intron-exon junctions of the gene were amplified by the polymerase chain reaction (PCR). The five exons of the gene were amplified to yield products of 306 bp (exon 1), 192 bp (exon 2), 209 bp (exon 3), 259 bp (exon 4), 292 bp (exon 5, 5'-terminal part) and 389 bp (exon 5, 3'-terminal part).

Amplification products of the expected size were obtained, but chemical mismatch detection showed the presence of mutations in exon 3 and in the 3'-terminal part of exon 5 of David's gene, together with the normal sequence. David's mother had only the mutation in exon 3, and his father had only the mutation in exon 5. Sequencing of the polymerase chain reaction (PCR) products showed two known mutations: the exon 3 mutation was a C → T transition converting Arg-83 in the polypeptide to cysteine, and the exon 5 mutation was a C → T transition converting the codon for Gln-347 to a stop codon.

Amniocentesis was performed as soon as these results were available, and after a 6-day culturing period the cells were sent to the laboratory for analysis. The fetus turned out to have the exon 5 mutation but not the exon 3 mutation. Five months later a healthy daughter was born to David's parents.

QUESTIONS

1. Describe in general terms the situations in which prenatal diagnosis is indicated.
2. What is the mode of inheritance for David's disease, and how high exactly is the risk that a next child of his parents is affected?
3. Why is a DNA-based method used for prenatal diagnosis in this case, rather than determination of the enzyme activity?
4. In which situations is chemical mismatch detection with subsequent sequencing performed?
5. PCR-based methods are preferred over Southern blotting for the prenatal diagnosis of genetic diseases. Why?
6. The two mutations found in David account for most cases of glucose 6-phosphatase deficiency in people of European ancestry. Try to design a routine diagnostic test for the detection of these two mutations that uses PCR and allele-specific probes. Do you expect that this test can be used for the diagnosis of glucose 6-phosphatase deficiency in patients from other ethnic backgrounds?

Suggested Readings

Hers H-G, van Hoof F, de Barsy T: Glycogen storage diseases. In: Scriver CR, Beaudet AL, Sly WS, Valle D, editors: *The metabolic basis of inherited disease*, vol. 1. McGraw-Hill, New York, 1989, pp. 425-452.

Lei KJ et al: Mutations in the glucose 6-phosphatase gene are associated with glycogen storage disease types Ia and IaSP and not Ib and Ic. *J Clin Invest* 95, 234-240, 1995.

The Missed Examination

Annemarie is a 22-year-old medical student who has been diabetic since the age of 14. She controls her diabetes with daily insulin injections, 20 U/day, and she has been free from complications so far. One Monday morning, however, she is rushed to the emergency room unconscious.

In the ambulance, Annemarie has the following vital signs: blood pressure 80/40; pulse 124; respiratory rate 35. The paramedics draw several tubes of blood and then administer 50 cc of 50% dextrose solution and 2 mg of naloxone.

Annemarie's parents, who arrive at the emergency room only a few minutes after the ambulance in their own car, report that their daughter spent the night in her room studying for a biochemistry exam. She had been extremely apprehensive about this exam for a number of days. Her mother was not able to wake her up in the morning for this exam, which was scheduled for 8 a.m. Although the paramedics in the ambulance had noticed a suspicious smell on her breath, the parents insist that their daughter has not touched any alcohol recently.

On physical exam, the patient is a thin, nonjaundiced, white female. She is in no obvious distress, but is breathing deeply and rapidly. Her blood pressure is 100/80 when she is lying down, but the systolic pressure falls to 40 in a sitting position. Examination of her chest reveals normal heart and breath sounds. The abdomen is normal. The only abnormal finding is inflammation of the vulva and deposits in the folds of the labia, suggestive of a fungus infection.

The laboratory reports the following results:

Urinalysis: 4+ glucose
             4+ ketones
             0+ blood
             1+ protein

Blood tests (normal ranges are in parentheses):

Sodium: 130 mEq/L (136-142)
Chloride: 95 mEq/L (95-103)
Potassium: 5.5 mEq/L (3.8-5.0)
Bicarbonate: 10.8 mEq/L (21-30)
Glucose: 720 mg/dL (70-110)
Creatinine: 1.7 mg/dL (0.6-1.2)
BUN: 35 mg/dL (8-23)
Osmolality: 340 mOsm/kg (275-295)
pH: 7.22 (7.35-7.45)

Complete blood count: mildly elevated WBCs.

Arterial blood gases:
pO_2:   102 mmHg (95-100)
pCO_2: 22 mmHg (35-40)

Treatment is started with regular insulin, 8 U/hr, and with isotonic saline. Annemarie receives 1.5 liters of saline during the first hour and another 1.0 L during the second hour, all IV. A blood sample taken at this time shows the following values:

Glucose: 540 mg/dL
Sodium: 142 mM
Potassium: 2.2 mM
pH: 7.25

Treatment is continued with the infusion of insulin, hypotonic saline (1 L/hr for another 2 hours), and potassium. Annemarie is fully conscious by this time and gradually regains her previous state of health. She is released the next day, with an increase in her insulin dose to 30 U/day, and with ketoconazole for the infection.

Three days later she is brought into the emergency room unconscious. After blood samples are drawn, she is given 50 cc of 50% dextrose and wakes up within a few minutes. She reports that over the 30 minutes before losing consciousness she had felt increasingly confused, cold, and sweaty.

The blood glucose at the time of the second admission is 15 mg/dL. A concerned ER physician immediately suspects an insulinoma and requests a serum C-peptide level.

QUESTIONS

1. What causes of unconsciousness do you know?
2. Can you propose physiological mechanisms for the patient's hypotension, tachycardia, and hyperventilation?
3. What biochemical and physiological abnormalities account for the patient's loss of consciousness at the time of the first and the second admission?
4. Why did the paramedics in the ambulance give Annemarie dextrose and naloxone?
5. A suspicious smell on Annemarie's breath was noted in the ambulance. What caused this smell? Are there any other situations in which an abnormal smell on the breath can point to the cause of unconsciousness?
6. Patients with diabetic coma suffer from dehydration. Why?
7. What metabolic aberrations account for Annemarie's markedly elevated serum glucose, although she had consumed no food for several hours?
8. The initial presentation of this patient included a reduced blood pH. Discuss the factors contributing to this and the metabolic pathways responsible for the acidosis.
9. Is ketoacidosis the only type of "diabetic coma"?
10. Why did the potassium level decrease within 2 hours after the treatment was started?
11. At the time of the patient's second visit, an insulin-secreting tumor was suspected, and this was investigated by measuring the levels of circulating C peptide. How is this peptide formed, and what controls its secretion? In which clinical situations might this be a useful test?
12. Diabetic ketoacidosis often is precipitated by an infection or some other stressful condition.

What counterregulatory hormones might be involved in this process? Do you know of other physiological situations that increase the insulin requirement of diabetic patients?

13. Some patients with type II diabetes have elevated levels of circulating insulin, despite displaying many classic signs of the disease. In some cases, cells taken from the individual display normal binding of insulin, yet the hormone does not induce an appropriate biological response. What biochemical defects might be the cause of such a problem?

Suggested Readings

Kahn CR, Goldstein BJ: Molecular defects in insulin action. *Science* 245, 13, 1989.

Rifkin H, Porte D, editors: *Diabetes mellitus*, 4th ed. Elsevier, Amsterdam, 1990.

Grant Application

This is not a clinical case study, but a grant application that has been submitted to the National Institutes of Health by a faculty member of your school. The project is currently under investigation by the institutional ethics board.

Project title: Cloning of human embryos from cultured cells.

Principal investigator: Frank N. Stein, M.D.

Amount requested: $75 million for a total period of 10 years.

Modern reproductive technology is devoted to the needs of infertile couples and of single women who wish to have children in the absence of a male partner. This is a large field because close to 10% of all married couples are unable to conceive naturally. Also, approximately half of all marriages in the United States end in divorce, and the situation is similar in most other developed countries. Therefore more and more women prefer having children without burdening themselves with a husband.

One important aspect in assisted reproduction is quality control: 2% of all naturally conceived children are born with congenital defects; approximately 1 in 200 has a single-gene disorder, and 1 in 160 has a chromosome aberration. In addition, many naturally conceived children are handicapped by genes for such multifactorial diseases as diabetes, high blood pressure, hay fever, and neuropsychiatric diseases, or by genes for undesirable physical or mental traits. It is therefore the obligation of the providers of assisted-reproduction technology to make sure that their own failure rates are lower than those in naturally conceived children.

OBJECTIVE

This project aims at the establishment of a cryobank for frozen embryos of reproducible quality. The project will apply the principles of modern molecular biology to ensure that the embryos will be of uniform, predictable quality, providing prospective parents with a wide choice of safe options for producing their children.

METHODS

The following procedure will be used for the production of frozen embryos:

1. Donor semen will be obtained from cooperating sperm banks whose donors are highly selected Nobel Prize winners. All of these sperm banks test their donors for transmissible diseases including AIDS, hepatitis, and gonorrhea, as well as for the presence of deleterious recessive mutations. Donor oocytes will be obtained from highly selected female medical students. Only students with a grade point average of A, attractive physical features, no police record, and without a family history of polygenic diseases will be accepted as donors. Each donor will be tested for the sickle cell mutation, Tay-Sachs (6 mutations), glucose 6-phosphate dehydrogenase deficiency (by electrophoresis), BRCA1 (5 mutations), and cystic fibrosis (12 mutations). In addition, typing for HLA, apoE, the dopamine D2 and D4 receptor genes, and the calcitriol receptor gene will be performed to evaluate the risk for, respectively, autoimmune diseases, Alzheimer's disease, unstable personality, and osteoporosis.

2. In vitro fertilization will be performed with sperm and ova that are likely to form favorable genotypes based on the donors' genetic profiles. Each zygote will be grown into a blastocyst that then will be fragmented into individual cells by treatment with trypsin and hyaluronidase. These cells will be transferred to a petri dish and cultured in the presence of a mixture of growth

factors obtained from fetal calf serum and sheep placenta. Under these conditions the cells will be maintained in an undifferentiated, totipotent state. These cells will be referred to as totipotent (TP) cells.

3. The major portion (more than 1 million cells) of each TP cell line will be quick-frozen in liquid nitrogen for possible later use. The rest will be used for cloning.

4. For cloning, an oocyte from a paid donor will be enucleated by micromanipulation, and the nucleus of a TP cell will be injected. The resulting "zygote" will be grown into a 16-cell embryo. At this point, a single cell will be removed from the embryo, and this cell will be cultured and subjected to karyotyping and further genetic testing. The embryo itself will be frozen in liquid nitrogen. Each embryo will be released for use only after the tests show freedom from karyotypic abnormalities and from potentially hazardous combinations of genes.

5. Several dozen embryos will be prepared from each TP cell line. These embryos, which are genetically identical, will be frozen and supplied to cooperating IVF (in vitro fertilization) clinics for implantation, free of charge.

6. Each child obtained by this procedure will be evaluated at regular intervals for physical and mental development, personality traits, and health. Additional genetic tests will be performed as they become available. This follow-up, known technically as "progeny testing," is essential for the production of trouble-free embryos in the future.

7. If gene-related problems appear in one or more children, their TP cell line will be destroyed. If the children show desirable traits, however, their cryopreserved TP cell line will be used to produce more embryos. These embryos will be sold to IVF clinics worldwide. The project will become financially self-supporting at this time.

ADVANTAGES FOR CLIENTS

This project will serve clients in situations in which donor insemination or IVF with donated oocytes otherwise would be required. In comparison with these alternative methods, the advantages are:

- Better quality control: both the sperm donor and the oocyte donor are highly selected, and

each embryo is tested for genetic abnormalities. This reduces the risk of genetic disease. The risk is reduced further by the use of embryos from progeny-tested cell lines.

- Client choice: clients can be provided with a detailed profile of their child, including physical characteristics, personality traits, and intellectual potential.

PUBLIC HEALTH IMPACT

This project impacts on two aspects of public health:

1. The health expectations of the general public have increased with increased quality of medical care. This has led to a new emphasis on the prevention of disease rather than treatment. Many diseases now are prevented rather effectively — for example, heart attacks, by eating more polyunsaturated fat; viral diseases, by immunizations; bad teeth, by the fluoridation of drinking water; AIDS, by the use of condoms. On the other hand, the only way currently to reduce the risk of congenital and genetic diseases is prenatal diagnosis, with the selective abortion of affected fetuses. Our embryo cryobank will greatly reduce the need for this crude and morally reprehensible practice. The use of cloned embryos will have a great impact in reducing the suffering caused by Mendelian disorders (except those caused by a new mutation), will essentially eliminate chromosome aberrations, and will significantly reduce the incidence of multifactorial disorders.

2. Medical costs have been exploding in the recent past. Although most of this is the result of overcharging by physicians, it also reflects the high incidence of chronic diseases in the population. Those diseases that can be prevented by the use of frozen embryos from progeny-tested TP cells are of a chronic nature, and they are a major burden on the health-care system. Therefore health-care costs will be reduced, for the benefit of all citizens.

POSSIBLE FUTURE DEVELOPMENTS

The use of cultured cell lines for embryo production will enable us to introduce targeted genetic alterations. It will be possible, in particular, to introduce genes obtained from other animals, plants, or microorganisms. One long-term prospect is the introduction of genes for enzymes of vitamin and amino acid synthesis, which will make human beings resistant to many nutritional deficiencies. These foreign genes are constructs of natural genes with flanking sequences that are complementary to endogenous DNA sequences. These flanking sequences permit a targeted incorporation of the foreign gene into the genome by homologous recombination. The proper incorporation of the gene into the genome will be assessed in subcultured embryonic cells by Southern blotting.

ECONOMIC IMPACT

This project will create a major market for donated oocytes. Two types of oocyte donation are required: oocytes from highly selected donors, which will be obtained from only a small number of individuals, and mass donations from unselected donors for enucleation. The latter type of donation will create income opportunities for poor women, thereby reducing welfare dependence. Brochures offering opportunities for paid oocyte donation will be distributed through local welfare departments.

QUESTIONS

1. Do you think there will be a great market for Dr. Stein's frozen embryos?

2. The testing of semen donors for the AIDS virus (a retrovirus) is commonly performed by PCR. What advantage does this method offer over alternative immunological methods? Would you prefer white blood cells for AIDS testing by PCR, or can you use cell-free serum?

3. Dr. Stein wants to test his oocyte donors for a number of recessive mutations that possibly could cause disease in future generations. Describe the methods that can be used for this purpose. What are the limitations of these methods?

4. In which ethnic groups are genes for sickle cell disease, Tay-Sachs disease, and glucose 6-phosphate dehydrogenase deficiency common?

5. Can all cases of glucose 6-phosphate dehydrogenase deficiency be diagnosed by electrophoresis? Why not use Southern blotting with allele-specific probes?

6. The use of trypsin and hyaluronidase is proposed for dissociating embryonic cells. How can the enzymes achieve this?

7. Can embryos and cultured cells be kept frozen? What conditions are best for the freezing of these samples? Can human bodies be preserved in a viable state by freezing?

8. Dr. Stein wants to use a mixture of growth factors to keep cultured embryonic cells in an undifferentiated state. Give some examples of growth factors. Through which signaling pathways can growth factors affect cell growth and differentiation?

9. Many growth factor receptors autophosphorylate on tyrosine side chains upon ligand binding. In some cases, different growth factor receptors of the tyrosine protein kinase type can mediate different effects on the same target cell—for example, proliferation versus terminal differentiation—even though the first step in the signaling cascade (receptor autophosphorylation) is the same for the different growth factor receptors. How?

10. Dr. Stein wants to use enucleated oocytes from paid donors. Do these enucleated oocytes contribute any genes to the embryo?

11. Cloning has been performed even with the nuclei of cells from adult tissues. What does this imply for the interaction between nucleus and cytoplasm in the regulation of gene expression?

12. We do not know whether nuclei from any somatic cell can be used for cloning. Can you think of irreversible or poorly reversible changes in the DNA of some somatic cells that would make these cells unsuitable for cloning?

13. In the context of progeny testing, Dr. Stein wants to use additional genetic tests "as they become available." Can you realistically expect that many new DNA-directed genetic tests will become available in the next few years?

14. Dr. Stein wants to introduce new genes into the genome by homologous recombination. How does homologous recombination work?

15. Can attempts at introducing new genes into the genome result in dangerous mutations? Propose a method that uses Southern blotting to determine whether a foreign gene has been incorporated only in the intended target site or also (by nonhomologous recombination) in other genomic locations.

16. What would be a suitable source for a transgene if you wanted to introduce the ability for vita-

min C synthesis to cultured embryonic cells? What about genes for cobalamin synthesis?

17. What is the current status of cloning in humans and other mammalian species? Go to the library, and use the Science Citation Index to find references to the articles by K. H. Campbell et al. in Nature 380, pp. 64-66 (1996) and by I. Wilmut et al. in Nature 385, pp. 810-813 (1997).

18. In the past, attempts to reduce the risk of genetic and congenital diseases and to improve the genetic constitution of human populations were known as "eugenics." Should such measures as the testing of semen and oocyte donors for transmissible diseases and recessive disease genes be performed? Should this be mandatory? Such testing currently is performed by many sperm banks. How would you counsel a patient who is considering artificial insemination by donor? Would you donate your own sperm or oocytes for purposes of assisted reproduction?

19. Should gene transfer technology be used to improve the human genotype, along the lines proposed by Dr. Stein? If not, why not?

20. Does Dr. Stein's embryo factory violate any established principles of medical ethics? Or do you follow Dr. Stein's reasoning that this project should be performed for ethical reasons, namely because it reduces the suffering from avoidable genetic diseases? Are there any specific procedures in his proposal that can be considered unethical?

Suggested Readings

Brody H: *Ethical decisions in medicine*, 2nd ed. Little, Brown, Boston, 1981, pp. 161-184, 267-286.

Campbell KH, McWhir J, Ritchie WA, Wilmut I: Sheep cloned by nuclear transfer from a cultured cell line. *Nature* 380, 64-66, 1996.

Wilmut I, Schnieke AE, McWhir J, Kind AJ, Campbell KHS: Viable offspring derived from fetal and adult mammalian cells. *Nature* 385, 810-813, 1997.

Answers to Case Studies

The Mafia Boss

Sixty percent of the adult human body is water, and therefore the density of the body is close to 1 g/cm³. Protein-rich tissues and bones have densities greater than 1 g/cm³, whereas the fat in adipose tissue (typically 10–15 kg) has a density close to 0.9 g/cm³. Gas-filled spaces are present in the lungs and in the intestine. Shortly after death, a dead body will sink in water as much of the air is forced out of the lungs. Within 1 to 3 days after death, bacterial decomposition of the body is initiated by anaerobic intestinal bacteria, and a large amount of gas (carbon dioxide, methane, and hydrogen) is formed. The body floats to the surface at this time. According to the source of this case study (a popular book about organized crime in America), the doctor advised the Mafia boss to make a hole in the abdomen with an ice pick, so the trapped gas could be released.

Viral Gastroenteritis

Gastroenteritis is a common disease, especially in children. It usually is caused by a viral infection of the gastric and intestinal mucosa, leading to vomiting and diarrhea. Although the loss of water and electrolytes can lead to serious dehydration and general weakness, most cases are mild and self-limited. Breast-feeding provides some protection through maternal immunoglobulin A (IgA) antibodies. In some affected children the functions of the intestinal mucosa are impaired, resulting in abnormal nutrient digestion and absorption.

In this case, small amounts of a reducing substance were demonstrated in the urine. This probably was undigested lactose that entered the bloodstream through the damaged intestinal mucosa. Like other disaccharides, lactose is not metabolized in the tissues once it has entered the blood but is excreted in the urine.

Mono- and disaccharides with at least one free anomeric carbon, including all monosaccharides and most disaccharides (but not sucrose), have reducing properties. The nature of a reducing substance in the urine can be determined by enzymatic tests, for example, the glucose oxidase test for free glucose.

This patient seems to have an impaired ability of lactose digestion. The apparent lactose intolerance is secondary, caused by the infection. Primary lactose intolerance, caused by a recessively inherited gene, is uncommon in infants although it is very common in older children and adults.

Undigested lactose is fermented readily by intestinal bacteria. Bacterial fermentation produces acetic, propionic, and lactic acids, as well as the gases methane, hydrogen, and carbon dioxide. Diarrhea is caused at least partially by the osmotic effect of lactose and the irritant effects of the acids on the intestine. The reducing substance in this patient's stool most likely is lactose, and the low pH is caused by bacterially produced acids.

The beneficial effects of the therapeutic milk formula were most likely due to the absence of lactose. Another difference that may have contributed to the effect was the presence of casein hydrolysate instead of intact milk proteins. Immunologic responses to proteins in cow's milk can develop in infants, especially during the course of an intestinal infection. The peptides and amino acids in casein hydrolysate are too small to be immunogenic.

Death In Installments

This patient has metachromatic leukodystrophy. The disease is caused by a recessively inherited deficiency of sulfatidase, which leads to an accumulation of sulfatide (sulfated galactocerebroside). Sulfatide is one of the major membrane lipids of myelin. Like most other lipid storage diseases, metachromatic leukodystrophy leads to neurologic degeneration. A complete deficiency of the enzyme causes death in infancy or early childhood, but incomplete deficiencies result in a milder and more protracted course. The enzyme deficiency is present in all tissues, but the nervous system is affected most seriously because of its high sulfatide turnover. This patient seems to have an abnormal enzyme that acts poorly on its natural substrate, although it does act quite well on arylsulfates, phenolic sulfate esters that can be used for the assay of sulfatidase ("arylsulfatase") in the laboratory.

Lipid storage diseases are rare, therefore the diagnosis often is missed. Histologic examinations can be helpful because they show the abnormal accumulation of lipids in lysosomes, but a definitive diagnosis requires either the electrophoretic separation of lipids from biopsy samples or cultured cells, or enzyme determinations. These tests often are done with cultured leukocytes or fibroblasts. The cultured cells grow better on serum than on plasma because blood clotting is induced when serum is prepared from fresh blood. Blood clotting induces the activation and degranulation of platelets which release platelet-derived growth factor (PDGF), an excellent stimulus for the growth of cultured cells.

Many diseases can cause neurologic degeneration, therefore a broad range of diagnostic tests have to be applied to arrive at the correct diagnosis. This patient had been tested specifically for pernicious anemia (B_{12} level), Wilson's disease (ceruloplasmin level, liver function tests), and syphilis. Pneumoencephalography is an old-fashioned method for the diagnosis of ventricular dilatation and cerebral atrophy. Computed axial tomography (CAT scan) would be a more modern technique for this purpose. Lumbar puncture is performed most commonly for the diagnosis of central nervous system (CNS) infections: an elevated cerebrospinal fluid (CSF) protein concentration and reduced CSF glucose are typical for bacterial infections. CSF protein normally is very low compared with protein levels in the plasma (20 mg/dL vs. 7,000 mg/dL), and CSF glucose is approximately two thirds of the blood glucose concentration. Glucose is transported into the brain by facilitated diffusion, and it is consumed but not produced in the brain. Therefore its CSF level always is less than the plasma level.

A Mysterious Death

Methylmalonicacidemia (also called methylmalonicaciduria) is caused by a recessively inherited deficiency of the B_{12}-dependent enzyme methylmalonyl-CoA mutase, which converts methylmalonyl-CoA to succinyl-CoA. This reaction participates in the catabolism of valine, isoleucine, methionine, threonine, and odd-chain fatty acids. Methylmalonic acid accumulates and causes life-threatening acidosis. Methylmalonicacidemia can be mistaken for ethylene glycol poisoning because ethylene glycol is metabolized to oxalic acid, which also causes severe acidosis:

$$HO-CH_2-CH_2-OH \longrightarrow \longrightarrow {}^-OOC-COO^- + 2\ H^+$$

Ethylene glycol

Oxalate

Acidosis results in peripheral vasodilation and circulatory shock. This in turn triggers a massive release of epinephrine from the adrenal medulla and norepinephrine from sympathetic nerve terminals. Epinephrine and norepinephrine do not only upregulate the abnormally low blood pressure; they also induce fat breakdown in adipose tissue. Some of the adipose tissue-derived fatty acids are converted to ketone bodies in the liver. This amounts to a vicious cycle because the ketone bodies, being acidic, aggravate the acidosis.

In a substantial minority of patients, the disease is not caused by a deficiency of methylmalonyl-CoA mutase but by an inability to convert dietary B_{12} to the active coenzyme form, adenosylcobalamin. These patients can be treated with adenosylcobalamin. The possibilities for dietary treatment by the restriction of valine, isoleucine, methionine, and threonine are limited because these amino acids are nutritionally essential and cannot be excluded from the diet.

To Treat Or Not To Treat?

Nonketotic hyperglycinemia is caused by a recessively inherited deficiency of the glycine cleavage enzyme, the major enzyme of glycine degradation. Glycine serves important functions in the CNS. It is an inhibitory neurotransmitter in the spinal cord and brain stem, and it acts as coligand for the NMDA (N-methyl-D-aspartate) receptor, a receptor for the excitatory neurotransmitter glutamate in the brain. Therefore the abnormal accumulation of glycine in patients with nonketotic hyperglycinemia induces both CNS depression and CNS excitation. Untreated patients die of sudden apnea or status epilepticus within a few months after birth, and severe CNS dysfunction and mental deficiency develop in survivors.

Dietary treatment is not effective because glycine is formed endogenously from serine, which in turn is synthesized from a glycolytic intermediate. Benzoic acid is useful because it becomes conjugated with glycine, forming hippuric acid. Hippuric acid is excreted in the urine. The doses of benzoic acid required to reduce the blood and CSF levels of glycine are enormous, however, and the treatment does not prevent brain damage although it permits survival. Carnitine deficiency can develop because carnitine reacts enzymatically with many organic acids, including benzoic acid. The resulting conjugation product is excreted in the urine.

Ethical problems arise because the patient would not be viable without heroic treatment, his quality of life is dismal, and he cannot give informed consent to his treatment. The extent of the patient's suffering cannot be assessed because communication is not possible. In some cases, parents may request the discontinuation of any life-prolonging treatment. Conflicts also arise from the considerable expense of long-term treatment: insurance companies are reluctant to pay for continued treatment whereas the treating physician may derive substantial income from the patient.

Yellow Eyes

Jaundice in an adult can be caused by hemolytic conditions, liver disease, or obstructive biliary disease. In this patient, biliary obstruction was suggested by the abnormal color of stool and urine. In healthy individuals, the brown color of the stool is caused by stercobilin and other urobilins, colored products that are generated from bilirubin diglucuronide by intestinal bacteria. In patients with biliary obstruction, bilirubin diglucuronide fails to reach the intestine, and therefore urobilins cannot be formed and the stools are "clay-colored." The bilirubin diglucuronide that cannot be passed from the liver to the intestine "overflows" into the blood and eventually is excreted in the urine, to which it imparts a brownish color.

The suspicion of biliary obstruction was confirmed by the high blood level of alkaline phosphatase and by the high blood level of conjugated bilirubin with near-normal unconjugated bilirubin. Also, the absence of urobilinogen in stool and urine suggests cholestasis. Severe hemolysis could be excluded because urobilinogen was absent and the hematocrit normal, and acute liver disease could be excluded because the alanine transaminase level was normal.

The patient had a prolonged prothrombin time, almost certainly because of impaired vitamin K absorption. Like the other fat-soluble vitamins, vitamin K requires bile salts for efficient intestinal absorption. Therefore the impaired blood clotting would respond to vitamin K injection or to large doses of oral vitamin K.

Biliary obstruction can result from a number of diseases, including malignancies. This patient has cancer of the head of the pancreas. Approximately two thirds of pancreatic cancers originate in the head of the pancreas, and they often present with obstructive jaundice before other signs of malignant disease (weight loss, pain) are evident. Most pancreatic cancers are highly aggressive, and surgical resection rarely is possible. Cancer chemotherapy is based on the use of agents that are most damaging for rapidly dividing cells. Some antineoplastic drugs, including methotrexate (a folate antagonist) and fluorouracil (a base analog) inhibit nucleotide metabolism and DNA synthesis. Others, including vincristine, bind to tubulin and interfere with the formation of the mitotic spindle.

An Abdominal Emergency

Abdominal pain with acute onset can have many causes, including food poisoning, peptic ulcer, biliary disease, intestinal infarction, hernia, renal diseases, malignancies, and pancreatitis. Blood tests are essential for the diagnosis. This patient shows no evidence of liver or biliary disease (normal alanine transaminase, alkaline phosphatase, and bilirubin) or renal disease (normal urea and creatinine). α-Amylase, however, is elevated to a level typical for patients with acute pancreatitis.

Acute pancreatitis is a disease in which pancreatic zymogens, including proteases and phospholipases, become activated in the pancreas, rather than the duodenum. The activated enzymes destroy pancreatic tissue and spill over into the abdominal cavity and the bloodstream. The action of pancreatic lipase on intraabdominal adipose tissue produces free fatty acids that bind calcium, leading to hypocalcemia. Hypomagnesemia may result from excessive vomiting. Hyperglycemia can develop when the endocrine pancreas is affected by the disease, with a resulting impairment of insulin secretion.

The treatment of acute pancreatitis is based on the complete avoidance of food because food constituents, particularly fat and protein, stimulate pancreatic enzyme production and fluid secretion. These effects are mediated by the hormones cholecystokinin (pancreozymin) and secretin.

The immediate cause for an attack of acute pancreatitis rarely is known with certainty, but a dislodged gallstone may be the culprit in some cases. A gallstone lodged in the ampulla of Vater can impair the patency of the pancreatic duct and may, in patients with joint pancreatic and common bile ducts, lead to a reflux of bile into the pancreatic duct system.

Normal bile contains a substantial amount of bile salts (deprotonated bile acids) and a far smaller amount of free (unesterified) cholesterol in addition to phospholipid, inorganic ions, and "bile pigments" (bilirubin diglucuronide and its derivatives). Cholesterol is insoluble in water and must be kept in solution as a constituent of mixed bile salt-phospholipid micelles. Most gallstones consist of cholesterol, and they form when the cholesterol concentration of the bile is increased or when the concentration of bile salts and phospholipid is reduced ("lithogenic bile"). Gallstones usually form in the gallbladder where the bile becomes concentrated by the absorption of water and electrolytes across the gallbladder epithelium.

Gallstones are associated with obesity and with high-calorie diets, which appear to increase the concentration of biliary cholesterol. Obese patients usually have elevated biliary cholesterol. Bile acid-binding resins (such as cholestyramine), which sometimes are used for the treatment of hypercholesterolemia, may increase the risk of gallstones because they reduce the supply of bile salts through the enterohepatic circulation. Conversely, orally administered bile acids, such as chenodeoxycholic acid (chenodiol) and ursodeoxycholic acid, can be helpful because they enter the bile through the enterohepatic circulation where they help to dissolve the stones. However, these bile acids can cause elevations of low-density lipoprotein (LDL) cholesterol because they inhibit the conversion of cholesterol to bile salts by 7α-hydroxylase in the liver. This raises the level of free cholesterol in the liver, and free cholesterol inhibits the synthesis of LDL receptors.

Shortness of Breath

Although its incidence has been declining during the past 25 years, coronary heart disease still is the leading cause of death in the United States and in most other western countries. It is caused by atheromatous lesions in the coronary arteries, which encroach on the arterial lumen and impair blood flow to the myocardium. The sequence of events leading to these lesions is not well known, but several risk factors have been described. High levels of LDL are known to promote atherosclerosis whereas high levels of high-density lipoprotein (HDL) are protective. Also, elevated very low-density lipoprotein (VLDL) levels in patients with type IV hyperlipoproteinemia increase the risk of coronary heart disease. These lipid abnormalities promote the accumulation of cholesterol esters in the walls of large arteries to form fatty streaks. Fatty streaks are reversible lesions, but some appear to progress to full-blown atheromatous plaques.

Additional risk factors include smoking, hypertension, and diabetes mellitus. Smoking may promote atherosclerosis because cigarette smoke contains oxidants that damage LDL. Oxidized LDL is taken up more readily by macrophages than virgin LDL—an important first step in the formation of a fatty streak. Hypertension exposes the arteries to physical stress, which promotes vascular injury and triggers a fibroproliferative response. Diabetes mellitus is injurious to arterial walls as well, possibly because of diabetic microangiopathy affecting the vasa vasorum.

Coronary heart disease can result in acute myocardial infarction, typically after the formation of a thrombus (intravascular blood clot) on the surface of the lesion. The thrombus either blocks the artery at the site of the lesion, or it causes a smaller infarction after being carried into one of the terminal branches of the coronary system. The myocardium can survive acute ischemia for 30 to 60 minutes. After this time the cells die because of the failure of adenosine triphosphate (ATP)-dependent ion pumps and the excessive accumulation of lactic acid, which is formed by anaerobic glycolysis from stored glycogen. Other patients have chronic impairments: they show exercise intolerance, shortness of breath, and chest pain on exertion. This condition is called angina pectoris. This patient has angina pectoris associated with obesity, a sedentary lifestyle, smoking, and a type IV hyperlipoproteinemia.

The patient's hyperlipoproteinemia responded to dietary carbohydrate restriction rather than lipid restriction. This is not unusual because VLDL triglycerides are synthesized from excess carbohydrates in the well-fed liver. The reaction sequence involves glycolysis, fatty acid biosynthesis, and esterification of the fatty acids.

Nitroglycerin is used for the treatment of angina pectoris because it is a potent vasodilator; it is metabolized to nitric oxide, a short-lived product that activates the cytoplasmic guanylate cyclase in vascular smooth muscle cells. Nitric oxide also is an endogenous product that plays a key role in the regulation of the vascular tone; it is formed by endothelial cells in response to agents that raise the cytoplasmic calcium concentration in the endothelial cells, including histamine, bradykinin, and acetylcholine. Being small and lipid soluble, nitric oxide diffuses readily from the endothelium into the vascular smooth muscle, where it acts as "endothelium-derived relaxing factor."

There are several strategies to combat coronary heart disease. Smoking should be discouraged. Dietary recommendations for hyperlipidemic patients include a low-cholesterol diet with a high ratio of polyunsaturated/saturated fatty acids and a lot of dietary fiber, and a low-carbohydrate diet for patients with elevated VLDL. Antioxidant vitamins, particularly vitamins C and E, are recommended because they protect LDL from oxidation. Oxidatively damaged LDL is a preferred substrate for macrophage scavenger receptors. Therefore it tends to accumulate in macrophages, initiating the formation of a fatty streak. Coumarin-type anticoagulants can be used in coronary patients to prevent acute myocardial infarction, but they are dangerous; patients receiving long-term anticoagulant treatment have died of cerebral hemorrhages and other complications. Fibrinolytic treatments, either streptokinase or tissue-type plasminogen activator, can be used within 1 hour after acute myocardial infarction in an attempt to dissolve the existing clot and thereby limit the extent of tissue damage.

Several lipid-reducing drugs are available. Lovastatin (Mevinoline) is an inhibitor of HMG-CoA reductase, the rate-limiting enzyme of cholesterol biosynthesis. It leads initially to a reduced level of free cholesterol in the cells, both in the liver and in many extrahepatic tissues. The cells respond to this situation by increasing the synthesis of LDL receptors. Cholestyramine is a nonabsorbable ion exchange resin that binds bile salts and prevents their intestinal absorption. The reduced supply of bile salts to the liver through the enterohepatic circulation increases the conversion of cholesterol to bile acids, and the resulting decrease of the intracellular cholesterol pool induces the increased synthesis of LDL receptors in the liver.

Bypass surgery is a treatment of last resort for coronary patients. It consists of an autograft from the patient's own saphenous vein that bypasses the affected portion of the coronary artery.

This patient was enrolled in a double-blind,

placebo-controlled clinical study about the protective effects of antioxidant vitamins. A double-blind study is a study in which neither the patient nor the physician knows whether the patient is getting the active treatment or the placebo. A placebo — an inactive substance such as lactose or starch administered in the same form as the active treatment — is essential in clinical trials because the psychological effects of receiving treatment may cause a beneficial therapeutic outcome in the absence of any active ingredient at all. Our patient appears suitable for participation in the clinical trial because he had quit smoking and complied with dietary changes in the past; noncompliance is a major problem in long-term clinical trials, as it is in general medical practice. The patient's blood level of vitamin C was determined for the same reason: the plasma ascorbic acid level depends on the dietary intake, and noncompliance with the active treatment would be revealed by a low plasma level.

Itching

This patient has primary biliary cirrhosis, an autoimmune disease that leads to inflammation and degeneration of intrahepatic bile ducts. The diagnosis is established by the results of the liver biopsy and the presence of antimitochondrial antibodies. The biochemical abnormalities are those of biliary obstruction, with elevated serum levels of bilirubin, bile acids, alkaline phosphatase, and γ-glutamyltransferase. The serum cholesterol level is elevated because the biliary excretion of cholesterol and bile acids is impaired. The backlog of bile acids inhibits 7α-hydroxylase, the rate-limiting enzyme of bile acid synthesis. Bile acid synthesis is the major metabolic fate of cholesterol in the liver (other than incorporation in VLDL), and therefore the inhibition of bile acid synthesis results in an elevated cholesterol level in the liver. Free cholesterol downregulates the hepatic LDL receptors, and this leads to elevated levels of LDL cholesterol.

Copper accumulates in patients with cholestasis because the bile is the normal vehicle for copper excretion. Like other heavy metals, copper is toxic if it accumulates in the tissues. The copper accumulation in patients with chronic cholestasis resembles that in Wilson's disease, an inherited deficiency of a copper transporter in which copper accumulates because it cannot be excreted into the bile.

The initial symptom of itching in this patient probably is the result of elevated blood levels of bile acids that irritate free nerve endings in the skin. Unlike the itching of allergic reactions, itching in patients with biliary disease is not accompanied by pustular or erythematous changes ("hives"), and it does not respond to antihistamines. Itching also occurs in patients with uremia and in those with polycythemia vera, a neoplastic disease with excessive formation of erythrocytes. However, renal failure and uremia can be excluded in this patient because of normal blood urea nitrogen (BUN); polycythemia vera can be excluded because of her low to normal hematocrit.

There are several treatment strategies for primary biliary cirrhosis, none of them entirely satisfactory. The inflammatory process can be suppressed by antiinflammatory steroids. The accumulation of copper, which contributes to liver damage, can be treated with penicillamine. This copper chelator forms a soluble copper complex that is excreted in the urine. Cholestyramine is a nonabsorbable ion exchange resin that binds bile acids in the intestine, preventing their absorption. Thus it prevents the excessive accumulation of bile acids in liver and blood, at least as long as the bile flow is not interrupted entirely. By removing excess bile acids, it also permits an increased metabolism of cholesterol to bile acids.

Chronic cholestasis leads to liver cirrhosis, a condition in which normal hepatocytes gradually die out and are replaced by fibrous connective tissue. The proliferation of fibrous connective tissue is a typical response to injury that is otherwise seen in the context of scar formation and abscess formation. Liver cirrhosis is accompanied by capillary metaplasia of the sinusoids: the wide sinusoids are replaced by narrow capillaries that offer more resistance to blood flow. This leads to portal hypertension.

Biochemical changes in liver cirrhosis include abnormalities in plasma protein concentrations with an increased globulin/albumin ratio and reduced levels of prothrombin and other clotting factors. The liver is the principal source of most plasma proteins, including albumin and the clotting factors. The clotting disorder in cirrhotic patients is not likely to respond to vitamin K because it is caused by a reduced capacity for clotting factor synthesis, not by vitamin K malabsorption. The deficiency of clotting factors is important because cirrhotic patients are prone to hemorrhages from peptic ulcer disease and from dilated lower esophageal veins, which form part of a collateral circulation around the diseased liver.

In addition to hemorrhage, hepatic encephalopathy is a major complication of liver cirrhosis. Although its etiology is complex, hyperammonemia is an important factor. Ammonia accumulates in cirrhotic patients because its detoxification in the urea cycle is no longer possible. The liver is the only major organ with a complete urea cycle. These patients have to be kept on a low-protein diet because ammonia is produced from dietary protein.

Intestinal bacteria are important sources of ammonia: they degrade leftover dietary protein, and they cleave the urea in digestive secretions to carbon dioxide and ammonia. In acute episodes of hepatic encephalopathy, a mannitol enema can be helpful immediately because mannitol (a sugar alcohol) stimulates the growth of intestinal bacteria by providing them with a carbon source. It does not provide any nitrogen, and therefore the growing bacteria have to assimilate nitrogen from ambient ammonia. The eradication of intestinal bacteria by broad-spectrum antibiotics is an alternative strategy.

The removal of excess nitrogen from the body also can be achieved by the liberal use of benzoic acid or phenylacetic acid. These organic acids are conjugated with glycine and glutamine, respectively, and the conjugation products are excreted by the kidneys. These reactions actually are detoxification reactions that are "designed" to remove foreign organic acids, but in cirrhotic patients they can be exploited as an alternative route of nitrogen excretion, thereby reducing the need for urea synthesis.

Abdominal Pain

The most remarkable feature of this patient is the lack of gross abnormalities, both on physical examination and in blood chemistry. Although patients with somatic complaints who show no evidence of physical illness usually are diagnosed with psychiatric disorders, some do indeed have an identifiable physical disorder. The patient in this case did show evidence of neurologic dysfunction, including seizures, but no evidence of a physical disorder. There is no indication of an infection (normal white cells and globulins), infectious or inflammatory CNS disease (normal lumbar CSF), focal brain damage (no aphasia and apraxia), kidney disease (normal urea nitrogen, normal appearance of the urine), liver disease (normal aspartate transaminase and bilirubin), pancreatitis (normal/low amylase), muscle disease (normal/low creatine kinase), and anemia (normal hematocrit).

The patient finally was diagnosed with porphyria, most likely intermittent acute porphyria. Porphyrias can be caused by a partial deficiency of any of the heme-synthesizing enzymes other than δ-aminolevulinate (ALA) synthase. ALA synthase catalyzes the committed and rate-limiting step in heme biosynthesis. It is feedback inhibited by free heme.

The symptoms of porphyria are not caused by a deficiency of heme but by the accumulation of biosynthetic intermediates. In the hepatic porphyrias, the liver is the source of the accumulating intermediates but the symptoms are caused by actions of these intermediates on the nervous system: autonomic dysfunctions are caused by actions on the sympathetic, parasympathetic and enteric nervous systems; pain is caused by a stimulation of visceral pain fibers; and weakness, irritability, and seizures result from toxic effects on the CNS.

Patients with neuropsychiatric disorders usually are treated symptomatically with tranquilizers, sedative-hypnotics, or anticonvulsants. Many of these drugs are contraindicated in patients with hepatic porphyrias because they induce drug-metabolizing microsomal enzymes in the liver. One component of these enzyme systems is a family of heme-containing enzymes collectively known as cytochrome P-450. It is the synthesis of the P-450 apoproteins that is induced by many drugs. The apoproteins bind heme, thereby depleting the pool of free, unbound heme in the cell. Free heme but not protein-bound heme represses ALA synthase, the first enzyme of the heme biosynthetic pathway. By this mechanism, drugs can induce ALA synthase and cause the accumulation of biosynthetic intermediates.

Porphyrias are rare diseases, and therefore they often go undiagnosed. An abnormal color of the urine, caused by the accumulated biosynthetic intermediates, can give a clue to the diagnosis. Other conditions in which the color of the urine is abnormal include conjugated hyperbilirubinemia ("choluric jaundice"), as well as hemoglobinuria in massive hemolysis and myoglobinuria in some muscle diseases. The levels of porphobilinogen and other intermediates of the heme biosynthetic pathway can be determined in the urine whenever a porphyria is suspected.

The treatment of porphyria consists of measures to reduce the activity of ALA synthase and thereby curtail the supply of the offending biosynthetic intermediates. Drugs that induce hepatic enzyme synthesis must be withdrawn. Hematin (a chemically stable oxidized form of heme) can be given intravenously to repress ALA synthase. Also, intravenous glucose and a high-carbohydrate diet repress ALA synthase by unknown mechanisms.

Rheumatism

Most patients with joint pain can be placed into the two major diagnostic categories of rheumatoid arthritis and osteoarthritis, depending on the relative prominence of autoimmune/inflammatory reactions or of degenerative changes, respectively. The treatment of these major forms of arthritis is symptomatic and not very satisfactory. Aspirin is the mainstay of treatment for the painful inflammatory process of rheumatoid arthritis, but it can cause gastritis and gastric ulcers. Being a weak acid, it becomes protonated and uncharged in the acidic environment of the stomach. In this form, it readily diffuses into the cells of the gastric mucosa, where it becomes deprotonated and negatively charged at the cellular pH which is close to 7. The charged form penetrates membranes poorly; therefore the drug accumulates to high levels in the cells, causing toxicity.

The patient in this case study does not have one of the common forms of arthritis; he has hemochromatosis. The most important laboratory findings are the elevated level of serum ferritin and an abnormally high transferrin saturation. The transferrin concentration (total iron binding capacity, TIBC) is not a very useful diagnostic parameter because it may be either normal or increased in hemochromatosis.

Ferritin is the principal intracellular iron storage protein. It is present in many tissues, including the intestinal mucosa, the spleen, the liver, the pancreas, the heart, and bone marrow. Its synthesis is induced by the presence of free iron in the cells. Free iron is toxic because it binds to proteins and, in particular, because it catalyzes the formation of highly reactive free radicals from molecular oxygen and polyunsaturated fatty acids. Therefore the tissue levels of ferritin are low in iron deficiency and high in iron overload. Small amounts of ferritin normally enter the bloodstream during cell turnover in the liver and other ferritin-rich tissues. It can be determined in the serum by sensitive radioimmunoassays. Transferrin is the principal iron transport protein of the blood. It has two binding sites for ferric iron. In most people, approximately 30% of the iron-binding sites actually are occupied by iron. This percentage is reduced in iron deficiency and increased in iron overload.

Hemochromatosis develops only when iron absorption exceeds iron excretion for a very long time. Therefore abnormal iron accumulation is seen only in middle-aged and older people.

Patients usually are men because women are protected by menstruation and childbearing. Iron overload (hemosiderosis) can develop as a result of unusual dietary habits, for example, in alcoholics drinking large amounts of iron-rich wines. Most patients, however, are homozygous for a recessive gene that increases intestinal iron absorption. Approximately 1 in 500 individuals have this genotype.

The first signs of hemochromatosis are variable and may include liver dysfunction, heart failure, diabetes mellitus, reduced pituitary and testicular function, joint pain, and abnormal skin pigmentation. Unsatisfactory testicular androgen production in hemochromatosis is caused by pituitary dysfunction. Hormone determinations in these patients would show low levels of pituitary gonadotropins in addition to reduced androgen levels. Conversely, testicular failure would cause low levels of androgens but elevated levels of gonadotropins because the androgens normally inhibit gonadotropin secretion. The signs of hemochromatosis are so nonspecific that the condition usually is overlooked. A correct diagnosis requires biochemical determinations.

Specific treatment of hemochromatosis is aimed at the removal of the excess iron. Dietary restrictions are ineffective; daily iron excretion amounts to approximately 1 mg/day, but more than 20 g of iron may be stored in the patient's tissues. Therefore the removal of the excess iron stores by simply eliminating all dietary sources of iron (which would be hard to achieve) would take almost a century. Treatment with the iron chelator desferrioxamine is possible, but it is too cumbersome (the drug has to be administered with a subcutaneous infusion pump) and the removal of excess iron is too slow. Therefore desferrioxamine is reserved for those patients in whom iron overload develops in the course of severe anemia or after repeated blood transfusions, for example, those patients with thalassemia. Repeated phlebotomy is more effective than chelation therapy for patients with hemochromatosis. The removal of blood increases erythropoiesis via erythropoietin, and the iron for the increased hemoglobin synthesis is mobilized from stored ferritin and hemosiderin. Treatment has to be continued for a long time; for example, removing 1/2 to 1 L of blood per week for 1/2 year or more, until the excess iron stores are nearly depleted. Early clinical signs of hemochromatosis improve with treatment, but more advanced lesions, such as liver cirrhosis, advanced diabetes mellitus or cardiac damage, are irreversible. Therefore early diagnosis and prompt treatment are essential.

A Bank Manager In Trouble

This patient has an attack of gouty arthritis that was precipitated by alcohol abuse. Alcohol is metabolized in the liver. It is oxidized first to acetaldehyde by the cytosolic alcohol dehydrogenase, and the acetaldehyde is oxidized to acetic acid by a mitochondrial aldehyde dehydrogenase. The acetic acid either is activated to acetyl-CoA in the liver mitochondria or it is transported to other parts of the body for oxidation.

Alcohol metabolism is not feedback inhibited and therefore large amounts of the products acetyl-CoA, adenosine triphosphate (ATP), and reduced nicotinamide adenine dinucleotide (NADH) are formed in the liver of alcoholics. Hypoglycemia may develop in inebriated individuals because the high [NADH]/[NAD$^+$] ratio favors the conversion of pyruvate to lactate and of oxaloacetate to malate, thereby depleting the liver of gluconeogenic precursors. Lactate is elevated because of the high [NADH]/[NAD$^+$] ratio and because pyruvate dehy-

drogenase is inhibited by high-energy charge and by high levels of acetyl-CoA and NADH.

Alcohol abuse can precipitate attacks of gouty arthritis because it can lead to dehydration, and possibly because the elevated lactic acid level during alcohol intoxication interferes with the renal excretion of uric acid. Gout is the result of prolonged hyperuricemia: crystals of sodium urate precipitate in the joints where they cause an inflammatory response. Unlike rheumatoid arthritis and osteoarthritis, gouty arthritis typically presents with acute attacks of severe pain that are separated by asymptomatic intervals. Although most patients have an elevated serum uric acid level at the time of the acute attack, some do not. Therefore a definitive diagnosis requires synovial fluid analysis from the inflamed joint. An acute attack develops when phagocytic cells engulf the needle-sharp sodium urate crystals. This results in lysosomal damage and death of the cell, with the release of lysosomal enzymes. Gout has a predilection for the small joints of the toes or fingers because the low temperature in these peripheral joints reduces the solubility of sodium urate.

Dietary treatments of gout are not very effective, and most patients require drugs. The acute attack is treated with nonsteroidal antiinflammatory drugs. Colchicine is useful but is rarely used because of gastrointestinal side effects. Long-term treatment is aimed at reducing the hyperuricemia. Allopurinol inhibits the formation of uric acid from xanthine and hypoxanthine by xanthine oxidase. Alternatively, uricosuric agents (such as probenecid), which increase the renal excretion of uric acid, can be used.

Kidney Problems

This patient has type I diabetes, a severe chronic disease that is caused by the autoimmune destruction of pancreatic β-cells. This disease can be controlled only by regular insulin injections. Insulin is not active orally because it is a protein and therefore is susceptible to digestive proteases. Neither dietary management nor oral antidiabetics (which stimulate insulin release from the pancreas) are effective.

Although acute complications of type I diabetes, including ketoacidosis, can be prevented by insulin treatment, late complications are likely to develop in the course of many years. These late complications include microangiopathy, early atherosclerosis, peripheral neuropathy, retinopathy, and nephropathy. Diabetes is a major cause of cardiovascular disease, blindness, and renal failure.

This patient has diabetic nephropathy. The most important diagnostic test for this condition is the determination of urinary protein. Healthy urine is essentially protein free. Proteinuria develops gradually in patients with diabetic nephropathy, and the amount of protein in the 24-hour urine is proportional to the extent of renal damage.

Renal failure leads to the accumulation of all those substances that normally are excreted in the urine, including nitrogenous wastes (urea, uric acid, creatinine) and inorganic ions (sodium, potassium, magnesium, phosphate). There also is a mild chronic acidosis because the healthy kidney participates in acid-base regulation by excreting excess protons, mostly in the form of the ammonium ion (ammonia + proton). The normal urinary pH is below 7. In most patients, renal acidosis is compensated by hyperventilation. These patients may have a normal or near-normal blood pH with reduced serum carbon dioxide and bicarbonate concentrations.

Kidney patients also are prone to hypertension. This usually is the result of reduced diuresis leading to an increased blood volume, but it also may result from activation of the renin-angiotensin system.

Another common problem in renal failure is bone demineralization ("renal osteodystrophy"). In part, this problem is the result of chronic acidosis, which increases the solubility of the calcium phosphates in bone. Even a slight reduction of the pH causes a large increase in the solubility of the "bone salt." Another reason for renal osteodystrophy is the inability to convert 25-hydroxy-vitamin D to the active form 1,25-dihydroxy-vitamin D (calcitriol). Calcitriol is required for the intestinal absorption of dietary calcium. In its absence, the plasma calcium level has to be maintained by parathyroid hormone (PTH), which mobilizes calcium from the bones. Over time, the bones become depleted of calcium and phosphate. PTH can be measured by radioimmunoassay (RIA) in the clinical laboratory. Its plasma level is high in patients with renal failure whereas the calcium level either is normal or low. The bone isoenzyme of alkaline phosphatase may be elevated in the serum.

Anemia is another typical abnormality in kidney patients. It is caused by the inability of the diseased kidneys to produce adequate amounts of erythropoietin, a growth factor that stimulates erythropoiesis in the bone marrow.

The kidneys are responsible for the excretion of many drugs. Those drugs that normally are excreted in the urine should be used with caution to avoid toxicity. Also, some drugs have significant nephrotoxicity and therefore may aggravate the condition. Finally, some antacids contain magnesium. This ion is absorbed to varying extents, and it may accumulate in patients with renal failure.

The best way of treating incipient diabetic nephropathy is improved metabolic control of the disease. Supportive measures include the restriction of those dietary constituents that must be excreted by the kidneys. Excess electrolytes, in particular, should be avoided. Also dietary protein should be low because 1 g of urea is formed from every 3 g of protein, and urea must be excreted by the kidneys. Advanced renal failure necessitates the use of hemodialysis. This treatment is based on the diffusion of small molecules and ions through a system of semipermeable membranes; low-molecular weight waste products are removed, and plasma proteins and blood cells are retained.

A Sickly Child

The presenting problem of this patient is a respiratory infection with high fever and coughing. Although isolated respiratory infections are not unusual in infants, this patient had repeated bouts of infection, suggesting a "special reason" for his susceptibility.

The most remarkable finding of the physical examination was the presence of profound liver enlargement. The liver scan was performed to investigate the possibility of a tumor. Malignant liver tumors, known as hepatoblastoma, occasionally occur in this age group. The abnormally high heart rate suggests overactivity of the sympathetic nervous system. Also the mother's remark that "his skin becomes clammy and it tastes salty" suggests excessive sympathetic activity, with peripheral vasoconstriction and sweating. The slight cyanosis may indicate poor tissue oxygenation caused by the respiratory infection, or it may result from peripheral vasoconstriction. The patient apparently was given oxygen because his hyperventilation and cyanosis suggested an impairment of gas exchange in the lungs.

Laboratory test results show the presence of severe acidosis. The low level of carbon dioxide in the blood proves that the acidosis is metabolic, not respiratory. The low level of carbon dioxide in the blood also shows that there is no impairment of gas exchange in the lungs, therefore oxygen treatment is not indicated. The low level of carbon dioxide in the exhaled air simply is the result of hyperventilation. The hyperventilation is caused by a direct effect of the acidosis on the respiratory center in the brainstem, not by impaired gas exchange. The high blood lactate concentration and the presence of ketone bodies in the urine show that the patient has a mixed lactic acidosis and ketoacidosis.

In addition to metabolic acidosis, the other major finding is the presence of an abysmally low blood glucose level, suggesting a defect of the glucose-producing pathways in the liver. Both the hypoglycemia and the acidosis are so severe that they are immediately life threatening. There is no indication of acute liver failure, however, because the bilirubin concentration is normal and alanine transaminase is only mildly elevated. The nearly normal hematocrit suggests that the patient does not have a severe hemolytic condition either. The hematocrit of infants normally declines from 50% to 55% at birth to 30% to 40% at 6 months, partly because of the low iron content of breast milk. This decline does not reduce the efficiency of oxygen delivery because fetal hemoglobin is replaced by adult hemoglobin at the same time, and adult hemoglobin is the more effective oxygen transporter after birth.

Further investigations showed that the hypoglycemia was relieved by oral glucose, but the patient was unable to maintain a normal blood glucose level during fasting. The "twitching and jerking movements" that were noted were a seizure. Hypoglycemia can cause seizures both in infants and in adults. Insulin shock treatment has been used in psychiatry in place of electroconvulsive therapy. During fasting, glucose has to be synthesized by glycogen degradation and gluconeogenesis in the liver. Both of these pathways usually are stimulated by glucagon, and the complete unresponsiveness to

glucagon suggests that both pathways are blocked in the patient. The only reaction that is common to gluconeogenesis and glycogen degradation in the liver is the glucose 6-phosphatase reaction.

The biochemical determinations on the liver biopsy confirmed the absence of glucose 6-phosphatase and established a diagnosis of type I glycogen storage disease, also known as von Gierke's disease. A microsomal fraction, as used for these experiments, is obtained by mechanical disruption of the cells and centrifugation. The microsomal fraction is enriched in small membranous vesicles that are derived from the endoplasmic reticulum (ER). Glucose 6-phosphatase is in the ER, although the other enzymes of glycogen degradation and gluconeogenesis are cytoplasmic. Repeated freezing and thawing were performed to disrupt the ER membrane. In intact microsomes, the activity of the enzyme can be masked if either the glucose carrier or the carrier for glucose 6-phosphate in the ER membrane is defective. Some patients with type I glycogen storage disease have glucose 6-phosphatase, but one of the carriers is absent; glucose is not formed because either glucose 6-phosphate cannot reach the enzyme or glucose cannot leave the ER.

The absence of glucose 6-phosphatase explains the presence of fasting hypoglycemia. This hypoglycemia is more severe than that seen in other enzyme deficiencies (e.g., fructose 1,6-bisphosphatase or glycogen phosphorylase) because both glycogen breakdown and gluconeogenesis are interrupted. Hypoglycemia, in turn, inhibits insulin release and stimulates the release of glucagon, epinephrine, norepinephrine, and cortisol. Low insulin and high (nor)epinephrine stimulate the hormone-sensitive adipose tissue lipase. Large amounts of fatty acids are released into the blood, and some of these fatty acids are converted into ketone bodies by the liver. As in normal fasting, the products of β-oxidation (acetyl-CoA, NADH and ATP) inhibit the pyruvate dehydrogenase complex, thereby diverting glycolytic intermediates from mitochondrial oxidation to gluconeogenesis.

Gluconeogenesis, however, is interrupted in von Gierke's disease. Therefore the intermediates that cannot be converted to glucose or oxidized by pyruvate dehydrogenase are diverted into lactate, leading to lactic acidosis. Glycogen accumulates because the presumably very high level of glucose

6-phosphate in the patient's liver stimulates glycogen synthase, in addition to providing ample substrate for glycogen synthesis. Hyperuricemia is present because some of the accumulating glucose 6-phosphate is diverted into the pentose phosphate pathway to form ribose 5-phosphate, a precursor for purine biosynthesis. This results in an increased rate of de novo purine biosynthesis, which must be matched by an equally increased rate of purine degradation to uric acid.

The fat accumulation in the liver and the elevated level of plasma triglycerides suggest a high level of lipogenesis (fat synthesis) in the liver. The excess fat is synthesized from adipose tissue-derived fatty acids; although most of the excess fatty acids are used for ketogenesis, some are esterified into triglycerides by the liver.

Patients with von Gierke's disease can be kept alive and well only by continuous glucose feeding day and night. Hypoglycemia and the excessive accumulation of glycolytic intermediates in the liver must be avoided. The excessive accumulation of glucose 6-phosphate and other phosphorylated intermediates leads to lactic acidosis, hyperuricemia, and excessive glycogen deposition, and it also may deplete the cells of inorganic phosphate. This can damage the cells by interfering with ATP synthesis.

Why was the patient given lactose-free milk with extra glucose? In healthy adults, only 20% or 25% of the dietary glucose is metabolized in the liver after a carbohydrate-rich meal. This proportion is even lower in infants because of the relatively greater size of the brain in infants versus adults. The brain accounts for 70% of the basal metabolic rate in infants (25% in adults), and it subsists almost entirely on glucose. Moreover, in patients with von Gierke's disease, hypoglycemia is so severe and the insulin level so low that the use of glucose by the glucokinase reaction in the liver is minimal. The glucokinase activity of the liver can decrease to only 10% of its normal level in patients with extremely low insulin levels. However, approximately half of the dietary galactose is metabolized by the liver, forming glucose 6-phosphate and other glycolytic intermediates. Unlike glucose phosphorylation, hepatic galactose metabolism is not subject to tight controls. Therefore galactose will result in the excessive formation of glycolytic intermediates and aggravate lactic acidosis, hyperuricemia, and glycogen accumulation. Like galactose, fructose is converted rapidly to glycolytic intermediates in the liver and therefore should be avoided.

Glucose is absorbed very rapidly in the intestine; therefore it must be fed frequently to maintain an adequate blood glucose level. Also, some forms of starch are digested so rapidly that their effect on the blood glucose level is very similar to that of glucose—an important consideration in the design of diabetic diets. Conversely, some starchy foods are retained in the stomach for up to 3 or 4 hours, and some forms of starch are digested more slowly than others. Slowly digested forms of starch, such as cornstarch, are most suitable for the management of patients with von Gierke's disease because these starches maintain the blood glucose level for many hours.

Von Gierke's disease is inherited as an autosomal-recessive trait. This implies that the patient has inherited mutant forms of glucose 6-phosphatase from both the father and the mother. When both parents carry the disease gene in the heterozygous state, the risk of the disease in a child is 25%. Although the conception of an affected child cannot be prevented, the parents can be offered prenatal diagnosis; fetal cells are obtained by chorionic villus sampling at weeks 8 to 10, or by amniocentesis at weeks 14 to 16. The fetal cells are cultured, and the disease is diagnosed from the cultured cells. If the fetus is affected, the pregnancy is terminated. This procedure makes sense only if the disease is severe and if the parents agree to terminate the pregnancy if the fetus is affected.

Von Gierke's disease cannot be diagnosed by enzyme determination from cultured fetal cells because glucose 6-phosphatase is expressed only in liver, kidney, intestine, and pancreatic β-cells, but not in cells from the fetal membranes. DNA-directed methods can be used, however, because DNA is present in all nucleated cells. Allele-specific probes would be ideal for the diagnosis of a disease-producing mutation, but they require exact knowledge of the mutation. Most genetic diseases, however, including von Gierke's, can be caused by a large number of different mutations in the affected gene. In prenatal diagnosis, these disease genes can be tracked by linkage with highly informative VNTR (variable number of tandem repeats) polymorphisms, provided the genomic location of the gene is known. If the gene sequence also is known, a scanning method can be used to identify the exact mutation in each patient. Single-strand conformational polymorphism and chemical mismatch detection are the two most commonly used scanning methods. When combined with DNA sequencing, they can identify the exact mutation in the gene. Once the mutations in the parents are known, allele-specific probes can be used to test for these mutations in the fetus.

Prenatal diagnosis always is performed on a tight schedule because late pregnancy termination should be avoided. Therefore methods that do not require exceedingly long periods for cell culturing and testing are preferred. Polymerase chain reaction (PCR) is ideal because it requires only a minute amount of DNA that frequently can be obtained without cell culturing, and the amplification can be done in a single day. If the mutation is known, the relevant section of the fetal DNA can be amplified, the denatured amplification product applied to a nitrocellulose filter, and an allele-specific probe applied. This PCR/dot-blotting procedure obviates the need for gel electrophoresis, and it can be used for the detection of single-base substitutions that do not change the length of the PCR product.

Any inactivating mutation in the glucose 6-phosphatase gene can cause von Gierke's disease, therefore the number of theoretically possible mutations is huge. Nevertheless, in many genetic diseases, including von Gierke's, only a small number of mutations are common in the patients. Therefore effective heterozygote testing can be performed with allele-specific methods if probes for all the common mutations are available. This has been done, for example, for cystic fibrosis screening. The common disease-producing mutations may be extremely different in different ethnic groups, however. Therefore genetic screening technically is easier in ethnically homogeneous populations than in multi-ethnic "melting pots."

The Missed Examination

This patient has ketoacidosis, a life-threatening complication of type I diabetes. Ketoacidosis presents with coma, and it must be differentiated from other causes of unconsciousness. The emergency measures used in this case were the ad-

ministration of dextrose (glucose) and naloxone. Dextrose is effective only when the loss of consciousness is caused by hypoglycemia, and naloxone is an opiate antagonist that revives patients after an opiate overdose (and induces withdrawal signs in addicts). Neither dextrose or naloxone can do much harm. Even in patients with ketoacidosis, the injected glucose does not contribute much to the hyperglycemia.

In addition to the patient's history, which may or may not be known to the emergency room physician, there are some typical signs that suggest the presence of ketoacidosis. The patient's breath has a typical acetone smell that resembles the smell of alcohol. Acetone is produced by the nonenzymatic decarboxylation of acetoacetate. Hyperventilation is a response to the metabolic acidosis. Also signs of circulatory shock, with the patient's inability to maintain a normal blood pressure, are caused by acidosis. A reduced pH leads to peripheral vasodilation. This is a normal physiologic mechanism that increases the blood supply to hypoxic tissues where lactic acid is produced (e.g., vigorously contracting muscles). In generalized acidosis, however, the blood pressure drops, and this is a powerful stimulus for the sympathetic nervous system. Increased sympathetic activity results in sweating and tachycardia.

Patients with diabetic ketoacidosis have severe hyperglycemia. Hyperglycemia is caused both by the overproduction of glucose in the liver and its underuse in peripheral tissues. In the liver, insulin stimulates glycolysis and glycogen synthesis while inhibiting gluconeogenesis and glycogen degradation. Therefore patients with uncontrolled diabetes have rampant gluconeogenesis and glycogen degradation. Gluconeogenesis is more important than glycogen degradation for hyperglycemia because liver glycogen is depleted rapidly in severe diabetes.

Glucose use is impaired in diabetics. Muscle and adipose tissue have insulin-dependent glucose carriers and therefore become unable to take up glucose in severe diabetes. In other tissues, the glucose-metabolizing pathways are stimulated by insulin although glucose uptake is insulin independent. Only the brain and erythrocytes still consume normal amounts of glucose in diabetics because their glucose metabolism is insulin independent. Although hyperglycemia by itself is innocuous to the brain, it contributes to the development of "diabetic coma" by causing dehydration; it acts on the kidneys as an osmotic diuretic, impairing the reabsorption of water in the tubular system.

The excessive accumulation of ketone bodies is caused by uncontrolled fat breakdown in adipose tissue. Although the free fatty acids thus formed are a major fuel for most tissues, a substantial portion is converted to ketone bodies in the liver. Ketogenesis is useful during normal fasting when ketone bodies are a valuable energy source for many tissues, including even the brain. In diabetic ketoacidosis, however, ketogenesis gets out of hand and results in serious acidosis. The ketone bodies cause acidosis because they are acidic products (acetoacetic acid and β-hydroxybutyric acid) that are formed from a nonacidic precursor, namely, adipose tissue triglycerides. Acidosis, dehydration, and electrolyte imbalances combine to cause CNS depression and coma. Ketoacidosis is not the only type of "diabetic coma": in nonketotic hyperosmolar coma, massive hyperglycemia causes coma by inducing osmotic diuresis and dehydration.

Diabetic ketoacidosis is treated with intravenous fluids and insulin injections. Some patients have elevated plasma levels of potassium that are derived from intracellular sources. When the patient recovers, however, potassium is transported back into the cells and hypokalemia can develop.

An episode of diabetic ketoacidosis is the result of insufficient insulin treatment of an insulin-dependent diabetic. It also can be precipitated by psychological stress or physical illness because the "stress hormones," including epinephrine and the glucocorticoids, act as insulin antagonists, stimulating gluconeogenesis in the liver and lipolysis in adipose tissue. Also some cytokines, hormone-like products that are released by white blood cells during infections and other illnesses, have insulin-antagonistic metabolic effects. Therefore the insulin requirement of diabetic patients always is increased during even minor illnesses and psychological stress. Once the metabolic derangements of ketoacidosis develop, the patient is in a vicious cycle that can be broken only by vigorous treatment.

Whereas type I diabetics are unable to produce insulin, type II diabetics have either a reduced capacity for glucose-stimulated insulin release, or a reduced insulin responsiveness of the target tissues ("insulin resistance"), or both. Most patients with insulin resistance have a reduced number of insulin receptors, but some may have an abnormal receptor, or they may have an abnormality in the insulin-initiated signaling cascades. The insulin receptor is a tyrosine kinase that triggers intracellular phosphorylation cascades.

A few days after the first episode, our patient was admitted to the emergency room with hypoglycemia. Hypoglycemic spells can be caused by a combination of insulin overuse and fasting, and they respond immediately to intravenous dextrose. Hypoglycemia also is seen in patients with insulinoma, an insulin-secreting tumor of pancreatic β-cells. Clinical laboratories usually determine C-peptide rather than insulin for the investigation of pancreatic function and the diagnosis of insulinoma because C-peptide is released along with insulin. Unlike insulin, which may come from insulin injection, C-peptide is definitely derived from the patient's own pancreas. In this case, C-peptide determination was not justified because the patient's history (ketoacidosis only a few days ago) was incompatible with the presence of an insulinoma.

Dr. Stein's Grant Application

The first question we have to ask about Dr. Stein's project is about its feasibility. There are indeed no published reports about the cloning of human embryos, but the technology has been developed in animal experiments. It is valuable for two reasons: it can produce a large number of genetically identical animals, and it can be used to manipulate the genome of the cultured cells from which the nuclei are obtained.

Undifferentiated, totipotent embryonic cells are most suitable as a source of the nuclear genome because they are intrinsically able to form all specialized cell types of the adult body. This potential is realized naturally during the formation of monozygotic twins. Differentiated adult cells, however, may not be suitable because of cell-type specific DNA methylation or other poorly reversible chromatin changes. The cultured cell contributes the nuclear genome, and the oocyte donor contributes the mitochondrial genes. The initiation of embryogenesis appears to depend on factors in the cytoplasm of the oocyte that can "reprogram" the nucleus. The nature of these factors is not known. They may be DNA-binding proteins that regulate transcription or protein kinases that enter the nucleus to phosphorylate nuclear proteins.

A major technical problem in cloning is the maintenance of undifferentiated embryonic cells. The enzymes that Dr. Stein wants to use for obtaining embryonic cells are trypsin and hyaluronidase. When used under carefully controlled conditions, these enzymes can dissociate tissues into individual cells by degrading proteins and glycosaminoglycans of the extracellular matrix. Once obtained, these embryonic cells can be propagated in culture, but they tend to differentiate and lose their totipotentiality.

Normal embryonic development depends on interactions of the cells with other cells, with matrix constituents, and with soluble "growth factors." Some of these interactions favor the maintenance of the undifferentiated state whereas others induce the formation of specialized cell types. Most growth factor receptors autophosphorylate on tyrosine side chains after binding their ligand. Signaling cascades are initiated by the binding of cytoplasmic proteins to the autophosphorylated receptor. However, the autophosphorylation sites are different in different growth factor receptors. Therefore different growth factors can trigger different and often opposing responses in the same target cell. Therefore it is a reasonable expectation that some growth factors maintain embryonic cells in an undifferentiated state although others induce their differentiation into specialized cell types. Our knowledge of embryonic cell differentiation still is rudimentary.

The preservation of cell cultures and even embryos by freezing is common practice. Freezing must be done quickly, for example, by dropping the specimen into liquid nitrogen. Quick-freezing is essential to avoid osmotic stress in partially frozen cells and to prevent the growth of large ice crystals that would damage the cellular membranes. Approximately two thirds of embryos survive freezing and thawing, and children produced from frozen embryos have been shown to develop normally.

Dr. Stein proposes the use of several diagnostic tests for disease-producing mutations. Protein electrophoresis is an old-fashioned method that still is used to identify glucose 6-phosphate dehydrogenase deficiency and hemoglobinopathies. It works only if the mutation changes the pattern of electrical charges on the protein.

Specific mutations can be diagnosed by the use of allele-specific probes, either with electrophoretic separation of the restriction-digested DNA ("Southern blotting") or without ("dot blotting"). Probes can be constructed for known disease-causing mutations. However, most genetic diseases are characterized by extensive allelic heterogeneity: many different mutations in the same gene can cause the same disease. Therefore the usefulness of molecular probes often is quite limited. Probes for major disease-producing mutations have been used not only in affected families and for population screening, but they also are used for quality control by sperm banks; most major sperm banks test their donors routinely for dangerous mutations. This is facilitated by the fact that many genetic diseases are common only in certain ethnic groups. Tay-Sachs disease, for example, is common in Jews; sickle cell disease is common in Africans; and glucose 6-phosphate dehydrogenase deficiency is common in people from Africa, the Mediterranean region, and the Middle East.

DNA-directed methods even are suitable for the diagnosis of infectious diseases. Acquired immune deficiency syndrome (AIDS) can be diagnosed from cell-free serum by a combination of reverse transcription and PCR amplification; the genomic viral RNA is copied into a cDNA by reverse transcriptase in vitro. A segment of this cDNA then is amplified by PCR and identified either by electrophoresis or by dot-blotting with a probe for the amplified retroviral cDNA. Repeat AIDS testing of donors is mandatory for sperm banks: the donor is tested at the time of the donation, the sample is quarantined, and the donor is retested 6 months later. The sample is released for use only after both test results are negative.

The cloning of nonhumans is performed to facilitate gene manipulations. Genes can be introduced into the cultured cells from which the nucleus is taken. The integration of genes in specific genomic locations can be achieved by the use of artificial gene constructs whose flanking sequences match the sequence of the intended integration site. Such constructs can be incorporated into the genomic DNA by homologous recombination. The tissue-specific expression of the foreign gene can be controlled by introducing it with a suitable promoter and/or by inserting it next to a tissue-specific enhancer. This general procedure can be used, for example, to construct sheep and cattle that secrete valuable hormones, clotting factors, or other medically useful proteins in their milk.

The targeting of the foreign gene (or "transgene") by homologous recombination is very inefficient, and haphazard integration in unintended genomic locations is possible. This can cause disease if the integration of the foreign gene disrupts an important gene in the recipient cell. Proper integration of the transgene can be determined in a transformed cell clone by Southern blotting with a probe for the transgene: if the transgene is integrated in a single genomic site and the restriction enzyme used for Southern blotting does not cut within the transferred DNA, only one restriction fragment can be seen. The integration site can be verified by cloning this restriction fragment in a bacterium and sequencing the insert.

This type of gene manipulation is not very suitable for the treatment or prevention of genetic diseases in humans, but it can, in theory, be used for the production of humans with interesting biochemical capabilities. Natural evolution has provided us with a method to combine genes from different individuals of our own species. This method is called sexual reproduction. However, we do not have a naturally evolved ability to exchange genes with nonhumans. Genetic engineering can overcome this limitation. A gene for the synthesis of vitamin C, for example, could be obtained from almost any nonprimate mammalian species. Genes for the synthesis of other vitamins and the synthesis of essential amino acids, however, would have to be obtained from plants or bacteria. The genes for cobalamin synthesis are not even present in plants. They would have to be obtained from prokaryotic sources.

Ethical concerns about human cloning and gene manipulations are of two kinds: the first type of objection relates to the safety of the procedure and the possibility of causing serious harm, for example, by producing a diseased child; a second type of objection is based on general ethical principles rather than any possible harm done by the procedure.

The safety of human cloning has not been established. Most investigators agree that extensive experience in the cloning of nonhuman animals, including primates, should precede the first attempts at human cloning. Nevertheless it is likely that safe and effective procedures for the cloning of higher primates, including humans, can be developed. If this should be the case, Dr. Stein's claim that cloning from well-selected cell lines reduces the risk of disease in the offspring may well be valid. This would create a situation in which the ethical acceptability of the traditional reproductive method becomes questionable. Also germline gene manipulation can, potentially, improve the health and well-being of future generations if safety problems are addressed adequately.

There are many nontechnical objections to the proposed procedures. Most of these cannot be argued because they are based on arbitrary value judgments or traditional legal codes. These include, for example, notions about the protection of human or potentially human life (is a totipotent cultured cell a human being?) and about the relative merits of saving lives versus preventing suffering (which is worse: killing a cultured cell/zygote/embryo/fetus or producing a chronically ill child?). Also the notion that humans should be treated differently from nonhuman animals and that therefore new and potentially risky procedures should be tested in animals before being applied to humans is arbitrary and is not shared by all people (and certainly not by all nonhuman animals). More arguable than these theoretical/ethical concerns is the idea that although the potential benefits of cloning and gene manipulations may be great, human beings generally are either not sufficiently intelligent or too irresponsible to make acceptable use of major technologic advances. Historic examples for this contention could be cited easily.

Answers to Questions

Chapter 1
1. D
2. C
3. A

Chapter 2
1. C
2. D
3. A
4. D

Chapter 3
1. B
2. B
3. A

Chapter 4
1. E
2. C
3. E
4. A
5. D
6. B

Chapter 5
1. E
2. D
3. A

Chapter 6
1. B
2. D
3. C
4. E
5. B

Chapter 7
1. A
2. C
3. E

Chapter 8
1. B
2. C
3. E
4. D
5. A

Chapter 9
1. E
2. B
3. D
4. C

Chapter 10
1. B
2. E
3. C
4. D
5. D
6. A
7. C
8. C
9. A
10. E

Chapter 11
1. E
2. D
3. D
4. A

Chapter 12
1. E
2. B
3. C
4. A

Chapter 13
1. A
2. E
3. B
4. D
5. A

Chapter 14
1. C
2. D

Chapter 15
1. D
2. B

Chapter 16
1. A
2. E
3. C
4. B
5. C
6. D
7. E

Chapter 17
1. B
2. E
3. A
4. E
5. C

Chapter 18
1. D
2. C
3. B
4. A

Chapter 19
1. B
2. D
3. B

Chapter 20
1. E
2. D
3. B
4. E

Chapter 21
1. D
2. A
3. B
4. E
5. C

Chapter 22
1. D
2. B

Chapter 23
1. C
2. B

Chapter 24
1. B
2. C
3. E
4. A
5. B

Chapter 25
1. A
2. D
3. B
4. A
5. C
6. A

Chapter 26
1. E
2. B
3. C
4. E

Chapter 27
1. D
2. C
3. A
4. E

Chapter 28
1. C
2. B
3. D
4. C
5. E
6. B
7. E
8. A
9. D

Chapter 29
1. D
2. E
3. A
4. D
5. C
6. B

Glossary

Abetalipoproteinemia: An inherited inability to form chylomicrons and VLDL.

abl A (proto-)oncogene coding for a nuclear tyrosine protein kinase.

Acetal A bond between an aldehyde group and two hydroxy groups.

Acetyl-CoA carboxylase The rate-limiting enzyme of fatty acid biosynthesis.

Acetylcholinesterase An acetylcholine-degrading enzyme on the surface of the nerve terminal or the postsynaptic membrane.

Acid A proton donor.

Acid phosphatase A marker for prostatic cancer.

Actin A globular protein that polymerizes into microfilaments.

Actinomycin D An inhibitor of transcription that binds to double-stranded DNA.

Acute intermittent porphyria A hepatic porphyria, with abdominal pain and neurological symptoms.

Acute phase reactants Plasma proteins whose levels are elevated within 1 to 2 days of an acute stress.

Acyl-CoA The activated form of a fatty acid.

Acyl-CoA dehydrogenase The first enzyme of β-oxidation.

Adenylate cyclase The cyclic AMP synthesizing enzyme, located in the plasma membrane.

Adrenergic receptors Receptors for epinephrine and norepinephrine.

Adrenodoxin A mitochondrial iron-sulfur protein that participates in hydroxylation reactions of steroids.

Adrenogenital syndrome An inherited defect of steroid hormone synthesis; causes impaired corticosteroid synthesis and overproduction of adrenal androgens.

Agglutination Clumping of cells—for example, after exposure to an antibody directed at a cell surface component.

Aggrecan A large, aggregating proteoglycan in cartilage.

Agonist A stimulatory ligand for a receptor.

ALA synthase The regulated enzyme of heme biosynthesis.

Alanine transaminase Serum enzyme, elevated in liver diseases.

Albinism A condition that is caused by recessively inherited defects of melanin synthesis.

Albumin A plasma protein; accounts for approximately 60% of the total plasma protein.

Alcohol dehydrogenase A cytosolic liver enzyme that oxidizes ethanol to acetaldehyde.

Aldose Monosaccharide with an aldehyde group.

Alkaptonuria A rare inborn error of tyrosine metabolism, with accumulation of homogentisate.

Allele-specific oligonucleotide probes Probes that can distinguish between two different alleles (variants) of a gene.

Allelic heterogeneity Different mutations in the same gene leading to the same disease.

Allopurinol An inhibitor of xanthine oxidase; used to treat gout.

Allosteric effector A ligand that affects the equilibrium between the alternative conformations of an allosteric protein.

Allosteric protein A protein that can exist in alternative conformations (i.e., higher-order structures).

α-amanitin A mushroom poison that inhibits RNA polymerase II.

α-amylase A starch-degrading endoglycosidase in saliva and pancreatic juice.

α₁-antiprotease A circulating protease inhibitor. Deficiency causes lung emphysema.

α-fetoprotein A fetal plasma protein. Elevated in serum of patients with liver cancer, and in amniotic fluid if the fetus has an open neural tube defect.

α-helix A compact secondary structure in proteins that is stabilized by intrachain hydrogen bonds between peptide bonds.

7α-hydroxylase The regulated enzyme of bile acid synthesis.

α-lipoprotein High-density lipoprotein (HDL).

α₂-macroglobulin A circulating protease inhibitor, with a very high molecular weight (725,000 daltons).

α-oxidation A minor catabolic pathway that shortens fatty acids by one carbon.

α-thalassemia Underproduction of hemoglobin α chains.

α-tocopherol The most important form of vitamin E. An important lipid-soluble antioxidant.

Alu sequences A large family of short interspersed elements.

Amino acid oxidases H_2O_2-forming flavoproteins in peroxisomes that oxidatively deaminate amino acids.

Aminoacyl-tRNA A tRNA with an amino acid covalently bound to its 3′ terminus.

Aminoacyl-tRNA synthetases Cytoplasmic enzymes that attach an amino acid to a tRNA.

Ammonotelic Ammonia excreting.

Amphipathic Containing hydrophilic and hydrophobic portions in the same molecule.

Anabolic pathway Biosynthetic pathway.

Anaerobic Oxygen deficient.

Anaplerotic reactions Reactions that result in the net production of a TCA-cycle intermediate.

Anchorage dependence The inability of cultured cells to grow in the absence of a solid support.

Androgens 19-Carbon steroids derived from progestins by a side chain cleavage reaction.

Androstenedione The major adrenal androgen.

Anemia Abnormal decrease of the blood hemoglobin concentration.

Angiotensin II The active form of angiotensin, synthesized from angiotensinogen by the successive action of renin and converting enzyme.

Anhydride bond Bond between two acids.

Anion Negatively charged ion.

Annealing Formation of a double strand from two nucleic acid strands with complementary base sequences.

Anomers Monosaccharides that differ only in the orientation of substituents around their carbonyl carbons.

Antagonist An inhibitory ligand for a receptor.

Anticodon The base triplet of the tRNA that base-pairs with the codon during protein synthesis.

Antigen-antibody complex A noncovalent aggregate between antigen and antibody. Large complexes are insoluble.

Antiinflammatory steroids Glucocorticoids and their synthetic derivatives that inhibit the release of arachidonic acid from membrane lipids.

Antimycin A An inhibitor of electron flow through the QH_2–cytochrome c reductase complex.

Antiport The coupled transport of two substrates in opposite directions.

Antisense technology The use of synthetic nucleic acid analogs in an attempt to block the translation of a specific mRNA.

Antithrombin III A circulating inhibitor of thrombin and some other activated clotting factors.

AP endonuclease An endonuclease that cleaves a phosphodiester bond formed by a baseless ("apurinic") nucleotide in DNA.

APC Adenomatous polyposis coli, an inherited cancer susceptibility syndrome that is responsible for 1% of all colorectal cancers.

ApoA-I, apoA-II The major apolipoproteins of HDL.

ApoB-100 The major apolipoprotein of VLDL and LDL.

ApoB-48 The major apolipoprotein of chylomicrons.

ApoC-II An apolipoprotein that activates lipoprotein lipase.

ApoE receptor A receptor on hepatocytes that mediates the endocytosis of apoE-containing lipoproteins.

Apoprotein The polypeptide component of a conjugated protein.

Apoptosis Programmed cell death.

Arginase The urea-forming enzyme of the urea cycle.

Aromatase The enzyme that converts androgens to estrogens.

Arsenate A poison that competes with phosphate in many phosphate-dependent reactions.

Arsenite An inhibitor of pyruvate dehydrogenase that binds to dihydrolipoic acid.

Ascorbic acid Vitamin C, a water-soluble antioxidant.

Asialoglycoprotein Glycoprotein that has lost the terminal sialic acid residues from its oligosaccharides. Asialoglycoproteins are endocytosed by the liver.

Aspartate transaminase Serum enzyme. Elevated in liver diseases, muscle diseases, and acute myocardial infarction.

Atheromatous plaque The typical lesion of atherosclerosis.

ATP Adenosine triphosphate, a nucleotide that functions as the "energetic currency" of the cell.

Atrial natriuretic factor A hormone from the heart that stimulates a membrane-bound guanylate cyclase.

Autocrine signaling The action of an extracellular messenger on its cell of origin.

Autophosphorylation Self-phosphorylation of a protein kinase. Occurs with receptor tyrosine kinases and many other protein kinases.

Avidin A biotin-binding protein in egg white.

Azaserine An antineoplastic drug that inhibits the use of glutamine for nucleotide biosynthesis.

B lymphocyte A type of lymphocyte that produces membrane-bound immunoglobulin.

Bacteriophages "Phages"; bacteria-infecting viruses.

BARK β-adrenergic receptor kinase; desensitizes the β-adrenergic receptor.

Basal metabolic rate The energy consumed in the absence of physical activity.

Basal mutation rate The mutation rate in the absence of mutagens.

Base A proton acceptor.

Base pairing The specific interaction between two bases in opposite strands of a double-stranded nucleic acid.

Base stacking The noncovalent interaction between successive bases within a nucleic acid strand.

Basement membrane Synonym for basal lamina; an extracellular matrix structure beneath single-layered epithelia.

Belt desmosome A beltlike cell adhesion in epithelial cells that is connected with cytoplasmic actin microfilaments.

Bence Jones protein Immunoglobulin light chains overproduced by some patients with multiple myeloma (a malignant plasma cell dyscrasia).

Beriberi Thiamine deficiency, with severe neuromuscular weakness.

β-galactosidase A lactose-hydrolyzing enzyme.

β-lactamase Penicillinase; an enzyme that inactivates penicillin and related antibiotics.

β-lipoprotein Low-density lipoprotein (LDL).

β-oxidation The major pathway of fatty acid oxidation.

β-pleated sheet An extended higher-order structure in proteins stabilized by hydrogen bonds between parallel or antiparallel polypeptides.

β-thalassemia Underproduction of hemoglobin β chains.

Bile acids Emulsifiers in bile; required for lipid absorption.

Bilirubin A yellow pigment formed from biliverdin.

Biliverdin A green pigment formed from heme.

Biotin The prosthetic group of carboxylase enzymes.

Blood group substances Polymorphic constituents of the erythrocyte membrane.

Bohr effect Decrease in the oxygen-binding affinity of hemoglobin at low pH.

BPG 2,3-Bisphosphoglycerate, an allosteric effector that reduces the oxygen affinity of hemoglobin.

BRCA1, BRCA2 Two tumor suppressor genes associated with breast and ovarian cancers. Inherited defects of these genes account for 4% to 8% of all breast cancers.

Brush border enzymes Enzymes on the lumenal surface of intestinal mucosal cells.

Buffer A solution whose pH value is stabilized by the presence of ionizable groups.

Burkitt's lymphoma A B-cell malignancy in which the *myc* protooncogene has been translocated into an immunoglobulin locus.

C peptide A biologically inactive fragment of proinsulin that is released together with insulin.

C-reactive protein The most sensitive acute-phase reactant.

Cadherins Membrane-spanning cell adhesion proteins in belt desmosomes.

Calcitriol 1,25-Dihydroxycholecalciferol, the active form of vitamin D.

Calcium channel blockers Drugs that block voltage-gated calcium channels in excitable cells.

Calmodulin A calcium-binding protein that acts as a calcium-dependent enzyme activator.

Cap A methylguanosine-containing structure at the 5′ end of eukaryotic mRNA.

Capsid The protein coat of the virus particle.

Carbamino hemoglobin Hemoglobin with carbon dioxide covalently bound to its terminal amino groups.

Carbamoyl phosphate A metabolite formed from ammonia, carbon dioxide, and ATP; brings nitrogen into the urea cycle.

Carbohydrate loading A procedure aimed at the buildup of large muscle glycogen stores in endurance athletes.

Carbon monoxide A competitive inhibitor of oxygen binding to hemoglobin and myoglobin.

Carbonic anhydrase An enzyme in erythrocytes and other cells that establishes an equilibrium among carbon dioxide, water, and carbonic acid.

Carboxypeptidases A and B Two pancreatic carboxypeptidases.

Carcinoma Cancer of epithelial tissues.

Cardiotonic steroids A class of drugs that inhibit the sodium-potassium ATPase.

Carnitine A coenzyme that carries long-chain fatty acids into the mitochondrion.

Carnosine The dipeptide β-alanyl-histidine; used as a pH buffer in muscle tissue.

Carotenes Dietary precursors of vitamin A, in vegetables.

Carpal tunnel syndrome A peripheral nerve entrapment syndrome that can be treated with pyridoxine.

Catabolic pathway Degradative pathway.

Catabolite repression Repression of catabolic operons in the presence of glucose.

Catalase A hydrogen peroxide–degrading enzyme.

Catecholamines Biogenic amines derived from tyrosine: dopamine, norepinephrine, and epinephrine.

Cation Positively charged ion.

CDKs Cyclin-dependent kinases, important as positive regulators of cell cycle progression.

cDNA The double-stranded DNA copy of a single-stranded RNA.

cDNA library A collection of cDNA-containing bacterial clones.

CDP-diacylglycerol An activated form of phosphatidic acid for the synthesis of phosphoglycerides.

Ceramide A lipid consisting of sphingosine and a fatty acid.

Cerebrosides Sphingolipids containing a monosaccharide.

Ceruloplasmin A copper-containing plasma protein.

Cervical cancer Cancer of the uterine cervix.

Chemiosmotic hypothesis The hypothesis (now proved true) that mitochondrial electron flow and ATP synthesis are coupled through a proton gradient.

Chirality Optical isomerism, created by alternative configurations of substituents around an asymmetrical carbon.

Cholera toxin The enterotoxin of *Vibrio cholerae*. Causes cAMP accumulation in the intestinal mucosa by covalent modification of the G_s-protein.

Cholestasis Lack of bile flow.

Cholesterol The only important membrane steroid in humans.

Cholesterol ester transfer protein A protein that transfers cholesterol esters from HDL to other lipoproteins.

Cholesterol esters Esters of cholesterol with a fatty acid.

Cholestyramine A bile acid binding resin that is used as a cholesterol-lowering agent.

Choline-acetyltransferase An enzyme that synthesizes acetylcholine from acetyl-CoA and choline.

Cholinesterase A serum enzyme that participates in the metabolism of some drugs.

Choluric jaundice Jaundice accompanied by the urinary excretion of bilirubin diglucuronide.

Chondroitin sulfate The most abundant GAG (glycosaminoglycan) in many connective tissues.

Chromosome A large, double-stranded DNA molecule with associated proteins.

Chromosome walking A method for the sequencing of long, contiguous pieces of chromosomal DNA.

Chylomicrons Lipoproteins that carry triglycerides from the intestine to other tissues.

Chymotrypsin A serine protease from the pancreas.

Cirrhosis Fibrous degeneration of the liver.

Class switching A change in the class of the immunoglobulin expressed by a B lymphocyte.

Clonal selection Selective growth stimulation by an antigen of a B-cell clone carrying a matching surface antibody.

Clone A population of genetically identical cells that are all descended from the same ancestral cell.

Cloning vector A plasmid or bacteriophage into which cloned DNA is integrated.

Cobalamin Vitamin B_{12}.

Cockayne's syndrome Inherited defects of nucleotide excision repair, characterized by neurological degeneration and early senility.

Coding strand The strand of a gene whose base sequence corresponds to the base sequence of the RNA transcript.

Codon A base triplet on mRNA that specifies an amino acid.

Coenzyme A A cosubstrate that forms energy-rich thioester bonds with many organic acids, thereby activating them for biosynthetic reactions.

Cohesive ends The short, single-stranded ends of restriction fragments.

Coiled-coil Two or three α-helices coiled around each other.

Colchicine An alkaloid that inhibits the formation of microtubules.

Colloid-osmotic pressure The osmotic pressure of macromolecules.

Committed step The first irreversible reaction unique to a pathway.

Competitive inhibition Inhibition by an agent that binds noncovalently to the active site of the enzyme.

COMT Catechol-O-methyltransferase, a catecholamine-inactivating enzyme.

Condensation reaction Bond formation with release of a water molecule.

Conformation The noncovalent higher-order structure of a protein.

Conjugation Transfer of a selftransmissible plasmid from one cell to another.

Conjugation reactions Reactions in which a chemical becomes covalently linked to a hydrophilic molecule such as sulfate, glucuronic acid, or an amino acid.

Connexin A channel-forming transmembrane protein in gap junctions.

Consensus sequence The sequence of the most commonly encountered bases in a functionally defined nucleic acid sequence.

Constitutive proteins Proteins that are synthesized at all times.

Contact inhibition Inhibition of cell proliferation by contact with neighboring cells.

Contact-phase activation The very first reactions of the intrinsic pathway that require the binding of the clotting factors to subendothelial tissue.

Cooley's anemia Homozygous β-thalassemia.

Copper A trace mineral; present in many enzymes that use molecular oxygen as a substrate.

Cori cycle The shuttling of glucose and lactate between muscle and liver during physical exercise.

Corticosteroids Gluco- and mineralocorticoids; C-21 steroids that are derived from progestins by hydroxylation reactions.

Cortisol The most important glucocorticoid; a stress hormone.

Coumarin-type anticoagulants Vitamin K antagonists, which inhibit the posttranslational formation of γ-carboxyglutamate in some clotting factors.

Covalent bond Strong chemical bond formed by a binding electron pair.

Covalent catalysis A catalytic mechanism that involves the formation of a covalent bond between enzyme and substrate.

Creatine A metabolite in muscle that forms the energy-rich compound creatine phosphate.

Creatine kinase A serum enzyme that is elevated in muscle diseases and acute myocardial infarction.

CREB The cAMP response element binding protein; mediates effects of cAMP on gene transcription.

Cretinism The result of untreated congenital hypothyroidism; characterized by mental deficiency and growth retardation.

Cryoprecipitate A plasma protein preparation enriched in some clotting factors.

Curare An arrow poison that blocks acetylcholine receptors in the neuromuscular junction.

Cyanide A poison that prevents the reduction of molecular oxygen by cytochrome oxidase.

Cyanosis Blue discoloration of mucous membranes in patients with hypoxia.

Cyclic AMP A second messenger of many hormones.

Cyclic GMP Another second messenger of many hormones.

Cyclins The regulatory subunits of the CDKs.

Cyclooxygenase The key enzyme for the synthesis of prostaglandins, prostacyclin, and thromboxane.

Cystinuria An inherited defect in the transport of dibasic amino acids in kidney and intestine; causes kidney stones.

Cytochrome P-450 A large family of heme-containing proteins that participate in monooxygenase reactions.

Cytochromes Heme proteins that function as electron carriers.

Cytokines Biologically active protein products released by activated lymphocytes and monocytes/macrophages.

DCC Deleted in colon cancer; a tumor suppressor gene that is deleted or inactivated in 70% of all colorectal cancers.

7-dehydrocholesterol A steroid that is photochemically cleaved to cholecalciferol (vitamin D_3) in the skin.

Dehydrogenase reactions Hydrogen transfer reactions.

Delayed-response genes Genes whose expression is indirectly stimulated by growth factors.

Denaturation Destruction of a protein's higher-order structure.

Desaturases Enzymes that introduce double bonds into fatty acids.

Desmolase A mitochondrial enzyme system that cleaves the side chain of cholesterol, producing pregnenolone.

Desmosine A covalent crosslink in elastin.

1,2-diacylglycerol A second messenger.

Dialysis A method for the separation of proteins from low-molecular-weight contaminants.

Diastereomers Geometric isomers.

Diglyceride Structure formed from glycerol and two fatty acids.

Dihydrofolate reductase An enzyme that reduces dihydrofolate to tetrahydrofolate.

Dihydrotestosterone A potent androgen formed from testosterone by 5α-reductase in androgen target tissues.

Diphtheria toxin A bacterial toxin that inactivates an elongation factor of protein synthesis.

Diploid Containing two copies of each chromosome.

Dipole-dipole interaction Attractive force between the components of two polarized bonds.

Dissociation constant A measure for the affinity between a receptor and its ligand.

Disulfide bond A covalent bond formed by an oxidative reaction between two sulfhydryl groups.

DNA fingerprinting DNA-based methods for the identification of persons in criminal cases.

DNA glycosylases Enzymes that remove abnormal bases from DNA.

DNA ligase An enzyme linking two DNA strands.

DNA polymerases DNA-synthesizing enzymes.

Dominant Determining the phenotype in the heterozygous (as well as the homozygous) state.

Dot blotting A rapid screening method for mutations and DNA polymorphisms.

Down-regulation A long-term type of desensitization that can be overcome only by the synthesis of new protein.

Duchenne's muscular dystrophy A severe inherited muscle disease caused by defects of the structural protein dystrophin.

Dynein A microtubule-associated protein in cilia and flagella with ATPase activity; necessary for ciliary/flagellar motility.

E2F/DP A transcription factor that is negatively regulated by the retinoblastoma protein.

E6, E7 The oncogenes of the human papillomavirus; they bind and inactivate p53 and pRB, respectively.

Early-response genes Genes whose transcription is induced within approximately 15 minutes after mitogen treatment.

Edema Abnormal fluid accumulation in the interstitial tissue spaces.

Edman degradation A method for the sequencing of proteins.

EGF Epidermal growth factor; a growth factor that is mitogenic for many cell types.

Ehlers-Danlos syndrome A type of connective tissue disease characterized by stretchy skin and loose joints; some types are caused by abnormalities of collagen structure or biosynthesis.

Elastin The major component of elastic fibers.

Electronegativity The tendency of an atom to attract electrons.

Electrophoresis An analytical method that is based on the movement of charged molecules in an electrical field.

Electrostatic interaction "Salt bond"; the attractive force between oppositely charged ions.

Emphysema A degenerative lung disease.

Enantiomers Isomers that are mirror images.

Endergonic reaction Reaction with positive ΔG.

Endocytosis Cellular uptake of soluble macromolecules through an endocytotic vesicle.

Endonucleases Enzymes cleaving internal phosphodiester bonds in a nucleic acid.

Endorphins Peptides with agonist effects on opiate receptors.

Endosome An organelle derived from endocytotic vesicles.

Endosymbiont hypothesis The hypothesis that mitochondria (and chloroplasts) are derived from symbiotic prokaryotes.

Endothermic reaction Reaction with positive ΔH.

Energy charge A measure for the energy status of a cell.

Energy-rich bonds Bonds whose hydrolysis releases an unusually large amount of energy; examples are anhydride and thioester bonds.

Enhancement engineering Attempts to improve the genetic constitution of healthy people by DNA manipulations.

Enhancers DNA sequences that increase the rate of transcription by binding regulatory proteins.

Enterohepatic circulation The cycling of bile acids (and other compounds) through liver and intestine.

Enthalpy The energy content of a molecule.

Entropy The randomness of a thermodynamic system.

Envelope A membrane, acquired from the host cell, that surrounds many animal viruses.

Enzyme-substrate complex Enzyme with a noncovalently bound substrate.

Epidermolysis bullosa A group of inherited skin-blistering diseases, frequently caused by abnormalities of keratin.

Epimers Monosaccharides differing in the configuration of substituents around one of their asymmetrical carbons.

Epinephrine Synonym for adrenaline, a stress hormone from the adrenal medulla.

Equilibrium constant A thermodynamic constant that is defined as product concentration(s) divided by substrate concentration(s) at equilibrium.

ERKs Extracellular signal regulated kinases; serine/threonine kinases of the MAP kinase family.

Erythropoietin A kidney-derived growth factor that stimulates erythropoiesis in the bone marrow.

Escherichia coli An intestinal bacterium.

Estrogens 18-Carbon steroids, synthesized from androgens by the aromatization of ring A.

Euchromatin A dispersed, transcriptionally active form of chromatin.

Eukaryotes Cells with a membrane-bound nucleus.

Exergonic reaction Reaction with negative ΔG.

Exocytosis Secretion of water-soluble substances by fusion of an exocytotic vesicle with the plasma membrane.

Exons Those parts of the gene that are represented in the mature RNA.

Exonucleases Enzymes cleaving terminal phosphodiester bonds in a nucleic acid.

Exothermic reaction Reaction with negative ΔH.

Expression cloning Cloning of cDNA for the synthesis of the encoded protein.

F factor A selftransmissible plasmid in *E. coli*.

F_{ab} fragment The antigen-binding part of immunoglobulins.

Facilitated diffusion A passive type of carrier-mediated transport.

Familial combined hyperlipoproteinemia A genetic predisposition to type II and type IV hyperlipoproteinemia.

Familial hypercholesterolemia Inherited deficiency of LDL receptors.

Fatty streak Accumulation of cholesterol esters in arterial walls.

Favism Hemolysis caused by the ingestion of broad beans in people with glucose 6-phosphate dehydrogenase deficiency.

F_c fragment The crystallizable fragment of immunoglobulins, formed from the carboxy-terminal halves of the heavy chains.

Feedback inhibition Inhibition of a metabolic pathway by its own end product.

Feedforward stimulation Stimulation of a metabolic pathway by its own substrate.

Ferritin The principal intracellular iron storage protein; trace amounts also are present in the plasma.

Fibrinogen　The circulating precursor of fibrin.

Fibronectin　A multiadhesive glycoprotein with binding affinities for cell surfaces and extracellular matrix constituents.

First-order reaction　Reaction whose velocity is proportional to the concentration of one substrate.

Flavoproteins　Proteins containing FAD or FMN as a prosthetic group; participate in hydrogen transfer reactions.

Fluid-mosaic model　A model of membrane structure that assumes globular proteins embedded in a lipid bilayer.

Fluorouracil　A base analog used in cancer chemotherapy.

Foam cell　A macrophage filled with droplets of cholesterol esters.

Follicular hyperkeratosis　Gooseflesh; occurs in deficiency of vitamin C and vitamin A.

fos　A (proto-)oncogene coding for a nuclear transcription factor.

Frameshift mutation　Insertion or deletion that changes the reading frame of the mRNA.

Free energy　The "useful" energy in chemical reactions.

Fructokinase　The enzyme that phosphorylates fructose to fructose 1-phosphate.

Fructose 1,6-bisphosphatase　An important regulated enzyme of gluconeogenesis.

Fructose 2,6-bisphosphate　A regulatory metabolite that mediates hormonal effects on phosphofructokinase and fructose 1,6-bisphosphatase.

Fructose intolerance　Hereditary disorders caused by the deficiency of one of the fructose-metabolizing enzymes.

Furanose ring　Five-membered ring in monosaccharides.

Futile cycle　The simultaneous activity of two opposing metabolic reactions, leading to ATP hydrolysis.

G proteins　GTP-binding signal transducing proteins that mediate most hormone effects.

G_0 phase　The nondividing state of a cell.

G_1 phase　The time between mitosis and S phase.

G_2 phase　The time between S phase and mitosis.

GABA　Gamma-aminobutyric acid, an inhibitory neurotransmitter in the central nervous system that is synthesized from glutamate.

GAGs　Glycosaminoglycans; polysaccharides containing an amino sugar in every other position.

Galactokinase　The enzyme that phosphorylates galactose to galactose 1-phosphate.

Galactosemia　A hereditary disease caused by the deficiency of a galactose-metabolizing enzyme.

Gallstones　Calculi formed from cholesterol or other poorly soluble substances in the biliary system.

γ-carboxyglutamate　A posttranslationally formed amino acid in prothrombin and factors VII, IX, and X.

Gangliosides　Sphingolipids containing an acidic oligosaccharide.

Gap junction　A small aqueous channel connecting the cytoplasm of neighboring cells.

Gas gangrene　A severe type of wound infection caused by collagenase-producing anaerobic bacteria.

Gelatin　Denatured collagen.

Gene　A length of DNA directing the synthesis of a polypeptide.

Gene families　Structurally related genes with a common evolutionary origin.

Gene therapy　The introduction of a functional gene into the patient's cells.

Genomic library　A collection of bacterial clones containing fragments of genomic DNA.

Globosides　Sphingolipids containing a nonacidic oligosaccharide.

Glucagon　A pancreatic hormone that stimulates the glucose-producing pathways of the liver.

Glucogenic　Glucose forming.

Glucokinase　The liver isoenzyme of hexokinase.

Glucose oxidase test　An enzymatic method for the selective determination of glucose in the clinical laboratory.

Glucose 6-phosphatase　The glucose-producing enzyme of the liver.

Glucose 6-phosphate dehydrogenase　The first enzyme in the oxidative branch of the pentose phosphate pathway.

Glucose 6-phosphate dehydrogenase deficiency　A common enzyme deficiency that leads to hemolytic complications after exposure to certain drugs.

Glucose tolerance test　A laboratory test that determines the effect of glucose ingestion on the blood glucose level.

Glutamate dehydrogenase　An enzyme that catalyzes the oxidative deamination of glutamate and the reductive amination of α-ketoglutarate.

Glutaminase A hydrolytic enzyme that releases ammonia from glutamine.

Glutathione A tripeptide with reducing properties.

Glycerol phosphate shuttle The transfer of electrons from cytoplasmic glycerol phosphate to the respiratory chain.

Glycocalyx A carbohydrate coat formed by glycolipids and glycoproteins on the cell surface.

Glycogen phosphorylase The enzyme that cleaves glycogen to glucose 1-phosphate.

Glycogen synthase The enzyme that synthesizes glycogen from UDP-glucose.

Glycolipids Lipids whose hydrophilic head group contains carbohydrate.

Glycoprotein A protein that contains covalently bound carbohydrate.

Glycosidic bond Bond formed by the anomeric carbon of a monosaccharide.

Glycosyl transferases Biosynthetic enzymes that use activated monosaccharides.

Goiter Hypertrophy and/or hyperplasia of the thyroid gland; seen in iodine deficiency and many other forms of hypothyroidism.

Gouty arthritis Arthritis caused by sodium urate deposits in the joints.

Graves' disease An autoimmune disease leading to hyperthyroidism.

Growth factors Soluble extracellular messengers, usually proteins, that stimulate the proliferation or differentiation of cultured cells.

Guanylate cyclases cGMP-synthesizing enzymes.

Half-life The time that it takes to react half of the substrate molecules in a first-order reaction.

Haploid Containing one copy of each chromosome.

Haptoglobin A hemoglobin-binding protein in serum.

Hartnup disease An inherited defect in the renal and intestinal transport of large neutral amino acids, with pellagra-like symptoms.

Helicases Enzymes separating the strands of double-stranded DNA.

Hematin An oxidized derivative of heme containing a ferric iron.

Hematocrit The percentage of the blood volume that is occupied by blood cells.

Hemiacetal Bond between an aldehyde group and a hydroxy group.

Hemochromatosis An iron overload syndrome.

Hemoglobin A$_{1c}$ Hemoglobin A modified by a reaction between terminal amino groups and glucose.

Hemoglobin Bart's A γ_4 tetramer, in patients with α-thalassemia.

Hemoglobin H A β_4 tetramer, in patients with α-thalassemia.

Hemoglobin S Sickle cell hemoglobin.

Hemopexin A heme-binding protein in serum.

Hemophilia A group of inherited clotting disorders. The most common is factor VIII deficiency.

Hemorrhagic disease of the newborn A neonatal bleeding disorder caused by vitamin K deficiency.

Hemosiderin A partially denatured form of ferritin.

Hemosiderosis Abnormal accumulation of hemosiderin.

Heparan sulfate A GAG in many cell surface and connective tissue proteoglycans.

Heparin A sulfated GAG made by mast cells and basophils.

Hepatic coma The result of hyperammonemia in patients with advanced liver cirrhosis.

Hepatic lipase An enzyme in the space of Disse that hydrolyzes triglycerides and phospholipids in remnant particles and HDL.

Hereditary persistence of fetal hemoglobin γ-Chain production in an adult.

Heterochromatin A condensed, transcriptionally inactive form of chromatin.

Heterotropic effects Interactions between different ligands of an allosteric protein.

Heterozygous Carrying two different variants of a gene.

Hexokinase The enzyme that phosphorylates glucose to glucose 6-phosphate.

Hinge region The portion of the immunoglobulin heavy chain between the first and second constant domains.

Histidinemia A relatively benign inborn error of histidine metabolism.

Histones Small, basic proteins that are tightly associated with DNA in chromatin.

HMG-CoA reductase The regulated enzyme of cholesterol synthesis.

HNPCC Hereditary non-polyposis colon cancer. An inherited defect of postreplication mismatch repair, responsible for 5% of all colorectal cancers.

Homocystinuria An inborn error in the metabolism of the sulfur amino acids; causes skeletal deformities and mental deficiency.

Homologous recombination A reciprocal exchange of DNA between two DNA molecules of related sequence.

Homotropic effects Interactions between identical ligands of an allosteric protein.

Homozygous Carrying two identical variants of a gene.

Hormone-sensitive lipase An enzyme in adipose cells that hydrolyzes stored triglycerides.

Hyaluronic acid A large, unsulfated GAG, not bound to a core protein.

Hydrogen bond Dipole-dipole interaction involving a hydrogen atom.

Hydrogen peroxide A toxic product of some oxidative reactions.

Hydrolase Enzyme catalyzing hydrolytic cleavage reactions.

Hydrolysis Cleavage of a bond by the addition of water.

Hydroxyapatite The major inorganic component of bone.

Hyperammonemia Too much ammonia in the blood.

Hyperbilirubinemia Too much bilirubin in the blood.

Hyperlipidemia Too much lipid in the blood.

Hyperuricemia Too much uric acid in the blood.

Hypervariable regions The most variable parts of the variable domains in the immunoglobulins. Sites of contact with the antigen.

Hypoglycemic shock Brain dysfunction resulting from lack of blood glucose.

Hypoxanthine-guanine phosphoribosyltransferase HGPRT, the most important salvage enzyme for purine bases.

I-cell disease A lysosomal storage disease caused by the misrouting of lysosomal enzymes.

Immotile cilia syndrome A type of inherited disease caused by abnormalities of structural proteins in cilia and flagella.

Induced-fit model A model that assumes a flexible substrate-binding site in the enzyme.

Inducible proteins Proteins whose synthesis is regulated.

Inositol 1,4,5-trisphosphate A second messenger that releases calcium from the endoplasmic reticulum. Produced by phospholipase C.

Insertion sequence A mobile element in prokaryotes that contains a gene for transposase.

Insulin Pancreatic hormone that stimulates the utilization of dietary nutrients.

Insulinoma An insulin-secreting tumor of pancreatic β cells.

Integrases Enzymes that catalyze site-specific recombination.

Integrins Integral membrane proteins that function as receptors for components of the extracellular matrix.

Intermediate filament A type of cytoskeletal fiber formed from proteins in a coiled-coil conformation.

International unit (IU) The enzyme activity that converts one micromole of substrate to product per minute.

Intrinsic factor A glycoprotein from parietal cells in the stomach; required for efficient B_{12} absorption.

Introns Those parts of a gene that do not appear in the mature, functional RNA product.

Ion channel A pore in the membrane that is selectively permeable for specific ions.

Ion-dipole interaction Attractive force between an ion and a component of a polarized bond.

Irreversible inhibition Inhibition by the formation of a covalent bond with the enzyme.

Irreversible reaction A reaction that proceeds in only one direction under physiological conditions.

Ischemia Interruption of the blood supply.

Isoelectric point The pH value at which the number of positive charges on the molecule equals the number of negative charges.

Isoenzymes Enzymes catalyzing the same reaction but composed of different polypeptides.

Isoforms Tissue-specific variants of a protein.

Isoniazid A tuberculostatic that can induce B_6 deficiency.

J chain A polypeptide in polymeric immunoglobulins.

J gene A small gene that participates in the assembly of an immunoglobulin gene in developing B lymphocytes.

Janus kinase A type of nonreceptor tyrosine kinase that associates with activated receptors for cytokines, growth hormone, prolactin, and erythropoietin.

Jaundice Yellow discoloration of skin and sclera in patients with hyperbilirubinemia.

jun A (proto-)oncogene coding for a nuclear transcription factor.

Junk DNA Noncoding DNA of unknown function.

Keratin A type of intermediate filament protein in epithelial cells.

Kernicterus Brain damage caused by the deposition of bilirubin in the basal ganglia.

Ketoacidosis A metabolic emergency in insulin-dependent diabetics, with hyperglycemia, acidosis, dehydration, and electrolyte imbalances.

Ketogenesis Synthesis of ketone bodies.

Ketogenic Ketone body forming.

Ketone bodies Acetoacetate, β-hydroxybutyrate, and acetone.

Ketose Monosaccharide with a keto group.

Kinase An enzyme that transfers a phosphate group from a nucleotide.

Knockout mouse A mouse in which a gene has been disrupted by genetic manipulations.

Lactate dehydrogenase The enzyme that interconverts pyruvate and lactate.

Lactic acidosis Decrease of the blood pH resulting from lactic acid accumulation.

Lactose intolerance Digestive disturbances after the ingestion of milk or milk products, caused by low activity of intestinal lactase.

Lactose operon An operon in *E. coli* that codes for enzymes of lactose metabolism.

Lagging strand The strand that is synthesized piecemeal during DNA replication.

Laminin The most abundant multiadhesive glycoprotein in basement membranes.

LDL receptor A lipoprotein receptor that mediates the endocytosis of LDL.

Leading strand The strand that is synthesized continuously during DNA replication.

Lecithin Synonym for phosphatidylcholine, a phosphoglyceride.

Lecithin-cholesterol acyltransferase LCAT, an enzyme in HDL that converts free cholesterol into cholesterol esters.

Leptin A hormonelike polypeptide from overfed adipose cells that reduces appetite.

Leucine zipper proteins A type of DNA-binding protein.

Leukotrienes Biologically active products formed in the lipoxygenase pathway.

Li-Fraumeni syndrome A rare cancer susceptibility syndrome with germline mutations of the p53 gene.

Ligand-gated ion channels Ion channels that are regulated by the direct binding of a neurotransmitter.

LINEs Long interspersed elements, a type of moderately repetitive DNA.

Linoleic acid An ω^6-polyunsaturated fatty acid.

Linolenic acid An ω^3-polyunsaturated fatty acid.

Lipase Triglyceride-degrading enzyme.

Lipoic acid A prosthetic group of pyruvate dehydrogenase.

Lipolysis Triglyceride hydrolysis.

Lipoprotein A protein with noncovalently bound lipid.

Lipoprotein lipase An endothelial enzyme that hydrolyzes triglycerides in lipoproteins.

Liposome A bilayer-surrounded vesicle.

Lipoxygenase The key enzyme for the synthesis of leukotrienes and HETEs.

Lock-and-key model A model that assumes a rigid substrate-binding site in the enzyme.

Long terminal repeats The terminal repeat sequences of retroviral cDNAs.

Lovastatin A lipid-lowering drug that inhibits HMG-CoA reductase.

Lung surfactant A lipid secretion that reduces the surface tension in the lung alveoli.

Lyase An enzyme that removes a group nonhydrolytically from its substrate.

Lysogenic bacterium A bacterium that harbors a prophage.

Lysogenic pathway A reproductive strategy of some bacteriophages that involves the integration of the viral DNA into the host-cell chromosome.

Lysophosphoglyceride A phosphoglyceride with one fatty acid missing.

Lysozyme An enzyme that cleaves a bacterial cell wall polysaccharide.

Lysyl oxidase An enzyme that produces allysyl residues in collagen; required for crosslinking.

Lytic pathway The reproductive strategy of bacteriophages that destroys their host cell.

Macromolecule Large molecule.

Malate-aspartate shuttle The reversible shuttling of hydrogen, in the form of malate, across the inner mitochondrial membrane.

MAO Monoamine oxidase, a flavoprotein enzyme catalyzing the oxidative deamination of catecholamines and 5-hydroxytryptamine.

MAP kinases Mitogen-activated protein kinases. A family of protein kinases that are activated in response to growth factors or stress.

Maple syrup urine disease An inborn error of branched chain amino acid metabolism; causes mental and neurological problems.

Maxam-Gilbert method A method for DNA sequencing.

McArdle's disease Deficiency of glycogen phosphorylase in muscle, causing muscle weakness.

Megaloblastic anemia A type of anemia characterized by oversized red blood cells. Occurs in deficiency of folic acid and vitamin B_{12}. Related to impaired DNA synthesis.

MEK MAP kinase/ERK kinase. A protein kinase that activates MAP kinases by dual phosphorylation on threonine and tyrosine residues.

Melanin The dark pigment of skin and hair.

Metastatic calcification Abnormal calcification of soft tissues.

Methemoglobin A nonfunctional hemoglobin in which the heme iron is oxidized to the ferric state.

Methotrexate An anticancer drug that inhibits dihydrofolate reductase.

Methylation reaction Transfer of a methyl group from one molecule (often SAM) to another.

Methylmalonic aciduria Excretion of methylmalonic acid in the urine; caused by an inherited enzyme deficiency or by B_{12} deficiency.

Micelle Small globule formed from amphipathic lipids.

Michaelis constant A kinetic constant that is related to the affinity between enzyme and substrate.

Microfilaments Cytoskeletal fibers formed by the polymerization of actin.

Microsatellites Very small tandem repeats giving rise to RFLPs.

Microsomes Fragments of the endoplasmic reticulum obtained by cell fractionation.

Microtubules Cytoskeletal fibers formed by the polymerization of tubulin.

Minisatellites Small tandem repeats giving rise to RFLPs.

Mismatch repair A methyl-directed DNA repair system that corrects base mismatches and small insertions/deletions after DNA replication.

Mitochondrial diseases Diseases caused by mutations in the mitochondrial genome.

Mitogen Mitosis-inducing agent.

Monoclonal gammopathy Overproduction of a single immunoglobulin by a plasma cell clone in plasma cell dyscrasias.

Monoglyceride Structure formed from glycerol and one fatty acid.

Monosaccharide Polyalcohol containing a carbonyl group.

Monounsaturated fatty acid Fatty acid with one double bond.

mRNA Messenger RNA; specifies the amino acid sequence during protein synthesis.

Mucopolysaccharidoses Lysosomal storage diseases caused by deficiencies of GAG-degrading enzymes.

Muscarinic receptors G-protein–linked receptors for acetylcholine.

Mutagen Mutation-inducing agent.

Mutarotation Spontaneous interconversion of anomeric forms in a monosaccharide.

myc A (proto-)oncogene coding for a nuclear transcription factor. Amplified in many spontaneous cancers.

Myoglobin An oxygen-binding protein in muscle tissue.

Myosin The protein of the thick filaments in muscle.

Myxedema Hypothyroidism in adults.

N-linked oligosaccharides Oligosaccharides bound to asparagine side chains in glycoproteins.

NAD, NADP Nicotinamide adenine dinucleotide (phosphate); two cosubstrates that accept or donate electrons (+ proton) in many dehydrogenase reactions.

Negative control Inhibition of transcription by the binding of a regulatory protein to DNA.

Neoplasia Abnormal growth of either a benign or a malignant nature.

Nephrotic syndrome A type of kidney disease with massive proteinuria.

Niacin Nicotinic acid; also used as a generic name for nicotinic acid and nicotinamide.

Nicotinic receptors Acetylcholine-operated cation channels.

Nitric oxide An unstable, diffusible messenger molecule produced in endothelial cells and some other tissues.

Nitrogen balance The difference between ingested nitrogen and excreted nitrogen.

Noncompetitive inhibition Inhibition by an agent that binds the enzyme noncovalently outside its active site.

Nonketotic hyperosmolar coma A metabolic emergency in non−insulin-dependent diabetics; with hyperglycemia and dehydration but no acidosis.

Nonsense mutation A mutation that creates a stop codon.

Nonviral retroposons DNA sequences produced by the reverse transcription of a cellular RNA.

Northern blotting A method for the identification of RNA after gel electrophoresis, using a probe.

NSAIDs Nonsteroidal antiinflammatory drugs; act as inhibitors of cyclooxygenase.

Nucleocapsid The particle formed from viral nucleic acid and protein coat.

Nucleoside A structure formed from a pentose sugar and a base.

Nucleosome The structural unit of chromatin; formed from DNA and histones.

Nucleotide A structure formed from pentose sugar, base, and a variable number of phosphate groups.

Nucleotide excision repair A DNA repair system for bulky lesions.

O-linked oligosaccharides Oligosaccharides bound to hydroxy groups in proteins.

Okazaki fragments Pieces of DNA synthesized in the lagging strand during DNA replication.

Oleic acid A C-18 monounsaturated fatty acid.

Oligomycin An inhibitor of the mitochondrial ATP synthase.

Omega-oxidation Oxidation of the last carbon in the fatty acid.

Oncogene A growth-promoting gene in cancer cells.

Operator A repressor-binding regulatory DNA sequence in bacterial operons.

Operon The unit of promoter, operator, and structural genes in bacteria.

Opsonization The stimulation of phagocytosis by an antibody or other protein bound to the surface of a particle.

Oriental flush Hypersensitivity to alcohol, caused by the deficiency of a mitochondrial aldehyde dehydrogenase in many Asians.

Orotic acid An intermediate of pyrimidine biosynthesis.

Osteogenesis imperfecta Brittle bones; caused by inherited defects of type I collagen.

Osteomalacia Rickets in adults.

Osteoporosis A common bone disorder in old people.

Oxalic acid A component of kidney stones that can be formed from glycine.

Oxidoreductase Enzyme catalyzing oxidation-reduction reactions.

Oxygenase Enzyme using molecular oxygen as a substrate.

p53 A tumor suppressor gene (and its encoded protein) that is mutated in at least half of all spontaneous cancers.

Palindrome A type of symmetrical DNA sequence.

Palmitic acid A saturated C-16 fatty acid.

Pancreatic lipase The major enzyme of fat digestion.

Pantothenic acid A nutritionally essential constituent of coenzyme A.

Papillomavirus A DNA virus associated with cervical cancer.

PAPS Phosphoadenosine phosphosulfate, the "activated sulfate" used for sulfation reactions.

Para-aminobenzoic acid A constituent of folic acid.

Paracrine signaling The action of an extracellular messenger on neighboring cells within its tissue of origin.

Passive diffusion Diffusion across the lipid bilayer.

Pasteur effect The stimulation of glycolysis under anaerobic conditions.

PCR Polymerase chain reaction, a method for the amplification of selected DNA sequences.

PDGF Platelet-derived growth factor. Released from activated platelets during blood clotting.

Pellagra Niacin deficiency. Symptoms include dermatitis, diarrhea, dementia.

Penicillamine A metal chelator used to treat Wilson's disease and rheumatoid arthritis. Can cause B_6 deficiency.

PEP-carboxykinase A gluconeogenic enzyme that is induced by glucagon and glucocorticoids.

Pepsin An endopeptidase in gastric juice.

Peptide bond Amide bond between two amino acids.

Peptidyl transferase The enzymatic activity of the large ribosomal subunit that forms the peptide bond.

Pernicious anemia Megaloblastic anemia and neuropathy caused by B_{12} malabsorption.

Peroxidases Enzymes that consume hydrogen peroxide or organic peroxides.

Peroxidation The nonenzymatic, free radical–mediated oxidation of polyunsaturated fatty acids.

Pertussis toxin A toxin produced by *Bordetella pertussis*; causes cAMP accumulation by covalent modification of the G_i protein.

Phenylalanine tolerance test A diagnostic test for PKU heterozygotes.

Phenylketonuria PKU, an inherited deficiency of phenylalanine hydroxylase, causing mental retardation.

Phenylpyruvate A phenylalanine-derived metabolite in PKU.

Phorbol esters Tumor promoters from croton oil. Stimulate protein kinase C.

Phosphatase-1 The enzyme that dephosphorylates glycogen synthase, glycogen phosphorylase, and phosphorylase kinase.

Phosphatidic acid Glycerol + two fatty acids + phosphate.

Phosphodiester bond Bond between phosphate and two hydroxy groups.

Phosphodiesterases Enzymes that hydrolyze cyclic AMP, cyclic GMP, or both.

Phosphofructokinase The enzyme that catalyzes the committed step of glycolysis.

Phosphoglycerides Lipids structurally related to phosphatidic acid.

Phospholipase C A type of enzyme that cleaves phosphoglycerides between glycerol and phosphate.

Phospholipases Phosphoglyceride-hydrolyzing enzymes.

Phospholipids Lipids with phosphate in their hydrophilic head group.

Phosphopantetheine A prosthetic group of fatty acid synthase.

Phosphoprotein A protein containing covalently bound phosphate.

Phosphoribosyl pyrophosphate PRPP, the precursor of the ribose in the purine and pyrimidine nucleotides.

Phosphorylase kinase A protein kinase that phosphorylates glycogen phosphorylase.

Phosphorylation reactions Reactions in which a phosphate group becomes covalently attached to an acceptor molecule.

Physiological jaundice The common jaundice of newborns.

Phytosterols Steroids from plants.

Pinocytosis Nonselective uptake of fluid droplets into the cell.

Plasmids Circular, double-stranded DNAs that function as "accessory chromosomes" in bacteria.

Plasmin The principal fibrin-degrading enzyme.

Platelet activation A change in shape and membrane structure of platelets, accompanied by the release of various mediators.

Platelet-activating factor PAF, a soluble, biologically active phosphoglyceride released from white blood cells.

PLC-γ An isoenzyme of phospholipase C that is tyrosine phosphorylated and activated by growth factor receptors.

Point mutation Change in a single base pair.

Poly-A tail A structure at the 3′ end of eukaryotic mRNA.

Polyadenylation signal A conserved sequence at the 3′ end of eukaryotic genes.

Polyamines Polycations synthesized from ornithine and SAM.

Polyclonal gammopathy Nonspecific overproduction of immunoglobulins; seen in many diseases.

Polymer A macromolecule consisting of many covalently bonded units (monomers).

Polyol pathway A pathway that synthesizes fructose from glucose.

Polyp A benign tumor of mucous membranes.

Polypeptide Polymer of amino acids.

Polysaccharide Polymer of monosaccharides.

Polyunsaturated fatty acids Fatty acids with more than one double bond.

Porphyria cutanea tarda A common porphyria, characterized by cutaneous photosensitivity.

Porphyrias Diseases caused by an impairment of heme biosynthesis, with the accumulation of biosynthetic intermediates.

Porphyrinogens Biosynthetic precursors of the porphyrins.

Positive control Stimulation of transcription by the binding of a regulatory protein to DNA.

Postprandial thermogenesis Metabolic heat production in response to food intake.

Postreplication mismatch repair   A repair system that corrects replication errors.

Posttranscriptional processing   Chemical modification of RNA.

Posttranslational processing   Chemical modification of proteins.

Pre-β-lipoprotein   Very-low-density lipoprotein (VLDL).

Preimplantation diagnosis   Diagnosis of genetic diseases in the early embryo after in vitro fertilization.

Prenatal diagnosis   Also called antenatal diagnosis; the diagnosis of genetic (and other) diseases in the fetus during early pregnancy.

Preprocollagen   The earliest precursor of collagen.

Primary bile acids   Those bile acids that are synthesized by the liver.

Primary structure   The covalent structure of a protein.

Primary transcript   The product of RNA polymerase.

Primase   A specialized RNA polymerase that synthesizes a primer during DNA replication.

Probe   A labeled oligo- or polynucleotide that is used to identify a specific base sequence in DNA.

Processed pseudogenes   Nonviral retroposons derived by the reverse transcription of an mRNA.

Processivity   The ability of a DNA or RNA polymerase to synthesize long strands without interruption.

Procollagen   Preprocollagen minus the signal sequence.

Progestins   21-Carbon steroids derived from cholesterol; used as precursors for the other steroid hormones.

Prohormone   The inactive or less-active biosynthetic precursor of an active hormone.

Prokaryotes   Cells without nucleus.

Promoter   A regulatory DNA sequence at the upstream end of a gene or operon.

Proopiomelanocortin   A prohormone in the anterior pituitary gland.

Propeptides   The N- and C-terminal extensions in procollagen.

Prophage   The DNA of a temperate bacteriophage after its integration into the host-cell chromosome.

Prostanoids   The products of the cyclooxygenase pathway: prostaglandins, prostacyclin, and thromboxane.

Prosthetic group   A nonpolypeptide component in a protein.

Protein kinase A   The cAMP-activated protein kinase.

Protein kinase C   The diacylglycerol-activated protein kinase.

Protein kinase G   The cGMP-activated protein kinase.

Proteoglycans   Products consisting of core protein and covalently bound sulfated GAGs.

Protonation/deprotonation   The reversible binding and release of a proton by an ionizable (acidic or basic) group.

Protoporphyrin IX   The organic portion of the heme group.

Proximal histidine   A histidine residue in hemoglobin and myoglobin that is bound to the heme iron.

Pseudogenes   Degenerate, nonfunctional genes that are related to functional genes.

Pseudohypoparathyroidism   Reduced responsiveness to parathyroid hormone.

Pyranose ring   Six-membered ring in monosaccharides.

Pyridoxal phosphate   The coenzyme form of vitamin B_6; used as a prosthetic group in many enzymes of amino acid metabolism.

Pyrimidine dimer   A DNA lesion caused by UV radiation.

Pyruvate carboxylase   The mitochondrial enzyme that turns pyruvate into oxaloacetate.

Pyruvate dehydrogenase   The mitochondrial enzyme complex that turns pyruvate into acetyl-CoA.

Pyruvate kinase   The glycolytic enzyme that turns phosphoenolpyruvate (PEP) into pyruvate.

Quaternary structure   The subunit interactions of an oligomeric protein.

R factor   A plasmid that carries genes for antibiotic resistance.

raf   A (proto-)oncogene coding for a serine/threonine protein kinase.

ras   A (proto-)oncogene coding for the Ras protein, a membrane-associated, growth factor–activated G protein.

Reading frame   The frame in which the codons on the mRNA are translated.

Receptor   A cellular protein to which an extracellular agent binds and that mediates the physiological effects of this agent.

Recommended daily allowances Dietary intakes considered optimal under ordinary conditions.

Reduction potential A measure for the tendency of a redox couple to donate electrons in a redox reaction.

Remnant particles Lipoproteins that are produced by the action of lipoprotein lipase on VLDL or chylomicrons.

Respiratory chain A system of electron carriers (and electron + proton = hydrogen carriers) in the inner mitochondrial membrane.

Respiratory distress syndrome The result of insufficient lung surfactant in newborns.

Respiratory quotient The ratio of respiratory CO_2 produced to O_2 consumed.

Response element A regulatory DNA sequence that mediates the effects of a hormone, second messenger, or metabolite on gene transcription.

Restriction endonucleases Bacterial enzymes that cleave specific palindromic sequences in double-stranded DNA.

Restriction fragment DNA fragment produced by a restriction endonuclease.

Retinoblastoma A rare tumor of immature retinal cells in children. Occurs in spontaneous and heritable forms.

Retinoblastoma protein pRB, a negative regulator of cell cycle progression. Encoded by the retinoblastoma (*Rb*) tumor suppressor gene.

Retinoids The active forms of vitamin A retinol, retinal, and retinoic acid.

Retinol binding protein A plasma protein that brings retinol from the liver to other tissues.

Reverse cholesterol transport The transport of cholesterol from extrahepatic tissues to the liver.

Reverse transcriptase A retroviral enzyme that transcribes RNA into a double-stranded DNA.

RFLP Restriction fragment length polymorphism; DNA sequence variations that can be identified by Southern blotting.

Rhodopsin The light-sensing protein in retinal rod cells.

RIA Radioimmunoassay, a highly sensitive method for the quantitation of hormones and other substances.

Riboflavin Vitamin B_2, a constituent of FAD and FMN.

Ribonucleotide reductase The enzyme that reduces ribose to 2-deoxyribose in the nucleoside diphosphates.

Ribozyme Catalytic RNA.

Rickets Vitamin D deficiency in children, resulting in bone demineralization.

Rifampicin An inhibitor of bacterial RNA polymerase.

RNA polymerases RNA-synthesizing enzymes.

RNA replicase A viral enzyme that synthesizes RNA on an RNA template.

Rotenone A fish poison that inhibits electron flow through NADH-Q reductase.

Rous sarcoma virus A retrovirus that causes sarcomas in chickens.

rRNA Ribosomal RNA, a major constituent of the ribosome.

S phase The phase of DNA replication.

Salvage reactions Reactions that convert free bases to nucleotides.

Sanger dideoxy method A method for DNA sequencing.

Sarcoma Malignant connective-tissue tumor.

Sarcomere A functional compartment of the muscle fiber.

Sarcoplasmic reticulum The endoplasmic reticulum of muscle cells, specialized as a calcium-storage organelle.

Satellite DNA The tandemly repeated simple-sequence DNA of the centromeric and telomeric regions.

Saturated fatty acids Fatty acids without C=C double bond.

Scanning methods Methods for the detection of unspecified mutations.

Scavenger receptors Lipoprotein receptors with broad substrate specificity that mediate the uptake of LDL by macrophages.

Scurvy Vitamin C deficiency; causes impaired collagen synthesis and connective tissue abnormalities.

Second messengers Small, diffusible molecules that mediate the intracellular effects of hormones.

Secondary bile acids Those bile acids that are synthesized from the primary bile acids by intestinal bacteria.

Secondary structure The repetitive folding pattern of a polypeptide.

Secretory pathway The organelles through which secreted proteins are processed: ER, Golgi, and secretory vesicles.

Semiconservative replication The mechanism of DNA replication that leads to a daughter molecule with one old and one new strand.

Serotonin 5-Hydroxytryptamine (5-HT), the major indolamine.

Severe combined immunodeficiency Inherited diseases with combined B-cell and T-cell defects.

SH2 domain A regulatory domain of many signal-transducing proteins that binds to specific phosphotyrosine-containing proteins.

Shine-Delgarno sequence A ribosome-binding sequence in the 5'-untranslated region of bacterial mRNAs.

Sickle cell trait Heterozygosity for hemoglobin S.

Sideroblastic anemia A microcytic anemia in the presence of high iron stores; seen in B_6 deficiency.

σ subunit A subunit of bacterial RNA polymerase required for promoter recognition.

Signal peptidase An enzyme in the ER that cleaves off the signal sequence.

Signal recognition particle A cytoplasmic ribonucleoprotein that binds the signal sequence.

Signal sequence An amino acid sequence at the amino end of secreted proteins that directs them to the ER.

Simple-sequence DNA Short DNA sequences that are tandemly repeated many times.

SINEs Short interspersed elements, a form of moderately repetitive DNA.

Site-directed mutagenesis The production of specific mutations in the test tube.

7SL RNA A component of the signal recognition particle and the grandfather of the Alu sequences.

Slow-reacting substance of anaphylaxis A mixture of leukotrienes that causes bronchoconstriction in asthmatic patients.

Snurps Small nuclear ribonucleoprotein particles; components of the spliceosome.

Sodium cotransport A symport system that brings a substrate into the cell together with a sodium ion.

Sodium urate The poorly soluble uric acid salt that deposits in the joints of gouty patients.

Southern blotting A method for the identification of DNA fragments after gel electrophoresis, using a probe.

Spectrin A membrane-associated cytoskeletal protein in erythrocytes.

Spectrin repeat A structural element in spectrin and dystrophin, consisting of a three-stranded coiled-coil.

Spherocytosis A group of inherited diseases characterized by sphere-shaped erythrocytes; caused by defects in the membrane skeleton of RBCs.

Sphingolipidosis Lipid storage disease, a type of disease caused by the deficiency of a sphingolipid-degrading lysosomal enzyme.

Sphingomyelin A phosphosphingolipid.

Sphingosine A long-chain, hydrophobic amino-alcohol.

Spike proteins Viral proteins associated with the viral envelope.

Spliceosomes Nuclear ribonucleoproteins that remove introns from primary transcripts.

Spot desmosome A spotlike cell-cell adhesion that is linked to intermediate filaments.

src A (proto-)oncogene coding for a nonreceptor tyrosine protein kinase.

Stearic acid A saturated C-18 fatty acid.

Storage disease A type of inborn error of metabolism in which a nonmetabolizable macromolecule accumulates.

Stress fibers Actin microfilaments underlying the plasma membrane.

Structural gene Gene coding for a functional, nonregulatory protein product.

Substrate-level phosphorylation The use of an energy-rich metabolic intermediate for the synthesis of ATP or GTP.

Sulfonamides Bacteriostatic agents that inhibit bacterial folate synthesis.

Superoxide dismutase An enzyme that turns superoxide into oxygen and hydrogen peroxide.

Superoxide radical A highly reactive product of oxidative reactions, made by the transfer of a single electron to molecular oxygen.

Supertwisting Over- or underwinding of double-helical DNA.

Symport Coupled transport of two substrates in the same direction.

T lymphocytes Lymphocytes possessing no surface antibody but an antigen-recognizing T-cell receptor.

Credits

Figure 2.4 Based on illustration ©Irving Geis from Dickerson/Geis: *The structure and action of proteins*. W.A. Benjamin & Co., 1969. Permission, The Estate of Irving Geis.

Figure 2.5 Redrawn from Pauling L: *The nature of the chemical bond*, 3rd ed., Cornell University Press, Ithaca, 1960. Used with permission of the publisher, Cornell University Press.

Figure 2.8 Redrawn from Richardson JS: The anatomy and taxonomy of protein structure. *Adv Protein Chem* 34: 264-265, 1981.

Figure 3.2 Redrawn from Dickerson RE: *The proteins*, 2nd ed. Academic Press, 1964.

Figure 6.9 Redrawn from Devlin TM: *Textbook of biochemistry with clinical correlations*, 4th ed. ©1997 Wiley-Liss. Reprinted with permission of Wiley-Liss, Inc., a subsidiary of John Wiley & Sons, Inc.

Figure 6.27 Redrawn with permission from Quigley GJ, Rich A: Structural domains of transfer RNA molecules. *Science* 194: 797, 1976. ©1976 American Association for the Advancement of Science.

Figure 8.1 **A,** Adapted from Kornberg: *DNA replication* ©1980 W. H. Freeman and Company, used with permission. **B,** Modified from Devlin TM: *Textbook of biochemistry*, 4th ed., ©1997 Wiley-Liss. Reprinted with permission of Wiley-Liss, Inc., a subsidiary of John Wiley & Sons, Inc.

Figure 8.7 **C,** Modified from Lamb P, McKnight SL: Diversity and specificity in transcriptional regulation: the benefits of heterotypic dimerization. *Trends Biochem Sci* 16(11): 421, 1991.

Figure 12.12 Modified from Stryer L: *Biochemistry*, 4th ed. New York, W. H. Freeman & Co., 1995, p. 406.

Figure 25.7 Redrawn from Stites PP, Terr AI, Parslow TG: *Basic and clinical immunology*, 8th ed. New York, 1994, Appleton & Lange.

Figure 25.8 **A,** Modified from Branden C, Tooze J: *Introduction to protein structure*, New York, 1991, Garland Publishing, Inc., p. 185. **B,** Modified from Silverton EW, Navia MA, Davies DR: *Proc Natl Acad Sci USA* 74: 5142, 1977.

Figure 25.10 Redrawn from Stites PP, Terr AI, Parslow TG: *Basic and clinical immunology*, 8th ed., New York, 1994, Appleton & Lange.

Figure 25.11 Redrawn from Stites PP, Terr AI, Parslow TG: *Basic and clinical immunology*, 8th ed, New York, 1994, Appleton & Lange.

Figure 27.3 Redrawn from Unwin N: *Cell 72 Neuron* 10(suppl): 31-41, 1993. ©Cell Press.

Case Study, Viral Gastroenteritis Adapted from Montgomery R, et al: *Biochemistry: a case-oriented approach*. St. Louis, 1996, Mosby−Year Book.

Case Study, A Mysterious Death Adapted with permission from Hoffman M: *Science* 254: 931, 1991. © 1991 American Association for the Advancement of Science.

Case Studies, A Sickly Child; The Missed Examination Adapted from Folkman J, D'Amore P, Karnovsky M: *MAF case 3.91-1, Matthew's feeding difficulties*; Birnbaum M: *MAF case 8.91-1, Mr. Minkowski's lack of response*. Boston, 1990, President and Fellows of Harvard College.

Index

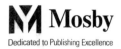

Mosby
Dedicated to Publishing Excellence

WE WANT TO HEAR FROM YOU!

To help us publish the most useful materials for students, we would appreciate your comments on this book. Please take a few moments to answer the questions below, and then tear it out and mail to us. Thank you for your input.

Meisenberg: PRINCIPLES OF MEDICAL BIOCHEMISTRY

1. What year and course of study are you in?

   _____medical school   _____ 1st year
   _____osteopathic school   _____ 2nd year
   _____dental school   _____ 3rd year
   _____pharmacy school   _____ 4th year
   _____physician assistant program   _____ other _____
   _____nursing school
   _____other _____

2. How are you using this book? Please be specific: as a textbook for a course, to refresh the material before a Board exam, etc. If you are using the book for a course, what is the name of the course are you using it for?

3. Was this book useful to you? Why or why not?

4. What features of textbooks are important to you?

   _____color figures   _____ self-assessment questions
   _____summary tables and boxes   _____ price
   _____summaries   _____ concept-type headings
   _____other _____

5. What influenced your decision to buy this text?

   _____required/recommended by instructor
   _____recommendation by student
   _____bookstore display
   _____other _____

6. What other instructional materials did/would you find useful in this course?

   _____computer-assisted instruction
   _____slides
   _____other _____

Are you interested in doing in-depth reviews of our textbooks?   _____ yes   _____ no

NAME:_____

ADDRESS:_____

_____

TELEPHONE:_____

FAX:_____

E-MAIL:_____

THANK YOU!

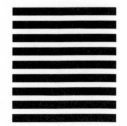